Snell's Clinical Anatomy by Regions

ELEVENTH EDITION

Snell's Clinical Anatomy by Regions

ELEVENTH EDITION

LAWRENCE E. WINESKI, PHD
Professor and Chair
Department of Pathology and Anatomy
Morehouse School of Medicine
Atlanta, Georgia

Wolters Kluwer

Philadelphia • Baltimore • New York • London
Buenos Aires • Hong Kong • Sydney • Tokyo

Acquisitions Editor: Crystal Taylor
Development Editors: Deborah Bordeaux, Kelly Horvath
Editorial Coordinator: Erin E. Hernandez
Editorial Assistant: Parisa Saranj
Marketing Manager: Danielle Klahr
Production Project Manager: Catherine Ott
Manager, Graphic Arts & Design: Stephen Druding
Art Director, Illustration: Jennifer Clements
Manufacturing Coordinator: Margie Orzech
Prepress Vendor: Lumina Datamatics Ltd.

Eleventh Edition

9 8 7 6 5 4 3 2 1

Printed in Mexico

Library of Congress Cataloging-in-Publication Data

ISBN-13: 978-1-9751-9409-3

Cataloging in Publication data available on request from publisher.

shop.lww.com

QUADM0124

To Karen

For your understanding, extraordinary patience,
and unconditional support. I couldn't do this without you.

To Anatomical Donors

With the deepest appreciation to our essential teachers
for your remarkable gifts.

Preface

I am honored to continue the authorship of this new edition of Dr. Richard S. Snell's textbook of anatomy. I hope this 11th edition meets Dr. Snell's high standards and will continue his legacy of scholarship and clinical relevance in teaching.

This book provides health science students with a review of basic anatomy in a strong clinical context. It includes the following changes:

1. The number of chapters has been reduced. Certain previously separate chapters (eg, Thoracic Wall and Thoracic Cavity) have been merged into single chapters without reducing content.
2. The progression of topics has been revised within certain chapters, beginning with foundational material and building more complex relations. For example, discussion of the joints of the upper limb now is in immediate proximity to the description of the bones.
3. The text has been largely reworked throughout and now includes new material and updated terminology. New tables provide succinct summaries of information.
4. Many new and/or updated illustrations better demonstrate points of anatomy, especially those related to organizational concepts.

Each chapter follows a similar format. This makes it easier to locate material and facilitates moving from one part of the book to another. Each chapter centers on the following categories:

1. **Clinical Example:** A short case report that dramatizes the relevance of anatomy in medicine introduces the chapter.
2. **Learning Objectives:** These enable the student to focus on the primary anatomy that is most important to learn and understand.
3. **Basic Clinical Anatomy:** The bulk of the chapter provides basic information on gross anatomic structures of clinical importance. Clinical and Embryology Notes supplement the core text, indicate clinical applications, and explain adult morphology and major congenital malformations.
4. **Radiographic Anatomy:** Each chapter includes numerous standard medical images (eg, radiographs, CT scans, MRI studies, and sonograms) to demonstrate normal anatomy in the manner most often observed by clinicians. Labeled photographs of cross-sectional anatomy stimulate students to think in terms of three-dimensional anatomy, which is so important in the interpretation of imaging studies.
5. **Surface Anatomy:** This outlines surface landmarks and palpation points of important anatomic structures fundamental to a thorough physical examination.
6. **Key Concepts:** This closing part of the chapter summarizes the major points of anatomy discussed in the chapter to reinforce the topics covered.
7. **Review Questions:** A collection of review questions is available online at https://thepoint.lww.com/student. The purpose of these questions is threefold: to focus attention on areas of importance, to enable students to assess their areas of strengths and weaknesses, and to provide a form of self-evaluation for questions asked under examination conditions. The questions are in the National Board format and center around a clinical problem that requires an anatomic answer.

As with previous editions, the book is heavily illustrated. Most figures have been kept simple in order to convey the fundamental floor plans that underlie the organization of body regions. Many new illustrations have been added. These include an emphasis on organizational schemes and diversity in patient populations.

L.E.W.

Acknowledgments

I thank my teachers and colleagues who have contributed directly and indirectly to the development and completion of this book, whether they are aware of their contributions or not. I very much appreciate the time, input, mentoring, and general support and encouragement of the following individuals.

Dr. Robert I. Bowman (deceased), Department of Biology, San Francisco State University, San Francisco, California

Dr. James F. Densler, Adjunct Professor, Department of Surgery, Morehouse School of Medicine, Atlanta, Georgia

Dr. Martha L. Elks, Professor and Associate Dean for Medical Education, Morehouse School of Medicine, Atlanta, Georgia

Dr. Noelle Granger, Professor Emeritus, Department of Cell and Developmental Biology, University of North Carolina School of Medicine, Chapel Hill, North Carolina

Dr. Joseph G. Hall (deceased), Department of Biology, San Francisco State University, San Francisco, California

Dr. Susan W. Herring, Professor, Department of Orthodontics, University of Washington, Seattle, Washington

Dr. Herbert C. Jones, Adjunct Professor, Department of Pathology and Anatomy, Morehouse School of Medicine, Atlanta, Georgia

Dr. James A. McCoy, Professor, Department of Medical Education, Morehouse School of Medicine, Atlanta, Georgia

Dr. Allan Muth (retired), Truckee, California

Dr. Douglas F. Paulsen, Professor, Department of Pathology and Anatomy, Morehouse School of Medicine, Atlanta, Georgia

Dr. Lawrence W. Swan (deceased), Department of Biology, San Francisco State University, San Francisco, California

I am grateful to Dr. H. Wayne Lambert (Professor of Neurobiology and Anatomy, West Virginia University School of Medicine) for his extensive contributions to the Review Questions.

Finally, I wish to express my deep gratitude to the staff of Wolters Kluwer for their great help and support in the preparation of this new edition. My special thanks to Crystal Taylor (Acquisitions Editor) for the opportunity of authorship and the freedom to revise as I felt was appropriate, to Kelly Horvath (Freelance Development Editor) for exceptional editing and concept discussions, and to Deborah Bordeaux (Development Editor) and Erin Hernandez (Editorial Coordinator) for steering this project to completion. I also thank Jennifer Clements for revisions to Dr. Snell's artwork. I especially thank Lionel Williams for his insight and artistry in developing and implementing the numerous original new illustrations in this edition.

Contents

1 Introduction

A 65-year-old male was admitted to the emergency department with the sudden onset of a severe crushing pain over the front of his chest, spreading down his left arm and up into his neck and jaw. On questioning, he said that he had had several attacks of pain before and that they had always occurred when he was climbing stairs or digging in the garden. Previously, he found that the discomfort disappeared with rest after about 5 minutes. However, on this occasion, the pain was more severe and had occurred spontaneously while he was sitting in a chair. Additionally, the pain had not abated.

See the Clinical Case Discussion at the end of this chapter for further insight.

CHAPTER OUTLINE

LEARNING OBJECTIVES

The purpose of this chapter is to introduce the primary terminology used in describing the position and movement of the human body, some of the basic structures that compose the body (eg, skin, fascia, muscles, and bones), and the principles of medical imaging.

1. Define the anatomic position, major planes of section, and primary terms of direction used in anatomic descriptions.
2. Define the primary movements utilized in anatomic descriptions.
3. Identify the components of the skin and its appendages.
4. Identify the types and distributions of the fasciae of the body.
5. Identify the main structural features of bone. Describe bone classification systems. Describe the developmental processes of bone formation.
6. Identify the major forms of cartilage and the locations where each form is generally found.
7. Identify the major categories of joints and the structures that characterize each type of joint. Provide examples of each type of joint. Identify the structures responsible for maintaining the stability of joints.
8. Define and differentiate a bursa versus a synovial sheath.
9. Identify the three types of muscle and describe the basic structure of each type. Define the terms used to describe the actions of skeletal muscles. Describe the pattern of innervation of skeletal muscles and the parameters used in naming them.
10. Identify the major subdivisions of the nervous system. Describe the components of a typical spinal nerve. Trace the distribution of a typical spinal nerve.

11. Describe the general organization of the autonomic nervous system. Differentiate between sympathetic and parasympathetic components and pathways, and preganglionic and postganglionic elements.
12. Define a dermatome. Contrast this with the cutaneous territory of a peripheral nerve.
13. Identify the main types of blood vessels and their functional roles in transporting blood.
14. Identify the components of the lymphatic system. Trace the major routes of lymph drainage in the body.
15. Identify and differentiate mucous and serous membranes.
16. Describe the general sex-, age-, and ethnicity-related differences in anatomic form.
17. Describe the major steps in embryonic development. Differentiate ectoderm, endoderm, and mesoderm, and identify the main derivatives of each.
18. Identify the primary forms of medical imaging and the characteristics of images formed by each technique.

GENERAL ORIENTATION

Anatomy is the science of the structure and function of the body. **Clinical anatomy** is the study of the macroscopic structure and function of the body as it relates to the practice of medicine and other health sciences.

Anatomic Terminology

It is essential to understand the terms used for describing the structures in different regions of the body because without these terms, it is impossible to describe the composition of the body in a meaningful way. Clinicians also need these terms so that anatomic abnormalities found on the clinical examination of a patient can be accurately recorded. The accurate use of anatomic terms by medical personnel enables them to communicate with their colleagues both nationally and internationally.

Understanding anatomic terminology (with the aid of a medical dictionary) rather than memorizing rote nomenclature greatly assists you in the learning process. Without anatomic terms, abnormal functions of joints, the actions of muscles, the alteration of position of organs, or the exact location of swellings or tumors cannot be accurately discussed or recorded.

Terms Related to Position

Spatial orientation and organization are crucial concepts in anatomy, and understanding the standard geometric references that allow uniform, clear descriptions of locations, relations, and movements of structures is important. All descriptions of the human body are based on a conventional reference posture termed the **anatomic position**. In this, a person is standing erect and facing forward, the upper limbs are by the sides, the palms of the hands are directed forward, the lower limbs are together, the soles of the feet are on the ground, and the toes are pointing forward (Fig. 1.1). All directional and movement descriptions are based on this body position. Four geometric planes, three of which are at right angles to the others, are applied to the body in the anatomic position.

- The **median plane** is a vertical plane passing through the center of the body, dividing it into equal right and left halves (see Fig. 1.1A).
- A **sagittal plane** is any plane parallel to the median plane that divides the body into unequal right and left portions.
- The **coronal** (**frontal**) **plane** is a vertical plane situated at a right angle to the median plane. The coronal plane divides the body into the anterior (front) and posterior (back) portions.
- The **horizontal plane** lies at right angles to both the median and the coronal planes. A horizontal plane divides the body into the upper and lower parts.
- A **transverse plane** lies perpendicular to the long axis of a given structure and divides that structure in a cross-sectional orientation. The terms "transverse plane" and "horizontal plane" are often used interchangeably. However, they are not necessarily equivalent. Consider the difference between the horizontal and transverse planes in the leg versus the foot and in the abdomen versus the gut tube. Understand that these planes in such regions produce very different orientations of the structures in question.

The terms **anterior** (**ventral**) and **posterior** (**dorsal**) are used to indicate the front and back of the body, respectively (see Fig. 1.1B). To describe the relationship of two structures, one is said to be anterior or posterior to the other, insofar as it is comparatively closer to the anterior or posterior body surface (eg, the nose is on the anterior side of the head, whereas the buttocks are on the posterior side of the body). In describing the hand, the terms **palmar** and **dorsal** surfaces are used in place of anterior and posterior, respectively. In describing the foot, the term **plantar** surface refers to the sole of the foot, and the **dorsal** surface indicates the upper (top) surface (see Fig. 1.1C).

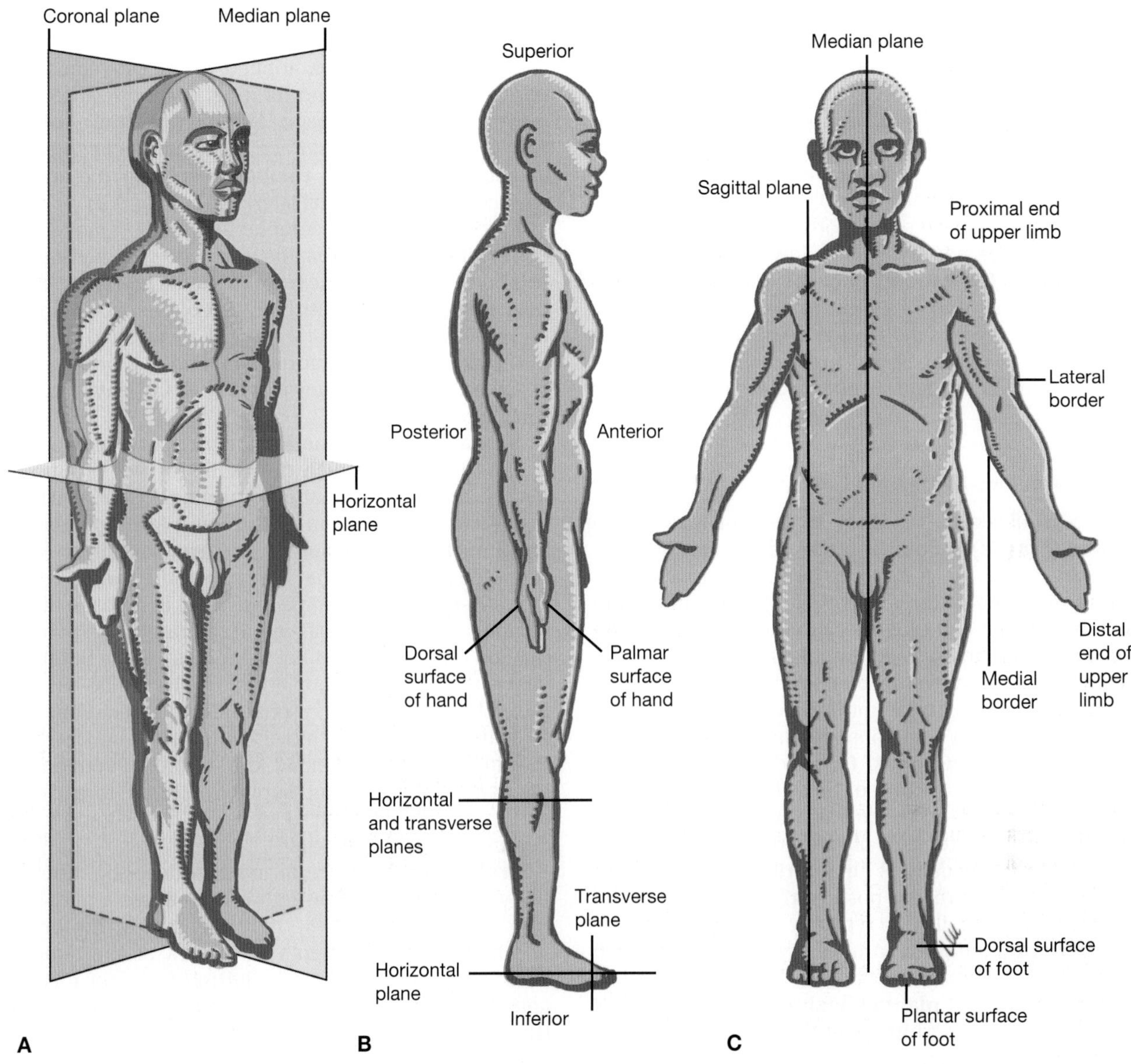

Figure 1.1 Anatomic terms used in relation to position. Note that the subjects are standing in the anatomic position. **A.** Illustration of the median, coronal, and horizontal planes. Note that these planes are aligned at 90° to one another. **B.** Lateral view, demonstrating anatomic planes and directional terms. Note that the horizontal and transverse planes may or may not be equivalent. **C.** Anterior view, showing planes of section and anatomic directions.

A structure situated nearer to the median plane of the body than another is said to be **medial** to the other. Similarly, a structure that lies farther away from the median plane than another is said to be **lateral** to the other (eg, in the head, the eyes are lateral to the nose, and the nose is medial to the eyes).

The terms **superior** (**cranial**; **cephalic**) and **inferior** (**caudal**) denote the levels relatively high or low with reference to the upper and lower ends of the body (eg, the head is at the superior end of the body, whereas the feet are at the inferior end of the body).

The terms **proximal** and **distal** describe positions relative to the core, root, or attached end of a reference point. Proximal is closer to the core, and distal is further away from the core (eg, in the upper limb, the shoulder is proximal to the elbow, and the hand is distal to the elbow).

The terms **superficial** and **deep** denote positions relative to the surface of the body or a given structure. Superficial is closer to the surface, whereas deep is farther away from the surface (eg, the skin is superficial to the ribs, but the heart is deep to the ribs).

The terms **internal** and **external** are used to describe locations relative to the center of a structure or space. Internal is inside the structure, and external is outside the structure (eg, the thoracic cavity is an internal space in the trunk of the body, whereas the skin is the external layer of the trunk).

Ipsilateral and **contralateral** are terms referring to positions relative to a reference side of the body. Ipsilateral is on the same side as the reference point, and contralateral is on the opposite side from the reference point (eg, the right eye is ipsilateral to the right ear; however, the right eye is contralateral to the left ear).

The **supine** position of the body is lying on the back. The **prone** position is laying face downward.

The terms **afferent** and **efferent** refer to the direction of flow relative to a reference point. Afferent is flow toward the reference point, whereas efferent is flow away from the reference point (eg, venous blood flow is afferent to the heart, and arterial blood flow is efferent to the heart).

Terms Related to Movement

In the musculoskeletal system, movement takes place at joints (Fig. 1.2). A joint is a site where two or more bones articulate, or come together. Some joints have no movement (eg, sutures of the skull), some have only slight movement (eg, superior tibiofibular joint), and some are freely movable (eg, shoulder joint).

Flexion is the movement in which a joint angle is decreased (closed) during motion occurring in a sagittal plane. **Extension** is the opposite movement in which the joint angle is increased (opened; straightened) in a sagittal plane (eg, flexion of the elbow approximates the anterior surface of the forearm to the anterior surface of the arm; extension of the elbow is the reverse motion). Flexion usually is an anterior movement, but it is occasionally directed posteriorly, as in the case of the knee joint. Also, flexion typically implies a relatively more powerful, antigravity movement directed toward the embryonic ventral aspect of the body.

Dorsiflexion and **plantar flexion** are special terms used to simplify descriptions of the movements of the foot. Dorsiflexion (the equivalent to extension) refers to lifting the top of the foot superiorly, toward the shin. Plantar flexion (the equivalent to flexion) refers to moving the sole of the foot inferiorly, as in standing on the toes. These points will become clearer in the following chapters on the back and limbs. "Lateral flexion" is an imprecise term sometimes used in clinical settings that refers to a sideways bending movement of the trunk in the coronal plane (Fig. 1.3). However, "abduction" is the more correct term and the one that should be used.

Abduction is movement away from the midline of the body in the coronal plane. **Adduction** is movement toward the midline of the body in the coronal plane (see Fig. 1.2). In the fingers and toes, abduction is applied to spreading apart the digits, and adduction is applied to drawing them together. The movements of the thumb, which are more complicated, are described in Chapter 3.

Inversion and **eversion** are the special terms used to describe certain movements of the foot (see Fig. 1.3). Inversion is turning the sole of the foot so that it faces in a medial direction, toward the midline, and eversion is the opposite movement of the foot so that the sole faces in a lateral direction.

Rotation is the term applied to the movement of a part of the body around its long axis, with little to no movement through space. **Medial (internal) rotation** results in the anterior surface of the part facing medially, and **lateral (external) rotation** results in the anterior surface of the part facing laterally (see Fig. 1.2).

Circumduction is a complex sequence of movements combining flexion, extension, abduction, adduction, and rotation. The overall movement results in transcribing a cone through space, with the apex of the cone being the more proximal articular cavity of a joint and the base of the cone being the more distal end of a bone or limb segment. Circumduction is most easily envisioned at the shoulder.

Pronation and **supination** are the special movements of the forearm in which the radius moves around the ulna (see Fig. 1.3). Pronation is turning the forearm medially such that the palm of the hand faces posteriorly, and supination is turning the forearm laterally from the pronated position so that the palm of the hand comes to face anteriorly. These movements are composed of both rotation (at the proximal end of the radius) and circumduction (at the distal end of the radius). Some references describe pronation/supination of the ankle and the foot. Clinically defined, pronation and supination of the foot are the complex movements of the ankle region that include plantar flexion, dorsiflexion, eversion, and inversion. Pronation and supination of the forearm and ankle are very different movements that should not be confused with one another.

Protraction is the term used to describe moving a body part forward. **Retraction** is to move a part backward. Examples of these movements are the forward and backward movements of the jaw at the temporomandibular joints (as when jutting the chin forward) and the forward/backward motion of the scapula across the rib cage (as when reaching forward).

Eponyms

International commissions reflecting the views of multiple professional anatomic societies determine official anatomic terminology. One of the guidelines used in producing this *Terminologica Anatomica* is that eponyms shall not be used. In a scientific context, an eponym is an identifying term formed from the name of a person (eg, ampere, volt, foramen of Winslow, and circle of Willis). However, eponyms are used randomly, conveying no information about the structure in question, and they are often historically misleading in that the person honored by the naming did not necessarily contribute the first description of the structure (eg, François Poupart was not the first to describe the inguinal ligament). Unfortunately, eponyms remain in wide use in the biomedical sciences, especially in clinical settings. Newer generations of anatomists and other health science professionals should adopt current official terminology and avoid eponyms whenever possible to reverse this trend.

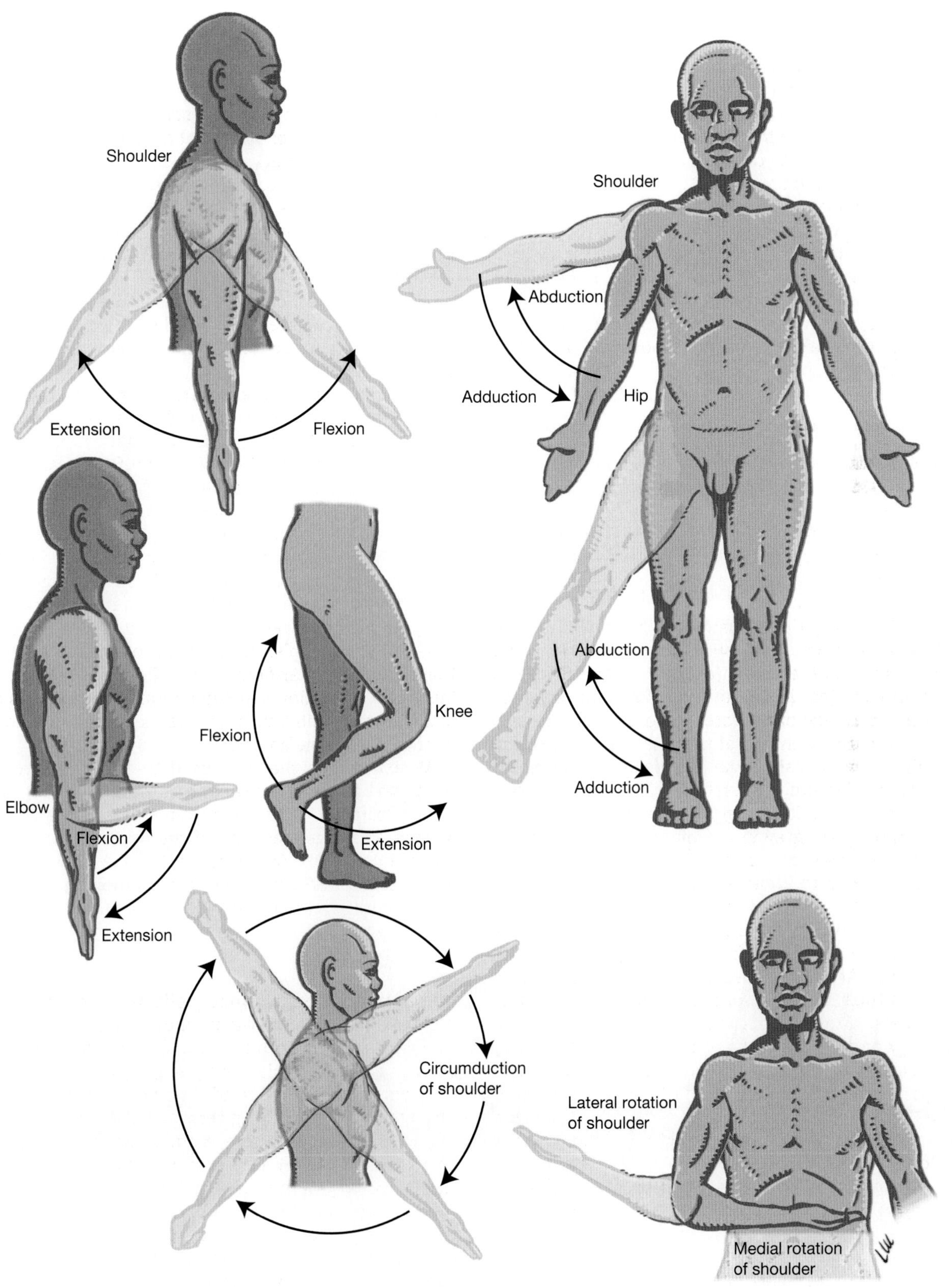

Figure 1.2 Some anatomic terms used in relation to movement. Note the difference between flexion of the elbow versus the knee.

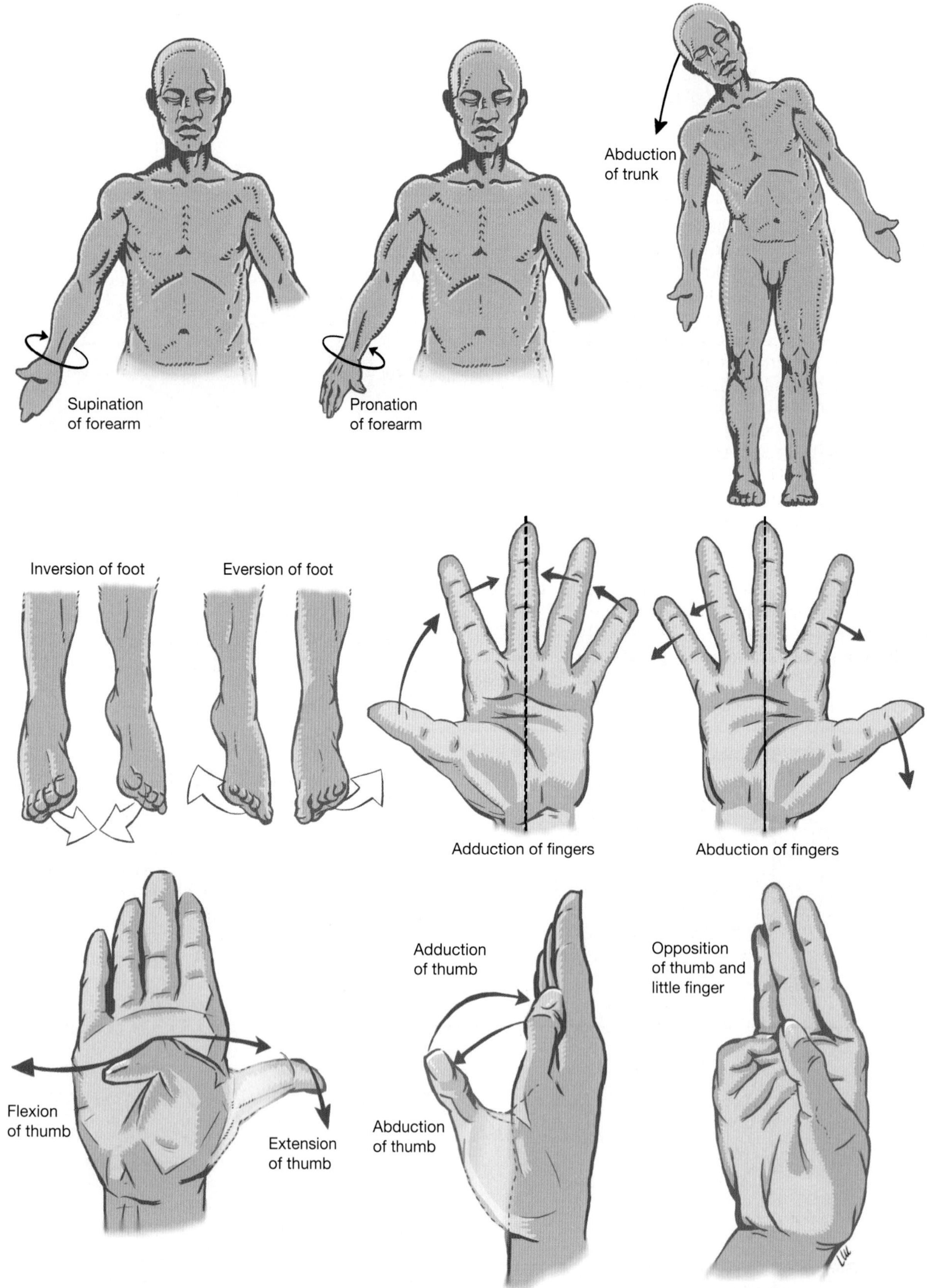

Figure 1.3 Additional anatomic terms used in relation to movement.

BASIC ANATOMY

Basic anatomy is the study of the minimal amount of anatomy consistent with the understanding of the overall structure and function of the body.

Skin

The skin is divided into two parts: the superficial part, the **epidermis**, and the deep part, the **dermis** (Fig. 1.4). The epidermis is a stratified epithelium with cells that flatten as they mature and rise to the surface. The epidermis is extremely thick on the palms of the hands and soles of the feet to withstand the wear and tear that occurs in these regions. It is thin on other areas of the body, such as on the anterior surface of the arm and the forearm. The dermis is composed of dense connective tissue containing many blood vessels, lymphatic vessels, and nerves. It shows considerable variation in thickness in different parts of the body, tending to be thinner on the anterior than on the posterior surface. It is thinner in women than in men. The dermis of the skin is connected to the underlying deep fascia or bones by the **superficial fascia**, otherwise known as **subcutaneous tissue**.

The skin over joints always folds in the same place, the **skin creases** (Fig. 1.5). At these sites, the skin is thinner than elsewhere and is firmly tethered to underlying structures by strong bands of fibrous tissue.

The appendages of the skin are the nails, hair follicles, sebaceous glands, and sweat glands.

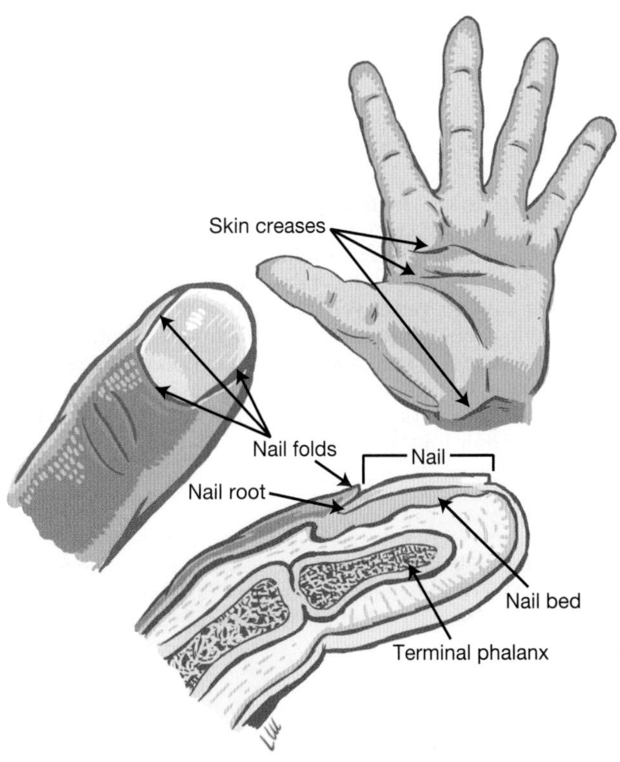

Figure 1.5 The various skin creases on the palmar surface of the hand and the anterior surface of the wrist joint. The relationship of the nail with other structures of the finger is also shown.

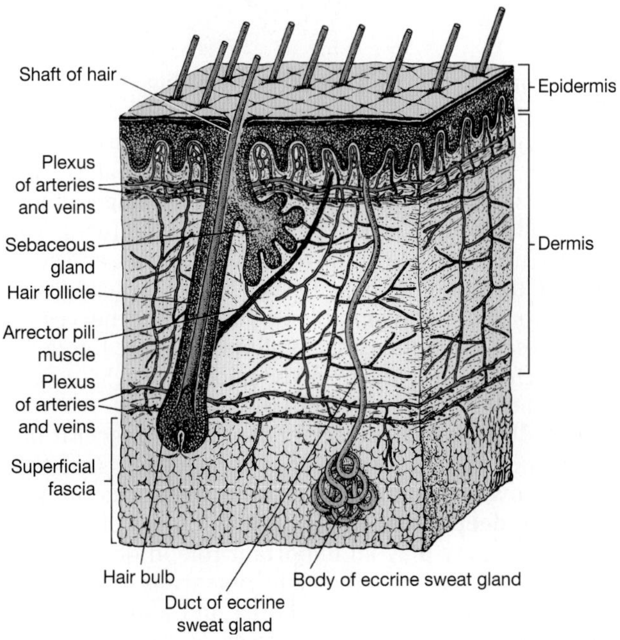

Figure 1.4 General structure of the skin and its relationship with the superficial fascia. Note that hair follicles extend into the deeper part of the dermis or into the superficial fascia, whereas sweat glands extend deeply into the superficial fascia.

The **nails** are keratinized plates on the dorsal surfaces of the tips of the fingers and toes. The proximal edge of the plate is the **root** of the nail. With the exception of the distal edge of the plate, the nail is surrounded and overlapped by folds of skin known as **nail folds**. The surface of skin covered by the nail is the **nail bed**.

Hairs grow out of **follicles**, which are invaginations of the epidermis into the dermis (see Fig. 1.4). The follicles lie obliquely to the skin surface, and their expanded extremities, called **hair bulbs**, penetrate to the deeper part of the dermis. Each hair bulb is concave at its end, and the concavity is occupied by the vascular connective tissue called the **hair papilla**. A band of smooth muscle, the **arrector pili**, connects the undersurface of the follicle to the superficial part of the dermis. The muscle is innervated by sympathetic nerve fibers, and its contraction causes the hair to move into a more vertical position; it also compresses the sebaceous gland and causes it to extrude some of its secretion. The pull of the muscle also causes dimpling of the skin surface, so-called **gooseflesh** ("goose bumps" and "goose pimples"). Hairs are distributed in various numbers over the whole surface of the body, except on the lips, palms, sides of the fingers, glans penis and clitoris, labia minora and the internal surface of the labia majora, the soles and sides of the feet, and the sides of the toes.

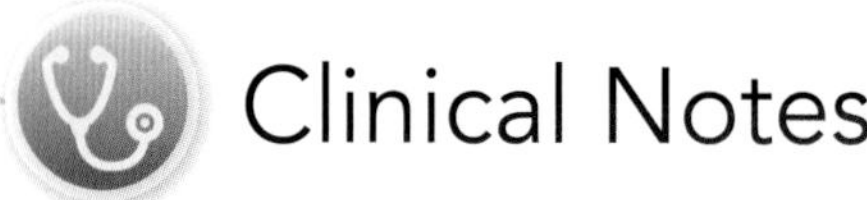

Clinical Notes

Skin Infections

The nail folds, hair follicles, and sebaceous glands are common sites for pathogenic organisms such as *Staphylococcus aureus* to enter into the underlying tissues. Infection occurring between the nail and the nail fold is called a **paronychia**. Infection of the hair follicle and sebaceous gland is responsible for the common **boil**. A **carbuncle** is a staphylococcal infection of the superficial fascia that commonly occurs in the nape of the neck and usually starts as an infection of a hair follicle or a group of hair follicles.

Sebaceous Cyst

A **sebaceous cyst** is caused by the obstruction of the mouth of a sebaceous duct. It may also be caused by the damage from a comb or by infection. It occurs most frequently on the scalp.

Shock

A patient who is in a state of **shock** may be pale and may have gooseflesh because of the overactivity of the sympathetic system, which causes vasoconstriction of the dermal arterioles and contraction of the arrector pili muscles. However, depending on the nature of the shock, dermal vessels may be dilated, resulting in more flushed skin tone.

Skin Burns

The depth of a **burn** determines the method and rate of healing. A partial-thickness burn heals from the cells of the hair follicles, sebaceous glands, and sweat glands as well as from the cells at the edge of the burn. A burn that extends deeper than the sweat glands heals slowly and from the edges only. The fibrous tissue at the margins of the burn causes considerable contracture of the wound. A deep burn often is grafted in order to speed up healing and reduce the incidence of contracture.

Skin Grafting

The two main types of skin grafts are split-thickness and full-thickness grafts. In a **split-thickness graft**, the greater part of the epidermis, including the tips of the dermal papillae, is removed from the donor site and placed on the recipient site. This leaves the epidermal cells on the sides of the dermal papillae and the cells of the hair follicles and sweat glands at the donor site for repair purposes.

A **full-thickness graft** includes both the epidermis and the dermis and requires rapid establishment of a new circulation within it at the recipient site to survive. The donor site is usually covered with a split-thickness graft. In certain circumstances, the full-thickness graft is made in the form of a pedicle graft, in which a flap of full-thickness skin is turned and stitched in position at the recipient site, leaving the base of the flap with its blood supply intact at the donor site. Later, when the new blood supply to the graft is established, the base of the graft is cut across.

Sebaceous glands secrete **sebum** onto the **shafts of the hairs** as they pass up through the necks of the follicles. They are situated on the sloping undersurface of the follicles and lie within the dermis. Sebum is an oily material that helps preserve the flexibility of the emerging hair. It also oils the surface epidermis around the mouth of the follicle.

Sweat glands are long, spiral, tubular glands distributed over the surface of the body, except on the red margins of the lips, nail beds, and the glans penis and clitoris. These glands extend through the full thickness of the dermis, and their extremities may lie in the superficial fascia. The sweat glands are therefore the most deeply penetrating structures of all the epidermal appendages.

Fascia

Fascia is the connective tissue that encloses the body deep to the skin and also envelops and separates individual muscles and groups of muscles as well as deeper organs. Think of fascia as the connective tissue sheaths that hold the structures of the body together in organized arrangements. There are two types of fasciae of the body: superficial and deep.

The **superficial fascia**, or **subcutaneous tissue**, is a mixture of loose areolar and adipose tissue that unites the dermis of the skin to the underlying deep fascia (Fig. 1.6). In most areas, superficial fascia allows the skin to move relatively easily over deeper structures. However, in the scalp, back of the neck, palms, and soles, it contains numerous bundles of collagen fibers that hold the skin firmly to the deeper structures. The eyelids, nose, auricle of the ear, clitoris, penis, and scrotum are devoid of adipose tissue. The superficial fascia transmits the cutaneous blood vessels and nerves. In some areas, it contains skeletal muscles (eg, the facial muscles in the face and neck) or smooth muscle (eg, the dartos muscle in the scrotum).

The **deep fascia** (muscular fascia and visceral fascia) is a denser, fibrous layer of connective tissue that closely covers the muscles and other deep structures as **investing deep fascia**. In the neck, it forms well-defined layers that may play an important role in determining the path taken by pathogenic organisms during the spread of infection. In the thorax and abdomen, it is merely a thin film of areolar tissue covering the muscles and aponeuroses. In the limbs, it forms a definite sheath around the muscles and other structures, holding them in place. **Fibrous septa** extend from the deep surface of the membrane down between the groups of muscles and, in many places, divide the interior of the limbs into **osseofascial compartments** (Fig. 1.6). These

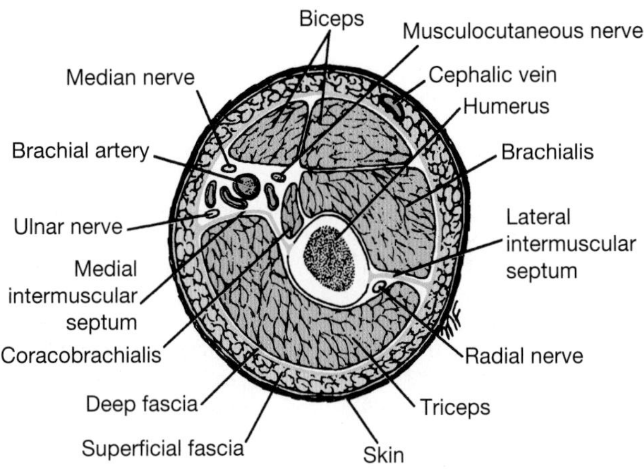

Figure 1.6 Section through the middle of the right arm showing the arrangement of the superficial and deep fascia. Note how deep extensions of the deep fascia extend between the groups of muscles and form intermuscular septa, which divide the arm into osseofascial compartments.

compartments organize muscles into functionally similar groups and assist in return of blood to the heart. In the region of joints, the deep fascia may be considerably thickened to form restraining bands called **retinacula** (Fig. 1.7). Their function is to hold underlying tendons in position and prevent "bowstringing" of the tendons during muscular contraction, or to serve as pulleys around which the tendons can move.

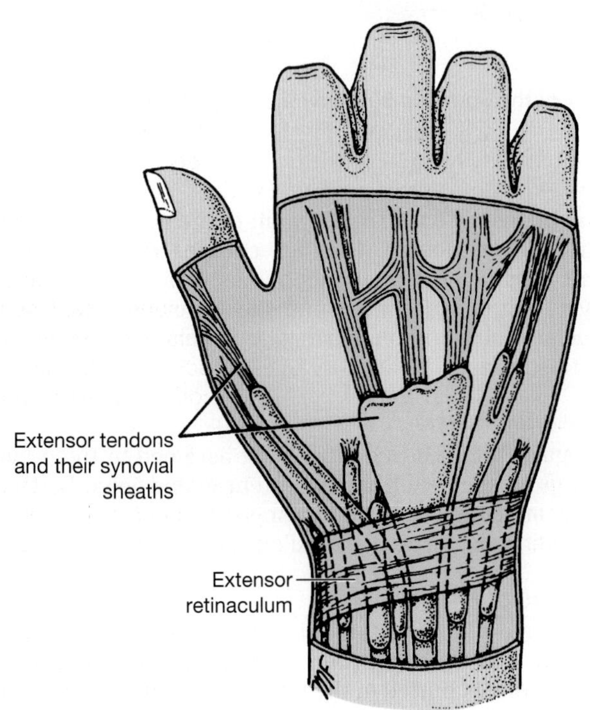

Figure 1.7 Extensor retinaculum on the posterior surface of the wrist holding the underlying tendons of the extensor muscles in position.

Bone

Bone is a living tissue capable of changing its structure when subjected to stresses. Like other connective tissues, bone consists of cells, fibers, and matrix. It is hard because of the calcification of its extracellular matrix and possesses a degree of elasticity because of the presence of organic fibers. Bone has a protective function; for example, the skull and vertebral column protect the brain and spinal cord from injury, and the sternum and ribs protect the thoracic and upper abdominal viscera (Fig. 1.8). It serves as a lever, as seen in the long bones of the limbs, and as an important storage area for calcium salts. Internally, bone houses and protects the delicate blood-forming bone marrow.

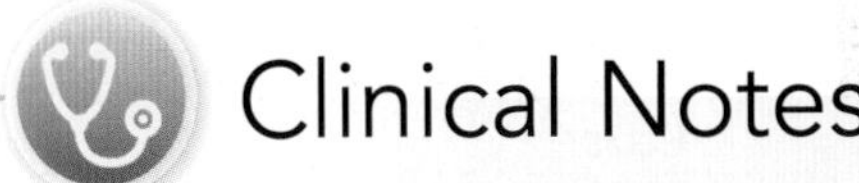

Fasciae and Infection

Knowledge of the arrangement of the deep fasciae often helps explain the path taken by an infection when it spreads from its primary site. For example, in the neck, the various fascial planes determine how infection can extend from the floor of the mouth to the larynx or from the base of the skull into the thoracic cavity.

A thick layer of fibrous tissue called the **periosteum** covers all bone surfaces, other than the articulating surfaces. The periosteum has an abundant vascular supply, and the cells on its deeper surface are osteogenic. The periosteum is particularly well united to bone at sites where muscles, tendons, and ligaments are attached to bone. Bundles of collagen fibers known as perforating (Sharpey's) fibers extend from the periosteum into the underlying bone. The periosteum receives a rich nerve supply and is very sensitive to trauma.

Bone exists in two forms: compact and cancellous. Compact bone appears as a solid mass; cancellous bone consists of a branching network of **trabeculae** (Fig. 1.9). The trabeculae are arranged so as to provide resistance against mechanical stresses and strains.

Bone Classification

Bones can be classified regionally or according to their general shape. In the regional classification scheme (Table 1.1), the bones are organized into two main groups: axial and appendicular skeletons. The **axial skeleton** consists of the elements forming the central axis of the body. The **appendicular skeleton** consists of the bones forming the upper and lower limb girdles and extremities.

In the general shape classification scheme, bones are organized into five categories: long, short, flat, irregular, and sesamoid.

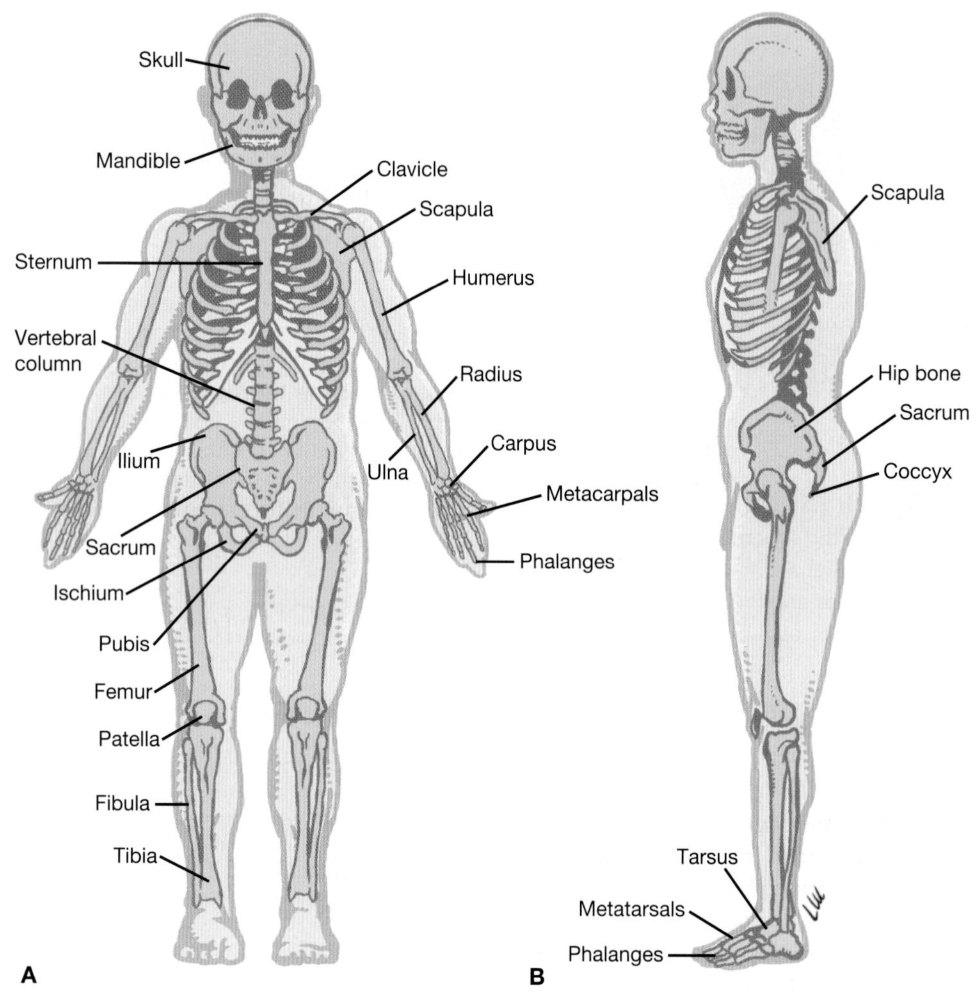

Figure 1.8 Skeleton. **A.** Anterior view. **B.** Lateral view with most of the upper limb removed.

Long Bones

Long bones are found in the limbs (eg, the humerus, femur, metacarpals, metatarsals, and phalanges). Their length is greater than their breadth (see Fig. 1.9A). They have a tubular shaft, the *diaphysis*, and usually an epiphysis at each end. During the growing phase, the diaphysis is separated from the epiphysis by an epiphyseal cartilage. The part of the diaphysis that lies adjacent to the epiphyseal cartilage is called the *metaphysis*. The shaft has a central marrow cavity containing bone marrow. The outer part of the shaft is composed of compact bone covered by periosteum. The ends of long bones are composed of cancellous bone surrounded by a thin layer of compact bone. The articular surfaces of the ends of the bones are covered by hyaline cartilage.

Short Bones

Short bones are found in the hand and foot (eg, the scaphoid, lunate, talus, and calcaneum). They are roughly cuboidal in shape and composed of cancellous bone surrounded by a thin layer of compact bone. Short bones are covered with periosteum, and the articular surfaces are covered by hyaline cartilage.

Flat Bones

Flat bones are found in the vault of the skull (eg, frontal and parietal bones). They are composed of thin inner and outer layers of compact bone, the **tables**, separated by a layer of cancellous bone, the **diploë** (see Fig. 1.9C). The scapulae, although irregular in shape, are included in this group.

Irregular Bones

Irregular bones include those not assigned to the previous groups (eg, skull bones, vertebrae, and pelvic bones). They are composed of a thin shell of compact bone with an interior made up of cancellous bone (see Fig. 1.9B).

Sesamoid Bones

A sesamoid bone is formed within a tendon where the tendon passes over a joint. The greater part of a sesamoid bone is buried in the tendon, and the free surface is covered with cartilage. The largest sesamoid bone is the patella ("kneecap"), which is located in the tendon of the quadriceps femoris (see Fig. 1.9D). Other examples are found in the tendons of the flexor pollicis brevis (in the thumb) and flexor hallucis brevis (in the

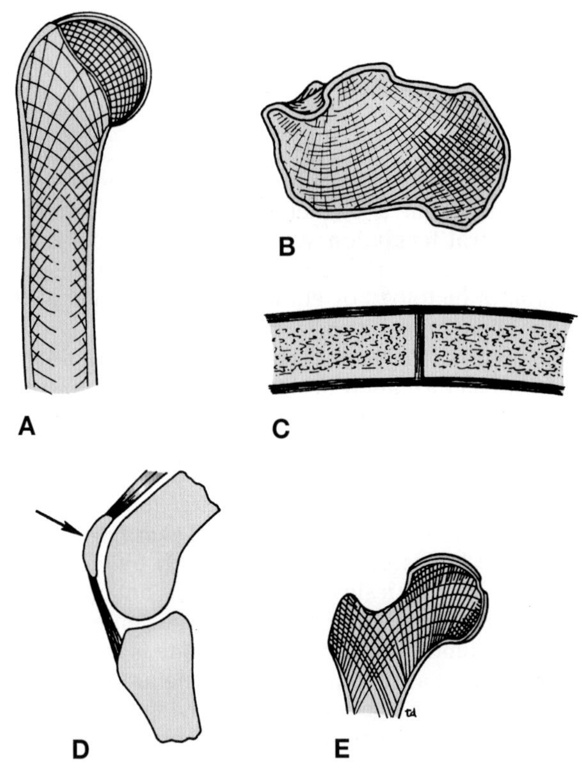

Figure 1.9 Sections of different types of bones. **A.** Long bone (humerus). **B.** Irregular bone (calcaneum). **C.** Flat bone (two parietal bones separated by the sagittal suture). **D.** Sesamoid bone (patella). **E.** Note the arrangement of trabeculae to act as struts to resist both compression and tension forces in the upper end of the femur.

big toe). Sesamoid bones protect tendons from stress and wear by relieving tension in tendons, altering the direction of pull of a tendon to increase leverage, and decreasing friction on tendons by redistributing weight-bearing forces.

Table 1.1 Regional Classification of Bones

REGION OF SKELETON	NUMBER OF BONES (ADULT)
I. Axial skeleton	
Skull	
Cranium	8
Face	14
Auditory ossicles	6
Hyoid	1
Vertebrae (including sacrum and coccyx)	26
Sternum	1
Ribs	24
II. Appendicular skeleton	
Shoulder girdles	
Clavicle	2
Scapula	2
Upper extremities	
Humerus	2
Radius	2
Ulna	2
Carpals	16
Metacarpals	10
Phalanges	28
Pelvic girdle	
Os coxae	2
Lower extremities	
Femur	2
Patella	2
Fibula	2
Tibia	2
Tarsals	14
Metatarsals	10
Phalanges	28
	206

Bone Surface Markings

The surfaces of bones typically show various surface markings or irregular features. The surface is raised or roughened where bands of fascia, ligaments, tendons, or aponeuroses are attached to bone. These roughenings are not present at birth. They appear at puberty and become progressively more obvious during adult life. The pull of these fibrous structures causes the periosteum to elevate and new bone to be deposited beneath. In certain situations, the surface markings are large and given special names. Some of the more important markings are summarized in Table 1.2.

Each of the following chapters provides a comprehensive description of the bones of that region and their significant features. Do not relegate learning this material to a painful exercise in rote memorization of meaningless words. Try to understand the terminology in order to better appreciate the application of the anatomy. Most importantly, ask yourself functional questions when you examine the bones themselves, such as: Is this a right or left element? What articulates with this structure/area? What attaches to this structure? Is this structure palpable? Can this structure be identified in a standard radiographic image? Are there any important neurovascular relations to this region/structure?

Bone Marrow

Bone marrow occupies the marrow cavity in long and short bones and the interstices of the cancellous bone in flat and irregular bones. The marrow of all bones is red and hematopoietic at birth. This blood-forming activity gradually lessens with age, and the red marrow is replaced by yellow marrow. Yellow marrow begins to appear in the distal bones of the limbs at about age 7 years. This replacement of marrow gradually moves proximally, so that by adulthood, red marrow is restricted to the skull

Table 1.2 Bone Surface Markings

BONE MARKING	EXAMPLE
Linear elevation	
Line	Superior nuchal line of the occipital bone
Ridge	Medial and lateral supracondylar ridges of the humerus
Crest	Iliac crest of the hip bone
Rounded elevation	
Tubercle	Pubic tubercle
Protuberance	External occipital protuberance
Tuberosity	Greater and lesser tuberosities of the humerus
Malleolus	Medial malleolus of the tibia, lateral malleolus of the fibula
Trochanter	Greater and lesser tuberosities of the humerus
Sharp elevation	
Spine or spinous process	Ischial spine, spine of the vertebra
Styloid process	Styloid process of temporal bone
Expanded ends for articulation	
Head	Head of humerus, head of femur
Condyle	Medial and lateral condyles of femur (knuckle-like process)
Epicondyle (a prominence situated just above condyle)	Medial and lateral epicondyles of femur
Small flat area for articulation	
Facet	Facet on head of rib for articulation with vertebral body
Depressions	
Notch	Greater sciatic notch of hip bone
Groove or sulcus	Bicipital groove of humerus
Fossa	Olecranon fossa of humerus, acetabular fossa of hip bone
Openings	
Fissure	Superior orbital fissure
Foramen	Infraorbital foramen of the maxilla
Canal	Carotid canal of temporal bone
Meatus	External acoustic meatus of temporal bone

bones, vertebral column, thoracic cage, girdle bones, and the head of the humerus and femur.

Bone Development

Bone develops by two processes: membranous and endochondral. In **membranous formation**, bone develops directly from a connective tissue membrane. In **endochondral formation**, a cartilaginous model is first laid down and is later replaced by bone. Consult a textbook of histology or embryology for details of the cellular changes involved.

The bones of the vault of the skull develop rapidly by membranous formation in the embryo, which protects the underlying developing brain. At birth, small areas of membrane persist between the bones. This is important clinically because it allows the bones a certain amount of mobility, so that the skull can undergo molding during its descent through the female genital passages.

The long bones of the limbs develop by endochondral ossification, in a slow process that is not completed until age 18 to 20 years or even later. The center of bone formation found in the shaft of the bone is the **diaphysis**; the centers at the ends of the bone are **epiphyses**. The plate of cartilage at each end, lying between the epiphysis and diaphysis in a growing bone, is the **epiphyseal plate**. The **metaphysis** is the part of the diaphysis that abuts onto the epiphyseal plate.

Cartilage

Cartilage is a form of connective tissue in which the cells and fibers are embedded in a gel-like matrix, the fibers lending firmness and resilience. A fibrous membrane called the **perichondrium** covers the cartilage except on the exposed surfaces in joints. Of the three types of cartilage, hyaline cartilage and fibrocartilage tend to calcify or even ossify in later life.

- **Hyaline cartilage** has a high proportion of amorphous matrix that has the same refractive index as the fibers embedded in it. Throughout childhood and adolescence, it plays an important part in the lengthening of long bones (epiphyseal plates are composed of hyaline cartilage). It has great resistance to wear and covers the articular surfaces of nearly all synovial joints. Hyaline cartilage is incapable of repair when fractured; the defect is filled with fibrous tissue.
- **Fibrocartilage** has many collagen fibers embedded in a small amount of matrix and is found in the discs within joints (eg, temporomandibular, sternoclavicular, and knee joints) and on the articular surfaces of the clavicle and mandible. Fibrocartilage, if damaged, repairs itself slowly in a manner similar to fibrous tissue elsewhere. Joint discs have a poor blood supply and therefore do not repair themselves when damaged.
- **Elastic cartilage** possesses large numbers of elastic fibers embedded in matrix, making it flexible. It is found in the auricle of the ear, external auditory meatus, auditory tube, and the epiglottis. Elastic cartilage, if damaged, repairs itself with fibrous tissue.

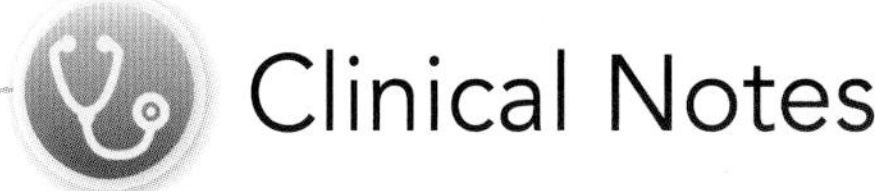

Clinical Notes

Bone Fractures

Immediately after a fracture, the patient experiences severe local pain and is not able to use the injured part. Deformity may be visible if the bone fragments have been displaced relative to each other. The degree of deformity and the directions taken by the bony fragments depend not only on the mechanism of injury but also on the pull of the muscles attached to the fragments. Ligamentous attachments also influence the deformity. In certain bones (eg, the ilium) fractures result in no deformity because the inner and outer surfaces are splinted by the extensive origins of muscles. In contrast, a fracture of the neck of the femur produces considerable displacement. The strong muscles of the thigh pull the distal fragment upward so that the leg is shortened. The very strong lateral rotators rotate the distal fragment laterally so that the foot points laterally.

Fracture of a bone is accompanied by considerable hemorrhage of blood between the bone ends and into the surrounding soft tissue. The blood vessels and the fibroblasts and osteoblasts from the periosteum and endosteum take part in the repair process.

Rickets

Rickets is a defective mineralization of the cartilage matrix in growing bones. This produces a condition in which the cartilage cells continue to grow, resulting in excess cartilage and a widening of the epiphyseal plates. The poorly mineralized cartilaginous matrix and the osteoid matrix are soft, and they bend under the stress of bearing weight. The resulting deformities include enlarged costochondral junctions, bowing of the long bones of the lower limbs, and bossing of the frontal bones of the skull. Deformities of the pelvis may also occur.

Epiphyseal Plate Disorders

Epiphyseal plate disorders affect only children and adolescents. The epiphyseal plate is the part of a growing bone concerned primarily with growth in length. Trauma, infection, diet, exercise, and endocrine disorders can disturb the growth of the hyaline cartilaginous plate, leading to deformity and loss of function. In the femur, for example, the proximal epiphysis can slip because of mechanical stress or excessive loads. The length of the limbs can increase excessively because of increased vascularity in the region of the epiphyseal plate secondary to infection or in the presence of tumors. Shortening of a limb can follow trauma to the epiphyseal plate resulting from diminished blood supply to the cartilage.

Joints

A site where two or more bones come together, whether or not movement occurs between them, is termed a **joint**.

Joint Classification

The three main types of joints are based on the tissues that lie in the **joint space** between the bones: fibrous joints, cartilage joints, and synovial joints (Fig. 1.10).

Fibrous Joints

In fibrous joints, the articulating surfaces of the bones are tightly linked by fibrous tissue that fills the joint space (see Fig. 1.10A). Thus, very little movement is possible at these joints. The sutures of the vault of the skull and the inferior tibiofibular joints are examples of fibrous joints.

Cartilage Joints

In cartilage joints, the space between the articulating bony surfaces is filled with a cartilaginous pad. The two types of cartilage joints are synchondroses and symphyses. A **synchondrosis** is a cartilaginous joint in which the articulating bones are united by a plate or bar of hyaline cartilage. The epiphyseal plate between the epiphysis and diaphysis of a growing bone is a temporary form of a synchondrosis. The first sternocostal joint between the first rib and the manubrium sterni is a permanent synchondrosis. No movement occurs in synchondroses.

A **symphysis** is a cartilage joint in which the bones are united primarily by a pad or plate of fibrocartilage. Symphyses are located along the midline of the body. The intervertebral joints between the vertebral bodies (see Fig. 1.10B), the manubriosternal joint, and the symphysis pubis are symphyseal joints. A small amount of movement is possible in symphyses.

Synovial Joints

In synovial joints, the articular surfaces of the bones are covered by a thin layer of hyaline cartilage and are separated by a fluid-filled joint cavity (see Fig. 1.10C). This arrangement permits a great degree of freedom of movement. The cavity of the joint is lined by a **synovial membrane**, which extends from the margins of one articular surface to those of the other. A tough fibrous membrane referred to as the **capsule** of the joint protects the exterior of the synovial membrane. A viscous fluid called **synovial fluid**, which is produced by the synovial membrane, fills the joint cavity and lubricates the articular surfaces. Synovial fluid has the consistency of about that of egg white, thus the *syn-ovum* terminology. In certain synovial joints (eg, knee and temporomandibular joints), discs or wedges of fibrocartilage are interposed between the articular surfaces of the bones. These are referred to as **articular discs**. Some synovial joints (eg, hip and knee

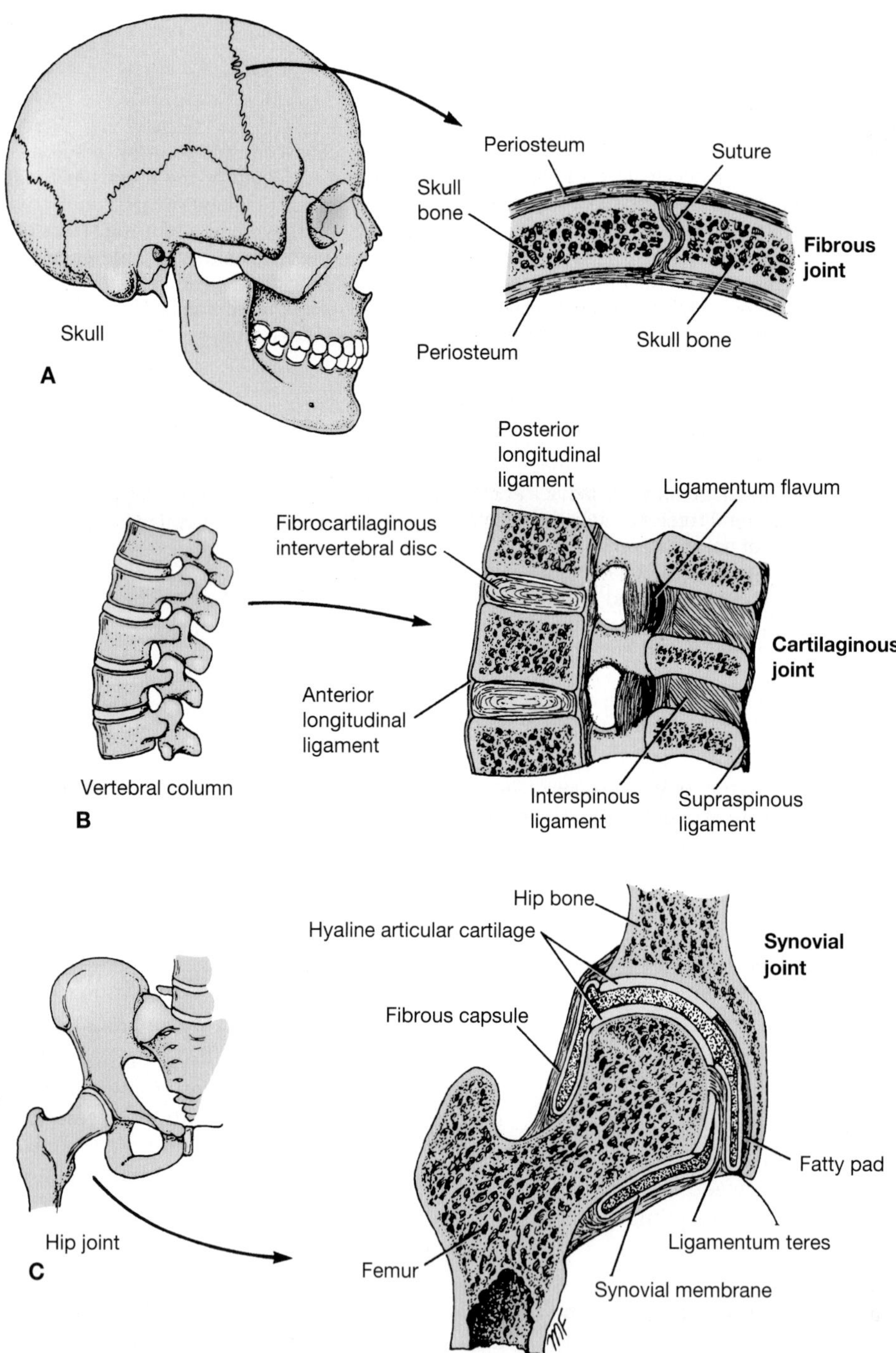

Figure 1.10 Examples of three types of joints. **A.** Fibrous joint (coronal suture of the skull). **B.** Cartilaginous joint (joint between two lumbar vertebral bodies). **C.** Synovial joint (hip joint).

joints) contain fatty pads lying between the synovial membrane and the fibrous capsule or bone.

The shape of the bones participating in the joint, the approximation of adjacent anatomic structures (eg, the thigh against the anterior abdominal wall on flexing the hip joint), and the presence of fibrous ligaments uniting the bones all contribute to limiting the degree of movement in a synovial joint. Most ligaments lay outside the joint capsule and are referred to as **extracapsular ligaments**. However, some important ligaments (eg, the cruciate ligaments in the knee) lie within the capsule and are termed **intracapsular ligaments**.

Synovial joints can be classified according to the shapes of the articular surfaces and the types of movements that are possible. Table 1.3 and Figure 1.11 summarize the

Table 1.3 Synovial Joint Types

JOINT TYPE	MORPHOLOGY	EXAMPLE(S)
Plane joint	Apposed articular surfaces are flat or almost flat, permitting the bones to slide on one another in multiple directions.	Joints between the articular processes of the vertebrae Sternoclavicular joint Acromioclavicular joint
Hinge joint	This resembles the hinge on a door, so that uniaxial flexion-extension movements are possible.	Humeroulnar joint in the elbow Interphalangeal joints in the hands and feet Ankle (talocrural) joint
Pivot joint	Central bony pivot is surrounded by a bony-ligamentous ring. Rotation is the only movement possible.	Median atlantoaxial joint Superior radioulnar joint
Condyloid joint	Two distinct convex surfaces that articulate with two concave surfaces. Biaxial movements (movements in two planes) are typical.	Metacarpophalangeal joints in the hands (knuckle joints) and feet
Ellipsoid joint	Elliptical convex articular surface fits into an elliptical concave articular surface. Mainly biaxial movements are allowed.	Radiocarpal (wrist) joint
Saddle joint	Articular surfaces are reciprocally concave-convex and resemble a saddle on a horse's back. This is a specialized biaxial joint that allows multiaxial movement.	Carpometacarpal joint of the thumb
Ball-and-socket joint	Ball-shaped head of one bone fits into a socket-like concavity of another, allowing multiaxial movement.	Glenohumeral (shoulder) joint Hip joint

types of synovial joints. The examples given are not necessarily the only joints of each type.

Joint Stability

The stability of a joint depends on three main factors: the morphology of the bony articular surfaces, the ligaments, and the tone of the muscles around the joint (Fig. 1.12).

Articular Surfaces

In certain joints, the shapes of the bones and their articulating surfaces cause the bones to form a relatively tight-fitting framework that imparts overall stability to the joint, such as the ball-and-socket arrangement of the hip joint (see Fig. 1.12A) and the mortise arrangement of the tarsal bones in the ankle joint. However, in some other joints, the shape of the bones contributes little or nothing to joint stability (eg, the acromioclavicular, calcaneocuboid, and knee joints).

Ligaments

Fibrous ligaments prevent excessive movement in a joint (see Fig. 1.12B), but if the stress is continued for an excessively long period, fibrous ligaments stretch. For example, the ligaments of the joints between the bones forming the arches of the feet will not support the weight of the body. If the tone of the muscles that normally supports the arches become impaired by fatigue, the ligaments stretch, and the arches collapse, producing flat feet. Elastic ligaments, conversely, return to their original length after stretching. The elastic ligaments of the auditory ossicles play an active part in supporting the joints and assisting in the return of the bones to their original position after movement.

Muscle Tone

In most joints, muscle tone is the major factor controlling stability. For example, the muscle tone of the short muscles around the shoulder joint keeps the hemispherical head of the humerus in the shallow glenoid cavity of the scapula. Without the action of these muscles, very little force would be required to dislocate this joint. The knee joint is very unstable without the tonic activity of the quadriceps femoris muscle. The joints between the small bones forming the arches of the feet are largely supported by the tone of the muscles of the leg, whose tendons are inserted into the bones of the feet (Fig. 1.12C).

Joint Nerve Supply

The joint capsule and ligaments receive an abundant sensory nerve supply. A sensory nerve supplying a joint also supplies the muscles moving the joint and the skin overlying the insertions of these muscles, a fact that has been codified as Hilton's law.

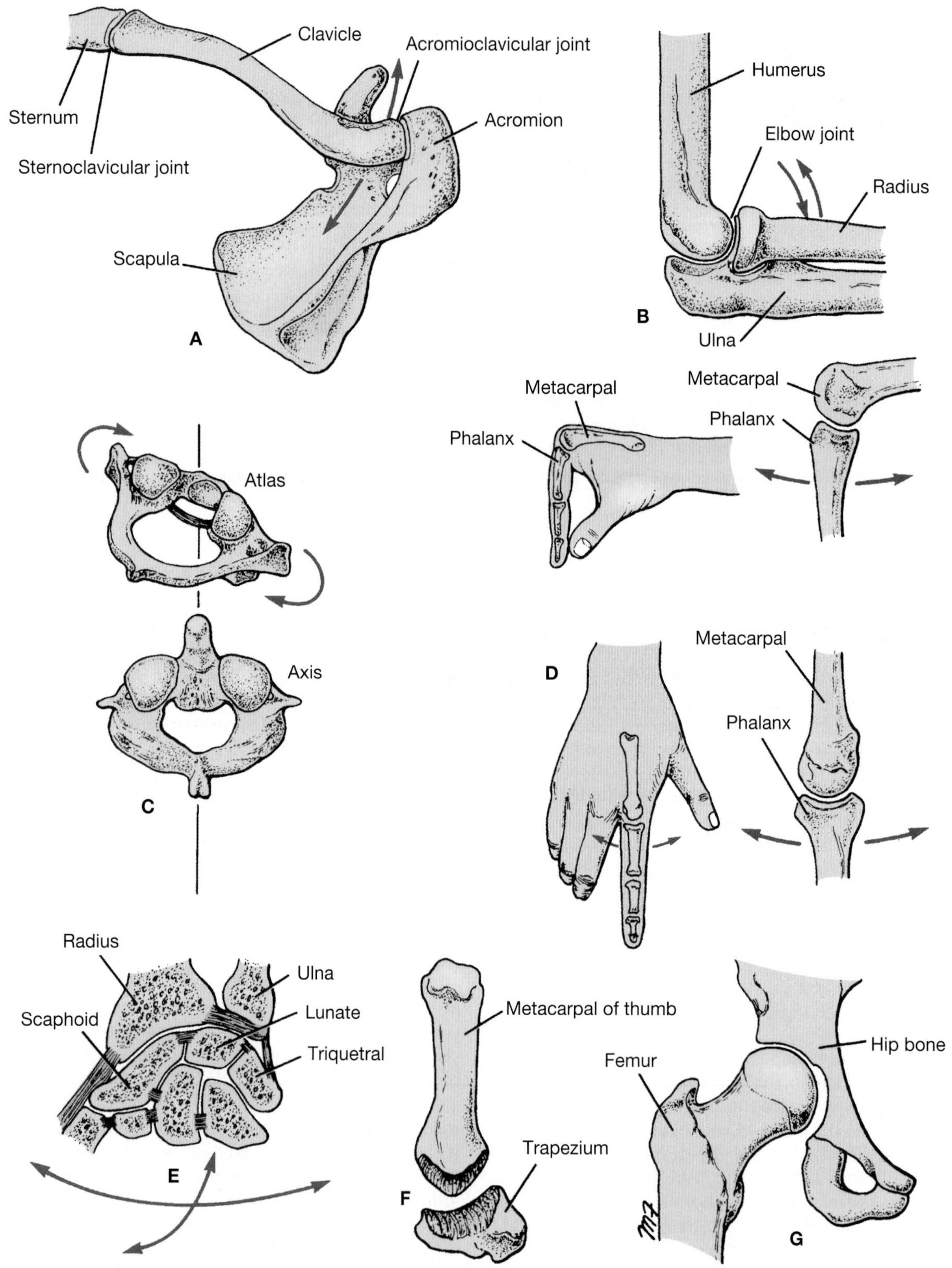

Figure 1.11 Examples of different types of synovial joints. **A.** Plane joints (sternoclavicular and acromioclavicular joints). **B.** Hinge joint (humeroulnar part of the elbow joint). **C.** Pivot joint (medial atlantoaxial joint). **D.** Condyloid joint (metacarpophalangeal joint). **E.** Ellipsoid joint (radiocarpal part of the wrist joint). **F.** Saddle joint (carpometacarpal joint of the thumb). **G.** Ball-and-socket joint (hip joint).

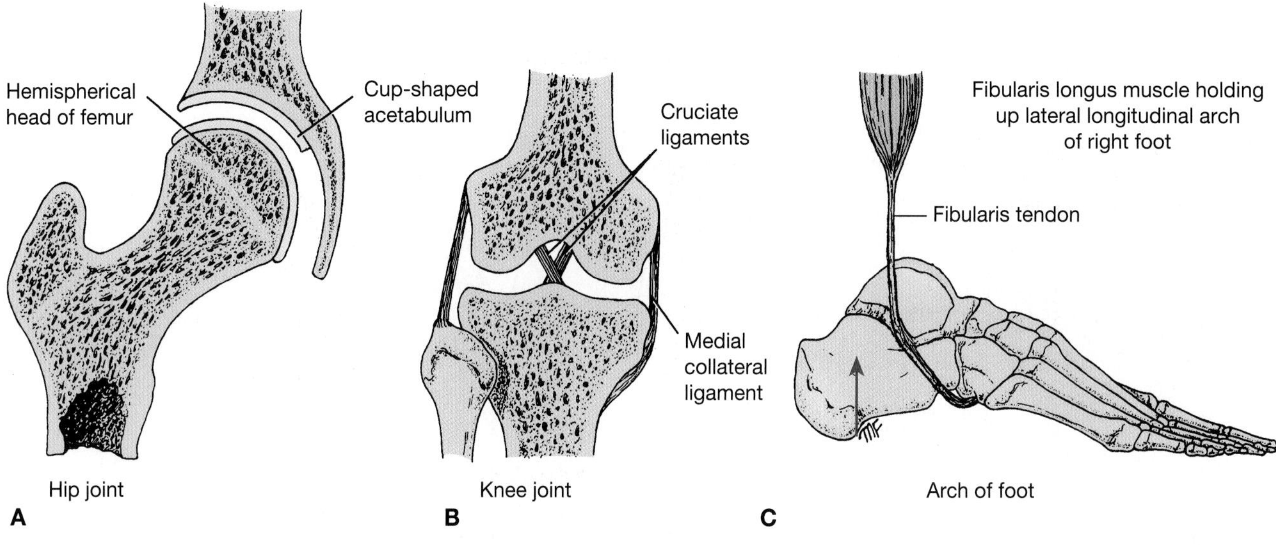

Figure 1.12 The three main factors responsible for stabilizing a joint. **A.** Shape of articular surfaces. **B.** Ligaments. **C.** Muscle tone.

Ligaments

A ligament is a cord or band of fibrous connective tissue uniting two or more structures. In the context of the musculoskeletal system, ligaments typically bind bones at joints. The two types of ligaments are fibrous and elastic. Most **fibrous ligaments** are composed of dense bundles of collagen fibers and are not stretchable under normal conditions (eg, iliofemoral ligament of the hip joint and collateral ligaments of the elbow joint). **Elastic ligaments** are composed largely of elastic tissues and can therefore regain their original length after stretching (eg, ligamentum flavum of the vertebral column and calcaneonavicular ligament of the foot).

Bursae and Synovial Sheaths

A **bursa** is a closed fibrous sac lined internally with synovial membrane. The synovial membrane secretes a film of viscous fluid that fills the sac. Bursae are typically found in areas subject to friction and serve to reduce friction (eg, wherever tendons rub against bones, ligaments, or other tendons). They are commonly found close to joints where the skin rubs against underlying bony structures such as the prepatellar bursa (Fig. 1.13). Occasionally, the cavity of a bursa communicates with the cavity of a synovial joint (eg, the suprapatellar bursa communicates with the knee joint, and the subscapularis bursa communicates with the shoulder joint).

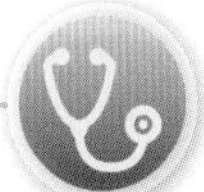

Clinical Notes

Joint Examination

When examining a patient, the clinician should assess the normal range of movement of all joints. When the bones of a joint are no longer in their normal anatomic relationship with one another, the joint is **dislocated**. Some joints are particularly susceptible to dislocation because of lack of support by ligaments, the poor shape of the articular surfaces, or the absence of adequate muscular support. The shoulder, temporomandibular, and acromioclavicular joints are good examples. Dislocation of the hip is usually congenital, being caused by inadequate development of the socket that normally holds the head of the femur firmly in position.

The presence of cartilaginous discs within joints, especially weight-bearing joints, as in the case of the knee, makes the disc particularly susceptible to injury in sports. During a rapid movement, the disc loses its normal relationship to the bones and becomes crushed between the weight-bearing surfaces.

In certain diseases of the nervous system (eg, syringomyelia), the sensation of pain in a joint is lost. This means that the warning sensations of pain felt when a joint moves beyond the normal range of movement are not experienced. This phenomenon results in the destruction of the joint.

Knowledge of the classification of joints is valuable because, for example, certain diseases affect only certain types of joints. Gonococcal arthritis affects large synovial joints such as the ankle, elbow, or wrist, whereas tuberculous arthritis also affects synovial joints and may start in the synovial membrane or in the bone.

Remember that more than one joint may receive the same nerve supply. For example, the obturator nerve supplies both the hip and knee joints. Thus, a patient with disease limited to one of these joints may experience pain in both.

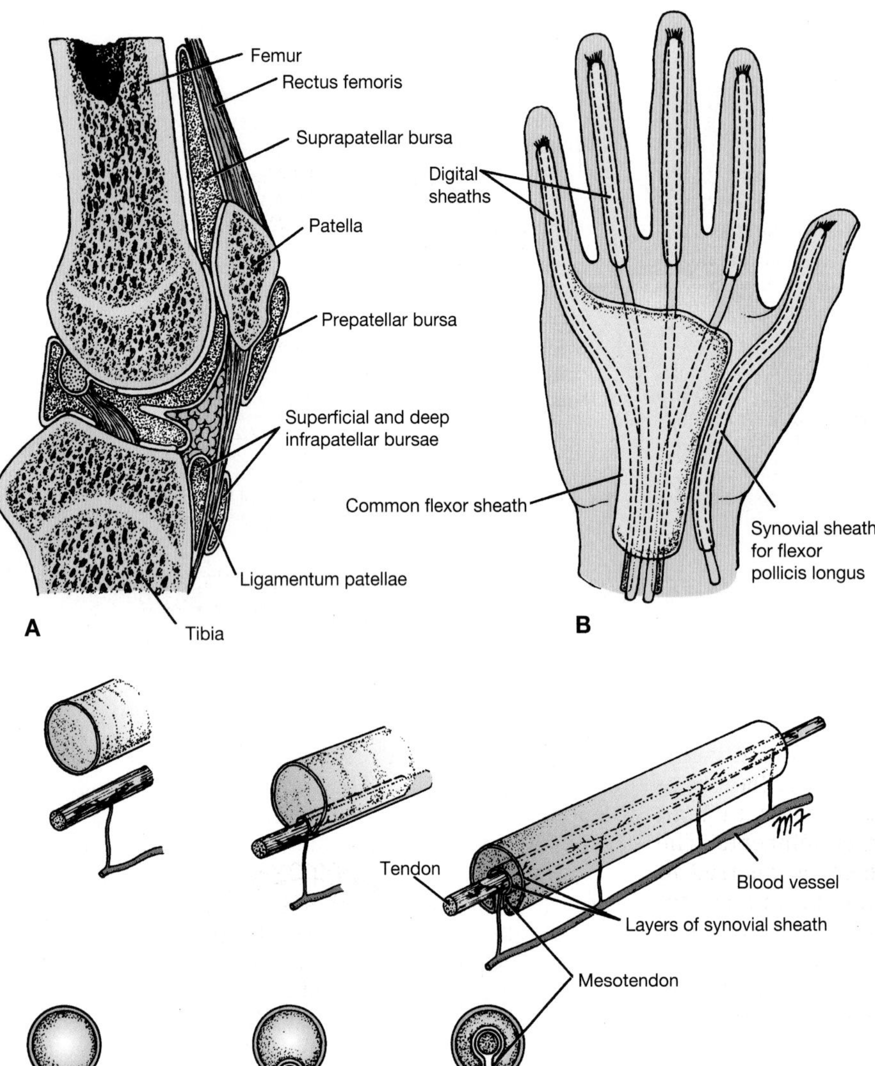

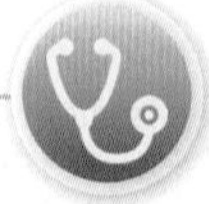

Figure 1.13 Examples of bursae and synovial sheaths. **A.** Four bursae related to the front of the knee joint. Note that the suprapatellar bursa communicates with the cavity of the joint. **B.** Synovial sheaths around the long tendons of the fingers. **C.** How a tendon indents a synovial sheath during development, and how blood vessels reach the tendon through the mesotendon.

Clinical Notes

Ligament Damage

Joint ligaments are very prone to excessive stretching, tearing, and rupture. A ligament **sprain** is an injury caused by abnormal or excessive force at a joint, but without dislocation of the joint or fracture of a bone. In treating damaged ligaments, if possible, the apposing damaged surfaces of the ligament are brought together by positioning and immobilizing the joint. In severe injuries, surgical approximation of the cut ends may be required. The blood clot at the damaged site is invaded by blood vessels and fibroblasts. The fibroblasts lay down new collagen and elastic fibers, which become oriented along the lines of mechanical stress.

A **synovial sheath** is a tubular bursa that surrounds a tendon (see Fig. 1.13B). The tendon invaginates the bursa from one side so that the tendon becomes suspended within the bursa by a **mesotendon** (see Fig. 1.13C). The mesotendon enables blood vessels to enter the tendon along its course. In certain situations, when the range of movement is extensive, the mesotendon disappears or remains in the form of narrow threads, the **vincula** (eg, on the long flexor tendons of the fingers and toes). Synovial sheaths occur where tendons pass under ligaments and retinacula and through osseofibrous tunnels. Their function is to reduce friction between the tendon and its surrounding structures.

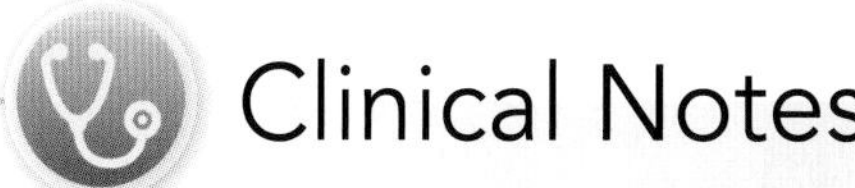

Clinical Notes

Bursae and Synovial Sheath Trauma and Infection

Bursae and synovial sheaths are commonly the site of traumatic or infectious disease. **Bursitis** is inflammation of a bursa (eg, inflammation of the prepatellar bursa, or "housemaid's knee," may occur as the result of trauma from repeated kneeling on a hard surface). **Tenosynovitis** is inflammation of a tendon and its synovial sheath (eg, the extensor tendon sheaths of the hand may become inflamed after excessive or unaccustomed use). Notable tenosynovitis may lead to contracture of the synovial sheath and obstruct efficient sliding of the tendon.

Muscle

The three types of muscle are skeletal, smooth, and cardiac.

Skeletal Muscle

Skeletal muscles generally act to produce the movements of the skeleton; they are sometimes called **voluntary muscles** and are made up of **striated muscle fibers**. A skeletal muscle has two or more attachments. The more proximal, less mobile attachment is referred to as the **origin**. The more distal, more mobile attachment is the **insertion** (Fig. 1.14). When a muscle contracts, the insertion is drawn proximally toward the origin. However, under varying circumstances, the degree of mobility of the attachments may be reversed; therefore, *origin* and *insertion* are relative terms.

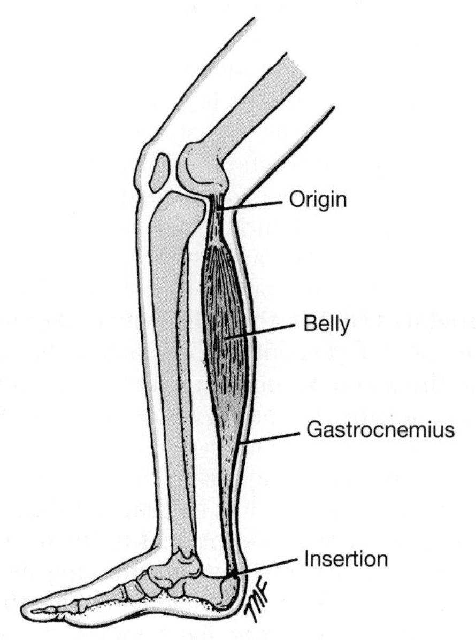

Figure 1.14 Origin, insertion, and belly of the gastrocnemius muscle.

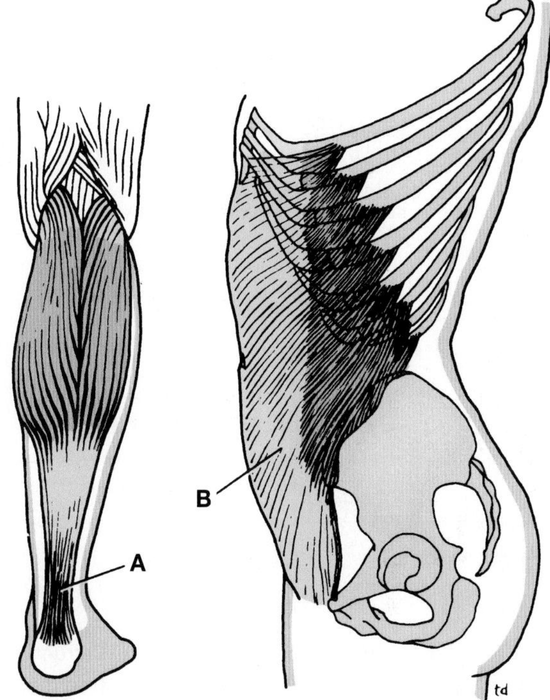

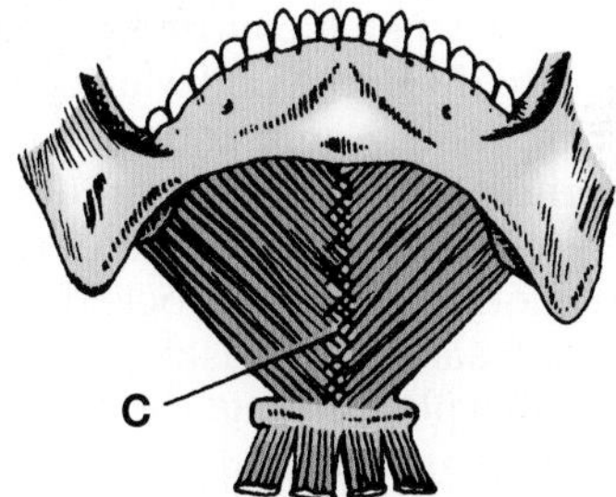

Figure 1.15 Examples of **(A)** a tendon, **(B)** an aponeurosis, and **(C)** a raphe.

The fleshy part of the muscle is referred to as its **belly**. The ends of a muscle are attached to supporting elements (bones, cartilage, ligaments, or other muscles) by cords of fibrous tissue called **tendons** (Fig. 1.15). Some tendons (eg, those belonging to the flat, wide abdominal oblique muscles) form a thin, strong sheet termed an **aponeurosis** (see Fig. 1.15B). Other tendons may form a **raphe**, which is an interdigitation of the tendinous ends of fibers of flat muscles (see Fig. 1.15C).

Skeletal Muscle Internal Structure

Individual muscle fibers are bound together with continuous, delicate sheaths of areolar tissue, which are condensed on the surface of the muscle to form a fibrous envelope, the **epimysium (investing deep fascia)**. The individual fibers of a muscle are arranged either parallel

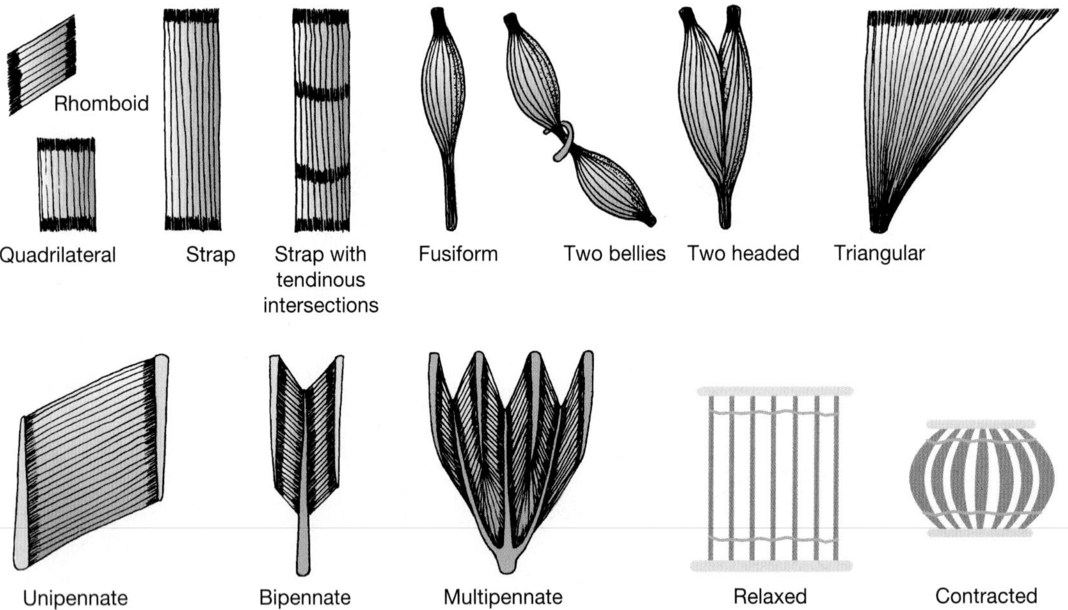

Figure 1.16 Different forms of the internal structure of skeletal muscle. A relaxed and a contracted muscle are also shown. Note how the muscle fibers, on contraction, shorten by one-third to one-half of their resting length. Note also how the muscle swells.

or oblique to the long axis of the muscle (Fig. 1.16). Because a muscle fiber shortens by one-third to one-half its resting length when it contracts, muscles whose fibers run parallel to the line of pull will act over a longer distance and bring about a greater degree of movement compared with those whose fibers run obliquely. That is, parallel-fibered muscles have a greater excursion (ie, greater range of motion). The sternocleidomastoid, rectus abdominis, and sartorius muscles are examples of muscles with parallel fiber arrangements.

Muscles whose fibers run obliquely to the line of pull are referred to as **pennate muscles** (ie, they resemble a feather). In a **unipennate muscle**, the tendon lies along one side of the muscle, and the muscle fibers pass obliquely to it (eg, extensor digitorum longus), whereas in a **bipennate muscle**, the tendon lies in the center of the muscle, and the muscle fibers pass to it from two sides (eg, rectus femoris). A **multipennate muscle** may be arranged as a series of bipennate muscles lying alongside one another (eg, acromial fibers of the deltoid) or may have the tendon lying within its center and the muscle fibers passing to it from all sides, converging as they go (eg, tibialis anterior).

The force (strength) that a muscle produces when it contracts is directly proportional to the physiologic cross-sectional area of the muscle (ie, total cross-sectional area of the muscle fibers). Pennate muscles have a greater number of fibers per given volume of muscle substance and thus a greater cross-sectional area compared to parallel-fibered muscles. Therefore, pennate muscles produce more force but have less excursion.

Skeletal Muscle Action

All movements are the result of the coordinated action of many muscles, but studying each muscle individually is necessary to understand their actions. A muscle may work in the following four ways:

Agonist (prime mover): A muscle is an agonist (prime mover) when it is the chief muscle or member of a chief group of muscles responsible for producing a particular movement. The quadriceps femoris, for example, is the agonist in the movement of extending the knee joint (Fig. 1.17A).

Antagonist: Any muscle that opposes the action of the agonist is an antagonist, such as the biceps femoris, which is an antagonist during knee extension because it opposes the action of the quadriceps femoris (see Fig. 1.17B). Before a prime mover can contract, the antagonist muscle must be equally relaxed; this is brought about by nerve reflex inhibition. Remember that these terms describe movements relative to each other. Therefore, the biceps femoris becomes an agonist and the quadriceps femoris becomes the antagonist during knee flexion.

Fixator: A fixator contracts isometrically (ie, contraction increases the tone but does not in itself produce movement) to stabilize the origin of the prime mover so that it can act efficiently. For example, the muscles attaching the shoulder girdle to the trunk contract as fixators to allow the deltoid to act on the shoulder joint (see Fig. 1.17C).

Synergist: In many locations in the body, the agonist muscle crosses multiple joints before it reaches the joint at which its main action takes place. To prevent unwanted movements in an intermediate joint, muscles called **synergists** contract and stabilize the intermediate joints. For example, the flexor and extensor muscles of the carpus contract to fix the wrist joint, which allows the long flexor and extensor muscles of the fingers to work efficiently (see Fig. 1.17D).

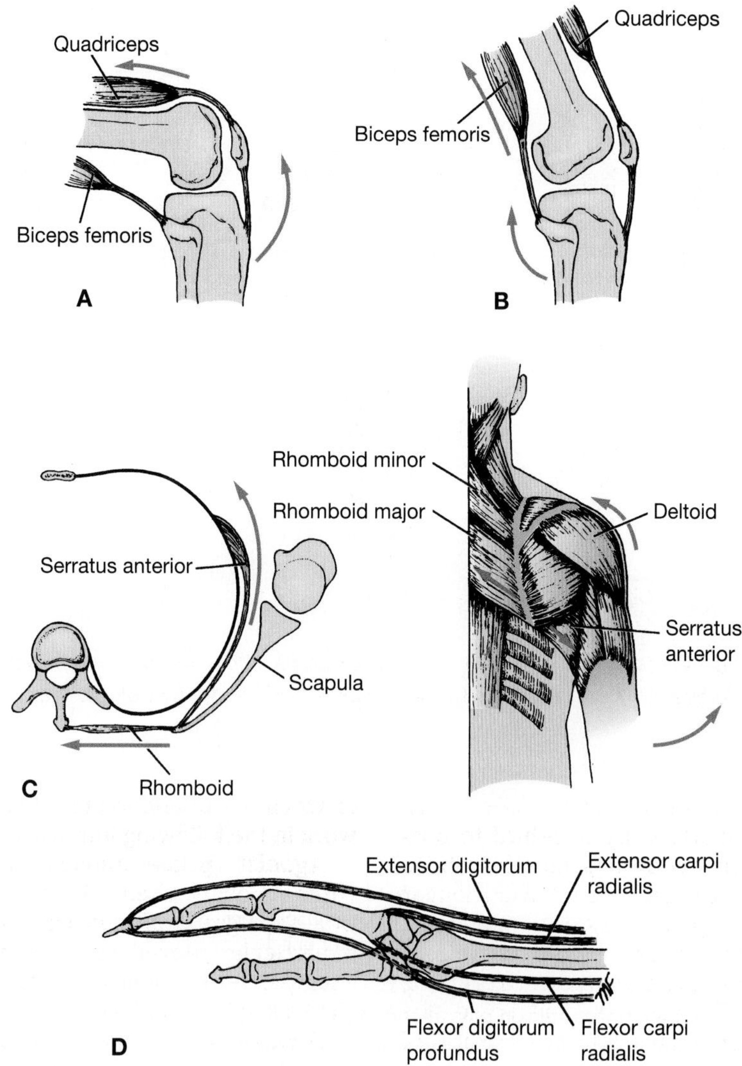

Figure 1.17 Different types of muscle action. **A.** Quadriceps femoris extending the knee as an agonist (prime mover) and biceps femoris acting as an antagonist. **B.** Biceps femoris flexing the knee as an agonist and quadriceps acting as an antagonist. **C.** Muscles around shoulder girdle fixing the scapula so that the movement of abduction can take place at the shoulder joint. **D.** Flexor and extensor muscles of the carpus acting as synergists and stabilizing the carpus so that the long flexor and extensor tendons can flex and extend the fingers.

Remember, these terms are applied to the role of a particular muscle during a particular movement. Many muscles can alter their roles and act as an agonist, an antagonist, a fixator, or a synergist, from moment to moment, depending on the movement to be accomplished. Muscles can also act paradoxically (eg, the biceps brachii, a flexor of the elbow joint, may contract and modulate the rate of extension of the elbow when the triceps brachii contracts).

Skeletal Muscle Nerve Supply

The nerve trunk to a muscle is a mixed nerve. About 60% of the nerve fibers are motor, and 40% are sensory. Also, the nerve contains some sympathetic autonomic fibers. The nerve enters the muscle at about the midpoint on its deep surface, often near the margin. The point of entrance is known as the **motor point**. This arrangement allows the muscle to both protect its nerve trunk and move with minimum interference with the nerve trunk.

The individual motor neurons within a muscle nerve supply a variable number of muscle fibers that are arranged in a variable spatial distribution. A single motor neuron plus all the muscle fibers innervated by that neuron constitute a **motor unit**. The size of a motor unit (ie, the number of muscle fibers supplied by a motor neuron) varies greatly from muscle to muscle, according to the size and function of the muscle (Fig. 1.18). Large motor units (up to several hundred muscle fibers per neuron) are characteristic of the large trunk and lower limb muscles. Small motor units (as few as 5 to 10 muscle fibers per neuron) are features of precision movement muscles such as the extraocular muscles and the small muscles in the hand.

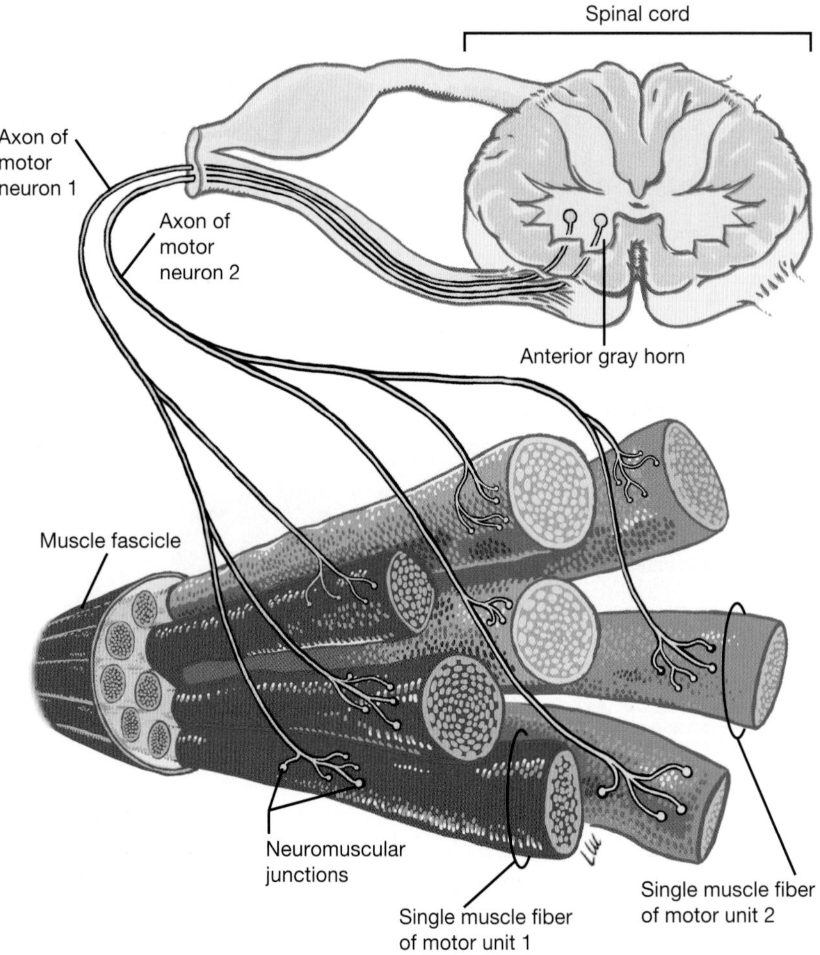

Figure 1.18 Two motor units. Each motor neuron plus all the muscle cells it supplies constitute a motor unit. In this example, motor unit 1 (in *red*) contains three muscle fibers, whereas motor unit 2 (in *blue*) has five fibers. Therefore, motor unit 1 is a smaller motor unit, and unit 2 is a larger motor unit.

Skeletal Muscle Naming

The names of muscles convey valuable information about their shape, size, number of heads or bellies, position, depth, attachments, actions, and other features. Some examples of muscle names are shown in Table 1.4. Pay attention to the names of muscles and try to understand them, as they provide meaningful information that enables better comprehension and reduces rote memorization.

Smooth Muscle

Smooth muscle consists of long, spindle-shaped cells closely arranged in bundles or sheets. In the tubes of the body, it provides the motive power for propelling the contents through the lumen. In the digestive system, it also mixes ingested food with digestive juices. A wave of contraction of the circularly arranged fibers passes along the tube, milking the contents onward. By their contraction, the longitudinal fibers pull the wall of the tube proximally over the contents. This method of propulsion is referred to as **peristalsis**.

In storage organs such as the urinary bladder and the uterus, the fibers are irregularly arranged and interlaced with one another. Their contraction is slow and sustained and brings about expulsion of the contents of the organs. In the walls of the blood vessels, the smooth muscle fibers are arranged circularly and serve to modify the caliber of the lumen. Depending on the organ, smooth muscle fibers may be stimulated to contract by local stretching of the fibers, by nerve impulses from autonomic nerves, or by hormonal stimulation.

Cardiac Muscle

Cardiac muscle consists of striated muscle fibers that branch and unite with each other. It forms the myocardium of the heart. Its fibers tend to be arranged in whorls and spirals, and they have the property of spontaneous and rhythmic contraction. Specialized cardiac muscle fibers form the **conducting system of the heart**. Cardiac muscle is supplied by autonomic nerve fibers that terminate in the nodes of the conducting system and in the myocardium.

Table 1.4 Skeletal Muscle Naming[a]

NAME	SHAPE	SIZE	NUMBER OF HEADS OR BELLIES	POSITION	DEPTH	ATTACHMENTS	ACTIONS
Deltoid	Triangular						
Teres	Round						
Rectus	Straight						
Major		Large					
Latissimus		Broadest					
Longissimus		Longest					
Biceps			Two heads				
Quadriceps			Four heads				
Digastric			Two bellies				
Pectoralis				Of the chest			
Supraspinatus				Above spine of scapula			
Brachii				Of the arm			
Profundus					Deep		
Superficialis					Superficial		
Externus					External		
Sternocleidomastoid						From sternum and clavicle to mastoid process	
Coracobrachialis						From coracoid process to arm	
Extensor							Extend
Flexor							Flex
Constrictor							Constrict

[a]These names are commonly used in combination, for example, flexor pollicis longus (long flexor of the thumb).

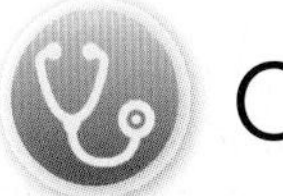

Clinical Notes

Muscle Tone

Determining the **tone** of a muscle is important in clinical examination. If a muscle is **flaccid**, the afferent, efferent, or both neurons involved in the reflex arc necessary to produce muscle tone have been interrupted (eg, if the nerve trunk to a muscle is severed, both neurons will have been interrupted). If poliomyelitis has involved the motor anterior horn cells at a level in the spinal cord that innervates the muscle, the efferent motor neurons will not function. Conversely, if the muscle is found to be hypertonic, the possibility exists of a lesion involving higher motor neurons in the spinal cord or brain.

Muscle Attachments

By knowing the main attachments of all the major muscles of the body, understanding the normal and abnormal actions of individual muscles or muscle groups becomes possible. Without this information, clinicians cannot even attempt to analyze, for example, a patient's abnormal gait.

Muscle Shape and Form

Also note the general shape and form of muscles. A paralyzed muscle or one that is not used (such as occurs when a limb is immobilized in a cast) quickly atrophies and changes shape. In the case of the limbs, remember that a muscle on the opposite side of the body can be used for comparison.

Cardiac Muscle Necrosis

Cardiac muscle receives its blood supply from the coronary arteries. A sudden block of one of the large branches of a coronary artery inevitably leads to necrosis of the cardiac muscle and often to the death of the patient.

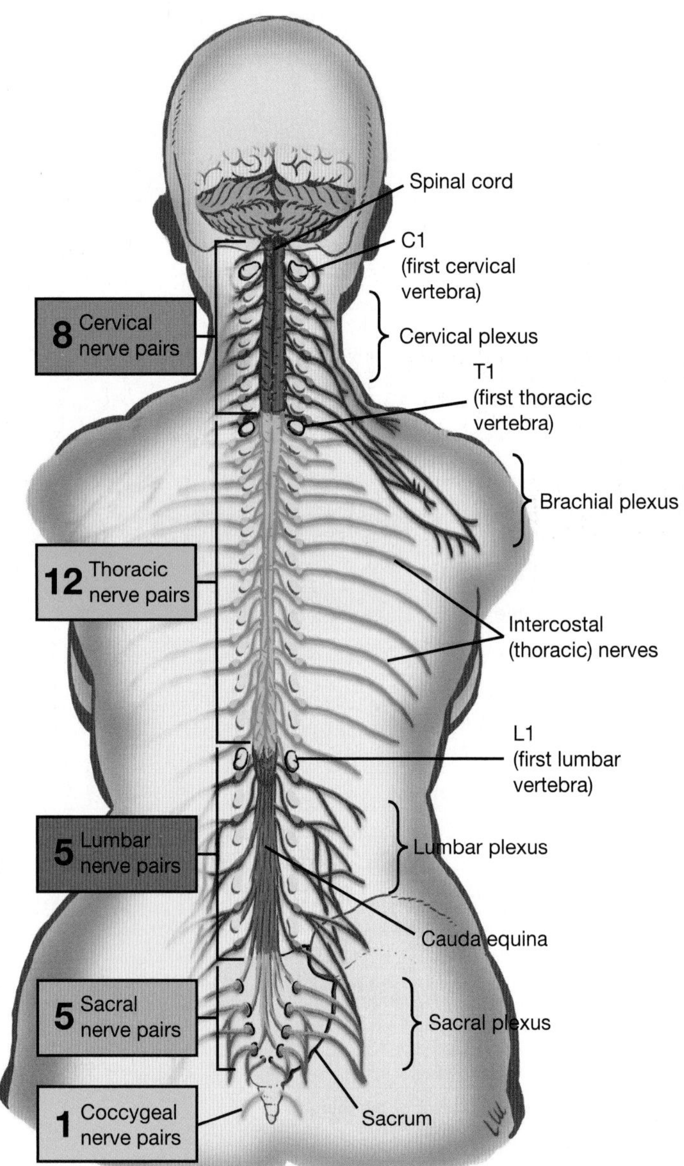

Figure 1.19 Components of the central and peripheral nervous systems: brain, spinal cord, spinal nerves, and plexuses.

Nervous System

The nervous system, together with the endocrine system, controls and integrates the activities of the different parts of the body. The nervous system is divided into two main parts: the **central nervous system (CNS)**, which consists of the brain and spinal cord, and the **peripheral nervous system (PNS)**, which consists of a paired series of cranial and spinal nerves and their associated ganglia (Fig. 1.19). Functionally, the nervous system can be further divided into the **somatic nervous system** and the **autonomic nervous system (ANS)**. The somatic nervous system acts on the body's external environment, primarily through the actions of skeletal muscles, and uses mostly voluntary responses to consciously perceived sensory signals from the body wall and limbs. The ANS acts on the body's internal environment, primarily through the actions of smooth muscle, cardiac muscle, and glands and uses mostly involuntary responses to sensory signals that are not consciously perceived.

Central Nervous System

The CNS is composed of large numbers of nerve cells and their processes, supported by specialized tissue called **neuroglia**. A **neuron** is an individual nerve cell, including all its processes. Each neuron has three main components: the cell body and two types of processes termed **dendrites** and an **axon**. Dendrites typically conduct nerve impulses toward the cell body and are the short processes of the cell body. The axon usually conducts impulses away from the cell body and dendrites and is the longest process of the cell body (Fig. 1.20A). Cell bodies within the CNS are mostly located in clusters termed **nuclei**.

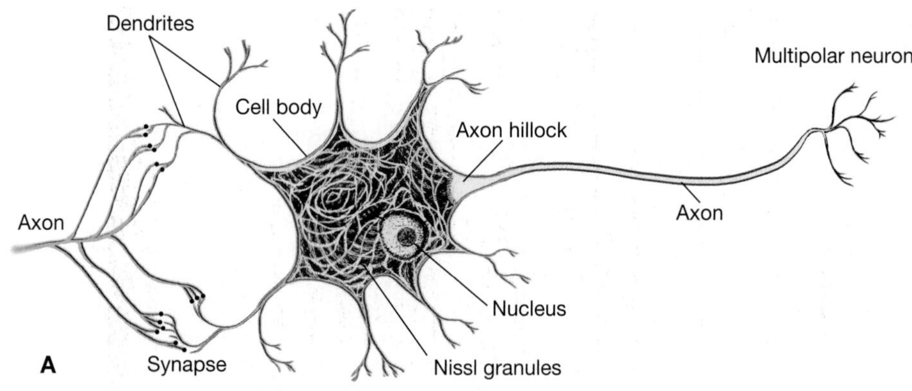

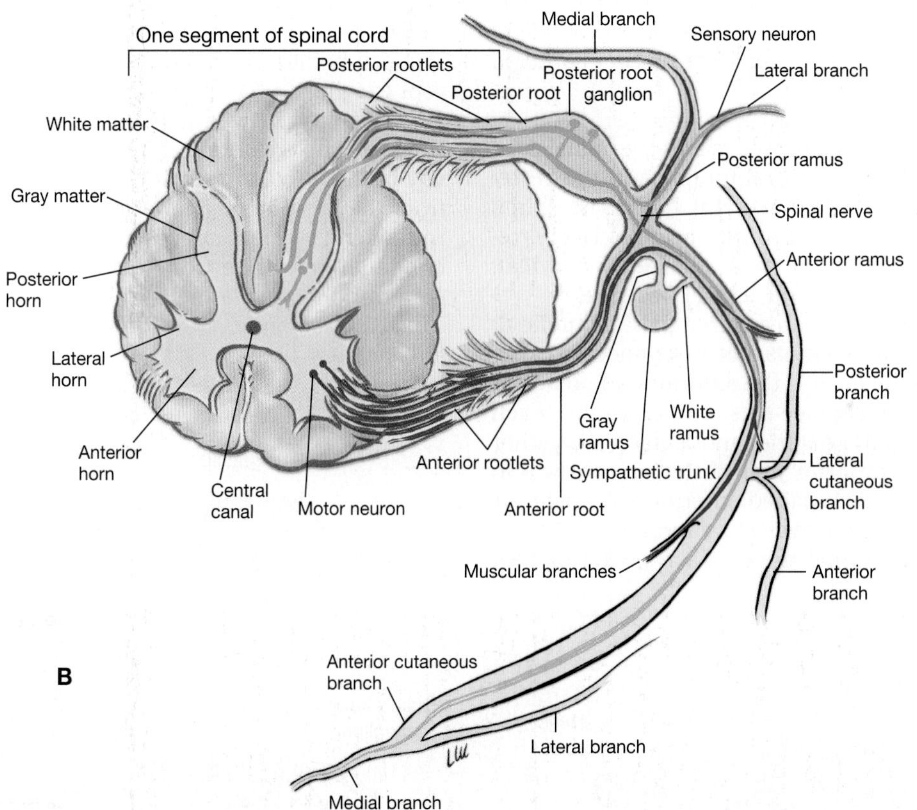

Figure 1.20 **A.** Multipolar motor neuron with connector neuron synapsing with it. **B.** Horizontal section through a thoracic segment of the spinal cord showing the segmental organization of a typical spinal nerve.

The interior of the CNS is organized into gray and white matter. **Gray matter** consists largely of nerve cell bodies embedded in neuroglia. **White matter** consists largely of nerve processes (axons) and blood vessels embedded in neuroglia. Gray matter and white matter are so named because of their relative color tones in fresh tissue. The large population of myelinated nerve processes in white matter gives that tissue a relatively white, glistening color. Conversely, the large population of nonmyelinated cell bodies in gray matter presents a relatively dull, grayish color. In the spinal cord, the gray matter is organized in a characteristic H-shaped (or butterfly-shaped) pattern (see Fig. 1.20B). Paired **posterior (dorsal)** and **anterior (ventral) gray horns** extend along the length of the cord. Paired **lateral gray horns** bulge out in the thoracic and upper lumbar portions of the cord. A **central canal** containing **cerebrospinal fluid** runs the internal length of the CNS.

Three membranes (**meninges**) surround the entire CNS (brain plus spinal cord): the **dura mater** is the most external membrane, the **arachnoid mater** is the middle membrane, and the **pia mater** is the innermost layer. The meninges serve to protect, anchor, and stabilize the CNS and also contain a surrounding sac of cerebrospinal fluid.

Peripheral Nervous System

The PNS consists of the cranial and spinal nerves and their associated ganglia. A **ganglion** is a cluster of neuron cell bodies located outside the CNS. In dissection, the cranial and spinal nerves appear as grayish white cords. They are made up of bundles of neuron processes (axons) supported by delicate areolar tissue.

Cranial Nerves

The 12 pairs of cranial nerves branch off the brain and upper spinal cord and pass through openings (foramina) in the skull. All the cranial nerves are distributed in the head and neck except cranial nerve (CN) X (vagus nerve), which also supplies structures in the thorax and abdomen. The cranial nerves are described in Chapter 9.

Spinal Nerves

A total of 31 pairs of spinal nerves leaves the spinal cord and pass through intervertebral foramina in the vertebral column (Fig. 1.21; also see Fig. 1.19). The spinal nerves are named according to the region of the vertebral column with which they are associated: 8 **cervical**, 12 **thoracic**, 5 **lumbar**, 5 **sacral**, and 1 **coccygeal**.

Each spinal nerve originates with a paired bundle of **anterior and posterior rootlets** that are connected to the spinal cord along the lines of the anterior and posterior gray horns, respectively (see Figs. 1.19 and 1.20). Each bundle of anterior and posterior rootlets joins together and forms a single **anterior and posterior root** within the vertebral canal. Each paired anterior and posterior root merges within an intervertebral foramen (IVF) and forms an individual **spinal nerve**. Each posterior root possesses a **posterior root ganglion**, which is located at the IVF. The spinal nerve passes through the IVF and immediately divides into a smaller **posterior ramus** and a larger **anterior ramus**.

The anterior rootlets and roots consist of bundles of **efferent (motor) nerve fibers** carrying nerve impulses away from the CNS (Fig. 1.21; also see Fig. 1.19). The cell bodies of somatic motor neurons that supply skeletal muscles and cause them to contract lie in the anterior gray horn of the spinal cord. Cell bodies of autonomic (visceral) motor neurons that supply smooth and cardiac muscle and glands and cause those to contract or secrete lie in the lateral gray horn.

The posterior rootlets and roots contain bundles of **afferent (sensory) nerve fibers** that carry impulses to the CNS (see Figs. 1.20 and 1.22). These fibers are concerned with conveying information about touch, pain, temperature, and other sensations from the periphery. The cell bodies of sensory neurons lie in the posterior root ganglion.

The spinal nerves and the anterior and posterior rami are mixed nerve components in that they convey both motor and sensory neuron processes to and from the periphery. Therefore, lesions of rootlets and roots versus spinal nerves and rami result in different combinations of sensory and motor deficits. Lesion of anterior roots affects only motor neuron fibers. However, lesion of anterior rami affects both motor and sensory fibers.

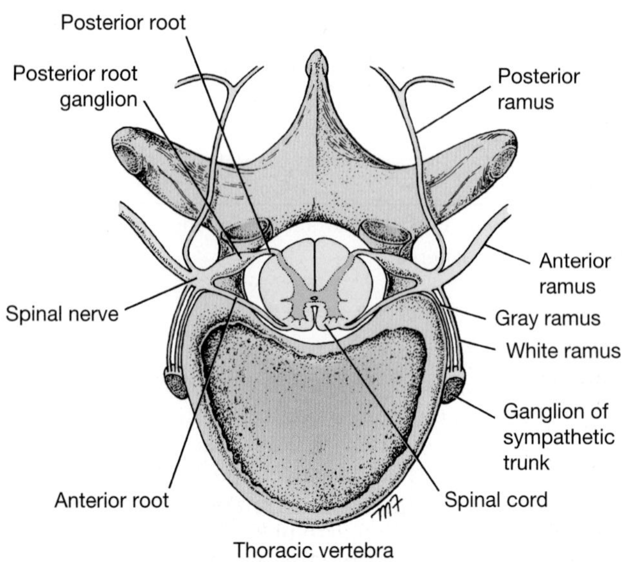

Figure 1.21 Association between spinal cord, spinal nerves, and sympathetic trunks.

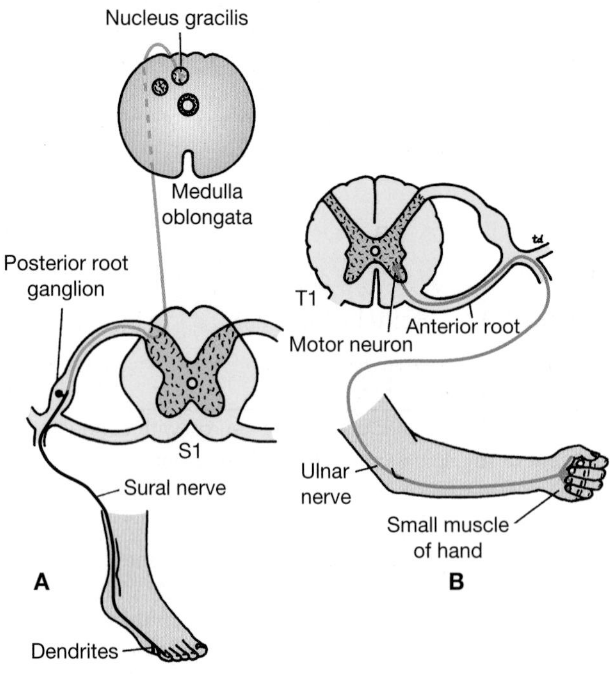

Figure 1.22 Two neurons that pass from the central to the peripheral nervous system. **A.** Afferent neuron that extends from the little toe to the brain. **B.** Efferent neuron that extends from the anterior gray horn of the first thoracic segment of spinal cord to a small muscle of the hand.

The anterior rami continue laterally and anteriorly to supply the muscles and skin over the anterolateral body wall and all the muscles and skin of the limbs. The posterior rami pass posteriorly around the vertebral column to supply the muscles and skin of the back. In addition to the anterior and posterior rami, the spinal nerves give a small meningeal branch that supplies the vertebrae and the spinal meninges. Thoracic and upper lumbar spinal nerves also have branches, called *rami communicantes*, which are associated with the sympathetic part of the ANS.

The anterior rami of spinal nerves distribute in one of two patterns: (1) via simple segmentation and (2) via plexuses (see Fig. 1.19). In **simple segmentation**, each anterior ramus remains an independent structure and wraps around the trunk separately from its neighboring anterior rami, such as with the intercostal nerves. In this system, each peripheral nerve retains its identity with the spinal nerve of origin (eg, intercostal nerve T5 is an identifiable branch of spinal nerve T5). However, adjacent anterior rami may have overlapping territories. In a **plexus**, several adjacent anterior rami join one another, intermix their neuron processes, and form complex networks that generate peripheral nerves. In this patterning, the nerves emerging from a plexus are formed from multiple spinal nerves, and the peripheral nerves lose their gross identity with the spinal nerves of origin (eg, the median nerve in the upper limb is formed by fibers derived from anterior rami of spinal nerves C5 to T1). Nerve plexuses form in the neck (**cervical plexus**), at the root of the upper limb (**brachial plexus**), and the root of the lower limb (**lumbosacral plexus**).

The classic division of the nervous system into central and peripheral parts is purely artificial and one of descriptive convenience because the processes of the neurons pass freely between the two. For example, a motor neuron located in the anterior gray horn of the first thoracic segment (T1) of the spinal cord gives rise to an axon that passes through the anterior root of the T1 nerve (see Fig. 1.22), passes through the brachial plexus, travels down the arm and forearm in the ulnar nerve, and finally reaches the motor endplates on several muscle fibers of a small muscle of the hand—a total distance of about 3 ft (90 cm).

As another example, consider the sensation of touch felt on the lateral side of the little toe. The first sacral segment of the spinal cord (S1) supplies this area of skin. The fine terminal nerve fibers leave the sensory organs of the skin and unite to form the axon of the sensory nerve. The axon passes up the leg in the sural nerve and then in the tibial and sciatic nerves to the lumbosacral plexus. It then passes through the posterior root of the S1 nerve to reach the cell body in the posterior root ganglion of the S1 nerve. The central axon now enters the posterior white column of the spinal cord and passes up to the nucleus gracilis in the medulla oblongata—a distance of about 5 ft (1.5 m). Thus, a single neuron extends from the little toe to the inside of the skull. Both these examples illustrate the potentially great length of a single neuron.

Autonomic Nervous System

The **ANS** is the part of the nervous system concerned with motor control of smooth muscle, cardiac muscle, and glands throughout the body. The hypothalamus of the brain controls the ANS and integrates the activities of the autonomic and neuroendocrine systems, thus preserving homeostasis in the body. The ANS is distributed throughout the central and peripheral nervous systems. The somatic and ANS differ in several significant ways, which are summarized in Table 1.5 and Figure 1.23. The major anatomic difference is that the peripheral part of the somatic nervous system (to skeletal muscle) is a

Table 1.5 Somatic Versus Autonomic Nervous Systems

	SOMATIC	AUTONOMIC
Target	Skeletal muscle	Smooth muscle, cardiac muscle, glands
Peripheral pathway	One-neuron pathway Single motor neuron runs the entire distance from the central nervous system (CNS) to the target muscles, through peripheral nerves, without intervening synapses.	Two-neuron pathway Two neurons, in series, run from the CNS to the target cells. Neuron #1 is the preganglionic neuron; neuron #2 is the postganglionic neuron. Preganglionic neurons generally do not innervate the target cells; instead, they synapse with postganglionic neurons in autonomic ganglia. Postganglionic neurons generally innervate the target cells.
Cell bodies	Within the CNS, in either brain stem motor nuclei or ventral gray horn of the spinal cord	*Preganglionic neurons*: within the CNS, in either brain stem autonomic nuclei or lateral gray horn of the spinal cord *Postganglionic neurons*: outside the CNS, within autonomic (visceral) ganglia
Termination	Motor endplate on each muscle cell	No motor endplates

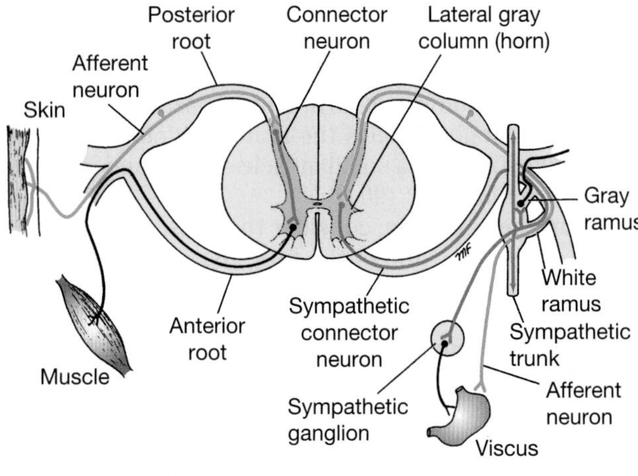

Figure 1.23 General arrangement of somatic part of the nervous system (*left*) compared to the autonomic part (*right*).

one-neuron pathway, whereas the peripheral part of the ANS is a two-neuron pathway.

The ANS is divided into two parts: the **sympathetic division** and the **parasympathetic division**. The general floor plan and functional aspects of each division are summarized in Figure 1.24 and Table 1.6. Overall, sympathetic activity prepares the body for emergency, whereas parasympathetic activity aids in recovery.

The sympathetic and parasympathetic divisions often function as antagonistic systems, that is, they produce activities in opposition to one another. For example, sympathetic activity produces accelerated heart rate, bronchodilation, decreased peristalsis in the gut tube, closing of the sphincters, relaxation of the general bladder wall, and dilation of the pupils. Conversely, parasympathetic activity results in decelerated heart rate, bronchoconstriction, increased gut peristalsis, opening of sphincters, contraction of the bladder wall, and constriction of the pupils. However, the two divisions may function as complementary (synergistic) systems. For example, in normal sexual function, parasympathetic activity produces erection, and sympathetic activity results in ejaculation. Additionally, one division may function independently of the other—sympathetic stimulation activates sweat gland secretion, but parasympathetics play no role in sweat gland activity.

Sympathetic Division

The sympathetic division supplies all parts of the body via a complex nerve network that can frustrate beginning students (and many instructors). Despite its complexity, sympathetic distribution is elegantly organized and comprehensible.

- Preganglionic neuron cell bodies are in the lateral gray horn of the spinal cord, from T1 to about the L2 levels (see Fig. 1.23). Preganglionic fibers exit the spinal cord via the T1 to L2 anterior roots and spinal nerves. Because of these levels of origin and departure from the spinal cord, the sympathetic division is traditionally referred to as the **thoracolumbar outflow**.
- These myelinated fibers exit their spinal nerves via **white rami communicantes** and enter the unilateral **sympathetic trunk** (see Figs. 1.23 and 1.24). Two sympathetic trunks lie along the vertebral column, one on each side. Each sympathetic trunk is a series of ganglia linked together in a segmental, roughly chainlike arrangement. Because of their location, the chain ganglia collectively are termed the **paravertebral ganglia**.
- The sympathetic trunks extend above and below the T1 to L2 levels, along the entire length of the vertebral column and sacrum (see Fig. 1.24). Typically, 11 to 12 thoracic chain ganglia exist, and only 3 cervical chain ganglia formed by fusions of segmental embryonic ganglia. Lumbar and sacral chain ganglia are variable in form and number, and fusions of ganglia are common. A single midline coccygeal ganglion, the **ganglion impar**, representing the fusion of the embryonic paired coccygeal ganglia, is the caudal end of the sympathetic trunks.
- Further sympathetic outflow emanates from the sympathetic chain ganglia and follows four general pathways to four specific target regions (Table 1.7; also see Fig. 1.24). Synapses between the pre- and postganglionic neurons occur in ganglia related to each pathway (eg, sympathetic outflow originating in spinal cord levels T1 to L2 enters the sympathetic chains, and synapses occur within the chain ganglia along the entire length of the sympathetic chain). Postganglionic fibers then exit the chain ganglia and follow branches of spinal nerves to reach the body wall and limbs. Further details on sympathetic distribution to the four target regions are provided in the appropriate chapters to come.

Parasympathetic Division

Compared with the sympathetic division, the parasympathetic division is more limited in scope and less complex in its geography. Parasympathetic distribution is focused on the head, body cavities, and external genitalia. The body wall and limbs do not receive parasympathetic innervation.

Preganglionic parasympathetic neurons originate in the brain and some sacral segments of the spinal cord (see Fig. 1.24). Those in the brain form parts of the nuclei of origin of CNs III (oculomotor), VII (facial), IX (glossopharyngeal), and X (vagus), and the axons emerge from the brain in the corresponding cranial nerves. The sacral preganglionic neurons originate in the lateral gray matter of the S2, S3, and S4 segments of the cord. However, because the number of cells here is insufficient to form a distinct bulge such as seen in the thoracolumbar region, a lateral gray horn does not exist. Myelinated axons leave the spinal cord in the anterior nerve roots of the corresponding spinal nerves, then leave the S2 to S4 spinal nerves, and form the **pelvic splanchnic nerves**. Because of these levels of origin and departure from the CNS, the parasympathetic division is traditionally referred to as the **craniosacral outflow**.

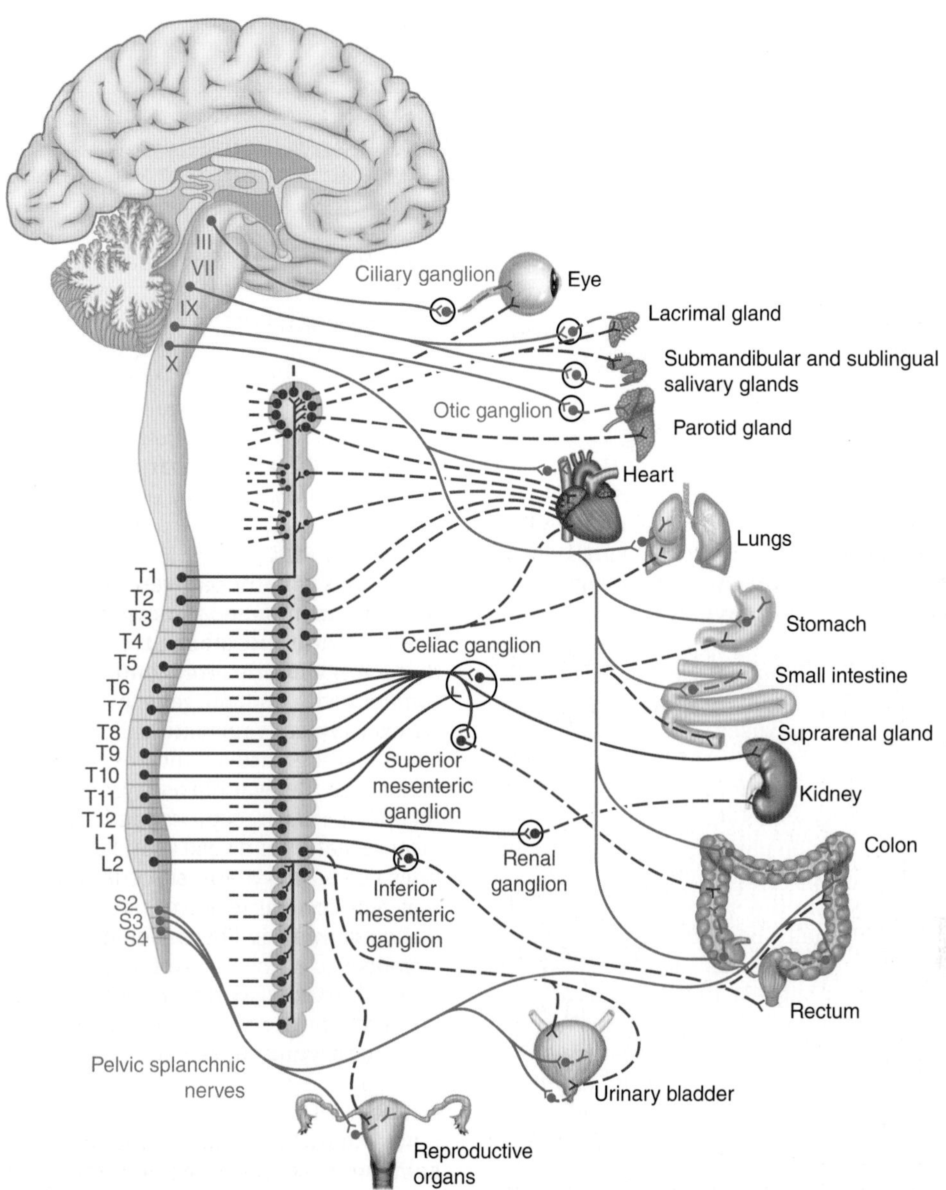

Figure 1.24 Schematic summary of the autonomic nervous system. Preganglionic parasympathetic fibers are shown in *solid blue*; postganglionic parasympathetic fibers are exhibited in *interrupted blue*. Preganglionic sympathetic fibers are shown in *solid red*; postganglionic sympathetic fibers in *interrupted red*. A sympathetic chain is indicated in *yellow*.

Table 1.6 General Functional Aspects of the Sympathetic and Parasympathetic Divisions

	SYMPATHETIC DIVISION	PARASYMPATHETIC DIVISION
Territory	Supplies all areas of the body	Does not supply all areas; no parasympathetic innervation in the body wall and limbs
Activity	More generalized and indirect; ratio of pre- to postganglionic neurons is ~1:15 or more	More specific and direct; ratio of pre- to postganglionic neurons is ~1:2
Functions	Emergency: This is the classic "fight-or-flight" response. Functions are associated with increased levels of activity or excitation and assistance in coping with stress and physical exertion.	Recovery: This is the classic "vegetative state" response. Functions are associated with homeostasis, restoration, recuperation, and relaxation.

Table 1.7 Sympathetic Distribution Routes

SPINAL CORD ORIGIN	SYNAPSE LOCATION	POSTGANGLIONIC PATHWAY	TARGET
T1 to L2	Sympathetic chain ganglia	Spinal nerves	Body wall and limbs
T1 to T4	Superior cervical ganglion	Cranial arteries	Head
T1 to T4	Cervical and upper thoracic sympathetic chain ganglia	Thoracic splanchnic nerves	Thoracic viscera
T5 to L2	Preaortic ganglia	Abdominopelvic splanchnic nerves	Abdominopelvic viscera External genitalia

Preganglionic neurons synapse with postganglionic cells in peripheral ganglia that are usually situated close to the viscera they innervate. The preganglionic fibers in CNs III, VII, and IX project to autonomic ganglia in the head, and their distributions are limited to the head. The preganglionic neurons in CN X have extensive distributions to ganglia near the viscera in the neck, thoracic cavity, and much of the abdominal cavity. The preganglionic fibers in the pelvic splanchnic nerves project to ganglia in the hypogastric plexuses or in the walls of the lower abdominal and pelvic viscera. Characteristically, the postganglionic fibers are nonmyelinated and are relatively short compared with sympathetic postganglionic fibers. Further details on parasympathetic distribution are provided in the appropriate chapters to follow.

Autonomic outflow from the sacral segments of the spinal cord has traditionally been considered part of the parasympathetic division, as described above. However, recent studies suggest that the sacral autonomics are, in fact, anatomically part of the sympathetic nervous system. Although these postganglionic cells, like those that activate sweat glands, express a cholinergic phenotype, they are anatomically sympathetic fibers. Thus, including all sacral autonomic fibers as components of the sympathetic division is more accurate. This rethinking of the sacral outflow is based on neurophysiologic factors and does not alter the basic anatomy described above. The current view is that the sacral components of the ANS should more properly be considered part of the sympathetic division. Therefore, the sympathetic division should be described as the **spinal outflow** (T1 to L2 plus S2 to S4) of the ANS and the parasympathetic division as the **cranial outflow** (CNs III, VII, IX, X) of the ANS.

VISCERAL AFFERENTS

The ANS is a motor pathway. However, sensory neurons do travel in intimate association with autonomic fibers. **Visceral afferent neurons** are the sensory neurons that supply information about the body's internal environment via visceral reflexes and sensation. Visceral reflexes typically regulate blood pressure and chemistry by mediating cardiac and respiratory rates and vessel resistance. Relevant sensory receptors include chemoreceptors, baroreceptors, and osmoreceptors. Normal visceral activity (eg, gut motility and distension) usually does not produce conscious sensation. However, abnormal activity (eg, extreme stretch, chemical irritation, ischemia) may evoke conscious sensations of pain and/or nausea.

Myelinated visceral afferent fibers from thoracic and abdominopelvic viscera travel with both sympathetic and parasympathetic nerves. These afferents pass through the various autonomic plexuses and ganglia but do not synapse within them. Many visceral afferents course into the sympathetic trunks, then course into spinal nerves via the white rami communicantes, then course into the posterior roots of spinal nerves, and finally enter the spinal cord (see Fig. 1.23). The cell bodies of visceral afferent neurons are located within the posterior root ganglia. Other visceral afferents travel with the vagus nerve and enter the brainstem. The cell bodies of these neurons are located within the vagal sensory ganglia at the base of the skull.

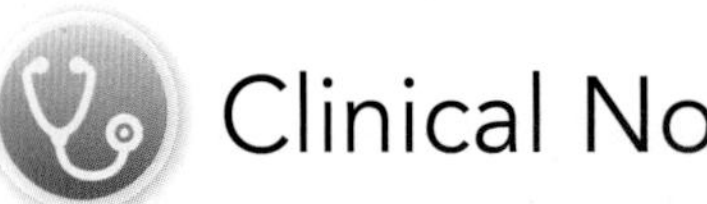

Clinical Notes

Dermatomes: Segmental Innervation of Skin

Each spinal nerve (and therefore each segment of the spinal cord) innervates a specific area of skin in a highly organized fashion. A **dermatome** is the area of skin supplied by the somatic sensory fibers of a single spinal nerve (Figs. 1.25 and 1.26). On the trunk, the dermatomes form a relatively simple bandlike pattern. In the limbs, arrangement of the dermatomes is more complicated because of the embryonic rotations that take place as the limbs grow out from the body wall. Adjacent dermatomes overlap considerably, especially on the trunk. At least three contiguous spinal nerves must be sectioned to produce complete anesthesia in any one dermatome.

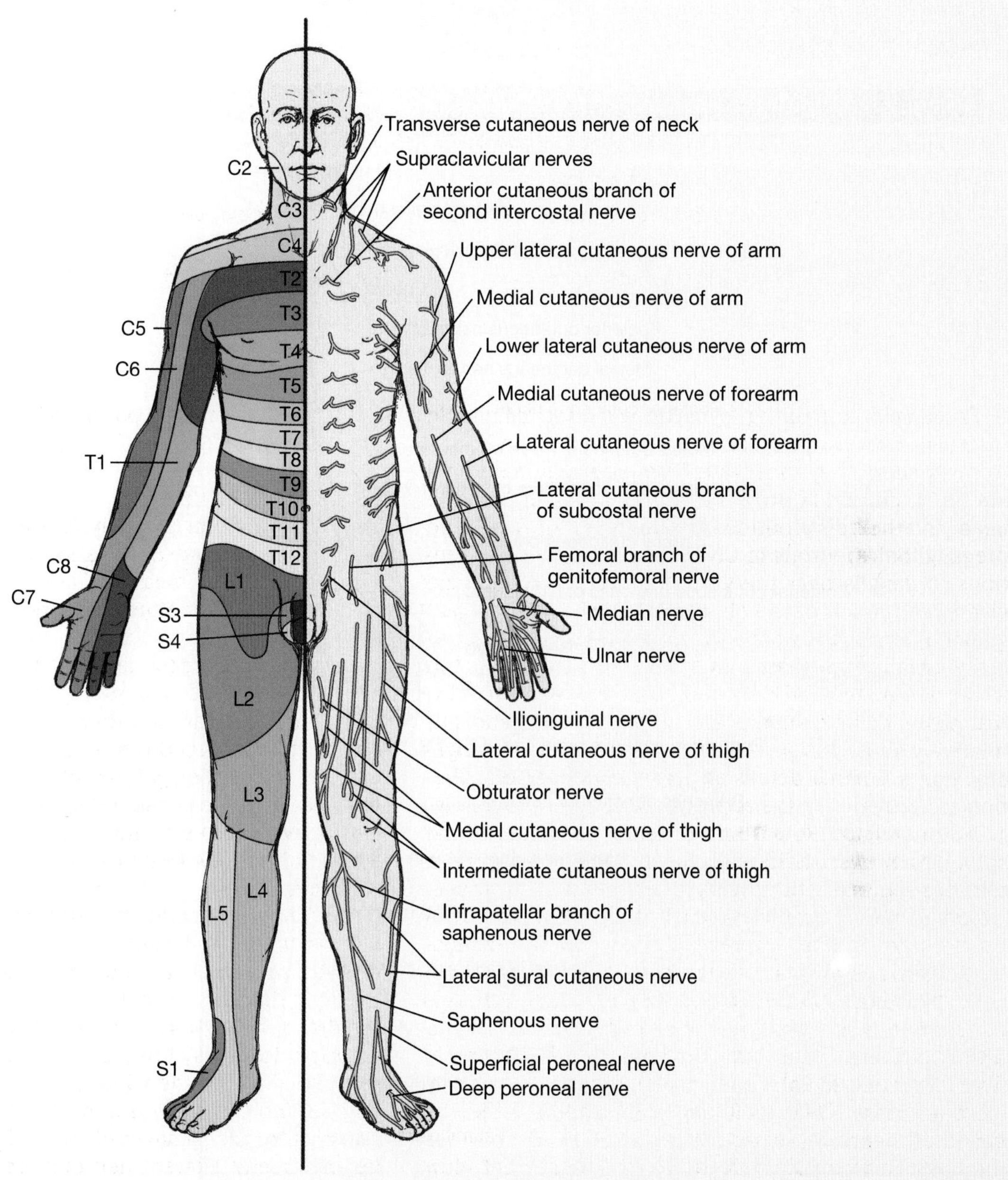

Figure 1.25 Dermatomes and distribution of cutaneous nerves on the anterior aspect of the body.

A clinician should have a working knowledge of the dermatomal (segmental) innervation of skin, because understanding the dermatome map can help determine whether the sensory component of a particular spinal nerve or segment of the spinal cord is functioning normally (eg, a sensory deficit in the skin over the nipple is likely related to a problem primarily with the T4 spinal nerve/posterior nerve root/spinal cord segment).

Segmental Innervation of Muscle

Skeletal muscle also receives a segmental innervation. Most muscles are innervated by two, three, or four spinal nerves (via plexuses) and thus by the same number of segments of the spinal cord. Therefore, several spinal nerves or several segments of the spinal cord must be lesioned to paralyze a muscle completely.

Learning the segmental innervation of all the muscles of the body is an impossible task. Nevertheless, the segmental innervation of the following muscles should be known because these muscles can be tested by eliciting simple muscle reflexes in the patient (Fig. 1.27):

- **Biceps brachii tendon reflex**: C5 and C6, flexion of the elbow joint by tapping the biceps tendon
- **Triceps tendon reflex**: C6 to C8, extension of the elbow joint by tapping the triceps tendon

(continued)

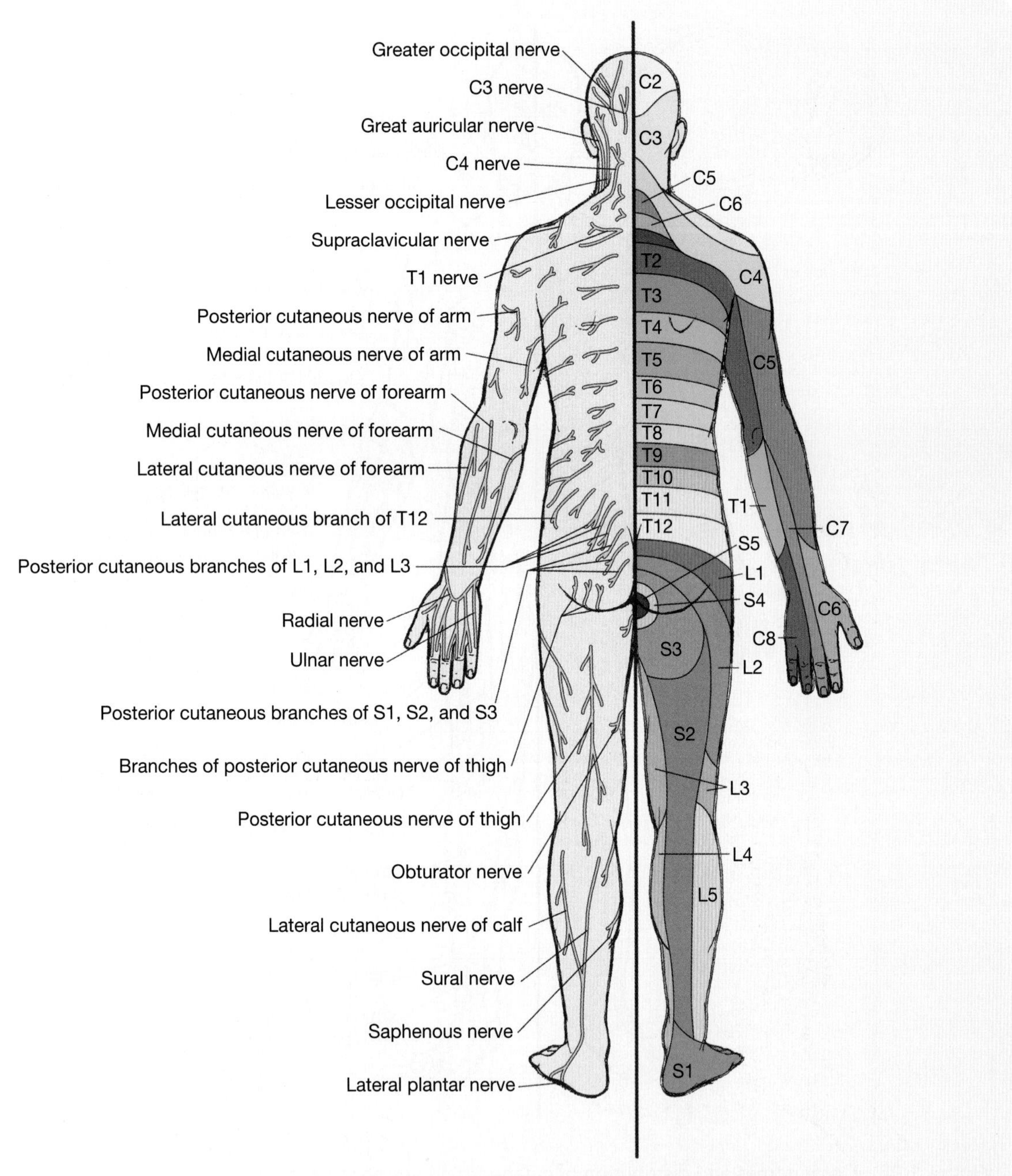

Figure 1.26 Dermatomes and distribution of cutaneous nerves on the posterior aspect of the body.

- **Brachioradialis tendon reflex**: C5 to C7, supination of the radioulnar joints by tapping the insertion of the brachioradialis tendon
- **Abdominal superficial reflexes**: Upper abdominal skin T6 to T7, middle abdominal skin T8 to T9, and lower abdominal skin T10 to T12; contraction of underlying abdominal muscles by stroking the skin
- **Patellar tendon reflex (knee jerk)**: L2 to L4, extension of the knee joint on tapping the patellar tendon
- **Achilles tendon reflex (ankle jerk)**: S1 and S2, plantar flexion of the ankle joint on tapping the Achilles tendon

Clinical Modification of Autonomic Nervous System Activities

Many drugs and surgical procedures can modify the activity of the ANS. For example, drugs can be administered to lower the blood pressure by blocking sympathetic nerve endings and causing vasodilation of peripheral blood vessels. In patients with severe arterial disease affecting the main arteries of the lower limb, sectioning the sympathetic innervation to the blood vessels can sometimes save the limb. This produces vasodilation and enables an adequate amount of blood to flow through the collateral circulation, thus bypassing the obstruction.

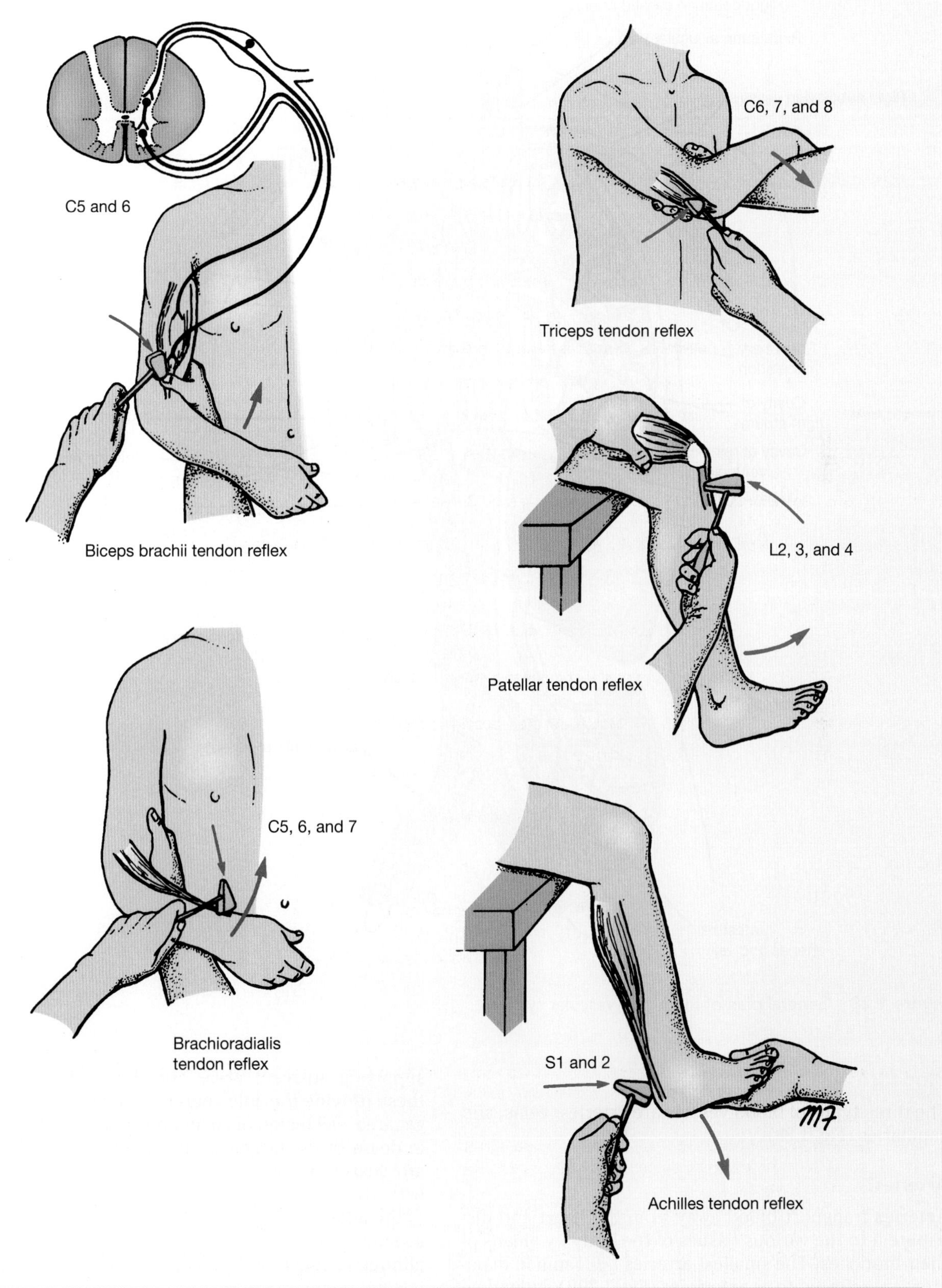

Figure 1.27 Some important tendon reflexes used in medical practice.

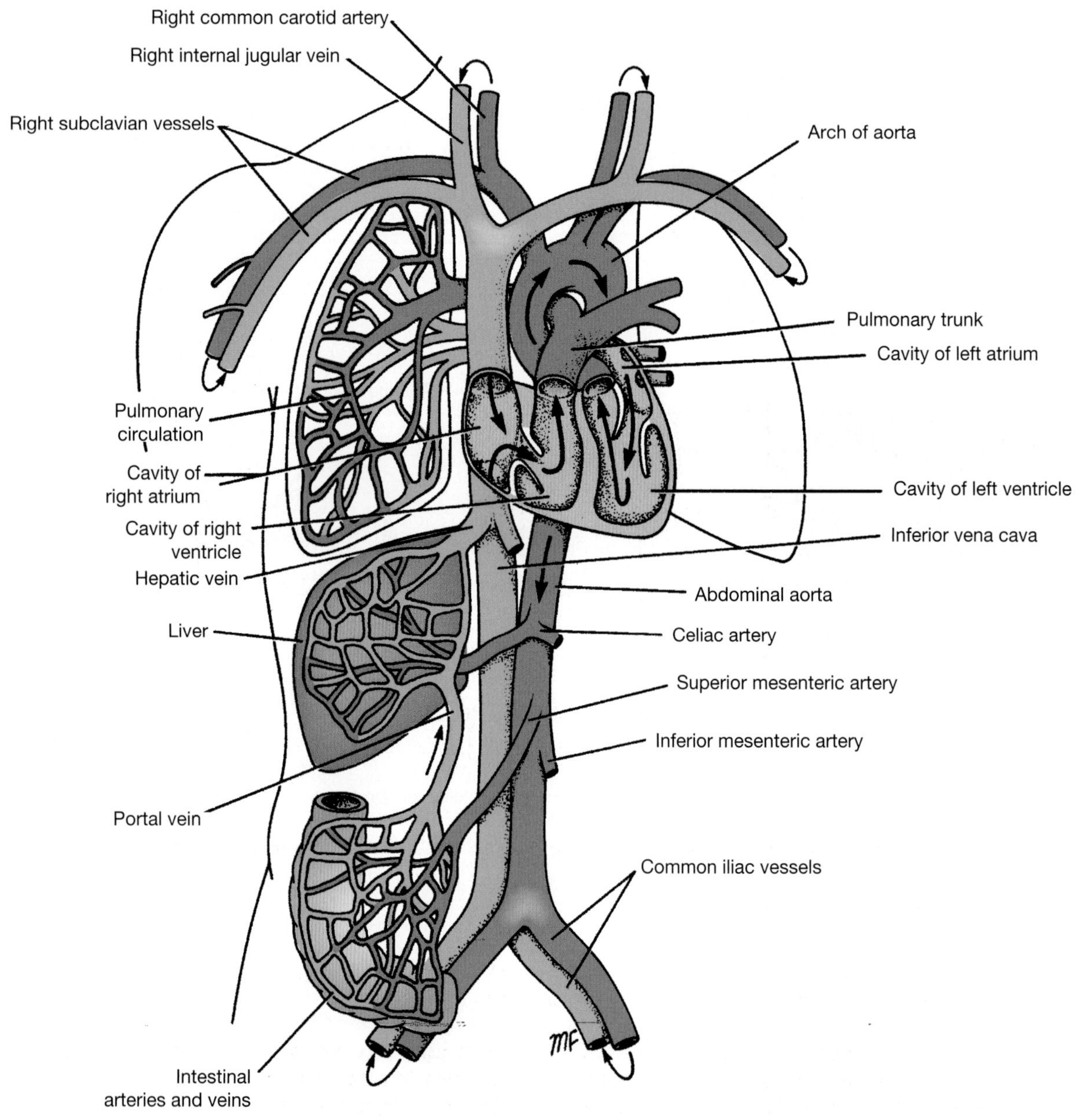

Figure 1.28 General plan of the blood vascular system.

Blood Vessels

The three types of blood vessels are arteries, veins, and capillaries (Fig. 1.28).

Arteries

Arteries transport blood away from the heart and distribute it to the various tissues of the body by means of their branches. The smallest arteries (<0.1 mm in diameter) are referred to as **arterioles** (Fig. 1.29B). Individual arteries may connect with other arteries via a communicating branch termed an **anastomosis** (see Fig. 1.29A). Arteries do not have valves.

Anatomic end arteries are vessels whose terminal branches do not anastomose with branches of arteries supplying adjacent areas (see Fig. 1.29C). Therefore, these provide the sole source of blood to a specific target area. Occlusion of an anatomic end artery will result in death of the target tissues. **Functional end arteries** are vessels whose terminal branches do anastomose with those of adjacent arteries; however, the caliber of the anastomosis is insufficient to keep the target tissue alive if one of the arteries becomes blocked. Thus, although some blood may enter a functional end artery, it is not enough blood to be functionally meaningful.

Veins

Veins are vessels that transport blood toward the heart. Many veins possess **valves**, which function to

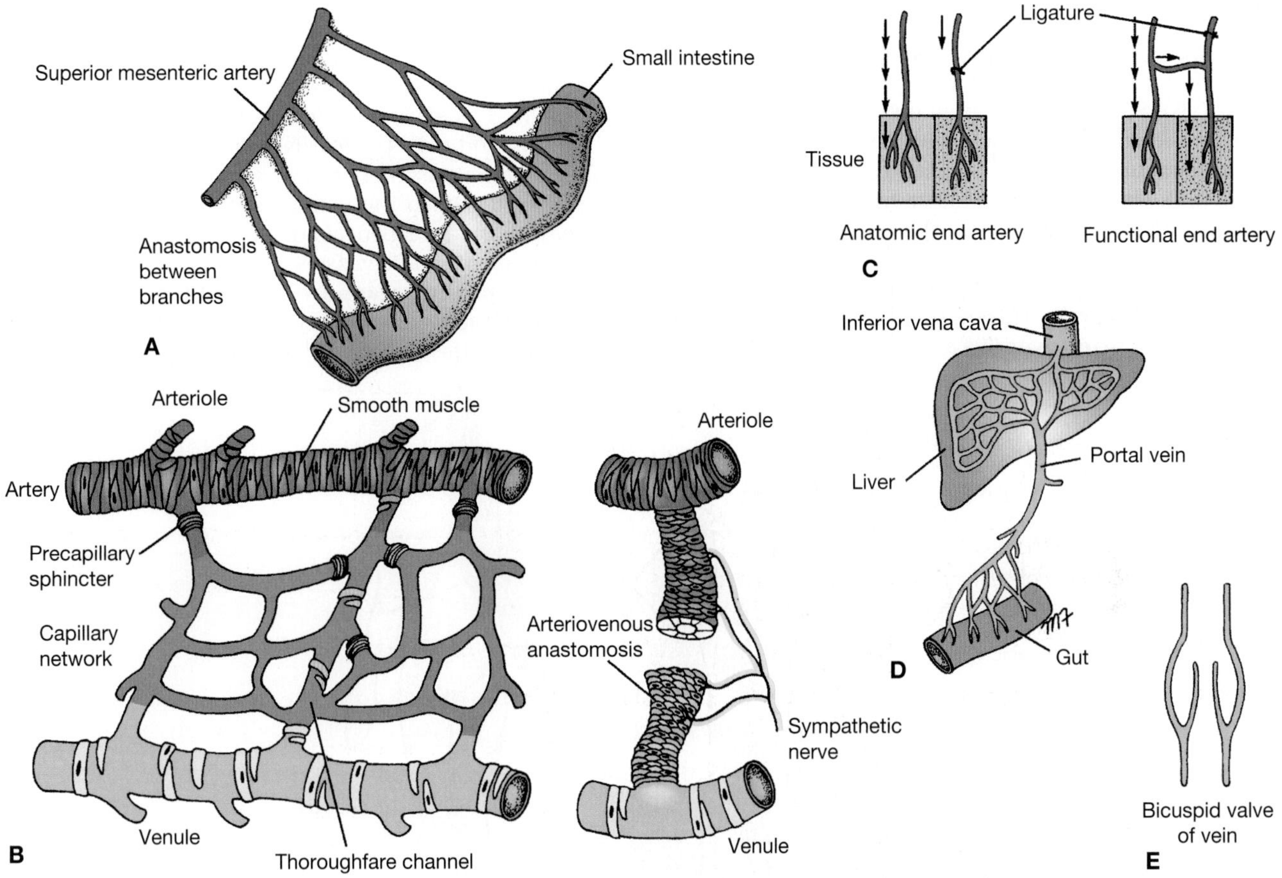

Figure 1.29 Different types of blood vessels and their methods of union. **A.** Anastomosis between the branches of the superior mesenteric artery. **B.** Capillary network and an arteriovenous anastomosis. **C.** Anatomic end artery and functional end artery. **D.** Portal system. **E.** Structure of the bicuspid valve in a vein.

prevent reflux of blood (see Fig. 1.29E). The smallest veins are called **venules** (see Fig. 1.29B). The smaller veins, or tributaries, unite to form larger veins, which commonly join together to form venous plexuses. Two veins often accompany medium-size deep arteries, one on each side of the artery. Such veins are called **venae comitantes**.

Veins leaving the gastrointestinal tract do not go directly to the heart but converge on the portal vein (see Figs. 1.28 and 1.29D). This vein enters the liver and breaks up again into veins of diminishing size, which ultimately join capillary-like vessels, termed **sinusoids**, in the liver. A **portal system** is thus a system of vessels interposed between two capillary beds.

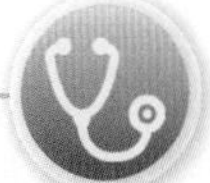

Clinical Notes

Blood Vessel Diseases

Diseases of blood vessels are common. The surface anatomy of the main arteries, especially those of the limbs, is discussed in the appropriate sections of this text. Know the collateral circulation of most large arteries as well as the distinction between anatomic end arteries and functional end arteries.

All large arteries that cross over a joint are liable to be kinked during movements of the joint. However, the distal flow of blood is not interrupted because an adequate anastomosis is usually formed between branches of the artery that arise both proximal and distal to the joint. The alternative blood channels, which dilate under these circumstances, form the **collateral circulation**. Knowing the existence and position of such a circulation may be of vital importance when it becomes necessary to tie off a large artery that has been damaged by trauma or disease.

Coronary arteries are functional end arteries, and, if they become blocked by disease (coronary arterial occlusion is common), the cardiac muscle normally supplied by that artery will receive insufficient blood and undergo necrosis. Blockage of a large coronary artery results in the death of the patient. (See the Clinical Case at the beginning of this chapter.)

Capillaries

Capillaries are microscopic vessels in the form of a network connecting the arterioles to the venules (see Fig. 1.29B). Sinusoids resemble capillaries in that they are thin-walled blood vessels, but they have an irregular cross diameter and are wider than capillaries. They are found in the bone marrow, spleen, liver, and some endocrine glands. In some areas of the body, principally the tips of the fingers and toes, direct connections occur between the arteries and the veins without the intervention of capillaries. The sites of such connections are referred to as **arteriovenous anastomoses**.

Lymphatic System

Lymph is a clear, colorless tissue fluid that is collected from tissues throughout the body. It consists of a liquid portion and a cellular portion that is composed mainly of white blood cells (primarily lymphocytes). Lymph is collected in a vast network of vessels and eventually mostly returned to the venous system. The lymphatic system consists of two major components: lymphatic organs and lymphatic vessels (Fig. 1.30).

The **lymphatic organs** are the **lymph nodes**, **tonsils**, **thymus**, and **spleen**. Additionally, localized aggregations of lymphatic tissue (**lymph nodules**) occur in various

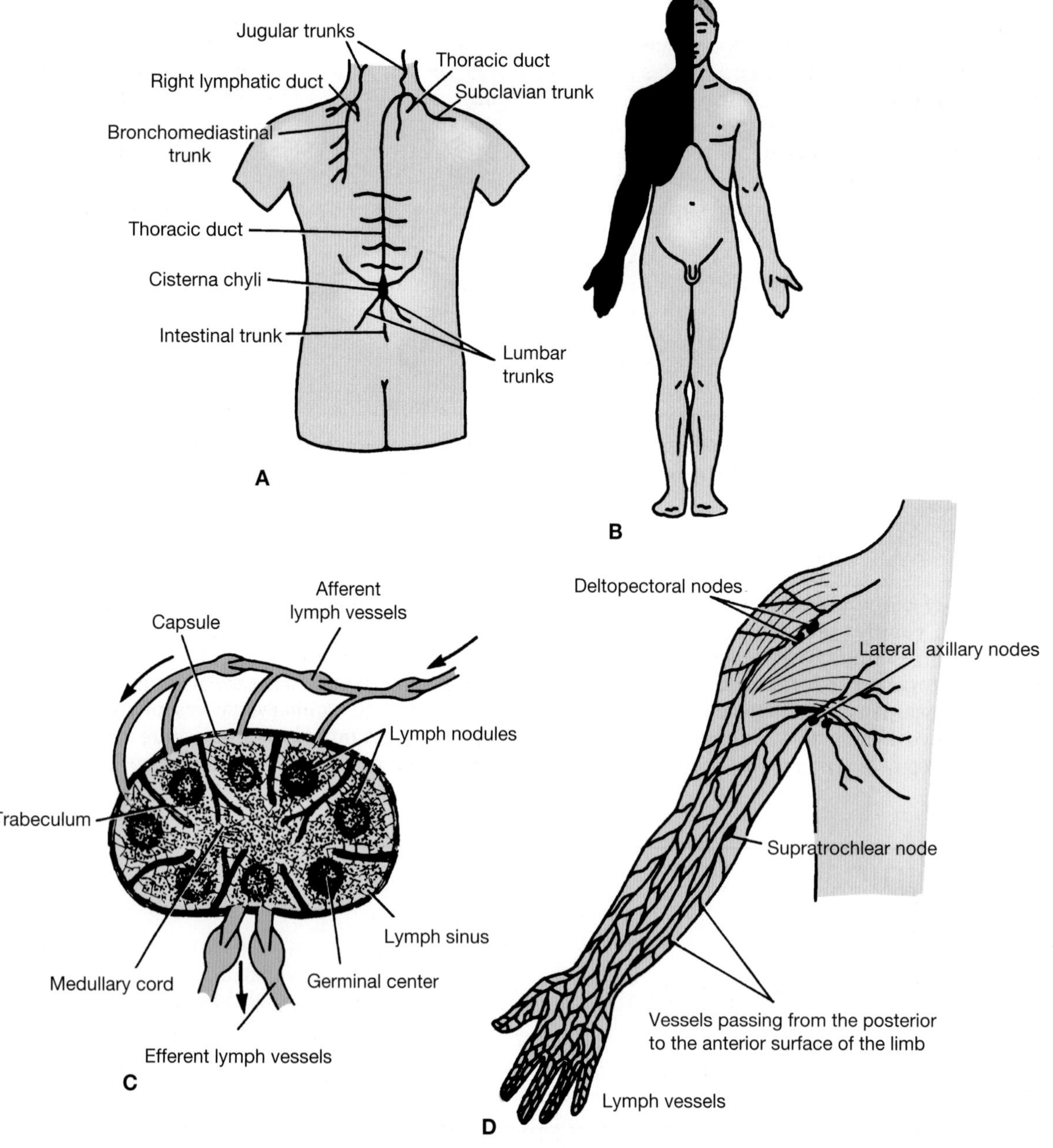

Figure 1.30 General plan of the lymphatic system. Frames A, B, and D are anterior view schematics. **A.** Thoracic duct and right lymphatic duct and their main tributaries. **B.** Areas of the body drained into the thoracic duct (*clear*) and right lymphatic duct (*black*). **C.** General structure of a lymph node. **D.** Lymph vessels and nodes of the upper limb.

places (eg, mucus membranes, intestinal nodules). However, the nodules are not sufficiently organized to be considered organs. Lymphatic organs are essential for the immunologic defenses of the body against bacteria and viruses. The organs serve to produce lymphocytes; act as barriers to pathogens; and, in the case of the spleen, filter the blood.

Lymphatic vessels are tubes that assist the cardiovascular system in the removal of tissue fluid from the tissue spaces of the body. These vessels then return the fluid to the blood. The lymphatic system is essentially a drainage system, with no circulation. Lymphatic vessels are found in all tissues and organs of the body except cartilage, bone, the CNS, eyes, internal ear, and the epidermis of the skin.

Lymph capillaries form a network of fine vessels that drain lymph from the tissues. The capillaries are larger and more irregular than blood capillaries, possess few valves, and are present in most locations where blood capillaries are found. **Lacteals** are blind-ending projections of lymph capillaries in the villi of the small intestine. The lacteals absorb chyle (emulsified fat), which is produced during digestion. The lymph capillaries are in turn drained by small lymphatic **collecting vessels**, which unite to form larger collecting vessels. The collecting vessels tend to run in multiples rather than as single channels and often accompany veins. The collecting vessels usually present a beaded or knotted appearance because of the presence of numerous **valves** along their course. The valve cusps are directed so as to allow lymph flow only toward the heart. The largest collecting vessels are termed the **lymphatic trunks** or **ducts**. These are the major lymphatic tubes that are most apparent at the gross dissection level (eg, the bronchomediastinal trunk and the thoracic duct). Before lymph is returned to the bloodstream, it passes through at least one lymph node and often through several. The lymph vessels that carry lymph to a lymph node are referred to as **afferent vessels**; those that transport it away from a node are **efferent vessels** (see Fig. 1.30C).

The flow of lymph is driven by extravessel forces, for example, the pressures produced by contractions of neighboring muscles, or the negative pressure produced during inspiration. Obstruction of lymph flow from a given area results in accumulation of tissue fluid in that area. An abnormally large accumulation of fluid is referred to as **lymphedema**. Almost all lymph eventually drains into the venous system at the junction of the internal jugular and subclavian veins in the root of the neck on each side of the body. Lymph from the upper right quadrant of the body (head, neck, upper limb, and the trunk above the umbilicus) drains into several trunks, which independently enter the venous system on the right side. Sometimes, these vessels unite to form a single **right lymphatic duct** that then drains into the venous system (see Fig. 1.30A). Lymph from the rest of the body eventually drains into the **thoracic duct**, which empties into the left side of the venous system. The arrangement of the lymphatic ducts is extremely variable. The **cisterna chyli** (described as a dilated sac forming the origin of the thoracic duct) may, in fact, be only a plexus of vessels in the upper lumbar region. Also, the thoracic duct typically possesses few, if any, valves.

The major lymphatic channels tend to run in parallel with blood vessel pathways, except in the thoracic cavity. Therefore, understanding the anatomy of the blood vascular system assists in following the main lymphatic drainage routes. The major lymph drainage channels are summarized in Table 1.8.

Mucous and Serous Membranes

A **mucous membrane** is the tissue layer that lines the luminal surface of an organ or passageway and communicates with the surface of the body. A mucous membrane consists essentially of a layer of epithelium supported by a layer of connective tissue, the lamina propria. Smooth muscle, called the muscularis mucosa, is sometimes present in the connective tissue. A mucous membrane may or may not secrete mucus on its surface.

Serous membranes line the thoracic and abdominopelvic cavities of the trunk and are reflected onto the mobile viscera lying within these cavities (Fig. 1.31). They consist of a smooth layer of mesothelium supported by a thin layer of connective tissue. The serous

Table 1.8 Major Lymphatic Channels and Drainage Routes

LYMPH CHANNEL	DRAINAGE ROUTE
Limbs	Lymph follows the main veins (eg, basilic vein to axillary vein to subclavian vein).
Superficial (subcutaneous) thoracoabdominal walls	Lymph follows the subcutaneous blood vessels (eg, lateral thoracic artery to axillary artery; superficial epigastric vein to femoral vein).
Deep thoracoabdominal walls	Lymph follows the main blood vessels (eg, intercostal vessels, internal thoracic vessels).
Thoracic viscera	Lymph follows the respiratory tree (eg, bronchopulmonary nodes to tracheobronchial nodes to bronchomediastinal trunk).
Abdominopelvic viscera	Lymph follows the arterial trees (eg, gastric nodes to celiac nodes to cisterna chyli).

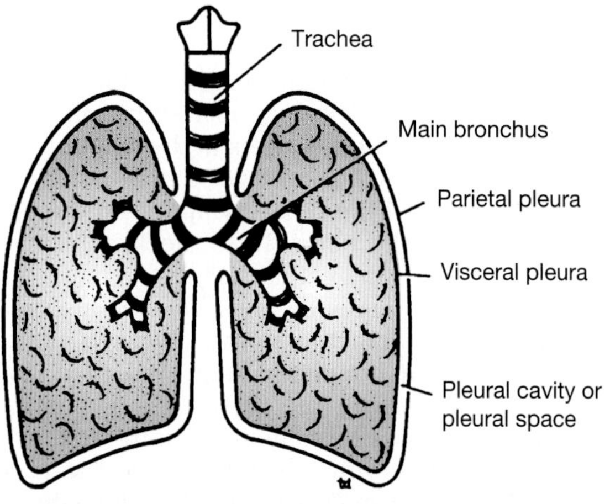

Figure 1.31 Arrangement of pleura within the thoracic cavity. Note that under normal conditions the pleural cavity is a slit-like space. The parietal and visceral layers of pleura are separated by a small amount of serous fluid.

membrane lining the wall of the cavity is referred to as the **parietal layer**, and that covering the viscera is the **visceral layer**. The narrow, slit-like interval that separates these layers forms the pleural, pericardial, and peritoneal cavities and contains a small amount of **serous fluid**, which is the exudate of the serous membrane. The serous fluid lubricates the surfaces of the membranes and allows the two layers to slide readily on each other. Connecting bridges of the serous membranes form mesenteries, omenta, and serous ligaments, which are described in other chapters.

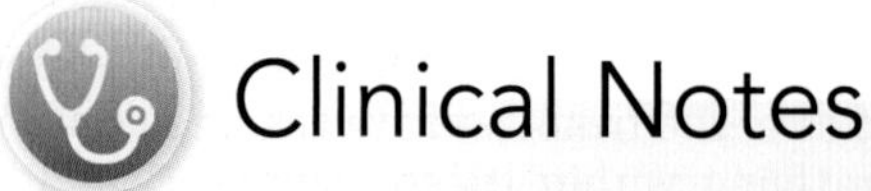

Lymphatic System Disease

The lymphatic system is commonly underemphasized in traditional anatomy courses because it is difficult to see on a cadaver. However, it is of vital importance to medical personnel, because lymph nodes may swell as the result of metastases, or primary tumor. For this reason, the lymphatic drainage of all major organs of the body, including the skin, should be known.

A patient may report a swelling produced by lymph node enlargement. Clinicians must know the areas of the body that drain lymph to a particular node if they are to be able to find the primary site of the disease. Often, the patient ignores the primary disease, which may be a small, painless cancer of the skin.

Conversely, the patient may report a painful ulcer of the tongue, for example, and the clinician must know the lymph drainage of the tongue to be able to determine whether the disease has spread beyond the limits of the tongue.

The parietal layer of a serous membrane is developed from the somatopleure (inner cell layer of mesoderm) and is richly supplied by spinal nerves. It is therefore sensitive to all common sensations such as touch and pain. The visceral layer is developed from the splanchnopleure (inner cell layer of mesoderm) and is supplied by visceral afferent nerves. It is insensitive to touch and temperature but very sensitive to stretch.

Effects of Sex, Age, and Ethnicity on Structure

Descriptive anatomy tends to concentrate on a fixed descriptive form. Medical personnel must always remember that sex and ethnic differences exist and that the body's structure and function change as a person grows and ages.

In general, the adult male tends to be taller than the adult female and to have longer legs. His bones are bigger and heavier, his muscles are larger, and he has less subcutaneous fat. His larynx is larger, and his vocal cords are longer so that his voice is deeper. He has facial hair and coarse body hair. He possesses axillary and pubic hair, the latter extending to the region of the umbilicus.

In general, the adult female tends to be shorter than the adult male and to have smaller bones and less bulky muscles. She has more subcutaneous fat and fat accumulations in the breasts, buttocks, and thighs. She has axillary and pubic hair, but the latter does not extend up to the umbilicus. The adult female has larger breasts and a proportionally wider pelvis than the male. She has a wider carrying angle at the elbow, which results in a greater lateral deviation of the forearm on the arm.

Until the age of ~10 years, males and females grow at about the same rate. Around age 12 years, males often start to grow faster, so that most males reach a greater adult height. Puberty begins between ages 10 and 14 years in females and between 12 and 15 years in males. In the female at puberty, the breasts enlarge, and the pelvis broadens. in the male, the penis, testes, and scrotum enlarge. Axillary hair and pubic hair appear in both sexes.

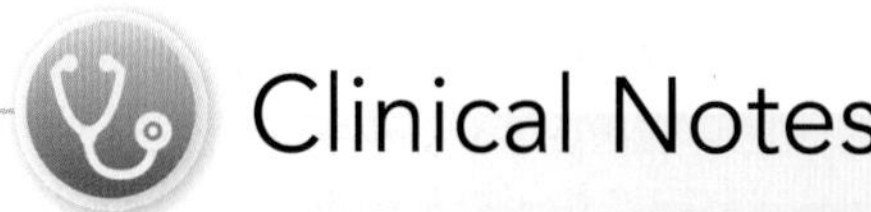

Mucous and Serous Membranes and Inflammatory Disease

Mucous and serous membranes are common sites for inflammatory disease. **Rhinitis**, or the common cold, is an inflammation of the nasal mucous membrane, and **pleurisy** is inflammation of the visceral and parietal layers of the pleura.

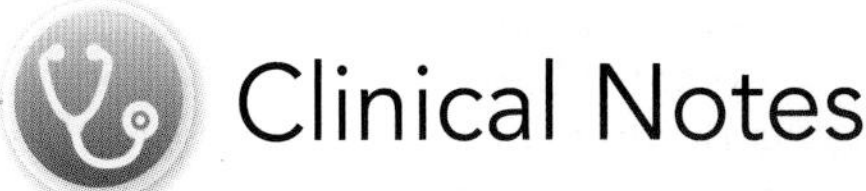

Clinical Notes

Clinical Significance of Age on Structure

The fact that the structure and function of the human body change with age may seem obvious, but it is often overlooked. A few examples of such changes are given here:

1. In the infant, the bones of the skull are more resilient than in the adult. For this reason, fractures of the skull are much more common in the adult than in the young child.
2. The liver is relatively much larger in the child than in the adult. In the infant, the lower margin of the liver extends inferiorly to a lower level than in the adult. This is an important consideration when making a diagnosis of hepatic enlargement.
3. The urinary bladder in the child cannot be accommodated entirely in the pelvis because of the small size of the pelvic cavity and thus is found in the lower part of the abdominal cavity. As the child grows, the pelvis enlarges, and the bladder sinks down to become a true pelvic organ.
4. At birth, all bone marrow is red. With advancing age, the red marrow recedes up the bones of the limbs so that, in the adult, it is largely confined to the bones of the head, thorax, and abdomen.
5. Lymphatic tissues reach their maximum degree of development at puberty and thereafter atrophy, so the volume of lymphatic tissue in older persons is considerably reduced.

Ethnic differences may be seen in the color of the skin, hair, and eyes and in the shape and size of the eyes, nose, and lips.

After birth and during childhood, bodily functions become progressively more efficient, reaching their maximum degree of efficiency during young adulthood. During late adulthood and old age, many bodily functions become less efficient.

MEDICAL IMAGING

Medical imaging is the suite of procedures used to visualize the body in ways applicable to medicine. **Radiology** is the field of medical imaging that uses high-energy radiation to diagnose and treat disease. Sources of the radiant energy may include ionizing radiation (x-rays), radionucleotides, nuclear magnetic resonance, ultrasound, and others. The most commonly used medical imaging techniques include:

1. Conventional radiography (x-ray imaging)
2. Computerized tomography (CT) scanning
3. Magnetic resonance imaging (MRI)
4. Ultrasonography (US)
5. Nuclear medicine imaging

Wilhelm Roentgen, a Dutch physicist, established the basis for medical imaging in 1895, when he discovered a new form of radiation while experimenting with the behavior of cathode ray tubes. He accidentally found that the radiation he produced could create an image showing the bones in his hand and that he could capture that image on photographic paper. Roentgen named this radiation "x-rays," and his work formed the foundation of the science of radiology. Later, x-rays were named "roentgen rays" and for many years radiology was referred to as "roentgenology."

X-rays are a form of electromagnetic energy similar in many respects to visible light. The fundamental difference between x-rays and other portions of the electromagnetic spectrum is their range of wavelengths. X-rays have a relatively short wavelength, produce greater energy, and have greater ability to penetrate various substances.

Conventional Radiography (X-Rays)

Radiography is the imaging technique that utilizes x-rays. In **conventional radiography** (**plain film**), a penetrating beam of x-rays is projected through the patient onto a film or other detection device (eg, a computer monitor) without any added special enhancement techniques (eg, contrast media). The x-rays transilluminate the patient and are differentially absorbed, reflected, or passed on according to the different densities and thickness of the tissues in the path of the beam.

More dense tissues/structures (eg, compact bone) absorb or reflect more x-rays than do less dense tissues/structures (eg, fat). Therefore, fewer x-rays penetrate the subject and reach the film/detector in more dense substances, whereas more x-rays penetrate the subject and reach the film/detector in less dense substances. The same principle holds true relative to the thickness of any given substance (eg, fewer x-rays penetrate thicker samples of compact bone compared to thinner specimens).

The x-ray film/detector is or acts as a photographic negative. Fewer x-rays reaching the film results in less reaction with the film coating. This results in a transparent, bright (white) area on the film. More x-rays reaching the film results in more reaction with the film, resulting in a darker area on the film. Denser substances (eg, compact bone) are termed **radiopaque** and appear whiter; less dense substances (eg, air) are **radiolucent** and appear darker (Fig. 1.32).

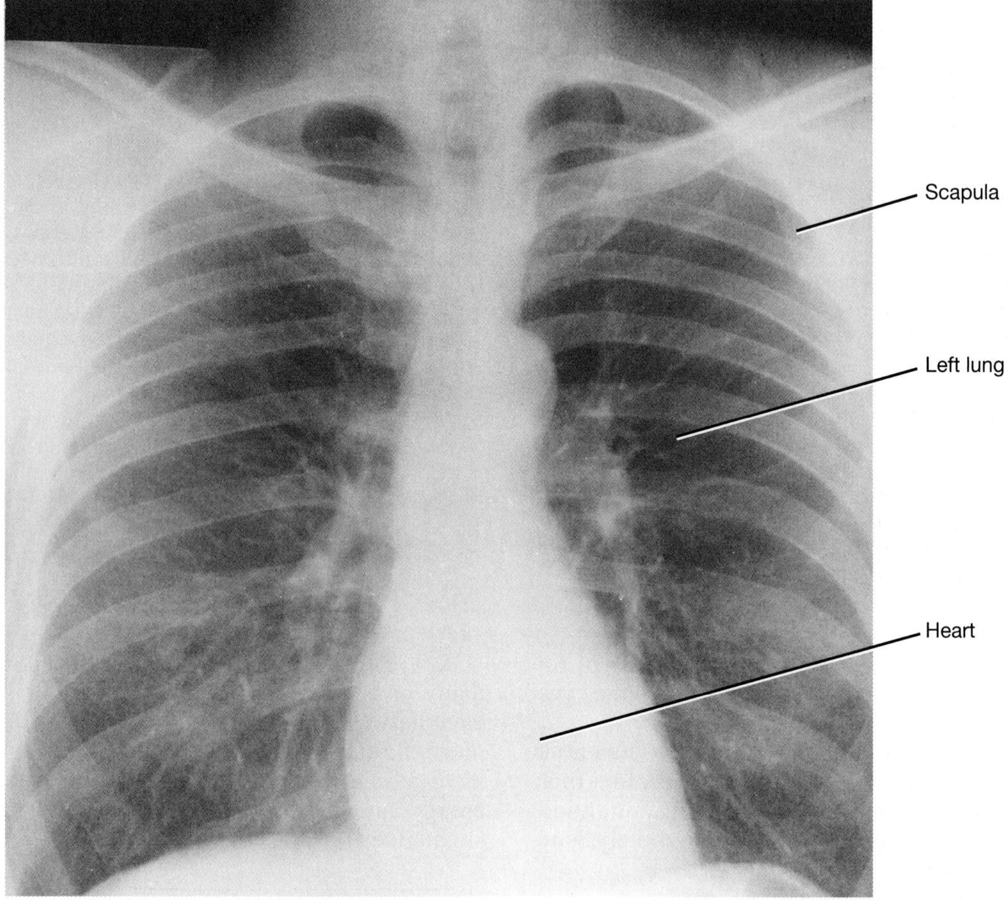

Figure 1.32 Conventional radiograph (plain film) of the thorax. This periapical (PA) projection demonstrates denser or thicker radiopaque tissues (eg, scapula, heart) appearing white versus less dense, less thick radiolucent structures (eg, lungs) appearing *black*.

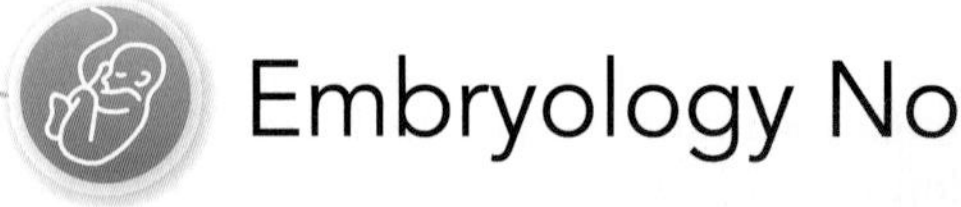

Embryology Notes

Embryology and Clinical Anatomy

Embryology provides a basis for understanding adult anatomy and an explanation of many of the congenital anomalies seen in clinical medicine. A very brief overview of the early development of the embryo follows. Where appropriate, a more detailed account of the development of different organs is given in subsequent chapters.

Once the spermatozoon has fertilized the ovum, a single cell is formed, called the **zygote**. This undergoes a rapid succession of mitotic divisions with the formation of smaller cells. The centrally placed cells are called the **inner cell mass** and ultimately form the tissues of the embryo. The **outer cell mass** forms the **trophoblast**, which plays an important role in the formation of the placenta and the fetal membranes.

The cells that form the embryo become defined in the form of a **bilaminar embryonic disc**, composed of two germ layers. The upper layer is called the **ectoderm** and the lower layer, the **endoderm** (**entoderm**). As growth proceeds, the embryonic disc becomes pear shaped, and a narrow streak formed of ectoderm termed the **primitive streak** appears on its dorsal surface. The further proliferation of the cells of the primitive streak forms a layer of cells that extends between the ectoderm and the endoderm to form the third germ layer, the **mesoderm**.

Ectoderm

Further thickening of the ectoderm gives rise to a plate of cells on the dorsal surface of the embryo called the **neural plate**. This plate sinks beneath the surface of the embryo to form the **neural tube**, which ultimately gives rise to the CNS. The remainder of the ectoderm forms the **cornea**, **retina**, and **lens** of the eye and the **membranous labyrinth** of the inner ear. The ectoderm also forms the **epidermis** of the skin; **nails** and **hair**; **epithelial cells** of the sebaceous, sweat, and mammary glands; the **mucous membrane** lining the mouth, nasal cavities, and paranasal sinuses; tooth

enamel; the **pituitary gland** and the **alveoli** and **ducts** of the parotid salivary glands; the **mucous membrane** of the lower half of the anal canal; and the terminal parts of the **genital tract** and the **male urinary tract**.

Endoderm

The endoderm eventually gives origin to the **epithelial lining of the alimentary tract** from the mouth cavity down to halfway along the anal canal and the **epithelium** of the glands that develop from it (**thyroid**, **parathyroid**, **thymus**, **liver**, and **pancreas**) and the epithelial linings of the **respiratory tract**, **pharyngotympanic tube** and **middle ear**, **urinary bladder**, parts of the female and male **urethras**, **greater vestibular glands**, **prostate gland**, **bulbourethral glands**, and **vagina**.

Mesoderm

The mesoderm differentiates into the paraxial, intermediate, and lateral mesoderm. The **paraxial mesoderm** is situated initially on either side of the midline of the embryo. It becomes segmented and forms the **bones**, **cartilage**, and **ligaments** of the **vertebral column** and part of the **base of the skull**. Some cells form the skeletal muscles of their own segment, and some of the cells migrate beneath the ectoderm and take part in the formation of the dermis and subcutaneous tissues of the skin.

The **intermediate mesoderm** is a column of cells on either side of the embryo that is connected medially to the paraxial mesoderm and laterally to the lateral mesoderm. It gives rise to portions of the **urogenital system**.

The **lateral mesoderm** splits into somatic and splanchnic layers associated with the ectoderm and the endoderm, respectively. It encloses a cavity within the embryo called the **intraembryonic coelom**. The coelom eventually forms the **pericardial**, **pleural**, and **peritoneal cavities**.

In addition, the embryonic mesoderm gives origin to **smooth**, **voluntary**, and **cardiac muscles**; all forms of **connective tissue**, including cartilage and bone; **blood vessel walls** and **blood cells**; **lymph vessel walls** and **lymphoid tissue**; the **synovial membranes** of joints and bursae; and the **suprarenal cortex**.

The part of the patient's body under study should be as close as possible to the film/detector. Structures closer to the film/detector (ie, further from the beam projector) receive greater resolution and are sharper and clearer. Structures further from the film/detector (ie, closer to the beam projector) are more greatly magnified and less sharp. Therefore, body parts under examination should be placed closer to the film/detector in order to maximize resolution and minimize magnification artifacts.

In standard terminology, the direction of the projected beam through the patient's body defines the view of the radiograph. In a **posteroanterior (PA) projection**, the x-ray projector is posterior to the patient, whereas the film/detector is anterior. The beam travels through the patient from the patient's posterior to anterior aspects (Fig. 1.33A). An **anteroposterior (AP) projection** is the opposite situation. In a **lateral or oblique projection**, the side of the patient placed closest to the film/detector defines the radiographic view (Fig. 1.33B). For example, in a left lateral radiograph of the chest, the left side of the patient's chest is placed closer to the film/detector, and the x-ray beam is projected from the patient's right to their left.

Because conventional radiographs produce two-dimensional images of three-dimensional structures, many structures overlap each other in any one projection. Thus, most radiographic exams consist of at least two projections made at right angles to one another (called **orthogonal views**) in order to better define and locate individual structures.

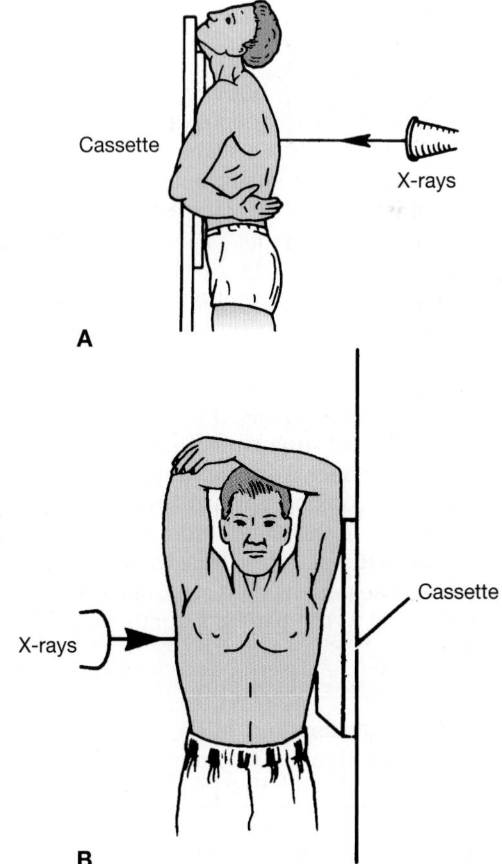

Figure 1.33 Directional orientation in conventional radiographs. Note the position of the patient in relation to the x-ray source and the cassette holder. **A.** Posteroanterior projection. **B.** Left lateral projection.

Computed Tomography

Both conventional radiography and **computed tomography (CT)** use a projected beam of x-rays to transilluminate the patient's body. In CT, the x-ray projector and

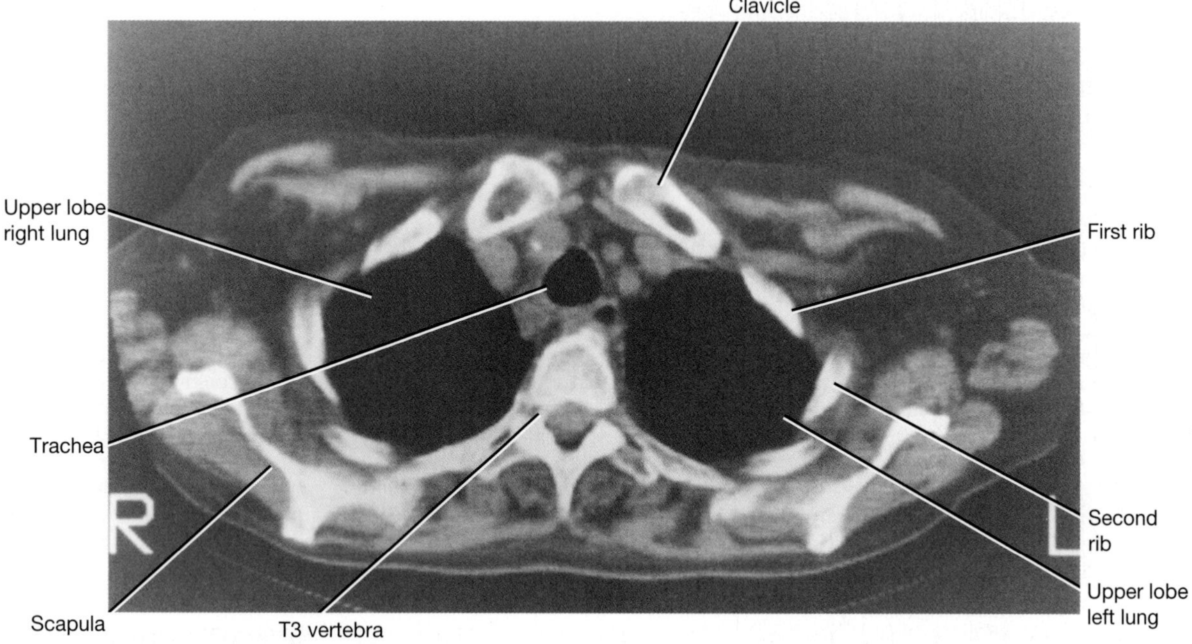

Figure 1.34 Axial CT of the upper thorax. The patient's left side is on the right side of the image. More dense tissue appears *white*, whereas less dense tissue appears *gray* to *black*.

detector rotate about the body axis, creating multiple overlapping scans of individual planes of the body. A computer reconstructs these scans and produces a single image of each plane. Usually, but not always, CTs are used to produce images of transverse sections along the long axis of the body trunk or limbs (Fig. 1.34). Such images are termed **axial CTs**. Because CTs use x-rays, they appear much like conventional radiographs, with structures of greater density appearing whiter, and structures of less density appearing darker.

In viewing axial CTs, each scan (image) is displayed from the inferior aspect. Thus, the orientation view is as if the patient is in the supine position (ie, lying on their back) and the examiner were standing at the foot of the patient's bed and looking upward toward the patient's head. Importantly, in this view, understand that orientation is relative to the patient. Thus, the examiner's right side is actually the patient's left side, and directions are applied according to the patient's anatomic position.

Magnetic Resonance Imaging

Magnetic resonance imaging (MRI) uses radiofrequency pulses projected within a strong magnetic field to excite free protons within a patient's tissues. Energy emitted by differential proton excitation and "relaxation" produces radiofrequency signals that are collected in the MRI scanner and reconstructed into images. Modifying the timing of the pulse projections and/or collection of the radiofrequency pulses can vary the appearance of the tissues in the images. Two basic types of signals typically are collected: T1-weighted (T1 signal) and T2-weighted (T2 signal). These are related to the realignment (T1 signal) and loss of resonance (T2 signal) of the excited protons. In an applied context, T1 images highlight fat tissue, whereas T2 images highlight fat and water within tissues. This makes the interpretation of images easier in that one tissue type (fat) is white in T1 images, whereas two tissue types (fat and water) are white in T2 images. MRI produces images that resemble anatomic sections more closely than any other imaging technique. MRI is particularly noteworthy in that it produces superior images of soft tissues without the use of ionizing radiation. MRI is very useful in diagnosing soft tissue abnormality/trauma such as intervertebral disc herniation (Fig. 1.35).

MRIs can be reconstructed in any plane of the body to produce a great variety of imaging views. The strong magnetic field used in MRI demands thorough safety checks (eg, for metallic objects) before imaging commences.

Ultrasonography

Ultrasound uses the reflections (echoes) of high-frequency sound waves (ultrasound) to reconstruct images of structures. A transducer in contact with a body surface transmits ultrasounds that penetrate the body and reflect off the interfaces between tissues of varying densities. These echoes are collected, converted to electrical energy, and reconstructed into images of structures (Fig. 1.36) and/or measurements of velocity (eg, rate of blood flow through vessels).

Ultrasound has several notable advantages over other imaging techniques: it produces real-time images of structures, motion, and flow; costs less than CT and MRI; is highly portable and noninvasive; and does not use dyes or radiation.

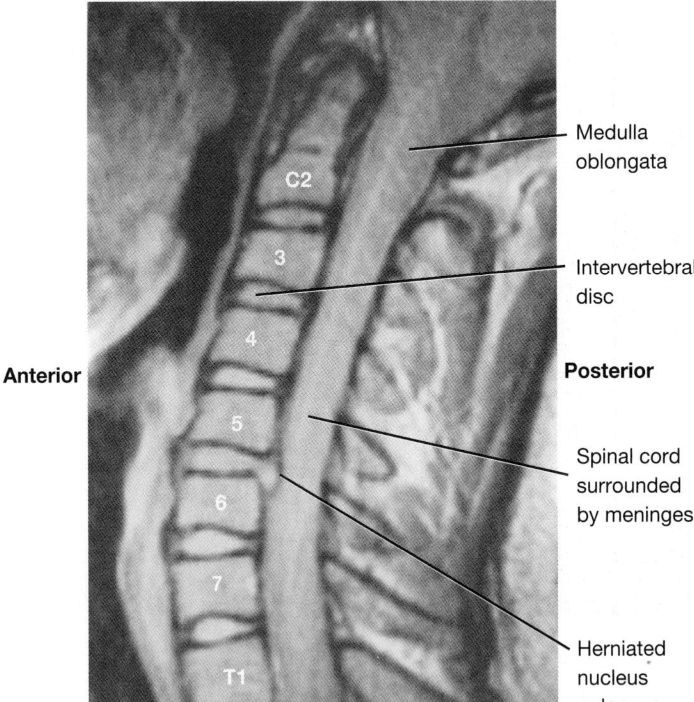

Figure 1.35 Sagittal MRI scan of the cervical region. Note the clearly seen herniated C5 intervertebral disc.

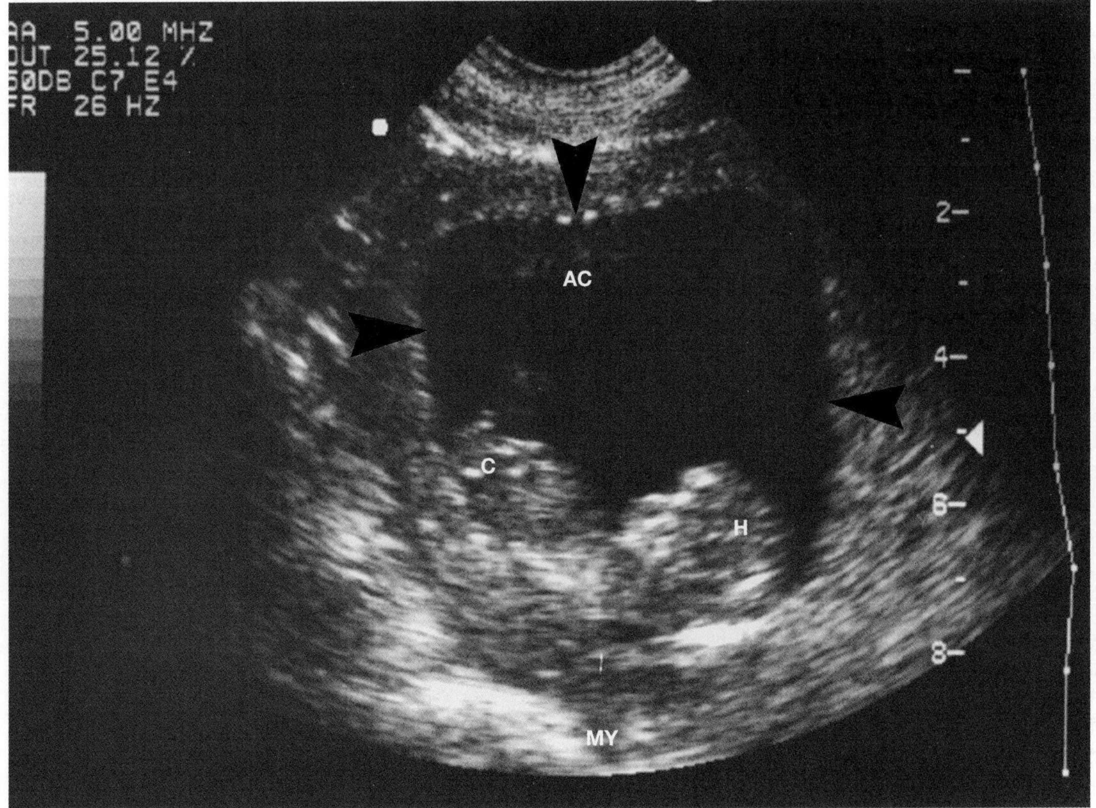

Figure 1.36 Longitudinal sonogram of a pregnant uterus at 11 weeks. The amniotic cavity (AC) is filled with amniotic fluid. The fetus is seen in longitudinal section with the head (H) and coccyx (C) well defined. The myometrium (MY) is also visible. (Courtesy of L. Scoutt.)

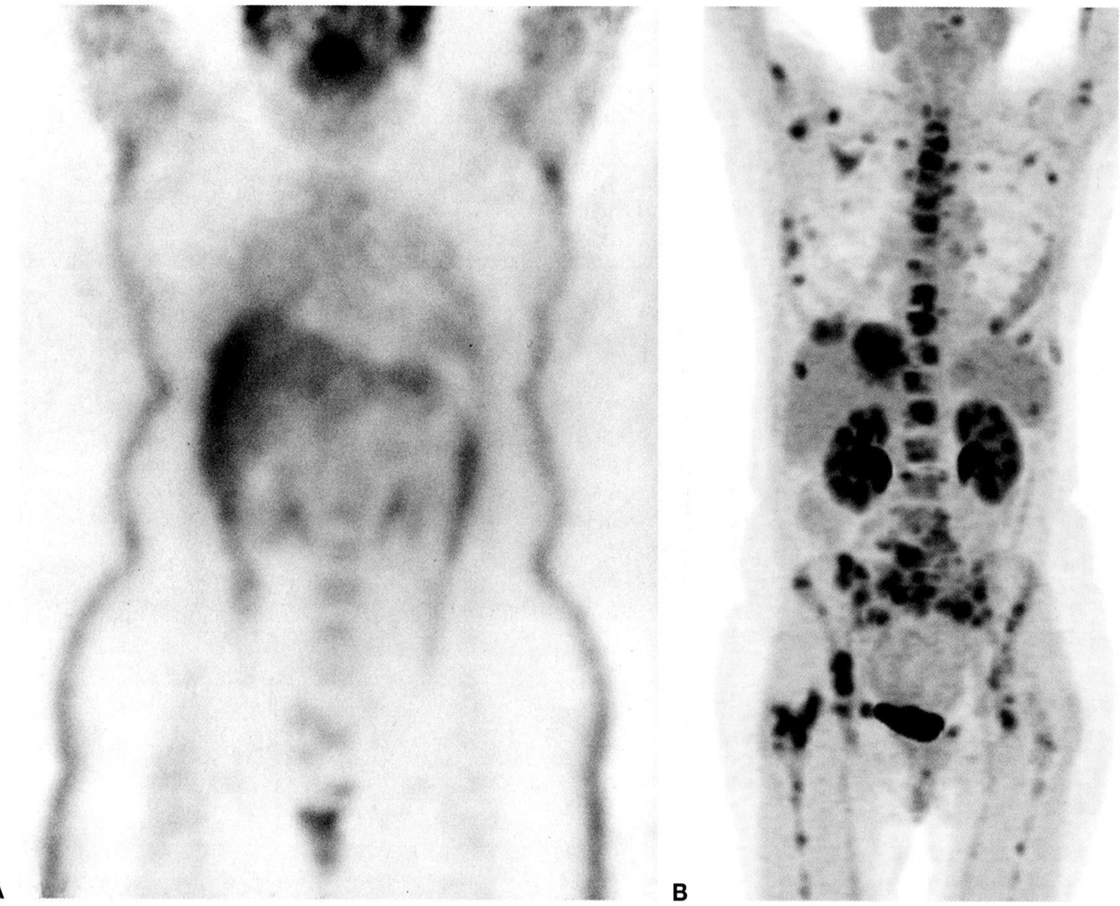

Figure 1.37 Whole body PET scans. **A.** A 62-year-old female suspected of having skeletal metastases secondary to recently treated breast cancer. **B.** A 65-year-old female diagnosed with stage IV adenocarcinoma of the lungs that developed widespread skeletal and internal organ metastases. (From Greenspan A, Beltran J. *Orthopaedic Imaging: A Practical Approach*, 7th ed. Wolters Kluwer: Baltimore, MD; 2021.)

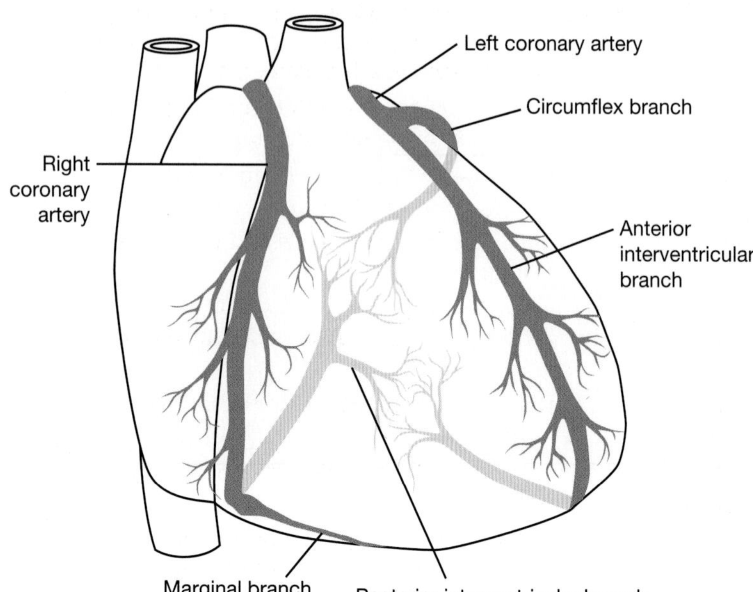

Figure 1.38 Major coronary arteries.

Nuclear Medicine Imaging

Nuclear medicine imaging uses intravenous (IV) injection of small doses of radioactive materials to construct images of specific structures and/or trace the distribution or concentration of the radioactive material. **Positron emission tomography** (PET) is a relatively common nuclear medicine imaging technique that uses very short half-life isotopes to monitor the physiologic functioning of organs such as the brain. In this, areas of increased activity show selective uptake of the injected isotope (Fig. 1.37).

Clinical Case Discussion

The initial episodes of pain were angina, a form of cardiac pain that occurs on exertion and disappears on rest. Insufficient blood flow to the cardiac muscle from narrowing of the coronary arteries causes the angina (Figs. 1.38 and 1.39). The patient has now experienced myocardial infarction (MI), in which the coronary blood flow is suddenly reduced or stopped, and the cardiac muscle degenerates or dies. Because MI is the major cause of death in industrialized nations, knowledge of the blood supply to the heart and the arrangement of the coronary arteries is of paramount importance in making the diagnosis and treating this patient.

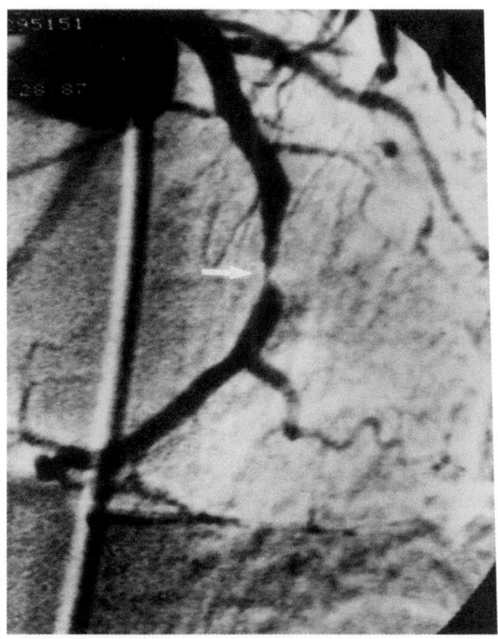

Figure 1.39 Coronary angiogram showing an area of extreme narrowing of the circumflex branch of the left coronary artery (*white arrow*).

Key Concepts

Anatomy Terms

- The anatomic position is the reference posture for all terms of direction and movement.
- Four geometric planes (median, coronal, horizontal, and transverse) are the references for descriptions of direction and movement.
- Eponyms are to be avoided when possible.

Basic Anatomy

- The skin has two main parts: epidermis and dermis.
- The main skin appendages are nails, hair follicles, and sebaceous and sweat glands.
- Fascia is connective tissue that ties the skin to underlying tissues and both unites and separates deeper lying structures.
- The two types of fascia are superficial fascia and deep fascia.
- Bone is hardened connective tissue that forms the framework of the body, protects many internal organs, and provides the mechanical base for movement.
- Bones can be classified according to regional layout or general shape.
- Cartilage is the form of connective tissue in which cells and fibers are embedded in a gel-like matrix.
- The three types of cartilage are hyaline, fibrocartilage, and elastic.
- Joints are the sites where two or more bones come together; they may or may not permit movement between the articulating elements.
- The three main types of joints are fibrous joints, cartilage joints, and synovial joints.
- Synovial joints are the most complex joints and normally permit the greatest degrees of movement.
- Ligaments bind bones to bones and limit movement between bones.
- Bursae are fluid-filled sacs that reduce friction and enhance movement between hard or soft tissue structures.
- Muscles are contractile tissues that cause movement.
- The three types of muscle are skeletal, cardiac, and smooth.
- Skeletal muscles act in antagonistic groups in which agonists produce a desired action and antagonists oppose the agonist(s).

- A motor unit is a single motor neuron plus all the skeletal muscle fibers supplied by that neuron.
- The nervous system controls and integrates the activities of the body.
- The CNS consists of the brain and spinal cord. The peripheral nervous system consists of the cranial and spinal nerves and their ganglia.
- The somatic nervous system acts upon the body's external environment, mainly via skeletal muscle actions. The visceral (autonomic) nervous system acts upon the body's internal environment, mainly via the actions of cardiac and smooth muscle and glands.
- Three membranes (meninges) surround the entire CNS: dura mater, arachnoid mater, and pia mater.
- The autonomic nervous system consists of two parts: the sympathetic division and the parasympathetic division. The sympathetic division prepares the body for emergency, whereas the parasympathetic division aids in recovery.
- Dermatomes are the areas of skin supplied by the somatic sensory fibers of a single spinal nerve.
- Arteries, veins, and capillaries are the three types of blood vessels.
- Arteries carry blood away from the heart, veins transport blood toward the heart, and capillaries connect the smallest arteries and veins.
- Lymph is clear tissue fluid that drains mainly into the venous system.
- Lymphatic organs (lymph nodes, tonsils, thymus, spleen) and lymphatic vessels (ducts and trunks) are the two major components of the lymphatic system.
- The structure and function of the body may vary according to sex, age, and ethnicity.

Medical Imaging

- Medical imaging is the suite of procedures used to visualize the body in ways applicable to medicine.
- The most commonly used medical imaging techniques include conventional radiography (x-rays), computerized tomography (CT), magnetic resonance imaging (MRI), ultrasonography, and nuclear medicine imaging.

2 Back

A 35-year-old female visited her clinician with severe pain in her lower back and leg. She described how she was helping her neighbor move his car, which was stuck in a snowdrift, when suddenly she experienced a sharp, shooting pain in her lower back. At the same time, she felt a deep, sharp pain down the back of her right leg. She tried to walk, but her back felt "locked," and any attempt to move intensified the pain. When the physician asked where it hurt, she pointed to her lower back as the site of maximum pain and then ran her finger down the back of her thigh and the outer side of her right leg.

On physical examination, the physician noted a decreased range of motion in the lumbosacral region of the spine. When asked to walk, the patient was reluctant to put her weight on the involved leg. The pain worsened when sitting and coughing. Further examination revealed weakness in flexion of the right big toe and slight weakness in plantarflexion of the foot. Muscle reflexes were normal in both lower limbs. A slight sensory deficit was present over the posterior part of the right leg and the sole of the foot down to the big toe. In further testing, with the patient lying down in the supine position and her pelvis stabilized, the clinician slowly raised her right leg by lifting her heel with the knee extended. This placed tension on the lumbosacral nerve roots. During this maneuver, the patient experienced severe pain down her leg below the knee.

See the Clinical Case Discussion at the end of this chapter for further insight.

CHAPTER OUTLINE

LEARNING OBJECTIVES

The purpose of this chapter is to review the basic anatomy of the vertebral column and related soft tissue structures in order to understand the basis for common back injuries, back pain, motor deficits, congenital defects, medical imaging, and general surface examination.

1. Identify the bones of the back and their major features. Describe the functional aspects of these structures.
2. Identify the regions of the vertebral column, giving the number of vertebrae and the

characteristics of typical and atypical vertebrae in each region.

3. Describe the normal curvatures of the vertebral column in pre- and postnatal conditions. Describe the features and the clinical significance of the major abnormal curvatures of the vertebral column.
4. Identify the components of a typical embryonic vertebra and their fate in each region of the adult vertebral column. Describe the embryonic basis of accessory ribs and spina bifida.
5. Identify the intervertebral joints and the major ligaments related to each joint. Identify the movements allowed in each case.
6. Describe the components of the intervertebral disc and the functional significance of each. Describe the anatomical basis of a herniated (slipped) disc.
7. Identify the major forms of fracture and dislocation of the vertebral column and the functional consequences of each.
8. Identify the muscles of the back according to their general topography. Describe their innervation and major actions. Differentiate the extrinsic and intrinsic muscles of the back. Predict the functional consequences of lesions of specific motor nerves and paralysis of the associated muscles.
9. Describe the boundaries and major contents of the auscultatory, lumbar, and suboccipital triangles.
10. Describe the blood supply and lymphatic drainage of the back. Note the topography and major anastomoses of the vertebral venous plexuses. Explain the significance of the venous network in collateral circulation and spread of disease.
11. Identify the major external features of the spinal cord. Describe the vascular supply of the spinal cord.
12. Describe the components of a typical spinal cord segment, including the formation of a typical spinal nerve. Trace the distribution of a typical spinal nerve.
13. Identify the spinal meninges, the spaces between them, and the major contents of each space. Describe the functions and clinical significance of each.
14. Describe the development of the spinal cord in relation to that of the vertebral column. Compare and contrast the length of the spinal cord, the location of spinal segments, and the relationship of spinal roots and nerves with the intervertebral spaces in pre- and postnatal states.
15. Describe the anatomical basis for and clinical significance of a lumbar puncture (spinal tap) versus caudal anesthesia.
16. Identify the major features of the vertebral column in standard radiographic images.
17. Identify the major features of the back in a standard surface anatomy examination.

OVERVIEW

The back, which extends from the skull to the tip of the coccyx, can be defined as the posterior surface of the trunk (Fig. 2.1). The scapulae and the muscles that connect the scapulae to the trunk are superimposed on the upper part of the back.

VERTEBRAL COLUMN

The vertebral column is the central, longitudinal bony pillar of the body. It supports the skull, pectoral girdle, upper limbs, and thoracic cage and, by way of the pelvic girdle, transmits the body weight to the lower limbs. The spinal cord, roots of the spinal nerves, and the covering meninges lie within the cavity of the vertebral column that provides great protection to those structures.

Composition

The vertebral column (Fig. 2.2; also see Fig. 2.1) is composed of 33 vertebrae organized in five regions—7 cervical, 12 thoracic, 5 lumbar, 5 sacral (fused to form the sacrum), and ~4 coccygeal (the lower 3 are commonly fused). Numerous joints connect these many individual segments, thus making the vertebral column quite flexible.

Vertebrae

The vertebrae within each region possess distinctive distinguishing features. However, all vertebrae share a common structural floor plan (Fig. 2.3).

A **typical vertebra** consists of a rounded **body** anteriorly and a **vertebral arch** posteriorly. These enclose a space termed the **vertebral foramen**. In

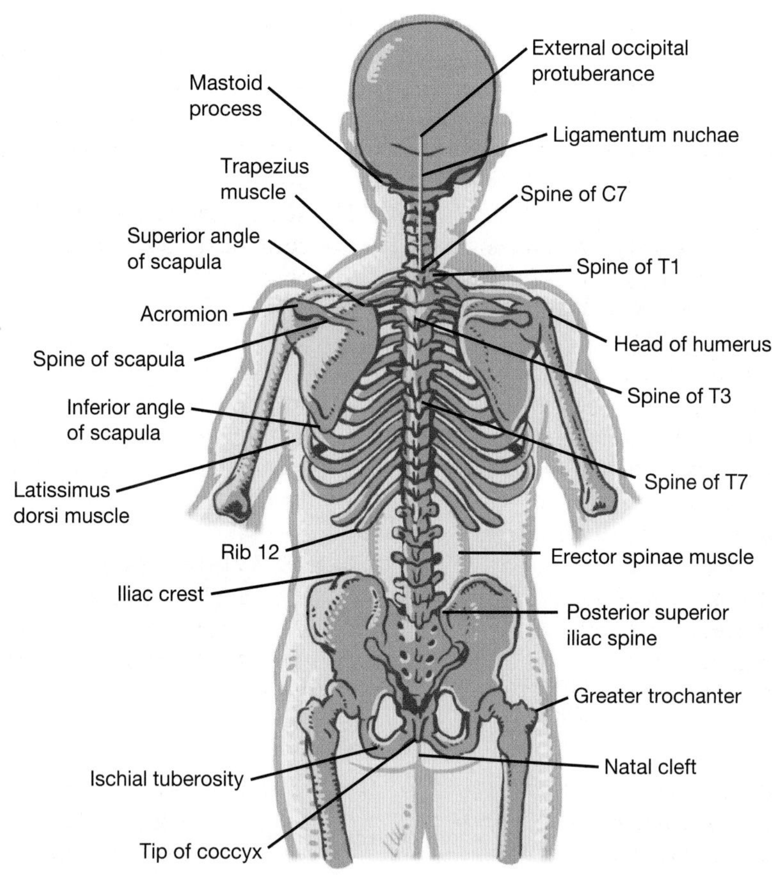

Figure 2.1 Posterior view of the back showing the vertebral column and related surface markings.

an articulated skeleton, the vertebral foramina are aligned to form a continuous passageway termed the **vertebral canal** that conveys the spinal cord and its coverings. The vertebral arch consists of a pair of cylindrical **pedicles**, which form the sides of the arch, and a pair of flattened **laminae**, which complete the arch posteriorly. The vertebral arch gives rise to seven processes: one spinous, two transverse, and four articular (see Fig. 2.2B).

The **spinous process** (**spine**) is directed posteriorly from the junction of the two laminae. The **transverse processes** are directed laterally from the junction of the laminae and the pedicles. Both the spinous and transverse processes serve as levers and receive attachments of muscles and ligaments.

The **articular processes** are vertically arranged and consist of two superior and two inferior processes. They arise from the junction of the laminae and the pedicles, and their articular surfaces (facets) are covered with hyaline cartilage.

The two superior articular processes of one vertebral arch articulate with the two inferior articular processes of the arch above, forming two synovial joints. Likewise, the two inferior articular processes of the vertebral arch articulate with the two superior articular processes of the arch below, forming two additional synovial joints. Thus, each vertebra possesses a total of four synovial articular joints.

The pedicles are notched on their superior and inferior borders, forming the **superior** and **inferior vertebral notches**. On each side in an articulated skeleton, the superior notch of one vertebra and the inferior notch of the adjacent vertebra above align and form an **intervertebral foramen**. These foramina serve to transmit the spinal nerves and blood vessels. The anterior and posterior nerve roots of a spinal nerve unite within these foramina with their meningeal coverings to form the segmental spinal nerves.

Typical Vertebrae Regional Characteristics

The distinguishing features of typical cervical, thoracic, and lumbar vertebrae are summarized in Table 2.1 and illustrated in Figures 2.2 through 2.12.

Atypical Vertebrae Characteristics

The C1, C2, and C7 (Fig. 2.12; also see Fig. 2.4) and T1, T10 to T12 vertebrae are atypical.

The **first cervical vertebra**, or **atlas**, does not possess a body or a spinous process. Instead, it has **anterior and posterior arches**. It has a **lateral mass** on each side with articular surfaces on its upper surface

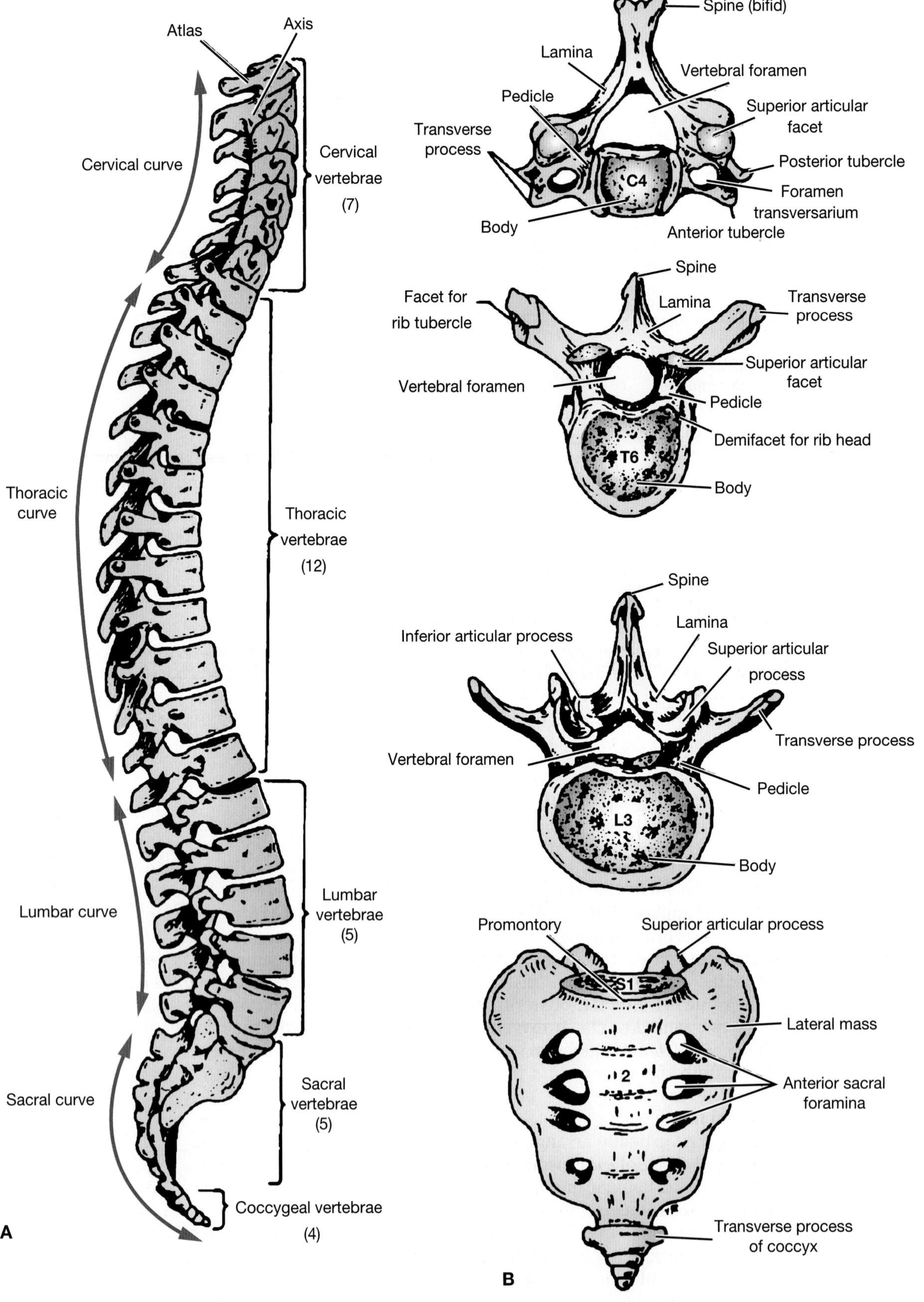

Figure 2.2 **A.** Lateral view of the vertebral column. **B.** General features of different kinds of vertebrae.

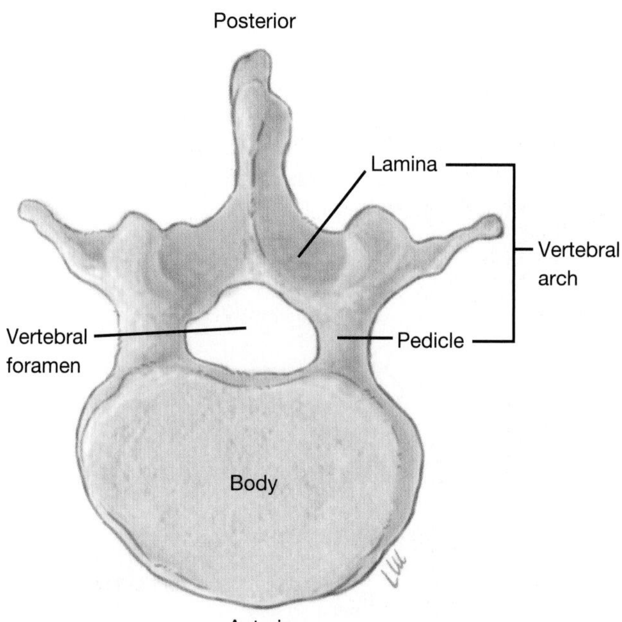

Figure 2.3 All vertebrae share a common floorplan organized around a body and a vertebral arch.

Table 2.1 Typical Vertebrae Regional Characteristics

	CERVICAL (C3–C6)	THORACIC (T2–T9)	LUMBAR (L1–L5)
Body	Small and transversely broad No costal facets	Medium sized and heart shaped Costal facets (demifacets) present on each side at the posterior superior and posterior inferior corner for articulation with the heads of the ribs	Large and kidney shaped No costal facets
Vertebral foramen	Large and triangular to accommodate the cervical enlargement of the spinal cord	Small and circular	Large and triangular to accommodate the lumbar enlargement of the spinal cord
Spinous process	Short, bifid, and inclined inferiorly	Long and inclined inferiorly Thoracic spines overlap in a shingle-like pattern	Short, flat, quadrangular, and projecting posteriorly
Transverse process	Possesses a foramen transversarium for passage of the vertebral artery and veins Note: vertebral artery passes through transverse processes of C1 to C6 but not C7 No costal facet	No foramen transversarium Possesses a costal facet for articulation with the tubercle of a rib Note: T11 and T12 do not have costal facets	No foramen transversarium No costal facet
Articular processes	Relatively flat facets Facets on superior articular processes face superiorly and posteriorly Facets on inferior processes face inferiorly and anteriorly	Relatively flat facets Facets on superior articular processes face posteriorly and laterally Facets on inferior processes face anteriorly and medially Note: facets on the inferior processes of T12 face laterally, in typical lumbar fashion	Curved facets Facets on superior articular processes are concave and face medially Facets on inferior processes are convex and face laterally
Interlaminar space	Small	Small	Short laminae in the vertical dimension produce large interlaminar spaces

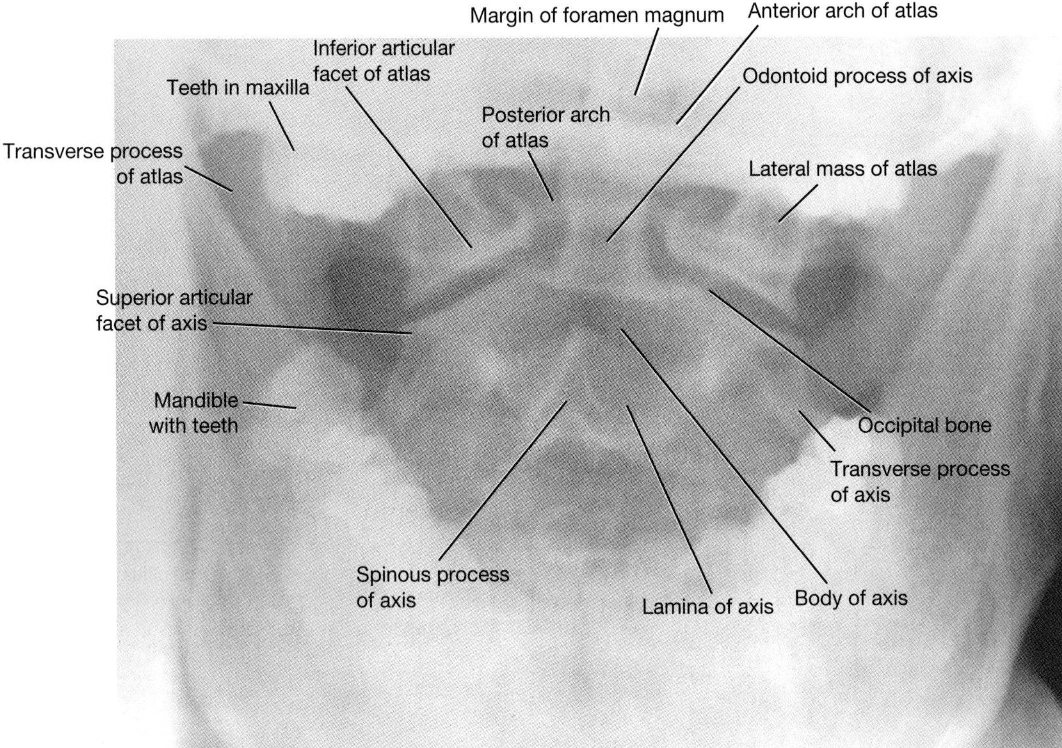

Figure 2.4 Anteroposterior (AP) radiograph of the upper cervical region of the vertebral column with the patient's mouth open to show the odontoid process of the axis.

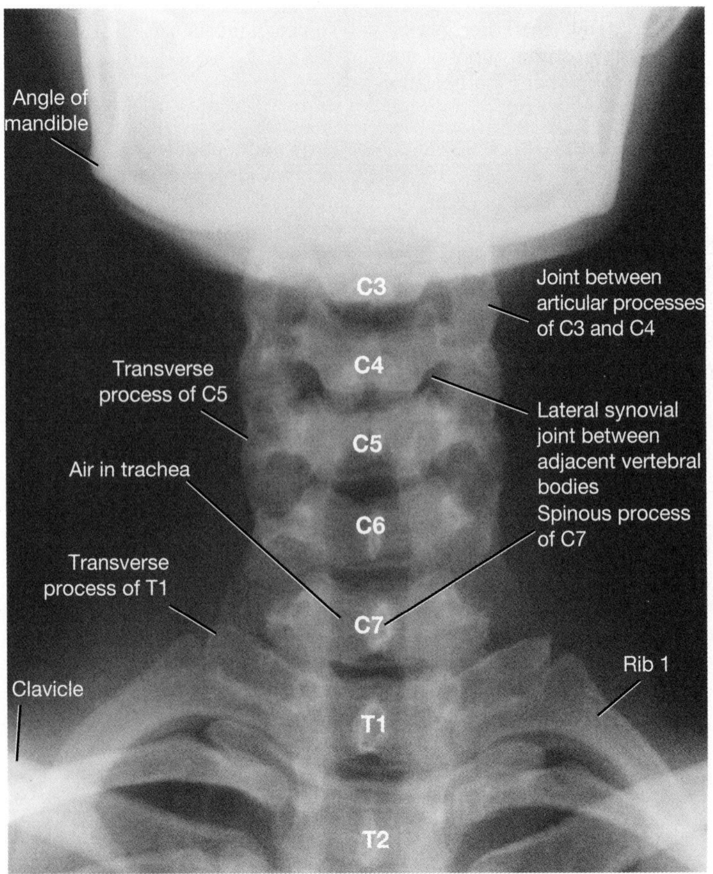

Figure 2.5 Anteroposterior (AP) radiograph of the cervical region of the vertebral column.

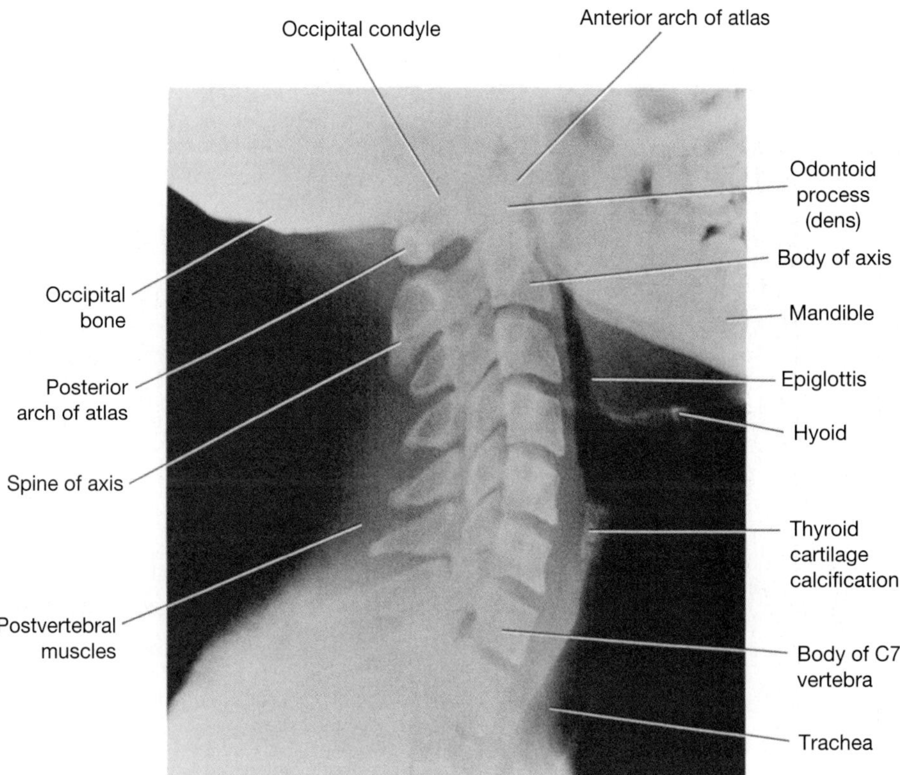

Figure 2.6 Lateral radiograph of the cervical region of the vertebral column.

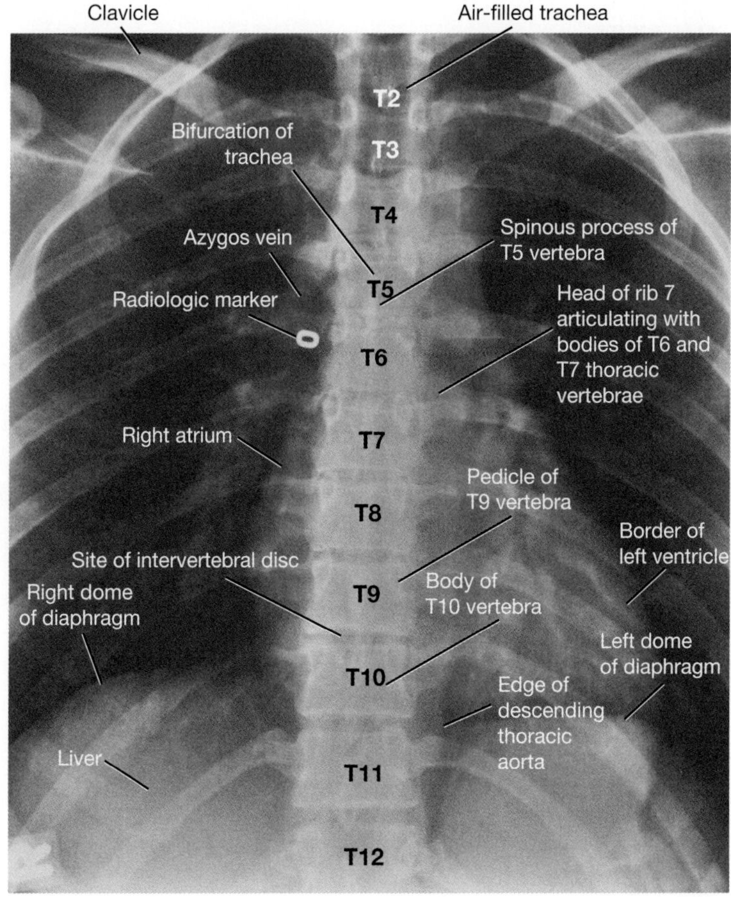

Figure 2.7 Anteroposterior (AP) radiograph of the thoracic region of the vertebral column.

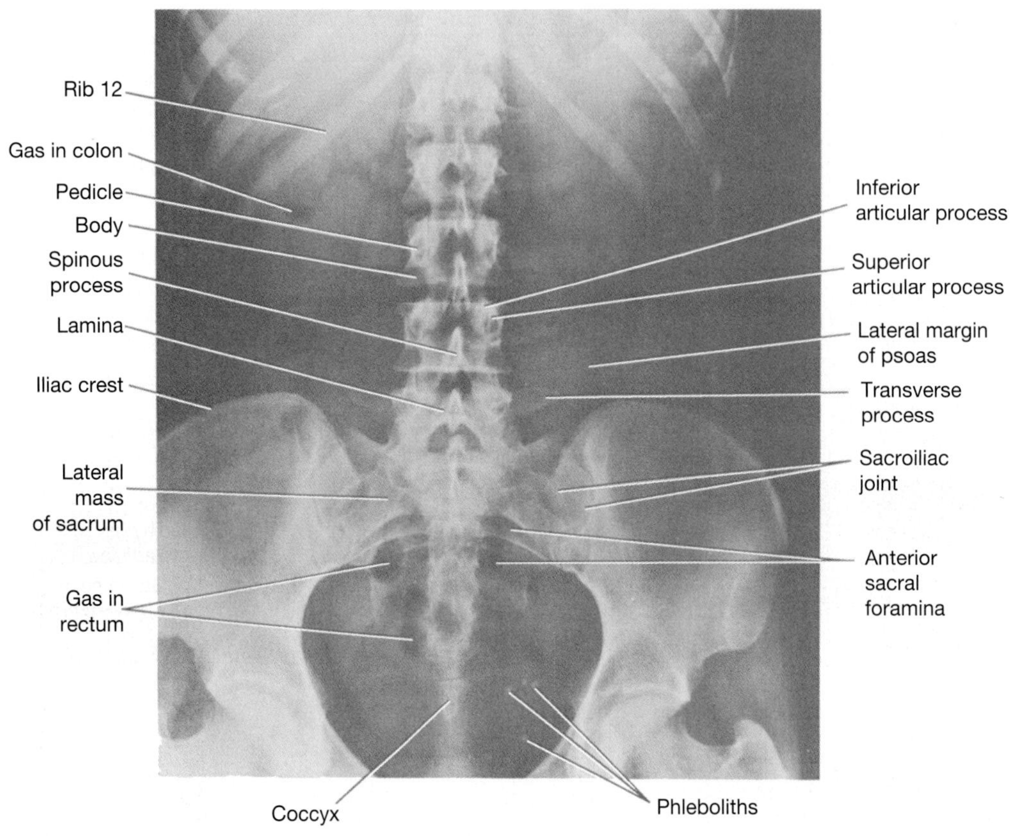

Figure 2.8 Anteroposterior (AP) radiograph of the lumbar and sacral regions of the vertebral column.

for articulation with the occipital condyles of the skull (**atlanto-occipital joints**) and articular surfaces on its inferior surface for articulation with the C2 vertebra (**atlantoaxial joints**).

The **second cervical vertebra**, or **axis**, has a peg-like **odontoid process** (**dens**) that projects upward from the superior surface of the body. The dens represents the body of the atlas that fused with the body of the axis during early development.

The **seventh cervical vertebra**, or **vertebra prominens**, is so named because it has the longest spinous process, and the process is not bifid. The transverse process is large, but the foramen transversarium is small and transmits the vertebral vein or veins.

T1 and T10 to T12 are atypical because of variations in the attachments of ribs to the bodies and/or transverse processes. Those details are described in Chapter 4.

Sacrum

The **sacrum** (see Fig. 2.2B) consists of five rudimentary vertebrae fused together to form a wedge-shaped bone, which is concave anteriorly. The upper border, or **base**, of the bone articulates with the L5 vertebra. The narrow inferior border, or **apex**, articulates with the coccyx. Laterally, the sacrum articulates with the two iliac bones to form the **sacroiliac joints** (see Fig. 2.1). The anterior and upper margin of the S1 vertebra bulges forward as the posterior margin of the pelvic inlet and is termed the **sacral promontory**. The sacral promontory in the female is of considerable obstetric importance and is used when measuring the size of the pelvis.

The vertebral canal continues into the sacrum where it forms the **sacral canal**. The sacral canal contains the cauda equina (composed mainly of the anterior and posterior roots of the sacral and coccygeal spinal nerves) and fibrofatty material. It also contains the lower part of the subarachnoid space down as far as the S2 vertebra. The laminae of the S5 vertebra, and sometimes those of S4, fail to meet in the midline, forming the **sacral hiatus** (see Fig. 2.45). At the sacral hiatus, the posterior inferior end of the sacral canal is devoid of a bony cover, making the canal easily accessible (see Chapter 6).

The anterior and posterior surfaces of the sacrum each have four foramina (**anterior** and **posterior sacral foramina**) for the passage of the anterior and posterior rami of the upper four sacral nerves.

The L5 vertebra may be incorporated into the sacrum, in a condition termed **sacralization of the L5 vertebra** (Fig. 2.13). This is usually incomplete and may be limited

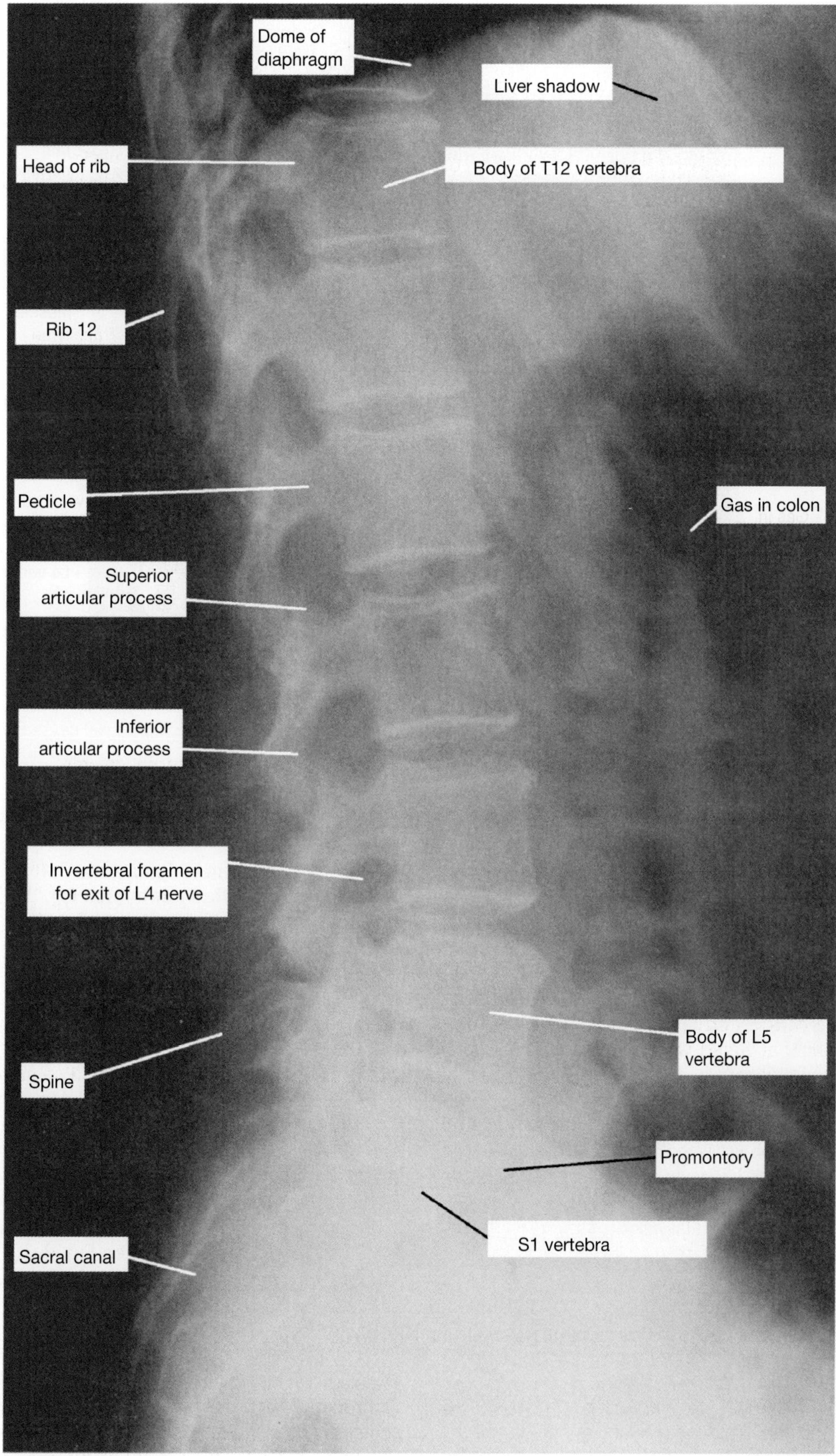

Figure 2.9 Lateral radiograph of the lower thoracic, lumbar, and sacral regions of the vertebral column.

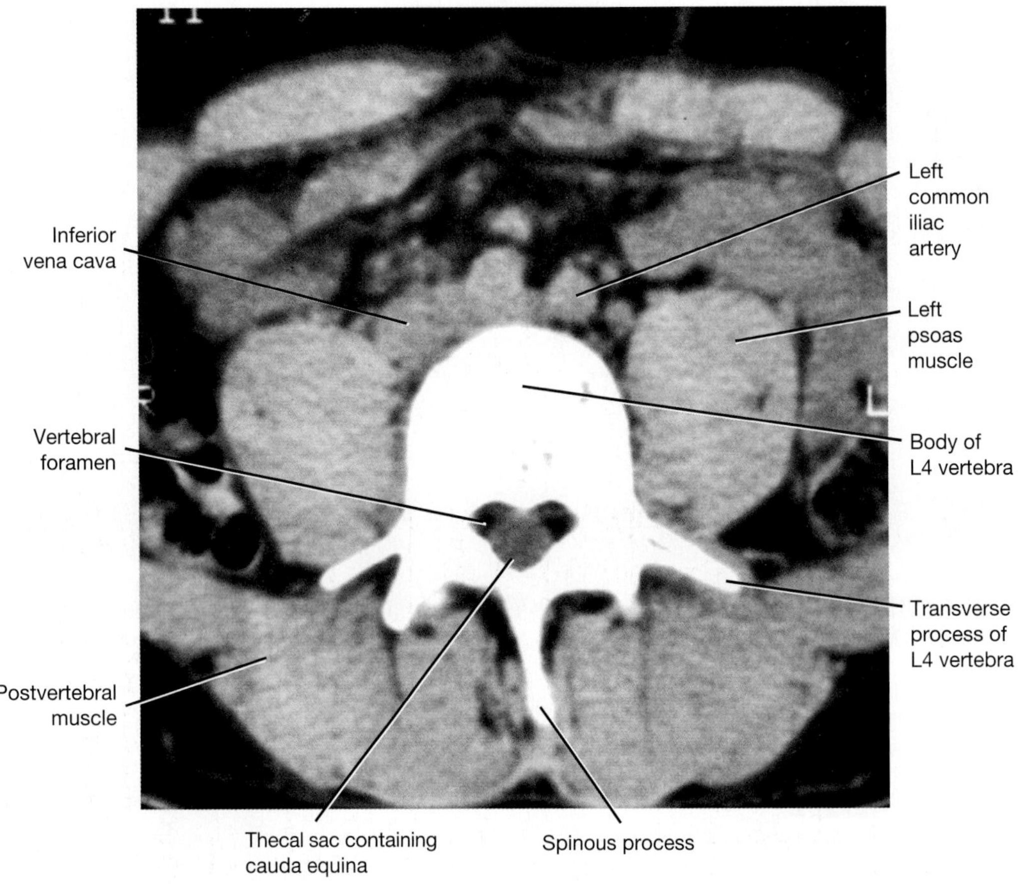

Figure 2.10 Axial CT scan of the L4 vertebra.

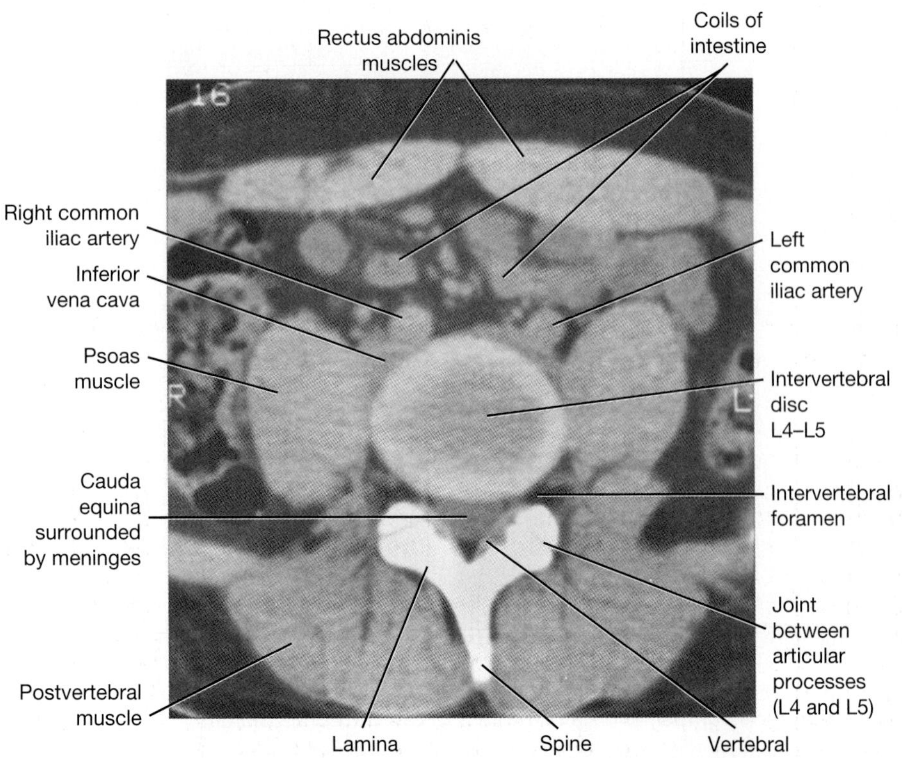

Figure 2.11 Axial CT scan through the vertebral column at the level of the intervertebral disc between the L4 and L5 vertebrae. The spine of L4 and the intervertebral foramen on each side are shown. Note the joints between the articular processes.

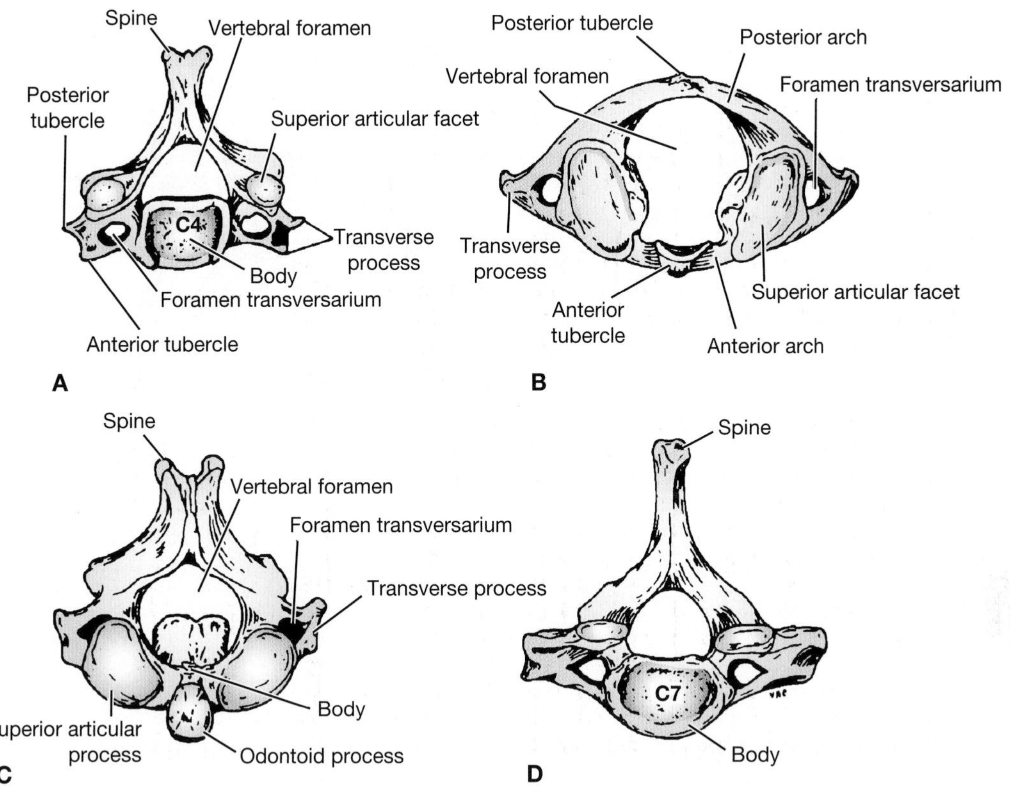

Figure 2.12 **A.** Typical cervical vertebra, superior aspect. **B.** Atlas, or C1 vertebra, superior aspect. **C.** Axis, or C2 vertebra, from above and behind. **D.** C7 vertebra, superior aspect; the foramen transversarium forms a passage for the vertebral vein but not for the vertebral artery.

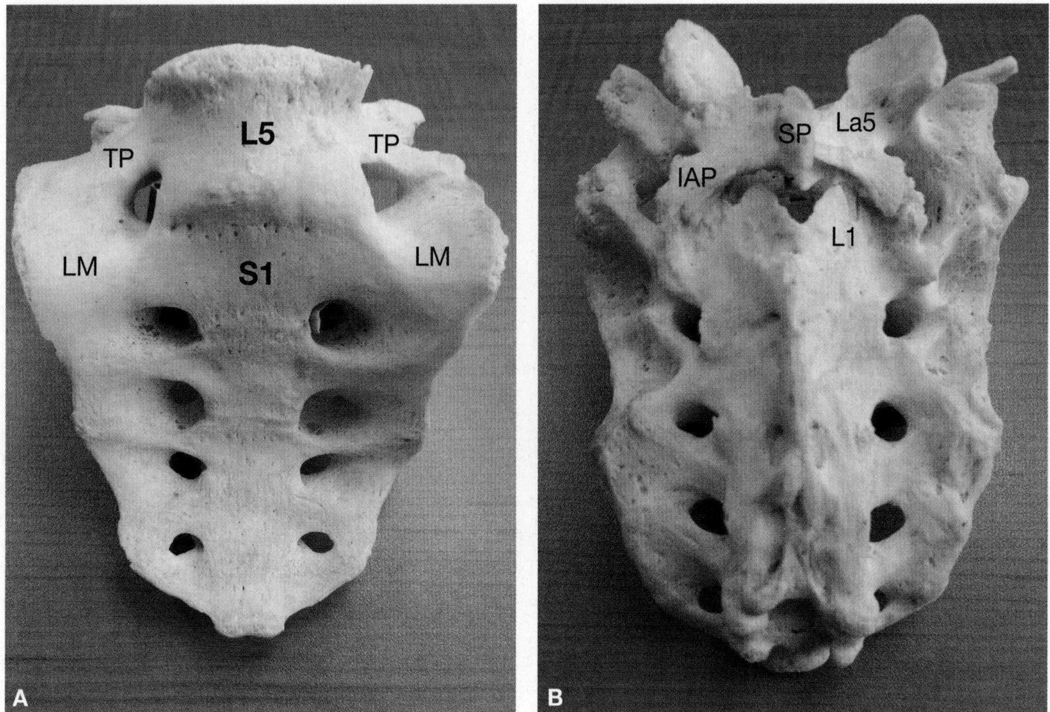

Figure 2.13 Incomplete sacralization of the L5 vertebra. **A.** Anterior aspect. **B.** Posterior aspect. IAP, inferior articular process of L5; L1, lamina of S1; La5, lamina of L5; LM, lateral mass of S1; SP; spinous process of L5; TP, transverse process of L5.

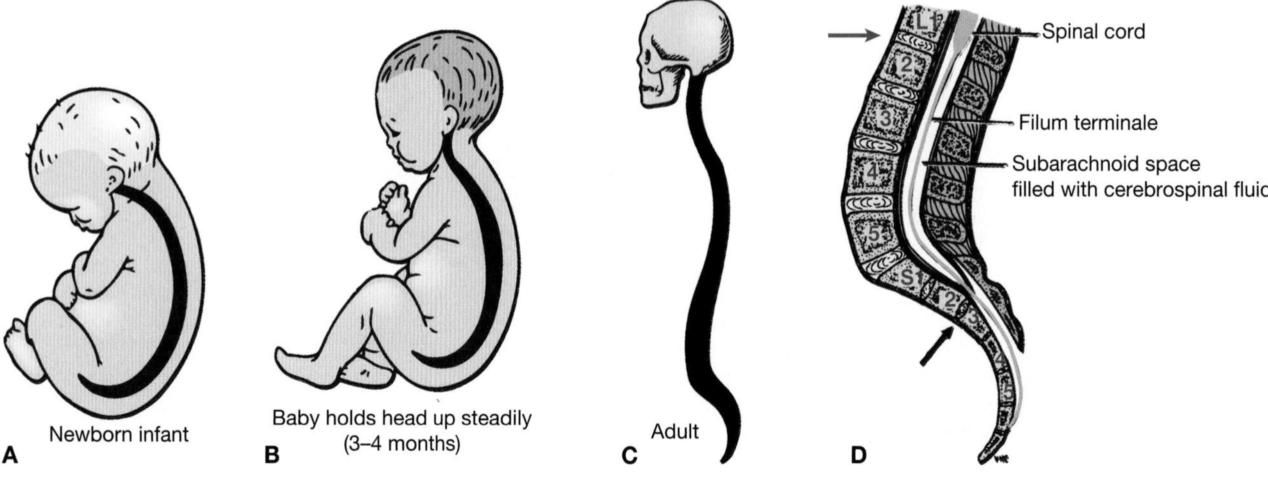

Figure 2.14 **A–C.** Curves of the vertebral column at different ages. **D.** In the adult, the lower end of the spinal cord lies at the level of the lower border of the body of the L1 vertebra (*top arrow*), and the subarachnoid space ends at the lower border of the body of the S2 vertebra (*bottom arrow*).

to one side. Conversely, the S1 vertebra may remain partially or completely separate from the sacrum and resemble the L6 vertebra (**lumbarization of the S1 vertebra**). A large extent of the posterior wall of the sacral canal may be absent because the laminae and spines fail to develop.

Coccyx

The **coccyx** usually consists of four vertebrae fused together to form a single, small triangular bone that articulates at its base with the lower end of the sacrum (see Fig. 2.2). The first coccygeal vertebra is usually not fused or is incompletely fused with the second vertebra. However, the coccyx may have only three or up to five vertebrae. The first coccygeal vertebra may be separate. In this condition, the free vertebra usually projects downward and anteriorly from the apex of the sacrum. Greater detail on the morphology of the sacrum and coccyx is provided in Chapter 6.

Knowledge of the preceding basic anatomy of the vertebral column is important when interpreting radiographs and when noting the precise sites of bony pathologic features relative to soft tissue injury.

Vertebral Column Curvatures

The adult vertebral column (in the standing position) is aligned to form four regional curvatures in the sagittal plane (see Figs. 2.2 and 2.14). The **thoracic** and **sacrococcygeal curves** have anterior concavities; the **cervical** and **lumbar curves** have posterior concavities. Collectively, the curves serve to align the center of gravity of the body through the pelvis, thereby counteracting the weight of the thoracoabdominal viscera, allowing the head to balance on top of the vertebral column and enabling upright posture (see Fig. 2.29). However, in the initial development, the fetal vertebral column has only one continuous anterior concavity (see Fig. 2.14A). As development proceeds, the **lumbosacral angle** appears at the junction of the L5 and S1 vertebrae, forming two anteriorly concave curves. After birth, the cervical curve forms in association with the child raising their head and keeping it poised on the vertebral column (Fig. 2.14B). Toward the end of the first year, the lumbar curve forms in association with the child beginning to sit up and stand upright. Because the thoracic and sacrococcygeal curves retain their initial prenatal anterior concavities, these curves are termed **primary curvatures**. Because the cervical and lumbar curves form mainly postnatally and take on posterior concavities, they are termed **secondary curvatures**. The development of the secondary curves results in a modification in the shape of the vertebral bodies and the intervertebral discs.

The lumbar curve is more pronounced in adult females than in males. During the later months of pregnancy, with the increase in size and weight of the fetus, females tend to increase the lumbar concavity to preserve their center of gravity. In old age, the intervertebral discs atrophy, resulting in a loss of height and a gradual return of the vertebral column to a continuous anterior concavity.

The development of minor lateral vertebral curves in the thoracic region is common in late childhood. This is normal and is usually caused by the predominant use of one of the upper limbs. For example, right-handed individuals will often have a slight right-sided thoracic convexity. Slight compensatory curves are always present superior and inferior to such a curvature.

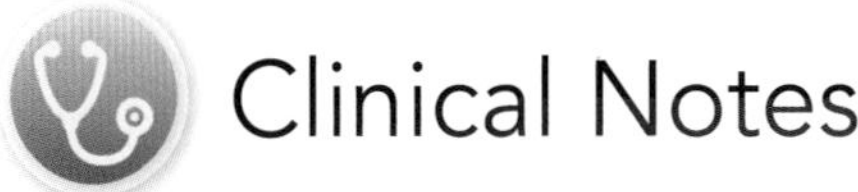

Clinical Notes

Abnormal Vertebral Column Curves

Kyphosis is severe exaggeration in the thoracic curvature of the vertebral column caused by structural changes in the vertebral bodies or intervertebral discs (Fig. 2.15). In **disease-based kyphosis**, conditions such as crush fractures or tuberculosis caused destruction of the vertebral bodies lead to acute angular kyphosis of the vertebral column. In **senile kyphosis** in the aged, osteoporosis and/or degeneration of the intervertebral discs and/or notable weakening of the intrinsic back muscles may lead to kyphosis involving the cervical, thoracic, and lumbar regions of the column. In adolescents with poor muscle tone, long hours of study, or work over a low desk can lead to a less severe, gently curved upper thoracic region. Such a "round-shouldered" condition may or may not be categorized as kyphosis.

Lordosis is an exaggeration of either of the secondary vertebral curvatures (Fig. 2.15). It is more often an accented lumbar curve; however, it may be a severe cervical curvature. Lumbar lordosis may be caused by an increase in the weight of the abdominal contents, as with the gravid uterus or a large ovarian tumor, or it may be caused by disease of the vertebral column such as spondylolisthesis. It is also possible that lumbar lordosis is a postural compensation for kyphosis in the thoracic region or a disease of the hip joint (eg, congenital dislocation).

Scoliosis is a lateral deviation of the vertebral column, usually including malrotation (Figs. 2.16 and 2.17). This is most commonly found in the thoracic region and has multiple possible causes. Paralysis of muscles caused by poliomyelitis or the presence of a congenital hemivertebra can cause scoliosis. Often, scoliosis is compensatory and may be caused by a short leg or hip disease. Scoliosis is more common in females, and its onset has a strong association with the adolescent growth spurt. However, most incidents of scoliosis are idiopathic (ie, of unknown cause).

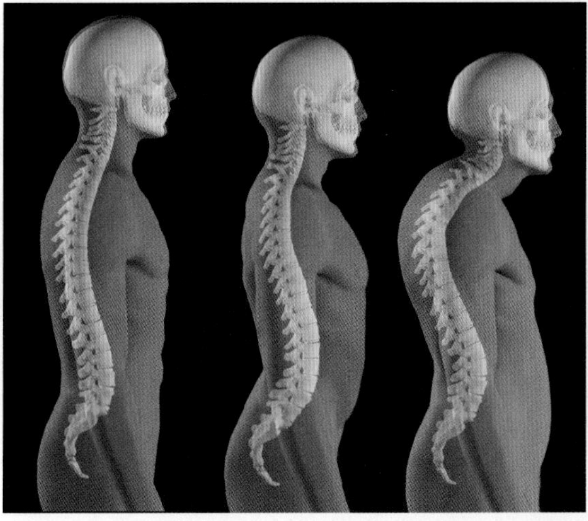

Figure 2.15 Lateral views of normal vertebral curves (*left*), lordosis (*middle*), and kyphosis (*right*). (LifeART image copyright © 2024 Lippincott Williams & Wilkins. All rights reserved.)

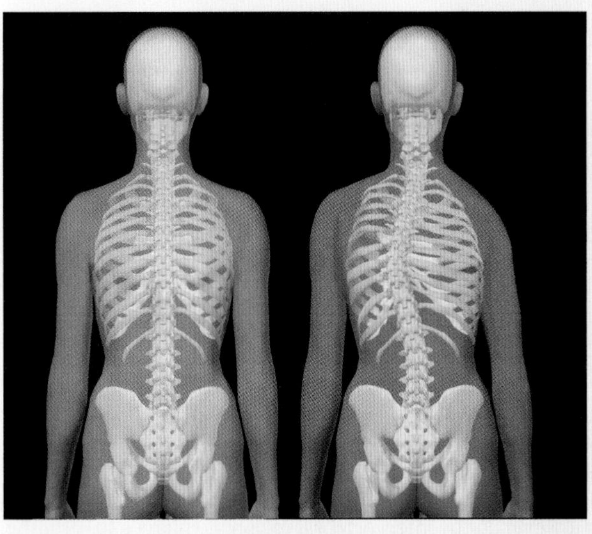

Figure 2.16 Posterior views of normal vertebral curves (*left*) and scoliosis (*right*). (LifeART image copyright © 2024 Lippincott Williams & Wilkins. All rights reserved.)

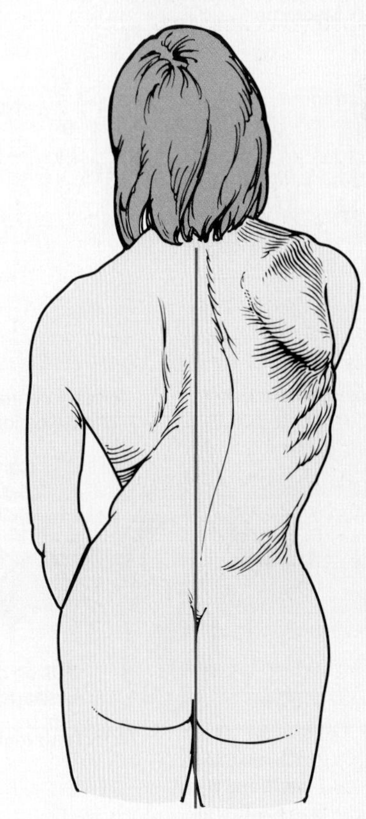

Figure 2.17 Posterior view of surface anatomy of a female with scoliosis. (LifeART image copyright © 2024 Lippincott Williams & Wilkins. All rights reserved.)

Embryology Notes

Vertebral Column Development

Early in development, the embryonic mesoderm differentiates into three distinct regions: **paraxial**, **intermediate**, and **lateral mesoderm**. The paraxial mesoderm is a column of tissue situated on either side of the midline of the embryo. At about the fourth week, it divides into blocks of tissue termed **somites**. Each somite differentiates into a ventromedial part (**sclerotome**) and a dorsolateral part (**dermatomyotome**). The dermatomyotome next further differentiates into the **myotome** and the **dermatome** (Fig. 2.18A).

The mesenchymal cells of the sclerotome rapidly divide and migrate medially during the fourth week of development and surround the **notochord**. The caudal half of each sclerotome now fuses with the cephalic half of the immediately succeeding sclerotome to form the mesenchymal vertebral body (Fig. 2.19; also see Fig. 2.18B). Each vertebral body is thus an intersegmental structure. The notochord degenerates completely in the region of the vertebral body. However, in the intervertebral region, it enlarges to form the **nucleus pulposus** of the **intervertebral disc** (see Fig. 2.19). The surrounding fibrocartilage, the **annulus fibrosus**, of the intervertebral disc is derived from sclerotomic mesenchyme situated between adjacent vertebral bodies.

Meanwhile, the mesenchymal vertebral body gives rise to posterior and lateral outgrowths on each side. The posterior outgrowths grow around the neural tube between the segmental nerves to fuse with their fellows of the opposite side and form the mesenchymal vertebral arch (see Figs. 2.19 and 2.20). The lateral outgrowths pass between the myotomes to form the mesenchymal **costal processes** or primordia of the ribs.

Costal Processes

The **costal processes** contribute to the final vertebral form in region-specific patterns (Table 2.2 and Fig. 2.20).

Abnormal enlargements of the costal processes may occur and form **accessory ribs**. This occurs most often at the L1 and C7 vertebrae. The most common occurrence is

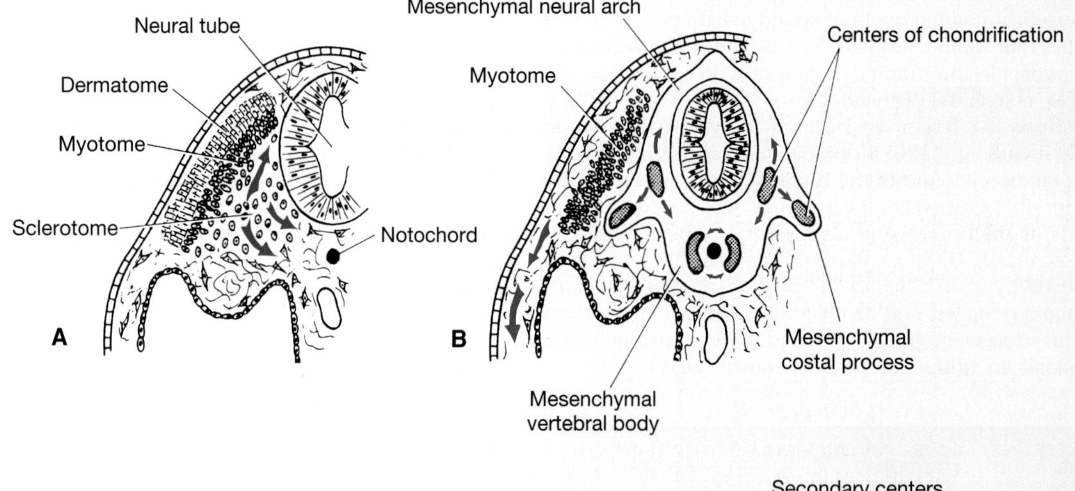

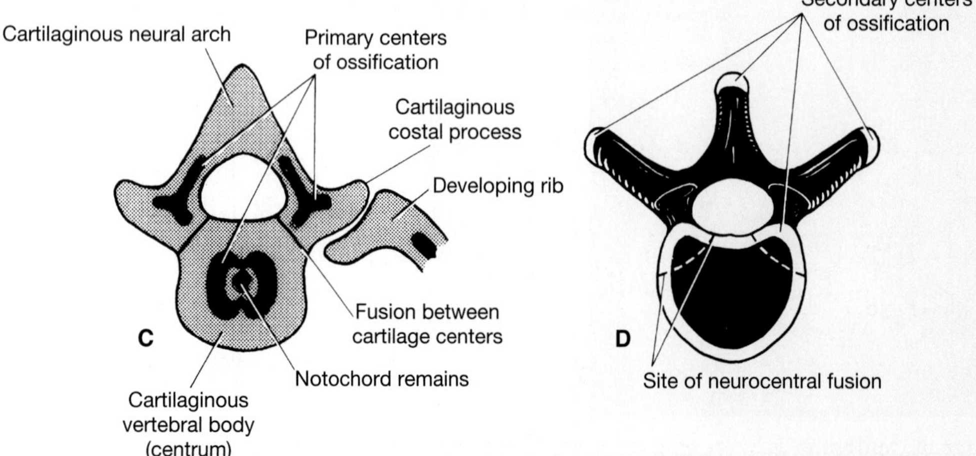

Figure 2.18 Stages in the formation of a thoracic vertebra. **A.** Differentiation of a somite into dermatome, myotome, and sclerotome. **B.** Differentiation of sclerotome into vertebral elements. **C, D.** Progressive formation of ossification centers.

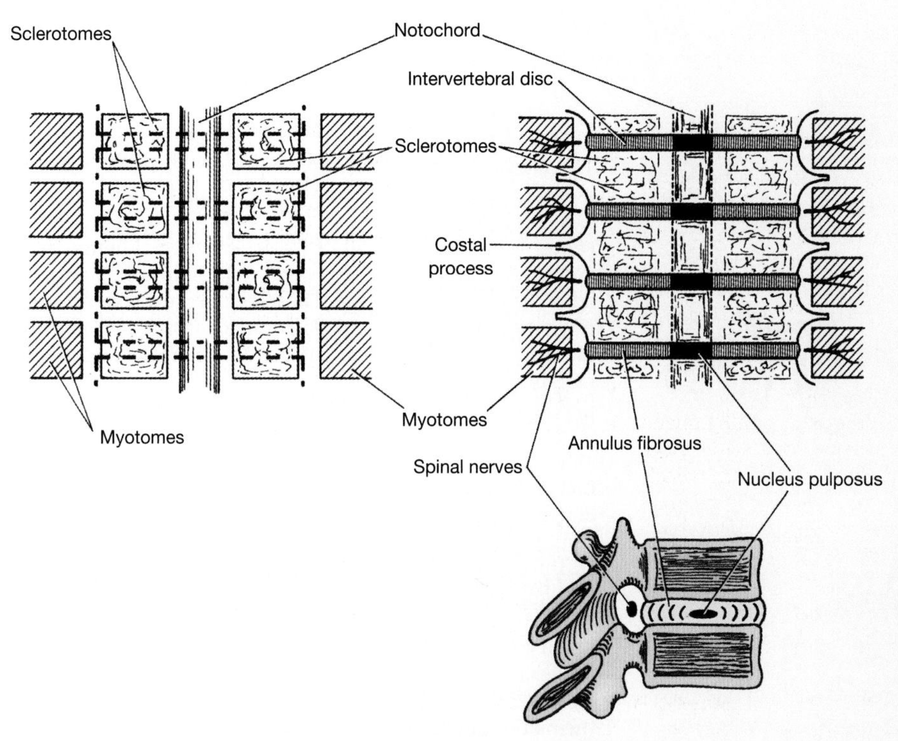

Figure 2.19 Formation of each mesenchymal vertebral body by the fusion of the caudal half of each sclerotome with the cephalic half of the immediately succeeding sclerotome. Each vertebral body is thus an intersegmental structure. The costal processes grow out between adjacent myotomes. Also shown is the close relationship that exists between each spinal nerve and each intervertebral disc.

Table 2.2 Derivatives of Embryonic Costal Processes

REGION	COSTAL PROCESS DERIVATIVE
Cervical	Normally remains small Forms the anterior and lateral boundary of the foramen transversarium
Thoracic	Ribs
Lumbar	Large part of the transverse process
Sacral	Fuse together to form much of the lateral masses (alae) of the sacrum

the formation of a lumbar rib at L1. This is usually an asymptomatic condition. Accessory ribs at C7 are termed **cervical ribs**. These may be unilateral or bilateral and can range from small fibrous bands to complete bony ribs. Cervical ribs may be asymptomatic, or they may produce neurovascular effects in the upper limb due to the compression of the subclavian artery and/or lower trunk of the brachial plexus. See Chapter 3 for further discussion of the cervical rib syndrome.

Vertebral Arch

The dorsal outgrowths from the vertebral body may fail to fuse in the posterior midline, leaving a gap in the vertebral arch of one or more adjacent vertebrae. This condition, termed **spina bifida**, occurs most frequently in the lower

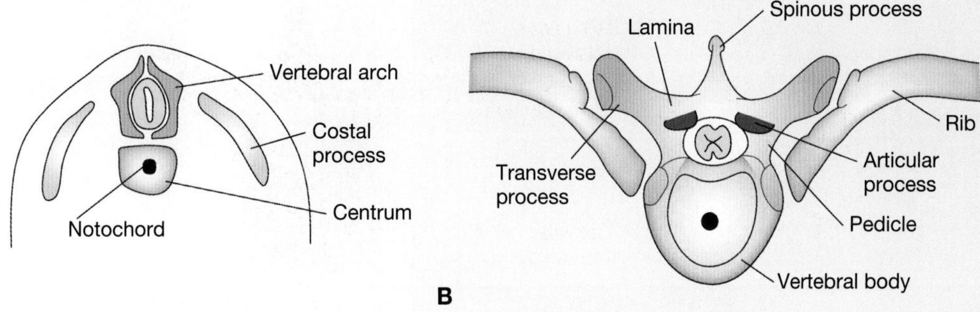

Figure 2.20 Schematic horizontal sections of thoracic vertebrae showing their main developmental components. Also see Table 2.2. **A.** Three distinct components are present at about 5 to 7 weeks: the centrum, vertebral arch, and costal process. **B.** Adult. Each component develops into distinct structures, as indicated by the shading. (From Dudek, RW. *BRS Embryology*; 6th ed. Baltimore, MD: Wolters Kluwer Health. 2014, with permission.)

(continued)

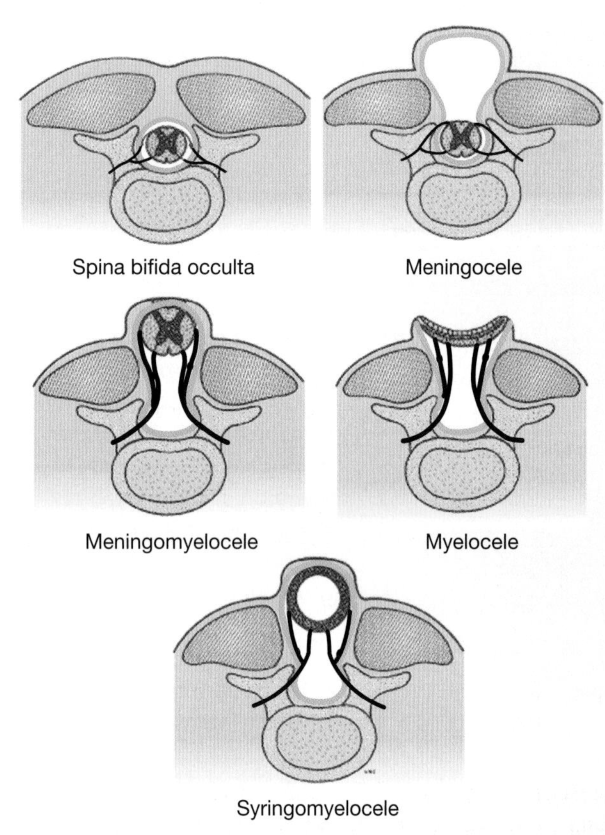

Figure 2.21 Different types of spina bifida.

thoracic, lumbar, and sacral regions. Underlying this defect, the meninges and spinal cord may or may not be involved to varying degrees. This condition is a result of failure of the mesenchyme, which grows in between the neural tube and the surface ectoderm, to form the vertebral arches in the affected region. The major types of spina bifida are shown in Figures 2.21 and 2.22.

Development Completion

Two centers of chondrification appear in the middle of each mesenchymal vertebral body. These quickly fuse to form a cartilaginous **centrum** (see Fig. 2.18). A chondrification center forms in each half of the mesenchymal neural arch and spreads dorsally to fuse behind the neural tube with its fellow of the opposite side. These centers also extend anteriorly to fuse with the cartilaginous centrum and laterally into the costal processes. The condensed mesenchymal or membranous vertebra has thus been converted into a cartilaginous vertebra.

At about the ninth week of development, primary ossification centers appear: two for each centum and one for each half of the neural arch. The two centers for the centrum usually unite quickly, but the complete union of all the primary centers does not occur until several years after birth.

During adolescence, secondary centers appear in the cartilage covering the superior and inferior ends of the vertebral body, and the epiphyseal plates are formed. A secondary center also appears at the tip of each transverse process and at the tip of the spinous process (see Fig. 2.18). By the 25th year, all the secondary centers have fused with the rest of the vertebra.

The atlas and axis develop somewhat differently. The centrum of the atlas fuses with that of the axis and becomes the **odontoid process**. This leaves only the vertebral arch remaining of the atlas, which grows anteriorly and finally fuses in the midline to form the characteristic ring shape of the atlas vertebra.

In the sacral region, the bodies of the individual vertebrae are separated from each other in early life by intervertebral discs. At about the 18th year, the bodies start to become united by bone. This process starts caudally. Usually by the 13th year, all the sacral vertebrae are united. In the coccygeal region, segmental fusion also takes place, and, in later life, the coccyx commonly fuses with the sacrum.

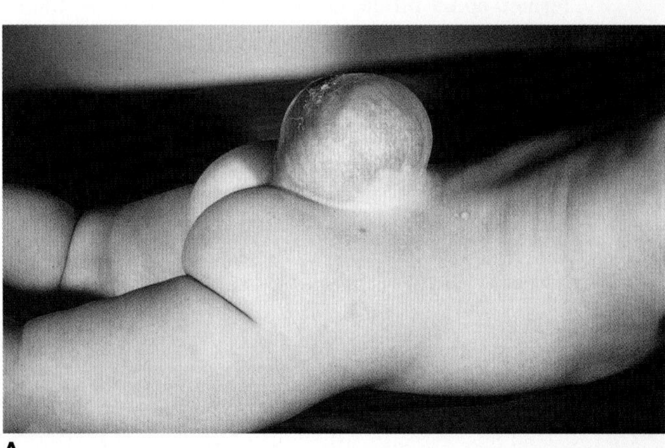
A

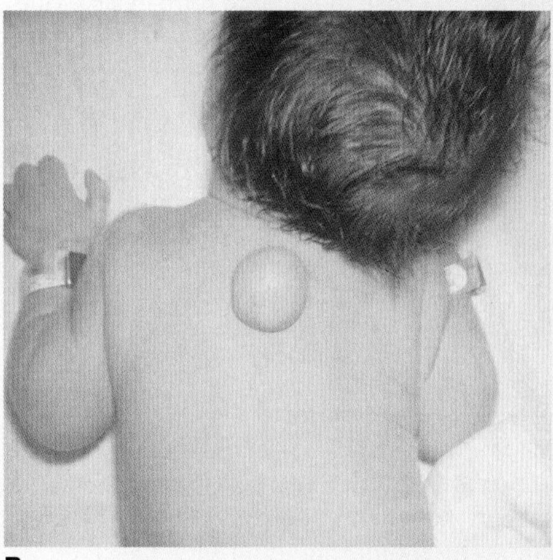
B

Figure 2.22 **A.** Meningocele in the lumbosacral region. (Courtesy of L. Thompson.) **B.** Meningomyelocele in the upper thoracic region. (Courtesy of G. Avery.)

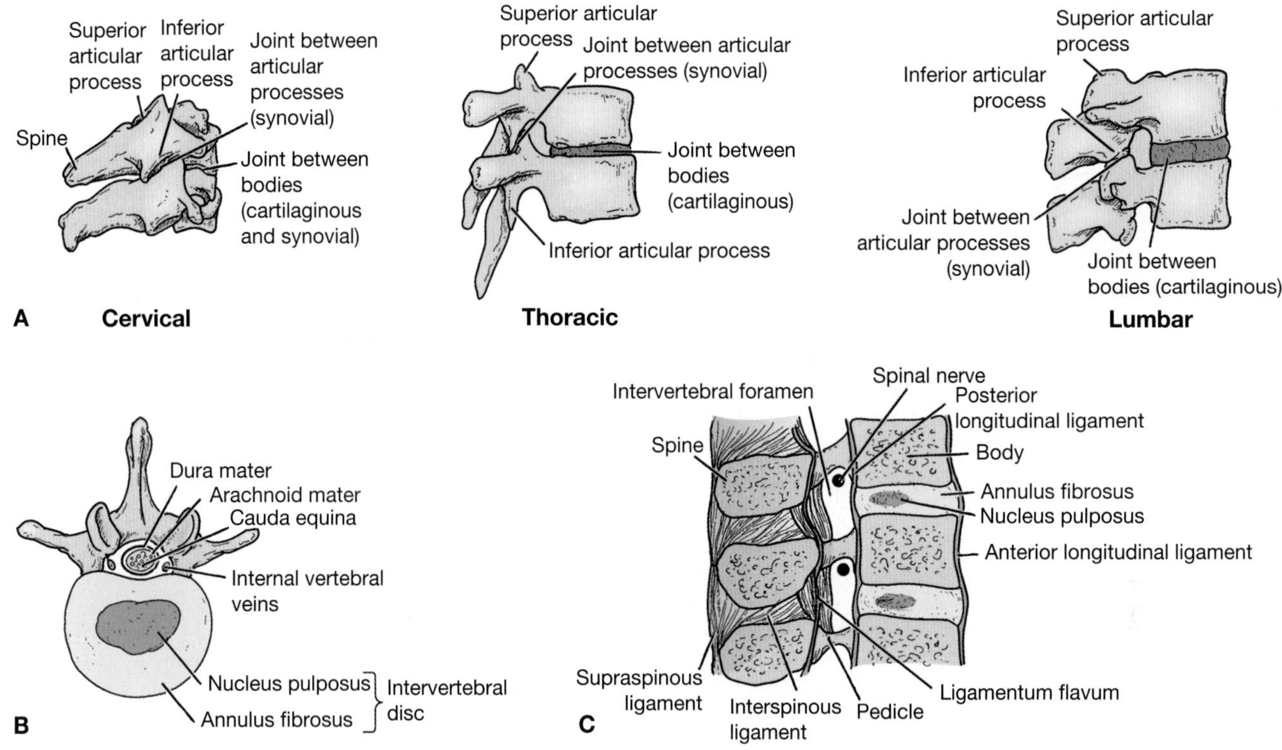

Figure 2.23 **A.** Joints in the cervical, thoracic, and lumbar regions of the vertebral column. **B.** L3 vertebra seen from above showing the relationship between the intervertebral disc and the cauda equina. **C.** Sagittal section through three lumbar vertebrae showing ligaments and intervertebral discs. Note the relationship between the emerging spinal nerve in an intervertebral foramen and the intervertebral disc.

Vertebral Column Joints

In general, the individual vertebrae from the levels C2 to L5 articulate with each other by means of cartilaginous joints between their bodies and by synovial joints between their articular processes (Fig. 2.23). The C1 vertebra (atlas) articulates with the base of the skull at the atlanto-occipital joints and with C2 (axis) at the atlantoaxial joints.

Atlanto-Occipital Joints

The **atlanto-occipital joints** are paired synovial joints formed between the occipital condyles, which are found on either side of the foramen magnum superiorly, and the facets on the superior surfaces of the lateral masses of the atlas inferiorly (Fig. 2.24A, B). A capsule encloses them.

Ligaments

- **Anterior atlanto-occipital membrane:** This is a continuation of the **anterior longitudinal ligament** that runs as a band down the anterior surface of the vertebral column. The membrane connects the anterior arch of the atlas to the anterior margin of the foramen magnum.
- **Posterior atlanto-occipital membrane:** This membrane is similar to the **ligamentum flavum** and connects the posterior arch of the atlas to the posterior margin of the foramen magnum.

Atlantoaxial Joints

The **atlantoaxial joints** are three synovial joints, one between the odontoid process (dens) and the anterior arch of the atlas, and the other two between the lateral masses of the bones (see Fig. 2.24C, D). Capsules enclose the joints.

Ligaments

- **Apical ligament:** This median-placed structure connects the apex of the odontoid process to the anterior margin of the foramen magnum.
- **Alar ligaments:** These two structures lie on each side of the apical ligament and connect the odontoid process to the medial sides of the occipital condyles.
- **Cruciate ligament:** This ligament consists of a **transverse part** and a **vertical part**. The transverse part (also termed the **transverse ligament of the atlas**) is attached on each side to the inner aspect of the lateral mass of the atlas and binds the odontoid process to the anterior arch of the atlas. The vertical part runs from the posterior surface of the body of the axis to the anterior margin of the foramen magnum.
- **Membrana tectoria:** This is an upward continuation of the posterior longitudinal ligament. It is attached above to the occipital bone just within the foramen magnum. It covers the posterior surface of the odontoid process and the apical, alar, and cruciate ligaments.

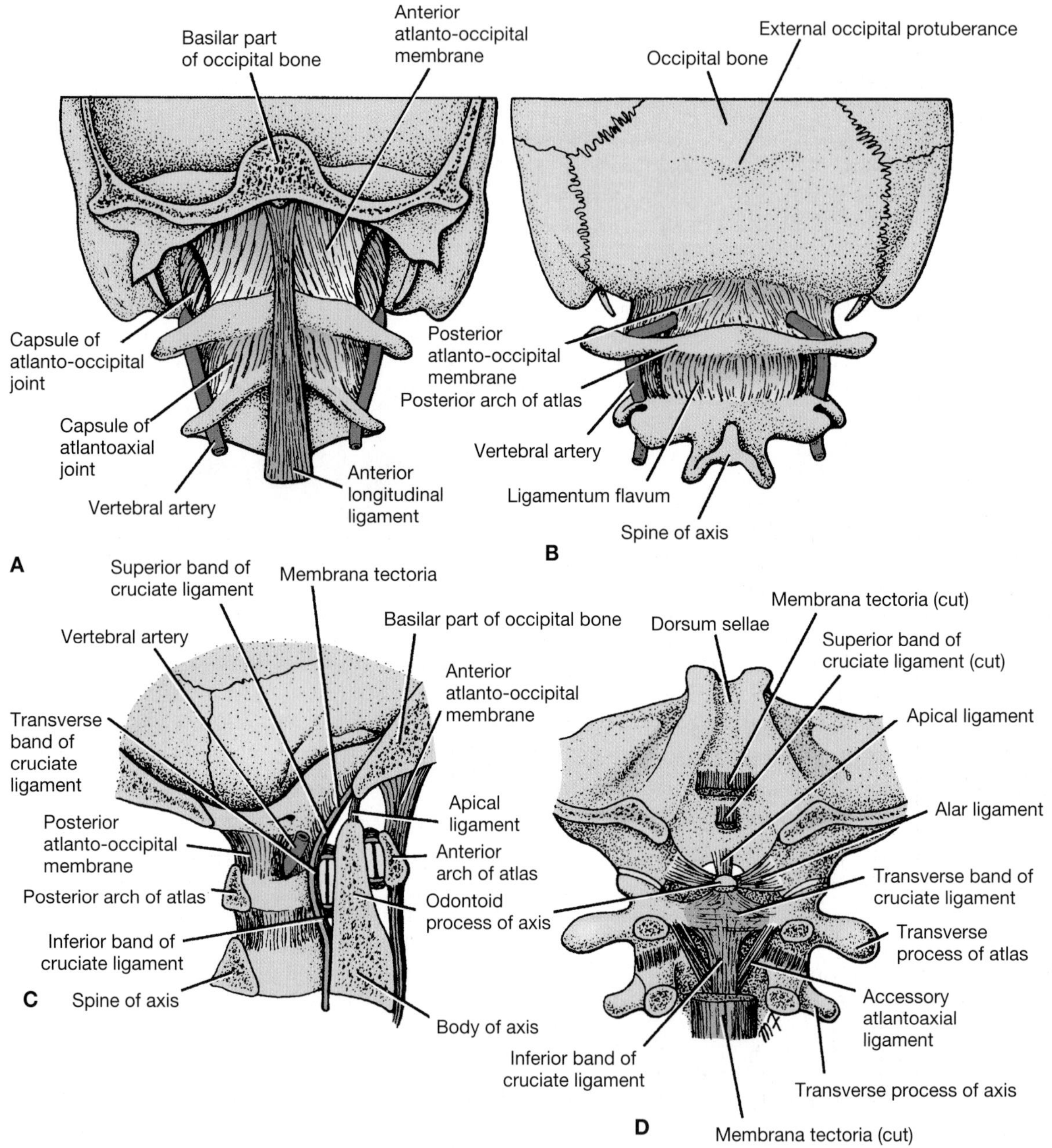

Figure 2.24 Anterior view **(A)** and posterior view **(B)** of the atlanto-occipital joints. Sagittal section **(C)** and posterior view **(D)** of the atlantoaxial joints. Note that the posterior arch of the atlas and the laminae and spine of the axis have been removed.

Joints between Vertebral Bodies

Thin plates of hyaline cartilage cover the superior and inferior surfaces of the bodies of adjacent vertebrae. Sandwiched between the plates of hyaline cartilage is an intervertebral disc composed mainly of fibrocartilage (see Fig. 2.23). The collagen fibers of the disc strongly unite the bodies of the two vertebrae. In the lower cervical region, small synovial joints (**uncovertebral joints**) may be present at the lateral sides of the intervertebral disc between the upper and lower margins of the bodies of the vertebrae.

Intervertebral Discs

Intervertebral discs are present from C2 to the sacrum and are the main structures that bind together the vertebral bodies (see Fig. 2.23). Because C1 has no body, intervertebral discs do not occur between C1 and the base of the skull and between C1 and C2. The adult sacrum and the coccyx also lack intervertebral discs. The vertebra located immediately above the disc identifies each disc (eg, the L2 disc is located between the L2 and L3 vertebrae, immediately below

Table 2.3 Intervertebral Disc Components

	NUCLEUS PULPOSUS	ANULUS FIBROSUS
Development	Remnant of the notochord	Anulus plus the bony vertebrae derived from sclerotome
Composition	Mucopolysaccharide gel with high (>80%) water content and small amount of collagen and cartilage	~14 concentric layers (lamellae) of fibrocartilage
Morphology	Ovoid mass in an eccentric location Normally under pressure and situated slightly closer to the posterior margin of the disc	Layers arranged in perpendicular, alternating angulations to one another, in a roughly onionskin-like morphology Fibers more numerous and thicker anteriorly and laterally More peripheral fibers strongly attached to anterior and posterior longitudinal ligaments of vertebral column

the L2 vertebral body). The discs are responsible for about one quarter of the length of the vertebral column below the level of C2. They are thickest in the cervical and lumbar regions, where the movements of the vertebral column are greatest. They may be regarded as semielastic pads that lie between the rigid bodies of adjacent vertebrae. Their physical characteristics permit them to serve as shock absorbers when the load on the vertebral column is suddenly increased, as when a person is jumping from a height. Their elasticity allows the rigid vertebrae to move one on the other. Unfortunately, their resilience is gradually lost with advancing age. Each disc consists of a peripheral part, the **annulus fibrosus**, and a central part, the **nucleus pulposus** (Table 2.3; also see Fig. 2.23B, C).

Intervertebral Disc Function

The semifluid nature of the nucleus pulposus allows it to change shape and permits one vertebra to rock on another, such as in the flexion and extension of the vertebral column. A sudden increase in the compression load on the vertebral column causes the nucleus pulposus to flatten; however, the resilience of the surrounding annulus fibrosus accommodates the resulting outward bulging of the nucleus. Sometimes, the outward thrust of the nucleus is too great for the annulus fibrosus, and it ruptures, allowing the nucleus pulposus to herniate and protrude into the vertebral canal, where it may press on spinal nerve roots, a spinal nerve, or even the spinal cord (see Clinical Notes on herniated discs).

With advancing age, the water content of the nucleus pulposus diminishes and is replaced by fibrocartilage. The collagen fibers of the annulus degenerate, and, as a result, it cannot always contain the nucleus pulposus under stress. In older adults, the result of such normal disc degeneration is that the discs become thinner, less elastic, and stiffer, and distinguishing the nucleus from the annulus is no longer possible. The shorter height of the discs leads to shortening of the vertebral column and decreased body height. Thus, we do shrink with age.

Ligaments

The **anterior** and **posterior longitudinal ligaments** run as continuous bands down the anterior and posterior surfaces of the vertebral column from the skull to the sacrum (see Fig. 2.23C). The anterior ligament is wide and strongly attached to the front and sides of the vertebral bodies and to the intervertebral discs. The posterior ligament is weaker and narrower and is attached to the posterior borders of the discs. These ligaments hold the vertebrae firmly together but also permit a small amount of movement to take place between them.

Joints between Vertebral Arches

The joints between the vertebral arches (**zygapophyseal joints**) consist of synovial joints between the superior and inferior articular processes of adjacent vertebrae (see Fig. 2.23A). The articular facets are covered with hyaline cartilage, and a capsular ligament surrounds the joints.

Ligaments

- **Supraspinous ligament** (see Fig. 2.23C): This runs between the tips of adjacent spines.
- **Interspinous ligament** (see Fig. 2.23C): This connects adjacent spines.
- **Intertransverse ligaments:** These run between adjacent transverse processes.
- **Ligamentum flavum** (see Fig. 2.23C): This connects the laminae of adjacent vertebrae.

In the cervical region, the supraspinous and interspinous ligaments are greatly thickened to form the strong **ligamentum nuchae**. The latter extends from the spine of C7 to the external occipital protuberance of the skull, with its anterior border being strongly attached to the cervical spines in between.

Vertebral Joint Nerve Supply

Small meningeal branches of each spinal nerve innervate the joints between the vertebral bodies (Fig. 2.25). The meningeal nerve arises from the spinal nerve as it exits from the intervertebral foramen. It then reenters the vertebral canal through the intervertebral foramen

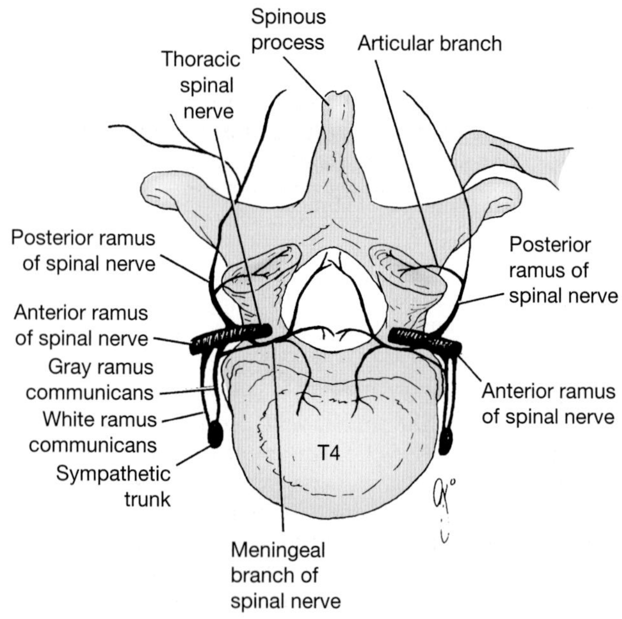

Figure 2.25 The innervation of vertebral joints. At any particular vertebral level, the joints receive nerve fibers from two adjacent spinal nerves.

and supplies the meninges, ligaments, and intervertebral discs. Branches from the posterior rami of the spinal nerves innervate the joints between the articular processes. Note that nerve fibers from two adjacent spinal nerves supply the joints at any particular level.

Vertebral Column Movement

As described earlier, the vertebral column consists of a series of separate vertebrae accurately positioned one on the other and separated by intervertebral discs. The vertebrae are held in position by strong ligaments that severely limit the degree of movement possible between adjacent vertebrae (Table 2.4). Nevertheless, the small degrees of movement allowed between individual vertebrae summate to large degrees of movement along the length of the vertebral column as a whole, resulting in a remarkable degree of mobility.

Table 2.4 Vertebral Column Major Ligaments

LIGAMENT	LOCATION	MOVEMENT RESISTED
Anterior longitudinal	Anterior sides of vertebral bodies and intervertebral discs	Extension
Posterior longitudinal	Posterior sides of vertebral bodies and intervertebral discs	Flexion
Ligamenta flava	Anterior sides of adjacent laminae	Flexion
Intertransverse	Between adjacent transverse processes	Contralateral abduction (lateral flexion)
Interspinous	Between adjacent spinous processes	Flexion
Supraspinous	Between tips of adjacent spinous processes	Flexion
Ligamentum nuchae	Cervical thickening of the interspinous and supraspinous ligaments	Flexion

The following movements are possible: flexion, extension, abduction (lateral flexion), rotation, and circumduction (Table 2.5). To best understand the mechanics of these movements, recognize that the longitudinal axis of movement of the vertebral column runs through the centers of the bodies of the vertebrae, not through the vertebral canal.

- **Flexion** is anterior bending of the vertebral column. Extension is posterior bending.

Table 2.5 Regional Intervertebral Movements

	CERVICAL	THORACIC	LUMBAR
Flexion/extension	Extensive ~50% of the cervical range of motion occurs at the atlanto-occipital joints	Limited	Extensive
Abduction (lateral flexion)	Extensive	Limited	Extensive
Rotation	Extensive ~50% of the cervical range of rotation occurs at the atlantoaxial joints No rotation occurs at the atlanto-occipital joints	Possible but very limited	Almost none Great mobility of the lumbar region mainly results from circumduction and pelvic tilting
Circumduction	Extensive	Limited	Extensive

- **Abduction** (lateral flexion) is the lateral bending of the body to one or the other side. Abduction is the proper anatomic descriptor for this movement (see Chapter 1). Unfortunately, lateral flexion has become fixated in clinical usage.
- **Rotation** is a twisting about the long axis of the vertebral column. Remember, the axis of rotation runs through the centers of the bodies of the vertebrae.
- **Circumduction** is a combination of all these movements.

The type and range of movements possible in each region of the column largely depend on the thickness of the intervertebral discs and the shape and direction of the articular processes. In the thoracic region, the ribs, costal cartilages, and sternum severely restrict range of movement (ROM). The atlanto-occipital joints permit extensive flexion and extension of the head. These joints permit most of the ROM associated with nodding the head up and down, as in saying, "yes." The atlanto-axial joints allow a wide range of rotation of the atlas and thus of the head on the axis. These joints permit most of the ROM associated with rotating the head side to side, as in saying, "no."

Numerous muscles move the vertebral column. Many are attached directly to the vertebrae, whereas others, such as the sternocleidomastoid and the abdominal wall muscles, are attached to the skull or to the ribs or fasciae.

In the cervical region, the longus cervicis, scalenus anterior, and sternocleidomastoid (SCM) muscles produce flexion, whereas the postvertebral muscles produce extension (see Back Muscles, later in this chapter). The scalenus anterior muscle and scalenus medius and the trapezius and SCM muscles produce abduction (lateral flexion). The SCM on one side and the contralateral splenius act together to produce rotation.

In the thoracic region, the unilateral semispinalis and rotatores muscles, assisted by the oblique muscles of the anterolateral abdominal wall, produce rotation.

In the lumbar region, the rectus abdominis and psoas muscles produce flexion, whereas the postvertebral muscles produce extension. The postvertebral muscles, quadratus lumborum, and the oblique muscles of the anterolateral abdominal wall produce abduction (lateral flexion). The psoas may also play a part in this movement. The rotatores muscles and the oblique muscles of the anterolateral abdominal wall produce rotation.

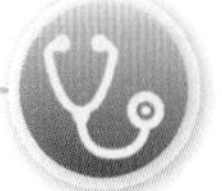

Clinical Notes

Vertebral Column Dislocation

Dislocations without fracture occur only in the cervical region because the obliquely oriented articular processes of the cervical vertebrae are not interlocked with one another and permit significant intervertebral movement (see Tables 2.1 and 2.5). In the thoracic and lumbar regions, dislocations can occur only if the vertically aligned and interlocking articular processes are fractured.

Dislocations commonly occur between C4 and C5 or C5 and C6 vertebrae, where mobility is greatest (Fig. 2.26). In unilateral dislocations, the inferior articular process on one side of one vertebra is forced forward over the anterior margin of the superior articular process of the vertebra below. Because the articular processes normally overlap, they become locked in the dislocated position. The spinal nerve on the same side is usually impinged in the intervertebral foramen, producing severe pain. Fortunately, the large size of the vertebral canal allows the spinal cord to escape damage in most cases.

Bilateral cervical dislocations are almost always associated with severe injury to the spinal cord. Death occurs immediately if the upper cervical vertebrae are involved because the respiratory muscles, including the diaphragm (phrenic nerves, C3 to C5), are paralyzed.

Vertebral Column Fracture

Anterior compression fractures of the vertebral bodies are usually caused by an excessive flexion-compression type of injury and take place at the sites of maximum mobility or at the junction of the mobile and fixed regions of the column. Interestingly, the body of a vertebra in such a fracture is crushed, whereas the strong posterior longitudinal ligament (which resists flexion) remains intact. The vertebral arches remain unbroken, and the intervertebral ligaments remain intact so that vertebral displacement and spinal cord injury do not occur. When injury causes excessive abduction (lateral flexion) in addition to excessive flexion, the lateral part of the body is also crushed.

Fracture-Dislocations

Fracture-dislocations are usually caused by a combination of a flexion and rotation type of injury, with the upper vertebra excessively flexed and twisted on the lower vertebra. Here again, the site is usually where maximum mobility occurs, as in the lumbar region, or at the junction of the mobile and fixed region of the column, as in the lower lumbar vertebrae. Because the articular processes are fractured and the ligaments are torn, the vertebrae involved are unstable, and the spinal cord is usually severely damaged or severed, with accompanying paraplegia.

Vertical Compression Fractures

Vertical compression fractures occur in the cervical and lumbar regions, where it is possible to fully straighten the vertebral column (see Fig. 2.26D). In the cervical region, with the neck straight, excessive vertical force applied from above will cause the ring of the atlas to be disrupted and the lateral masses to be displaced laterally (**Jefferson's fracture**). If the neck is slightly flexed, the lower cervical vertebrae remain in a straight line, and the compression

(continued)

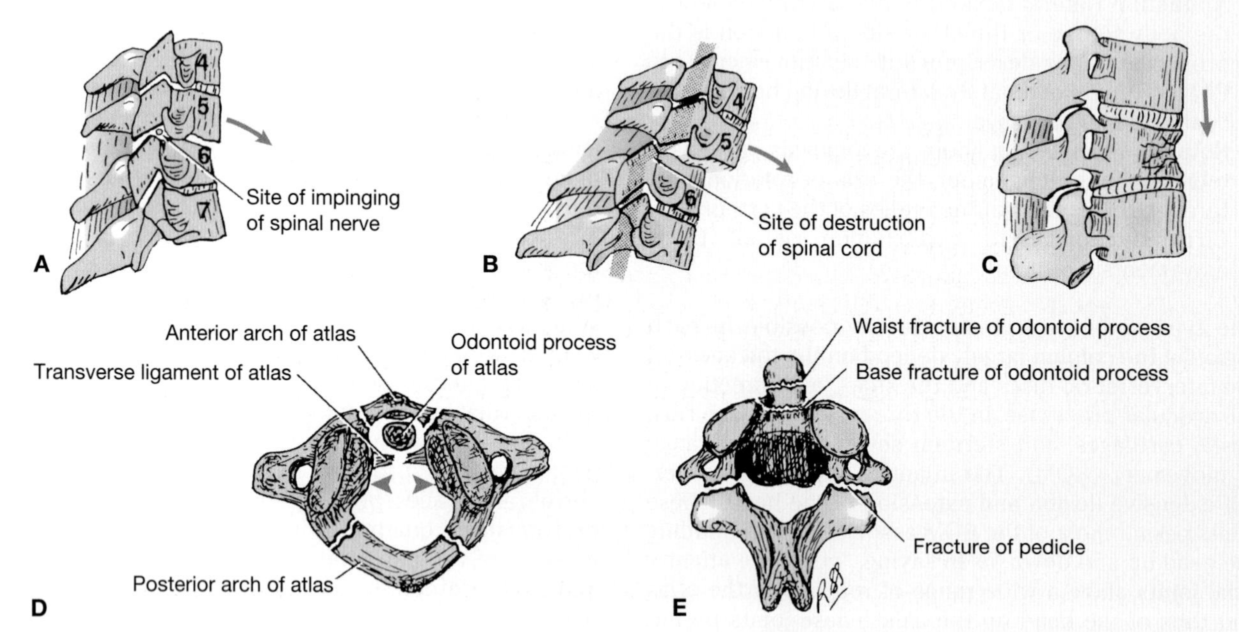

Figure 2.26 Dislocations and fractures of the vertebral column. **A.** Unilateral dislocation of the C5 or C6 cervical vertebra. Note the anterior displacement of the inferior articular process over the superior articular process of the vertebra below. **B.** Bilateral dislocation of the C5 or C6 cervical vertebra. Note that 50% of the vertebral body width has moved forward on the vertebra below. **C.** Flexion compression-type fracture of the vertebral body in the lumbar region. **D.** Jefferson-type fracture of the atlas. **E.** Fractures of the odontoid process and the pedicles (hangman's fracture) of the axis.

load is transmitted to the lower vertebrae, causing disruption of the intervertebral disc and breakup of the vertebral body. Pieces of the vertebral body are commonly forced back into the spinal cord. In the straightened lumbar region, excessive force from below can cause the vertebral body to break up, with protrusion of fragments posteriorly into the vertebral canal.

Nontraumatic compression fractures may occur as a result of severe disease states such as osteoporosis or tuberculosis (tuberculous spondylitis). In such cases, the diseased vertebral body may break down and collapse under the weight of the upper body.

Odontoid Process of Axis Fracture

Fractures of the odontoid process are relatively common and result from falls or blows on the head (see Fig. 2.26E). Excessive mobility of the odontoid fragment or rupture of the transverse ligament can result in compression injury to the spinal cord.

Pedicle of Axis Fracture (Hangman's Fracture)

Severe extension injury of the neck, such as might occur in an automobile accident or a fall, is the usual cause of hangman's fracture. Sudden overextension of the neck, as produced by the knot of a hangman's rope beneath the chin, is the reason for the common name. Because the vertebral canal is enlarged by the forward displacement of the vertebral body of the axis, the spinal cord is rarely compressed (see Fig. 2.26E).

Spondylolisthesis

In spondylolisthesis, the body of a lower lumbar vertebra (usually L5) slips forward on the body of the vertebra below (or upon the sacrum) and carries with it the whole of the upper portion of the vertebral column.

Congenital Spondylolisthesis

In this condition, the essential defect is in the pedicles of the migrating vertebra. Most believe that the pedicles are abnormally formed, and accessory centers of ossification are present and fail to unite. The spine, laminae, and inferior articular processes remain in position, whereas the remainder of the vertebra, having lost the restraining influence of the inferior articular processes, slips forward. Because the laminae are left behind, the vertebral canal is not narrowed, but the nerve roots may be pressed on, causing low backache and sciatica. In severe cases, the trunk becomes shortened, and the lower ribs contact the iliac crest.

Degenerative Spondylolisthesis

This condition is common in older adults and involves degeneration of the intervertebral discs in the lumbar region and osteoarthritis of the intervertebral joints. Anterior slippage of the L5 vertebra often occurs, and the lumbar nerves roots may be pressed on, causing low back pain and pain down the leg in the distribution of the involved nerve.

BACK MUSCLES

The muscles of the back may be divided into three groups:

- The **superficial group** (trapezius, latissimus dorsi, levator scapulae, rhomboid major, rhomboid minor): These muscles connect the shoulder girdle with the vertebral column (Fig. 2.27). Developmentally and functionally, these are upper limb muscles, and as such are described in Chapter 3.
- The **intermediate group** (serratus posterior superior, serratus posterior inferior): These two small muscles are involved with movements of the thoracic cage (Fig. 2.28). They are described in Chapter 4.
- The **deep group**: This is a complex of large and small muscles concerned with movement of the vertebral column, ribs, and skull.

Deep Muscles (Postvertebral Muscles)

In the standing position, the line of gravity (Fig. 2.29) passes through the odontoid process of the axis, posterior to the centers of the hip joints, and anterior to the knee and ankle joints. Thus, when the body is in this position, the greater part of its weight falls in front of the vertebral column. Not surprisingly, therefore, the postvertebral muscles of the back are well developed in humans. The postural tone of these muscles is the major factor responsible for the maintenance of the normal curves of the vertebral column.

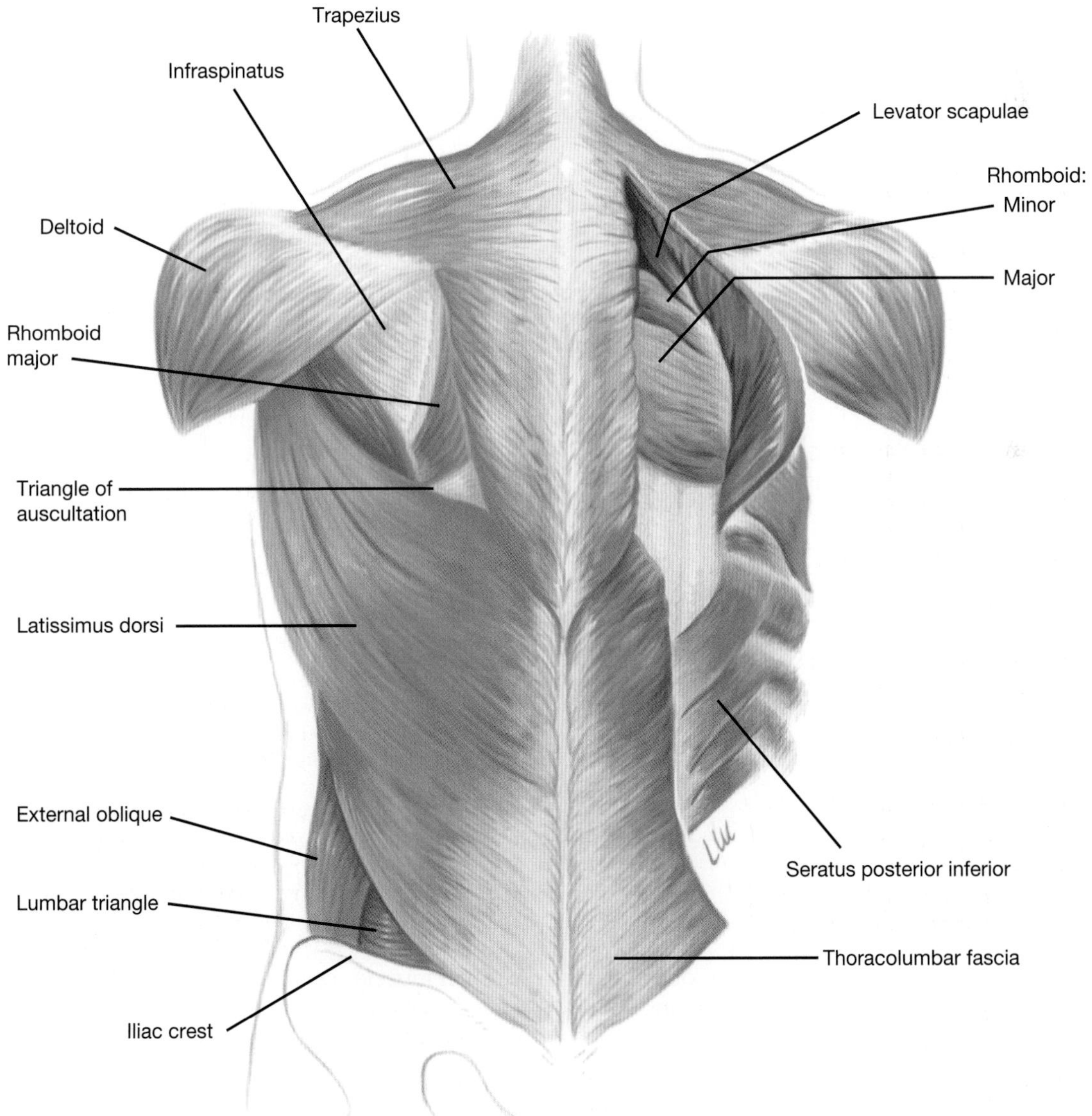

Figure 2.27 Superficial group of back muscles. The left side of the diagram shows the most superficial muscles: trapezius and latissimus dorsi. On the right side, the trapezius is reflected and the latissimus is removed to show the rhomboids and levator scapulae. Also note the triangle of auscultation and the lumbar triangle on the left side.

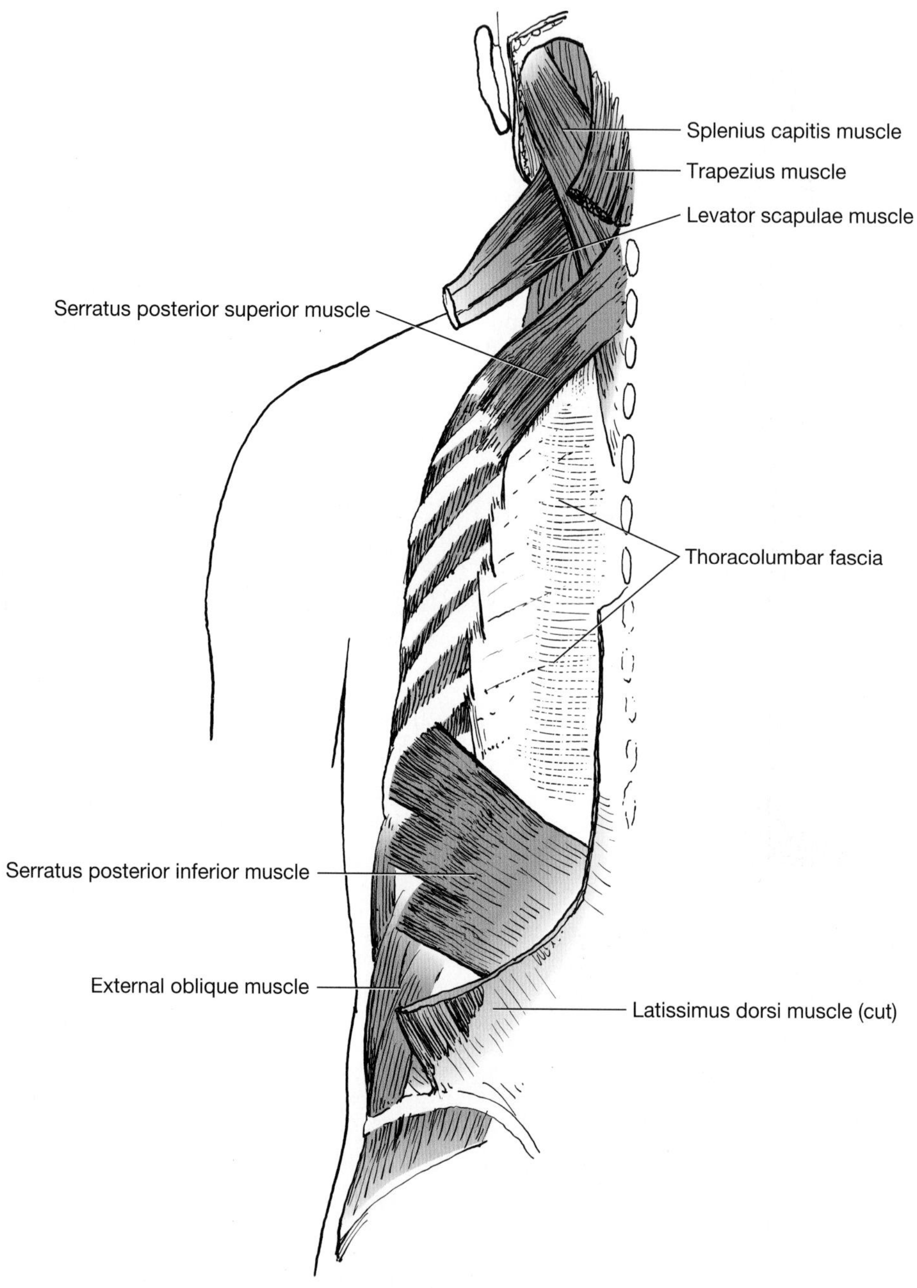

Figure 2.28 Intermediate group of back muscles. The superficial group muscles are removed for the clarity of the serratus posterior muscles.

In the lumbar region, the deep muscles of the back form a thick, heavy column, the **erector spinae**, which occupies the hollow on each side of the spinous processes of the vertebral column (Table 2.6; Fig. 2.30). As it ascends the back, the erector spinae divides into three main parts: iliocostalis, longissimus, and spinalis. Higher and deeper in the back, the deep muscles are a complex mass composed of many individual muscles of varying length that extend from the sacrum to the skull. Collectively, the deep group muscles may be organized as shown in Table 2.6.

Each muscle resembles a string, which, when pulled on, causes one or several vertebrae to move. Because the attachments of the muscles overlap, entire regions of the vertebral column can move smoothly. The spines and transverse processes of the vertebrae serve as levers that facilitate the muscle actions. The longest muscles lie superficially and run vertically from the sacrum to the rib angles, transverse processes, and upper vertebral spines. The intermediate length muscles run obliquely between the transverse processes and the spines. The shortest and deepest muscle fibers

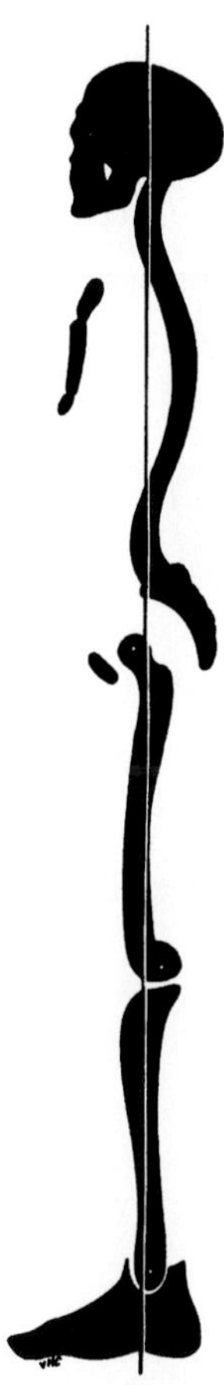

Figure 2.29 Lateral view of the skeleton showing the line of gravity. Because the greater part of the body weight lies anterior to the vertebral column, the deep back muscles are important in maintaining the normal postural curves of the vertebral column in the standing position.

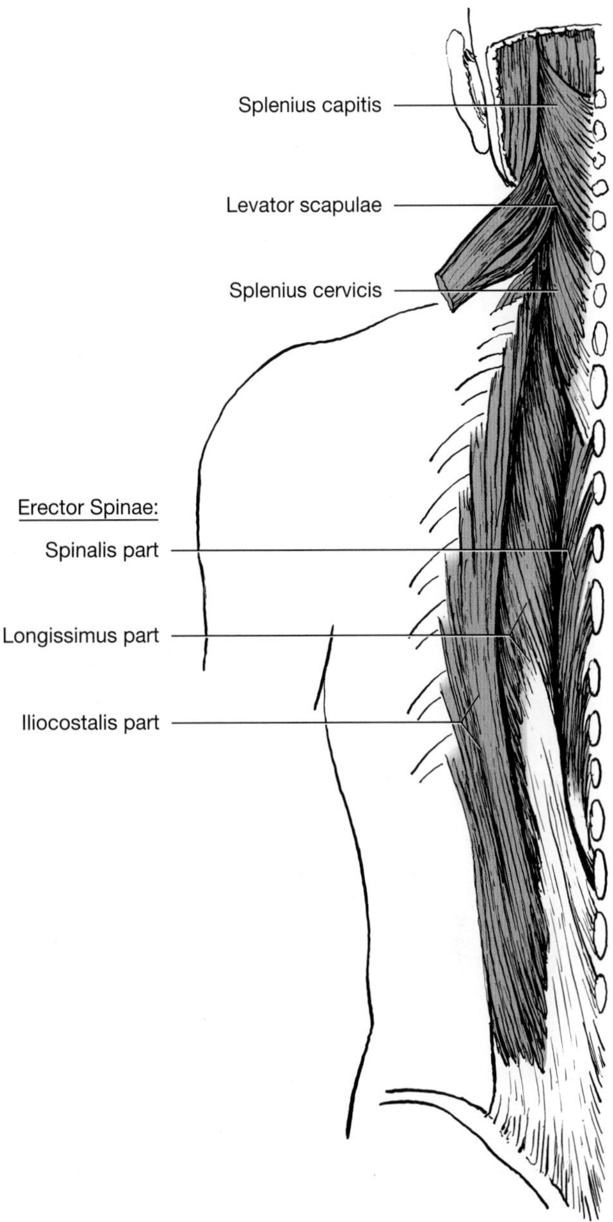

Figure 2.30 Some of the deep group of back muscles: splenius capitis, splenius cervicis, and erector spinae. Note the erector spinae divides into three main parts: iliocostalis, longissimus, and spinalis.

Table 2.6 Deep Group Back Muscles

SUPERFICIAL VERTICALLY RUNNING MUSCLES	INTERMEDIATE OBLIQUE RUNNING MUSCLES	DEEPEST MUSCLES
Iliocostalis Longissimus Spinalis	Splenius capitis and cervicis Transversospinalis group • Semispinalis • Multifidus • Rotatores	Interspinales Intertransversarii Levatores costarum Suboccipital muscles • Obliquus capitis superior • Obliquus capitis inferior • Rectus capitis posterior major • Rectus capitis posterior minor

run between the spines and transverse processes of adjacent vertebrae.

The deep muscles of the back generally act to produce varying degrees of extension of the vertebral column and skull. In addition, especially when acting unilaterally, they can produce varying degrees of abduction and/or rotation of the vertebrae and skull. Understanding the actions and innervation of the deep muscles is valuable in the biomedical professions. However, in-depth knowledge of the attachments of these muscles is more or less useful depending on the specific professional field. Therefore, the details of muscle attachments are omitted in this text.

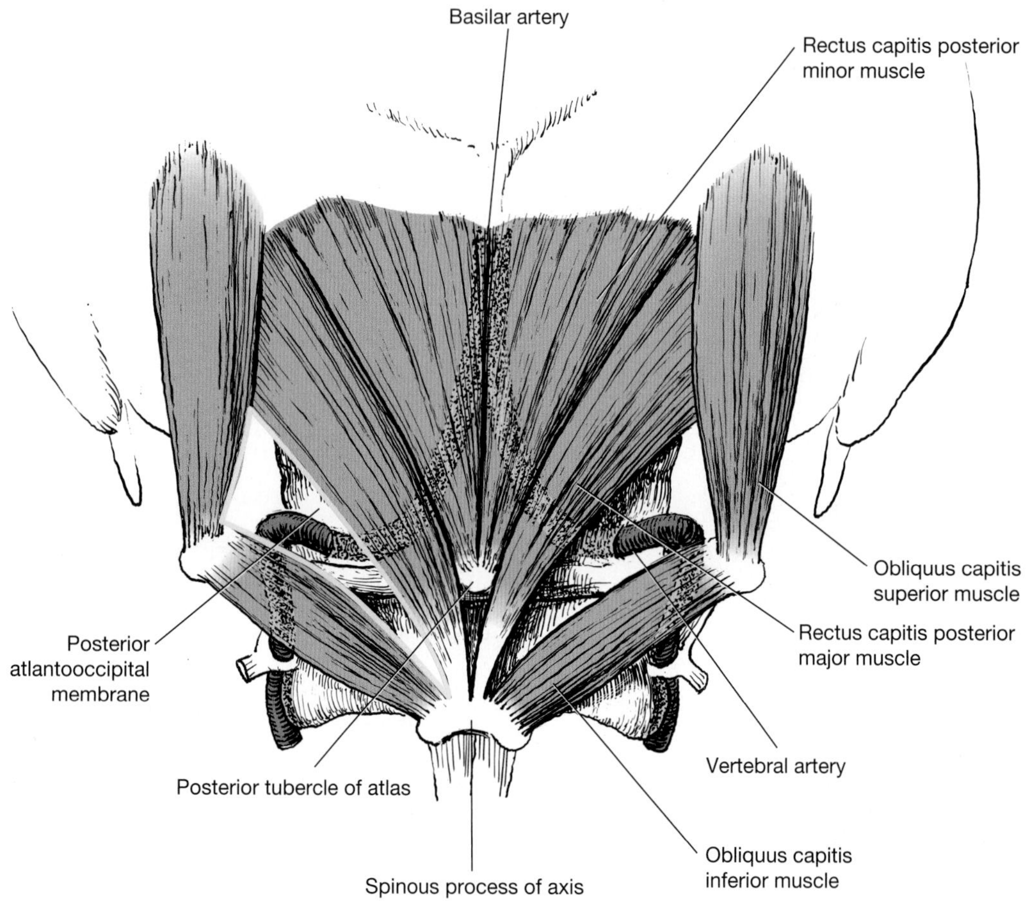

Figure 2.31 Suboccipital muscles and suboccipital triangle. The triangle is outlined in *yellow*.

Back Muscle Nerve Supply

All the muscles constituting the superficial and intermediate groups of muscles of the back, except one, are innervated by anterior rami of spinal nerves. The exception is the trapezius, which is supplied by the spinal accessory nerve (CN XI). All the deep group muscles of the back are innervated by posterior rami of spinal nerves.

Muscular Triangles

The margins of certain intersecting muscles and bones form three distinctive triangular spaces in the back.

Triangle of Auscultation

The auscultatory triangle is the site on the back where breath sounds may be most easily heard with a stethoscope because the space of the triangle has no covering muscles. The boundaries are the latissimus dorsi, trapezius, and rhomboid major (see Fig. 2.27).

Lumbar Triangle

The lumbar triangle is a site where pus or a lumbar hernia may emerge from the abdominal wall. The boundaries are the latissimus dorsi, posterior border of the external oblique muscle of the abdomen, and the iliac crest (see Fig. 2.27).

Suboccipital Triangle

The suboccipital triangle contains the suboccipital nerve (the posterior ramus of spinal nerve C1) and the vertebral artery. The boundaries are the rectus capitis posterior major, obliquus capitis inferior, and obliquus capitis superior (Fig. 2.31). Note that the rectus capitis posterior minor is included as one of the muscles in the suboccipital region but does not form a boundary of the suboccipital triangle. The four small suboccipital muscles produce significant motions at the atlanto-occipital and atlantoaxial joints.

DEEP FASCIA (THORACOLUMBAR FASCIA)

The lumbar part of the deep fascia is situated in the interval between the iliac crest and the 12th rib and is referred to as the **thoracolumbar fascia**. It forms a strong aponeurosis superficially with deeper running septa that enclose

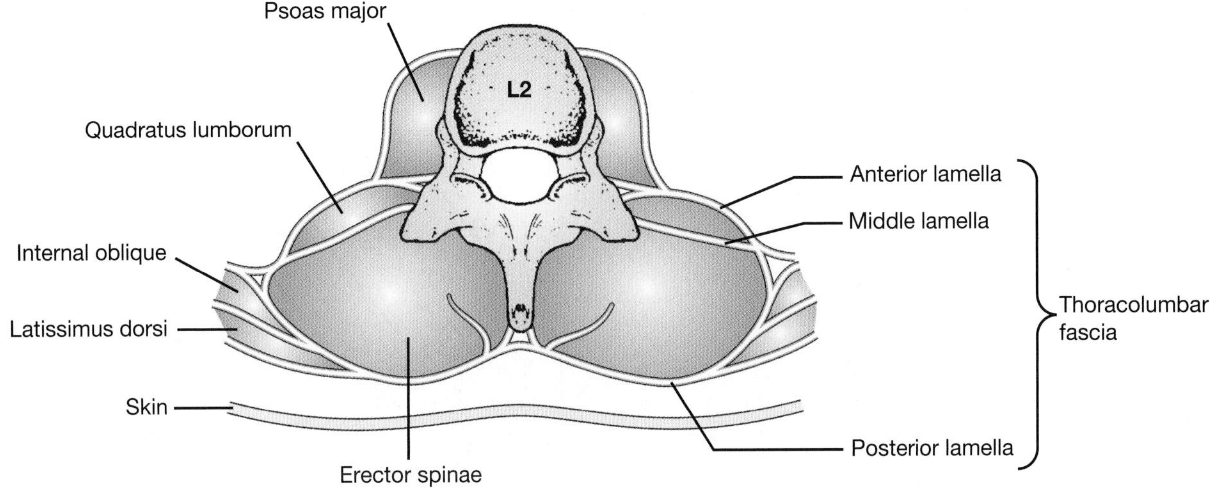

Figure 2.32 Schematic cross section of the lumbar region showing the organization of the thoracolumbar fascia. Note the three lamellae that enclose the erector spinae muscles and give origin to other muscles of the back and abdominal wall.

the main parts of the erector spinae muscles. Laterally, this fascia gives origin to the middle fibers of the transversus abdominis, upper fibers of the internal abdominal oblique, and the latissimus dorsi (Fig. 2.32).

The thoracolumbar fascia splits into three lamellae. The posterior lamella covers the deep muscles of the back and is attached to the lumbar spines. The middle lamella passes medially and attaches to the tips of the transverse processes of the lumbar vertebrae; it lies anterior to the deep muscles of the back and posterior to the quadratus lumborum. The anterior lamella passes medially and attaches to the anterior surface of the transverse processes of the lumbar vertebrae; it lies anterior to the quadratus lumborum muscle.

BACK BLOOD SUPPLY

The blood supply of the back is extensive and complex. Numerous branches connect the vertebral column and adnexa with vascular sources along the entire length of the back.

Arteries

The arterial supply to the back derives from multiple vessels along its length.

- In the **cervical region**, branches arise from the occipital artery (branch of the external carotid artery), from the vertebral artery (branch of the subclavian artery), and from the deep cervical artery (branch of the costocervical trunk).
- In the **thoracic region**, branches arise from the posterior intercostal arteries.
- In the **lumbar region**, branches arise from the subcostal and lumbar arteries.
- In the **sacral region**, branches arise from the iliolumbar and lateral sacral arteries, both of which are branches of the internal iliac artery.

Veins

The veins draining the back form plexuses extending along the vertebral column from the skull to the coccyx.

- The **external vertebral venous plexus** surrounds the external aspect of the vertebral column.
- The **internal vertebral venous plexus** lies within the vertebral canal but outside the dura mater of the spinal cord, in the extradural (epidural) space (Fig. 2.33).

The external and internal vertebral plexuses form a capacious network of thin-walled veins that have incompetent valves or are valveless. They communicate through the foramen magnum with the venous sinuses within the skull. Therefore, free venous blood flow may occur between the skull, neck, thorax, abdomen, pelvis, and the vertebral plexuses, with the direction of flow depending on the pressure differences that exist at any given time between the regions. This fact is of considerable clinical significance (see Clinical Notes, carcinoma of the prostate, below).

The internal vertebral plexus receives tributaries from the vertebrae by way of the **basivertebral veins** (see Fig. 2.33) and from the meninges and spinal cord. The internal plexus is drained by the **intervertebral veins**, which pass outward with the spinal nerves through the intervertebral foramina. Here, they are joined by tributaries from the external vertebral plexus and, in turn, drain into the vertebral, intercostal, lumbar, and lateral sacral veins.

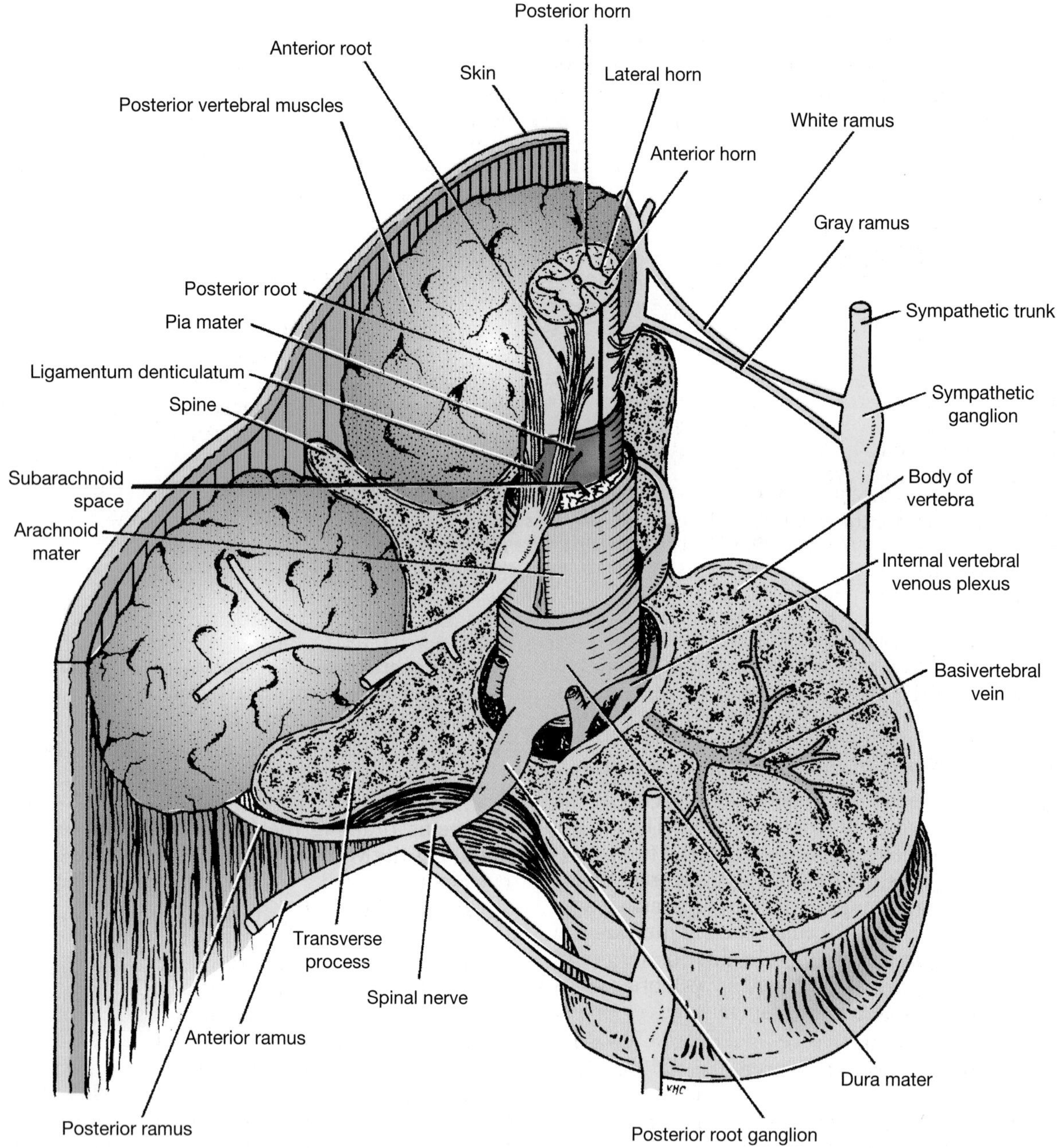

Figure 2.33 Oblique section through the L1 vertebra showing the spinal cord and its covering membranes. Note the relationship between the spinal nerve and the sympathetic trunk on each side. Note also the important internal vertebral venous plexus.

LYMPH DRAINAGE

The deep lymph vessels follow the veins and drain into the deep cervical, posterior mediastinal, lateral aortic, and sacral nodes. The lymph vessels from the skin of the neck drain into the cervical nodes, those from the trunk above the iliac crests drain into the axillary nodes, and those from below the level of the iliac crests drain into the superficial inguinal nodes (see Fig. 5.23).

SPINAL CORD

The spinal cord is the elongate, cylindrical part of the CNS below the head. It is completely enclosed within the vertebral canal of the vertebral column. At the gross anatomic level, the spinal cord begins above at the foramen magnum, where it is continuous with the medulla oblongata of the brain. In the adult, it terminates inferiorly at about the level of the L1 vertebra (see Fig. 2.14D). The spinal cord has a fusiform enlargement in the cervical region (**cervical enlargement**), where it gives origin to the brachial plexus, and another in the lower thoracic and lumbar region (**lumbar enlargement**), where it gives origin to the lumbosacral plexus.

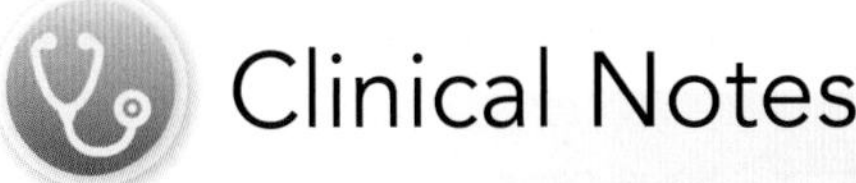

Vertebral Venous Plexus and Prostate Carcinoma

The longitudinal, thin-walled, valveless vertebral venous plexus is a clinically important structure because it communicates above with the intracranial venous sinuses and segmentally with the veins of the thorax, abdomen, and pelvis. Pelvic venous blood enters not only the inferior vena cava but also the vertebral venous plexus and, by this route, may also enter the skull. This is especially likely to occur if intra-abdominal pressure is increased. The internal vertebral venous plexus is not subject to external pressures when intra-abdominal pressure rises. A rise in pressure on the abdominal and pelvic veins tends to force the blood backward out of the abdominal and pelvic cavities into the veins within the vertebral canal. The morphology of this venous plexus explains how carcinoma of the prostate may metastasize to the vertebral column and the cranial cavity.

The external surface of the spinal cord is marked by several grooves of varying depths. The **anterior median fissure** is a deep cleft in the anterior midline. The **posterior median sulcus** is a comparatively shallow depression in the posterior midline. A bilateral pair of **posterolateral sulci** forms shallow grooves on the posterolateral aspects of the cord. Paired **anterolateral sulci** are shallow grooves on the anterior lateral sides of the cord.

The spinal cord ends inferiorly as a tapered cone termed the **conus medullaris**. A prolongation of the pia mater, the **filum terminale**, descends from the apex of the conus and attaches to the back of the coccyx (Fig. 2.34; also see Figs. 2.14D and 2.38).

Spinal Nerves

As described in Chapter 1, a total of 31 pairs of spinal nerves attach to the spinal cord (Figs. 2.33 through 2.38). They are named according to the region of the vertebral column and the specific vertebrae with which they are associated: 8 cervical, 12 thoracic, 5 lumbar, 5 sacral, and 1 coccygeal. Each spinal nerve originates with a paired series of **posterior and anterior rootlets**, which attach to the posterolateral and anterolateral sulci of the spinal cord, respectively, and extend the whole length of the corresponding segment of the cord (see Figs. 2.33 and 2.34). Each paired bundle of posterior and anterior rootlets joins together and forms a single **posterior and anterior root** within the vertebral canal. Each paired posterior and anterior root merges within an intervertebral foramen (IVF) and forms an individual **spinal nerve**. Each posterior root possesses a **posterior root ganglion**, which is located at the IVF. The spinal nerve passes through the IVF and immediately divides into a smaller **posterior ramus** and a larger **anterior ramus**. The posterior ramus divides into medial and lateral branches, which distribute to the back. The anterior ramus distributes initially to more lateral and anterior regions.

The posterior rami of all 31 pairs of spinal nerves supply the skin and muscles of the back in a segmental manner. However, the posterior rami of nerves C1, C6 to C8, and L4 to L5 supply the deep muscles of the back but do not supply the skin. The posterior ramus of the C2 nerve (**greater occipital nerve**) ascends over the back of the head and supplies the skin of the scalp.

Functionally, the posterior rootlets and roots carry sensory (afferent) impulses from the spinal nerves into the spinal cord, whereas the anterior rootlets and roots carry motor (efferent) impulses from the spinal cord to the spinal nerves. The spinal nerves and the posterior and anterior rami are mixed nerve components in that they convey both sensory and motor information to and from the periphery. Therefore, lesions of rootlets and roots versus spinal nerves and rami result in different combinations of sensory and motor deficits (eg, lesion of anterior roots affects only motor neuron fibers). However, lesion of anterior rami affects both motor and sensory fibers.

In adults, the spinal cord is significantly shorter than the vertebral column. Because of this disparity, the length of the spinal nerve roots increases progressively from above downward (Fig. 2.35; also see Figs. 2.34 and 2.38). In the upper cervical region, the spinal nerve roots are short and run almost horizontally to their respective IVFs. However, the roots of the lumbar, sacral, and coccygeal nerves inferior to the conus medullaris form a long, thick, vertical leash of nerves around the filum terminale in order to reach their distant IVFs. The collective bundle of the nerve roots below the conus plus the filum terminale is termed the **cauda equina** because of its resemblance to a horse's tail (see Figs. 2.34 and 2.38).

Note that because of the numerical mismatch from having eight cervical nerves but only seven cervical vertebrae, spinal nerve C1 passes through the space between the C1 vertebra and the base of the skull (ie, above the C1 vertebra). Likewise, spinal nerves C2 to C7 emerge through the IVF above the same-numbered vertebra (eg, nerve C5 passes through the IVF between vertebrae C4 and C5, above the C5 vertebra). However, this positional relationship changes at the C8 spinal nerve level, where nerve C8 must run through the IVF between vertebrae C7 and T1, below the C7 vertebra. Below the C8 spinal nerve, the number of spinal nerves matches the number of vertebrae, except for the single coccygeal nerve. Thus, all the thoracic, lumbar, and sacral spinal nerves emerge through the IVF below the same-numbered vertebra (eg, nerve L2 emerges from

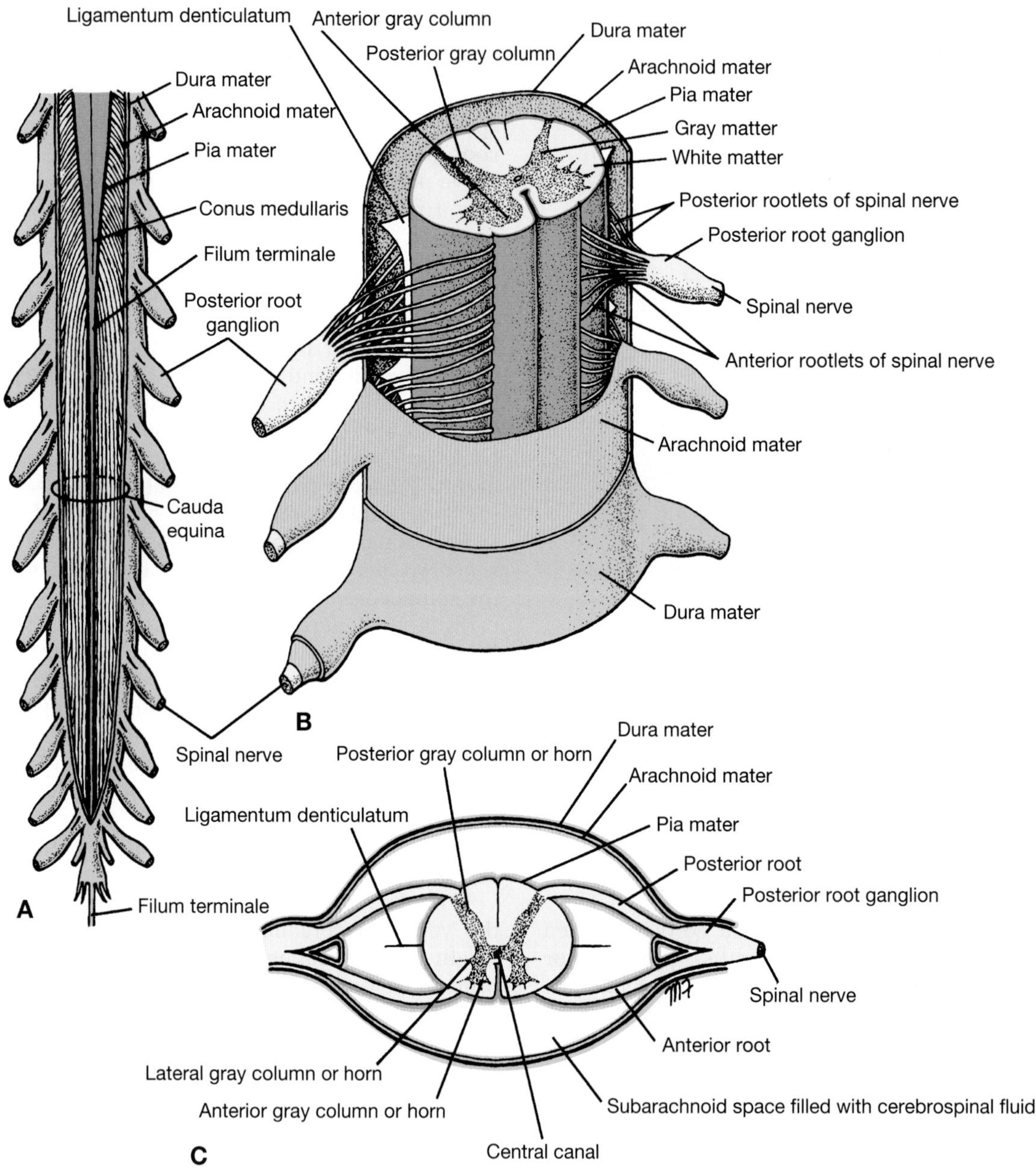

Figure 2.34 **A.** Lower end of the spinal cord and the cauda equina. **B.** Section through the thoracic part of the spinal cord showing the anterior and posterior roots of the spinal nerves and meninges. **C.** Transverse section through the spinal cord showing the meninges and the position of the cerebrospinal fluid.

the IVF between the L2 and L3 vertebrae, inferior to the L2 vertebra). These relations are important when considering the effect of a herniated intervertebral disc or narrowing of an IVF on specific spinal nerves (see Clinical Notes below).

Spinal Cord Blood Supply

The spinal cord receives its arterial supply from two primary sources: (1) **spinal arteries**, which originate from the vertebral arteries within the cranial cavity, and (2) **radicular (radiculomedullary) arteries**, which branch from segmental arteries alongside the vertebral column. Three small spinal arteries run longitudinally: two **posterior spinal arteries** and one **anterior spinal artery**. The posterior spinal arteries run inferiorly down the spinal cord, close to the attachments of the posterior spinal nerve rootlets. The anterior spinal artery runs down within the anterior median fissure. The posterior and anterior spinal arteries are reinforced by several radicular (radiculomedullary) arteries, which originate outside the vertebral column and along the entire length of the trunk. The radicular arteries enter the vertebral canal through the intervertebral foramina.

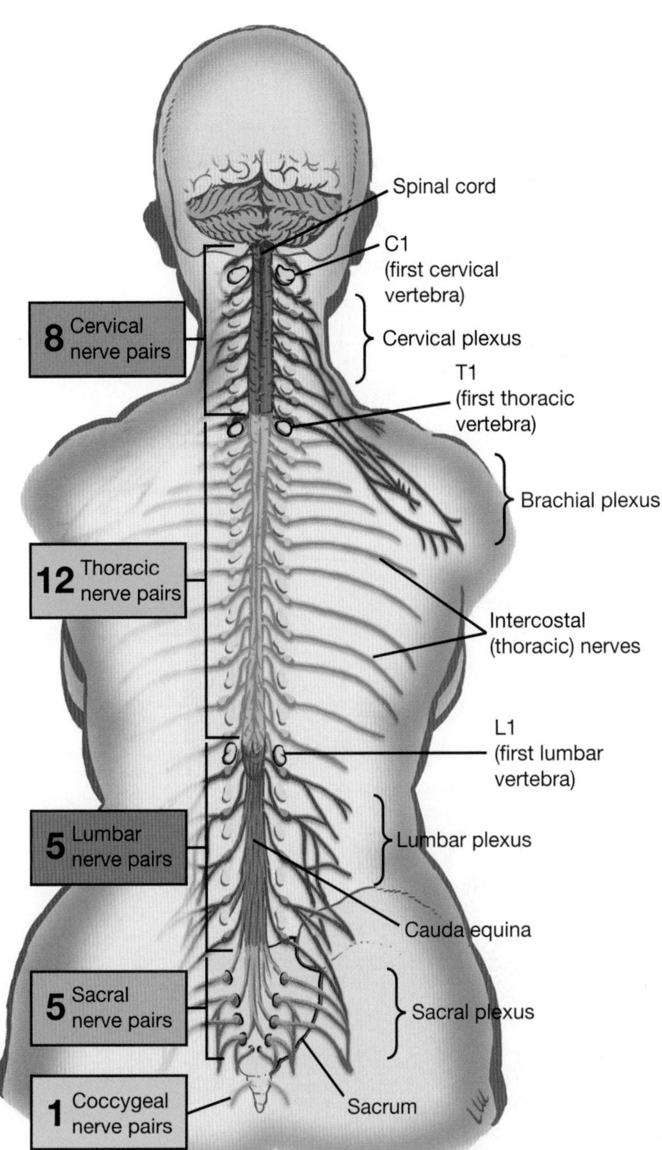

Figure 2.35 Posterior view of the spinal cord showing the origins of the roots of the spinal nerves and their relationship with the different vertebrae. The laminae have been removed to expose the spinal cord and the nerve roots.

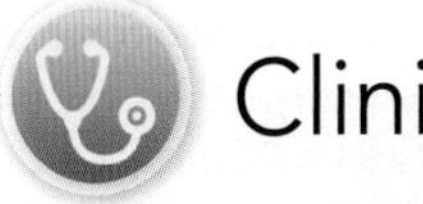

Clinical Notes

Spinal Cord Ischemia

The blood supply to the spinal cord is surprisingly meager, considering the importance of this organ. The anterior and posterior spinal arteries are of small and variable diameter, and the reinforcing segmental radicular arteries vary in number and in size. Ischemia of the spinal cord can easily follow minor damage to the arterial supply as a result of regional anesthesia, pain block procedures, or aortic surgery.

The venous system of the spinal cord is composed of a complex network of veins that all drain into the internal vertebral venous plexus.

Spinal Cord Meninges

The entire CNS (brain plus spinal cord) is surrounded by three meninges: the **dura mater**, **arachnoid mater**, and **pia mater** (see Figs. 2.33, 2.34, 2.37, and 2.38).

Dura Mater

The dura mater is the most external membrane. It is a dense, strong, fibrous sheet that encloses the spinal cord and cauda equina in a loose, sleeve-like fashion. Superiorly, it is continuous through the foramen magnum with the meningeal layer of dura covering the brain. Inferiorly, it ends on the filum terminale at the level of the S2 vertebra (see Fig. 2.14D). Laterally, the dura extends along each nerve root and becomes continuous with the connective tissue surrounding each spinal nerve (epineurium) at the intervertebral foramen. The dural sheath lies in the vertebral canal and upper sacral canal and is separated from the walls of the canal

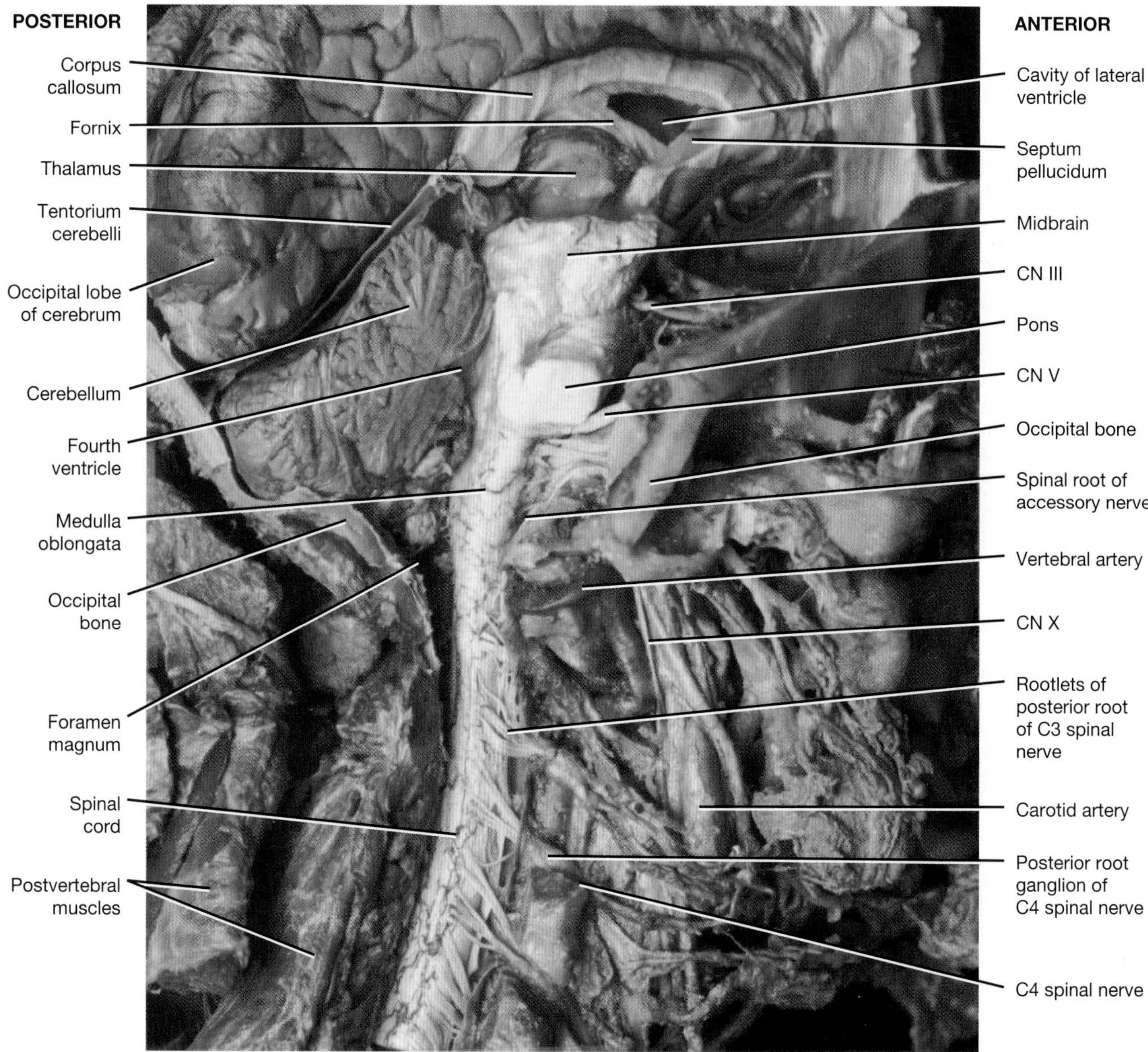

Figure 2.36 Dissection of the skull and the upper part of the cervical vertebral column showing the brain in the sagittal section and the intact spinal cord in situ. Note the continuity of the medulla oblongata and the spinal cord at the foramen magnum. Note also the roots of the cervical spinal nerves and the trunks of the spinal nerves as they emerge through the dissected intervertebral foramina. CN, cranial nerve.

by the **extradural (epidural) space**. This space contains loose connective tissue; extradural fat; the internal vertebral venous plexus; and small arteries, nerves, and lymphatics.

Arachnoid Mater

The arachnoid mater is the middle membrane layer. It is a delicate, impermeable sheet that intimately lines the deep aspect of the dura throughout its extent (see Figs. 2.33 and 2.34). Superiorly, the arachnoid is continuous through the foramen magnum with the arachnoid covering the brain. Inferiorly, it ends on the filum terminale at the level of the S2 vertebra (see Figs. 2.14D and 2.38). Laterally, the arachnoid continues along the spinal nerve roots and ends by merging with the perineurium of the spinal nerves at the intervertebral foramina.

The dura and arachnoid are a continuous series of cell layers that form a common **dura–arachnoid sac**. Current evidence indicates that a natural subdural space at the junction between the dural and arachnoid cell zones does not occur.

The arachnoid is separated from the underlying pia mater by a wide space, the **subarachnoid space**, which is filled with cerebrospinal fluid (CSF) (see Figs. 2.33 and 2.34). Small strands of tissue, the **subarachnoid**

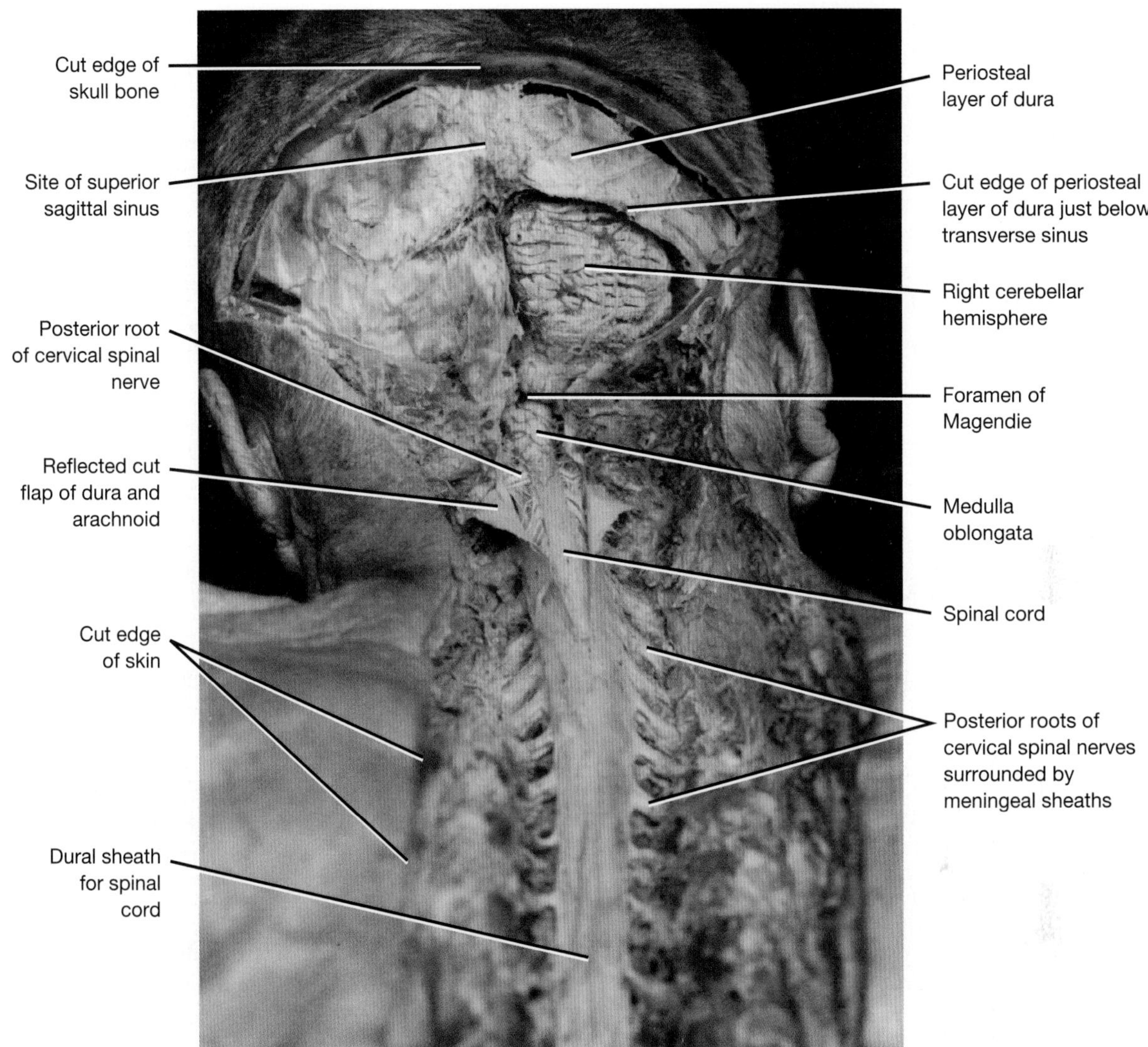

Figure 2.37 Dissection of the back of the head and the neck. The greater part of the occipital bone has been removed exposing the periosteal layer of the dura. On the right side, a window has been made in the dura below the transverse venous sinus to expose the cerebellum and the medulla oblongata in the posterior cranial fossa. In the neck, the dura and the arachnoid have been incised in the midline to expose the spinal cord and rootlets of the cervical spinal nerves. Note the cervical spinal nerves leaving the vertebral canal enveloped in a meningeal sheath.

trabeculae, span the subarachnoid space and link the arachnoid and pia. Because of the disparate lengths of the spinal cord and the dura–arachnoid sac, the subarachnoid space inferior to the conus medullaris is notably enlarged and is termed the **lumbar cistern**. Thus, the cauda equina effectively floats in a large pool of CSF within the lumbar cistern.

Pia Mater

The pia mater is the innermost layer of the meninges. It is a vascular membrane that tightly adheres to the external surface of the spinal cord and spinal nerve rootlets and roots. Superiorly, it is continuous through the foramen magnum with the pia covering the brain. Inferiorly, it fuses with the filum terminale. Laterally, the pia extends along the nerve roots and ends by merging with the epineurium of the spinal nerves at the intervertebral foramina.

The pia mater has two specialized components that serve to stabilize the spinal cord within the vertebral canal and subarachnoid space: (1) the ligamentum denticulatum and (2) the filum terminale (see Figs. 2.33, 2.34, and 2.38). The **ligamentum denticulatum** (**denticulate ligament**; **dentate ligament**) is a lateral extension of the pia off each side of the length of the spinal cord. Its serrated lateral edge forms a series of triangular-shaped ligaments that attach to the dura–arachnoid sac. The denticulate ligament is located between the rows of nerve rootlets and roots and divides the subarachnoid

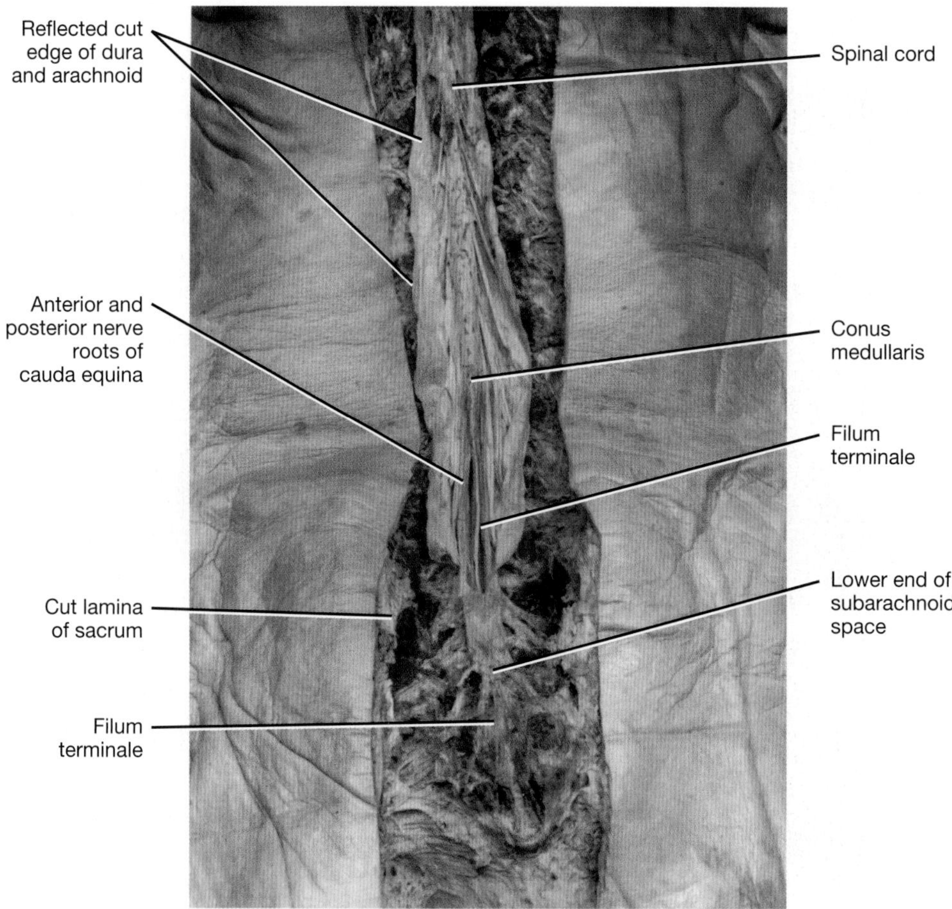

Figure 2.38 Dissection of the lower part of the back, including a complete laminectomy of the lumbar and sacral regions of the vertebral column. The meningeal sheath has been incised and reflected laterally exposing the subarachnoid space, lower end of the spinal cord, and the cauda equina. Note the filum terminale surrounded by the anterior and posterior nerve roots of the lumbar and sacral spinal nerves forming the cauda equina.

space into anterior and posterior compartments. The **filum terminale** is a long, slender filament of the pia that extends from the tip of the conus medullaris to the coccyx. It is located in the center of the cauda equina. The segment of the filum terminale from the conus medullaris to the end of the dura–arachnoid sac (at S2) is termed the **filum terminale internum**. The portion from the sac to the coccyx is termed the **filum terminale externum (coccygeal ligament)**.

Cerebrospinal Fluid

The **CSF** is a clear, colorless fluid formed mainly by the choroid plexuses, within the lateral, third, and fourth ventricles of the brain. CSF circulates through the ventricular system and enters the subarachnoid space through three foramina in the roof of the fourth ventricle. It circulates both upward over the surface of the cerebral hemispheres and downward around the spinal cord. The spinal part of the subarachnoid space extends inferiorly to the level of the S2 vertebra, where the arachnoid fuses with the filum terminale (see Fig. 2.14D).

In addition to removing waste products associated with neuronal activity, CSF provides a fluid medium that surrounds the spinal cord. This fluid, together with the bony and ligamentous walls of the vertebral canal, effectively protects the spinal cord from trauma.

The subarachnoid space can be studied radiographically by the injection of contrast media into the subarachnoid space by lumbar puncture. Iodized oil has been used with success. This technique is referred to as **myelography** (Fig. 2.39).

If the patient is sitting in the upright position, the oil sinks to the lower limit of the subarachnoid space at the level of the S2 vertebra. By placing the patient on a tilting table, the oil can be made to gravitate gradually to higher levels of the vertebral column. A normal myelogram will show pointed lateral projections at regular intervals at the intervertebral space levels. This appearance is caused by the opaque medium filling the lateral extensions of the subarachnoid space around each spinal nerve. The presence of a tumor or a prolapsed intervertebral disc may obstruct the movement of the oil from one region to another when the patient is tilted.

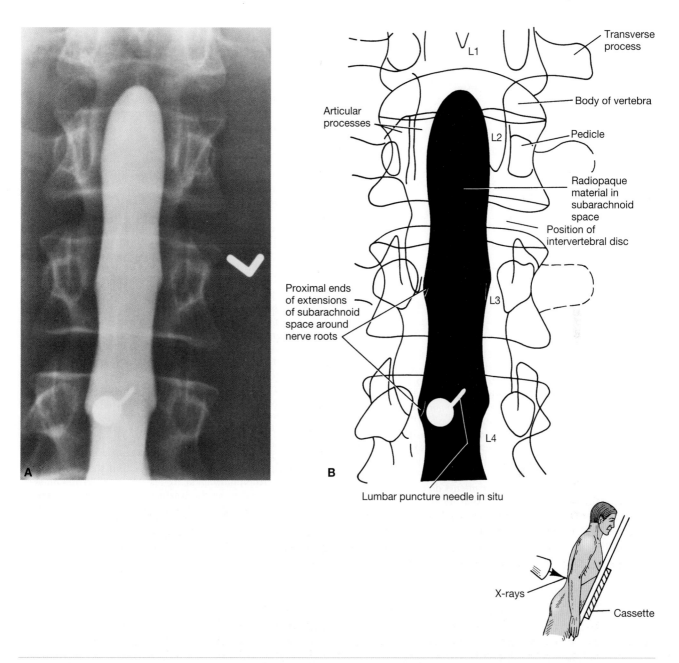

Figure 2.39 **A.** Posteroanterior myelogram of the lumbar region. **B.** Main features observable that can be seen in the myelogram in A.

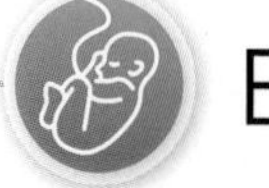

Embryology Notes

Spinal Cord and Spinal Nerve Development

Following neurulation, the spinal cord runs the entire length of the trunk of the body. The cord extends to the coccyx, and all the spinal nerve roots are short and nearly horizontal as they course to their respective intervertebral foramina (IVFs), with no cauda equina and no large lumbar cistern. As development proceeds, differential growth rates of the spinal cord, vertebral column, and trunk of the body cause the spinal cord to regress in length relative to the vertebral column. As a result, the conus medullaris shifts to higher vertebral positions, and the lower spinal nerve roots and filum terminale elongate and form the cauda equina. Simultaneously, the lumbar cistern forms as the dura–arachnoid sac separates from the pia mater. At birth, the conus lies at about the L3 vertebral level, and, by

(continued)

Table 2.7 Vertebral Level Versus Spinal Segmental Level

VERTEBRAL LEVEL	SPINAL CORD SEGMENT LEVEL
Cervical	Add 1 (eg, C5 vertebra corresponds with C6 cord segment)
Upper thoracic	Add 2 (eg, T3 vertebra corresponds with T5 cord segment)
Lower thoracic (T7 to T9)	Add 3 (eg, T8 vertebra corresponds with the T11 cord segment)
10th thoracic	L1 and L2 cord segments
11th thoracic	L3 and L4 cord segments
12th thoracic	L5 cord segment
First lumbar	Sacral and coccygeal cord segments

adulthood, it reaches about the L1 vertebral level. However, the normal length of the adult spinal cord varies significantly. The conus may extend to the T12 to L3 vertebral levels in normal conditions. The age-related changes in the position of the conus and the formation and enlargement of the cauda equina and lumbar cistern have critical implications for clinical procedures, such as lumbar puncture and the functional outcomes of herniated intervertebral discs (see Clinical Notes below).

Because the spinal cord is shorter than the vertebral column in adults, the spinal cord segments do not correspond numerically with the vertebrae that lie at the same level. Table 2.7 describes which spinal segment is contiguous with a given vertebral body in adults.

Tethered Spinal Cord

During development, the filum terminale may become abnormally thickened or infiltrated with other tissue. This may produce tension and/or traction on the caudal part of the spinal cord that interferes with the normal ascent of the cord and results in a low-lying conus medullaris. Such a condition is referred to as **tethered cord syndrome (TCS)**. TCS is associated with multiple possible disorders presenting from the lower back through the pelvis and lower limbs.

Back Muscle Development

All the muscles of the back (except the trapezius) develop from the segmental **myotomes**. Each myotome splits into two portions, the epimere and the hypomere. The **epimere** is smaller, forms posterior to the developing vertebral column (in the back of the body), and is innervated by the **posterior rami of spinal nerves** (Fig. 2.40). The **hypomere** is larger, forms lateral and anterior to the incipient vertebral column, and is supplied by the **anterior rami of spinal nerves**. The **pharyngeal (branchial) arches** in the head region also give rise to numerous muscles, all of which are innervated by cranial nerves.

The pattern of innervation seen in the adult reveals the developmental history of the muscles of the back. All the muscles of the superficial and intermediate groups (except for trapezius) are supplied by anterior rami of spinal nerves. All the muscles of the deep group are supplied by posterior rami of spinal nerves. The trapezius is innervated by cranial nerve XI (spinal accessory nerve). Therefore, the deep muscles originated in the epimeres, the superficial and intermediate muscles (except trapezius) formed from the hypomeres, and the trapezius developed from pharyngeal arches. The deep group muscles are referred to as the **intrinsic muscles of the back** because their developmental origins are from the epimeres, within the back proper. The superficial and intermediate group muscles are termed the **extrinsic muscles of the back** because their origins are from the hypomeres and pharyngeal arches, outside the back proper. The intrinsic muscles remain in their area of origin, whereas the extrinsic muscles secondarily grow into the back from other sites of origin.

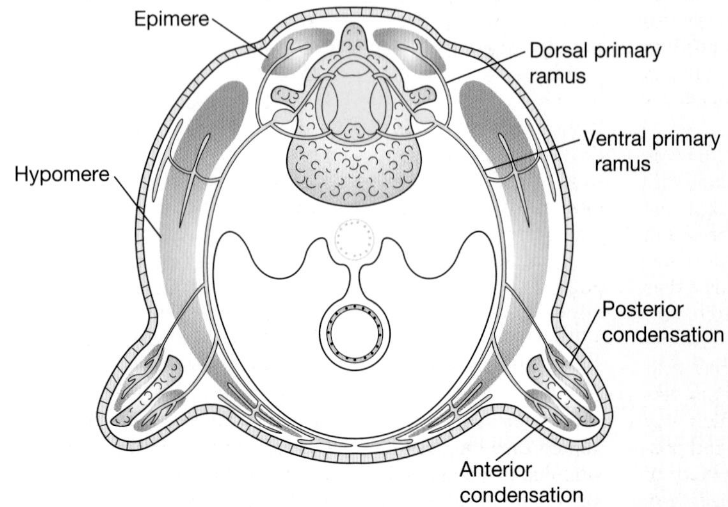

Figure 2.40 Schematic cross section through the thorax and the upper limb bud of an embryo showing the relations between the anterior and posterior primary rami of spinal nerves and the hypomere and epimere. (From Dudek RW. *BRS Embryology*, 6th ed. Baltimore, MD: Wolters Kluwer Health; 2014, with permission.)

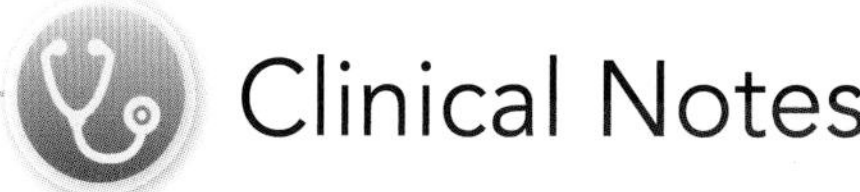

Clinical Notes

Nerve Pain and Intervertebral Foramina

The intervertebral foramina (IVFs) transmit the spinal nerves and the small segmental arteries and veins, all of which are embedded in areolar tissue (Figs. 2.23, 2.25, and 2.33). Each IVF is bounded superiorly and inferiorly by the pedicles of adjacent vertebrae, anteriorly by the lower part of the vertebral body and by the intervertebral disc, and posteriorly by the articular processes and the zygapophyseal joint between them. At this location, the spinal nerve is vulnerable to compression, stretching, and edematous forces produced by abnormalities of the surrounding structures. Such factors may give rise to dermatomal pain, muscle weakness, and diminished or absent reflexes.

One complication of osteoarthritis of the vertebral column is the growth of **osteophytes** (bony protrusions; bone spurs), which commonly encroach on the IVFs, pinch the spinal nerves, and cause pain along the distribution of those nerves. In the lumbar region, the largest IVF is between the L1 and L2 vertebrae, and the smallest is between the L5 and S1 vertebrae. The L5 spinal nerve is the largest of the lumbar spinal nerves, and it runs through the smallest IVF. For this reason, the L5 nerve is highly vulnerable at the IVF.

Remember the numerical relationships of the spinal nerves to the vertebrae (see the earlier description of Spinal Nerves). Because of this, stenosis of a cervical IVF would affect the spinal nerve one number higher than the IVF itself. However, narrowing of a thoracic or lumbar IVF would affect the spinal nerve of the same number as the affected IVF (eg, stenosis of the C6 IVF between the C6 and C7 vertebrae would influence the C7 spinal nerve, whereas narrowing of the L4 IVF between the L4 and L5 vertebrae would affect the L4 spinal nerve).

Osteoarthritis as a cause of back pain is suggested by the patient's age, its insidious onset, and a history of back pain of long duration. A prolapsed disc usually occurs in a younger age group and often has an acute onset.

Herniated Intervertebral Discs

The structure and function of the intervertebral discs were described earlier in this chapter. The discs are very effective in resisting compression forces, as seen, for example, in circus acrobats who can support four or more of their colleagues on their shoulders. Nevertheless, the discs are vulnerable to sudden shocks, particularly if the vertebral column is flexed and the disc is undergoing degenerative changes that favor displacement (herniation) of the nucleus pulposus.

The discs most prone to herniation are those in areas where a mobile part of the column joins a relatively immobile part (ie, cervicothoracic and lumbosacral junctions). In these areas, the posterior part of the annulus fibrosus ruptures, and the nucleus pulposus is forced posteriorly like toothpaste out of its tube. In such a herniation, the nucleus protrudes either posteriorly in the midline under the posterior longitudinal ligament or posterolaterally at the edge of the posterior longitudinal ligament close to the intervertebral foramen (Figs. 2.41 and 2.42). The escape of the nucleus pulposus produces narrowing of the space between the vertebral bodies, which may be visible on radiographs. Slackening of the anterior and posterior longitudinal ligaments results in abnormal mobility of the vertebral bodies, producing local pain and possible subsequent development of osteoarthritis.

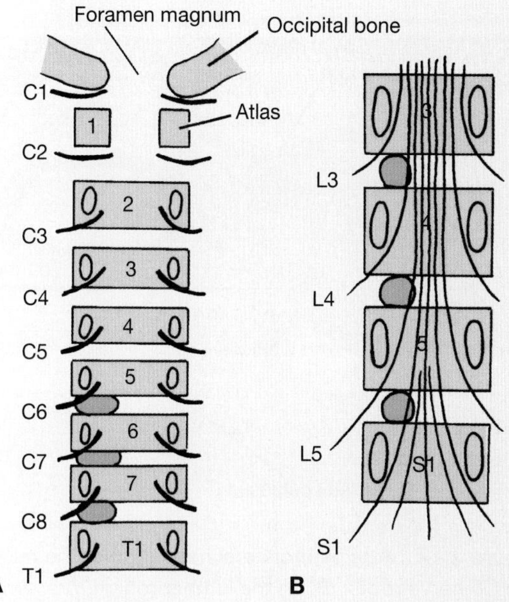

Figure 2.41 Posterior views of vertebral bodies in the cervical **(A)** and lumbar **(B)** regions showing the relationship that might exist between the herniated nucleus pulposus and the spinal nerve roots. Note that there are eight cervical spinal nerves but only seven cervical vertebrae. In the lumbar region, for example, the emerging L4 nerve roots pass out laterally close to the pedicle of the L4 vertebra and are not related to the intervertebral disc between the L4 and L5 vertebrae.

Cervical disc herniations (see Figs. 2.41 to 2.43) are less common than herniations in the lumbar region. The most susceptible discs are those between the C5 and C6 or C6 and C7 vertebrae. Posterolateral protrusions cause pressure on a spinal nerve or its roots. Again, remember the numerical relationships of the cervical nerves and vertebrae. Because each cervical spinal nerve emerges above the corresponding vertebra, a posterolateral disc protrusion affects the next higher numbered spinal nerve (see Fig. 2.41A). Thus, a protruding C5 disc (between the C5 and C6 vertebrae) can compress the C6 spinal nerve or its roots. Pain is felt near the lower part of the back of the neck and shoulder and along the area in the distribution of the spinal nerve involved. Posterior protrusions may press on the spinal cord and the anterior spinal artery and involve the various nerve tracts of the spinal cord.

Computed tomography (CT) and magnetic resonance imaging (MRI) are extensively used to detect lesions of the vertebral column, especially those involving the soft tissues. CT scans can concentrate on the intervertebral spaces and reveal the intervertebral disc in transverse slices. The disc has a higher density than the cerebrospinal fluid in the subarachnoid space and the surrounding fat. Fragments of a herniated disc can be identified beyond the boundaries of the annulus fibrosus. MRI easily defines the intervertebral disc on sagittal section and shows its relationship to the vertebral body and the posterior longitudinal ligament (Fig. 2.43).

(continued)

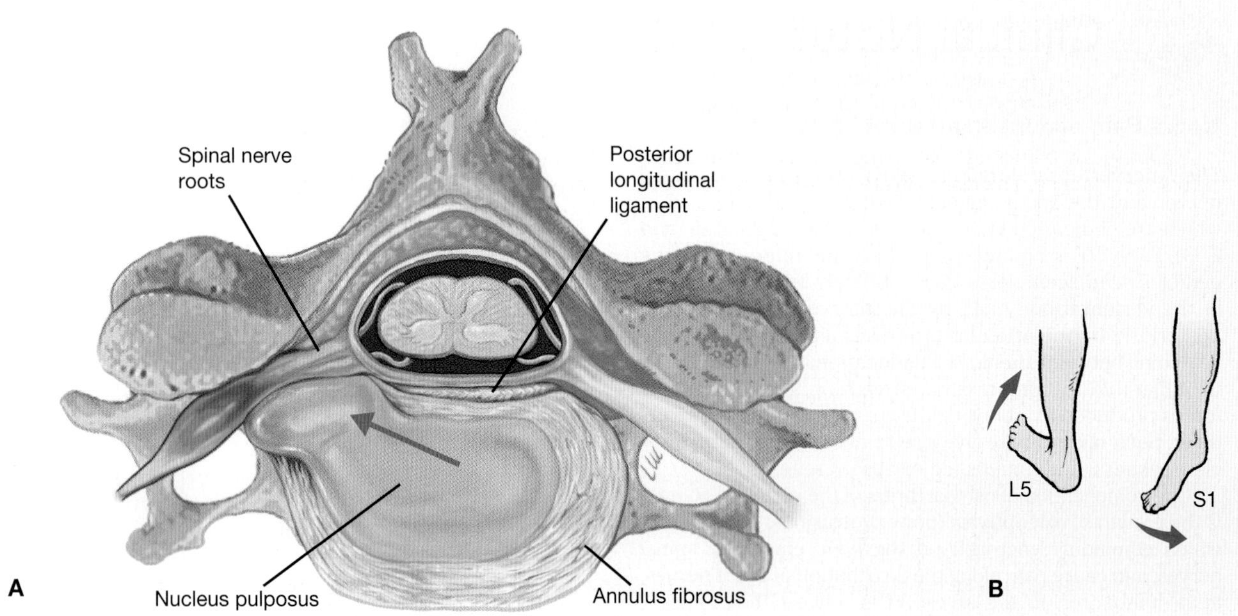

Figure 2.42 **A.** Posterolateral herniation of the nucleus pulposus (*red arrow*) of the C4 intervertebral disc pressing on the C5 nerve roots. **B.** In the lumbar region, pressure on the L5 motor nerve root produces weakness of dorsiflexion of the ankle; pressure on the S1 motor nerve root produces weakness of plantar flexion of the ankle joint.

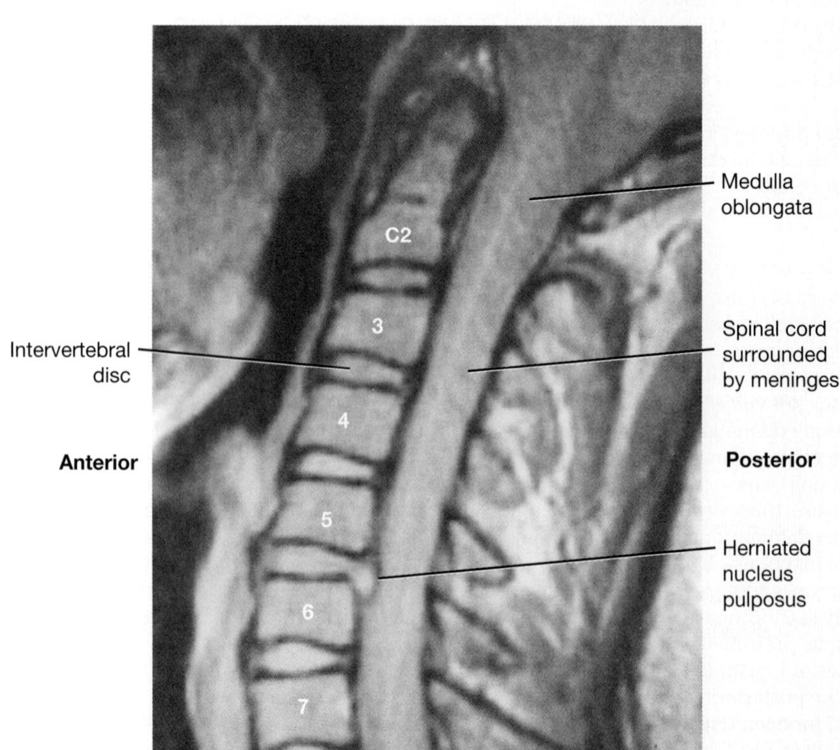

Figure 2.43 Sagittal MRI scan of the cervical part of the vertebral column. A herniated disc between the C5 and C6 vertebrae is shown. Note the position of the spinal cord and its meningeal coverings relative to the herniated disc. (Courtesy of Pait.)

In this image, a herniated disc can be identified bulging into the vertebral canal. The herniated nucleus pulposus and its relationship to the dural sac can be demonstrated easily. MRI is now largely replacing myelography or CT in imaging studies of the intervertebral disc.

Lumbar disc herniations are more common than cervical disc herniations. The discs affected most often are those between the L4 and L5 vertebrae or between the L5 vertebra and the sacrum. Recall again the numerical relationships of the spinal nerves and vertebrae. Each lumbar spinal nerve emerges through the IVF of the same-numbered vertebra (eg, the L4 spinal nerve roots enter the L4 IVF between the L4 and L5 vertebrae to form the L4 spinal nerve). In the lumbar region, the roots of the cauda equina descend vertically over the posterior aspects of several intervertebral discs (see Fig. 2.41B). The nerve roots must take an ~45° turn below the roofing pedicle of the IVF in order to enter the appropriate IVF. This acute turn places the nerve roots and spinal nerve above the corresponding disc. Thus, a typical posterolateral herniation often misses the corresponding nerve roots and, instead, affects the nerve roots going to the IVF immediately below (eg, a posterolateral herniation of the L4 disc between the L4 and L5 vertebrae often impinges upon the L5 spinal nerve roots rather than the L4 roots). As a result, the symptoms are referable to the L5 nerve roots, even though the L5 nerve exits via the L5 IVF. The nucleus pulposus occasionally herniates directly posteriorly and may displace or disrupt the posterior longitudinal ligament. If the herniation is large, the whole cauda equina may be compressed, producing paraplegia.

When dealing with typical posterolateral disc herniations in the cervical and lower lumbar regions, remember the formula "N+1." That is, N = the number of the intervertebral disc in question; +1 = the number of the spinal nerve roots affected by the herniation (eg, a herniated C5 disc will influence the C6 nerve roots, and a protruding L4 disc will affect the L5 nerve roots). In the cervical region, this formula works because each numbered spinal nerve runs through the IVF above the matching numbered vertebra. The formula also works in the low lumbar region because of the acute angles the nerve roots take in entering the IVFs.

Injury of a disc usually produces an initial period of back pain that is referred down the leg and foot in the distribution of the affected nerve. Because the posterior (sensory) roots of L5 and S1 are most commonly compressed, pain is usually felt down the back and lateral side of the leg, radiating to the sole of the foot. This condition is commonly known as **sciatica**. In severe cases, paresthesia or actual sensory loss may be present.

Pressure on the anterior (motor) roots causes muscle spasm and/or weakness, especially on the side of the herniation. Consequently, the vertebral column shows scoliosis, with its concavity on the side of the lesion.

Involvement of the L5 motor root produces weakness in dorsiflexion of the ankle, whereas pressure on the S1 motor root causes weakness in plantar flexion. The ankle jerk reflex may be diminished or absent (see Fig. 2.42B).

A large, centrally placed protrusion may give rise to bilateral pain and muscle weakness in both legs. Acute retention of urine may also occur.

Correlations between disc lesions, the nerve roots involved, pain dermatomes, muscle weakness, and missing or diminished reflexes are shown in Table 2.8.

Table 2.8 Cervical and Lumbosacral Root Syndromes: Summary of Important Features

ROOT INJURY	DERMATOME PAIN	MUSCLE SUPPLIED	MOVEMENT WEAKNESS	REFLEX INVOLVED
C5	Lower lateral aspect of upper arm	Deltoid and biceps	Shoulder abduction, elbow flexion	Biceps
C6	Lateral aspect of forearm	Extensor carpi radialis longus and brevis	Wrist extensors	Brachioradialis
C7	Middle finger	Triceps and flexor carpi radialis	Extension of elbow and flexion of wrist	Triceps
C8	Medial aspect of forearm	Flexor digitorum superficialis and profundus	Finger flexion	None
L1	Groin	Iliopsoas	Hip flexion	Cremaster
L2	Anterior aspect of thigh	Iliopsoas, sartorius, hip adductors	Hip flexion, hip adduction	Cremaster
L3	Medial aspect of knee	Iliopsoas, sartorius, quadriceps, hip adductors	Hip flexion, knee extension, hip adduction	Patellar
L4	Medial aspect of calf	Tibialis anterior, quadriceps	Foot inversion, knee extension	Patellar
L5	Lateral part of lower leg and dorsum of foot	Extensor hallucis longus, extensor digitorum longus	Toe extension, ankle dorsiflexion	None
S1	Lateral edge of foot	Gastrocnemius, soleus	Ankle plantar flexion	Ankle jerk
S2	Posterior part of thigh	Flexor digitorum longus, flexor hallucis longus	Ankle plantar flexion, toe flexion	None

(continued)

Vertebral Canal Stenosis

The vertebral canal undergoes age-related narrowing after about the fourth decade of life. Osteoarthritic changes in the zygapophyseal joints with the formation of osteophytes, together with degenerative changes in the intervertebral discs and the formation of large osteophytes between the vertebral bodies, can all contribute to stenosis. In individuals in whom the vertebral canal was originally small, significant stenosis in the area of the cauda equina can lead to neurologic compression. Symptoms vary from mild discomfort in the lower back to severe pain radiating down the leg with the inability to walk.

Sacroiliac Joint Disease

The sacroiliac joint is described in Chapter 6. The clinical aspects of this joint are referred to here because disease of this joint can cause low back pain and may be confused with disease of the lumbosacral joints. Essentially, the sacroiliac joint is a synovial joint that has irregular elevations on one articular surface that fit into corresponding depressions on the other articular surface. It is a strong joint and is responsible for the transfer of weight from the vertebral column to the hip bones. The lower lumbar and sacral nerves innervate the joint, thus explaining the low back pain and sciatica commonly associated with sacroiliac disorders.

The sacroiliac joint is inaccessible to clinical examination. However, a small area located just medial to and below the posterior superior iliac spine is where the joint comes closest to the surface. In disease of the lumbosacral region, movements of the vertebral column in any direction cause pain in the lumbosacral part of the column. In sacroiliac disease, pain is extreme on rotation of the vertebral column and is worst at the end of flexion. The latter movement causes pain because the hamstring muscles hold the hip bones in position while the sacrum is rotating forward as the vertebral column is flexed.

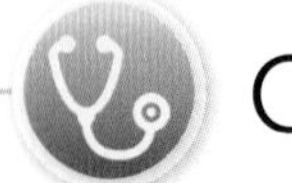

Clinical Notes

Spinal Cord Injuries

The degree of spinal cord injury at different vertebral levels is largely governed by regional anatomic factors. In the cervical region, dislocation or fracture dislocation of the vertebrae is common, but the large size of the vertebral canal often results in the spinal cord escaping severe injury. However, when considerable displacement occurs, the cord is sectioned, and death occurs immediately. Respiration ceases if the lesion occurs above the segmental origin of the phrenic nerves (C3, C4, and C5).

In fracture dislocations in the thoracic region, vertebral displacement is often considerable, and the small size of the vertebral canal results in severe injury to the spinal cord.

In fracture dislocations in the lumbar region, two anatomic facts aid the patient. First, the spinal cord in the adult extends inferiorly only to the level of about the L1 vertebra. Second, the large size of the vertebral canal and the lumbar cistern in this region gives the roots of the cauda equina ample room. Nerve injury may therefore be minimal in this region.

Injury to the spinal cord can produce partial or complete loss of function at the level of the lesion and partial or complete loss of function of afferent and efferent nerve tracts below the level of the lesion. The symptoms and signs of spinal shock and paraplegia are beyond the scope of this book. Please consult a textbook of neurology for further information.

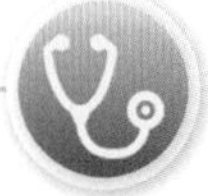

Clinical Notes

Lumbar Puncture (Spinal Tap)

Lumbar puncture is a clinical procedure designed to insert a needle into the subarachnoid space in the low lumbar region. The purpose may be to withdraw a sample of cerebrospinal fluid (CSF) for examination, administer anesthetic, or inject a radiographic medium. The large interlaminar spaces between the low lumbar vertebrae afford relatively open access to the vertebral canal. In adults, the spinal cord terminates inferiorly at the level of the T12 to L3 vertebrae. In infants, the cord ends at about the L3 vertebra. Thus, puncture inferior to the L3 vertebra minimizes the possibility of impaling the spinal cord. The lower lumbar part of the vertebral canal (inferior to L3) contains the cauda equina floating within the large subarachnoid space (lumbar cistern). Thus, a sizable pool of CSF is available in this region. Also, a needle introduced into the lumbar cistern usually pushes the nerve roots to one side without causing damage.

With the patient lying on the side with the vertebral column well flexed, the lumbar interlaminar spaces are opened to a maximum (Fig. 2.44). An imaginary line joining the highest points on the iliac crests passes over the L4 spine. With careful aseptic technique and under local anesthesia, the lumbar puncture needle, fitted with a stylet, is passed into the vertebral canal immediately above or below the L4 spine. The needle passes through the following anatomic structures before it enters the subarachnoid space: skin, superficial fascia, supraspinous ligament, interspinous ligament, ligamentum flavum, areolar

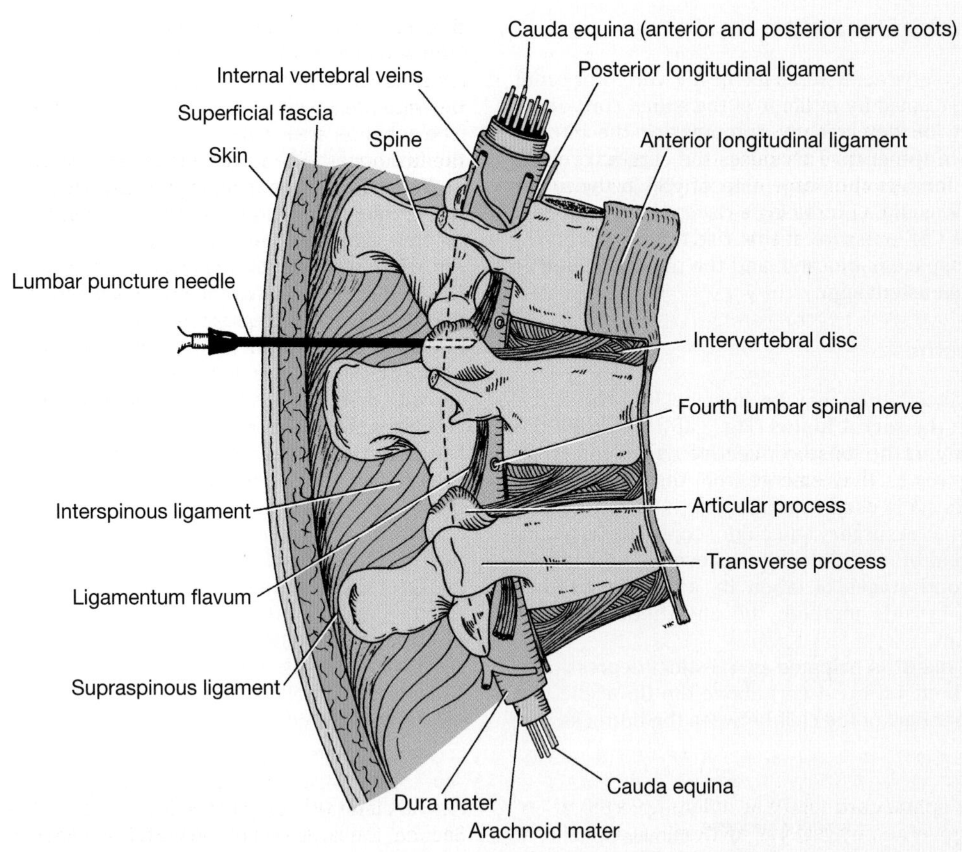

Figure 2.44 Sagittal section through the lumbar part of the vertebral column in flexion. Note that the spines and laminae are well separated in this position, enabling one to introduce a lumbar puncture needle into the subarachnoid space.

tissue (containing the internal vertebral venous plexus in the epidural space), dura mater, and arachnoid mater. The depth to which the needle will have to pass varies from 1 in. (2.5 cm) or less in a child to as much as 4 in. (10 cm) in obese adults.

As the stylet is withdrawn, a few drops of blood commonly escape. This usually indicates that the point of the needle is situated in one of the veins of the internal vertebral plexus and has not yet reached the subarachnoid space. If the entering needle should stimulate one of the nerve roots of the cauda equina, the patient will experience a fleeting discomfort in one of the dermatomes, or a muscle will twitch, depending on whether a sensory or a motor root is impaled. If the needle is pushed too far anteriorly, it may hit the body of the L3 or L4 vertebra.

CSF pressure can be measured by attaching a manometer to the needle. In the recumbent position, the normal pressure is about 60 to 150 mm H_2O. Note that CSF pressure normally fluctuates slightly with the heartbeat and with each phase of respiration.

Anatomy of "Not Getting In"

If the spinal needle encounters bone, it should be withdrawn as far as the subcutaneous tissue, and the angle of insertion should be changed. The most common bone encountered is the spinous process of the vertebra above or below the path of insertion. If the needle is directed laterally rather than in the midline, it may hit the lamina or an articular process.

Anatomy of Complications

- **Postlumbar puncture headache**: This headache starts after the procedure and lasts 24 to 48 hours. The cause is a leak of CSF through the dural puncture, especially after using a wide-bore needle. The leak reduces the volume of CSF, which, in turn, causes a downward displacement of the brain and stretches the nerve-sensitive meninges. Assuming the recumbent position relieves the headache. Using small-gauge styletted needles and avoiding multiple dural holes reduces the incidence of headache.
- **Brain herniation**: Lumbar puncture is contraindicated in cases in which intracranial pressure is significantly raised (eg, a large tumor above the tentorium cerebelli with a high intracranial pressure may result in a caudal displacement of the uncus through the tentorial notch or a dangerous displacement of the medulla through the foramen magnum, when the lumbar CSF pressure is reduced).

(continued)

Subarachnoid Space Block

A block of the subarachnoid space in the vertebral canal, which may be caused by a tumor of the spinal cord or the meninges, can be detected by compressing the internal jugular veins in the neck. This raises the cerebral venous pressure and inhibits the absorption of CSF in the arachnoid granulations, thus producing a rise in the manometric reading of the CSF pressure. If this rise fails to occur, the subarachnoid space is blocked, and the patient exhibits a positive **Queckenstedt sign**.

Caudal Anesthesia

Solutions of anesthetics may be injected into the sacral canal through the **sacral hiatus** (Fig. 2.45). The solutions pass superiorly in the loose connective tissue and bathe the spinal nerves as they emerge from the dural sheath. Caudal anesthesia is used in surgery in the sacral region, including anorectal surgery and culdoscopy. Obstetricians use this method of nerve block to relieve pain during the first and second stages of labor. Its advantage is that, administered by this method, the anesthetic does not affect the infant.

The sacral hiatus is palpated as a distinct depression in the midline about 1.6 in. (4 cm) above the tip of the coccyx in the upper part of the cleft between the buttocks. The hiatus is triangular or U shaped and is bounded laterally by the **sacral cornua**.

The size and shape of the hiatus depend on the number of laminae that fail to fuse in the midline posteriorly. The common arrangement is for the hiatus to be formed by nonfusion of the S5 and sometimes the S4 vertebrae.

With careful aseptic technique and under local anesthesia, the needle, fitted with a stylet, is passed into the vertebral (sacral) canal through the sacral hiatus. The needle pierces the skin and fascia and the **sacrococcygeal membrane** that fills in the sacral hiatus. The membrane is formed of dense fibrous tissue and represents the fused supraspinous and interspinous ligaments as well as the ligamentum flavum. A distinct feeling of "give" is felt when the ligament is penetrated.

Note that the sacral canal is curved and follows the general curve of the sacrum. The anterior wall, formed by the fusion of the bodies of the sacral vertebrae, is rough and ridged. The posterior wall, formed by the fusion of the laminae, is smooth. The average distance between the sacral hiatus and the lower end of the subarachnoid space at the S2 vertebra is about 2 in. (5 cm) in adults.

Note also that the sacral canal contains the dural sac (containing the cauda equina), which is tethered to the coccyx by the filum terminale. Their dural sheath surrounds the sacral and coccygeal nerves as they emerge from the dural sac. Also, thin-walled veins of the internal vertebral venous plexus are located in the sacral canal.

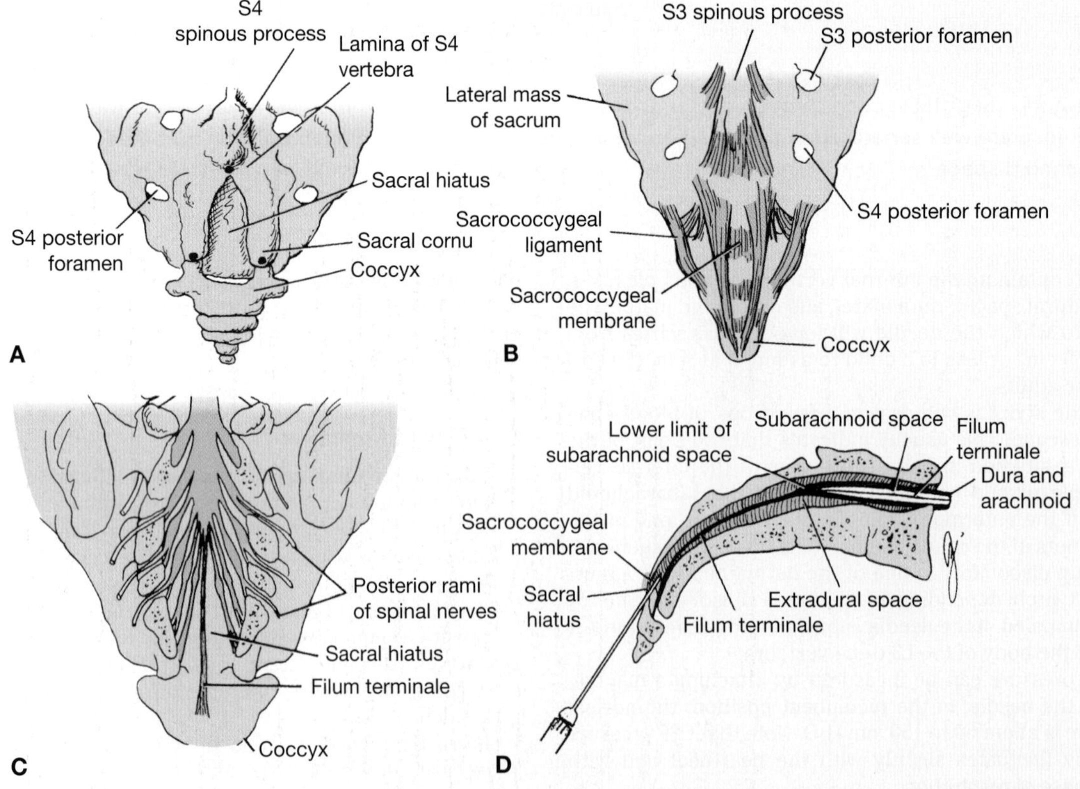

Figure 2.45 **A.** The sacral hiatus. *Black dots* indicate the position of important bony landmarks. **B.** Posterior surface of the lower end of the sacrum and the coccyx showing the sacrococcygeal membrane covering the sacral hiatus. **C.** The dural sheath (thecal sac) around the lower end of the cauda equina and spinal nerves in the sacral canal; the laminae have been removed. **D.** Longitudinal section through the sacrum showing the anatomy of caudal anesthesia.

SURFACE ANATOMY

Examine the whole area of the back and legs with the patient's shoes removed, and their arms hanging loosely at their side. Unequal length of the legs or disease of the hip joints can lead to abnormal curvatures of the vertebral column. The patient should be asked to walk up and down the examination room so that the normal tilting movement of the pelvis can be observed. As one side of the pelvis is raised, a coronal lumbar convexity develops on the opposite side, with a compensatory thoracic convexity on the same side. When a person assumes the sitting position, the normal lumbar curvature flattens, with an increase in the interval between the lumbar spines.

Test the normal range of movements of the different parts of the vertebral column. In the cervical region, flexion, extension, lateral rotation, and abduction (lateral flexion) are possible. Remember that about half of the movement referred to as flexion is carried out at the atlanto-occipital joints. In flexion, the patient should be able to touch their chest with their chin, and, in extension, they should be able to look directly upward. In lateral rotation, the patient should be able to place the chin nearly in line with the shoulder. Half of lateral rotation occurs between the atlas and the axis. In abduction (lateral flexion), the head can normally be tilted 45° to each shoulder. Importantly, the shoulder is not raised when this movement is being tested.

In the thoracic region, movements are limited by the presence of the ribs and sternum. When testing for rotation, make sure the patient does not rotate the pelvis.

In the lumbar region, flexion, extension, and abduction (lateral flexion) are possible. Flexion and extension are fairly free. Test abduction (lateral flexion) in the thoracic and lumbar regions by asking the patient to slide, in turn, each hand down the lateral side of the thigh.

Midline Structures

In the midline, the following structures can be palpated from above downward.

External Occipital Protuberance

The external occipital protuberance lies at the junction of the head and neck (see Fig. 2.1). An index finger placed on the skin in the midline can be drawn inferiorly from the protuberance in the nuchal groove.

Cervical Vertebrae

The spine of the C7 vertebra (vertebra prominens) is the most prominent spinous process that can be felt in the neck (Fig. 2.46). C1 to C6 spines are covered by the ligamentum nuchae and are difficult to palpate.

The transverse processes are short but easily palpable from the lateral side in a thin neck. The anterior tubercle of the C6 transverse process can be palpated medial to the sternocleidomastoid muscle, and the common carotid artery can be compressed against it.

Thoracic and Lumbar Vertebrae

The nuchal groove is continuous inferiorly with a furrow that runs down the middle of the back over the tips of the spines of all the thoracic and the L1 to L4 vertebrae. The most prominent spine is that of the T1 vertebra; the others may be easily recognized when the trunk is flexed.

Sacrum

The spines of the sacrum are fused with each other in the midline to form the median sacral crest. The crest can be felt beneath the skin in the uppermost part of the cleft between the buttocks.

The sacral hiatus (see Fig. 2.45) is situated on the posterior aspect of the lower end of the sacrum. The extradural (epidural) space terminates here. The hiatus lies about 2 in. (5 cm) above the tip of the coccyx and beneath the skin of the groove between the buttocks.

Coccyx

The inferior surface and tip of the coccyx can be palpated in the groove between the buttocks about 1 in. (2.5 cm) behind the anus (see Fig. 2.1). The anterior surface of the coccyx can be palpated with a gloved finger in the anal canal.

Upper Lateral Part of Thorax

The scapula and its associated muscles cover the upper lateral part of the thorax. The scapula lies posterior to the first through seventh ribs (see Figs. 2.1 and 2.46).

Scapula

The medial border of the scapula forms a prominent ridge, which ends above at the superior angle and below at the inferior angle (see Figs. 2.1 and 2.46).

The superior angle can be palpated opposite the first thoracic spine, and the inferior angle can be palpated opposite the seventh thoracic spine.

The crest of the spine of the scapula can be palpated and traced medially to the medial border of the scapula, which it joins at the level of the third thoracic spine.

The acromion of the scapula forms the lateral extremity of the spine of the scapula. It is subcutaneous and easily located.

Lower Lateral Part of Back

The posterior aspect of the upper part of the bony pelvis (false pelvis), and its associated gluteal muscles form the lower lateral part of the back.

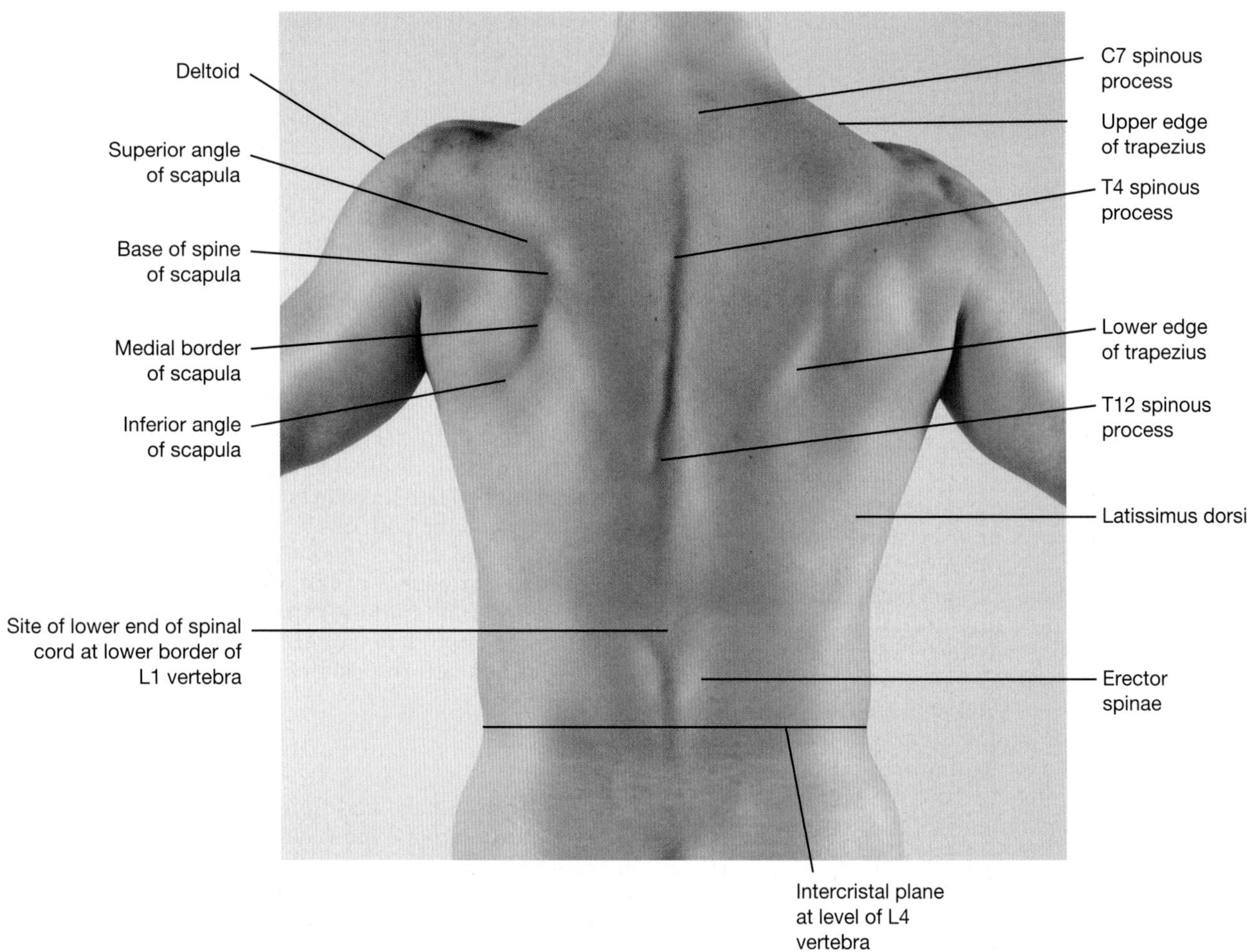

Figure 2.46 Surface anatomy of the back.

Iliac Crests

The iliac crests are easily palpable along their entire length (see Fig. 2.1). They lie at the level of the L4 spine and are used as a landmark when performing a lumbar puncture. Each crest ends in front at the anterior superior iliac spine and behind at the posterior superior iliac spine; the latter lies beneath a skin dimple at the level of the S2 vertebra and the middle of the sacroiliac joint. The iliac tubercle is a prominence felt on the outer surface of the iliac crest about 2 in. (5 cm) posterior to the anterior superior iliac spine. The iliac tubercle lies at the level of the L5 spine.

Spinal Cord and Subarachnoid Space

The spinal cord in adults extends inferiorly to approximately the level of the spine of the L1 vertebra (see Fig. 2.14D). In young children, it may extend to the L3 spine.

The subarachnoid space extends inferiorly to the S2 vertebra, which lies at the level of the posterior superior iliac spine.

Back Symmetry

Observe the back as a whole and compare the two sides with reference to an imaginary line passing inferiorly from the external occipital protuberance to the cleft between the buttocks.

The posterior vertebral musculature, which mainly controls the movements of the vertebral column and maintains the postural curves of the column, can be palpated. The muscles are large and lie on either side of the spines of the vertebrae (see Figs. 2.1, 2.30, and 2.46). They should be examined with the flat of the hand. If they exhibit normal tone, they are firm to the touch. A spastic muscle feels harder than normal; it is also shorter than normal, which produces a concavity of the vertebral column on the side of the muscular contraction.

The curves of the vertebral column can be examined by inspecting the lateral contour of the back. Normally, the posterior surface is concave in the cervical region, convex in the thoracic region, and concave in the lumbar region (see Fig. 2.2A). The posterior surface of the sacrum and coccyx together has a convex surface. The lumbar region meets the sacrum at a sharp angle, the lumbosacral angle.

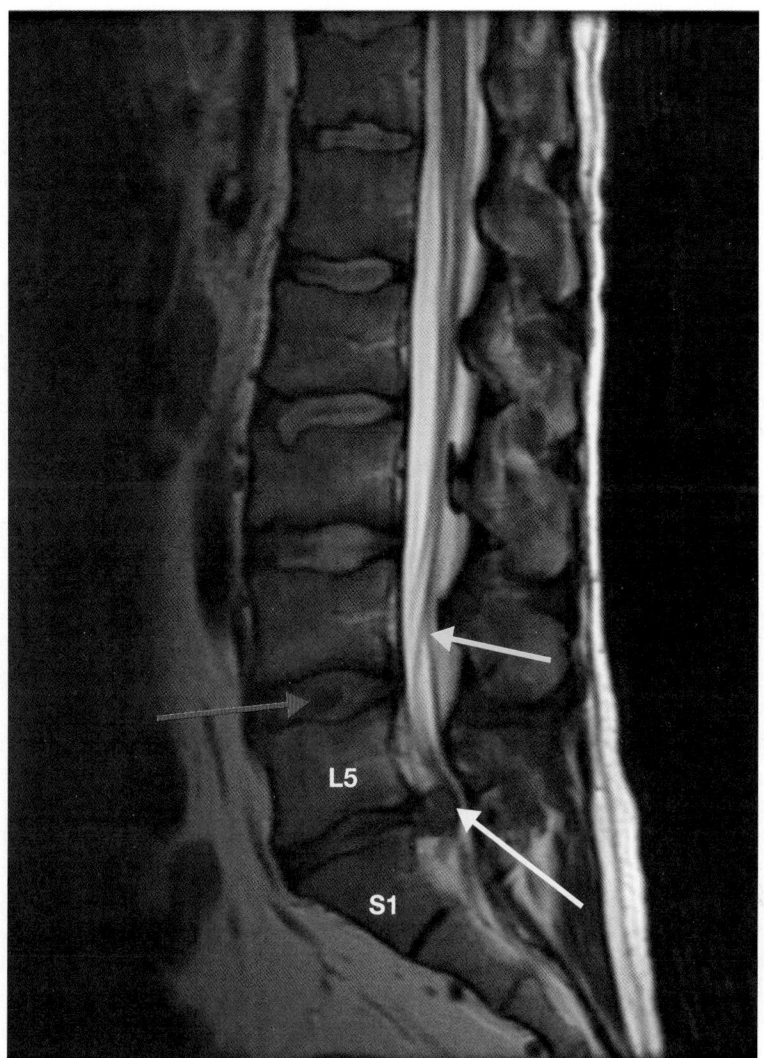

Figure 2.47 Sagittal MRI of the lumbosacral part of the vertebral column. Note the herniated L5 disc (*white arrow*) impinging upon the cauda equina (*yellow arrow*). Also note the normal L4 disc (*red arrow*).

Inspection of the posterior surface of the back, with particular reference to the vertical alignment of the vertebral spines, reveals a slight lateral curvature in most normal individuals. Right-handed people, especially those whose work involves extreme and prolonged muscular effort, usually exhibit a lateral thoracic curve to the right; left-handed people usually exhibit a lateral thoracic curve to the left.

Clinical Case Discussion

Radiographic and computed tomography examination of this patient revealed nothing abnormal. However, a magnetic resonance imaging (MRI) study showed a herniated disc between the L5 and S1 vertebrae (Fig. 2.47). A protruding nucleus pulposus, pressing on the S1 nerve root, would explain her symptoms and signs.

Low back pain is a common complaint in clinical practice and may be caused by a wide spectrum of diseases. The anatomy of the region is complex, and many structures have the potential to cause pain. The clinician can identify the cause and start treatment only by having a sound knowledge of the anatomy and the pathologic processes involving the area.

Key Concepts

Vertebral Column

- The vertebral column is composed of 31 individual vertebrae organized into five regions: cervical, thoracic, lumbar, sacral, and coccygeal.
- All vertebrae share several general features, and all vertebrae within each region share common regional features.
- The adult vertebral column has four natural curvatures: two primary curves (thoracic and sacrococcygeal) and two secondary curves (cervical and lumbar).
- Abnormal curvatures of the vertebral column include kyphosis (exaggerated thoracic curve), lordosis (exaggerated cervical or lumbar curves), and scoliosis (lateral and rotational deviations).
- All vertebrae share a common developmental floor plan that stems from a body, a vertebral arch, and paired costal processes. Maldevelopment of these elements may result in accessory ribs (from the costal processes) or spina bifida (from failure in the vertebral arch).
- The individual vertebrae from levels C2 to L5 articulate with one another via cartilage joints between the bodies (intervertebral discs) and synovial joints between the articular processes (zygapophyseal joints).
- Intervertebral discs have two components: the central nucleus pulposus and the peripheral annulus fibrosus. Abnormal displacement of the nucleus results in a herniated disc.

Back Muscles

- The muscles of the back are organized into three groups.
- The superficial group consists of upper limb muscles (trapezius, latissimus dorsi, rhomboids, and levator scapulae).
- The intermediate group consists of two small muscles of the thoracic wall (serratus posterior superior and serratus posterior inferior).
- The deep group consists of several large and small muscles that move the vertebral column, ribs, and skull.

Spinal Cord

- The spinal cord is the elongate, cylindrical part of the central nervous system below the head.
- Spinal nerves (31 pairs) branch off the sides of the spinal cord. The successive merging of anterior and posterior rootlets and anterior and posterior roots forms each spinal nerve. Each spinal nerve passes through an intervertebral foramen and divides into an anterior and posterior primary ramus.
- The spinal nerve rootlets and roots convey only motor (anterior elements) or sensory (posterior elements) neuron processes. The spinal nerves and the primary rami convey mixed populations of both motor and sensory fibers.
- The end of the spinal cord (the conus medullaris) reaches approximately the L1 vertebral level in adults.
- The cauda equina is the long bundle of spinal nerve roots that extends below the conus medullaris.
- Three membranes (meninges) surround the spinal cord and brain. The dura mater is the most external membrane; the arachnoid mater is the middle layer; the pia mater is the innermost layer.
- Cerebrospinal fluid fills the subarachnoid space between the arachnoid and the pia mater. Lumbar puncture (spinal tap) is the procedure in which a needle is inserted into the subarachnoid space in the low lumbar region.

Medical Imaging

- Numerous features of the back are readily visible and palpable in standard modes of medical imaging and in surface anatomy examination.

3 Upper Limb

A 64-year-old female fell down from the stairs and was admitted to the emergency department with severe right shoulder pain. While she was sitting up, her right arm was by her side, and her right elbow was flexed and supported by her left hand. Inspection of the right shoulder showed loss of the normal rounded curvature and evidence of a slight swelling below the right clavicle. The clinician then systematically tested the cutaneous sensibility of the right upper limb and found severe sensory deficits involving the skin of the back of the arm down as far as the elbow, the lower lateral surface of the arm down to the elbow, the middle of the posterior surface of the forearm as far as the wrist, the lateral half of the dorsal surface of the hand, and the dorsal surface of the lateral three and a half fingers proximal to the nail beds. What are the primary anatomical features underlying this patient's condition?

See the Clinical Case Discussion at the end of this chapter for further insight.

CHAPTER OUTLINE

LEARNING OBJECTIVES

The purpose of this chapter is to review the basic anatomy of the upper limb, including the breast, to understand normal functional relationships and the basis for common limb injuries, pain, motor deficits, congenital defects, medical imaging, and general surface examination.

1. Identify the bones of the upper limb and their major features. Describe the functional aspects of these structures. Identify these structures in standard medical imaging.
2. Identify the bony components, major ligaments, key accessory structures (eg, intra-articular discs), and movements permitted at the shoulder, elbow, and wrist joints. Describe the characteristic features of the major traumas to each joint.
3. Identify the specific anatomical regions of the upper limb.
4. Describe the general structure of the female breast and its relationship to the thoracic wall. Describe the lymphatic drainage of the breast and the anatomical bases for various degrees of mastectomy.
5. Define the boundaries of the axilla and identify its contents.
6. Define the boundaries of the cubital fossa and identify its contents.
7. Define the components of the shoulder complex. Identify the muscles of the shoulder, indicating their attachments, innervation, and major actions.
8. Identify the muscles composing the "rotator cuff." Describe the functional significance of this group.
9. Identify the quadrangular and triangular spaces of the shoulder. Describe the functional significance of each.
10. Define the osseofascial compartments of the upper limb. Identify the muscles contained in each compartment. Describe the attachments, innervation, and major actions of each muscle. Describe the innervation of each compartment and the major actions governed by that innervation. Predict the functional consequences of loss of action of each muscle and each compartment.
11. Describe the mechanisms of pronation and supination. Note the muscles involved, their sites of attachment, and their innervation.
12. Define the carpal tunnel. Note the relationships of tendons, nerves, and blood vessels to the carpal tunnel. Describe the clinical significance of this arrangement in the context of carpal tunnel syndrome.
13. Define the movements of the thumb and fingers. Describe the interaction of extrinsic and intrinsic muscles, retinacula, and fibrous digital sheaths in producing precision hand movement. Describe the relationship between the extensors of the digits and the lumbrical and interosseous muscles. Define the role of this arrangement in the production of precision hand movement.
14. Describe the arrangement of synovial sheaths in the wrist and hand. Explain the clinical significance of such a patterning.
15. Define the "anatomical snuffbox" and identify its major contents.
16. Identify the brachial plexus and its component parts, from spinal segmental sources to terminal branches.
17. Trace the course of motor and cutaneous innervation in the upper limb. Identify the spinal segmental level(s) of origin and relationship to the brachial plexus of each major peripheral nerve. Predict the functional consequences of lesions to specific spinal levels, parts of the brachial plexus, and individual peripheral nerves.
18. Trace the flow of blood from the subclavian artery to and through the upper limb by describing the courses and branching patterns of the major arteries and veins. Identify the territories supplied and drained by the major vessels. Note the main collateral routes around the shoulder and elbow. Describe the composition and anastomoses of the palmar arterial arches.
19. Describe the pattern of lymphatic drainage of the upper limb, including the relationship of this drainage to that of the axilla and breast.
20. Describe the major steps in the development of the upper limb.
21. Identify the major features of the upper limb in standard medical images.
22. Locate the surface projections and palpation points of the major structures of the upper limb in a basic surface examination.

OVERVIEW

The upper limb is a multijointed lever that is freely movable on the trunk at the shoulder joint. Its primary function is to maneuver the hand into positions in which the hand can manipulate objects. The hand is a highly evolved organ with the unique ability to grasp items in both coarse and fine ways. Much of the importance of the hand centers on the pincer-like opposable action of the thumb, which enables the tip of the thumb to contact the tips of the other digits.

The upper limb is organized into the **shoulder region**, **arm**, **cubital fossa**, **forearm**, **wrist**, and **hand**. The arm, forearm, and hand are compartmentalized into working units. Each compartment has its own muscles that perform both group and individual functions and its own distinct nerve and blood supply.

The physician commonly encounters pain, fractures, dislocations, and nerve injuries of the upper limb. Wrist and hand injuries deserve particular attention because of the importance of preserving as much function of the thumb as possible.

OSTEOLOGY

The upper limb is a component of the appendicular skeleton. The bones included here are the clavicle, scapula, humerus, ulna, radius, carpal bones, metacarpal bones, and phalanges. The clavicle and the scapula form the shoulder girdle. The humerus defines the arm, whereas the radius and the ulna delineate the forearm. The carpal bones form the wrist, and the metacarpals and phalanges constitute the hand. This section provides a comprehensive description of the bones of the upper limb and their significant features. Rather than relegating learning this material to an exercise in rote memorization of meaningless words, try to understand the terminology (eg, what is the difference between a tubercle and a tuberosity?) to better appreciate the application of the anatomy. Most importantly, ask yourself functional questions when you examine the bones themselves, such as, is this a right or left element? What articulates with this structure/area? What attaches to this structure? Is this structure palpable? Can this structure be identified in a standard radiographic image? Are there any important neurovascular relations to this region/structure?

Clavicle

Also known as the "collar bone," the clavicle (*clavicul* is Latin for "key") is located between the sternum and the scapula and lies horizontally across the root of the neck. It is roughly S-shaped and resembles a large key. The clavicle forms a light strut that connects the upper limb to the thorax and allows the limb to move freely from the trunk. It is the first bone to begin ossification. The clavicle is subcutaneous and easily palpable along its entire length.

The **sternal extremity** (Fig. 3.1) is the blunt, thickened, proximal (medial) end of the clavicle. It articulates

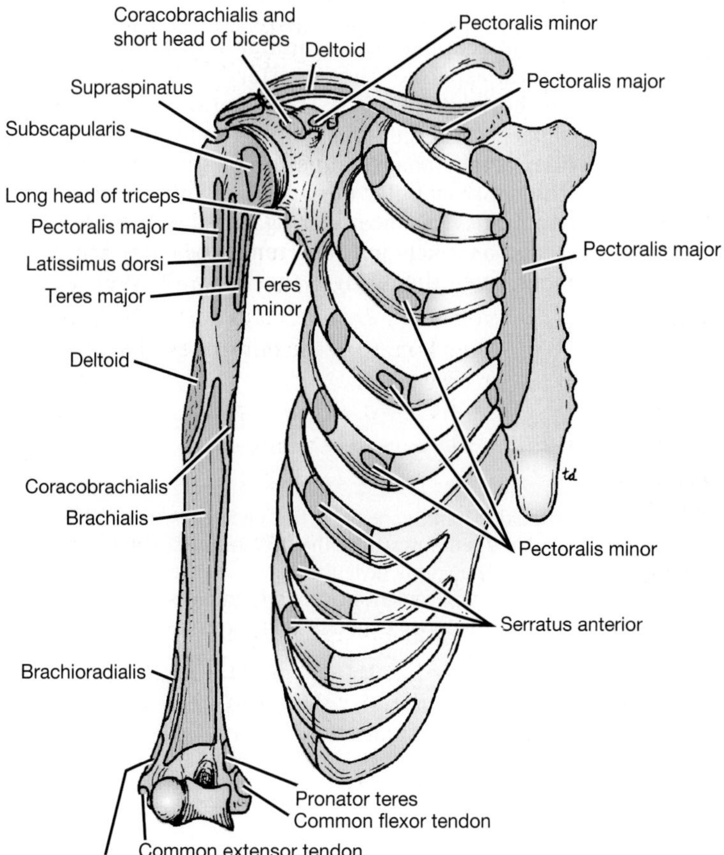

Figure 3.1 Muscle attachments to the bones of the thorax, clavicle, scapula, and humerus.

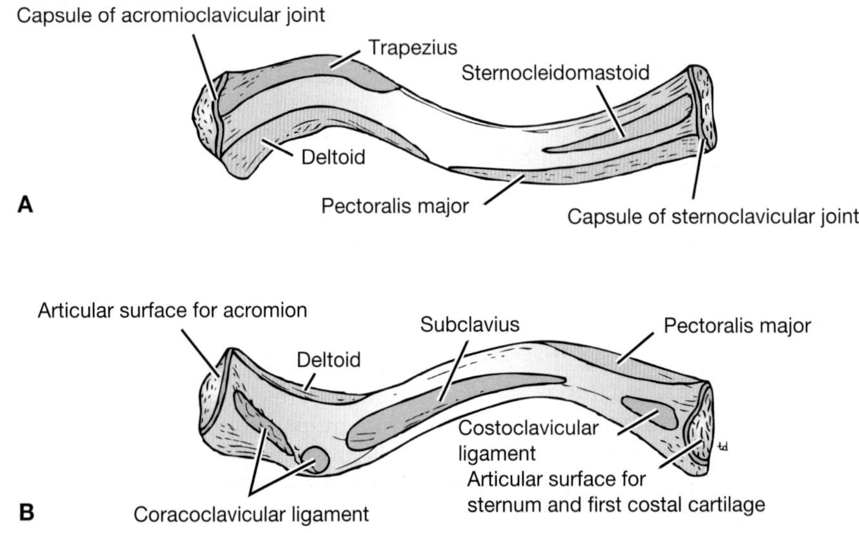

Figure 3.2 Important muscular and ligamentous attachments to the right clavicle. **A.** Superior surface. **B.** Inferior surface.

with the clavicular notch of the sternum through a compound synovial joint containing an articular disc. The **acromial extremity** is the flattened distal (lateral) end of the clavicle. It articulates with the acromion process of the scapula. The **conoid tubercle** (*cono* is Greek for "pinecone") is a small, roughened elevation on the inferior surface, near the acromial end. This serves as the attachment area for the conoid ligament part of the coracoclavicular ligament. The important muscle and ligament attachments to the clavicle are shown in Figures 3.1 and 3.2.

Scapula

Also known as the "shoulder bone," the scapula (*scapul* is Latin for "shoulder blade") is a large, flat, triangular bone that lies on the posterior chest wall between ribs 2 and 7. It articulates with the acromial extremity of the clavicle and the head of the humerus. The major defining features of the scapula are its three borders (superior, medial, and lateral), three angles (superior, inferior, and lateral), two surfaces (dorsal and costal), and three large bony processes (spine, acromion, and coracoid), as shown in Figure 3.3.

The **superior border** is the short, thin, superior edge of the scapula. The **scapular notch** is located on the lateral aspect of the superior border, near the base of the coracoid process. The superior transverse scapular ligament bridges the notch. Normally, the suprascapular artery passes superior to this ligament, whereas the suprascapular nerve passes inferior to it. Think of the transverse scapular ligament as a bridge over the scapular notch and then remember: the **A**rmy (**A**rtery) goes over the bridge; the **N**avy (**N**erve) goes under

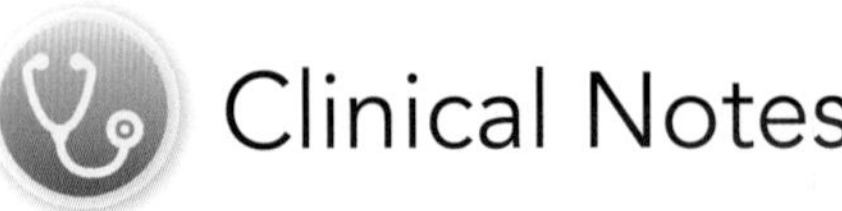

Clinical Notes

Clavicle Fracture

The clavicle is a strut that holds the arm laterally so that it can move freely on the trunk. It is the sole link between the upper limb and the axial skeleton, so it transmits all forces from the upper limb to the trunk. Because of its position, it is easily exposed to trauma: *it is the most fractured bone in the body*. The fracture usually occurs because of a fall on the shoulder or outstretched hand. Force is transmitted along the clavicle, which breaks at its weakest point, the junction of the middle and outer thirds. After the fracture, the lateral fragment is depressed by the weight of the arm and is pulled medially and forward by the strong adductor muscles of the shoulder joint, especially the pectoralis major. The medial end is tilted upward by the SCM muscle. The close relationship of the supraclavicular nerves to the clavicle may result in their involvement in callus formation after fracture. This may be the cause of persistent pain over the side of the neck.

Clavicular Compression of the Brachial Plexus, Subclavian Artery, and Subclavian Vein

The interval between the clavicle and rib 1 in some patients may become narrowed and compress nerves and blood vessels. (See the discussion of thoracic outlet syndrome in Chapter 4.)

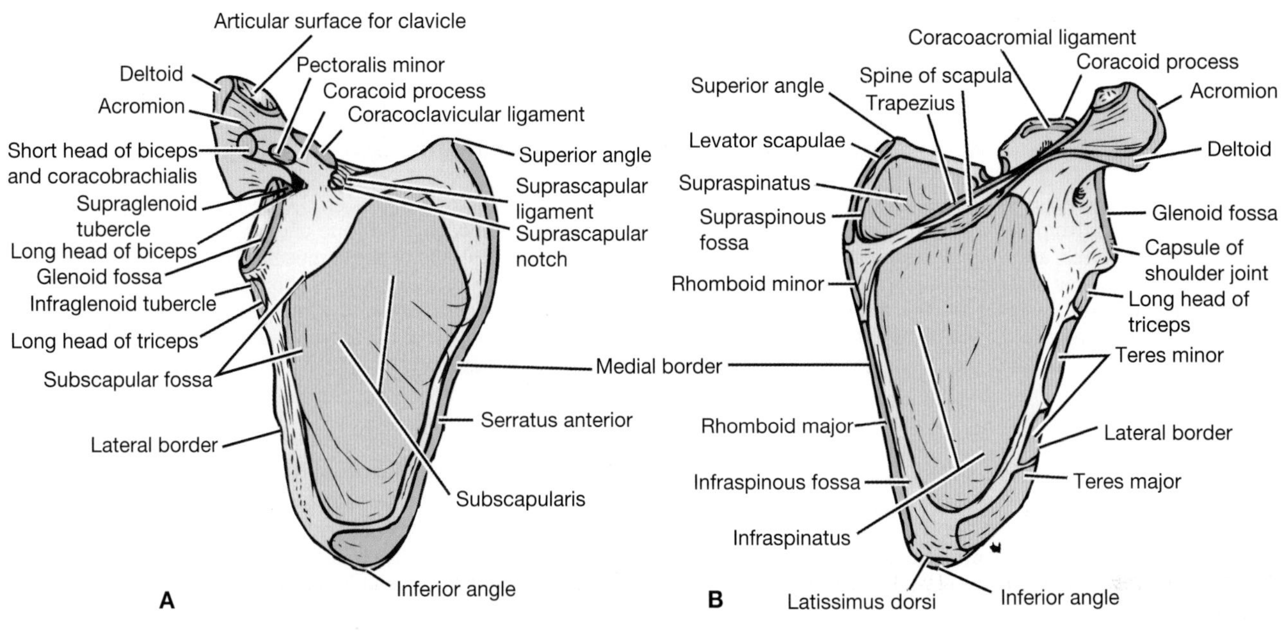

Figure 3.3 Important muscular and ligamentous attachments to the right scapula. **A.** Anterior surface. **B.** Posterior surface.

the bridge. The **medial (vertebral) border** is the long, medial edge of the scapula, located closest to the vertebral column. The **lateral (axillary) border** is the thickened, lateral edge of the scapula, located closest to the axilla. The junction of the superior and medial borders forms the **superior angle** of the scapula. The junction of the medial and lateral borders forms the **inferior angle**. The inferior angle of the scapula can be palpated easily and marks the level of rib 7 and the spine of the T7 vertebra. The junction of the superior and lateral borders forms the **lateral angle**.

The lateral angle of the scapula is the thickest and most complex part of the scapula. It is composed mainly of a broadened process (**head of the scapula**) that is connected to the rest of the bone by a slight constriction (**neck of the scapula**). The lateral surface of the head forms a shallow articular surface, the **glenoid cavity** or **fossa** (*glen* is Greek for "pit" or "socket"), for the head of the humerus. A fibrocartilage ring (**glenoid labrum**) rims the margin of the glenoid cavity and serves to broaden and deepen the joint cavity. A small elevation (**supraglenoid tubercle**) is located at the apex of the glenoid cavity, near the base of the coracoid process. A roughened area (**infraglenoid tubercle**) is located immediately inferior to the glenoid cavity.

The **dorsal (posterior) surface** of the scapula is subdivided into two unequal-sized regions by the spine of the scapula. The **spine** is the large, triangular ridge that runs laterally from the medial border of the scapula to merge into the acromion process. The smaller, troughlike area superior to the spine is the **supraspinous fossa**. The much larger area inferior to the spine is the **infraspinous fossa**. The lateral border of the spine blends into the neck of the scapula and forms a notch-like passageway (**spinoglenoid**, or **greater scapular**, **notch**) that connects the **supraspinous** fossa with the infraspinous fossa. This allows the suprascapular nerve and vessels to pass between these fossae. The **acromion** (*acromi* is Greek for "point of the shoulder") is the broad, flat lateral extension of the spine of the scapula. This forms the easily palpable tip of the shoulder. It partly roofs over the glenoid cavity and provides an articulation with the clavicle at the acromioclavicular joint.

The **costal (ventral** and **anterior) surface** of the scapula lies against the posterior aspect of the rib cage. A large part of this surface forms a shallow concavity, the **subscapular fossa**. The **coracoid process** (*coraco* is Greek for "like a crow's beak") is a thick, beaklike structure that projects anterolaterally from the junction of the neck and lateral end of the superior border of the scapula. It can be palpated via deep pressure through the anterior part of the deltoid muscle, inferior to the lateral end of the clavicle. The main muscle and ligament attachments to the scapula are shown in Figures 3.1 and 3.3.

Humerus

The humerus (*humer* is Latin for "shoulder") is in the arm (brachium) and is the longest bone of the upper limb. Proximally, the humerus articulates with the glenoid cavity of the scapula, at the glenohumeral (shoulder) joint. Distally, it articulates with the head of the radius and the trochlear notch of the ulna, at the elbow joint. The humerus can be divided into three main regions: (1) proximal extremity, (2) body or shaft, and (3) distal extremity. The major muscle and ligament attachments to the humerus are shown in Figures 3.1 and 3.4.

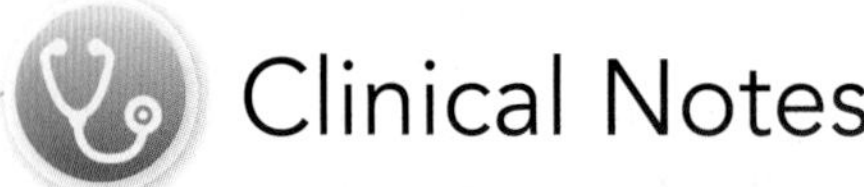

Clinical Notes

Scapular Fractures

Fractures of the scapula are usually the result of severe trauma, such as from being run over or from a motor vehicle crash. Injuries are usually associated with fractured ribs. Most fractures of the scapula require little direct treatment because the muscles on the anterior and posterior surfaces adequately splint the fragments.

Dropped Shoulder and Winged Scapula

The position of the scapula on the posterior wall of the thorax is maintained by the tone and balance of the muscles attached to it. If one of these muscles is paralyzed, the balance is disrupted, as in dropped shoulder, which occurs with paralysis of the trapezius, or winged scapula (see Fig. 3.85), caused by paralysis of the serratus anterior. Such imbalance can be detected by careful physical examination.

Proximal Extremity

The **head** is the round, smooth, proximal end of the humerus. It forms about one third of a sphere and is oriented medially, superiorly, and slightly posteriorly. It articulates with the glenoid cavity of the scapula to form the glenohumeral joint in the shoulder joint complex. The **greater tubercle** is the large, roughened elevation on the lateral proximal end of the humerus, lateral to the head. The **lesser tubercle** is the small, roughened elevation on the anterior proximal end of the humerus, inferior to the head and medial to the greater tubercle. The **anatomic neck** is the slightly constricted region surrounding the articular surface of the head. The articular capsule of the glenohumeral joint attaches along the inferior edge of the anatomic neck. Fractures here are generally rare but may be more frequent in the elderly. The **surgical neck** is the constricted area immediately inferior to the greater and lesser tubercles. This forms the interface between the proximal extremity and the shaft of the humerus. The

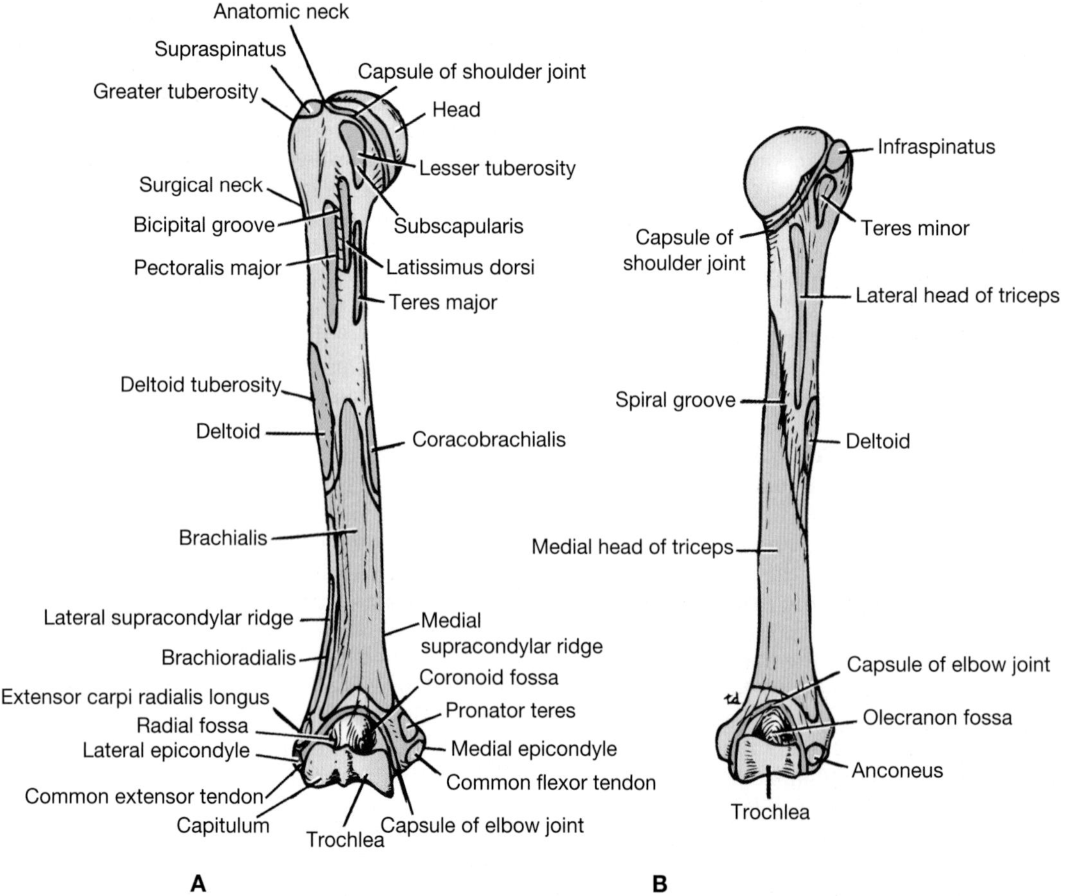

Figure 3.4 Important muscular and ligamentous attachments to the right humerus. **A.** Anterior surface. **B.** Posterior surface.

surgical neck has important relations with the axillary nerve and the anterior and posterior circumflex humeral vessels. Fractures here are common. The **intertubercular (bicipital) groove** is the deep groove on the anterior surface of the humerus that separates the greater and lesser tubercles. It houses the tendon of the long head of the biceps brachii muscle and extends into the upper third of the shaft of the humerus.

Body/Shaft

The **deltoid tuberosity** (*delt* as in the triangular Greek letter delta) is the roughened triangular elevation on the anterolateral surface of the midshaft of the humerus. This serves as the attachment area for the deltoid muscle. The posterior edge of the tuberosity defines the groove for the radial nerve. The **groove** (**sulcus**) for the **radial nerve** (**radial groove**; **spiral groove**) is the shallow depression that spirals around the posterior and lateral aspects of the midshaft of the humerus. The groove is most distinct where it lies between the deltoid tuberosity and the upper end of the lateral supracondylar ridge. It has important relations with the radial nerve and the profunda brachii vessels. Fractures of the midshaft humerus are common, especially inferior to the deltoid tuberosity, and may affect the radial groove and its contents. The **medial supracondylar ridge** is the narrow ridge running proximally from the medial epicondyle, forming the lower medial border of the humerus. The **lateral supracondylar ridge** is the narrow ridge running proximally from the lateral epicondyle, forming the lower lateral border of the humerus.

Distal Extremity

The **lateral epicondyle** is the small, roughened projection on the distal, lateral side of the humerus, proximal to the capitulum. It is readily palpable. The common extensor tendon (tendon of origin for several superficial forearm extensor muscles) attaches here. Inflammation of this tendon is termed "lateral epicondylitis" (tennis elbow). The **medial epicondyle** is the large, knoblike projection on the distal, medial side of the humerus, proximal to the trochlea. It is easily palpable and forms an important surface landmark in the arm. The ulnar nerve crosses the posterior surface of this epicondyle in the shallow **ulnar sulcus** and is susceptible to injury here (eg, via blunt trauma or bony fracture). The nerve can be palpated and rolled against the epicondyle. Stimulation of the nerve by contact against the epicondyle elicits the characteristic "funny bone" response of tingling sensations in the medial border of the hand and fifth digit. (So, why is the funny bone funny? Because it borders on the "humerus.") The **capitulum** (*capit* is Latin for "head"—in this case, "little head") is the rounded, half-spherical, articular process at the distal, lateral end of the humerus. It lies immediately lateral to the trochlea. The capitulum articulates with the head of the radius. The shapes of these structures allow both flexion/extension and rotation at the humeroradial joint. The **trochlea** (*trochle* is Greek for "pulley") is the pulley-shaped articular process at the distal, medial end of the humerus. It lies immediately medial to the capitulum. The trochlea articulates with the trochlear notch of the ulna. The shapes of the articulated trochlea and trochlear notch (plus the presence of the humeroradial joint) limit lateral movements of the ulna, resulting in essentially a hinge action at the humeroulnar joint. The **coronoid fossa** is the depression on the distal, anterior end of the humerus, immediately proximal to the trochlea. This receives the coronoid process of the ulna when the elbow is fully flexed. The **radial fossa** is the shallow depression on the distal, anterior end of the humerus, immediately proximal to the capitulum. This receives the margin of the head of the radius when the elbow is fully flexed. The **olecranon fossa** is the deep depression on the distal, posterior end of the humerus, immediately proximal to the trochlea. This holds the apex of the olecranon process of the ulna when the elbow is extended.

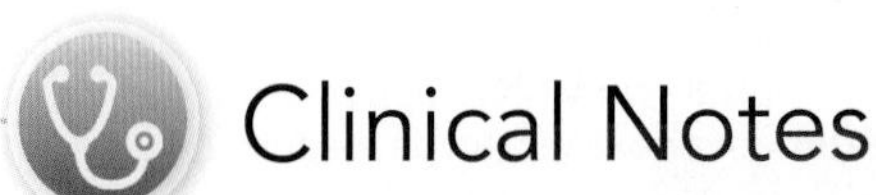

Proximal End of Humerus Fracture

Refer to Figure 3.5A to visualize the fractures described here.

Humeral Head Fracture

Fractures of the humeral head can occur during the process of anterior and posterior dislocations of the shoulder joint. The fibrocartilaginous glenoid labrum of the scapula produces the fracture, and the labrum can become jammed in the defect, making reduction of the shoulder joint difficult.

Greater Tuberosity Fracture

The greater tuberosity of the humerus can be fractured by direct trauma, displaced by the glenoid labrum during dislocation of the shoulder joint, or avulsed by violent contractions of the supraspinatus muscle. The bone fragment will hold the attachments of the supraspinatus, teres minor, and infraspinatus muscles, whose tendons form part of the rotator cuff. When associated with a shoulder dislocation, severe tearing of the rotator cuff with the fracture can result in the greater tuberosity remaining displaced posteriorly after the shoulder joint has been reduced. In this situation, open reduction of the fracture is necessary to attach the rotator cuff back into place.

Lesser Tuberosity Fracture

Occasionally, a lesser tuberosity fracture accompanies posterior dislocation of the shoulder joint. The bone fragment receives the insertion of the subscapularis tendon, a part of the rotator cuff.

(continued)

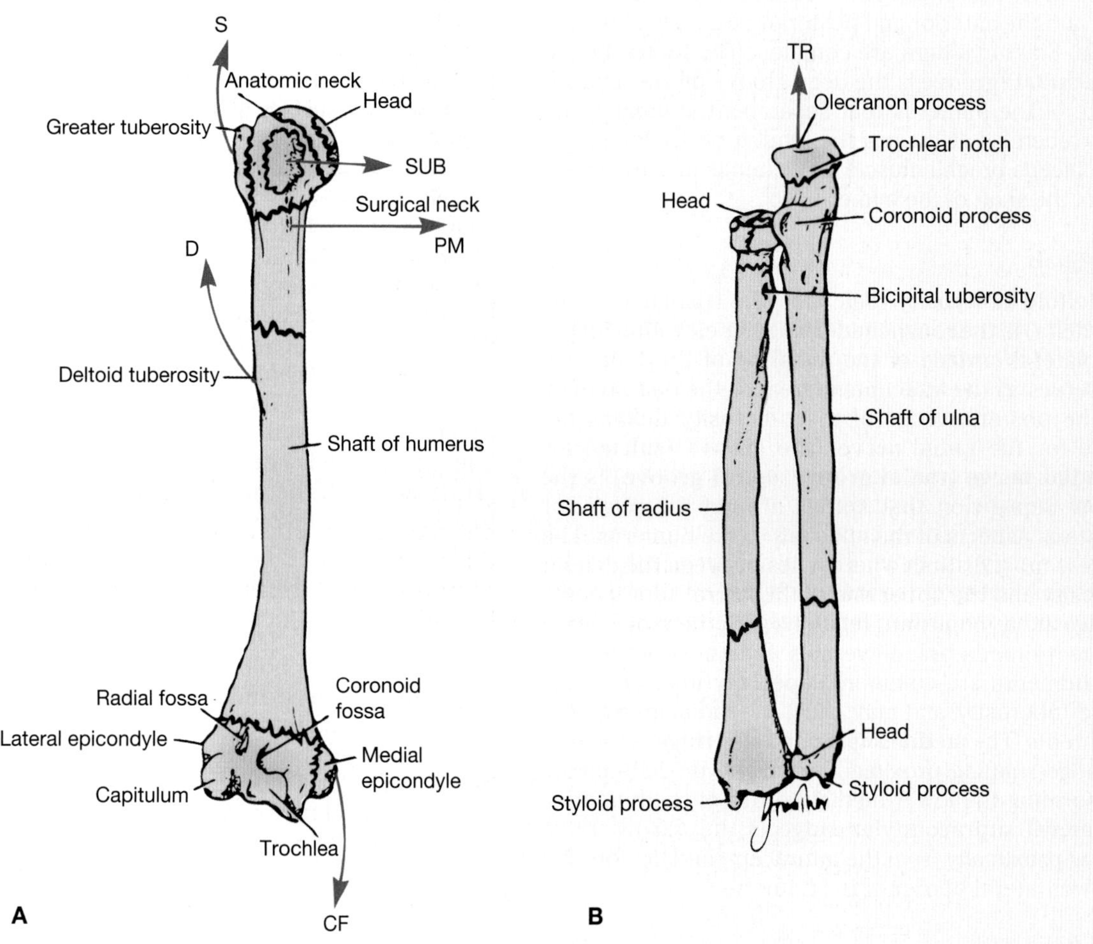

Figure 3.5 **A.** Common fractures of the humerus. **B.** Common fractures of the radius and ulna. The *red arrows* indicate the direction of displacement of the bony fragments on the site of the fracture line and the pull of the responsible muscles. CF, pull of common flexure muscles; D, deltoid; PM, pectoralis major; S, supraspinatus; SUB, subscapularis; TR, triceps.

Surgical Neck Fracture

The surgical neck of the humerus, which lies immediately distal to the lesser tuberosity, can be fractured by a direct blow on the lateral aspect of the shoulder or indirectly by falling on the outstretched hand. The axillary nerve and circumflex humeral blood vessels have close relations to the surgical neck and can be readily damaged in association with a fracture here.

Shaft of Humerus Fracture

Fractures of the humeral shaft are common; displacement of the fragments depends on the relation of the site of fracture to the insertion of the deltoid muscle. When the fracture line is proximal to the deltoid insertion, the pectoralis major, latissimus dorsi, and teres major muscles adduct the proximal fragment; the deltoid, biceps, and triceps pull the distal fragment proximally. When the fracture is distal to the deltoid insertion, the proximal fragment is abducted by the deltoid, and the biceps and triceps pull the distal fragment proximally. The radial nerve can be damaged where it lies in the spiral groove on the posterior surface of the humerus under cover of the triceps muscle.

Distal End of Humerus Fracture

Supracondylar fractures are common in children and occur when falling on the outstretched hand with the elbow partially flexed. Injuries to the median, radial, and ulnar nerves are not uncommon, although function usually quickly returns after reduction of the fracture. Damage to or pressure on the brachial artery can occur at the time of the fracture or from swelling of the surrounding tissues; the circulation to the forearm may be interfered with, leading to Volkmann ischemic contracture (see the Clinical Notes on the forearm).

The medial collateral ligament of the elbow can avulse the medial epicondyle if the forearm is forcibly abducted. The ulnar nerve can be injured at the time of the fracture, can become involved later in the repair process of the fracture (in the callus), or can undergo irritation on the irregular bony surface after the bone fragments are reunited.

Radius

The radius (*radi* is Latin for "spoke" or "ray") is the bone on the lateral side of the forearm (antebrachium). Proximally, it articulates with both the capitulum of the humerus and the radial notch of the ulna in the elbow joint. Distally, it articulates with the head of the ulna and the scaphoid and lunate bones in the wrist. During pronation and supination, the radius rotates on its long axis at its proximal end and circumducts the ulna at its distal end. The major muscle and ligament attachments to the radius are shown in Figure 3.6.

The **head** is the expanded, round, proximal end of the radius. Its proximal surface is a shallow concavity for articulation with the capitulum of the humerus. Its periphery articulates with the radial notch of the ulna. The head is held in place against the ulna by the encircling annular ligament. Note that the head of the radius is at its proximal end, whereas the head of the ulna is at its distal end. The **neck** is the constricted area immediately distal to the head. The **radial tuberosity** is the raised, mostly roughened area on the anteromedial, proximal aspect of the radius, just distal to the neck. This is the insertion site of the biceps brachii muscle. The **body** (**shaft**) is the elongated midportion of the radius. It widens along its proximal to distal extent. The medial border of the shaft forms a sharp crest (**interosseous border**) for the attachment of the interosseous membrane that binds together the radius and ulna. The **ulnar notch** is the shallow depression on the distal, medial aspect of the radius. This is the articular surface for the head of the ulna. The **styloid process** (*styl* is Greek for "pointed instrument") is the distal projection from the lateral, distal aspect of the radius. This extends lateral to the proximal row of carpal bones. The **carpal articular surface** forms the distal surface of the radius. This area articulates with the scaphoid (laterally) and lunate (medially) bones.

Ulna

The ulna (*ulna* is Latin for "elbow") lies on the medial side of the forearm (antebrachium). Proximally, the ulna articulates with both the trochlea of the humerus and the head of the radius, in the elbow joint. Distally, it articulates with the ulnar notch of the radius. Its large, hook-shaped proximal end characterizes the bone. The

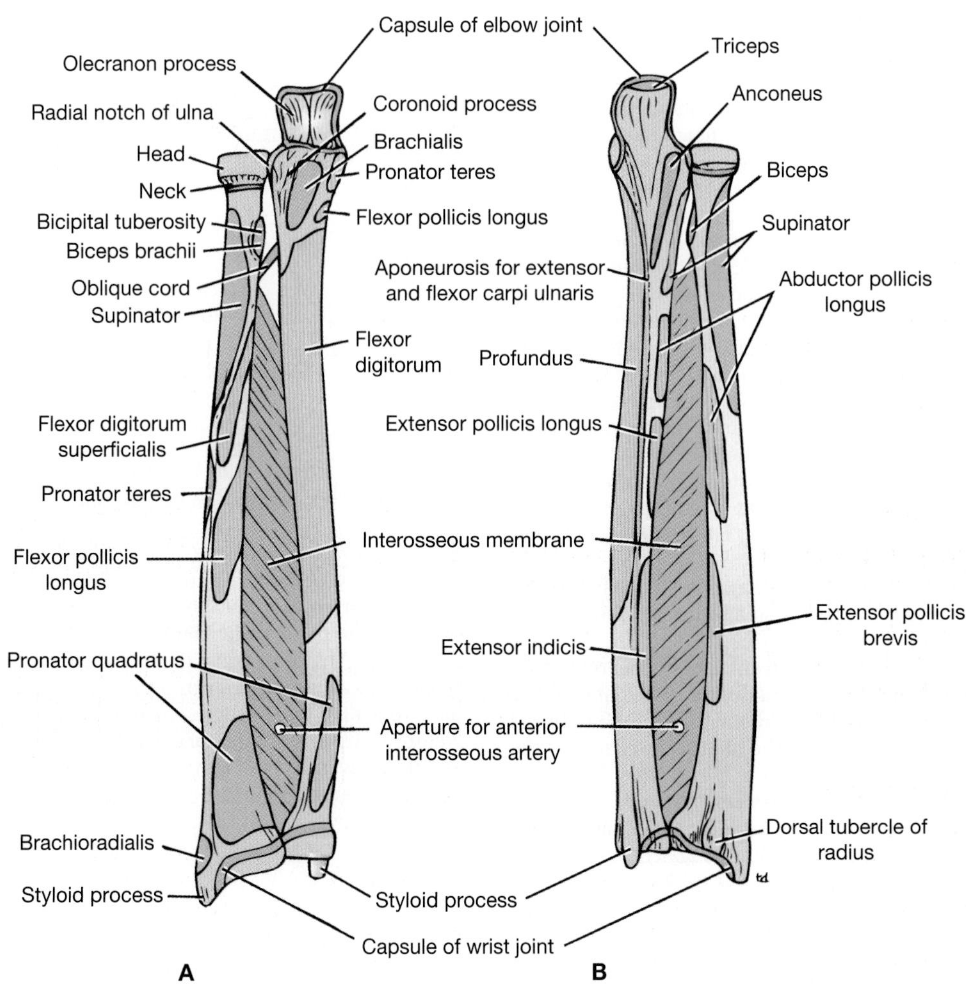

Figure 3.6 Important muscular and ligamentous attachments to the radius and the ulna. **A.** Anterior surface. **B.** Posterior surface.

major muscle and ligament attachments to the ulna are shown in Figure 3.6.

The **olecranon** (*olecran* is Greek for "elbow") is the easily palpable proximal end of the ulna that forms the "point" of the elbow. It is the insertion site of the triceps brachii muscle. The beaklike tip of the olecranon fits into the olecranon fossa of the humerus when the elbow is extended. The **coronoid process** (*coron* is Greek for "resembling a crow") is the anterior projection forming the inferior end of the hooklike proximal end of the ulna. It contributes to the formation of the trochlear notch. The **trochlear notch** is the large, crescent-shaped notch on the anterior aspect of the proximal end of the ulna. It is formed by the articular surfaces of the olecranon and the coronoid process and articulates with the trochlea of the humerus. The **radial notch** is the shallow, smooth notch on the lateral aspect of the coronoid process, immediately distal to the trochlear notch. It is the articular surface for the head of the radius. The **ulnar tuberosity** is the anterior, distal, roughened aspect of the coronoid process. This serves as the insertion area for the brachialis muscle. The **body** (**shaft**) is the elongated midportion of the ulna. In contradistinction to the radius, the body of the ulna tapers along its proximodistal length. The posterior aspect of the body is rounded and subcutaneous and easily palpable along its entire length. The lateral border of the shaft forms a sharp crest (**interosseous border**) for the attachment of the interosseous membrane. The **head** is the small, rounded distal end of the ulna. This has an articular surface on its lateral side for contact with the ulnar notch of the radius. However, the distal end of the head is separated and excluded from the wrist joint by an articular disc. The **styloid process** is a small projection from the posteromedial, distal end of the ulna.

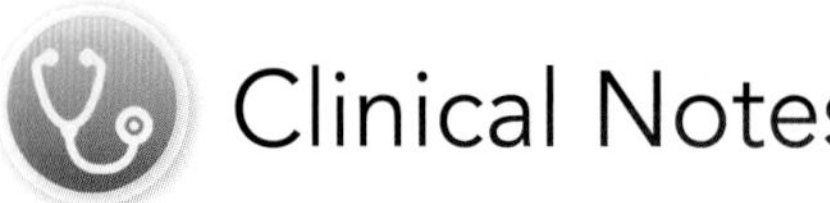

Clinical Notes

Ulnar and Radial Fractures

Fractures of the head of the radius can occur from falls on the outstretched hand. As the force is transmitted along the radius, the head of the radius is driven sharply against the capitulum, splitting or splintering the head (see Fig. 3.5B).

Fractures of the neck of the radius occur more often in young children from falls on the outstretched hand (see Fig. 3.5B).

Fractures of the shafts of the radius and ulna may or may not occur together (see Fig. 3.5B). Displacement of the fragments is usually considerable and depends on the pull of the attached muscles. The supinator and biceps brachii muscles supinate the proximal fragment of the radius. The pronator quadratus muscle pronates and medially deviates the distal fragment of the radius. The strength of the brachioradialis and extensor carpi radialis longus and brevis muscles shortens and angulates the forearm. In fractures of the ulna, the ulna angulates posteriorly. To restore the normal movements of pronation and supination, the normal anatomic relationship of the radius, ulna, and interosseous membrane must be regained.

A fracture of one forearm bone may be associated with a dislocation of the other bone. In a **Monteggia fracture**, a force applied from behind fractures the shaft of the ulna. The ulnar shaft bows forward and anterior dislocation of the radial head occurs with rupture of the annular ligament. In a **Galeazzi fracture**, the middle to distal third of the radius is fractured, and the distal end of the ulna is dislocated at the distal radioulnar joint.

Fractures of the olecranon process can result from a fall on the flexed elbow or from a direct blow. Depending on the location of the fracture line, the bony fragment may be displaced by the pull of the triceps muscle, which is inserted on the olecranon process (see Fig. 3.5). Avulsion fractures of part of the olecranon process can be produced by the pull of the triceps muscle. Return of function after any of these fractures depends on accurate anatomic reduction of the fragment.

The **Colles fracture** is a fracture of the distal end of the radius resulting from a fall on the outstretched hand. It commonly occurs in patients older than age 50 years. The force drives the distal fragment posteriorly and superiorly, and the distal articular surface is inclined posteriorly (Fig. 3.7A). This posterior displacement produces a posterior bump, sometimes referred to as the "dinner-fork deformity" because the forearm and wrist resemble that shape. Failure to restore the distal articular surface to its normal position severely limits the range of flexion of the wrist joint. The **Smith fracture** is a fracture of the distal end of the radius and occurs from a fall on the back of the hand (see Fig. 3.7B). It is a reversed Colles fracture because the distal fragment is displaced anteriorly.

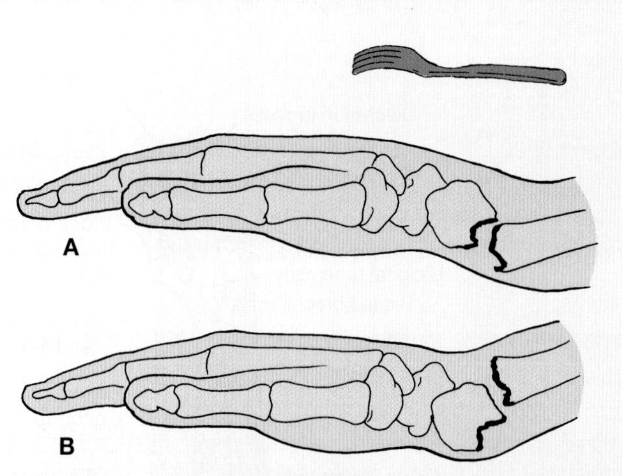

Figure 3.7 Fractures of the distal end of the radius. **A.** Colles fracture. **B.** Smith fracture.

Olecranon Bursitis

A small subcutaneous bursa is present over the olecranon process of the ulna, and repeated wear or trauma often produces chronic bursitis.

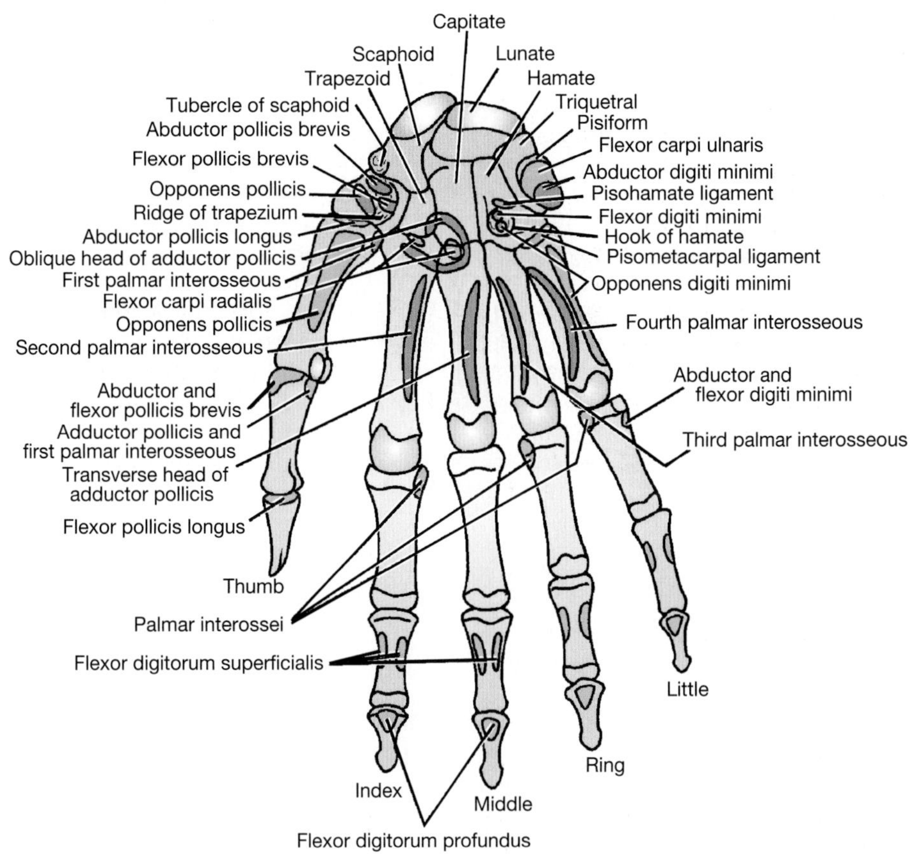

Figure 3.8 Important muscular attachments to the anterior surfaces of the bones of the hand.

Carpal Bones

The carpal (*carp* is Greek for "wrist") bones are the eight small bones comprising the wrist (Figs. 3.8 and 3.9). They are arranged in two rows (proximal and distal), with four bones in each row. The arrangement of the bones forms a deep concave groove on the anterior (ventral) aspect of the wrist. This groove is roofed over by a strong ligamentous band (**flexor retinaculum**), thus forming the osseofascial **carpal tunnel**. The carpal tunnel conveys several flexor tendons and the median nerve into the hand. Compression of the tunnel space and/or trauma to its contents results in **carpal tunnel syndrome**. The bones of the hand are cartilaginous at birth. The capitate begins to ossify during the 1st year, and the others begin to ossify at intervals thereafter until the 12th year, when all the bones are ossified.

Learn the carpal bones as an articulated group, rather than as individually separate items. A mnemonic helpful for remembering the carpal bones is "Some lovers try positions that they cannot handle." The first letter of each word represents the first letter of each carpal bone, arranged by row (proximal row first), from lateral to medial.

Proximal Row

From lateral to medial: scaphoid, lunate, triquetrum, and pisiform. The scaphoid and lunate bones articulate with the carpal articular surface of the radius.

The **scaphoid** (*scaph* is Greek for "something hollowed out," such as a bowl, boat, or trough) is the largest, most lateral carpal bone of the proximal row. The scaphoid is in the floor of the anatomical snuffbox. It is fractured frequently by impact on the base of the hand when the wrist is hyperextended and abducted, as when trying to break a fall with the outstretched hand. The **lunate** (*lun* is Latin for "moon") is the roughly semilunar-shaped carpal bone located between the scaphoid and the triquetrum. The **triquetrum** (*triquetr* is Latin for "triangular") is the roughly pyramid-shaped, most medial bone in the proximal carpal row. The pisiform lies anterior to the triquetrum. The **pisiform** (*pis* is Greek for "pea") is the small, pea-shaped, sesamoid bone formed in the tendon of the flexor carpi ulnaris muscle.

Distal Row

From lateral to medial, the trapezium, trapezoid, capitate, and hamate articulate distally with the metacarpal bones of the hand.

The **trapezium** (*trapez* is Greek for "table") is the most lateral carpal bone of the distal row. It forms a saddle joint with the first metacarpal bone, thus allowing the great mobility of the thumb. Remember: "the thumb swings on the trapezium." The **trapezoid** is the bone located between the trapezium and the capitate and is

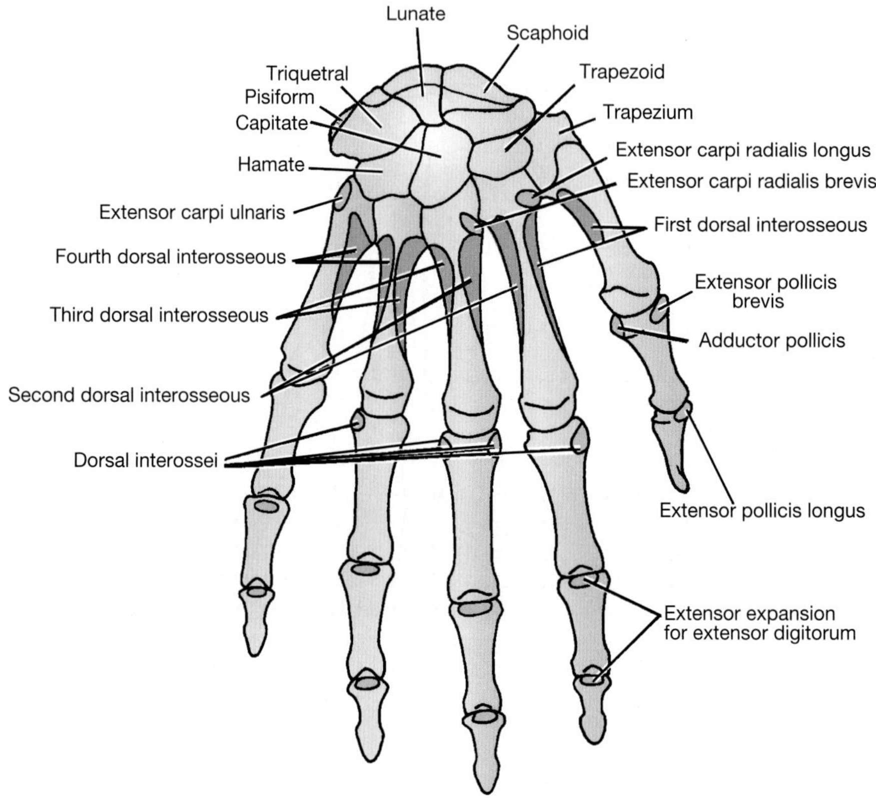

Figure 3.9 Important muscular attachments to the posterior surfaces of the bones of the hand.

named for its trapezoid shape. The **capitate** (recall that *capit* means "head") is the central and largest carpal bone, located between the trapezoid and the hamate. It is named for its rounded head, which sits in the concavity formed by the scaphoid and lunate bones. Forces generated in the hand (as during a punch with the fist) are transmitted through the third metacarpal bone to the capitate, then proximally through the lunate to the radius. The **hamate** (*hamat* is Latin for "hooked") is the most medial bone in the distal carpal row. Its distinguishing feature is the **hamulus** (hook), which is one of the attachment points of the flexor retinaculum.

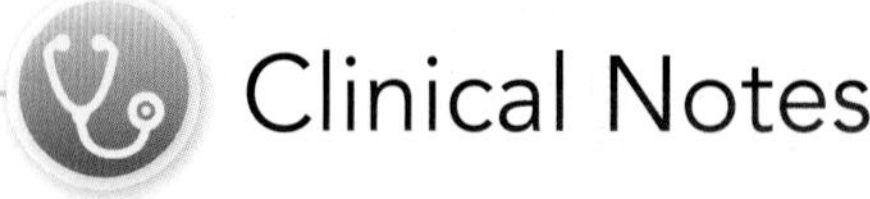

Clinical Notes

Hand Bone Injury

Fracture of the scaphoid bone is common in young adults; unless treated effectively, the fragments will not unite, and permanent weakness and pain of the wrist will result, with the subsequent development of osteoarthritis. The fracture line usually goes through the narrowest part of the bone, which, because of its location, is bathed in synovial fluid. The blood vessels to the scaphoid enter its proximal and distal ends, although the blood supply is occasionally confined to its distal end. If the latter occurs, a fracture deprives the proximal fragment of its arterial supply, and this fragment undergoes avascular necrosis. Deep tenderness in the anatomic snuffbox (see the following discussion of the wrist) after a fall on the outstretched hand in a young adult is suspicious for a fractured scaphoid.

Dislocation of the lunate bone occasionally occurs in young adults who fall on the outstretched hand in a way that causes hyperextension of the wrist joint. Involvement of the median nerve is common.

Fractures of the metacarpal bones can occur because of direct trauma, such as a clenched fist striking a hard object. The fracture always angulates dorsally. The "boxer's fracture" commonly produces an oblique fracture of the neck of the fifth and sometimes the fourth metacarpal bones. The distal fragment is commonly displaced proximally, thus shortening the finger posteriorly. The **Bennett fracture** is a fracture of the base of the metacarpal of the thumb caused when trauma occurs along the long axis of the thumb, or the thumb is forcefully abducted. The fracture is oblique and enters the carpometacarpal joint of the thumb, causing joint instability.

Fractures of the phalanges are common and usually follow direct injury.

Metacarpal Bones

The metacarpal bones are the five bones located between the carpal bones and the phalanges of the hand (see Figs. 3.8 and 3.9). These comprise the body of the hand, whereas the phalanges make up the fingers. The bones are identified by number (1 to 5), starting with the most lateral unit (ie, metacarpal #1 aligns with the thumb). Each bone has a base, body, and head. The **base** is the expanded proximal end that articulates with the distal row of carpal bones. The **body (shaft)** is the elongate, slender midportion that is slightly concave anteriorly and triangular in transverse section. It has posterior, lateral, and medial surfaces. The **head** is the rounded distal end that articulates with the proximal phalanx of the corresponding digit and forms a knuckle. The first metacarpal bone of the thumb is the shortest and most mobile. It does not lie in the same plane as the others but occupies a more anterior position. It is also rotated medially through a right angle so that its extensor surface is directed laterally rather than posteriorly.

Phalanges

The phalanges (*phalan* is Greek for "battle line"; the singular is "phalanx") are the bones that comprise the digits (see Figs. 3.8 and 3.9). As with the metacarpals, each has a base, body (shaft), and head. The thumb has two phalanges (proximal and distal), whereas each other digit has three phalanges (proximal, middle, and distal). Thus, each hand has 14 phalanges in total. The base of each proximal phalanx articulates with the head of the corresponding metacarpal bone. The base of the middle or distal phalanx articulates with the head of the next most proximal phalanx. The body of each distal phalanx is very short.

The head of each proximal and middle phalanx articulates with the base of the next most distal phalanx.

JOINTS

Numerous, mostly synovial, joints allow the great mobility of the upper limb. The shoulder and elbow regions each contain three individual joints. Likewise, the wrist and hand contain multiple joints.

Sternoclavicular Joint

- **Articulation:** Occurs between the sternal end of the clavicle, manubrium sterni, and the first costal cartilage (Fig. 3.10A).
- **Type:** Synovial double-plane joint.
- **Capsule:** Surrounds the joint and is attached to the margins of the articular surfaces.
- **Ligaments:** Capsule is reinforced in front of and behind the joint by the strong **sternoclavicular ligaments**.
- **Articular disc:** A flat fibrocartilaginous disc lies within the joint and divides the joint's interior into two compartments, medial and lateral. Its circumference is attached to the interior of the joint capsule, but it is also strongly attached to the superior margin of the articular surface of the clavicle above and to the first costal cartilage below.
- **Accessory ligament:** The **costoclavicular ligament** is a strong ligament that runs from the junction of rib 1 with the first costal cartilage to the inferior surface of the sternal end of the clavicle.
- **Synovial membrane:** Lines the joint capsule and is attached to the margins of the cartilage covering the articular surfaces.
- **Nerve supply:** Supraclavicular nerve and the nerve to the subclavius muscle.

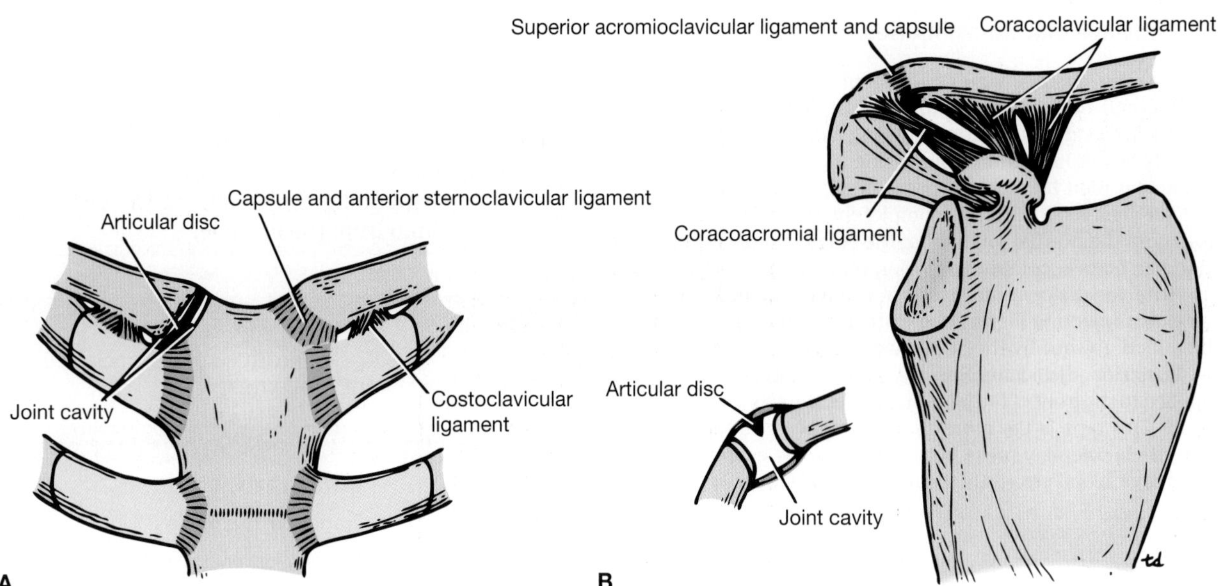

Figure 3.10 **A.** Sternoclavicular joint. **B.** Acromioclavicular joint.

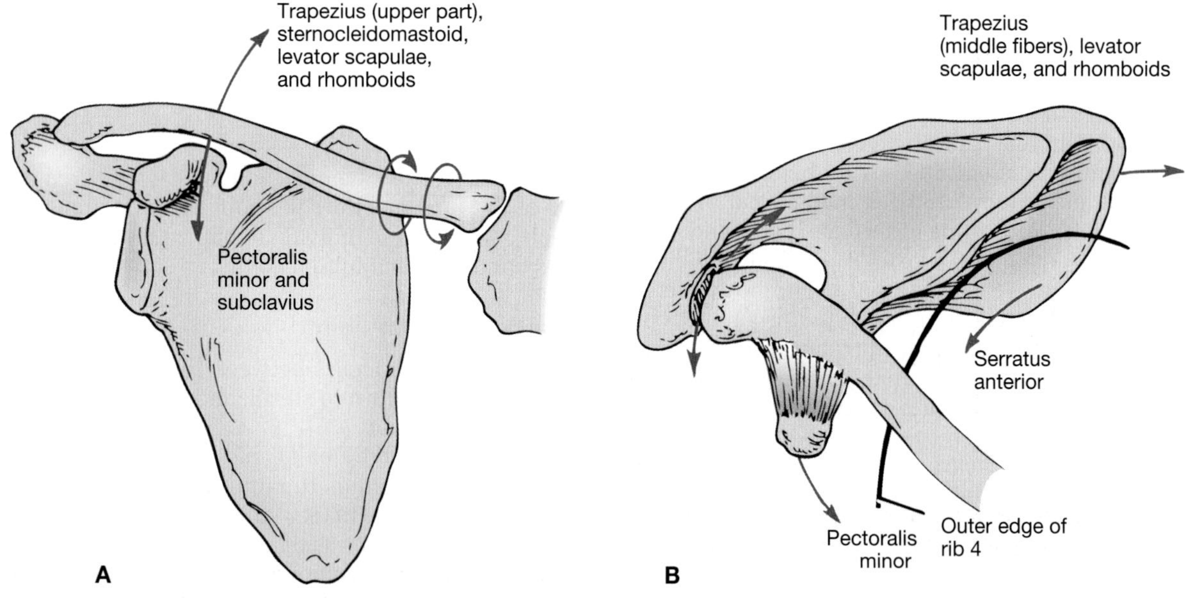

Figure 3.11 Wide range of movements possible at the sternoclavicular and the acromioclavicular joints gives great mobility to the clavicle and the upper limb. **A.** Movements at the sternoclavicular joint. **B.** Movements at the acromioclavicular joint.

Movements

Forward and backward movement of the clavicle takes place in the medial joint compartment. Elevation and depression take place in the lateral compartment (Fig. 3.11A). Multiple muscles act to produce movement at this joint (Table 3.1).

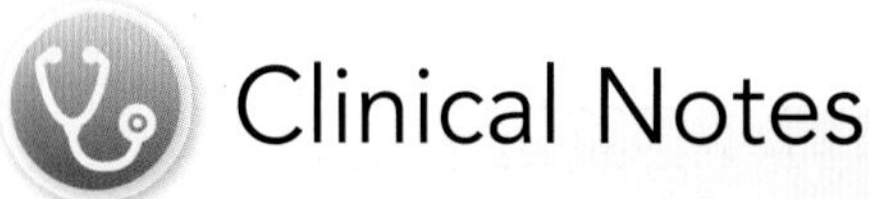

Clinical Notes

Sternoclavicular Joint Injuries

The strong costoclavicular ligament firmly holds the medial end of the clavicle to the first costal cartilage. Strong forces directed along the long axis of the clavicle usually result in fracture, but dislocation of the sternoclavicular joint takes place occasionally. If the costoclavicular ligament ruptures completely, it is difficult to maintain the normal position of the clavicle once reduction has been accomplished.

Anterior dislocation results in the medial end of the clavicle projecting forward beneath the skin; it may also be pulled upward by the SCM muscle.

Posterior dislocation usually follows direct trauma applied to the front of the joint that drives the clavicle backward. This type is the more serious one because the displaced clavicle may press on the trachea, the esophagus, and major blood vessels in the root of the neck.

Important Relations

- **Anteriorly:** Skin and some fibers of the SCM and pectoralis major muscles
- **Posteriorly:** Sternohyoid muscle; on the right, the brachiocephalic artery; on the left, the left brachiocephalic vein and the left common carotid artery

Acromioclavicular Joint

- **Articulation:** Occurs between the acromion of the scapula and the lateral end of the clavicle (see Fig. 3.10B).
- **Type:** Synovial plane joint.
- **Capsule:** Surrounds the joint and is attached to the margins of the articular surfaces.
- **Ligaments: Superior** and **inferior acromioclavicular ligaments** reinforce the capsule. A wedge-shaped fibrocartilaginous disc projects into the joint cavity from the capsule, from above.
- **Accessory ligament:** The very strong **coracoclavicular ligament** extends from the coracoid process to the undersurface of the clavicle and is largely responsible for suspending the weight of the scapula and the upper limb from the clavicle.

Table 3.1 Muscles Producing Sternoclavicular Joint Movement

MOVEMENT	MUSCLES
Forward	Serratus anterior
Backward	Trapezius, rhomboids
Elevation	Sternocleidomastoid, trapezius, rhomboids, levator scapulae
Depression	Pectoralis minor, subclavius

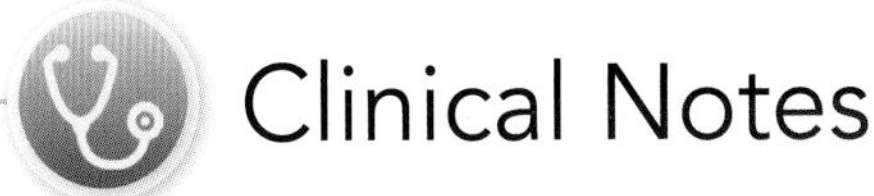

Clinical Notes

Acromioclavicular Joint Injuries

The plane of the articular surfaces of the acromioclavicular joint passes downward and medially so that the lateral end of the clavicle tends to ride up over the upper surface of the acromion. The strength of the joint depends on the strong coracoclavicular ligament, which binds the coracoid process to the undersurface of the lateral part of the clavicle. The greater part of the weight of the upper limb is transmitted to the clavicle through this ligament, and rotary movements of the scapula occur at this important ligament.

Acromioclavicular Dislocation

A severe blow on the point of the shoulder, as is incurred during blocking or tackling in football or any severe fall, can result in the acromion being thrust beneath the lateral end of the clavicle, tearing the coracoclavicular ligament. This condition is known as **shoulder separation**. The displaced outer end of the clavicle is easily palpable. As in the case of the sternoclavicular joint, the dislocation is easily reduced, but withdrawal of support results in immediate redislocation.

- **Synovial membrane:** Lines the capsule and is attached to the margins of the cartilage covering the articular surfaces.
- **Nerve supply:** Suprascapular nerve.

Movements

A gliding movement takes place when the scapula rotates or when the clavicle is elevated or depressed (see Fig. 3.11B).

Important Relations

- **Anteriorly:** Deltoid muscle
- **Posteriorly:** Trapezius muscle
- **Superiorly:** Skin

Glenohumeral Joint (Shoulder Joint)

- **Articulation:** This occurs between the rounded head of the humerus and the shallow, pear-shaped glenoid cavity of the scapula (Figs. 3.12 and 3.13). The articular surfaces are covered by hyaline articular cartilage, and the glenoid cavity is deepened by the presence of a fibrocartilaginous rim termed the **glenoid labrum** (Figs. 3.12B and 3.14).
- **Type:** Synovial ball-and-socket joint.
- **Capsule:** This surrounds the joint and is attached medially to the margin of the glenoid cavity outside the labrum; laterally, it is attached to the anatomic neck of the humerus. The capsule is thin and lax, allowing a wide range of movement. Fibrous slips from the tendons of the subscapularis, supraspinatus, infraspinatus, and teres minor muscles (rotator cuff muscles) strengthen the capsule.
- **Ligaments:** The **glenohumeral ligaments** are three weak bands of fibrous tissue that strengthen the front of the capsule. The **transverse humeral ligament** strengthens the capsule, bridges the gap between the two tuberosities, and holds the tendon of the long head of the biceps muscle in place. The **coracohumeral ligament** strengthens the capsule above and stretches from the root of the coracoid process to the greater tuberosity of the humerus.
- **Accessory ligaments:** The **coracoacromial ligament** extends between the coracoid process and the acromion. Its function is to protect the superior aspect of the joint.
- **Synovial membrane:** This lines the capsule and is attached to the margins of the cartilage covering the articular surfaces (see Figs. 3.12A and 3.14). It forms a tubular sheath around the tendon of the long head of the biceps brachii. It extends through the anterior wall of the capsule to form the subscapularis bursa beneath the subscapularis muscle.
- **Nerve supply:** Axillary and suprascapular nerves.

Movements

The shoulder joint has a wide range of movement, and the stability of the joint has been sacrificed to permit this. (Compare with the hip joint, which is stable but limited in its movements.) The strength of the joint depends on the tone of the short rotator cuff muscles that cross in front, above, and behind the joint—namely, the subscapularis, supraspinatus, infraspinatus, and teres minor. When the joint is abducted, the lower surface of the head of the humerus is supported by the long head of the triceps, which bows downward because of its length and gives little actual support to the humerus. In addition, the inferior part of the capsule is the weakest area.

As shown in Figure 3.15, the following movements are possible:

- **Flexion:** Normal flexion is about 90° and is performed by the anterior fibers of the deltoid, pectoralis major, biceps, and coracobrachialis muscles.
- **Extension:** Normal extension is about 45° and is performed by the posterior fibers of the deltoid, latissimus dorsi, and teres major muscles.
- **Abduction:** Abduction of the upper limb occurs both at the shoulder joint and between the scapula and the thoracic wall (see the Scapular–Humeral Mechanism section). The middle fibers of the deltoid, assisted by the supraspinatus, are involved. The supraspinatus muscle initiates the movement of abduction and holds the head of the humerus against the glenoid fossa of the scapula; this latter function allows the deltoid muscle to contract and abduct the humerus at the shoulder joint.

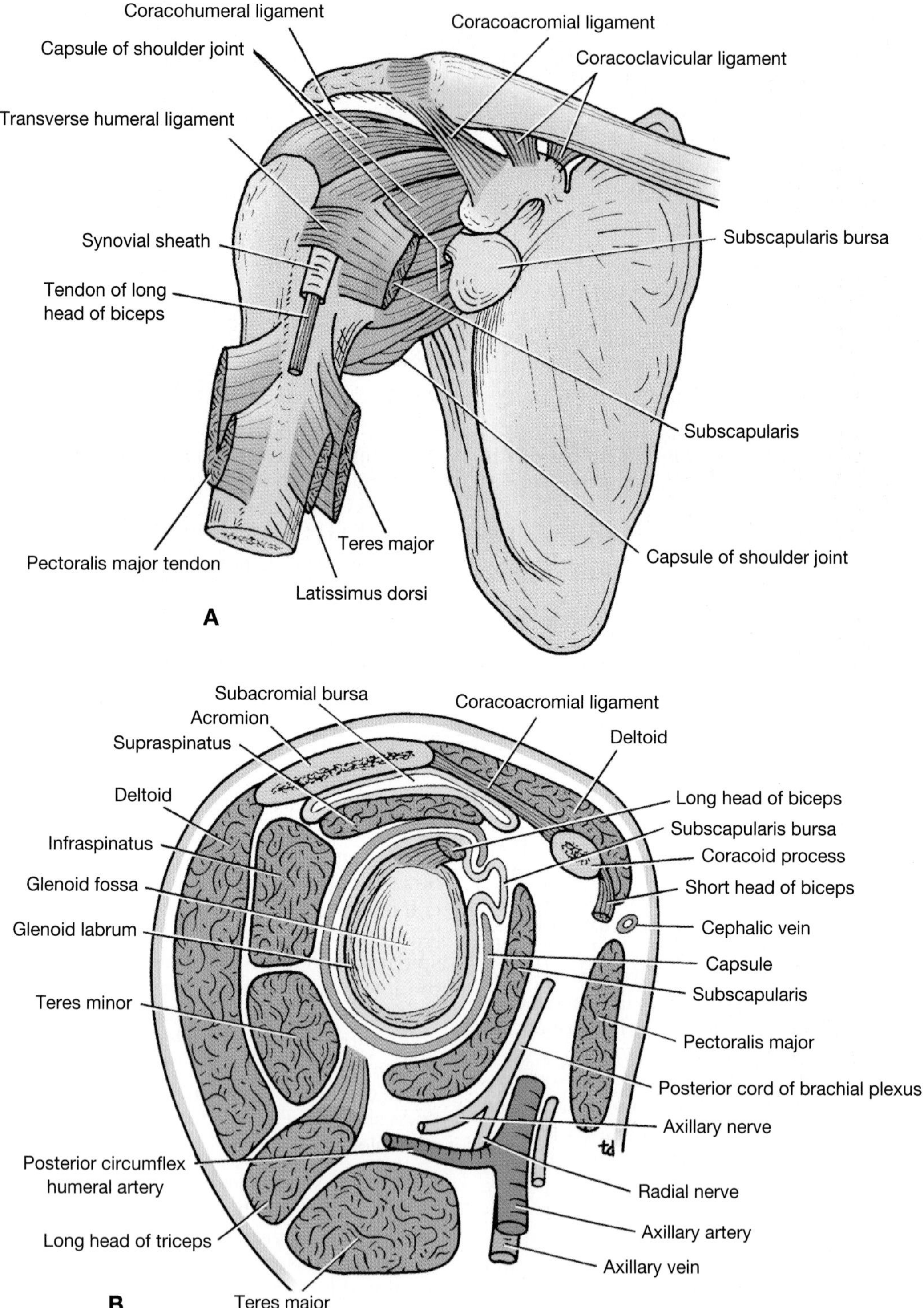

Figure 3.12 Shoulder joint and its relations. **A.** Anterior view. **B.** Sagittal section.

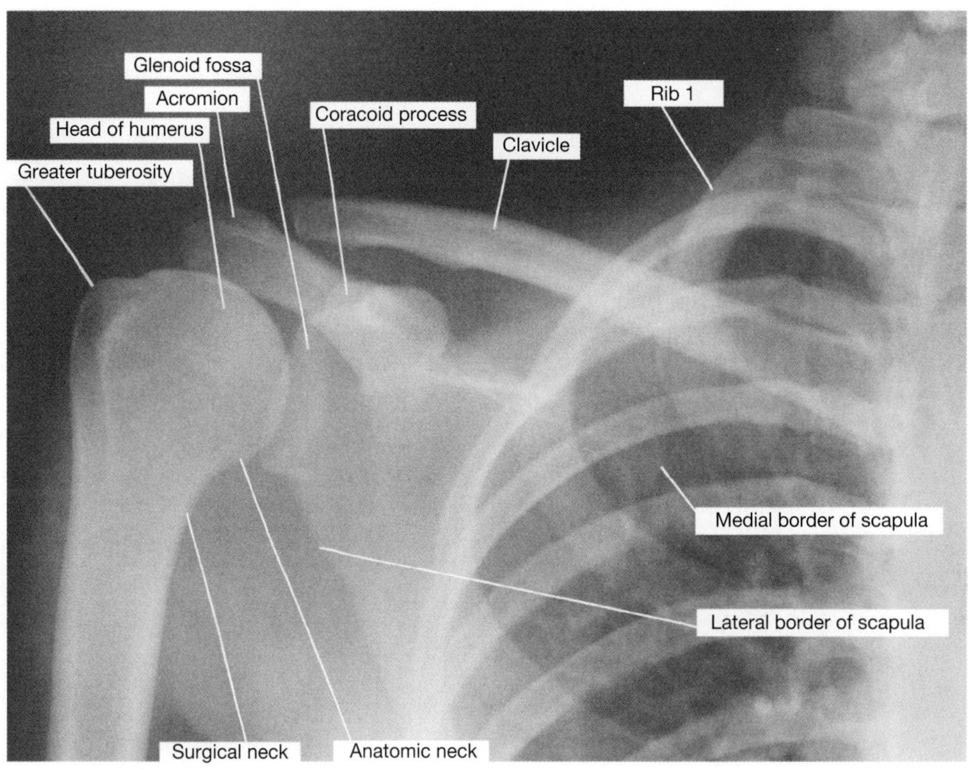

Figure 3.13 Anteroposterior radiograph of the shoulder region in the adult.

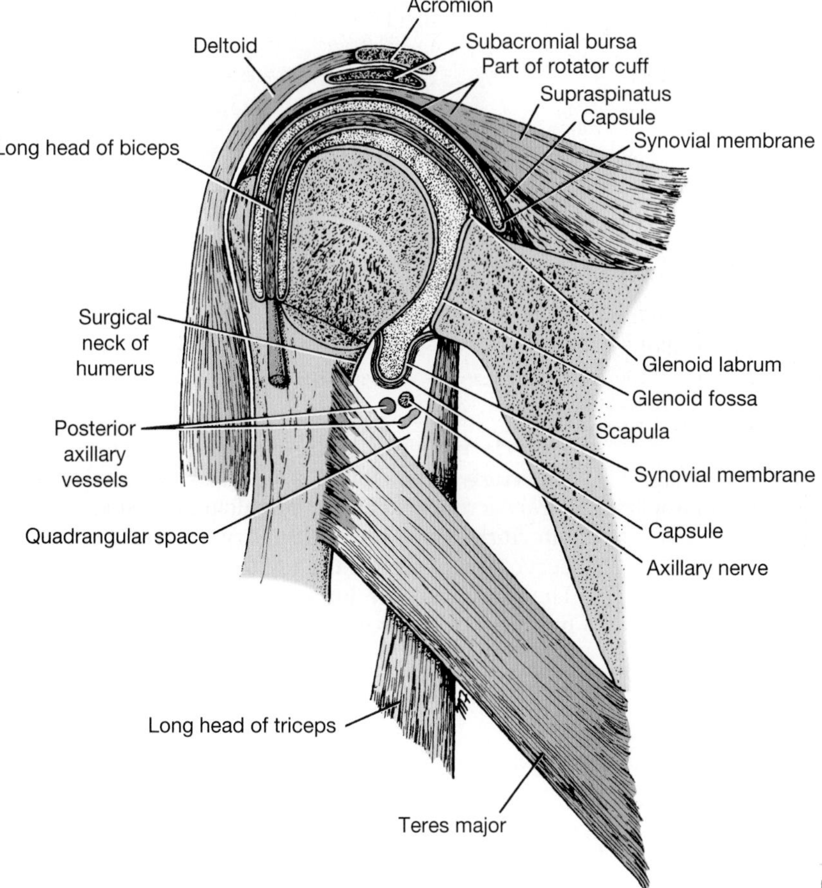

Figure 3.14 Interior of the shoulder joint.

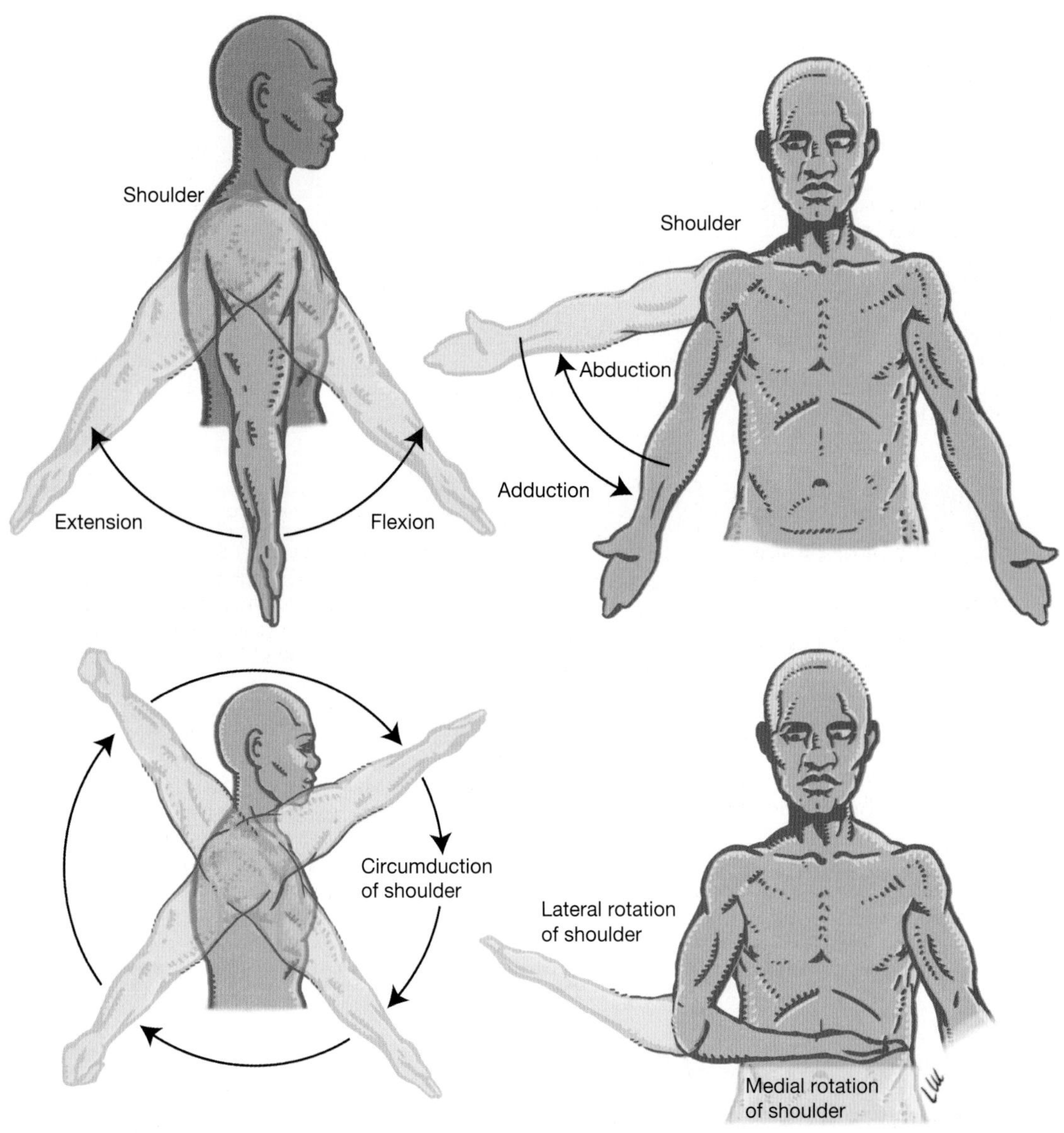

Figure 3.15 Movements possible at the shoulder joint. Pure glenohumeral abduction is possible only as much as about 120°; further movement of the upper limb above the level of the shoulder requires rotation of the scapula (see text).

- **Adduction:** Normally, the upper limb can be swung 45° across the front of the chest by the pectoralis major, latissimus dorsi, teres major, and teres minor muscles.
- **Lateral rotation:** Normal lateral rotation is 40° to 45° by the infraspinatus, teres minor, and the posterior fibers of the deltoid muscle.
- **Medial rotation:** Normal medial rotation is about 55° by the subscapularis, latissimus dorsi, teres major, and the anterior fibers of the deltoid muscle.
- **Circumduction:** This is a combination of the above movements.

Important Relations

- **Anteriorly:** Subscapularis muscle, axillary vessels, and brachial plexus.
- **Posteriorly:** Infraspinatus and teres minor muscles.
- **Superiorly:** Supraspinatus muscle, subacromial bursa, coracoacromial ligament, and deltoid muscle.
- **Inferiorly:** Long head of the triceps muscle, axillary nerve, and posterior circumflex humeral vessels.
- The **tendon of the long head of the biceps brachii muscle** passes through the joint and emerges beneath the transverse humeral ligament (see Figs. 3.12 and 3.14).

Scapular–Humeral Mechanism

The scapula and upper limb are suspended from the clavicle by the strong coracoclavicular ligament assisted by the tone of muscles. When the scapula rotates on the chest wall so that the position of the glenoid fossa is

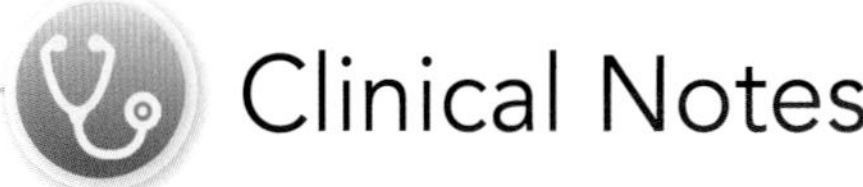

Clinical Notes

Shoulder Joint Stability

The shallowness of the glenoid fossa of the scapula and the lack of support provided by weak ligaments make this joint an unstable structure. Its strength almost entirely depends on the tone of the short muscles that bind the upper end of the humerus to the scapula—namely, the subscapularis in front, supraspinatus above, and infraspinatus and teres minor behind. The tendons of these muscles are fused to the underlying capsule of the shoulder joint. Together, they form the rotator cuff. The least supported part of the joint lies in the inferior location, where it is unprotected by muscles.

Shoulder Joint Dislocation

The shoulder joint is the most dislocated large joint.

Anterior–Inferior Dislocation

Sudden violence applied to the humerus with the joint fully abducted tilts the humeral head downward onto the inferior weak part of the capsule, which tears, and the humeral head comes to lie inferior to the glenoid fossa. During this movement, the acromion has acted as a fulcrum. The strong flexors and adductors of the shoulder joint now usually pull the humeral head forward and upward into the **subcoracoid position**.

Posterior Dislocations

Posterior dislocations are rare and are usually caused by direct trauma to the front of the joint.

On inspection of the patient with shoulder dislocation, the rounded appearance of the shoulder is seen to be lost because the greater tuberosity of the humerus is no longer bulging laterally beneath the deltoid muscle. A subglenoid displacement of the head of the humerus into the quadrangular space can cause damage to the axillary nerve, as indicated by paralysis of the deltoid muscle and loss of skin sensation over the lower half of the deltoid (see Figs. 3.12B and 3.14). Downward displacement of the humerus can also stretch and damage the radial nerve (see Fig. 3.12B).

Shoulder Pain

The axillary and suprascapular nerves innervate the synovial membrane, capsule, and ligaments of the shoulder joint. The joint is sensitive to pain, pressure, excessive traction, and distention. The muscles surrounding the joint undergo reflex spasm in response to pain originating in the joint, which, in turn, immobilizes the joint and thus reduces the pain.

Injury to the shoulder joint is followed by pain, limitation of movement, and muscle atrophy from disuse. However, note that pain in the shoulder region can be caused by disease elsewhere, and the shoulder joint may be normal. For example, diseases of the spinal cord and vertebral column and the pressure of a cervical rib can cause shoulder pain. Irritation of the diaphragmatic pleura or peritoneum can produce referred pain via the phrenic and supraclavicular nerves.

altered, the axis of rotation may be considered to pass through the coracoclavicular ligament.

Abduction of the arm involves rotation of the scapula as well as movement at the shoulder joint. For every 3° of abduction of the arm, a 2° abduction occurs in the shoulder joint, and a 1° abduction occurs by rotation of the scapula. At about 120° of abduction of the arm, the greater tuberosity of the humerus contacts the lateral edge of the acromion. Further elevation of the arm above the head is accomplished by rotating the scapula. Figure 3.16 summarizes the movements of abduction of the arm and shows the direction of pull of the muscles responsible for these movements.

Elbow Joint

The elbow joint is a complex of three individual articulating sets that share a common synovial cavity. They are the humeroulnar, humeroradial, and proximal radioulnar joints. Hyaline cartilage covers all the articular surfaces.

- **Articulation:** The humeroulnar joint occurs between the trochlea of the humerus and the trochlear notch of the ulna, the humeroradial joint occurs between the capitulum of the humerus and the head of the radius, and the proximal radioulnar joint occurs between the head of the radius and the radial notch of the ulna (Figs. 3.17 to 3.19).
- **Type:** The humeroulnar joint is a uniaxial hinge joint, the humeroradial joint is a biaxial condyloid joint, and the proximal radioulnar joint is a pivot joint.
- **Capsule:** Anteriorly, it is attached above to the humerus along the upper margins of the coronoid and radial fossae and to the front of the medial and lateral epicondyles and below to the margin of the coronoid process of the ulna and to the annular ligament, which surrounds the head of the radius. Posteriorly, it is attached above to the margins of the olecranon fossa of the humerus and below to the upper margin and sides of the olecranon process of the ulna and to the annular ligament.
- **Ligaments:** The **lateral (radial) collateral ligament** (see Fig. 3.17) is triangular and is attached by its apex to the lateral epicondyle of the humerus and by its base to the upper margin of the **annular ligament**. The **medial (ulnar) collateral ligament** is also triangular and consists principally of three strong bands: the anterior band, which passes from the medial epicondyle of the humerus to the medial margin of the coronoid process; the posterior band, which passes

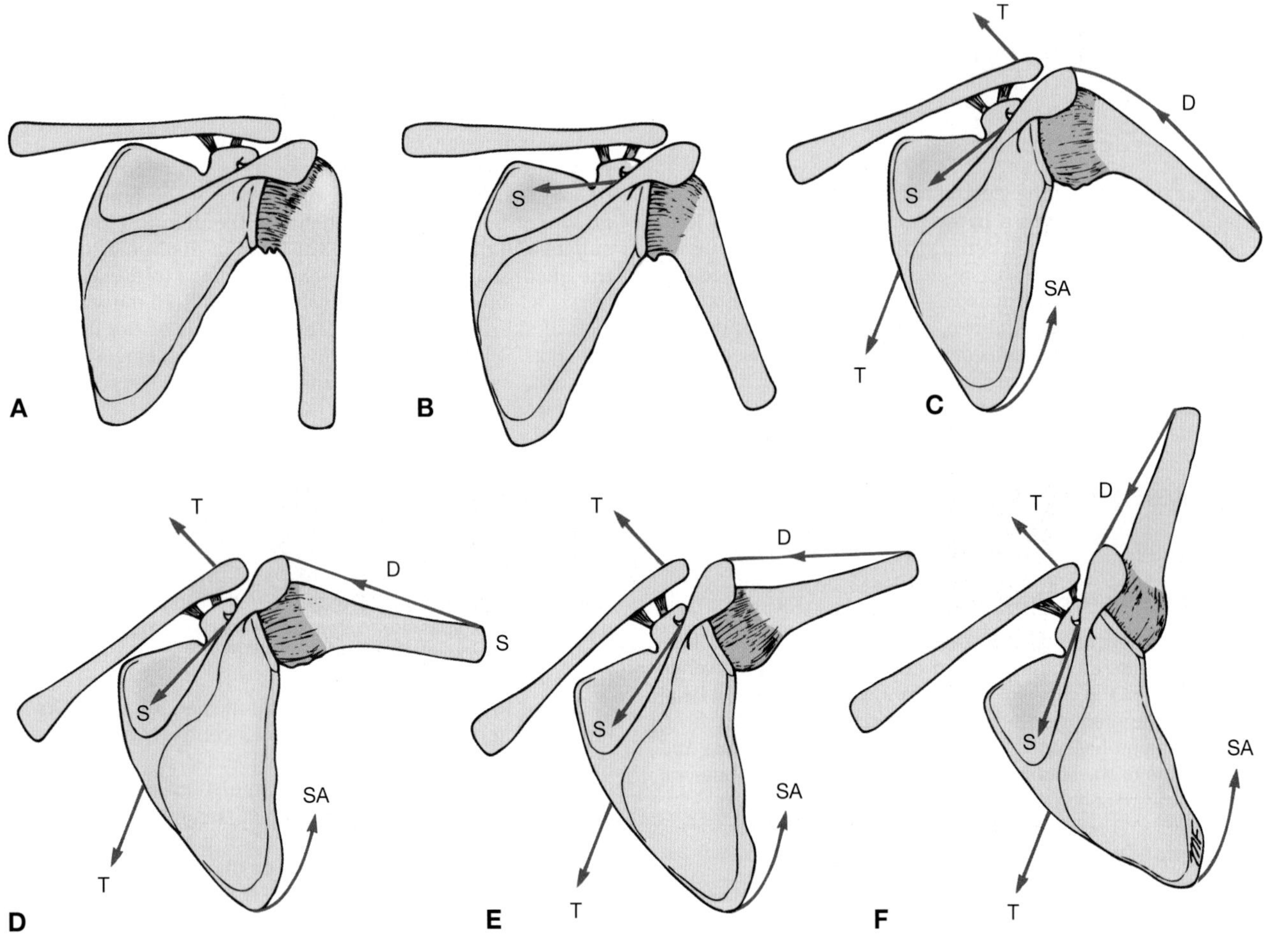

Figure 3.16 Progressive stages **(A–F)** in abduction of the shoulder joint and rotation of the scapula and the muscles producing these movements. **A.** Rest position. **B.** Initiation of abduction. **C–F.** Increasing abduction of humerus plus rotation of scapula. Note that for every 3° of abduction of the arm, a 2° abduction occurs in the shoulder joint, and 1° occurs by rotation of the scapula. At about 120° of abduction, the greater tuberosity of the humerus hits the lateral edge of the acromion. Elevation of the arm above the head is accomplished by rotating the scapula. D, deltoid; S, supraspinatus; SA, serratus anterior; T, trapezius.

from the medial epicondyle of the humerus to the medial side of the olecranon; and the transverse band, which passes between the ulnar attachments of the two preceding bands.

- **Synovial membrane:** This lines the capsule and covers fatty pads in the floors of the coronoid, radial, and olecranon fossae; it is continuous below with the synovial membrane of the proximal radioulnar joint.
- **Nerve supply:** Branches from the median, ulnar, musculocutaneous, and radial nerves.

Movements

The humeroulnar joint is capable of flexion and extension. Flexion is limited by the anterior surfaces of the forearm and arm coming into contact. Extension is checked by the tension of the anterior ligament and the brachialis muscle. The brachialis, biceps brachii, brachioradialis, and pronator teres muscles perform flexion. The triceps and anconeus muscles perform extension. The humeroradial joint permits flexion and extension as just described as well as pivoting of the head of the radius. See the description of the proximal radioulnar joint below for discussion of this movement.

It should be noted that the long axis of the extended forearm lies at an angle to the long axis of the arm. This angle, which opens laterally, is called the **carrying angle** and is about 170° in the male and 167° in the female. The angle disappears when the elbow joint is fully flexed.

Important Relations

- **Anteriorly:** Brachialis, tendon of the biceps, median nerve, and brachial artery.
- **Posteriorly:** Triceps muscle, a small bursa intervening.
- **Medially:** The ulnar nerve passes behind the medial epicondyle and crosses the medial collateral ligament of the joint.
- **Laterally:** Common extensor tendon and the supinator muscle.

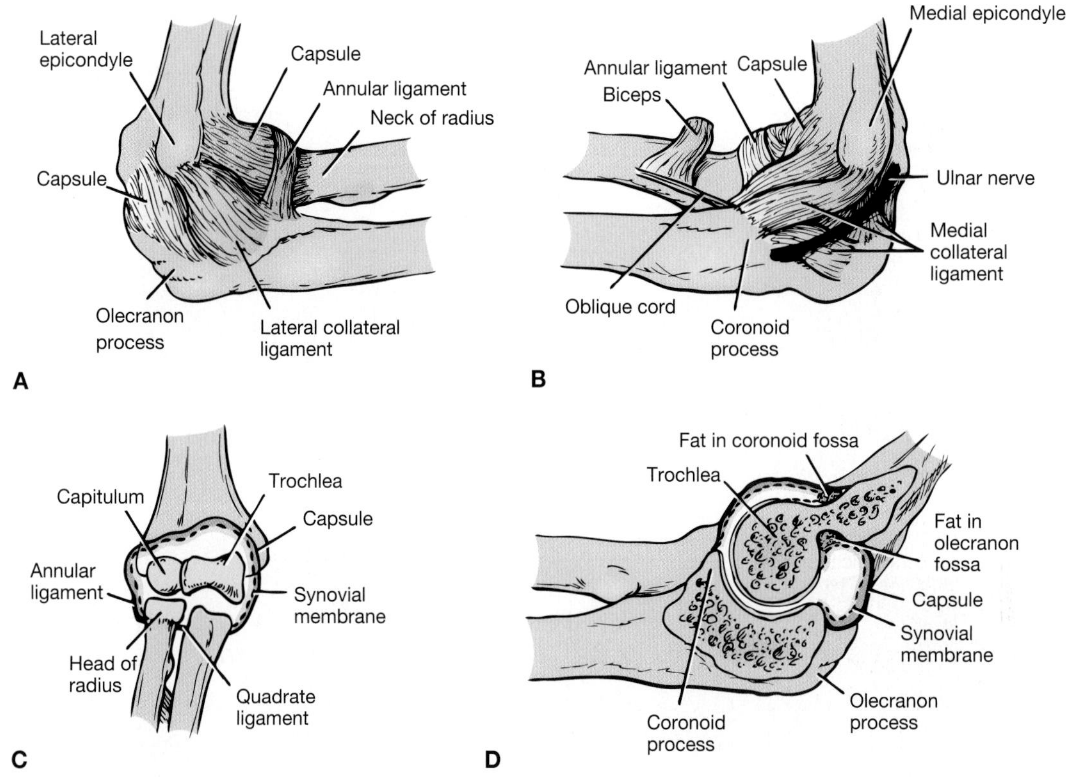

Figure 3.17 Right elbow joint. **A.** Lateral view. **B.** Medial view. **C.** Anterior view of the interior of the joint. **D.** Sagittal section.

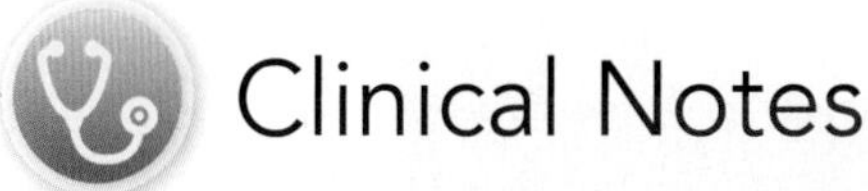

Clinical Notes

Elbow Joint Stability

The elbow joint is stable because of the wrench-shaped articular surface of the olecranon and the pulley-shaped trochlea of the humerus; it also has strong medial and lateral ligaments. When examining the elbow joint, clinicians must remember the normal relations of the bony points. In extension, the medial and lateral epicondyles and the top of the olecranon process are in a straight line; in flexion, the bony points form the boundaries of an equilateral triangle.

Elbow Joint Dislocation

Elbow dislocations are common, and most are posterior displacements of the olecranon. Posterior dislocation usually follows falling on an outstretched hand. Posterior dislocations of the joint are common in children because the parts of the bones that stabilize the joint are incompletely developed. Avulsion of the epiphysis of the medial epicondyle is also common in childhood because the medial ligament is much stronger than the bond of union between the epiphysis and the diaphysis.

Elbow Joint Arthrocentesis

The anterior and posterior walls of the capsule are weak, so when the joint is distended with fluid, the posterior aspect of the joint swells. Aspiration of joint fluid can easily be performed through the back of the joint on either side of the olecranon process.

Ulnar Nerve Damage with Elbow Joint Injuries

The close relationship of the ulnar nerve to the medial side of the humeroulnar joint often results in damage in dislocations of the joint or in fracture dislocations in this region (see Fig. 3.17B). The nerve lesion can occur at the time of injury or weeks, months, or years later. The nerve can be involved in scar tissue formation or can become stretched from lateral deviation of the forearm in a badly reduced supracondylar fracture of the humerus. During movements of the elbow joint, continued friction between the medial epicondyle and the stretched ulnar nerve may eventually result in ulnar palsy.

Radiology of Elbow Region after Injury

In examining lateral radiographs of the elbow region, remember that the lower end of the humerus is normally angulated forward 45° on the shaft; when examining a patient, the clinician should see that the medial epicondyle, in the anatomic position, is directed medially and posteriorly and faces in the same direction as the head of the humerus.

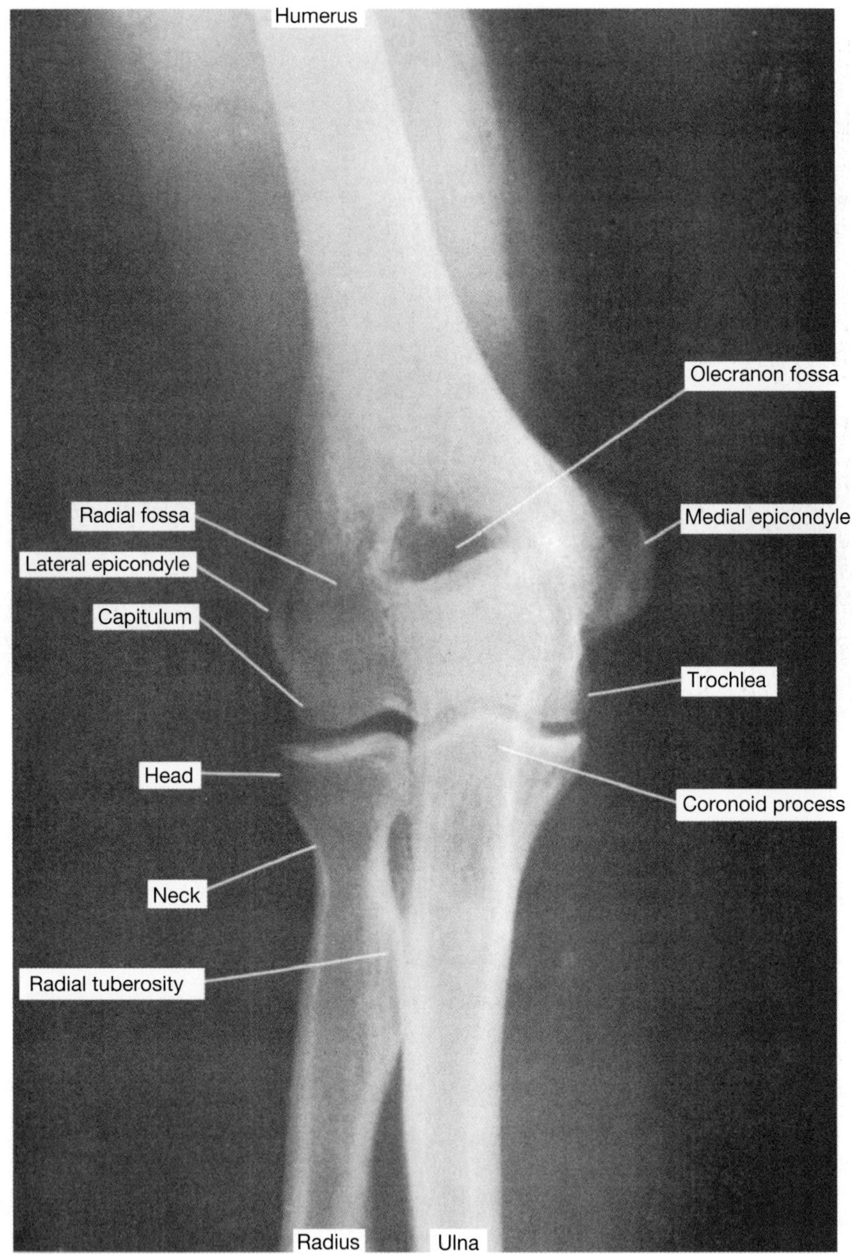

Figure 3.18 Anteroposterior radiograph of the elbow region in the adult.

Proximal Radioulnar Joint

- **Articulation:** Between the circumference of the head of the radius and the annular ligament and the radial notch on the ulna (Fig. 3.20A; see also Fig. 3.17). This constitutes the third joint in the elbow.
- **Type:** Synovial pivot joint.
- **Capsule:** Encloses the joint and is continuous with that of the elbow joint.
- **Ligament:** The **annular ligament** is attached to the anterior and posterior margins of the radial notch on the ulna and forms a collar around the head of the radius (see Fig. 3.20A). It is continuous above with the capsule of the elbow joint and is not attached to the radius.
- **Synovial membrane:** This is continuous above with that of the elbow joint. Below, it is attached to the inferior margin of the articular surface of the radius and the lower margin of the radial notch of the ulna.
- **Nerve supply:** Branches of the median, ulnar, musculocutaneous, and radial nerves.

Movements

The proximal radioulnar joint produces pronation and supination of the forearm (see below).

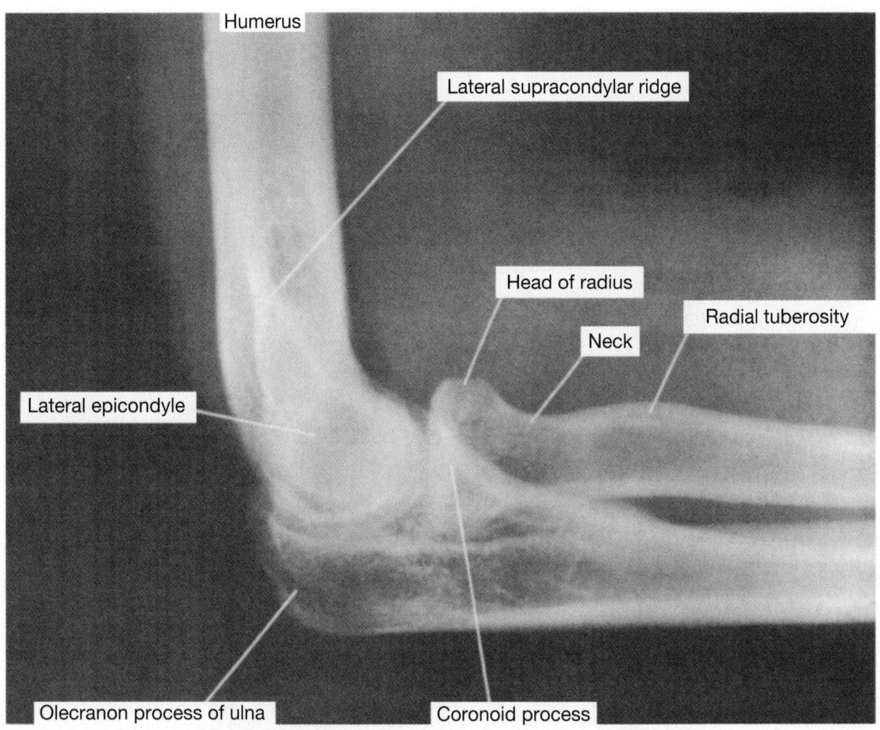

Figure 3.19 Lateral radiograph of the elbow region in the adult.

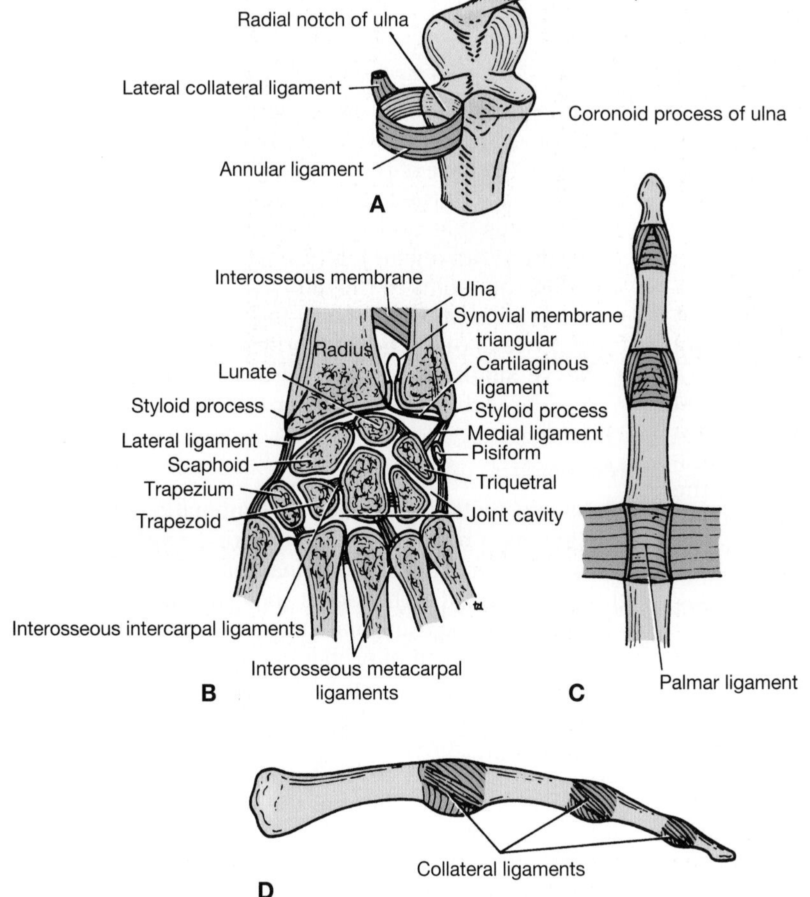

Figure 3.20 Ligaments of the proximal and distal radioulnar joints, wrist joint, carpal joints, and joints of the fingers. **A.** Anterior view of the proximal radioulnar joint. **B.** Anterior view of the distal radioulnar, radiocarpal, and intercarpal joints. **C.** Anterior view of metacarpophalangeal and interphalangeal joints. **D.** Lateral view of metacarpophalangeal and interphalangeal joints.

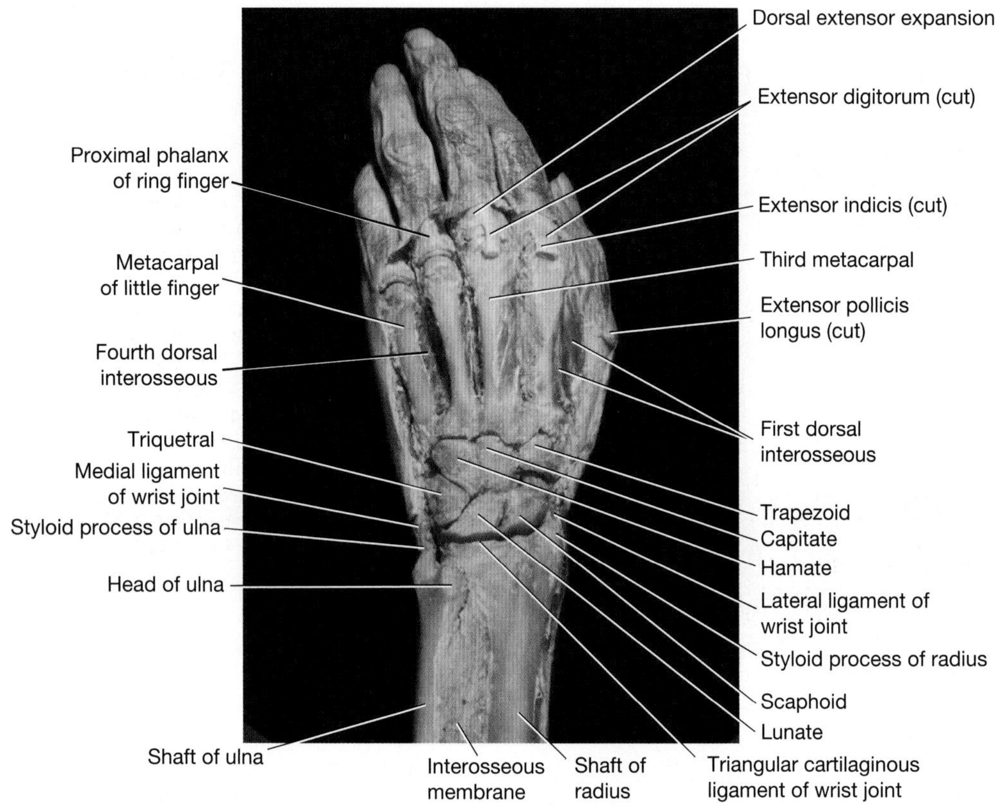

Figure 3.21 Dissection of the dorsal surface of the left hand and distal end of the forearm. Note the carpal bones and the intercarpal joints; also note the wrist (radiocarpal) joint.

Important Relations

- **Anteriorly:** Supinator muscle and the radial nerve
- **Posteriorly:** Supinator muscle and the common extensor tendon

Interosseous Membrane

The interosseous membrane is a strong ligament that attaches to the interosseous border of the radius and ulna and unites the shafts of these bones (see Fig. 3.6). Its fibers run obliquely downward and medially and resist proximal displacement of the radius so that a force applied to the lower end of the radius (eg, falling on the outstretched hand) is transmitted from the radius to the ulna and from there to the humerus and scapula. Its fibers are taut when the forearm is in the midprone position—that is, the position of function. The interosseous membrane also provides attachment for neighboring muscles.

Distal Radioulnar Joint

- **Articulation:** Between the rounded head of the ulna and the ulnar notch on the radius (see Fig. 3.20B).
- **Type:** Synovial pivot joint.
- **Capsule:** Encloses the joint but is deficient superiorly.
- **Ligaments:** Weak **anterior and posterior ligaments** strengthen the capsule.
- **Articular disc:** This is triangular and composed of fibrocartilage. It is attached by its apex to the lateral side of the base of the styloid process of the ulna and by its base to the lower border of the ulnar notch of the radius (Fig. 3.21; see also Fig. 3.20B). It shuts off the distal radioulnar joint from the wrist and strongly unites the radius to the ulna.
- **Synovial membrane:** Lines the capsule passing from the edge of one articular surface to that of the other.
- **Nerve supply:** Anterior interosseous nerve and the deep branch of the radial nerve.

Movements

The movements of pronation and supination of the forearm involve a rotary movement around a vertical axis at the proximal and distal radioulnar joints. The axis passes through the head of the radius above and the attachment of the apex of the triangular articular disc below.

In the movement of pronation, the head of the radius rotates at the capitulum and within the annular ligament, whereas the distal end of the radius with the hand moves bodily forward, the ulnar notch of the radius moving around the circumference of the head of the ulna (Fig. 3.22). In addition, the distal end of the ulna moves laterally so that the hand remains in line with the upper limb and is not displaced medially. This movement of the ulna is important when using an instrument

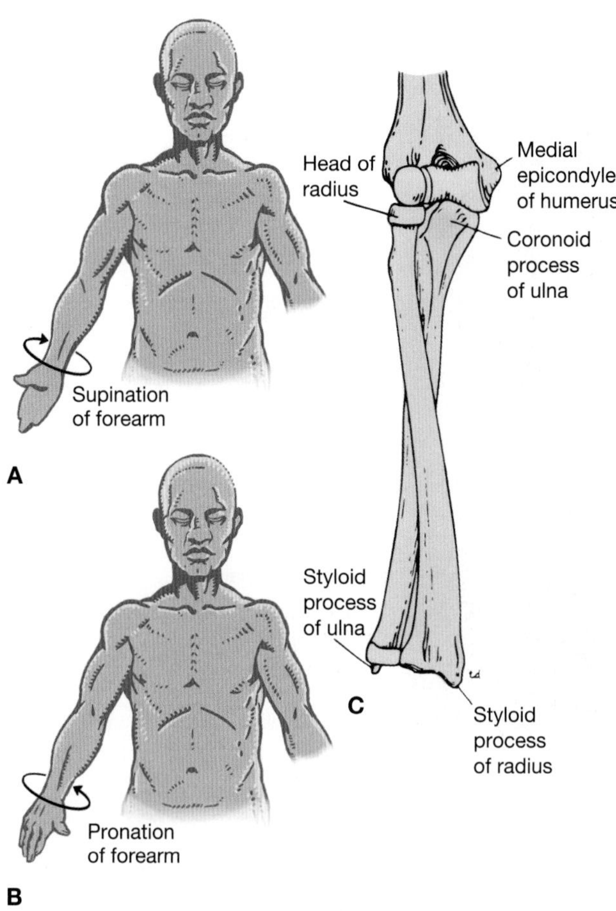

Figure 3.22 Movements of supination **(A)** and pronation **(B)** of the forearm that take place at the proximal and distal radioulnar joints. **C.** Relative positions of the radius and the ulna when the forearm is fully pronated.

such as a screwdriver because it prevents side-to-side movement of the hand during the repetitive movements of supination and pronation.

The movement of pronation results in the hand rotating medially in such a manner that the palm comes to face posteriorly, and the thumb lies on the medial side (see Fig. 3.22). The movement of supination is a reversal of this process so that the hand returns to the anatomic position, and the palm faces anteriorly.

The pronator teres and pronator quadratus muscles perform pronation. The biceps brachii and supinator muscles perform supination. Supination is the more powerful of the two movements because of the strength of the biceps muscle. Because supination is the more powerful movement, screw threads and the spiral of corkscrews are made so that the screw and corkscrews are driven inward by the movement of supination in right-handed people.

Important Relations

- **Anteriorly:** Tendons of flexor digitorum profundus
- **Posteriorly:** Tendon of extensor digiti minimi

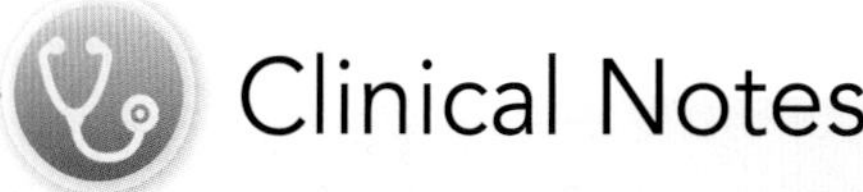

Clinical Notes

Radioulnar Joint Disease

The proximal radioulnar joint communicates with the elbow joint, whereas the distal radioulnar joint does not communicate with the wrist joint. In practical terms, this means that infection of the elbow joint invariably involves the proximal radioulnar joint. The strength of the proximal radioulnar joint depends on the integrity of the strong annular ligament. Rupture of this ligament occurs in cases of anterior dislocation of the head of the radius on the capitulum of the humerus. In young children, in whom the head of the radius is still small and undeveloped, a sudden jerk on the arm can pull the radial head down through the annular ligament. This condition is termed **transient subluxation of the head of the radius**, or **nursemaid's elbow**.

Wrist Joint (Radiocarpal Joint)

- **Articulation:** This joint is between the distal end of the radius and the articular disc proximally and the scaphoid, lunate, and triquetral bones distally (Figs. 3.23 and 3.24; see also Figs. 3.20B and 3.21). The proximal articular surface forms an ellipsoid concave surface, which is adapted to the distal ellipsoid convex surface.
- **Type:** Synovial ellipsoid joint.
- **Capsule:** Encloses the joint and is attached above to the distal ends of the radius and ulna and below to the proximal row of carpal bones.
- **Ligaments: Anterior** and **posterior ligaments** strengthen the capsule. The **medial ligament** is attached to the styloid process of the ulna and to the triquetral bone. The **lateral ligament** is attached to the styloid process of the radius and to the scaphoid bone (see Figs. 3.20B and 3.21).
- **Synovial membrane:** This lines the capsule and is attached to the margins of the articular surfaces. The joint cavity does not communicate with that of the distal radioulnar joint or with the joint cavities of the intercarpal joints.
- **Nerve supply:** Anterior interosseous nerve and the deep branch of the radial nerve.

Movements

The following movements are possible: flexion, extension, abduction, adduction, and circumduction. Rotation is not possible because the articular surfaces are ellipsoid shaped. The movements of pronation and supination of the forearm compensate for the lack of rotation.

Flexion is performed by the flexor carpi radialis, flexor carpi ulnaris, and palmaris longus. These muscles are assisted by the flexor digitorum superficialis, flexor digitorum profundus, and flexor pollicis longus.

Extension is performed by the extensor carpi radialis longus, extensor carpi radialis brevis, and extensor

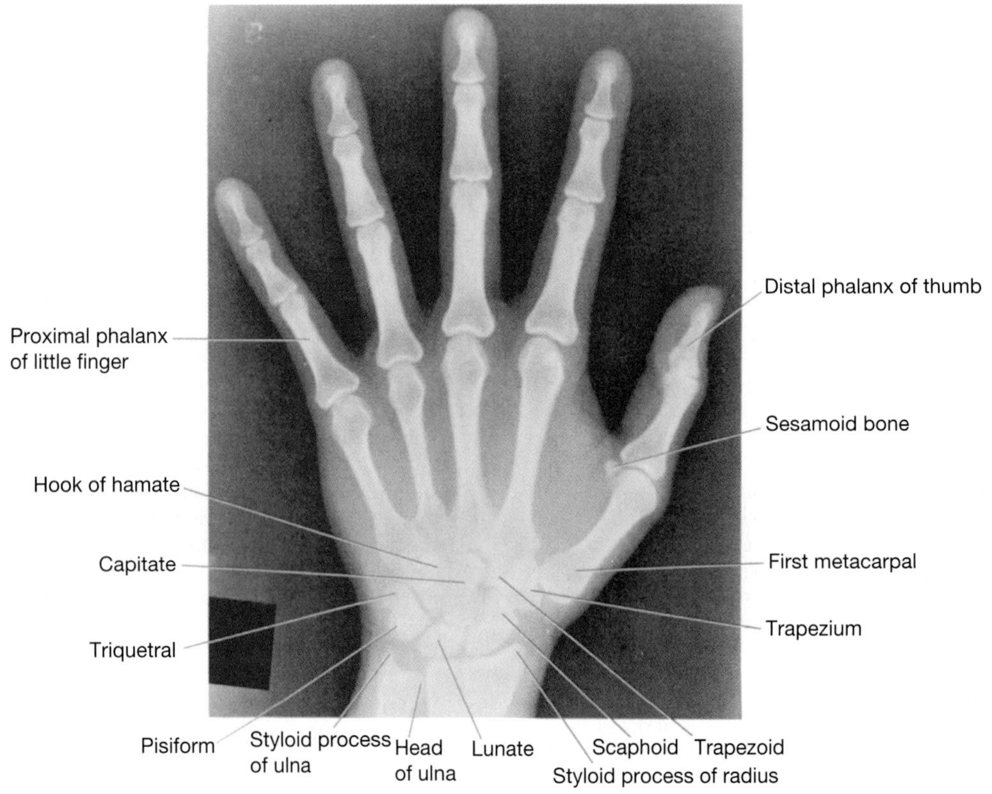

Figure 3.23 Posteroanterior radiograph of an adult wrist and hand.

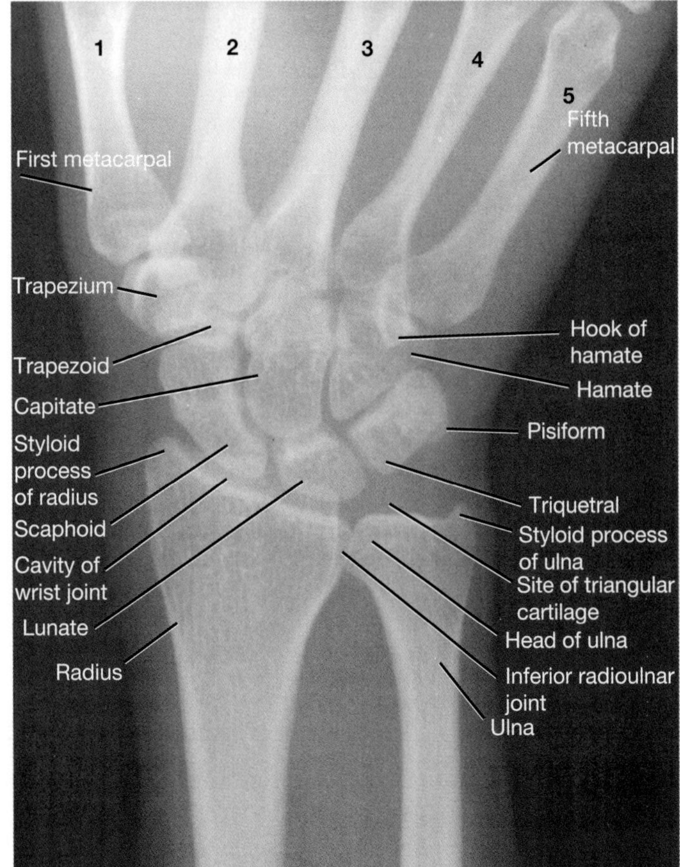

Figure 3.24 Posteroanterior radiograph of the wrist with the forearm pronated.

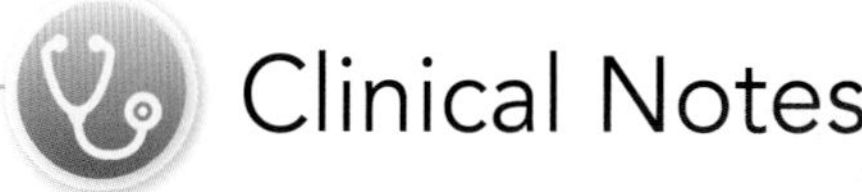

Wrist Joint Injuries

The wrist joint is essentially a synovial joint between the distal end of the radius and the proximal row of carpal bones. The head of the ulna is separated from the carpal bones by the strong triangular fibrocartilaginous disc, which separates the wrist joint from the distal radioulnar joint. The strong medial and lateral ligaments stabilize the joint.

Because the styloid process of the radius is longer than that of the ulna, abduction of the wrist joint is less extensive than adduction. In flexion–extension movements, the hand can be flexed about 80° but extended to only about 45°. Movement at the midcarpal joint (between the proximal and distal rows of carpal bones) increases the range of flexion.

A fall on an outstretched hand can strain the anterior ligament of the wrist joint, producing synovial effusion, joint pain, and limitation of movement. These symptoms and signs must not be confused with those produced by a fractured scaphoid or dislocation of the lunate bone, which are similar.

Falls on an Outstretched Hand

In falls on an outstretched hand, forces are transmitted from the scaphoid to the distal end of the radius, from the radius across the interosseous membrane to the ulna, and from the ulna to the humerus; from there, through the glenoid fossa of the scapula to the coracoclavicular ligament and the clavicle; and finally, to the sternum. If the forces are excessive, different parts of the upper limb give way under the strain. The area affected seems to be related to age. In a young child, for example, posterior displacement of the distal radial epiphysis may occur; in a teenager, the clavicle might fracture; in the young adult, the scaphoid is commonly fractured; and, in the elderly, the distal end of the radius is fractured about 1 in. (2.5 cm) proximal to the wrist joint (Colles fracture; see Fig. 3.7A).

carpi ulnaris. These muscles are assisted by the extensor digitorum, extensor indicis, extensor digiti minimi, and extensor pollicis longus.

Abduction is performed by the flexor carpi radialis and the extensor carpi radialis longus and brevis. These muscles are assisted by the abductor pollicis longus and extensor pollicis longus and brevis.

Adduction is performed by the flexor and extensor carpi ulnaris.

Important Relations

- **Anteriorly:** Tendons of the flexor digitorum profundus and superficialis, flexor pollicis longus, flexor carpi radialis, flexor carpi ulnaris, and median and ulnar nerves
- **Posteriorly:** Tendons of the extensor carpi ulnaris, extensor digiti minimi, extensor digitorum, extensor indicis, extensor carpi radialis longus and brevis, extensor pollicis longus and brevis, and abductor pollicis longus
- **Medially:** Posterior cutaneous branch of the ulnar nerve
- **Laterally:** Radial artery

Hand and Finger Joints

Five sets of synovial joints comprise the hand and fingers: intercarpal, carpometacarpal, intermetacarpal, metacarpophalangeal, and interphalangeal joints (Figs. 3.25 to 3.27; see also Figs. 3.20, 3.21, 3.23, and 3.24).

Intercarpal Joints

- **Articulation:** Between the individual bones of the proximal row of the carpus; between the individual bones of the distal row of the carpus; and, finally, the **midcarpal joint** between the proximal and distal rows of carpal bones (see Figs. 3.20B, 3.21, and 3.24).
- **Type:** Synovial plane joints.
- **Capsule:** Surrounds each joint.
- **Ligaments:** Strong **anterior**, **posterior**, and **interosseous ligaments** unite the bones.
- **Synovial membrane:** This lines the capsule and is attached to the margins of the articular surfaces. The joint cavity of the midcarpal joint extends not only between the two rows of carpal bones but also proximally between the individual bones forming the proximal row and distally between the bones of the distal row.
- **Nerve supply:** Anterior interosseous nerve, deep branch of the radial nerve, and deep branch of the ulnar nerve.

Movements

A small amount of gliding movement is possible.

Carpometacarpal and Intermetacarpal Joints

The carpometacarpal and intermetacarpal joints are synovial plane joints possessing **anterior**, **posterior**, and **interosseous ligaments**. They have a common joint cavity. A small amount of gliding movement is possible (see Figs. 3.20B and 3.21).

Carpometacarpal Joint of Thumb

- **Articulation:** Between the trapezium and the saddle-shaped base of the first metacarpal bone (see Figs. 3.20B and 3.23 to 3.25)
- **Type:** Synovial saddle-shaped joint
- **Capsule:** Surrounds the joint
- **Synovial membrane:** Lines the capsule and forms a separate joint cavity

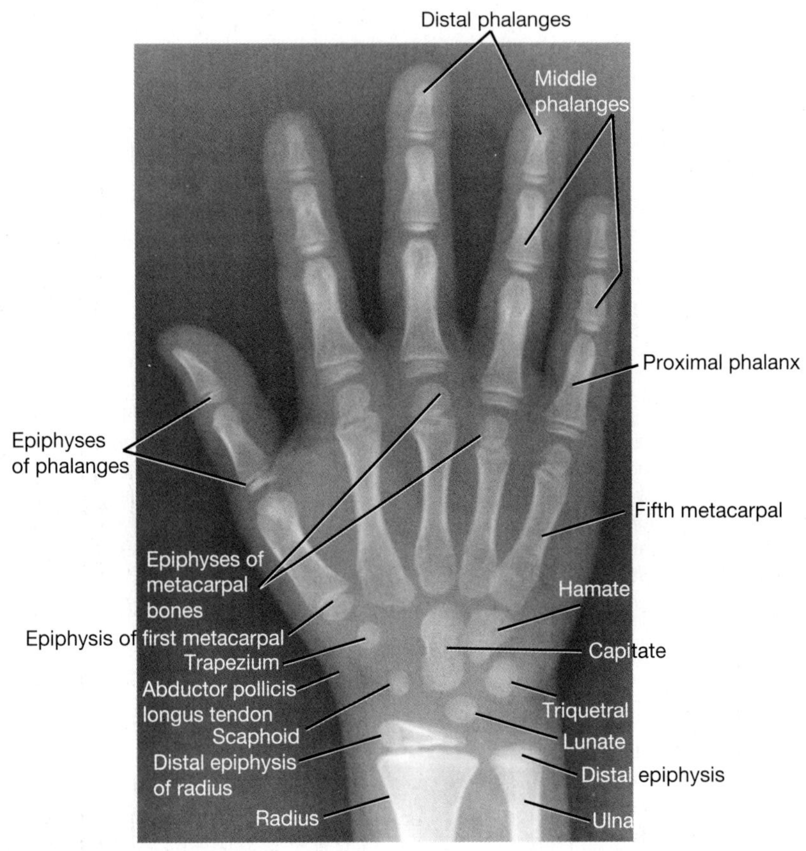

Figure 3.25 Posteroanterior radiograph of the wrist and hand of an 8-year-old male.

Movements

The following movements are possible:

- **Flexion:** Flexor pollicis brevis and opponens pollicis.
- **Extension:** Extensor pollicis longus and brevis.
- **Abduction:** Abductor pollicis longus and brevis.
- **Adduction:** Adductor pollicis.
- **Rotation (opposition):** The thumb is rotated medially by the opponens pollicis.

Metacarpophalangeal Joints

- **Articulation:** Between the heads of the metacarpal bones and the bases of the proximal phalanges (see Figs. 3.20 and 3.23 to 3.27).
- **Type:** Synovial condyloid joints.
- **Capsule:** Surrounds the joint.
- **Ligaments:** The **palmar ligaments** are strong and contain some fibrocartilage. They are firmly attached to the phalanx but less so to the metacarpal bone.

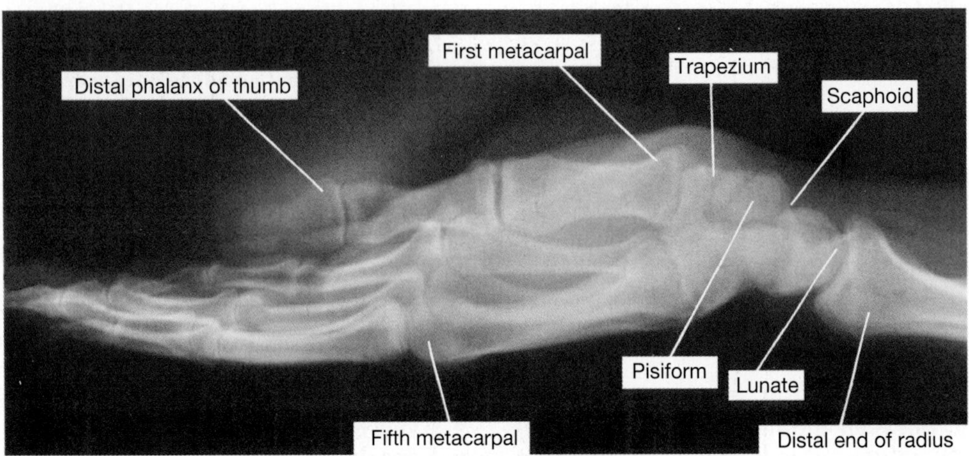

Figure 3.26 Lateral radiograph of an adult wrist and hand.

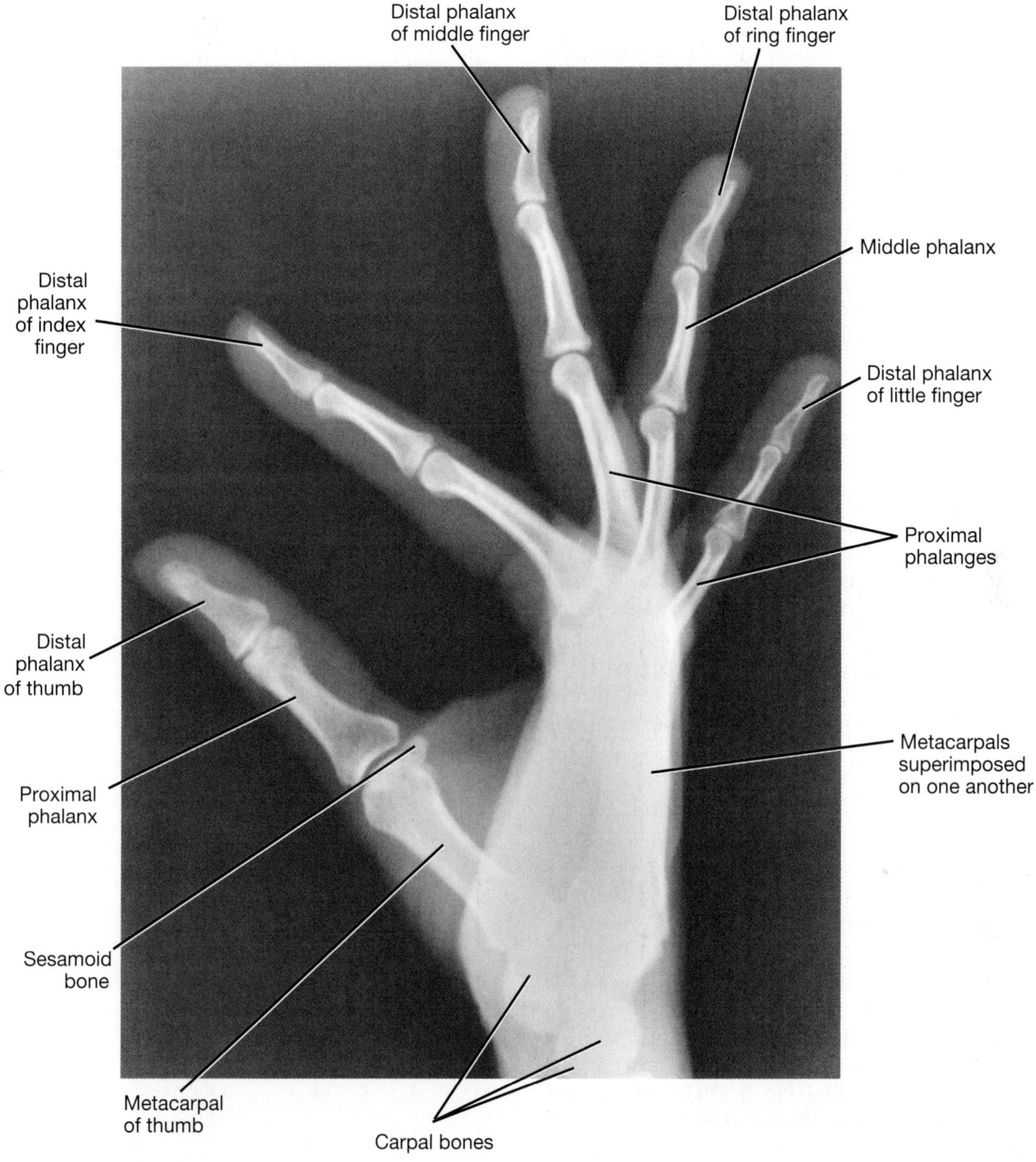

Figure 3.27 Lateral radiograph of an adult wrist and hand with the fingers at different degrees of flexion.

The palmar ligaments of the second through fifth joints are united by the **deep transverse metacarpal ligaments**, which hold the heads of the metacarpal bones together. The **collateral ligaments** are cordlike bands present on each side of the joints. Each passes downward and forward from the head of the metacarpal bone to the base of the phalanx. The collateral ligaments are taut when the joint is in flexion and lax when the joint is in extension (see Fig. 3.20).

- **Synovial membrane:** Lines the capsule and is attached to the margins of the articular surfaces.

Movements

The following movements are possible:

- **Flexion:** Lumbricals and interossei, assisted by flexor digitorum superficialis and profundus.
- **Extension:** Extensor digitorum, extensor indicis, and extensor digiti minimi.
- **Abduction:** Movement away from the midline of the third finger performed by the dorsal interossei.
- **Adduction:** Movement toward the midline of the third finger is performed by the palmar interossei. In the case of the metacarpophalangeal joint of the thumb, flexion is performed by the flexor pollicis longus and brevis, and extension is performed by the extensor pollicis longus and brevis. The movements of abduction and adduction are performed at the carpometacarpal joint.

Interphalangeal Joints

Interphalangeal joints are synovial hinge joints that have a structure similar to that of the metacarpophalangeal joints (see Figs. 3.20 and 3.23 to 3.27).

Hand as a Functional Unit

The upper limb is a multijointed lever freely movable on the trunk at the shoulder joint. At the distal end of the upper limb is the important prehensile organ—the hand. Much of the importance of the hand depends on the pincer action of the thumb, which enables us to grasp objects between the thumb and the index finger. The extreme mobility of the first metacarpal bone makes the thumb functionally as important as all the remaining fingers combined.

To comprehend fully the important positioning and movements of the hand described in this section, closely observe the movements in your own hand.

Hand Position

For the hand to be able to perform delicate movements (eg, those used in holding small instruments in watch repairing), the forearm is placed in the semiprone position, and the wrist joint is partially extended. Note that the forearm bones are most stable in the midprone position, when the interosseous membrane is taut. In other positions of the forearm bones, the interosseous membrane is lax. With the wrist partially extended, the long flexor and extensor tendons of the fingers are working to their best mechanical advantage. At the same time, the flexors and extensors of the carpus can exert a balanced fixator action on the wrist joint, ensuring a stable base for the movements of the fingers.

The **position of rest** is the posture adopted by the hand when the fingers are at rest and the hand is relaxed (Fig. 3.28A). The forearm is in the semiprone position; the wrist joint is slightly extended; the second through fifth fingers are partially flexed, although the index finger is not flexed as much as the others; and the plane of the thumbnail lies at a right angle to the plane of the other fingernails.

The **position of function** is the posture adopted by the hand when it is about to grasp an object between the thumb and the index finger (see Fig. 3.28B). The forearm is in the semiprone position, the wrist joint is partially extended (more so than in the position of rest), and the fingers are partially flexed, the index finger being flexed as much as the others. The metacarpal bone of the thumb is rotated in such a manner that the plane of the thumbnail lies parallel with that of the index finger and the pulp of the thumb and index finger are in contact.

The following movements are described with the hand in the anatomic position.

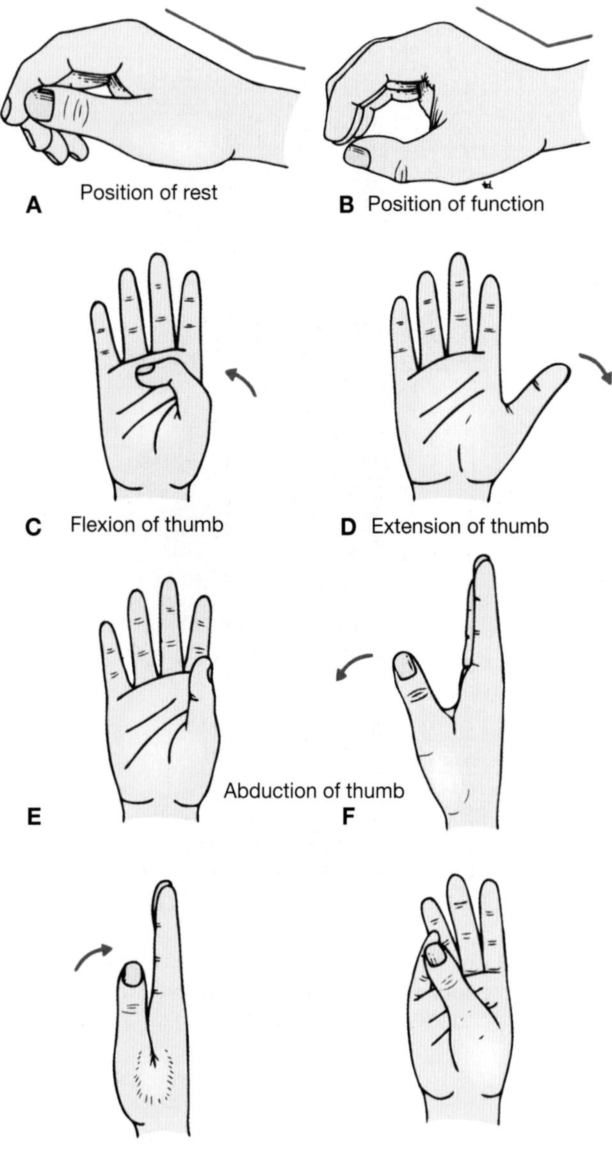

Figure 3.28 Various positions of the hand and movements of the thumb. **A, B.** Lateral views showing the hand in its position of rest **(A)** and function **(B)**. **C–H.** Anterior views showing movements of the thumb.

Thumb Movements

Flexion is the movement of the thumb across the palm to maintain the plane of the thumbnail at right angles to the plane of the other fingernails (see Fig. 3.28C). It takes place between the trapezium and the first metacarpal bone at the metacarpophalangeal and interphalangeal joints and is produced by the flexor pollicis longus and brevis and opponens pollicis muscles.

Extension is the movement of the thumb in a lateral or coronal plane away from the palm to maintain the plane of the thumbnail at right angles to the plane of the other fingernails (Fig. 3.29A; see also Fig. 3.28D). It takes place between the trapezium and the first metacarpal bone at the metacarpophalangeal and interphalangeal joints and is produced by the extensor pollicis longus and brevis muscles.

Abduction is the movement of the thumb in an anteroposterior plane away from the palm, the plane of the thumbnail being kept at right angles to the plane of the other nails (Fig. 3.30A; see also Figs. 3.28F and 3.29A). It takes place mainly between the trapezium and the first metacarpal bone, with a small movement occurring at the metacarpophalangeal joint. The abductor pollicis longus and brevis muscles produce this movement.

Adduction is the movement of the thumb in an anteroposterior plane toward the palm, the plane of the

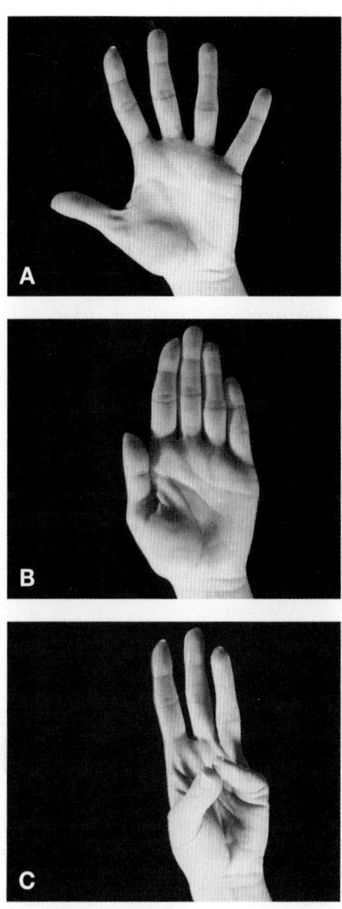

Figure 3.29 Left hand with the fingers abducted and the thumb extended **(A)**, with the fingers adducted and the thumb adducted **(B)**, and with the thumb in the position of opposition **(C)**.

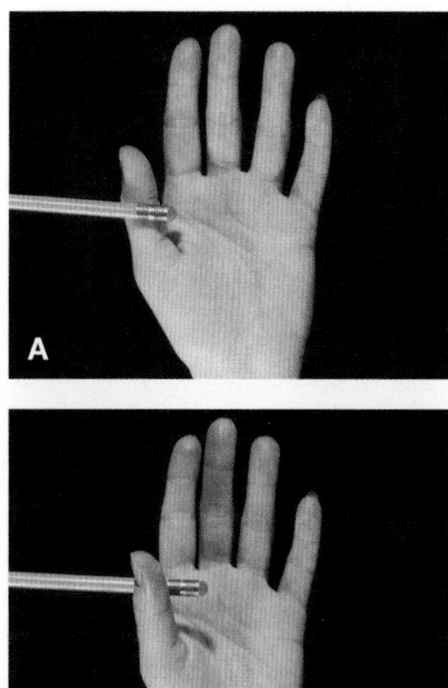

Figure 3.30 Left hand with the thumb about to move the pencil away from the palm to demonstrate abduction **(A)** and with the thumb about to move the pencil in the direction of the palm to demonstrate adduction **(B)**.

thumbnail being kept at right angles to the plane of the other fingernails (see Figs. 3.28G, 3.29B, and 3.30B). It takes place between the trapezium and the first metacarpal bone and is produced by the adductor pollicis muscle.

Opposition is the movement of the thumb across the palm so that the anterior surface of the tip contacts the anterior surface of the tip of any of the other fingers (see Figs. 3.28H and 3.29C). It is accomplished by the medial rotation of the first metacarpal bone and the attached phalanges on the trapezium. The plane of the thumbnail comes to lie parallel with the plane of the nail of the opposed finger. The opponens pollicis muscle produces this movement.

Index, Middle, Ring, and Little Finger Movements

Flexion is the movement forward of the finger in an anteroposterior plane. It takes place at the interphalangeal and metacarpophalangeal joints. The distal phalanx is flexed by the flexor digitorum profundus, the middle phalanx by the flexor digitorum superficialis, and the proximal phalanx by the lumbricals and the interossei.

Extension is the movement backward of the finger in an anteroposterior plane. It takes place at the interphalangeal and metacarpophalangeal joints. The distal phalanx is extended by the lumbricals and interossei, the middle phalanx by the lumbricals and interossei, and the proximal phalanx by the extensor digitorum (in addition, by the extensor indicis for the index finger and the extensor digiti minimi for the little finger).

Abduction is the movement of the fingers (including the middle finger) away from the imaginary midline of the middle finger (see Figs. 3.29A and 3.72). It takes place at the metacarpophalangeal joint and is produced by the dorsal interossei; the abductor digiti minimi abducts the little finger.

Adduction is the movement of the fingers toward the midline of the middle finger (see Fig. 3.29B). It takes place at the metacarpophalangeal joint and is produced by the palmar interossei muscle.

Abduction and adduction of the fingers are possible only in the extended position. In the flexed position, the articular surface of the base of the proximal phalanx lies in contact with the flattened anterior surface of the head of the metacarpal bone. The two bones are held in close contact by the collateral ligaments, which are taut in this position. In the extended position of the metacarpophalangeal joint, the base of the phalanx is in contact with the rounded part of the metacarpal head, and the collateral ligaments are slack.

Cupping the Hand

In the cupped position, the palm is formed into a deep concavity. To achieve this, the thumb is abducted and placed in a partially opposed position and is also slightly flexed. This has the effect of drawing the thenar eminence forward.

The fourth and fifth metacarpal bones are flexed and slightly rotated at the carpometacarpal joints. This has the effect of drawing the hypothenar eminence forward. The palmaris brevis muscle contracts and pulls the skin over the hypothenar eminence medially; it also puckers the skin, which improves the gripping ability of the palm.

The four fingers are partially flexed and rotated slightly at the metacarpophalangeal joints to increase the general concavity of the cupped hand.

Making a Fist

Making a fist is accomplished by flexing the metacarpophalangeal joints and the interphalangeal joints of the fingers and thumb. It is performed by the contraction of the long flexor muscles of the fingers and thumb. For this movement to be carried out efficiently, a synergic contraction of the extensor carpi radialis longus and brevis and the extensor carpi ulnaris muscles must occur to extend the wrist joint. (Trying to make a "strong fist" with the wrist joint flexed is very difficult.)

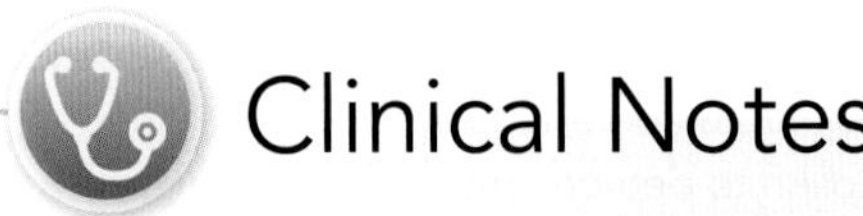

Clinical Notes

Hand Diseases and Preservation of Function

From the clinical standpoint, the hand is one of the most important organs of the body. Without a normally functioning hand, the patient's livelihood is often in jeopardy. (Place one of your hands in a pocket for 24 hours—you will be astonished at the number of times you would have liked to use it.)

From the purely mechanical point of view, the hand is a pincer-like mechanism between the thumb and the fingers, situated at the end of a multijointed lever. The most important part of the hand is the thumb, and preserving the thumb, or as much of it as possible, is the clinician's responsibility, so that the pincer-like mechanism can be maintained. This action largely depends on the thumb's unique ability to be drawn across the palm and opposed to the other fingers. This movement alone, although important, is insufficient for the mechanism to work effectively. The opposing skin surfaces must have tactile sensation—and this explains why median nerve palsy is so much more disabling than ulnar nerve palsy.

If the hand requires immobilization for the treatment of disease of any part of the upper limb, it should be immobilized (if possible) in the position of function. This means that if loss of movement occurs at the wrist joint or at the joints of the hand or fingers, the patient will at least have a hand that is in a position of mechanical advantage and can serve a useful purpose.

Clinicians should also remember that when a finger (excluding the thumb) is normally flexed into the palm, it points to the tubercle of the scaphoid; individual fingers requiring immobilization in flexion, on a splint or within a cast, should therefore always be placed in this position.

Always refer to the patient's fingers by name: thumb, index, middle, ring, and little finger. Referring to the fingers by number can be confusing to the patient.

UPPER LIMB REGIONS

The upper limb is divided into the shoulder, arm, elbow, forearm, wrist, and hand (Fig. 3.31). The **shoulder** is a complex region connecting the trunk with the upper limb and can be considered as three parts: pectoral region, scapular region, and axilla. The **arm (upper arm, brachium)** is the proximal segment of the upper limb from the shoulder to the elbow. In contrast, in the lower limb, the leg is the more distal segment from the knee to the ankle. Remember, spelling *does* matter because sometimes one or two letters can make a major difference in the location you are describing (eg, "brachial" vs. "bronchial" vs. "branchial"). The **elbow** is the area connecting the arm with the forearm. The **cubital fossa** is a depression across the front of the elbow. The **forearm (lower arm, antebrachium)** is the segment of the

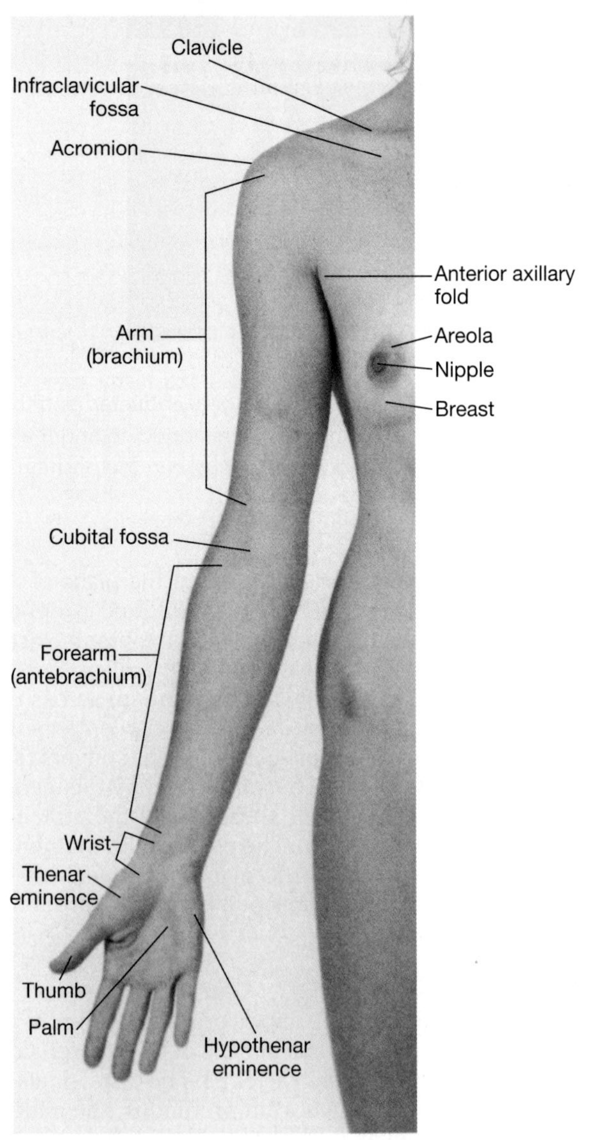

Figure 3.31 Photograph of the breast and upper limb in a young female.

upper limb from the elbow to the wrist. The **wrist** (**carpus**) is a complex of small bones connecting the forearm and hand. The **hand** (**manus**), a very important organ, is located at the distal end of the upper limb.

Pectoral Region

The pectoral region is the anterior aspect of the shoulder and chest. Although this area may be considered part of the anterior thoracic wall, several structures here (eg, pectoral muscles) connect with and function as part of the upper limb, thus uniting these areas. The pectoral region also houses the breasts. The general topography of the pectoral region is shown in Figures 3.32 through 3.34 as well as in 3.104 to 3.106.

Breasts

Strictly speaking, the breasts are not anatomically part of the upper limb. However, they are situated in the pectoral region, and their blood supply and lymphatic drainage are largely related to the armpit. The clinical importance of the breasts cannot be overemphasized.

Location and Description

The breasts are specialized accessory glands of the skin that secrete milk. They are present in both sexes and share similar structure in males and immature females. The nipples are small and surrounded by a colored area of skin called the **areola** (Fig. 3.35; see also Figs. 3.31 and 3.104). The breast tissue consists of a system of ducts embedded in connective tissue that does not extend beyond the margin of the areola.

PUBERTY

At puberty in females, the breasts gradually enlarge and assume their hemispherical shape under the influence of ovarian hormones. The ducts elongate, but the increased size of the glands is mainly from the deposition of fat. The base of the breast extends from rib 2 to rib 6 and from the lateral margin of the sternum to the midaxillary line. The greater part of the gland lies in the superficial fascia. An extension of the gland called the **axillary tail** (see Fig. 3.35C) continues upward and laterally, pierces the deep fascia at the lower border of the pectoralis major muscle, and enters the axilla.

Each breast consists of 15 to 20 **lobes**, which radiate out from the nipple (see Fig. 3.35A). The main duct from each lobe opens separately on the summit of the nipple and possesses a dilated **ampulla** just before its termination. The base of the nipple is surrounded by the areola. The underlying **areolar glands** produce tiny tubercles on the areola. The lobes of the gland are separated by fibrous septa that serve as **suspensory ligaments** (see Fig. 3.35A,B). A space filled by loose connective tissue called the **retromammary space** lies deep to the breast and superficial to the underlying pectoral muscles.

YOUNG WOMEN

In young women, the breasts tend to protrude forward from a circular base.

PREGNANCY

Early

In the early months of pregnancy, the duct system rapidly increases in length and branching (Fig. 3.36). The secretory alveoli develop at the ends of the smaller

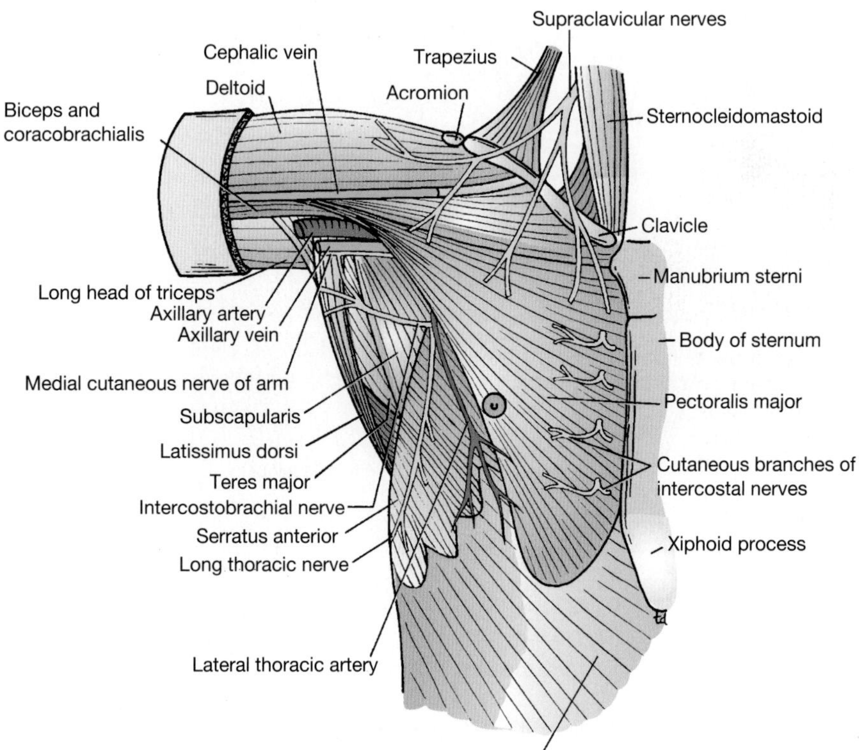

Figure 3.32 Pectoral region and axilla.

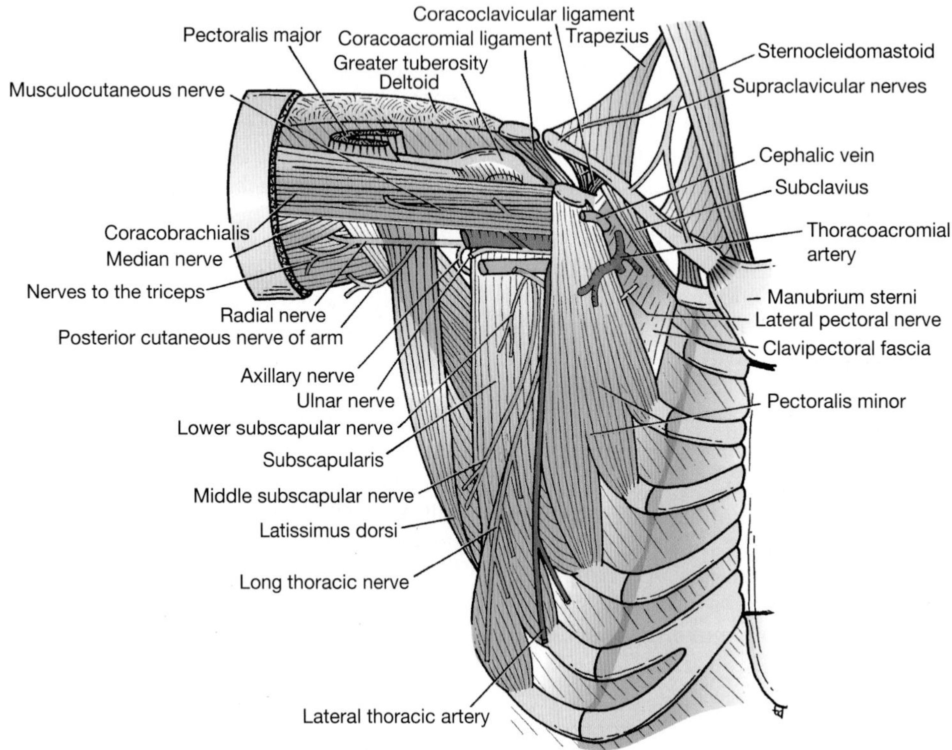

Figure 3.33 Pectoral region and axilla; the pectoralis major muscle has been removed to display the underlying structures.

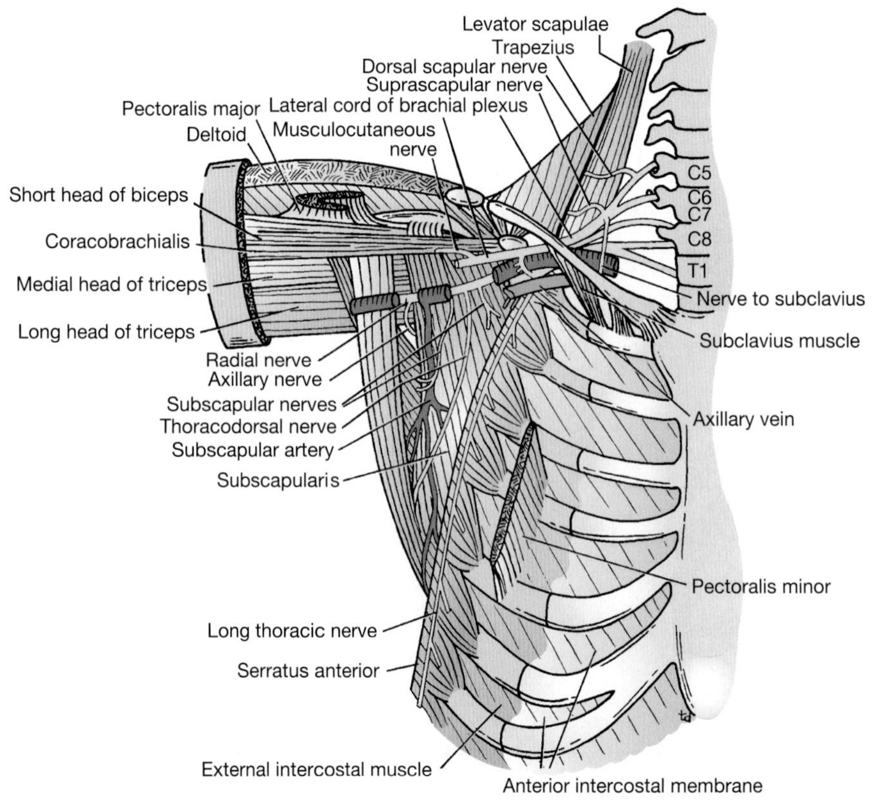

Figure 3.34 Pectoral region and axilla; the pectoralis major and minor muscles and the clavipectoral fascia have been removed to display the underlying structures.

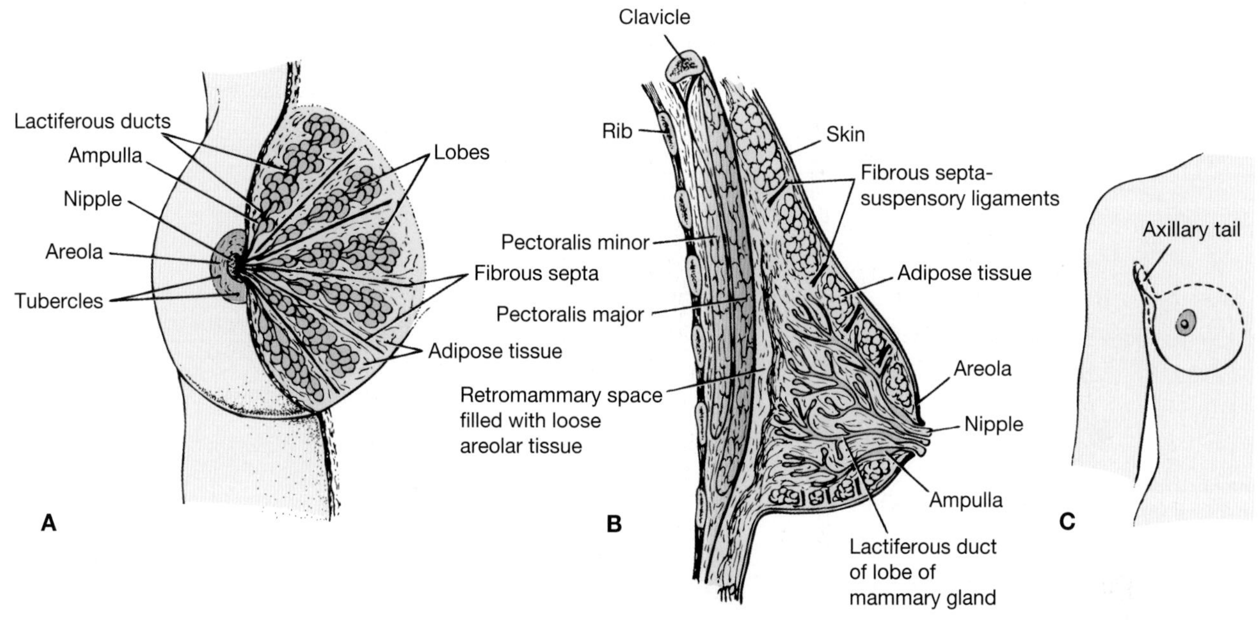

Figure 3.35 Mature female breast. **A.** Anterior view with skin partially removed to show internal structure. **B.** Sagittal section. **C.** Axillary tail, which pierces the deep fascia and extends into the axilla.

ducts, and the connective tissue becomes filled with expanding and budding secretory alveoli. The vascularity of the connective tissue also increases to provide adequate nourishment for the developing gland. The nipple enlarges, and the areola becomes darker and more extensive from increased deposits of melanin pigment in the epidermis. The areolar glands enlarge and become more active.

Late

During the second half of pregnancy, the growth process slows. However, the breasts continue to enlarge,

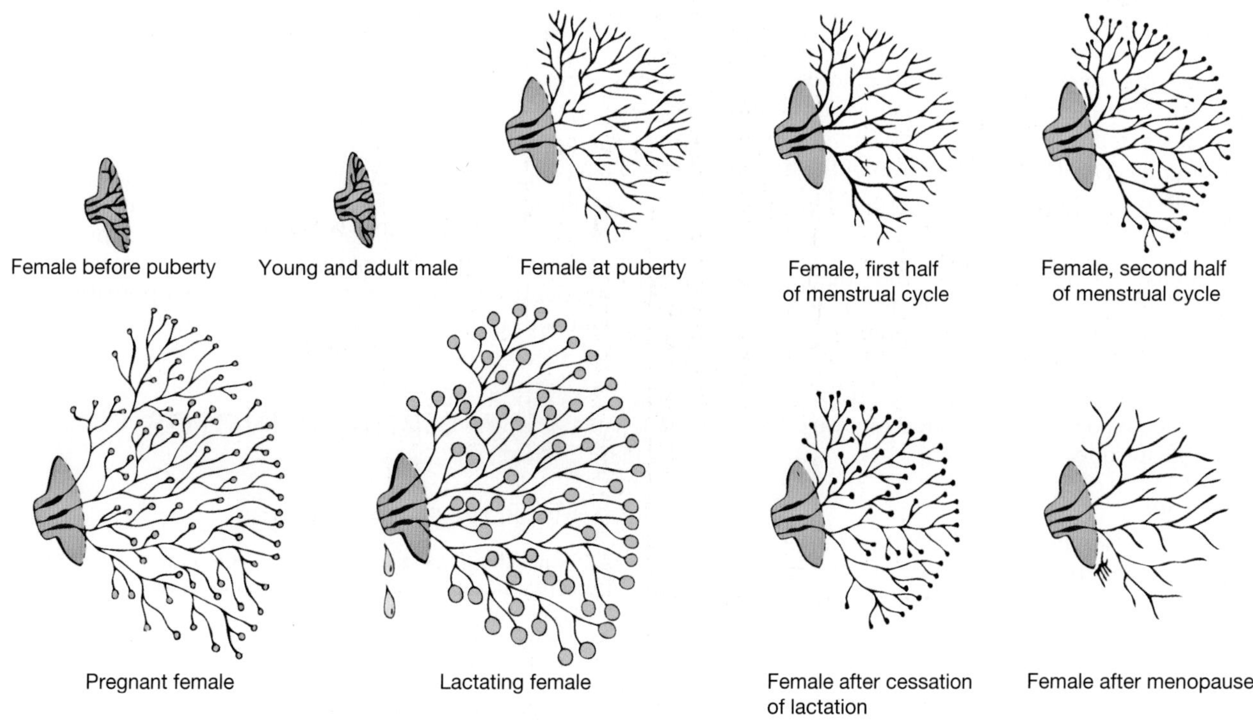

Figure 3.36 Extent of the development of the ducts and secretory alveoli in the breasts in both sexes at different stages of activity.

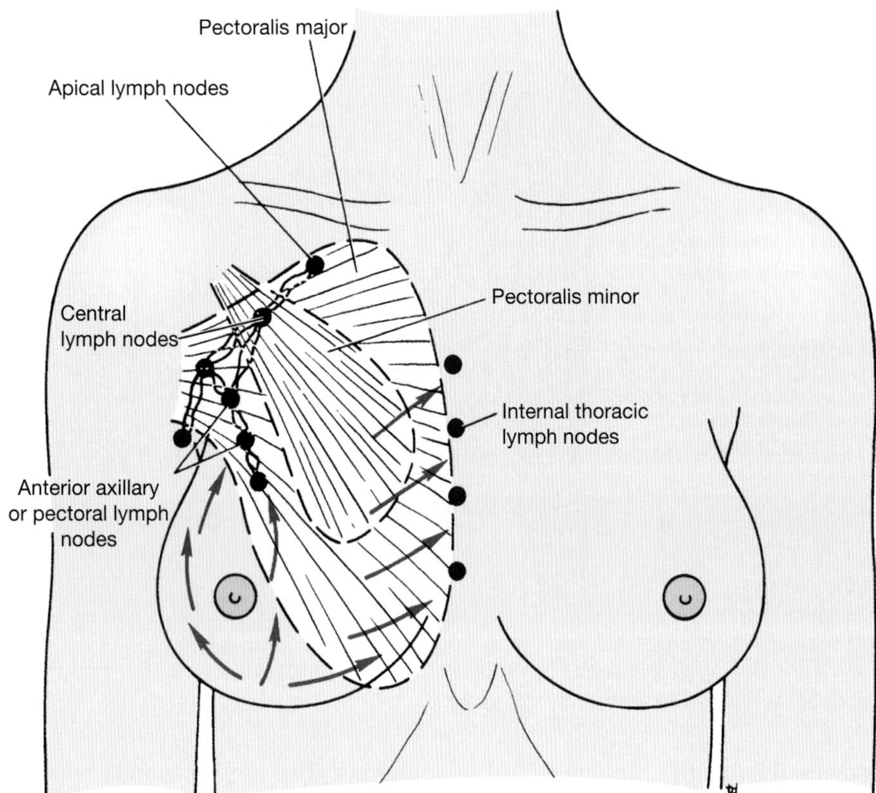

Figure 3.37 Lymph drainage of the breast.

mostly because of the distention of the secretory alveoli with the fluid secretion called **colostrum**.

Post-parturition

The breasts return to their inactive state if breastfeeding does not occur or once it stops. The remaining milk is absorbed; the secretory alveoli shrink, and most of them disappear. The interlobular connective tissue thickens. The breasts and the nipples shrink and return nearly to their original size. The pigmentation of the areola fades, but the area never lightens to its original color.

POSTMENOPAUSE

The breast atrophies after the menopause (see Fig. 3.36). Most of the secretory alveoli disappear, leaving behind the ducts. The amount of adipose tissue may increase or decrease. The breasts tend to shrink in size and become more pendulous. The atrophy after menopause is caused by the absence of ovarian estrogens and progesterone.

Blood Supply

The arterial supply to the breasts includes the perforating branches of the internal thoracic artery and the intercostal arteries. The axillary artery also supplies the gland via its lateral thoracic and thoracoacromial branches. The veins correspond to the arteries.

Lymph Drainage

The lymph drainage of the mammary gland is of great clinical importance because of the frequent development of cancer in the gland and the subsequent dissemination of the malignant cells along the lymph vessels to the lymph nodes.

The lateral quadrants of the breast drain into the anterior axillary or pectoral group of nodes (Fig. 3.37) (situated just posterior to the lower border of the pectoralis minor muscle). The medial quadrants drain by means of vessels that pierce the intercostal spaces and enter the internal thoracic group of nodes (situated within the thoracic cavity along the course of the internal thoracic artery). A few lymph vessels follow the posterior intercostal arteries and drain posteriorly into the posterior intercostal nodes (situated along the course of the posterior intercostal arteries); some vessels communicate with the lymph vessels of the opposite breast and with those of the anterior abdominal wall.

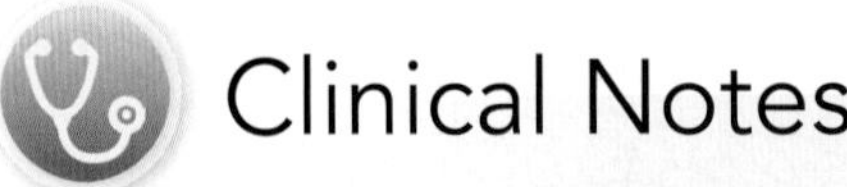

Clinical Notes

Milk in Newborns

While the fetus is in the uterus, the maternal and placental hormones cross the placental barrier and cause proliferation of the duct epithelium and the surrounding connective tissue. This proliferation may cause swelling of the mammary glands in both sexes during the first week of life. In some cases, a milky fluid called **"witch's milk"** may be expressed from the nipples. The condition is resolved spontaneously as the maternal hormone levels in the child fall.

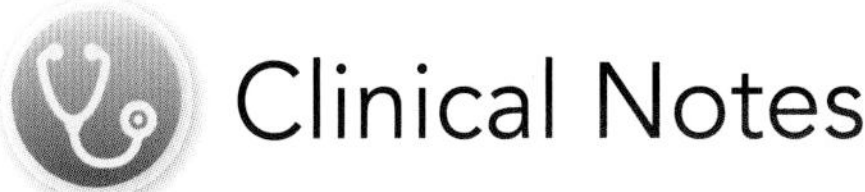

Clinical Notes

Breast Examination

The breast is one of the common sites of cancer in women. It is also the site of different types of benign tumors and may be subject to acute inflammation and abscess formation. For these reasons, clinical personnel must be familiar with the development, structure, and lymph drainage of this organ.

With the patient undressed to the waist and sitting upright, first inspect the breasts for symmetry. Some degree of asymmetry is common and is the result of unequal breast development. Any swelling should be noted. An underlying tumor, cyst, or abscess formation can cause a swelling. Carefully examine the nipples for evidence of retraction. A carcinoma within the breast substance can retract the nipple by pulling on the lactiferous ducts. Next, ask the patient to lie down so that their breasts can be palpated against the underlying thoracic wall. Finally, ask the patient to sit up again and raise both arms above their head. With this maneuver, a carcinoma tethered to the skin, suspensory ligaments, or lactiferous ducts produces skin dimpling or nipple retraction.

Mammography

Mammography is a radiographic examination of the breast (Fig. 3.38). This technique is extensively used for screening the breasts for benign and malignant tumors and cysts. Extremely low doses of x-rays are used so that the dangers are minimal, and the examination can be repeated often.

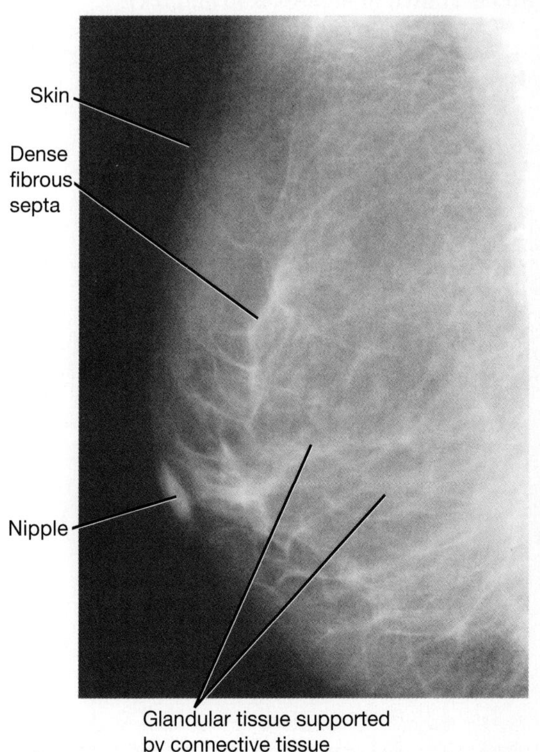

Figure 3.38 Mediolateral mammogram showing the glandular tissue supported by the connective tissue septa.

Its success is because a lesion measuring only a few millimeters in diameter can be detected long before it is felt by clinical examination.

Supernumerary and Retracted Nipples

Supernumerary nipples occasionally occur along a line extending from the axilla to the groin; they may or may not be associated with breast tissue (see Embryology Notes below). This minor congenital anomaly may result in a mistaken diagnosis of warts or moles. A longstanding retracted nipple is a congenital deformity caused by a failure in the complete development of the nipple. A retracted nipple of recent occurrence is usually caused by an underlying carcinoma pulling on the lactiferous ducts.

Importance of Fibrous Septa

The interior of the breast is divided into 15 to 20 compartments by fibrous septa (suspensory ligaments) that radiate from the nipple and extend from the deep surface of the skin. Each compartment contains a lobe of the gland. Normally, the skin feels completely mobile over the breast substance. However, a scirrhous carcinoma or a breast abscess may apply traction to the fibrous septa that causes skin dimpling.

Breast Abscess

Acute infection of the mammary gland may occur during lactation. Pathogenic bacteria gain entrance to the breast tissue through a crack in the nipple. Because of the presence of the fibrous septa, the infection remains localized to one compartment or lobe to begin with. Abscesses should be drained through a radial incision to avoid spreading of the infection into neighboring compartments; a radial incision also minimizes damage to the radially arranged ducts.

Lymph Drainage and Breast Carcinoma

The importance of knowing the lymph drainage of the breast in relation to the spread of cancer from that organ cannot be overemphasized. The lymph vessels from the medial quadrants of the breast pierce the second, third, and fourth intercostal spaces and enter the thorax to drain into the lymph nodes alongside the internal thoracic artery. The lymph vessels from the lateral quadrants of the breast drain into the anterior or pectoral group of axillary nodes. Therefore, a cancer occurring in the lateral quadrants of the breast tends to spread to the axillary nodes. Thoracic metastases are difficult or impossible to treat, but the lymph nodes of the axilla can be removed surgically.

Approximately 60% of carcinomas of the breast occur in the upper lateral quadrant. The lymphatic spread of cancer to the opposite breast, abdominal cavity, or into the lymph nodes in the root of the neck is caused by obstruction of the normal lymphatic pathways by malignant cells or destruction of lymph vessels by surgery or radiotherapy. The cancer cells are swept along the lymph vessels and follow the lymph stream. The entrance of cancer cells into the blood vessels accounts for the metastases in distant bones.

(continued)

In patients with localized cancer of the breast, most surgeons do a simple mastectomy or a lumpectomy, followed by radiotherapy to the axillary lymph nodes and/or hormone therapy. In patients with localized cancer of the breast with early metastases in the axillary lymph nodes, most authorities agree that radical mastectomy offers the best chance of cure. In patients in whom the disease has already spread beyond these areas (eg, into the thorax), simple mastectomy, followed by radiotherapy or hormone therapy, is the treatment of choice.

Radical mastectomy is designed to remove the primary tumor and the lymph vessels and nodes that drain the area. This means that the breast and associated structures containing the lymph vessels and nodes must be removed en bloc. The excised mass is therefore made up of the following: a large area of skin overlying the tumor and including the nipple; all the breast tissue; the pectoralis major and associated fascia through which the lymph vessels pass to the internal thoracic nodes; the pectoralis minor and associated fascia related to the lymph vessels passing to the axilla; all the fat, fascia, and lymph nodes in the axilla; and the fascia covering the upper part of the rectus sheath, serratus anterior, subscapularis, and latissimus dorsi muscles. The axillary blood vessels, brachial plexus, and the nerves to the serratus anterior and the latissimus dorsi are preserved. Some degree of postoperative edema of the arm is likely to follow such a radical removal of the lymph vessels draining the upper limb.

A modified form of radical mastectomy for patients with clinically localized cancer is also a common procedure and consists of a simple mastectomy in which the pectoral muscles are left intact. The axillary lymph nodes, fat, and fascia are removed. This procedure removes the primary tumor and permits pathologic examination of the lymph nodes for possible metastases.

Male Breast Carcinoma

Carcinoma in the male breast accounts for about 1% of all carcinomas of the breast. This fact tends to be overlooked when examining the male patient. Because the amount of breast tissue in the male is small, the tumor can usually be felt with the flat of the examining hand in the early stages. However, the prognosis is relatively poor in the male, because the carcinoma cells can rapidly metastasize into the thorax through the small amount of intervening tissue.

Scapular Region

The scapular region is the posterior aspect of the shoulder. Although this area may be considered part of the back and/or posterior thoracic wall, several structures here (eg, trapezius and latissimus dorsi muscles) connect with and function as part of the upper limb, thus uniting these areas.

Musculoskeletal and Neurovascular Structures

The underlying bones of the back are shown in Figure 3.39 and are described in detail in Chapter 2 (Back). Details of the scapula were described earlier in this chapter. The general topography of the scapular region is shown in Figures 3.40 and 3.41.

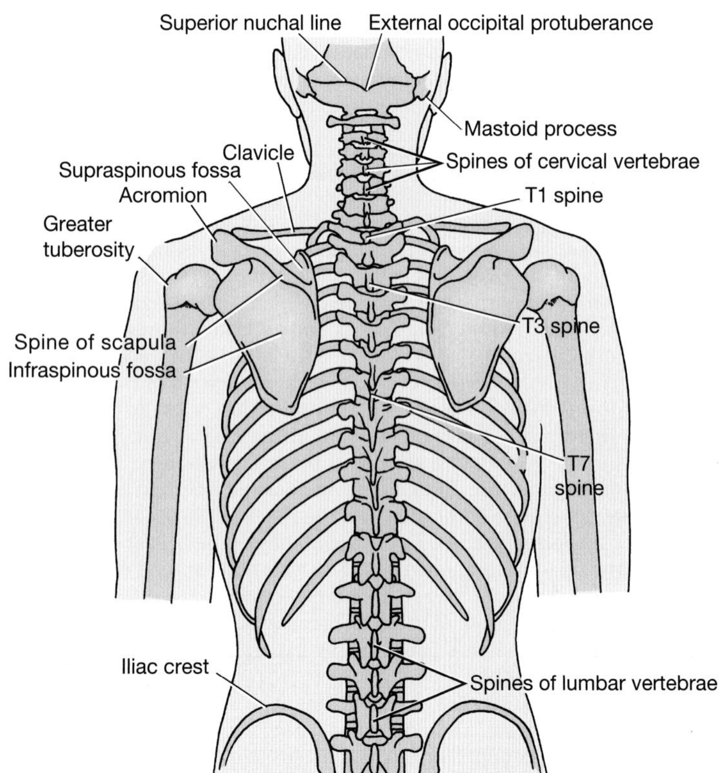

Figure 3.39 Bones of the back.

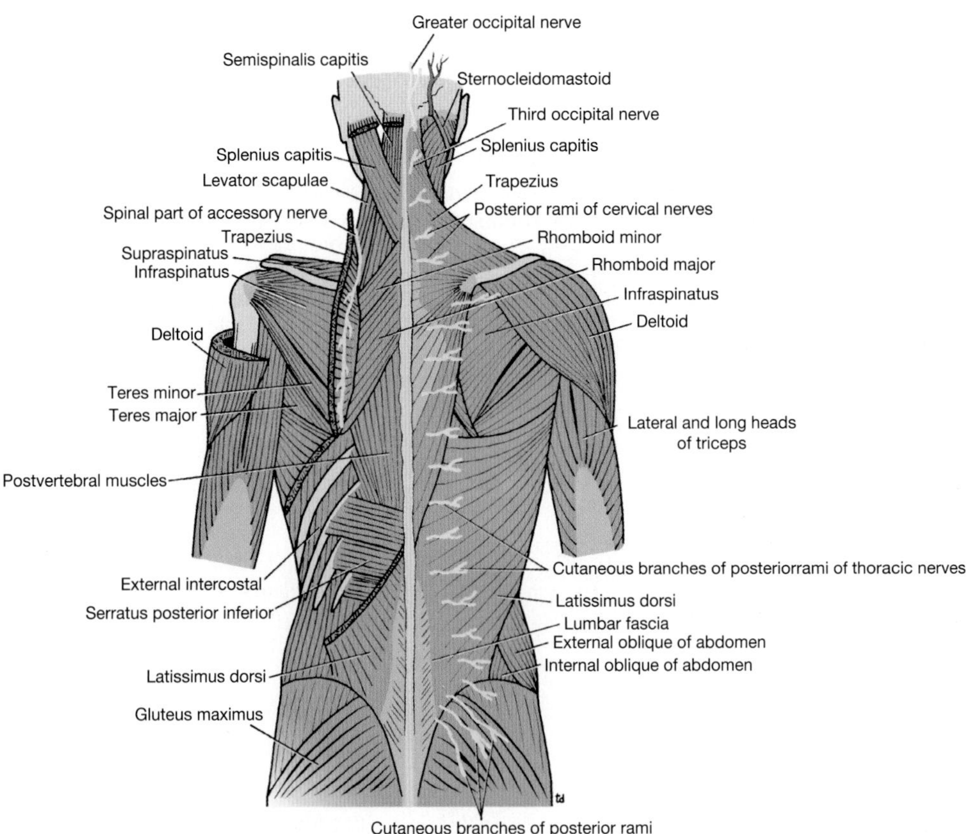

Figure 3.40 Superficial and deep muscles of the back.

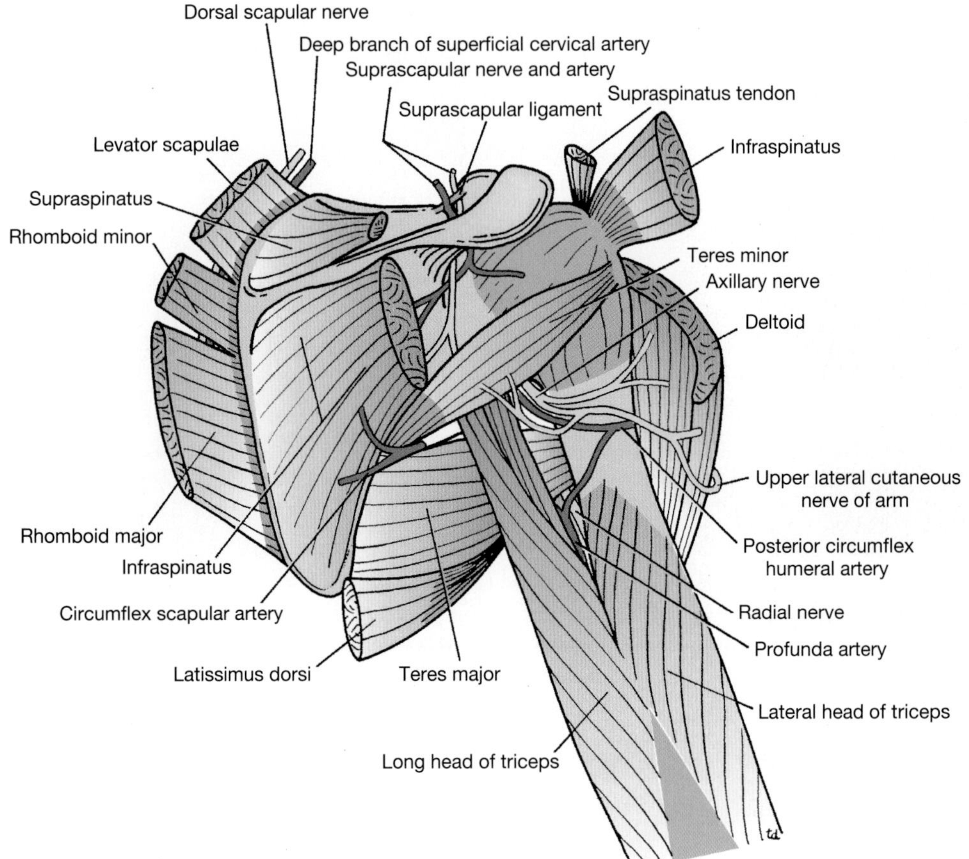

Figure 3.41 Muscles, nerves, and blood vessels of the scapular region. Note the close relation of the axillary nerve to the shoulder joint.

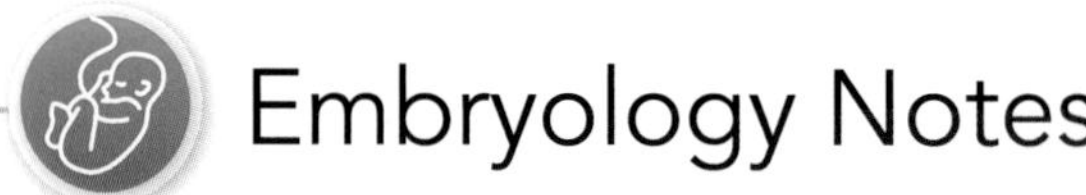

Embryology Notes

Breast Development

In the early embryo, a linear thickening of ectoderm appears called the **milk ridge**, which extends from the axilla obliquely to the inguinal region (Fig. 3.42). In many mammals, several mammary glands are formed along this ridge. In humans, the ridge disappears except for a small part in the pectoral region. This localized area thickens, becomes slightly depressed, and sends off 15 to 20 solid cords, which grow into the underlying mesenchyme. Meanwhile, the underlying mesenchyme proliferates, and the depressed ectodermal thickening becomes raised to form the nipple. At month 5, the areola is recognized as a circular pigmented area of skin around the future nipple.

Polythelia

Supernumerary nipples occasionally occur along a line corresponding (Fig. 3.43) to the position of the milk ridge. They are liable to be mistaken for moles or warts.

Retracted or Inverted Nipple

Retracted nipple is a failure in the development of the nipple during its later stages. It is important clinically, because breastfeeding cannot take place, and the nipple is prone to infection (see also the Clinical Notes section).

Micromastia

An excessively small breast on one side occasionally occurs, resulting from lack of development.

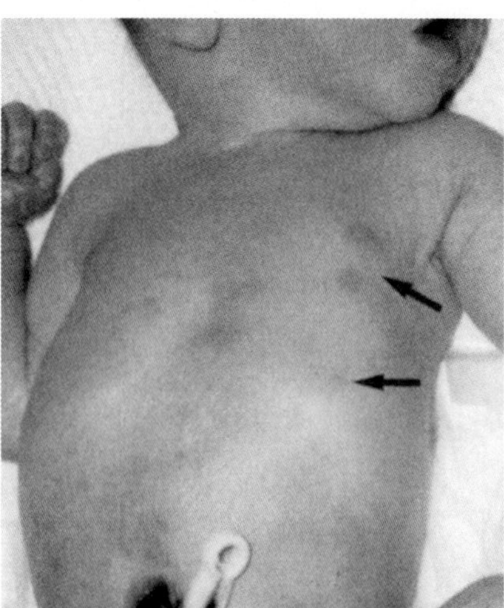

Figure 3.42 Example of polythelia in which two supernumerary nipples (*black arrows*) appear along the milk (mammary) line.

Macromastia

Diffuse hypertrophy of one or both breasts occasionally occurs at puberty in otherwise normal females.

Gynecomastia

Unilateral or bilateral enlargement of the male breast occasionally occurs, usually at puberty. The cause is unknown, but the condition is probably related to some form of hormonal imbalance.

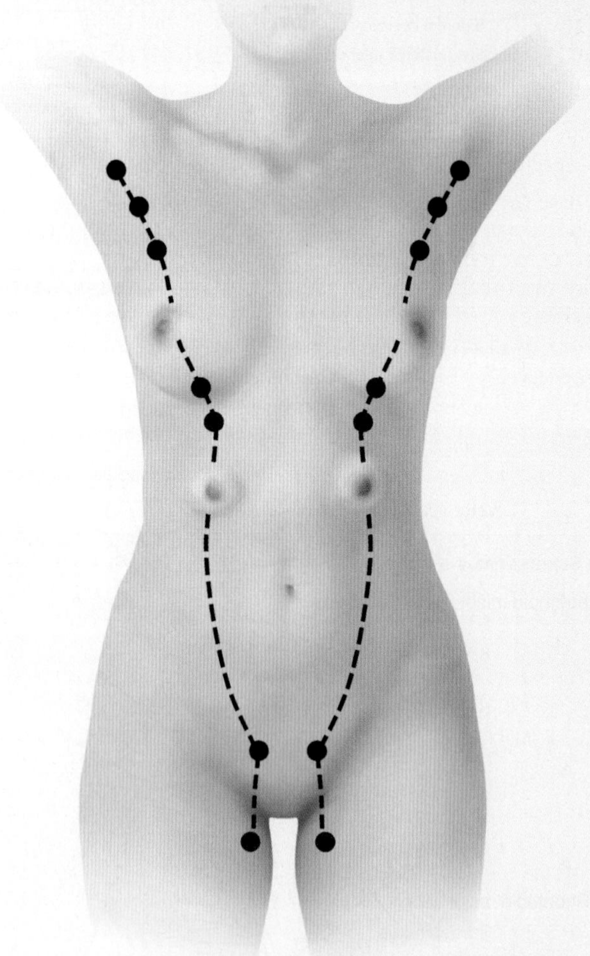

Figure 3.43 Milk (mammary) line extending from the axilla to the groin.

Quadrangular Space

The quadrangular space is an intermuscular space, located immediately below the glenohumeral (shoulder) joint (see Fig. 3.41). Its boundaries are as follows:

- **Superior:** Subscapularis and teres minor muscles and the capsule of the shoulder joint
- **Inferior:** Teres major muscle
- **Medial:** Long head of the triceps muscle
- **Lateral:** Surgical neck of the humerus

The significance of the quadrangular space is that the axillary nerve and the posterior circumflex humeral vessels emerge through this space to reach their terminal destinations in the shoulder.

Axilla

The axilla, or armpit, is a pyramid-shaped space between the upper part of the arm and the side of the chest (Fig. 3.44). It forms an important passage for nerves, blood vessels, and lymph channels as they travel between the root of the neck and the upper limb. The upper end of the axilla, or **apex**, is directed into the root of the neck and is bounded in front by the clavicle, behind by the upper border of the scapula, and medially by the outer border of rib 1. The lower end, or **base**, is bounded in front by the **anterior axillary fold** (formed by the lower border of the pectoralis major muscle), behind by the **posterior axillary fold** (formed by the tendons of the latissimus dorsi and teres major muscles), and medially by the chest wall.

Axillary Walls

The four walls of the axilla are constructed as follows (Figs. 3.45 and 3.46; see also Figs. 3.32 to 3.34):

- **Anterior wall:** By the pectoralis major, subclavius, and pectoralis minor muscles
- **Posterior wall:** By the subscapularis, latissimus dorsi, and teres major muscles
- **Medial wall:** By ribs 1 to 4 or 5 and the intercostal spaces covered by the serratus anterior muscle
- **Lateral wall:** By the coracobrachialis and biceps brachii muscles in the bicipital groove of the humerus

The skin stretching between the anterior and posterior walls forms the base of the axilla (see Figs. 3.44 and 3.45). Details of the muscles forming the walls of the axilla are summarized later in this chapter in Tables 3.4 through 3.6.

The axilla contains the axillary artery and its branches, which supply blood to the upper limb; the axillary vein and its tributaries, which drain blood from the upper limb; and lymph vessels and lymph nodes, which drain lymph from the upper limb, the breast, and the skin of the trunk as far down as the level of the umbilicus. The brachial plexus, an important nerve network that innervates the upper limb, lies among these structures. The contents of the axilla are embedded in fat.

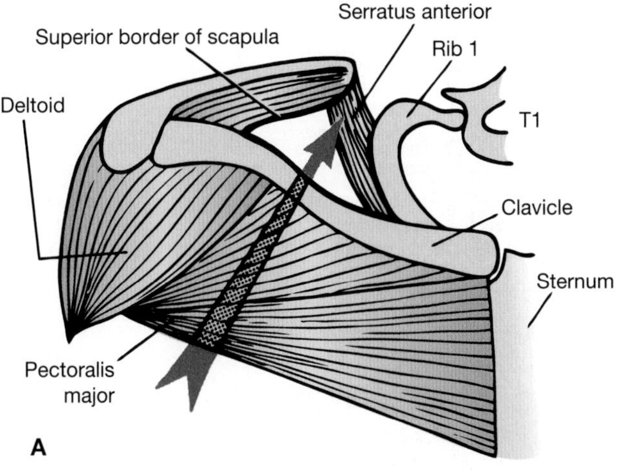

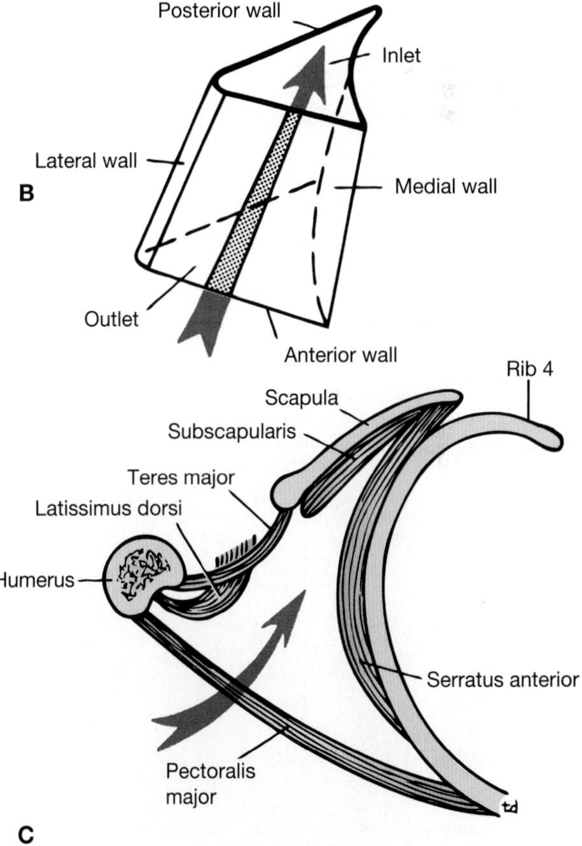

Figure 3.44 Right axilla. **A.** Axillary inlet from above. **B.** Axillary walls. **C.** Axillary outlet.

Pectoralis Minor

The pectoralis minor is a thin triangular muscle that lies deep to the pectoralis major (see Fig. 3.33). It arises from ribs 3 to 5 and runs upward and laterally to insert into the coracoid process of the scapula. Thus, it crosses the axilla and divides the area into three subregions (proximal, deep, and distal to the muscle) that are useful in describing the course of the axillary artery and the lymph drainage of the area (see the

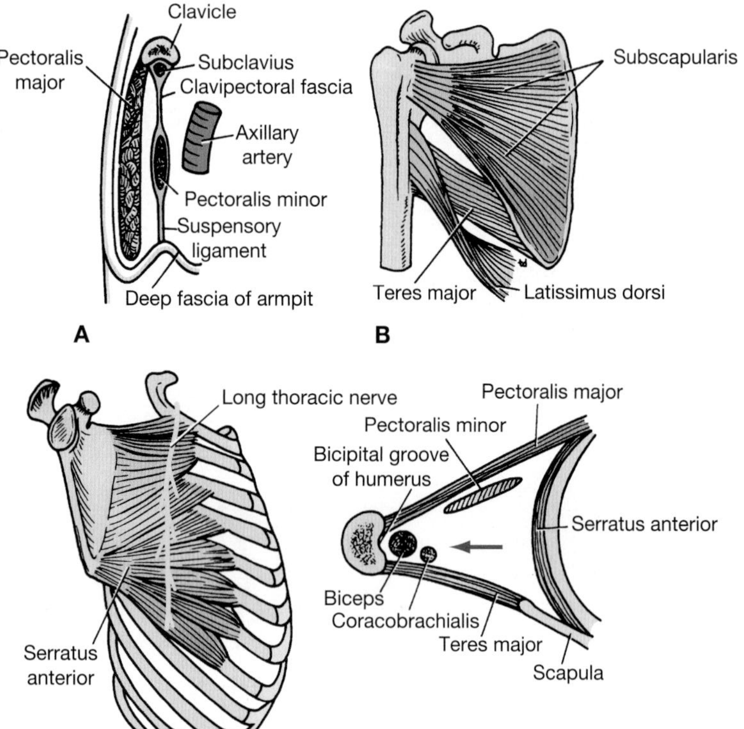

Figure 3.45 Structures that form the walls of the axilla. The *red arrow* indicates the lateral wall. **A.** Anterior wall. **B.** Posterior wall. **C.** Medial wall. **D.** Lateral wall.

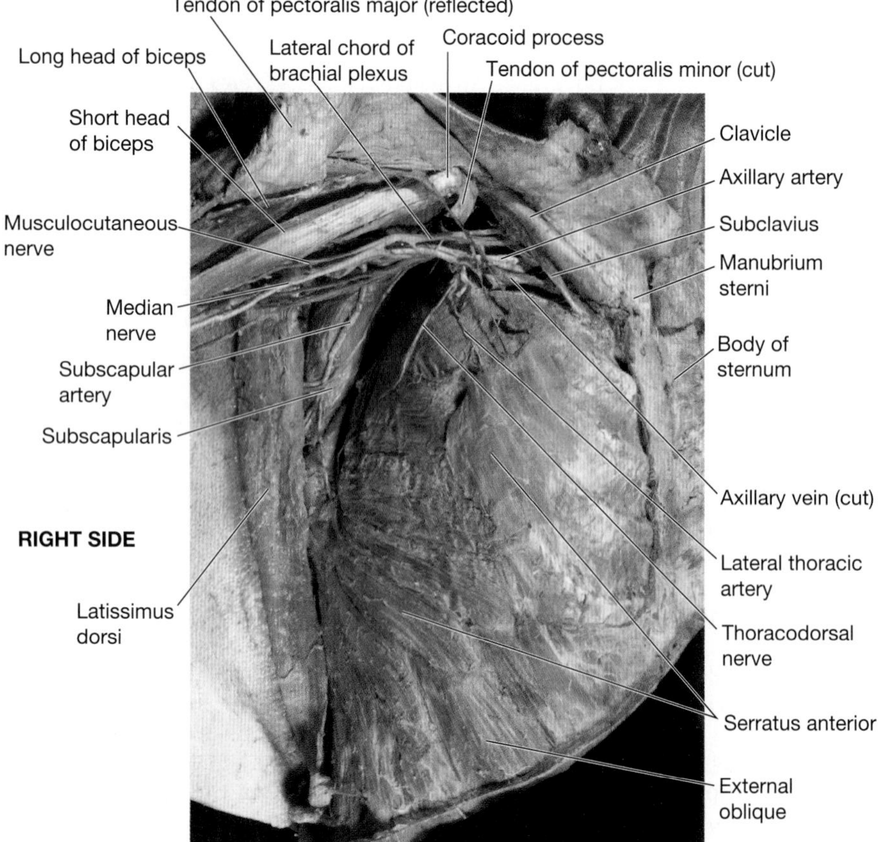

Figure 3.46 Dissection of the right axilla. The pectoralis major and minor muscles and the clavipectoral fascia have been removed to display the underlying structures.

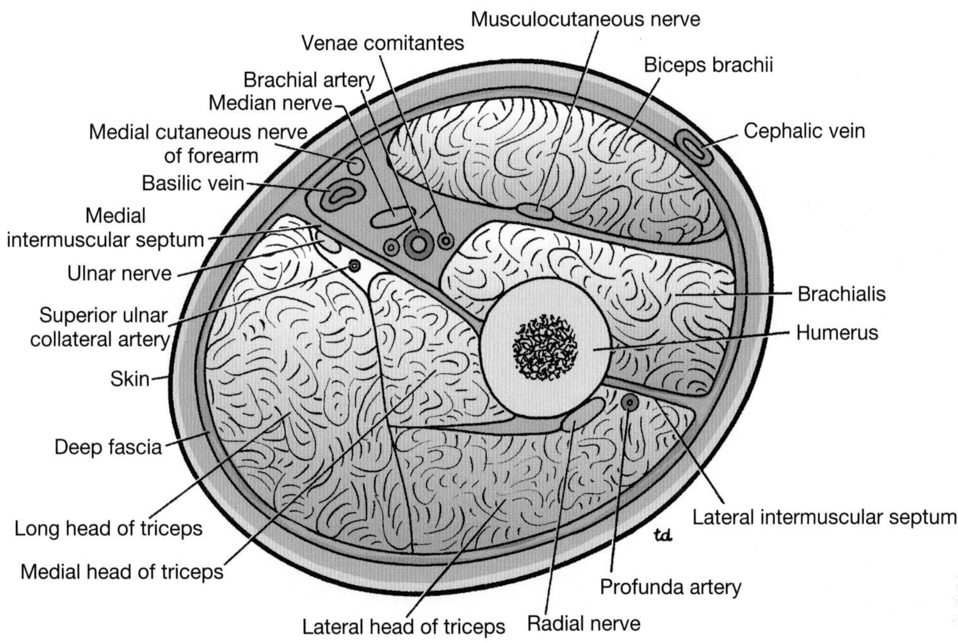

Figure 3.47 Cross section of the upper arm just below the level of insertion of the deltoid muscle. Note the division of the arm into anterior and posterior compartments by the humerus and the medial and lateral intermuscular septa.

descriptions of the axillary artery and lymph drainage below).

Clavipectoral Fascia

The clavipectoral fascia is a strong sheet of connective tissue lying immediately deep to the pectoralis major muscle (see Figs. 3.33 and 3.45). Superiorly, it attaches to the clavicle. Inferiorly, it splits to enclose the subclavius and pectoralis minor muscles and then continues downward as the **suspensory ligament of the axilla** and joins the fascial floor of the armpit. The lateral pectoral nerve, cephalic vein, branches of the thoracoacromial artery, and lymphatic channels from the infraclavicular nodes pierce the clavipectoral fascia to make their superficial–deep connections.

Arm

The arm (upper arm; brachium) is the proximal segment of the upper limb from the shoulder to the elbow.

Osseofascial Compartments

The arm is enclosed in a sheath of deep fascia (Fig. 3.47; see also the Introduction section of Chapter 1). Two fascial intermuscular septa, one on the medial side and one on the lateral side, extend inward from this sheath and are attached to the medial and lateral supracondylar ridges of the humerus, respectively. In this way, the upper arm is divided into anterior and posterior osseofascial compartments, each having a set of muscles, nerves, and arteries (Figs. 3.48 to 3.50; see also Fig. 3.47 and Table 3.2). Also, these and additional structures pass through each compartment en route to more distal areas.

Structures Passing through the Anterior Osseofascial Compartment

The musculocutaneous, median, and ulnar nerves; brachial artery; and basilic vein pass through this region. The radial nerve is present in the lower part of the compartment.

Structures Passing through the Posterior Osseofascial Compartment

The radial and ulnar nerves and profunda brachii vessels pass through this region.

Elbow and Cubital Fossa

The elbow is the area connecting the arm with the forearm. The cubital fossa is a triangular depression that lies in the anterior aspect of the elbow (Figs. 3.51 and 3.52). This fossa is important because it conveys several major structures between the arm and the forearm.

Cubital Fossa Boundaries

- **Laterally:** Medial border of brachioradialis muscle
- **Medially:** Lateral border of pronator teres muscle
- **Base:** Imaginary line drawn between the two epicondyles of the humerus forming the base of the triangle
- **Floor:** Supinator muscle laterally; brachialis muscle medially
- **Roof:** Skin and fascia, reinforced by the bicipital aponeurosis

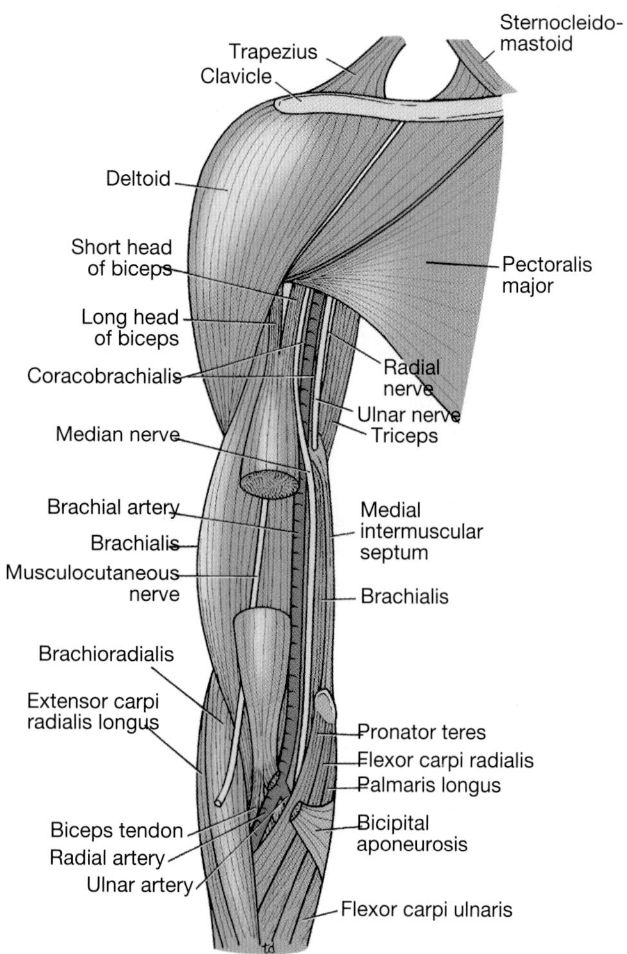

Figure 3.48 Anterior view of the upper arm. The middle portion of the biceps brachii has been removed to show the musculocutaneous nerve lying in front of the brachialis.

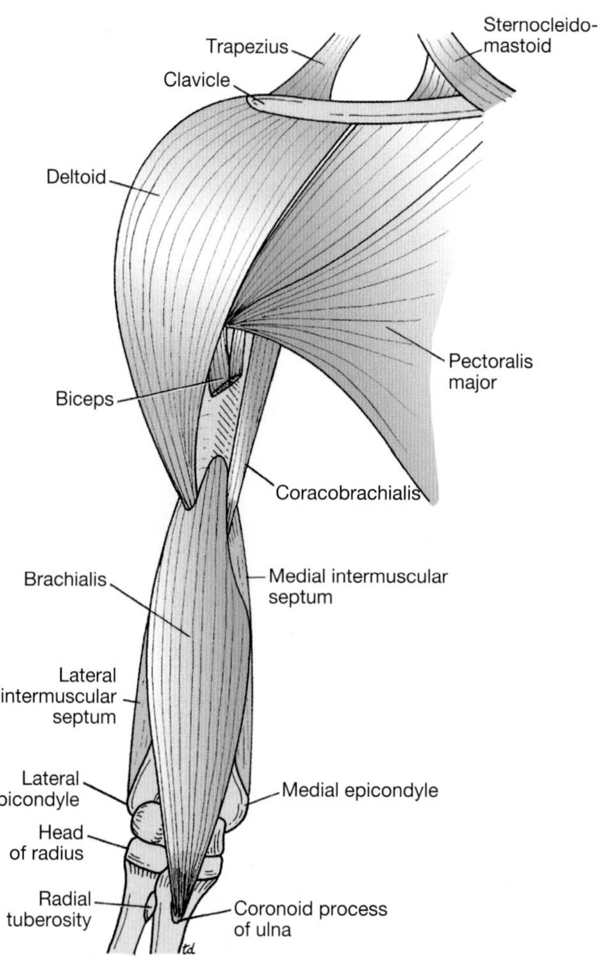

Figure 3.49 Anterior view of the upper arm showing the insertion of the deltoid and the origin and insertion of the brachialis.

Cubital Fossa Contents

The cubital fossa (see Fig. 3.52) contains the following structures from the medial to the lateral side: median nerve, bifurcation of the brachial artery into the ulnar and radial arteries, tendon of the biceps muscle, and radial nerve and its deep branch.

Forearm

The **forearm** (**lower arm**; **antebrachium**) is the segment of the upper limb from the elbow to the wrist.

Osseofascial Compartments

The forearm is enclosed in a sheath of deep fascia, which is attached to the periosteum of the posterior subcutaneous border of the ulna (Fig. 3.53). The **interosseous membrane** (Figs. 3.54, 3.57, and 3.59) is a strong ligamentous band that unites the shafts of the radius and the ulna and provides additional surface area for the attachments of neighboring muscles. This wrapping sheet of deep fascia, together with the interosseous membrane and fibrous intermuscular septa, divides the forearm into three osseofascial compartments: anterior, lateral, and posterior. Each compartment contains a set of muscles, nerves, and arteries (Figs. 3.53 to 3.59; Table 3.3).

Wrist

The **wrist** (**carpus**) is a complex of the eight small carpal bones that connect the forearm and hand (see Figs. 3.8 and 3.9). Before learning the anatomy of the hand, having a sound knowledge of the arrangement of the tendons, arteries, and nerves in the region of the wrist is essential. From a clinical standpoint, the wrist is a common site for injury.

Flexor and Extensor Retinacula

The flexor and extensor retinacula are strong bands of deep fascia that hold the long flexor and extensor tendons in position at the wrist.

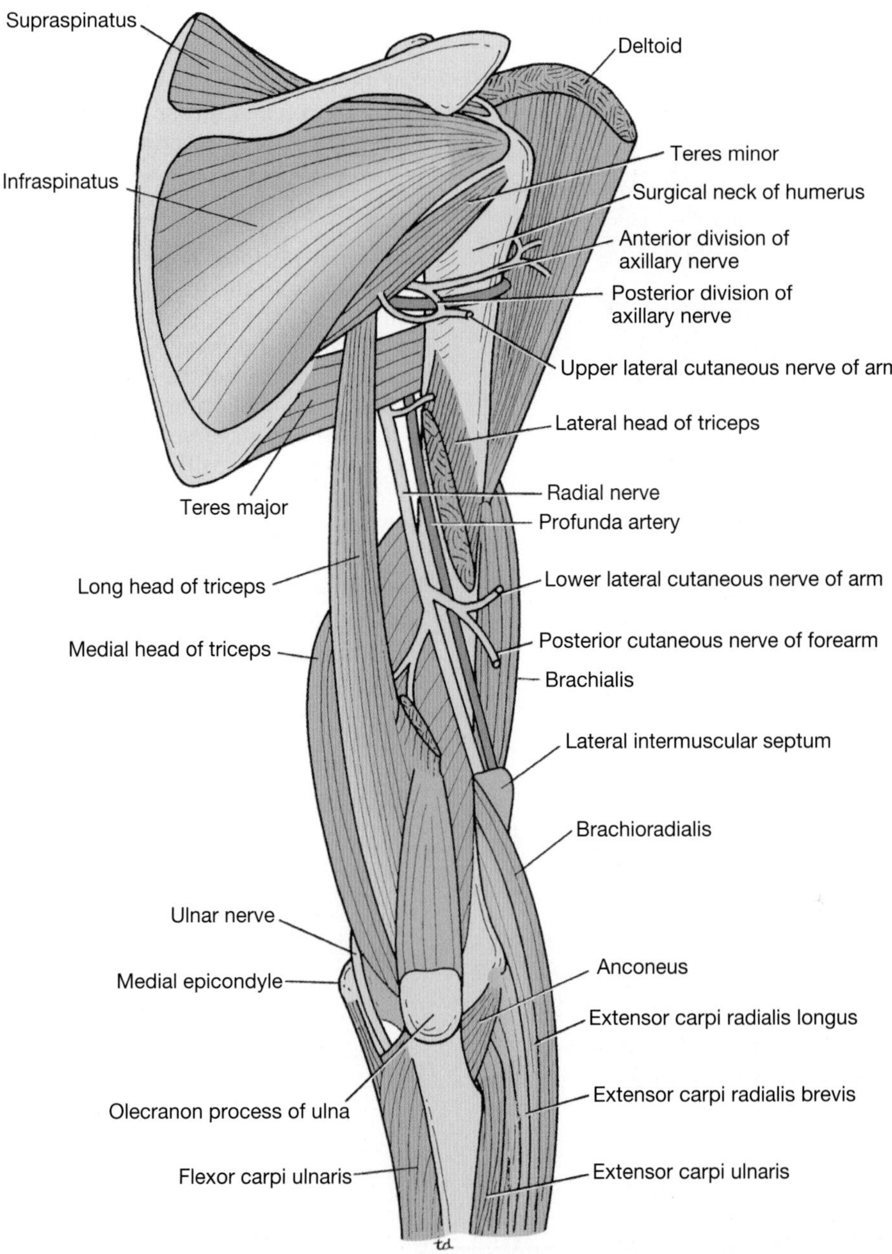

Figure 3.50 Posterior view of the upper arm. The lateral head of the triceps has been divided to display the radial nerve and the profunda artery in the spiral groove of the humerus.

Table 3.2 Contents of Arm Osseofascial Compartments

	ANTERIOR COMPARTMENT	POSTERIOR COMPARTMENT
MUSCLES	Biceps brachii Coracobrachialis Brachialis	Triceps brachii
MOTOR NERVE SUPPLY	Musculocutaneous nerve	Radial nerve
BLOOD SUPPLY	Brachial artery	Profunda brachii artery Ulnar collateral arteries

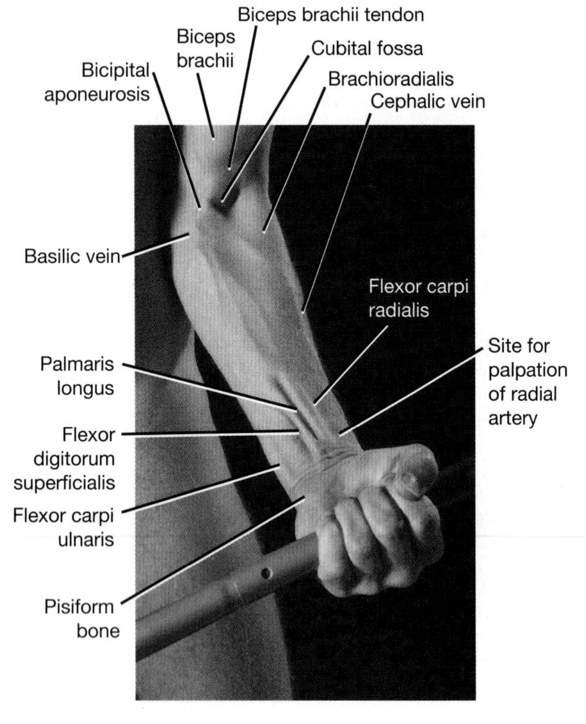

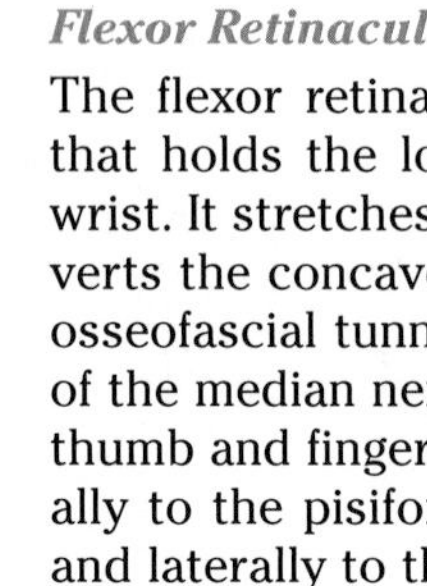

Figure 3.51 Cubital fossa and anterior surface of the forearm in a young male.

Flexor Retinaculum

The flexor retinaculum is a thickening of deep fascia that holds the long flexor tendons in position at the wrist. It stretches across the front of the wrist and converts the concave anterior surface of the wrist into an osseofascial tunnel, the **carpal tunnel**, for the passage of the median nerve and the long flexor tendons of the thumb and fingers (Figs. 3.60 to 3.62). It attaches medially to the pisiform bone and the hook of the hamate and laterally to the tubercle of the scaphoid and trapezium bones. The attachment to the trapezium consists of superficial and deep parts and forms a synovial-lined tunnel for passage of the tendon of the flexor carpi radialis. The proximal border of the retinaculum corresponds to the distal transverse skin crease in front of the wrist and is continuous with the deep fascia of the forearm. The distal border is attached to the palmar aponeurosis (see Fig. 3.61).

Extensor Retinaculum

The extensor retinaculum is a thickening of deep fascia that stretches across the back of the wrist and holds the long extensor tendons in position (Figs. 3.63 and 3.64; see also Figs. 3.58 and 3.60). It converts the grooves on the posterior surface of the distal ends of the radius and ulna into six separate tunnels for the passage of the long extensor tendons. Each tunnel is

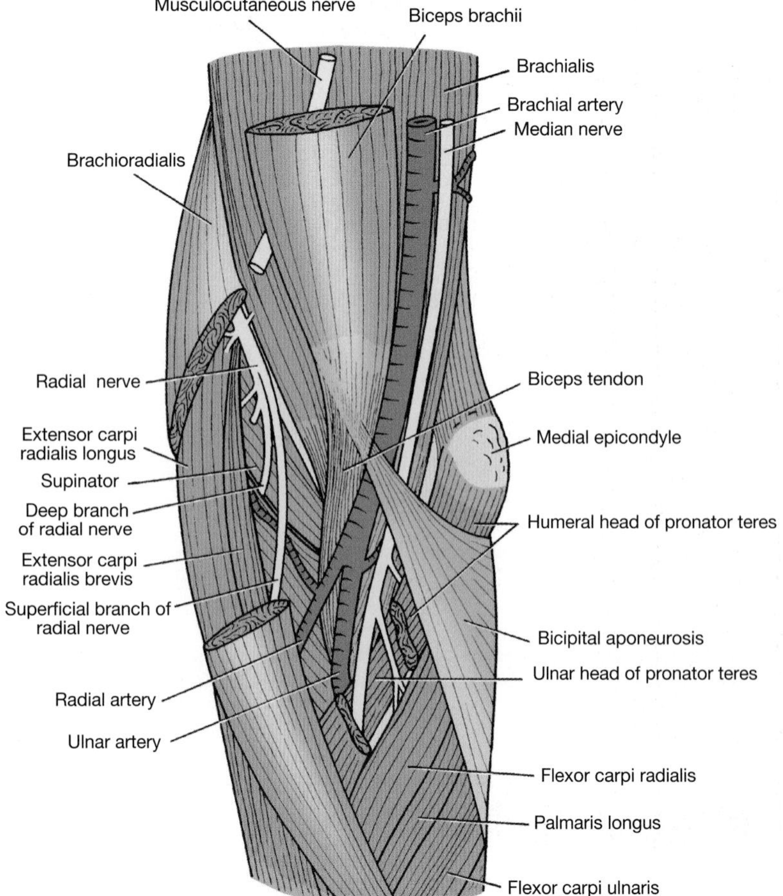

Figure 3.52 Right cubital fossa.

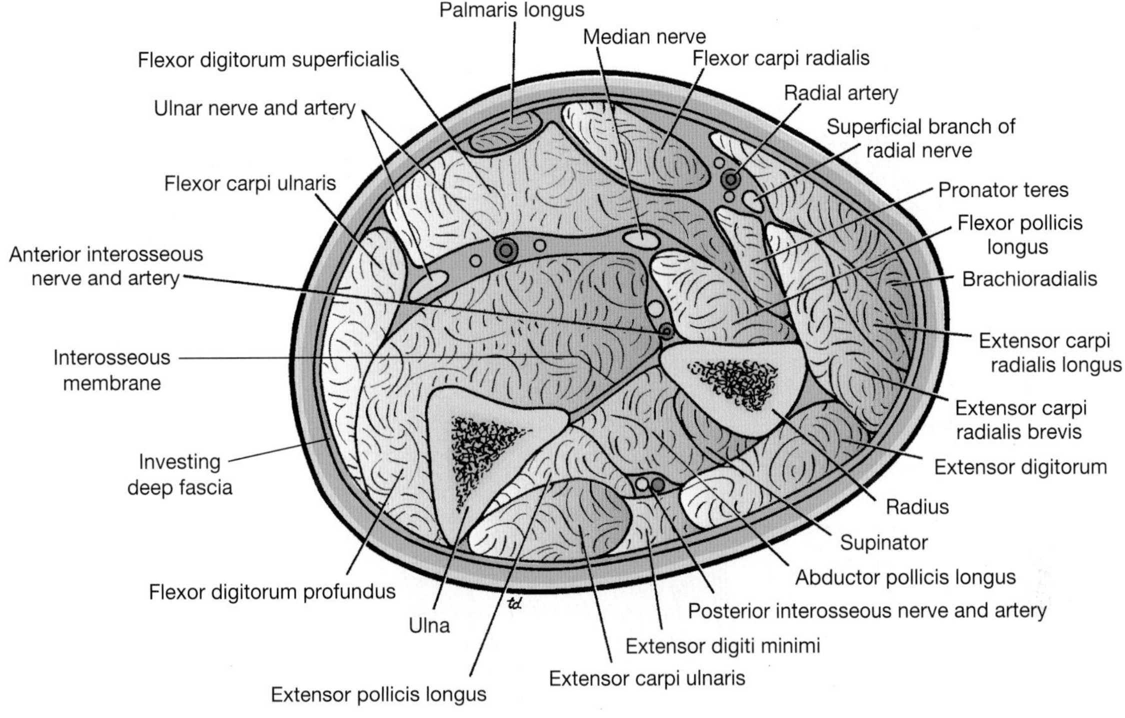

Figure 3.53 Cross-section of the forearm at the level of insertion of the pronator teres muscle.

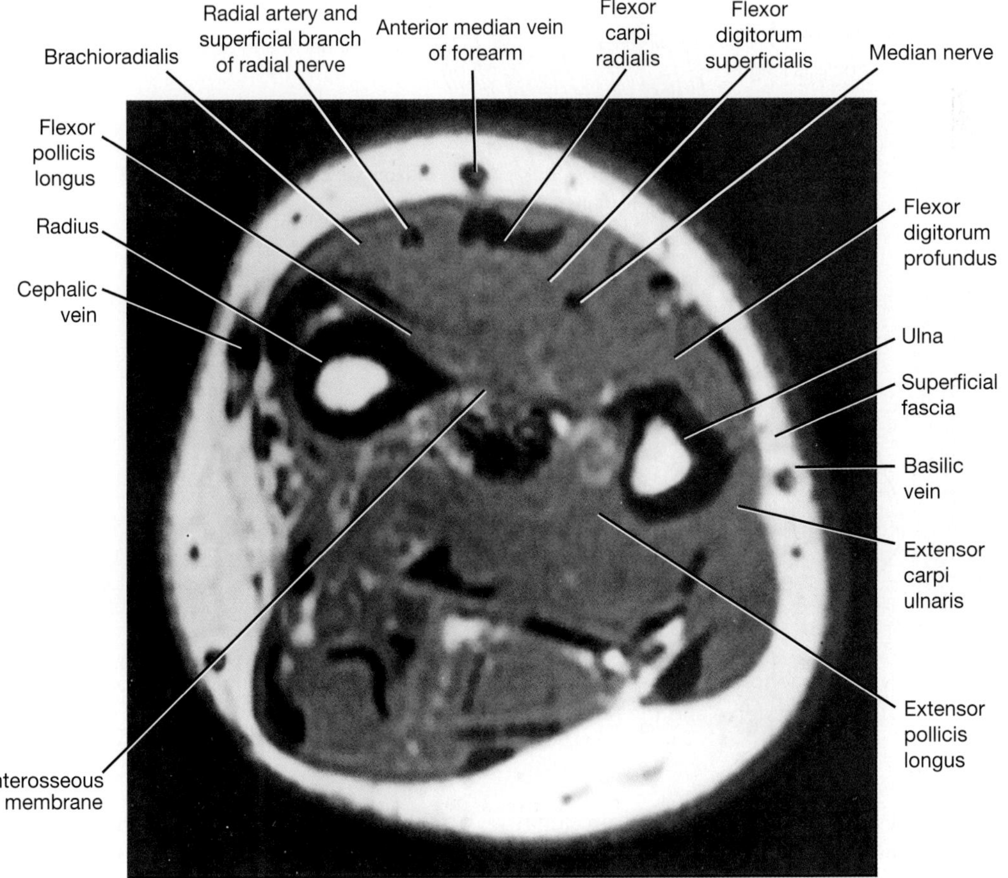

Figure 3.54 Transverse (axial) magnetic resonance image of the upper part of the right forearm (as seen from below).

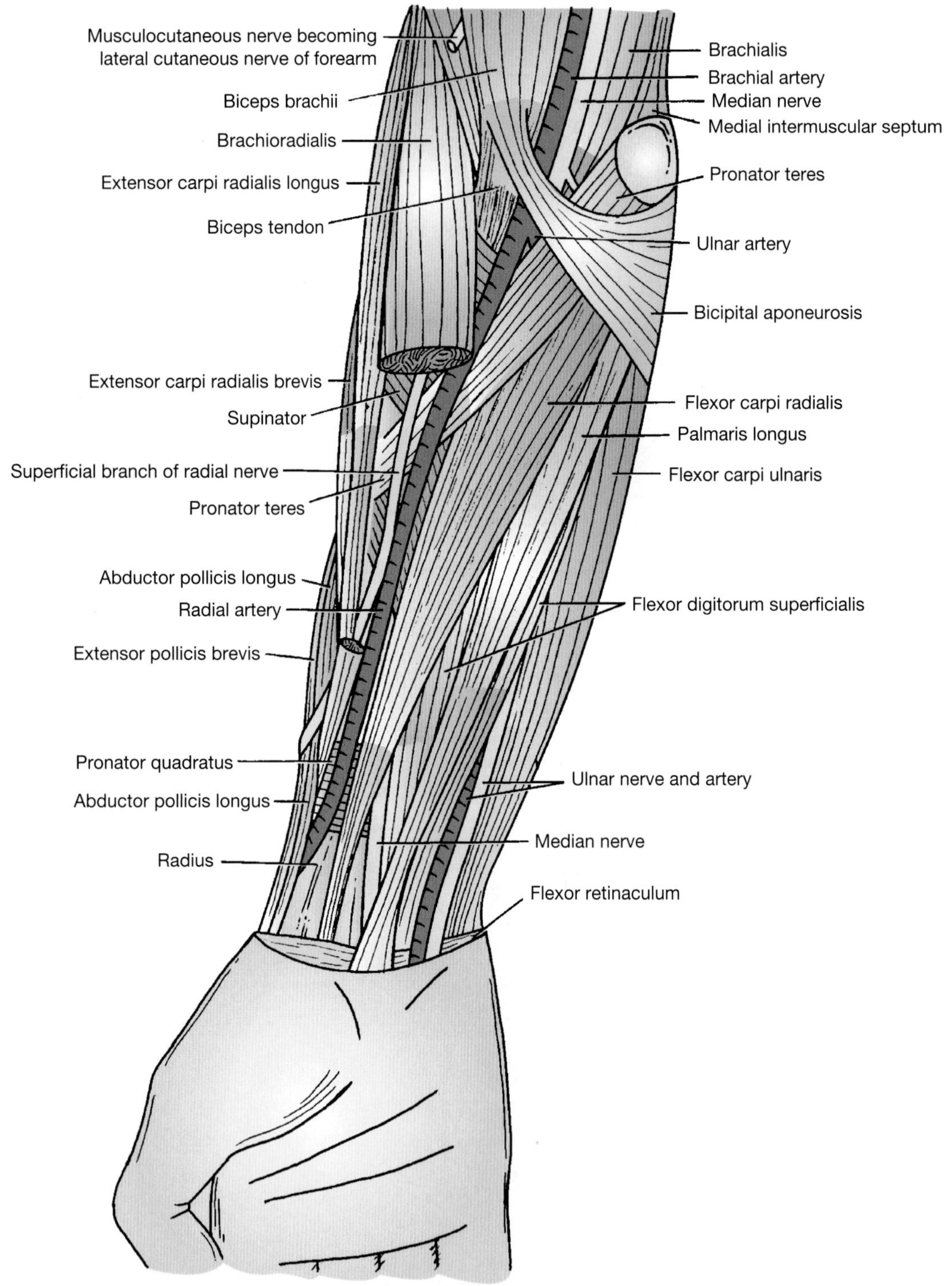

Figure 3.55 Anterior view of the forearm. The middle portion of the brachioradialis muscle has been removed to display the superficial branch of the radial nerve and the radial artery.

lined with a synovial sheath, which extends proximal and distal to the retinaculum on the tendons. The tunnels are separated from one another by fibrous septa that extend from the deep surface of the retinaculum to the underlying bones (see Fig. 3.60). The retinaculum attaches medially to the pisiform bone and the hook of the hamate and laterally to the distal end of the radius. The proximal and distal borders of the retinaculum are continuous with the deep fascia of the forearm and hand, respectively.

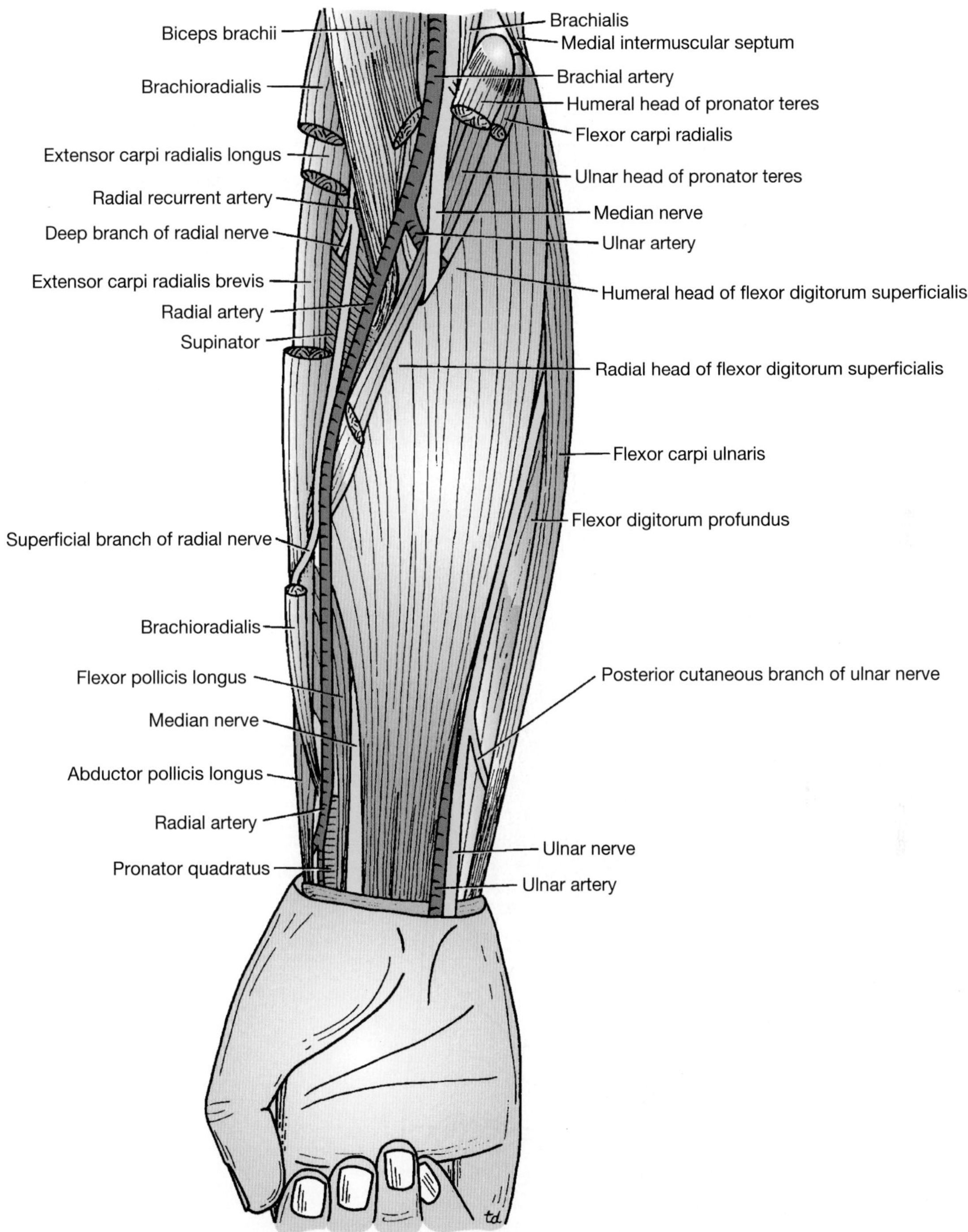

Figure 3.56 Anterior view of the forearm. Most of the superficial muscles have been removed to display the flexor digitorum superficialis, median nerve, superficial branch of the radial nerve, and radial artery. Note that the ulnar head of the pronator teres separates the median nerve from the ulnar artery.

Anterior Wrist Structures

A critical concept in wrist anatomy is recognizing the structures contained within the carpal tunnel vs. those located outside the tunnel (ie, which structures pass superficial vs. deep to the flexor retinaculum). The following structures pass superficial to the flexor retinaculum (outside the carpal tunnel), in medial to lateral sequence (see Fig. 3.60):

- **Flexor carpi ulnaris tendon**, ending on the pisiform bone (this tendon does not actually cross the flexor retinaculum but is included for the sake of completeness)

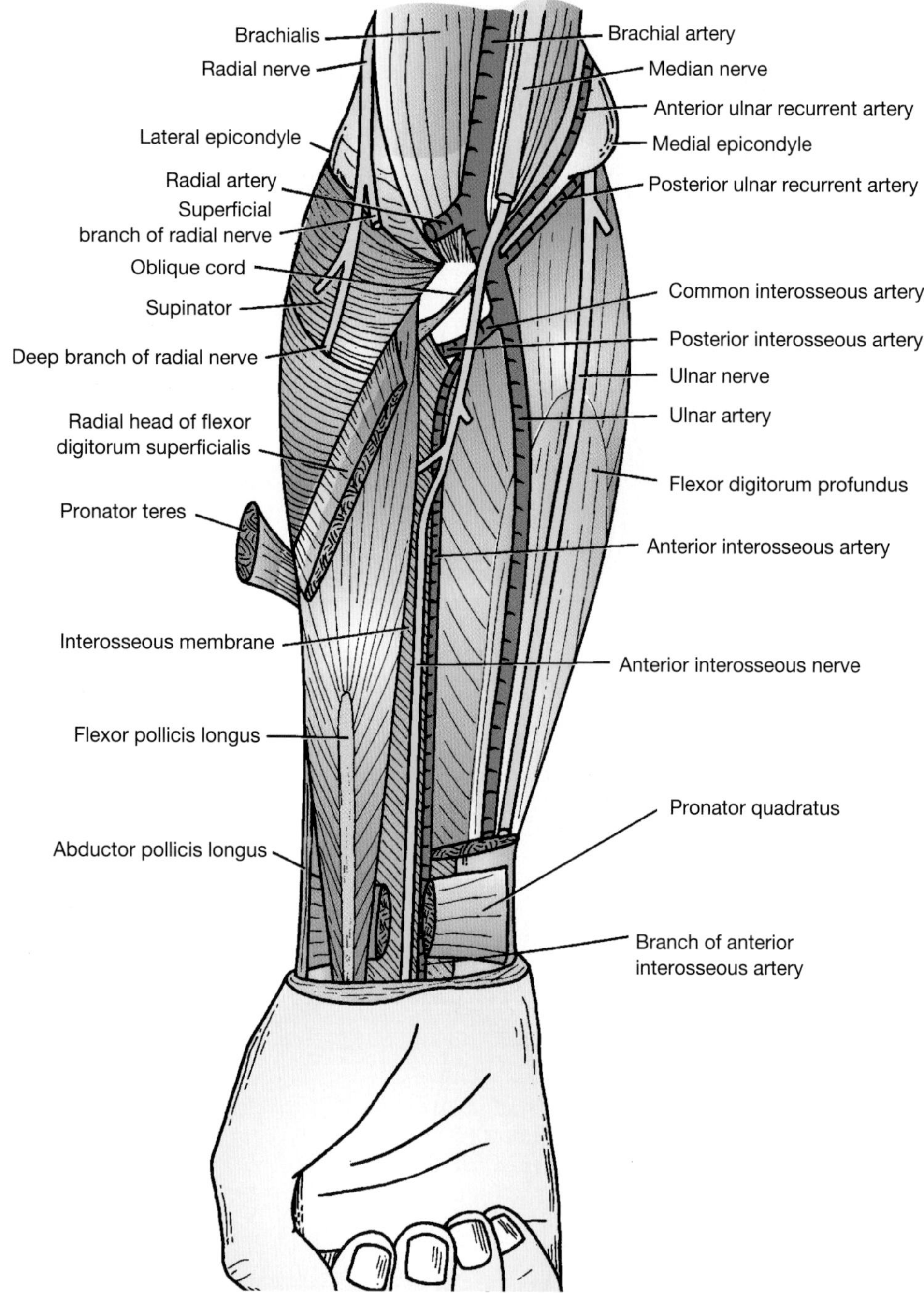

Figure 3.57 Anterior view of the forearm showing the deep structures.

- **Ulnar nerve**, lying lateral to the pisiform bone
- **Ulnar artery**, lying lateral to the ulnar nerve
- **Palmar cutaneous branch of the ulnar nerve**
- **Palmaris longus tendon** (if present), passing to its insertion into the flexor retinaculum and the palmar aponeurosis
- **Palmar cutaneous branch of the median nerve**

The following structures pass deep to the flexor retinaculum (within the carpal tunnel), from medial to lateral (Fig. 3.65; see also Fig. 3.60):

- **Flexor digitorum superficialis tendons** and, deep to these, the **tendons of the flexor digitorum profundus** (both groups of tendons share a common synovial sheath)
- **Median nerve**
- **Flexor pollicis longus tendon**, surrounded by a synovial sheath
- **Flexor carpi radialis tendon**, going through a split in the flexor retinaculum (synovial sheath surrounds the tendon; thus, this tendon is not contained within the carpal tunnel)

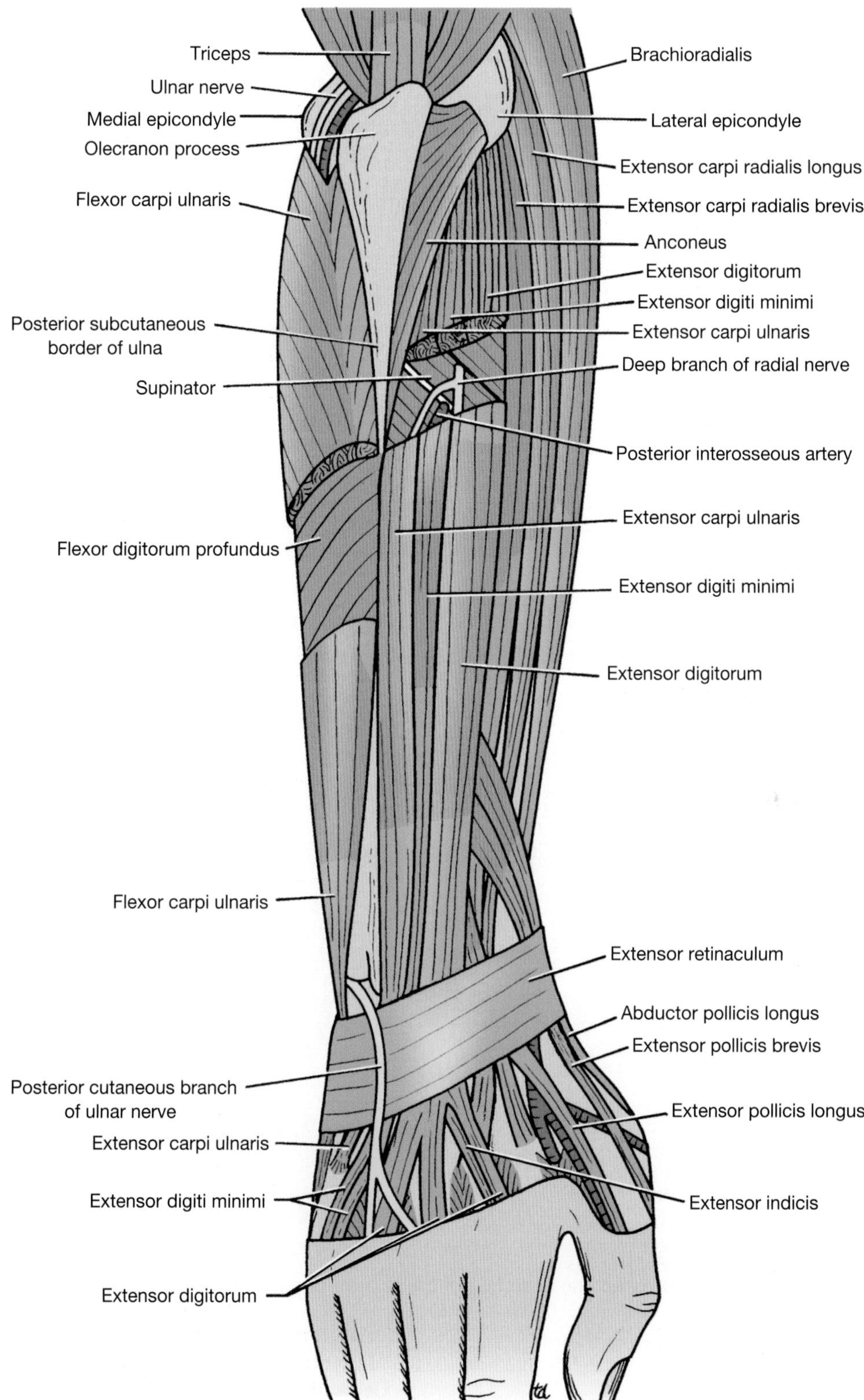

Figure 3.58 Posterior view of the forearm. Parts of the extensor digitorum, extensor digiti minimi, and extensor carpi ulnaris have been removed to show the deep branch of the radial nerve and the posterior interosseous artery.

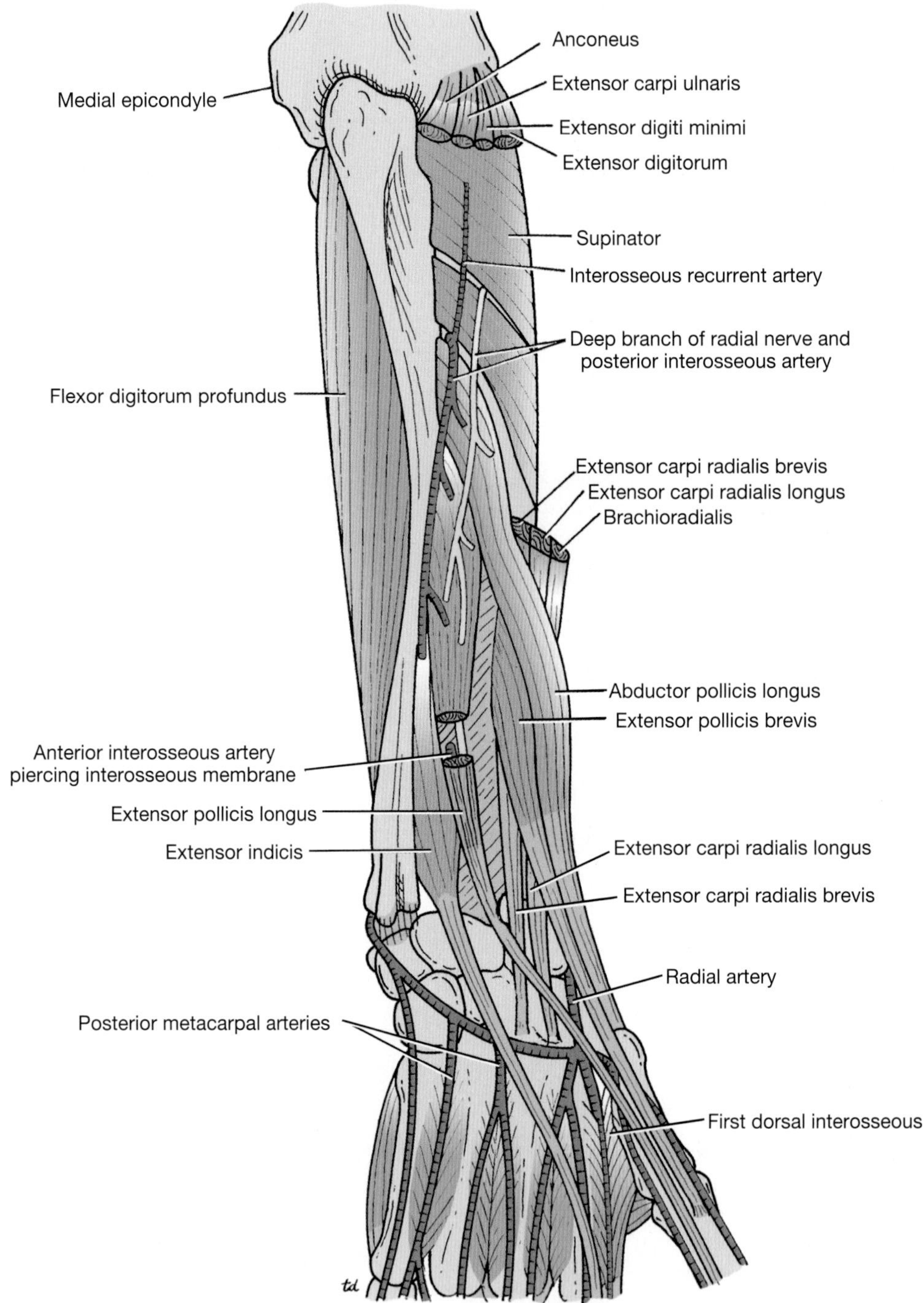

Figure 3.59 Posterior view of the forearm. The superficial muscles have been removed to display the deep structures.

Posterior Wrist Structures

The following structures pass superficial to the extensor retinaculum, from medial to lateral (see Fig. 3.60; notice there are no muscle tendons running in this plane):

- **Dorsal (posterior) cutaneous branch of the ulnar nerve**
- **Basilic vein**
- **Cephalic vein**
- **Superficial branch of the radial nerve**

The following structures pass deep to the extensor retinaculum from medial to lateral, within the six extensor tunnels of the retinaculum (see Figs. 3.58, 3.60, 3.63, and 3.64):

- **Extensor carpi ulnaris tendon**, which grooves the posterior aspect of the head of the ulna

Table 3.3 Contents of Forearm Osseofascial Compartments

	ANTERIOR COMPARTMENT	LATERAL COMPARTMENT	POSTERIOR COMPARTMENT
MUSCLES	*Superficial Group*: Pronator teres Flexor carpi radialis Palmaris longus Flexor carpi ulnaris *Intermediate Group*: Flexor digitorum superficialis *Deep Group*: Flexor digitorum profundus Flexor pollicis longus Pronator quadratus	Brachioradialis Extensor carpi radialis longus	*Superficial Group*: Extensor carpi radialis brevis Extensor digitorum Extensor digiti minimi Extensor carpi ulnaris Anconeus *Deep Group*: Supinator Abductor pollicis longus Extensor pollicis brevis Extensor pollicis longus Extensor indicis
MOTOR NERVE SUPPLY	Median nerve (all muscles except the one and a half supplied by the ulnar nerve) Ulnar nerve (flexor carpi ulnaris + medial half of flexor digitorum profundus)	Radial nerve	Radial nerve (deep branch)
BLOOD SUPPLY	Radial artery Ulnar artery	Brachial artery Radial artery	Ulnar artery (posterior interosseous artery)

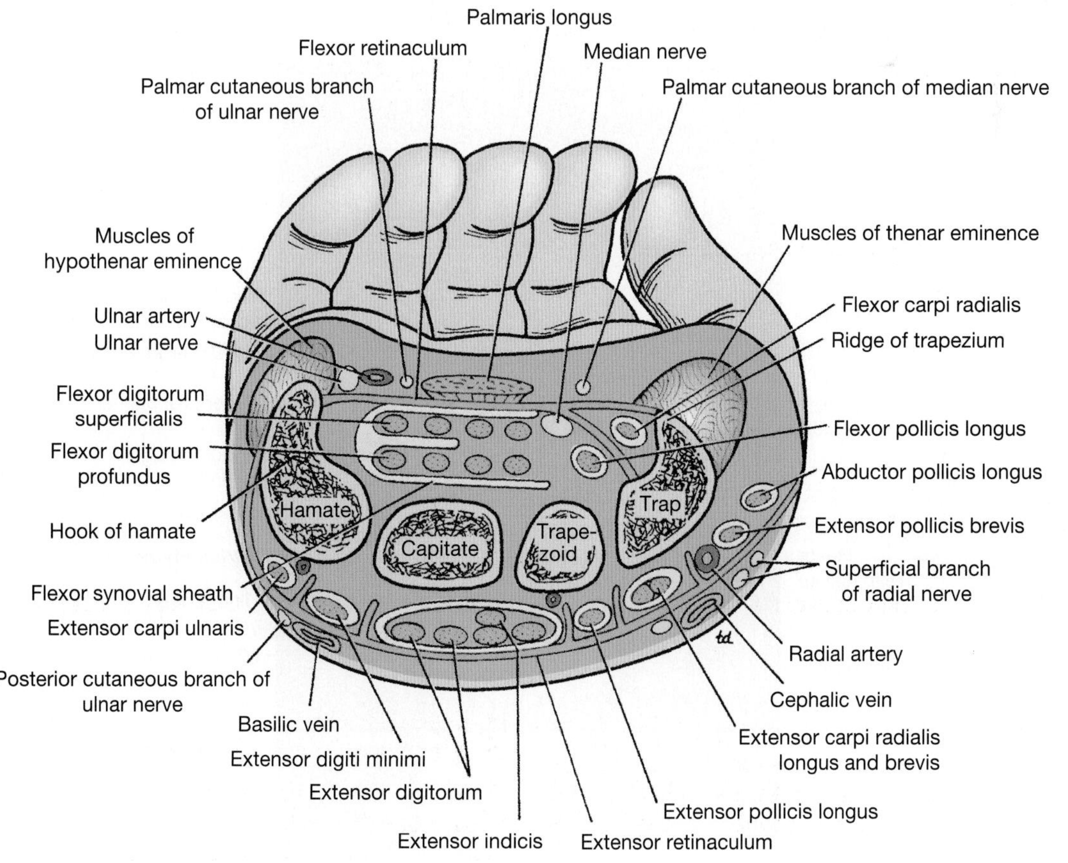

Figure 3.60 Cross section of the hand showing the relation of the tendons, nerves, and arteries to the flexor and extensor retinacula.

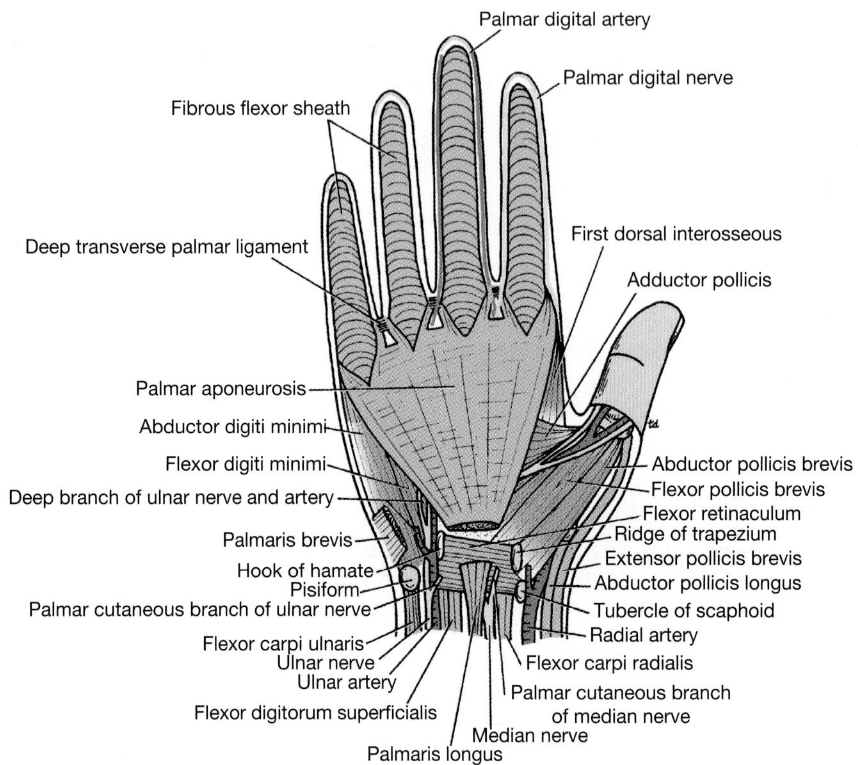

Figure 3.61 Anterior view of the palm of the hand. The palmar aponeurosis has been left in position.

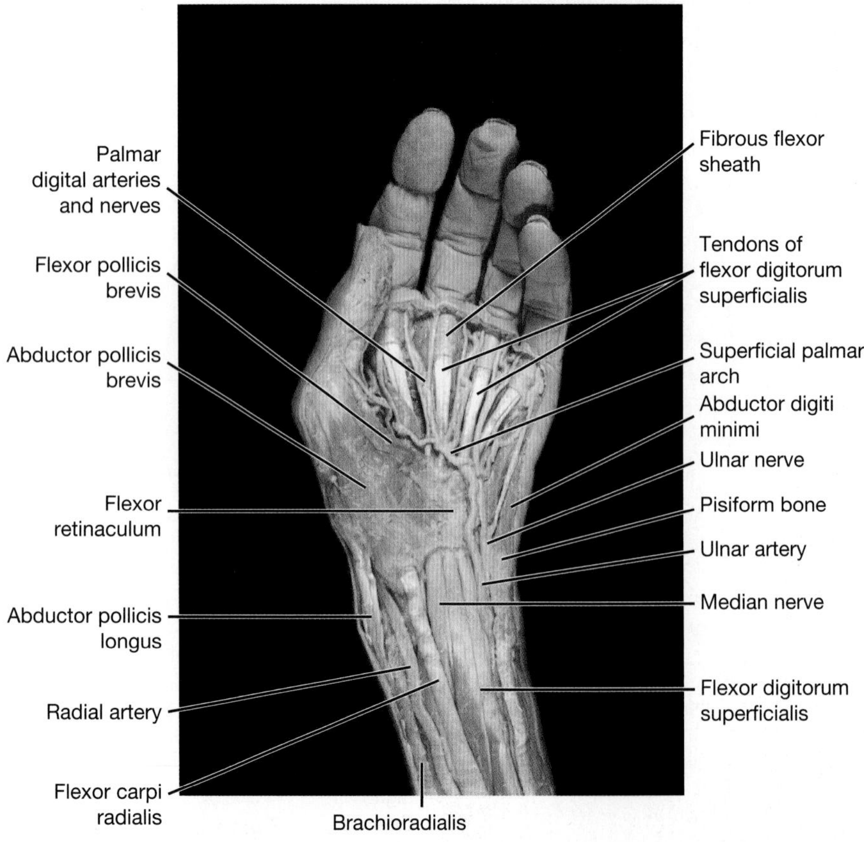

Figure 3.62 Dissection of the front of the left forearm and hand showing the superficial structures.

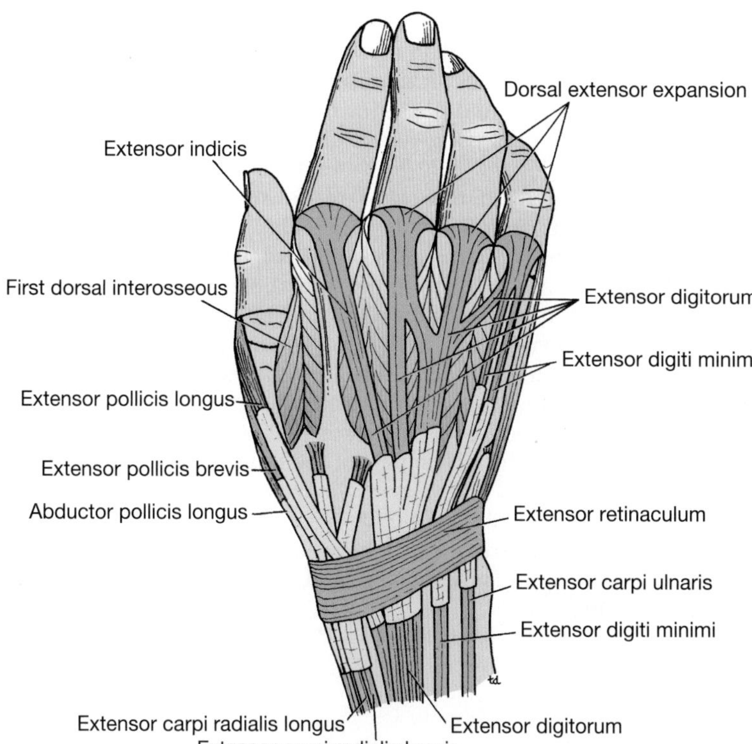

Figure 3.63 Dorsal surface of the hand showing the long extensor tendons and their synovial sheaths.

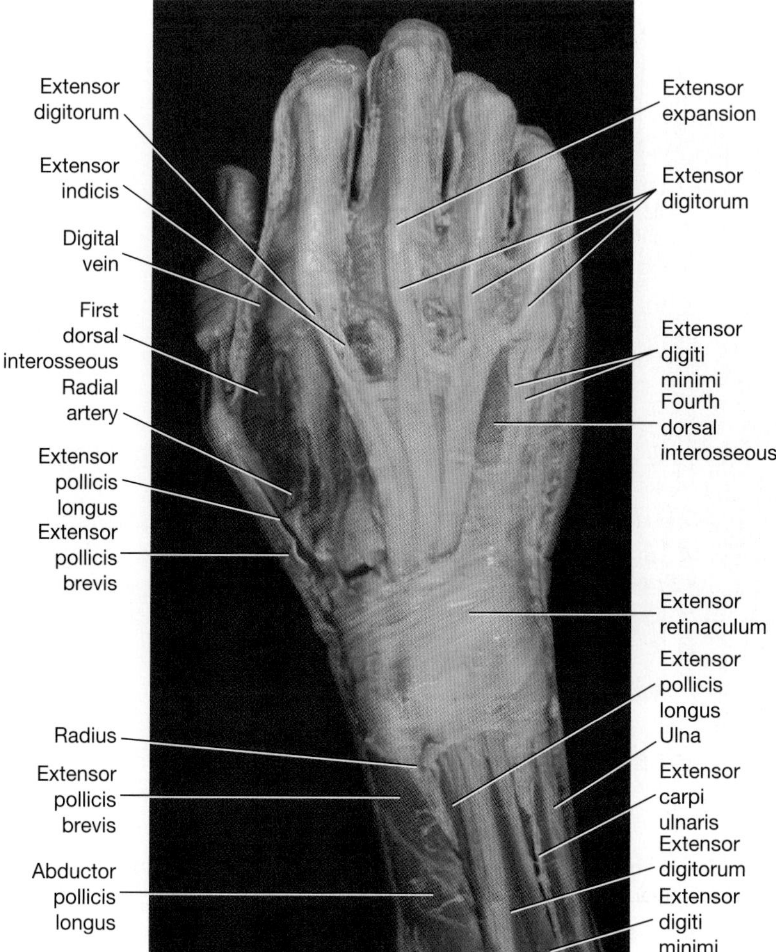

Figure 3.64 Dissection of the dorsal surface of the right hand showing the long extensor tendons and the extensor retinaculum.

- **Extensor digiti minimi tendon**, situated posterior to the distal radioulnar joint
- **Extensor digitorum and extensor indicis tendons**, sharing a common synovial sheath and situated on the lateral part of the posterior surface of the radius
- **Extensor pollicis longus tendon**, winding around the medial side of the dorsal tubercle of the radius
- **Extensor carpi radialis longus and brevis tendons**, sharing a common synovial sheath and situated on the lateral part of the posterior surface of the radius
- **Abductor pollicis longus and extensor pollicis brevis tendons**, having separate synovial sheaths but sharing a common compartment

Carpal Tunnel

The carpus is deeply concave on its anterior surface and forms a bony gutter. The gutter is converted into the carpal tunnel by the covering flexor retinaculum (see Fig. 3.60). The long flexor tendons to the fingers and thumb pass through the tunnel and are accompanied by the median nerve. The four separate tendons of the flexor digitorum superficialis muscle are arranged in anterior and posterior rows, those to the middle and ring fingers lying superficial to those of the index and little fingers. The four tendons diverge and become arranged on the same plane at the distal border of the flexor retinaculum (see Fig. 3.65). The tendons of the flexor digitorum profundus muscle are on the same plane and lie deep to the superficialis tendons. All eight tendons of the flexor digitorum superficialis and profundus invaginate a common synovial sheath from the lateral side (see Fig. 3.60). This allows the arterial supply to the tendons to enter from the lateral side.

The tendon of the flexor pollicis longus muscle runs through the lateral part of the tunnel in its own synovial sheath.

The median nerve passes deep to the flexor retinaculum in a narrow space between the tendons of the flexor digitorum superficialis and the flexor carpi radialis muscles.

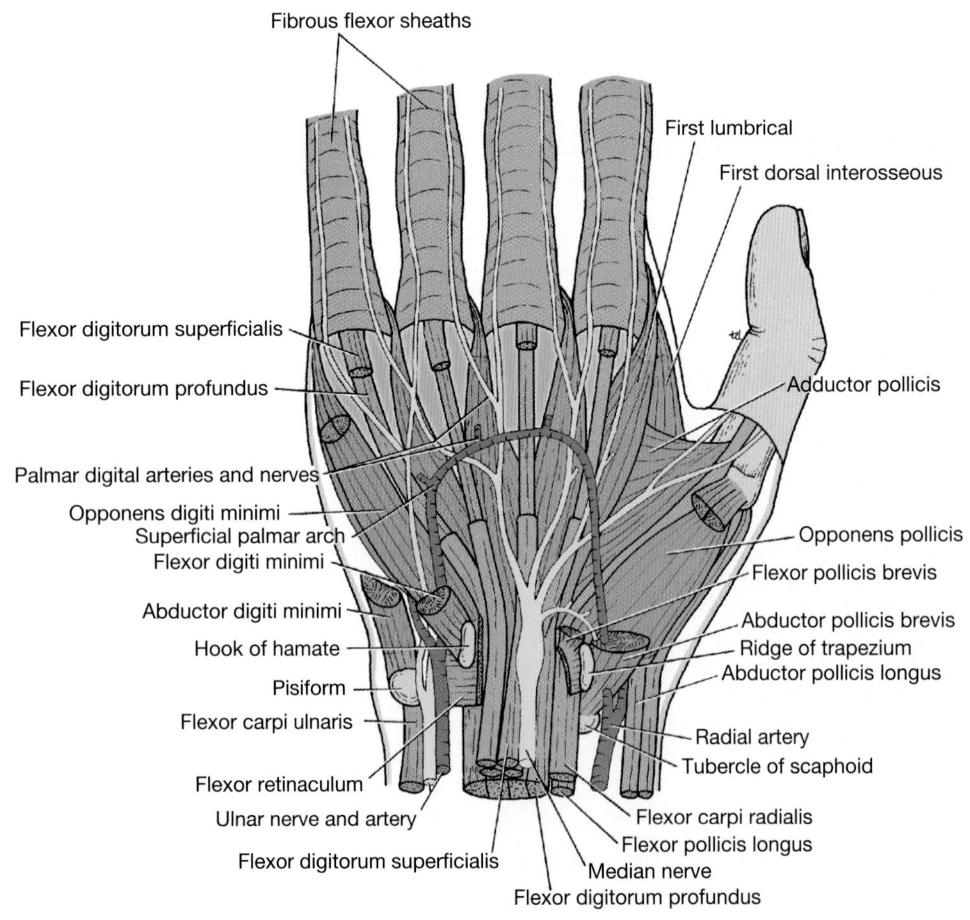

Figure 3.65 Anterior view of the palm of the hand. The palmar aponeurosis and the greater part of the flexor retinaculum have been removed to display the superficial palmar arch, the median nerve, and the long flexor tendons. Segments of the tendons of the flexor digitorum superficialis have been removed to show the underlying tendons of the flexor digitorum profundus.

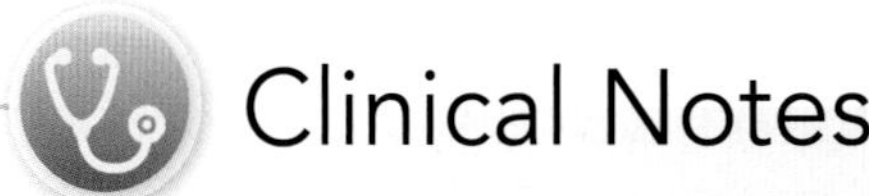

Carpal Tunnel Syndrome

The carpal tunnel is tightly packed with the long flexor tendons of the fingers, with their surrounding synovial sheaths, and with the median nerve (see Fig. 3.60). Any condition that significantly decreases the size of the carpal tunnel and compresses its contents is a carpal tunnel syndrome. See the Clinical Notes on the median nerve for further details.

"Anatomic Snuffbox"

The anatomic snuffbox is a small triangular skin depression on the posterolateral side of the wrist that is bounded medially by the tendon of the extensor pollicis longus and laterally by the tendons of the abductor pollicis longus and extensor pollicis brevis (see Figs. 3.58 and 3.109). Its clinical importance lies in the fact that the scaphoid bone is most easily palpated here and that the pulsations of the radial artery can be felt here (see Fig. 3.109).

Hand

The **hand** (**manus**), a very important organ, is located at the distal end of the upper limb. Much of the importance of the hand depends on the pincer-like action of the thumb, which enables us to grasp objects between the tips of the thumb and the index finger. The anterior (ventral) side of the hand is its **palmar** (**volar**) **surface**. The posterior aspect is the **dorsal surface**. The individual digits are identified in lateral to medial sequence. The **thumb** (**pollux**) is digit #1, the index finger is digit #2, the middle finger is digit #3, the ring finger is digit #4, and the little finger is digit #5.

Skin

The skin of the palm of the hand is thick and hairless. It is bound down to the underlying deep fascia by numerous fibrous bands. The skin shows many flexure creases at the sites of skin movement, which are not necessarily placed at the site of joints. Sweat glands are present in large numbers. The skin on the dorsum of the hand is thin, hairy, and freely mobile on the underlying tendons and bones.

Deep Fascia

The deep fascia of the wrist and palm is thickened to form the flexor retinaculum (described previously) and the palmar aponeurosis.

Palmar Aponeurosis

The palmar aponeurosis is triangular and occupies the central area of the palm (see Fig. 3.61). The apex is attached to the distal border of the flexor retinaculum and receives the insertion of the palmaris longus tendon. The base divides at the bases of the fingers into four slips. Each slip divides into two bands, one passing superficially to the skin, and the other passing deeply to the root of the finger. Here, each deep band divides into two, which diverge around the flexor tendons and fuse with the fibrous flexor sheath and the deep transverse ligaments.

The medial and lateral borders of the palmar aponeurosis are continuous with the thinner deep fascia covering the hypothenar and thenar muscles. From each of these borders, fibrous septa pass deeply into the palm and take part in the formation of the palmar fascial spaces (see below).

The function of the palmar aponeurosis is to give firm attachment to the overlying skin and so improve the grip and to protect the underlying tendons.

Fascial Spaces of Palm

Normally, the fascial spaces of the palm are potential spaces filled with loose connective tissue. Their boundaries are important clinically because they may limit the spread of infection in the palm.

The triangular palmar aponeurosis fans out from the distal border of the flexor retinaculum (see Fig. 3.61). From its medial border, a fibrous septum passes backward and is attached to the anterior border of the fifth metacarpal bone (Fig. 3.66C). Medial to this septum is a fascial compartment containing the three hypothenar muscles. From the lateral border of the palmar aponeurosis, a second fibrous septum passes obliquely

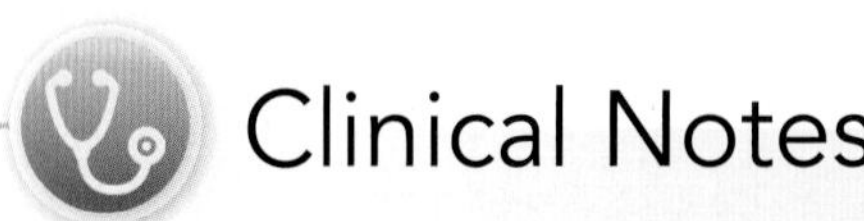

Palmar Fibromatosis

Palmar fibromatosis (Dupuytren contracture) is a localized thickening and contracture of the palmar aponeurosis, which limits hand function and may eventually disable the hand. It commonly starts near the root of the ring finger and draws that finger into the palm, flexing it at the metacarpophalangeal joint. Later, the condition involves the little finger in the same manner. In long-standing cases, the pull on the fibrous sheaths of these fingers results in flexion of the proximal interphalangeal joints. The distal interphalangeal joints are not involved and are instead extended by the pressure of the fingers against the palm. The posture of the affected hand may resemble that of claw hand, which is an ulnar nerve disorder (see the Clinical Notes on the ulnar nerve later in this chapter).

Surgical division of the fibrous bands followed by physiotherapy to the hand is the usual form of treatment. The alternative treatment of injection of the enzyme collagenase into the contracted bands of fibrous tissue has been shown to significantly reduce the contractures and improve mobility.

backward to the anterior border of the third metacarpal bone. Usually, the septum passes between the long flexor tendons of the index and the middle fingers. This second septum divides the palm into the **thenar space**, which lies lateral to the septum (and must not be confused with the fascial compartment containing the thenar muscles), and the **midpalmar space**, which lies medial to the septum. Proximally, the thenar and midpalmar spaces are closed off from the forearm by the walls of the carpal tunnel. Distally, the two spaces are continuous with the appropriate lumbrical canals (Fig. 3.66A).

The **thenar space** contains the first lumbrical muscle and lies deep to the long flexor tendons to the index finger and superficial to the adductor pollicis muscle (Fig. 3.66A,C).

The **midpalmar space** contains the second through fourth lumbrical muscles and lies posterior to the long flexor tendons to the middle, ring, and little fingers. It lies superficial to the interosseous muscles and the third through fifth metacarpal bones.

The **lumbrical canal** is a potential space surrounding the tendon of each lumbrical muscle and is normally filled with connective tissue. Proximally, it is continuous with one of the palmar spaces.

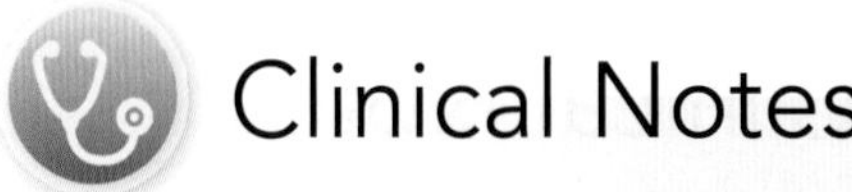

Fascial Spaces of the Palm and Infection

The fascial spaces of the palm (see Fig. 3.66A,C) are clinically important because they can become infected and distended with pus as a result of the spread of infection in acute suppurative tenosynovitis. Rarely, they can become infected after penetrating wounds such as from a dirty nail.

Finger Pulp Spaces

The deep fascia of the pulp of each finger fuses with the periosteum of the terminal phalanx just distal to the insertion of the long flexor tendons and closes off a fascial compartment known as the **pulp space** (see Fig. 3.66B). Each pulp space is subdivided by the presence of numerous septa, which pass from the deep fascia to the periosteum. The terminal branch of the digital artery that supplies the diaphysis of the terminal phalanx runs through the pulp space, which is filled with fat. The digital artery branch to the epiphysis of the distal phalanx does so proximal to the pulp space.

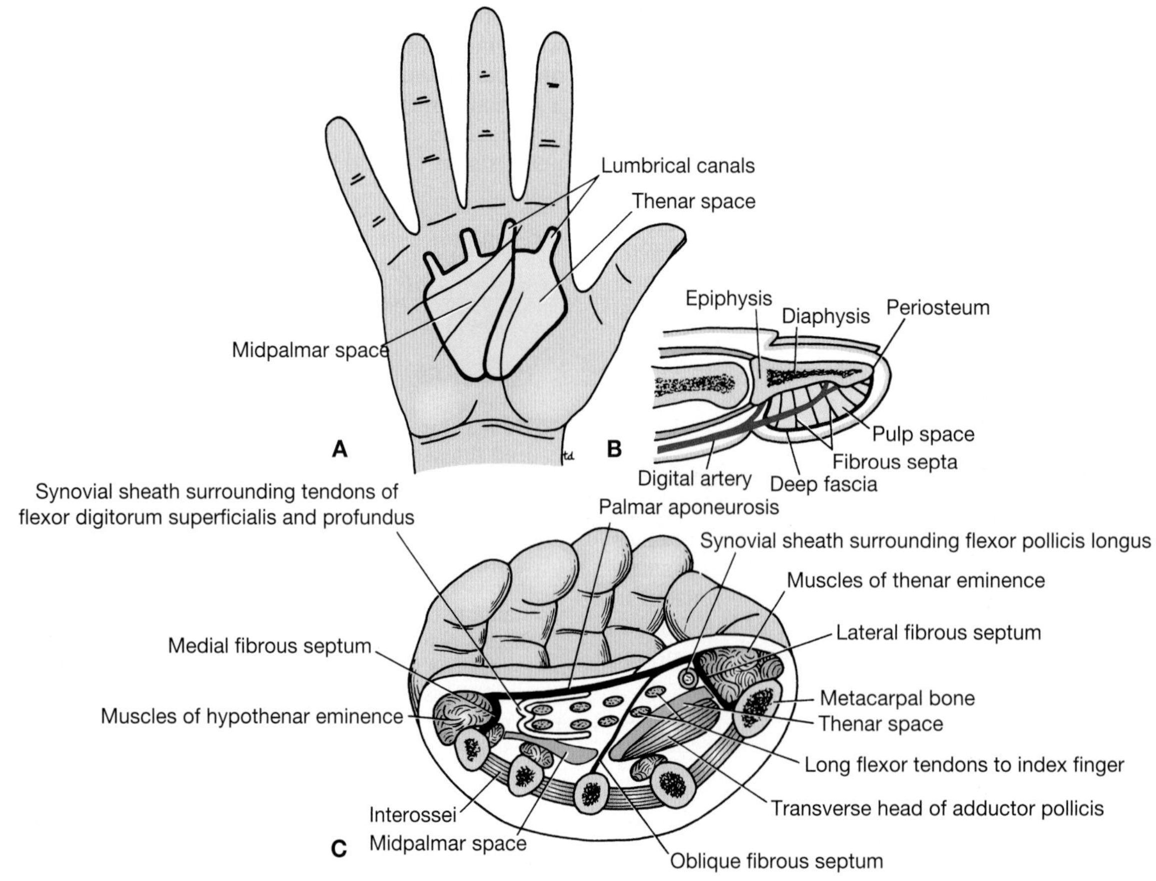

Figure 3.66 Palmar and pulp fascial spaces. **A.** Anterior view of the hand showing the positions of the thenar and midpalmar spaces and their continuities with the lumbrical canals. **B.** Sagittal section through a finger showing the pulp space and arterial supply to the distal phalanx. **C.** Transverse section through the hand showing the fascial spaces of the palm.

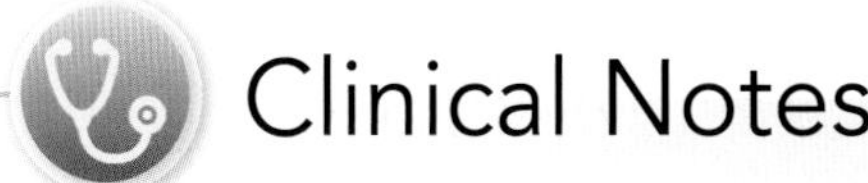

Pulp Space Infection (Felon)

The pulp space of the fingers is a closed fascial compartment situated anterior to the terminal phalanx of each finger (see Fig. 3.66B). Infection of such a space is common and serious, occurring most often in the thumb and index finger. Bacteria are usually introduced into the space by pinpricks or sewing needles. Because each space is subdivided into numerous smaller compartments by fibrous septa, the accumulation of inflammatory exudate within these compartments causes the pressure in the pulp space to quickly rise. If the infection is left without decompression, infection of the terminal phalanx can occur. In children, the blood supply to the diaphysis of the phalanx passes through the pulp space, and pressure on the blood vessels could result in necrosis of the diaphysis. The proximally located epiphysis of this bone is spared because it receives its arterial supply just proximal to the pulp space.

The close relationship of the proximal end of the pulp space to the digital synovial sheath accounts for the involvement of the sheath in the infectious process when the pulp space infection has been neglected.

MUSCLES

Pectoral Region

The muscles and major neurovascular structures of the pectoral region are shown in Figures 3.32 through 3.34. The muscles of the pectoral region are summarized in Table 3.4.

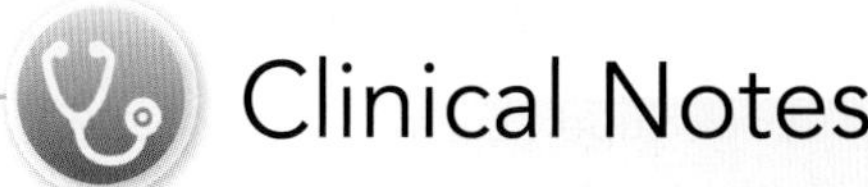

Absent Pectoralis Major

Occasionally, parts of the pectoralis major muscle may be absent. The sternocostal origin is the most commonly missing part, and this causes weakness in adduction and medial rotation of the shoulder joint.

Back and Scapular Region

The superficial group of muscles of the back (trapezius, latissimus dorsi, levator scapulae, rhomboid major, rhomboid minor; see Chapter 2, Back) connects the shoulder girdle with the vertebral column. However, developmentally (except for the trapezius) and functionally, these are upper limb muscles so are included here (Table 3.5; see also Fig. 3.40).

The muscles of the scapular region connect the shoulder girdle with the upper part of the humerus and are largely concerned with abduction and rotation of the arm. The muscles and major neurovascular structures of the scapular region are shown in Figures 3.40, 3.41, and 3.50. The muscles are summarized in Table 3.6.

Rotator Cuff

The tendons of the supraspinatus, infraspinatus, teres minor, and subscapularis muscles blend into and reinforce the underlying capsule of the glenohumeral (shoulder) joint, thus forming a musculotendinous cuff around the joint. All the muscles except the supraspinatus act to rotate the humerus. Because of these relationships,

Table 3.4 Pectoral Region Muscles

MUSCLE	ORIGIN	INSERTION	NERVE SUPPLY	NERVE ROOTS[a]	ACTION
Pectoralis major	Clavicle, sternum, and upper six costal cartilages	Lateral lip of bicipital groove of humerus	Medial and lateral pectoral nerves	C5, **C6** to **C8**, T1	Adducts arm and rotates it medially; clavicular fibers also flex arm
Pectoralis minor	Ribs 3 to 5	Coracoid process of scapula	Medial pectoral nerve (mainly); Lateral pectoral nerve (variable)	**C8** to T1 C5 to C7	Depresses point of shoulder; if the scapula is fixed, it elevates the ribs of origin
Subclavius	First costal cartilage	Clavicle	Nerve to subclavius	**C5**, C6	Depresses the clavicle and steadies this bone during movements of the shoulder girdle
Serratus anterior	Ribs 1 to 8	Medial border and inferior angle of scapula	Long thoracic nerve	C5, **C6**, **C7**	Draws the forward anterior around the thoracic wall; rotates scapula

[a]The predominant nerve root supply is in bold.

Table 3.5 Back Superficial Muscles

MUSCLE	ORIGIN	INSERTION	NERVE SUPPLY	NERVE ROOTS[a]	ACTION
Trapezius	Occipital bone, ligamentum nuchae, spine of C7, spines of all thoracic vertebrae	Upper fibers into lateral third of clavicle; middle and lower fibers into acromion and spine of scapula	Cranial nerve XI (spinal part) (motor); C3 and C4 (sensory)	**Cranial nerve XI** (spinal part)	Upper fibers elevate the scapula; middle fibers pull scapula medially; lower fibers pull medial border of scapula downward
Latissimus dorsi	Iliac crest, lumbar fascia, spines of T7 to T12 vertebrae, ribs 9/10 to 12, and inferior angle of scapula	Floor of bicipital groove of humerus	Thoracodorsal nerve	C6, **C7**, C8,	Extends, adducts, and medially rotates the arm
Levator scapulae	Transverse processes of C1 to C4 vertebrae	Medial border of scapula	C3 and C4 and dorsal scapular nerve	C3 to C5	Raises medial border of scapula
Rhomboid minor	Ligamentum nuchae and spines of C7 and T1 vertebrae	Medial border of scapula	Dorsal scapular nerve	**C4**, C5	Raises medial border of scapula upward and medially
Rhomboid major	T2 to T5 spines	Medial border of scapula	Dorsal scapular nerve	**C4**, C5	Raises medial border of scapula upward and medially

[a]The predominant nerve root supply is in bold.

Table 3.6 Scapular Region Muscles

MUSCLE	ORIGIN	INSERTION	NERVE SUPPLY	NERVE ROOTS[a]	ACTION
Deltoid	Lateral third of clavicle, acromion, spine of scapula	Middle of lateral surface of shaft of humerus	Axillary nerve	**C5**, C6	Abducts arm; anterior fibers flex and medially rotate arm; posterior fibers extend and laterally rotate arm
Supraspinatus	Supraspinous fossa of scapula	Greater tuberosity of humerus; capsule of shoulder joint	Suprascapular nerve	C**5**, C6	Abducts arm and stabilizes shoulder joint
Infraspinatus	Infraspinous fossa of scapula	Greater tuberosity of humerus; capsule of shoulder joint	Suprascapular nerve	C**5**, C6	Laterally rotates arm and stabilizes shoulder joint
Teres major	Lower third of lateral border of scapula	Medial lip of bicipital groove of humerus	Lower subscapular nerve	C5, C**6**, C7	Medially rotates and adducts arm and stabilizes shoulder joint
Teres minor	Upper two thirds of lateral border of scapula	Greater tuberosity of humerus; capsule of shoulder joint	Axillary nerve	C**5**, C6	Laterally rotates arm and stabilizes shoulder joint
Subscapularis	Subscapular fossa	Lesser tuberosity of humerus	Upper and lower subscapular nerves	C5, **C6**, C7	Medially rotates arm and stabilizes shoulder joint

[a]The predominant nerve root supply is in bold.

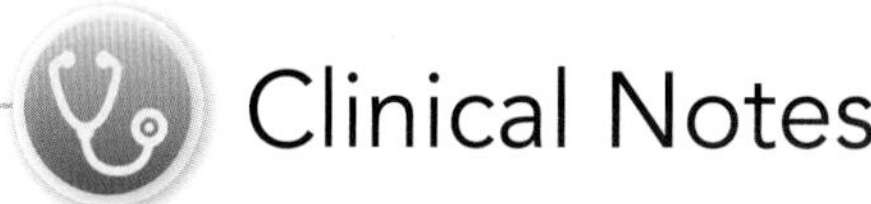

Clinical Notes

Rotator Cuff Tendinitis

Lesions of the rotator cuff are a common cause of pain in the shoulder region. Failure of the cuff is due to either wear or tear. Wear is age related. Inflammation or tearing is associated with excessive repetitive use. Overused overhead movements of the upper limb, such as seen in baseball pitchers, tennis players, and swimmers, may be the cause of tendinitis, although many cases appear spontaneously. The supraspinatus is the most injured muscle in the rotator cuff. During abduction of the shoulder joint, the supraspinatus tendon is exposed to friction against the acromion (Fig. 3.67). Under normal conditions, the amount of friction is reduced to a minimum by the large subacromial bursa, which extends laterally beneath the deltoid. Degenerative changes in the bursa are followed by degenerative changes in the underlying supraspinatus tendon, and these may extend into the other tendons of the rotator cuff. Clinically, the condition is known as **subacromial bursitis**, **supraspinatus tendinitis**, or **pericapsulitis**. It is characterized by the presence of a spasm of pain in the middle range of abduction, when the diseased area impinges on the acromion. Extensive acute traumatic tears are best repaired surgically as soon as possible. Small chronic cuff injuries are best managed without surgery using nonsteroidal anti-inflammatory drugs and muscle exercises.

Supraspinatus Tendon Rupture

In advanced cases of rotator cuff tendinitis, the necrotic supraspinatus tendon can become calcified or rupture. Rupture of the tendon seriously interferes with the normal abduction movement of the shoulder joint. Recall that the main function of the supraspinatus muscle is to hold the head of the humerus in the glenoid fossa at the commencement of abduction. The patient with a ruptured supraspinatus tendon is unable to initiate abduction of the arm. However, if the arm is passively assisted for the first 15° of abduction, the deltoid can then take over and complete the movement to a right angle.

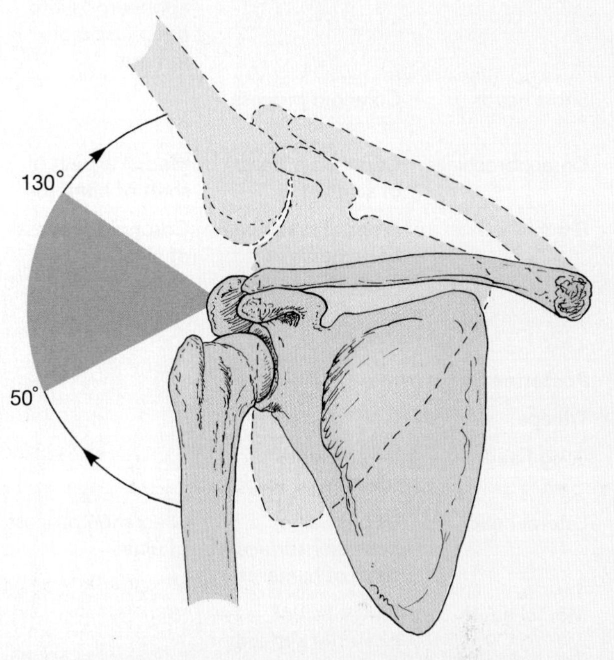

Figure 3.67 Subacromial bursitis, supraspinatus tendinitis, or pericapsulitis showing the painful arc in the middle range of abduction, when the diseased area impinges on the lateral edge of the acromion.

the four muscles collectively are referred to as the "rotator cuff." They are also referred to as the SITS muscles: **s**upraspinatus, **i**nfraspinatus, **t**eres minor, **s**ubscapularis. The rotator cuff plays an important role in stabilizing the glenohumeral joint. The tone of these muscles assists in holding the head of the humerus in the shallow glenoid cavity of the scapula during movements at the shoulder joint. The cuff covers the anterior, superior, and posterior aspects of the joint; it is deficient inferiorly, and this is a site of potential weakness. The supraspinatus works with the other three muscles to support the joint and acts to initiate the first 10° to 15° of abduction of the arm. (See the earlier discussion in this chapter of movements of the shoulder joint and Fig. 3.16.)

Arm

The muscles and major neurovascular structures of the arm are shown in Figures 3.47 through 3.50. The muscles are summarized in Table 3.7.

Osseofascial Compartments

The muscles of the arm are organized in two osseofascial compartments, anterior and posterior. The muscles influence the shoulder and/or elbow joints, with the anterior compartment muscles acting mainly as flexors and the posterior compartment muscle producing mainly extension. The musculocutaneous nerve supplies the anterior compartment, whereas the radial nerve innervates the posterior compartment.

Biceps Brachii Muscle

The **biceps brachii** is a component of the anterior compartment of the arm. It is a powerful flexor of the elbow joint and a weak flexor of the shoulder joint. Additionally, the biceps brachii is a powerful supinator, especially during supination against resistance. You can test the supination action when using a corkscrew to penetrate a cork or a screwdriver to drive a screw into wood. Interestingly, this test works only when using the right arm and not the left.

Table 3.7 Arm Muscles

MUSCLE	ORIGIN	INSERTION	NERVE SUPPLY	NERVE ROOTS[a]	ACTION
Anterior Compartment					
Biceps brachii					
Long head	Supraglenoid tubercle of scapula	Tuberosity of radius and bicipital aponeurosis into deep fascia of forearm	Musculocutaneous nerve	C5, **C6**	Supinator of forearm and flexor of elbow joint; weak flexor of shoulder joint
Short head	Coracoid process of scapula				
Coracobrachialis	Coracoid process of scapula	Medial aspect of shaft of humerus	Musculocutaneous nerve	C5, **C6**, C7	Flexes arm and also is a weak adductor
Brachialis	Front of lower half of humerus	Coronoid process of ulna	Musculocutaneous nerve (most of muscle); Radial nerve (small part of muscle)	C5, **C6**	Flexor of elbow joint
Posterior Compartment					
Triceps					
Long head	Infraglenoid tubercle of scapula				
Lateral head	Upper half of posterior surface of shaft of humerus	Olecranon process of ulna	Radial nerve	C6, C7, **C8**	Extensor of elbow joint
Medial head	Lower half of posterior surface of shaft of humerus				

[a]The predominant nerve root supply is in bold.

Forearm

The muscles and major neurovascular structures of the forearm are shown in Figures 3.53 through 3.59. The muscles are summarized in Tables 3.8 to 3.10.

Osseofascial Compartments

The muscles of the forearm are organized in three osseofascial compartments: anterior, lateral, and posterior. Some authors include the lateral compartment in the posterior compartment. The muscles influence the elbow, wrist, and digits. The anterior compartment muscles produce mainly flexion or pronation, whereas the lateral and posterior compartment muscles produce mainly extension or supination. The median and ulnar nerves supply the anterior compartment, and the radial nerve innervates the lateral and posterior compartments.

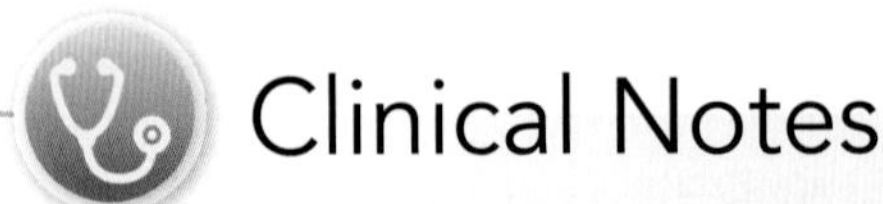

Biceps Brachii and Shoulder Joint Osteoarthritis

The tendon of the long head of biceps is attached to the supraglenoid tubercle within the shoulder joint. Advanced osteoarthritic changes in the joint can lead to erosion and fraying of the tendon by osteophytic outgrowths, and rupture of the tendon can occur.

Anterior Osseofascial Compartment Muscles

The muscles of the anterior osseofascial compartment (see Table 3.8) are arranged in three groups: superficial, intermediate, and deep. Note that the superficial group muscles possess a common tendon of origin that is attached to the medial epicondyle of the humerus.

- **Superficial group:** Pronator teres, flexor carpi radialis, palmaris longus, flexor carpi ulnaris
- **Intermediate group:** Flexor digitorum superficialis
- **Deep group:** Flexor pollicis longus, flexor digitorum profundus, pronator quadratus

Lateral Osseofascial Compartment Muscles

The brachioradialis and extensor carpi radialis longus muscles are the two members of the lateral osseofascial

Table 3.8 Muscles of Anterior Forearm Osseofascial Compartment

MUSCLE	ORIGIN	INSERTION	NERVE SUPPLY	NERVE ROOTS[a]	ACTION
Pronator Teres					
Humeral head	Medial epicondyle of humerus	Lateral aspect of shaft of radius	Median nerve	C6, **C7**	Pronation and flexion of forearm
Ulnar head	Medial border of coronoid process of ulna				
Flexor carpi radialis	Medial epicondyle of humerus	Bases of second and third metacarpal bones	Median nerve	C6, **C7**	Flexes and abducts hand at wrist joint
Palmaris longus	Medial epicondyle of humerus	Flexor retinaculum and palmar aponeurosis	Median nerve	C7, C8	Flexes hand
Flexor Carpi Ulnaris					
Humeral head	Medial epicondyle of humerus	Pisiform bone, hook of the hamate, base at fifth metacarpal bone	Ulnar nerve	C8; T1	Flexes and adducts hand at wrist joint
Ulnar head	Medial aspect of olecranon process and posterior border of ulna				
Flexor Digitorum Superficialis					
Humeroulnar head	Medial epicondyle of humerus, medial border of coronoid process of ulna	Middle phalanx of medial four fingers	Median nerve	C7, **C8**; T1	Flexes middle phalanx of fingers and assists in flexing proximal phalanx and hand
Radial head	Oblique line on anterior surface of shaft of radius				
Flexor pollicis longus	Mainly anterior surface of shaft of radius	Distal phalanx of thumb	Anterior interosseous branch of median nerve	**C8**; T1	Flexes distal phalanx of thumb
Flexor digitorum profundus	Anteromedial surface of shaft of ulna	Distal phalanges of medial four fingers	Ulnar (medial half) and median (lateral half) nerves	**C8**; T1	Flexes distal phalanx of fingers; then assists in flexion of middle and proximal phalanges and wrist
Pronator quadratus	Anterior surface of shaft of the ulna	Anterior surface of shaft of radius	Anterior interosseous branch of median nerve	**C8**; T1	Pronates forearm

[a]The predominant nerve root supply is in bold.

Table 3.9 Muscles of Lateral Forearm Osseofascial Compartment

MUSCLE	ORIGIN	INSERTION	NERVE SUPPLY	NERVE ROOTS[a]	ACTION
Brachioradialis	Lateral supracondylar ridge of humerus	Base of styloid process of radius	Radial nerve	C5, **C6**, C7	Flexes forearm at elbow joint; rotates forearm to the midprone position
Extensor carpi radialis longus	Lateral supracondylar ridge of humerus	Posterior surface of base of second metacarpal bone	Radial nerve	C6, C7	Extends and abducts hand at wrist joint

[a]The predominant nerve root supply is in bold.

compartment (see Table 3.9). Some authors regard this group as part of the posterior osseofascial compartment because of their common innervation by the radial nerve.

Note that the brachioradialis is an exception to the general functional theme of the lateral and posterior forearm compartments in that it is a significant flexor of the elbow rather than an extensor.

Posterior Osseofascial Compartment Muscles

The muscles of the posterior osseofascial compartment (see Table 3.10) are arranged in two groups: superficial

Table 3.10 Muscles of Posterior Forearm Osseofascial Compartment

MUSCLE	ORIGIN	INSERTION	NERVE SUPPLY	NERVE ROOTS[a]	ACTION
Extensor carpi radialis brevis	Lateral epicondyle of humerus	Posterior surface of base of third metacarpal bone	Deep branch of radial nerve	**C7**, C8	Extends and abducts hand at wrist joint
Extensor digitorum	Lateral epicondyle of humerus	Middle and distal phalanges of medial four fingers	Deep branch of radial nerve	**C7**, C8	Extends fingers and hand (see text for details)
Extensor digiti minimi	Lateral epicondyle of humerus	Extensor expansion of little finger	Deep branch of radial nerve	**C7**, C8	Extends metacarpal phalangeal joint of little finger
Extensor carpi ulnaris	Lateral epicondyle of humerus	Base of fifth metacarpal bone	Deep branch of radial nerve	C7, **C8**	Extends and adducts hand at wrist joint
Anconeus	Lateral epicondyle of humerus	Lateral surface of olecranon process of ulna	Radial nerve	C7, C8; T1	Extends elbow joint
Supinator	Lateral epicondyle of humerus, annular ligament of proximal radioulnar joint, and ulna	Neck and shaft of radius	Deep branch of radial nerve	C5, C6	Supination of forearm
Abductor pollicis longus	Posterior surface of shafts of radius and ulna	Base of first metacarpal bone	Deep branch of radial nerve	C7, **C8**	Abducts and extends thumb
Extensor pollicis brevis	Posterior surface of shaft of radius	Base of proximal phalanx of thumb	Deep branch of radial nerve	C7, **C8**	Extends metacarpophalangeal joints of thumb
Extensor pollicis longus	Posterior surface of shaft of ulna	Base of distal phalanx of thumb	Deep branch of radial nerve	C7, **C8**	Extends distal phalanx of thumb
Extensor indicis	Posterior surface of shaft of ulna	Extensor expansion of index finger	Deep branch of radial nerve	C7, **C8**	Extends metacarpophalangeal joint of index finger

[a]The predominant nerve root supply is in bold.

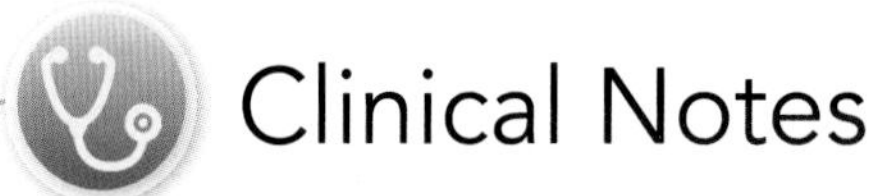

Clinical Notes

Forearm Compartment Syndrome

The forearm compartments are tightly packed spaces with very little extra room. Any edema can cause secondary compression of the blood vessels; the veins are first affected and later the arteries. Soft tissue injury is a common cause, and early diagnosis is critical. Early signs include altered skin sensation (caused by ischemia of the sensory nerves passing through the compartment), pain disproportionate to any injury (caused by pressure on nerves within the compartment), pain on passive stretching of muscles that pass through the compartment (caused by muscle ischemia), tenderness of the skin over the compartment (late sign caused by edema), and absence of capillary refill in the nail beds (caused by pressure on the arteries within the compartment). Once the diagnosis is made, the deep fascia must be incised surgically to decompress the affected compartment. Even short delays in treatment can cause irreversible damage to the muscles.

Volkmann Ischemic Contracture

Volkmann ischemic contracture is a contracture of the muscles of the forearm that commonly follows fractures of the distal end of the humerus or fractures of the radius and ulna. In this syndrome, a localized segment of the brachial artery goes into spasm, reducing the arterial flow to the flexor and the extensor muscles, inducing ischemic necrosis. The flexor muscles are larger than the extensor muscles and are therefore mainly affected. The muscles are replaced by fibrous tissue, which contracts, producing the deformity. An overtight cast may cause the arterial spasm, but in some cases, the fracture itself may be responsible. The deformity can be explained only by understanding the anatomy of the region. Three types of deformity exist:

- The long flexor muscles of the carpus and fingers are more contracted than the extensor muscles, and the wrist joint is flexed; the fingers are extended. If the wrist joint is extended passively, the fingers become flexed.
- The long extensor muscles to the fingers, which are inserted into the extensor expansion attached to the proximal phalanx, are greatly contracted; the metacarpophalangeal joints and the wrist joint are extended, and the interphalangeal joints of the fingers are flexed.
- Both the flexor and extensor muscles of the forearm are contracted. The wrist joint is flexed, the metacarpophalangeal joints are extended, and the interphalangeal joints are flexed.

Absent Palmaris Longus

The palmaris longus muscle may be absent on one or both sides of the forearm in about 10% of people. Others show variation in form, such as a centrally or distally placed muscle belly in the place of a proximal one. Because the muscle is relatively weak, its absence produces no disability.

Lateral Epicondylitis

A partial tearing or degeneration of the origin of the superficial extensor muscles from the lateral epicondyle of the humerus causes **lateral epicondylitis** (**tennis elbow**). It is characterized by pain and tenderness over the lateral epicondyle of the humerus, with pain radiating down the lateral side of the forearm; it is common in tennis players and violinists.

Stenosing Synovitis of the Abductor Pollicis Longus and Extensor Pollicis Brevis Tendons

As a result of repeated friction between these tendons and the styloid process of the radius, they sometimes become edematous and swell. Later, fibrosis of the synovial sheath produces **stenosing tenosynovitis** in which the movement of the tendons becomes restricted. Advanced cases require surgical incision along the constricting sheath.

Extensor Pollicis Longus Tendon Rupture

Rupture of this tendon can occur after fracture of the distal third of the radius. Roughening of the dorsal tubercle of the radius by the fracture line can cause excessive friction on the tendon, which can then rupture. Rheumatoid arthritis can also cause rupture of this tendon.

and deep. The superficial group muscles possess a common tendon of origin that is attached to the lateral epicondyle of the humerus.

- **Superficial group**: Extensor carpi radialis brevis, extensor digitorum, extensor digiti minimi, extensor carpi ulnaris, anconeus
- **Deep group**: Supinator, abductor pollicis longus, extensor pollicis brevis, extensor pollicis longus, extensor indicis

Hand

The muscles and major neurovascular structures of the hand are shown in Figures 3.68 and 3.69 (see also Figs. 3.58, 3.59, and 3.61 to 3.65). The compartments of the hand are outlined in Table 3.11. The intrinsic (small) muscles are summarized in Table 3.12.

Osseofascial Compartments

The muscles of the hand can be described as extrinsic or intrinsic. Extrinsic muscles originate outside of the hand proper (in the forearm) and insert within the hand via long tendons. Intrinsic muscles (small muscles) originate and insert within the hand. Both the extrinsic and intrinsic muscles are organized in five osseofascial compartments. Four compartments (thenar, hypothenar, central [midpalmar], and interosseous) are in the palmar aspect of the hand. One compartment (dorsal/extensor) is related to the dorsum of the hand.

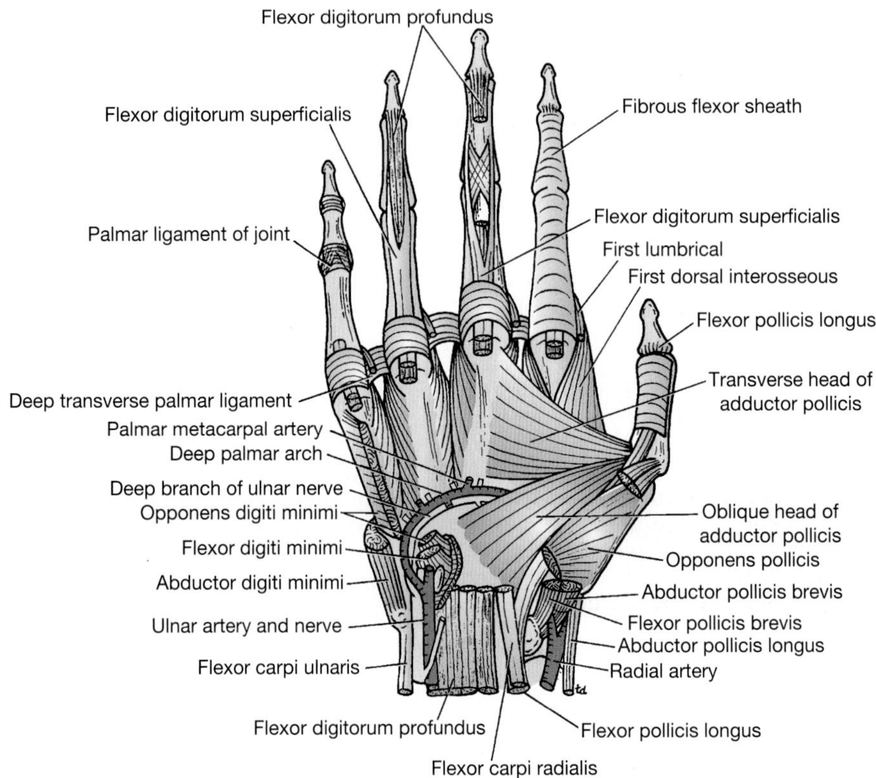

Figure 3.68 Anterior view of the palm of the hand. The long flexor tendons have been removed from the palm, but their method of insertion into the fingers is shown.

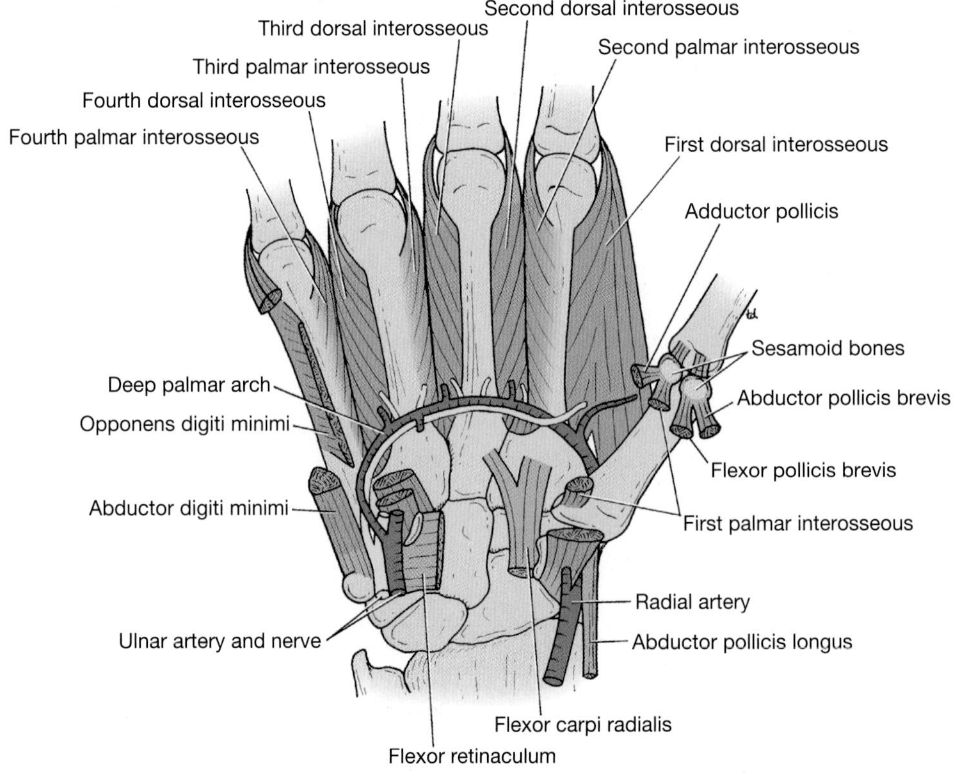

Figure 3.69 Anterior view of the palm of the hand showing the deep palmar arch and the deep terminal branch of the ulnar nerve. The interossei are also shown.

Table 3.11 Osseofascial Compartments of the Hand

COMPARTMENT	MUSCLES	MOTOR NERVE(S)
Thenar	Flexor pollicis brevis Abductor pollicis brevis Opponens pollicis	Median nerve (recurrent branch)
Hypothenar	Flexor digiti quinti Abductor digiti quinti Opponens digiti quinti	Ulnar nerve (deep branch)
Central (midpalmar)	Tendons of long extrinsic digital flexors (flexor digitorum superficialis, flexor digitorum profundus, flexor pollicis longus) Lumbrical muscles	Median nerve Ulnar nerve (deep branch)
Interosseous	Adductor pollicis Palmar interossei Dorsal interossei	Ulnar nerve (deep branch)
Dorsal (extensor)	Tendons of long digital extensors	No intrinsic motor nerves

Table 3.12 Intrinsic Hand Muscles

MUSCLE	ORIGIN	INSERTION	NERVE SUPPLY	NERVE ROOTS[a]	ACTION
Palmaris brevis	Flexor retinaculum, palmar aponeurosis	Skin of palm	Superficial branch of ulnar nerve	C8; **T1**	Corrugates skin to improve grip of palm
Lumbricals (4)	Tendons of flexor digitorum profundus	Extensor expansion of medial four fingers	First and second (ie, lateral two), median nerve; third and fourth deep branch of ulnar nerve	C8; **T1**	Flex metacarpophalangeal joints and extend interphalangeal joints of fingers except thumb
Interossei (8)					
Palmar (4)	First arises from base of first metacarpal; remaining three from anterior surface of shafts of second, fourth, and fifth metacarpals	Proximal phalanges of thumb and index, ring, and little fingers and dorsal extensor expansion of each finger	Deep branch of ulnar nerve	C8; **T1**	Palmar interossei adduct fingers toward center of third finger
Dorsal (4)	Contiguous sides of shafts of metacarpal bones	Proximal phalanges of index, middle, and ring fingers and dorsal extensor expansion	Deep branch of ulnar nerve	C8; **T1**	Dorsal interossei abduct fingers from center of third finger; both palmar and dorsal flex metacarpophalangeal joints and extend interphalangeal joints
Short Muscles of Thumb					
Abductor pollicis brevis	Scaphoid, trapezium, flexor retinaculum	Base of proximal phalanx of thumb	Median nerve	**C8**; T1	Abduction of thumb
Flexor pollicis brevis	Flexor retinaculum	Base of proximal phalanx of thumb	Median nerve	C8; T1	Flexes metacarpophalangeal joint of thumb

(continued)

Table 3.12 Intrinsic Hand Muscles *(Continued)*

MUSCLE	ORIGIN	INSERTION	NERVE SUPPLY	NERVE ROOTS[a]	ACTION
Opponens pollicis	Flexor retinaculum	Shaft of metacarpal bone of thumb	Median nerve	**C8**; T1	Pulls thumb medially and forward across palm
Adductor pollicis	Oblique head; second and third metacarpal bones; transverse head; third metacarpal bone	Base of proximal phalanx of thumb	Deep branch of ulnar nerve	C8; **T1**	Adduction of thumb
Short Muscles of Little Finger					
Abductor digiti minimi	Pisiform bone	Base of proximal phalanx of little finger	Deep branch of ulnar nerve	C8; **T1**	Abducts little finger
Flexor digiti minimi	Flexor retinaculum	Base of proximal phalanx of little finger	Deep branch of ulnar nerve	C8; **T1**	Flexes little finger
Opponens digiti minimi	Flexor retinaculum	Medial border of the fifth metacarpal bone	Deep branch of ulnar nerve	C8; **T1**	Pulls fifth metacarpal forward as in cupping the palm

[a]The predominant nerve root supply is in bold.

Fibrous Flexor Sheaths

The anterior surface of each finger, from the head of the metacarpal to the base of the distal phalanx, is provided with a strong fibrous sheath that is attached to the sides of the phalanges (Fig. 3.70; see also Fig. 3.68). The proximal end of the fibrous sheath is open, whereas the distal end of the sheath is closed and attached to the base of the distal phalanx. The sheath and the bones form a blind

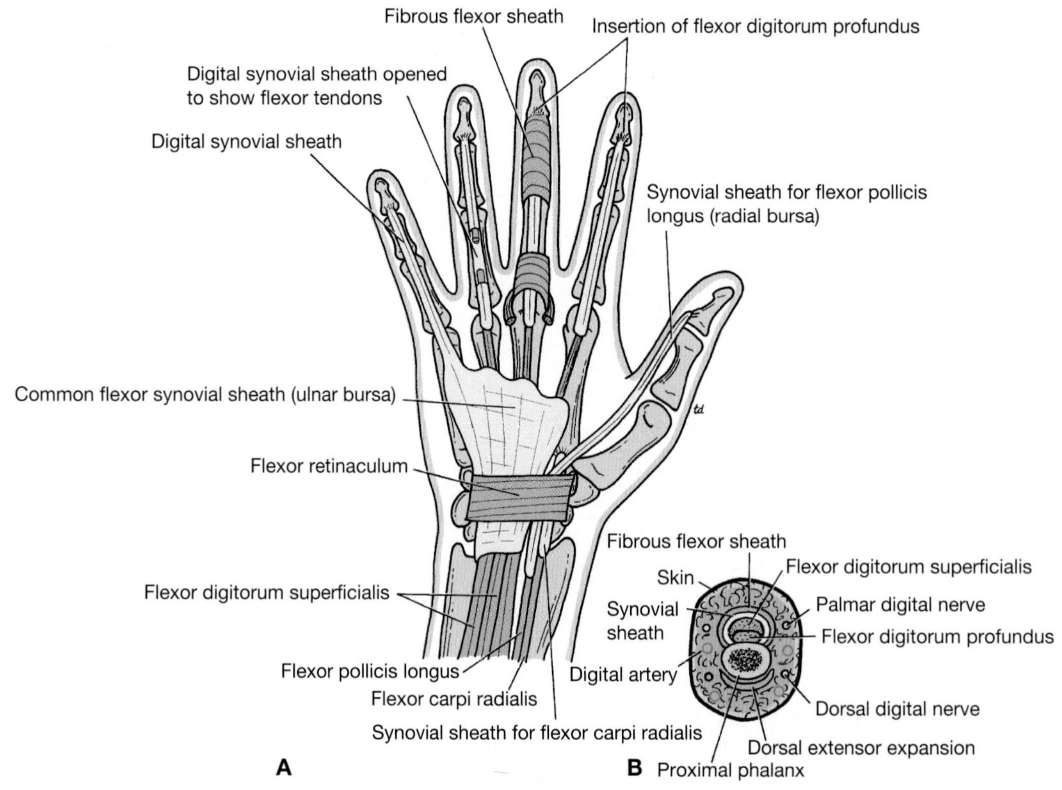

Figure 3.70 Fibrous and synovial flexor sheaths in the hand. **A.** Anterior view of the palm of the hand. **B.** Cross section of a finger.

tunnel, which contains the flexor tendons of the finger. In the thumb, the osseofibrous tunnel contains the tendon of the flexor pollicis longus. In the four medial fingers, the tunnels are occupied by the tendons of the flexor digitorum superficialis and profundus (see Fig. 3.70B). The fibrous sheath is thick over the phalanges but thin and lax over the joints.

Synovial Flexor Sheaths

In the hand, the tendons of the flexor digitorum superficialis and profundus muscles invaginate a **common synovial sheath** from the lateral side (see Fig. 3.60). The medial part of this common sheath extends distally without interruption on the tendons of the little finger (see Fig. 3.70A). The lateral part of the sheath stops abruptly on the middle of the palm, and the distal ends of the long flexor tendons of the index, the middle, and the ring fingers acquire digital synovial sheaths as they enter the fingers. The flexor pollicis longus tendon has its own synovial sheath that passes into the thumb. These sheaths allow the long tendons to move smoothly, with a minimum of friction, beneath the flexor retinaculum and the fibrous flexor sheaths.

The synovial sheath of the flexor pollicis longus (sometimes called the **radial bursa**) communicates with the common synovial sheath of the superficialis and profundus tendons (sometimes called the **ulnar bursa**) at the level of the wrist in about 50% of people.

The **vincula longa** and **brevia** are small vascular folds of synovial membrane that connect the tendons to the anterior surface of the phalanges (Fig. 3.71C). They resemble a mesentery and convey blood vessels to the tendons.

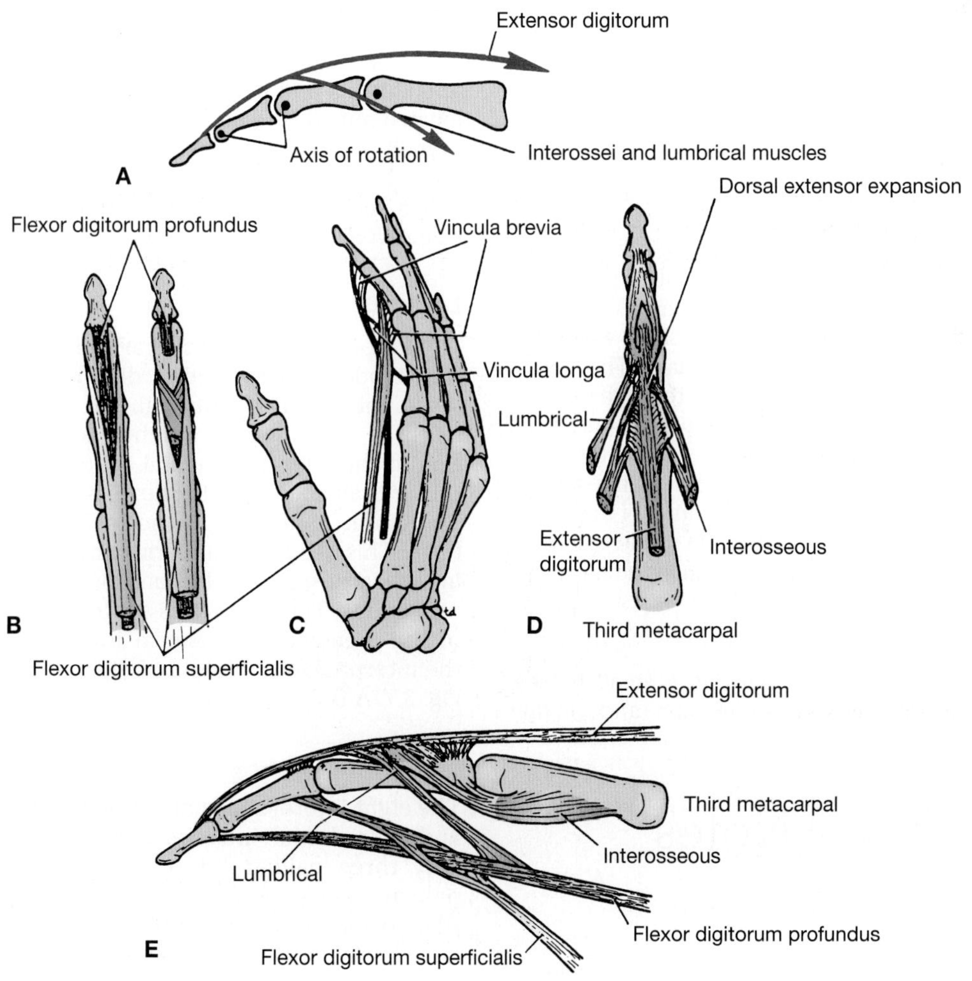

Figure 3.71 Insertions of long flexor and extensor tendons and lumbrical and interosseous muscles in the fingers. **A.** Lateral view showing the action of the lumbrical and interosseous muscles in flexing the metacarpophalangeal joints and extending the interphalangeal joints. **B.** Anterior view showing the arrangement of the tendons of the flexor digitorum superficialis and profundus muscles. **C.** Oblique view showing the vincula brevia and longa. **D.** Posterior view showing the relation of the lumbrical and interosseous muscles to the dorsal expansion. **E.** Lateral view showing the relations of the long flexor tendons, lumbricals, interossei, and dorsal expansion.

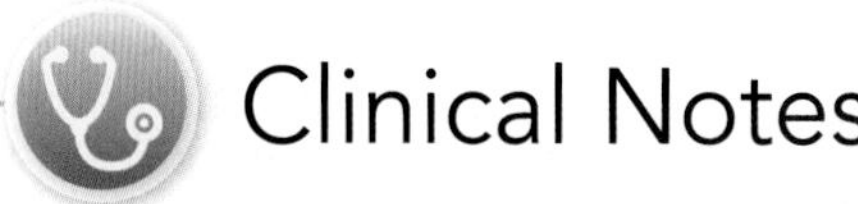

Clinical Notes

Tenosynovitis of the Flexor Tendon Synovial Sheaths

Tenosynovitis is an infection of a synovial sheath. It most commonly results from the introduction of bacteria through a small penetrating wound, such as from a needle or thorn. Rarely, the sheath may become infected by extension of a pulp space infection.

Infection of a digital sheath results in distention of the sheath with pus; the finger is held semiflexed and is swollen. Any attempt to extend the finger is accompanied by extreme pain because the distended sheath is stretched. As the inflammatory process continues, the pressure within the sheath rises and may compress the blood supply to the tendons that travel in the vincula longa and brevia (see Fig. 3.71C). Rupture or later severe scarring of the tendons may follow.

A further increase in pressure can cause the sheath to rupture at its proximal end. Anatomically, the digital sheath of the index finger is related to the thenar space, whereas that of the ring finger is related to the midpalmar space. The sheath for the middle finger is related to both the thenar and midpalmar spaces. These relationships explain how infection can extend from the digital synovial sheaths and involve the palmar fascial spaces.

In the case of infection of the digital sheaths of the little finger and thumb, the ulnar and radial bursae are quickly involved. If neglected, pus may burst through the proximal ends of these bursae and enter the fascial space of the forearm between the flexor digitorum profundus superficially and the pronator quadratus and the interosseous membrane deeply. This fascial space in the forearm is commonly referred to clinically as the **space of Parona**.

Long Flexor Tendon Insertion

Each tendon of the flexor digitorum superficialis enters its appropriate fibrous flexor sheath and then divides into two halves opposite the proximal phalanx (see Figs. 3.68 and 3.71B). The half tendons pass around the profundus tendon and then reunite deep to the profundus tendon, where partial decussation of the fibers takes place (see Fig. 3.71B,E). The superficialis tendon, having united again, divides almost at once into two further slips, which are attached to the borders of the middle phalanx. The tendon of the flexor digitorum profundus passes through the division of the superficialis tendon and continues distally, to be inserted into the anterior surface of the base of the distal phalanx (see Figs. 3.68 and 3.71B,E). The overall result is a "buttonhole effect," in which the split tendon of the superficialis serves as the buttonhole, and the single tendon of the profundus is the button passing through the hole.

Palmaris Brevis Muscle

The palmaris brevis (see Fig. 3.61) is a small muscle that arises from the flexor retinaculum and palmar aponeurosis and inserts into the skin of the palm. It is located outside the hand compartments. The superficial branch of the ulnar nerve supplies it. Its function is to corrugate the skin at the base of the hypothenar eminence and so improve the grip of the palm in holding a rounded object.

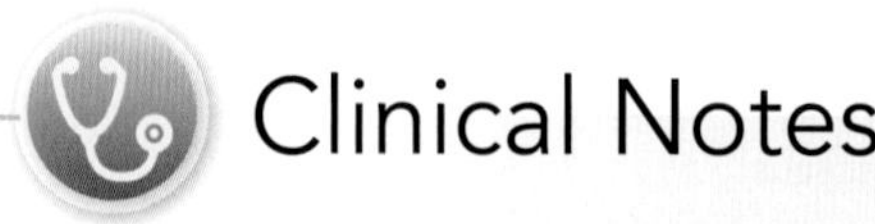

Clinical Notes

Trigger Finger

In trigger finger, a palpable and even audible snapping happens when a patient flexes and extends their fingers. It is caused by the presence of a localized swelling of one of the long flexor tendons that catches on a narrowing of the fibrous flexor sheath anterior to the metacarpophalangeal joint. A similar condition occurring in the thumb is called **trigger thumb**. The situation can be relieved surgically by incising the fibrous flexor sheath.

Lumbrical Muscles

The four lumbrical muscles arise in the hand from the four tendons of the flexor digitorum profundus and insert into digits #2 through #5. However, each lumbrical is identified by number according to its position in the lateral to medial sequence of the muscles rather than according to the digit to which it attaches. Therefore, lumbrical 1 inserts into digit #2 and so forth. This offset of numbers sometimes can be confusing when describing the lumbricals and their individual actions. The lumbricals act to produce both flexion of the metacarpophalangeal joints and extension of the interphalangeal joints of digits #2 through #5 (see Fig. 3.71A,D,E).

Interosseous Muscles

The eight interosseous muscles comprise four palmar and four dorsal interossei. Some authors describe only three palmar interossei, considering the first palmar interosseous as a second head to the flexor pollicis brevis or as part of the adductor pollicis muscle. In any case, the interossei (along with the lumbricals) act to produce both flexion of the metacarpophalangeal joints and extension of the interphalangeal joints of digits #2 through #5 (Fig. 3.72; see also Fig. 3.71A,D,E). Additionally, the interossei have significant actions in producing adduction (palmar) and abduction (dorsal) of the digits (see Fig. 3.72). A useful way to remember this is with PAD vs. DAB: **p**almars **ad**duct; **d**orsals **ab**duct.

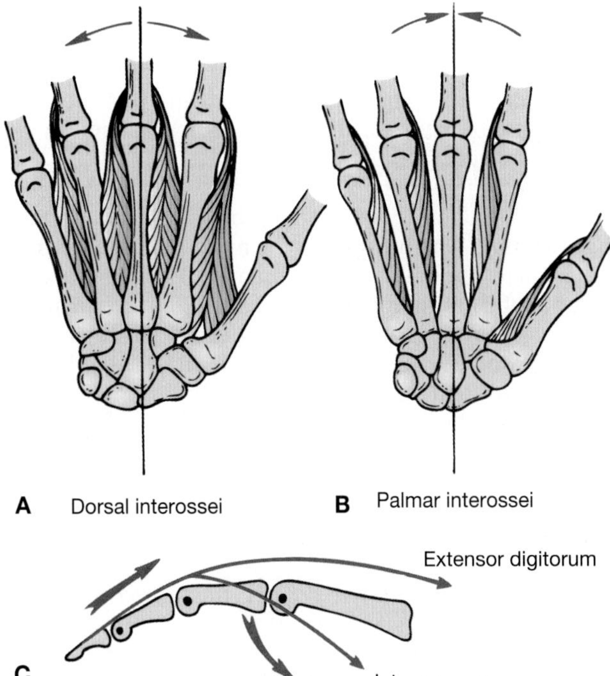

Figure 3.72 Attachments and actions of the palmar and dorsal interosseous muscles. **A.** Anterior view of the dorsal interossei showing their role in abduction. **B.** Anterior view of the palmar interossei showing their role in adduction. **C.** Lateral view showing the role of the interossei in flexion and extension.

Long Extensor Tendon Insertion

The four tendons of the extensor digitorum emerge from under the extensor retinaculum and fan out over the dorsum of the hand (see Figs. 3.63 and 3.64). The tendons are embedded in the deep fascia; together, they form the roof of a subfascial space, which occupies the whole width of the dorsum of the hand. Strong oblique fibrous bands connect the tendons to the little, ring, and middle fingers, proximal to the heads of the metacarpal bones. The tendon to the index finger is joined on its medial side by the tendon of the extensor indicis, and the tendon to the little finger is joined on its medial side by the two tendons of the extensor digiti minimi (see Fig. 3.63).

On the posterior surface of each finger, the extensor tendon joins the fascial expansion called the **extensor expansion** (Fig. 3.73A; see also Figs. 3.63 and 3.64). Near the proximal interphalangeal joint, the extensor expansion splits into a central part, which is inserted into the base of the middle phalanx, and two lateral parts, which converge to insert into the base of the distal phalanx (see Figs. 3.71D and 3.73A).

The dorsal extensor expansion receives the tendon of insertion of the corresponding interosseous muscle on each side and farther distally receives the tendon of the lumbrical muscle on the lateral side (see Figs. 3.71D,E and 3.73A). This arrangement, in which the tendons of the lumbricals and interossei emerge from the palmar aspect of the hand and cross the axes of rotation of the digits to attach onto the dorsal side of the digits, is the mechanism by which these muscles perform the

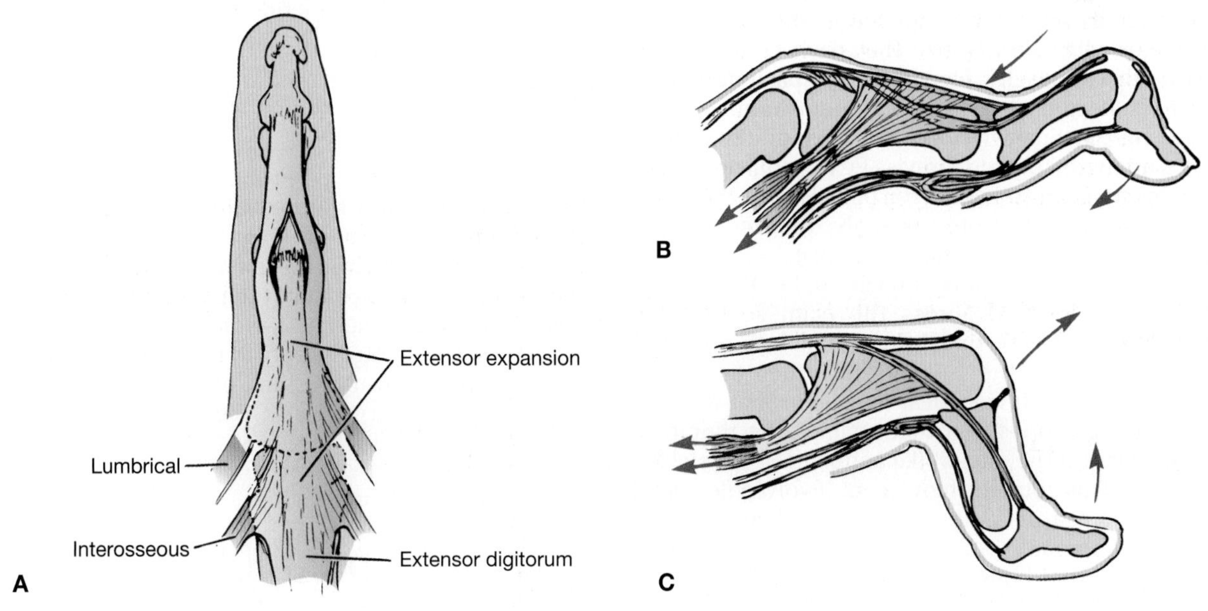

Figure 3.73 **A.** Posterior view of normal dorsal extensor expansion. The extensor expansion near the proximal interphalangeal joint splits into three parts: a central part, which is inserted into the base of the middle phalanx, and two lateral parts, which converge to be inserted into the base of the distal phalanx. **B.** Mallet or baseball finger. The insertion of the extensor expansion into the base of the distal phalanx is ruptured; sometimes, a flake of bone on the base of the phalanx is pulled off. **C.** Boutonnière deformity. The insertion of the extensor expansion into the base of the middle phalanx is ruptured. The *arrows* indicate the direction of the pull of the muscles and the deformity.

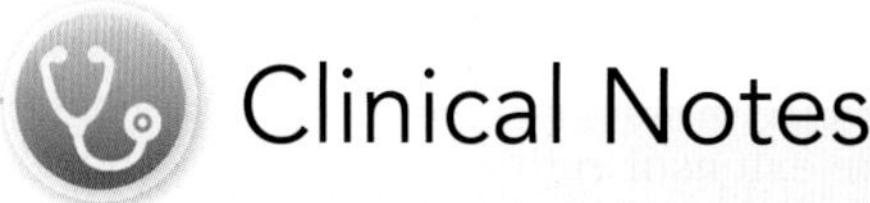

Clinical Notes

Mallet Finger

Avulsion of the insertion of one of the extensor tendons into the distal phalanges can occur if the distal phalanx is forcibly flexed when the extensor tendon is taut. The last 20° of active extension is lost, resulting in a condition known as mallet finger or baseball finger (see Fig. 3.73B).

Boutonnière Deformity

Avulsion of the central slip of the extensor tendon proximal to its insertion into the base of the middle phalanx causes a characteristic deformity (see Fig. 3.73C). The deformity results from flexing of the proximal interphalangeal joint and hyperextension of the distal interphalangeal joint. This injury can result from direct end-on trauma to the finger, direct trauma over the back of the proximal interphalangeal joint, or laceration of the dorsum of the finger.

seemingly contradictory actions of flexion of the metacarpophalangeal joints and extension of the interphalangeal joints (see Figs. 3.71A and 3.72C).

Thumb and Little Finger Muscles

The thenar compartment makes up the **thenar eminence**, which is the fleshy mound at the base of the thumb (digit #1). The hypothenar compartment forms the smaller **hypothenar eminence** at the base of the little finger (digit #5). Notice that each compartment contains three muscles named for the basic functions they share: flexion, abduction, and opposition.

The four intrinsic (short) muscles of the thumb are the abductor pollicis brevis, flexor pollicis brevis, opponens pollicis, and adductor pollicis (see Figs. 3.62, 3.65, 3.68, and 3.69). Note that only the first three of these muscles form the thenar eminence.

The opponens pollicis muscle pulls the thumb medially and forward across the palm so that the palmar surface of the tip of the thumb can meet the palmar surface of the tips of the other fingers in true opposition. It is a critical muscle in that it is the sole muscle of opposition that enables the thumb to form one claw in the pincer-like action used for picking up objects. This complex movement involves flexion of the carpometacarpal and metacarpophalangeal joints and a small amount of abduction and medial rotation of the metacarpal bone at the specialized first carpometacarpal joint.

Abduction of the thumb may be described as a forward movement in the anteroposterior plane taking place at the carpometacarpal and metacarpophalangeal joints.

Adduction of the thumb can be described as a backward movement of the abducted thumb in the anteroposterior plane. It restores the thumb to its anatomic position, which is flush with the palm. The adductor pollicis in association with the flexor pollicis longus and the opponens pollicis muscles is largely responsible for the power of the pincers grip of the thumb. Adduction of the thumb occurs at the carpometacarpal and metacarpophalangeal joints.

The short muscles of the little finger are the abductor digiti minimi, flexor digiti minimi brevis, and opponens digiti minimi, which together form the hypothenar eminence. The opponens digiti minimi is the only muscle capable of rotating the fifth metacarpal bone to a slight degree. However, it mainly assists the flexor digiti minimi in flexing the carpometacarpal joint of the little finger, thereby pulling the fifth metacarpal bone forward and cupping the palm (see the earlier text on Hand as a Functional Unit).

NERVES

Most of the nerves that supply the upper limb are derived from anterior (ventral) primary rami of spinal nerves (see Chapter 1, Introduction). Most of the spinal nerve derivatives are branches of the brachial plexus.

Spinal Accessory Nerve (Cranial Nerve XI)

The spinal accessory nerve is the only cranial nerve (CN) that supplies the upper limb. It runs downward in the posterior triangle of the neck on the levator scapulae muscle and is accompanied by branches from the anterior rami of the C3 and C4 nerves. The accessory nerve runs along the deep aspect of the belly of the trapezius muscle at the junction of its middle and lower thirds (see Fig. 3.40). The accessory nerve provides motor fibers to the trapezius, whereas the cervical nerves supply sensory innervation.

Brachial Plexus

The nerves entering the upper limb provide the following important functions: sensory innervation to the skin and deep structures, such as the joints; motor innervation to the muscles; influence over the diameters of the blood vessels by the sympathetic vasomotor nerves; and sympathetic secretomotor supply to the sweat glands.

The anterior (ventral) rami of the C5 to C8 and T1 spinal nerves intermingle in the posterior triangle of

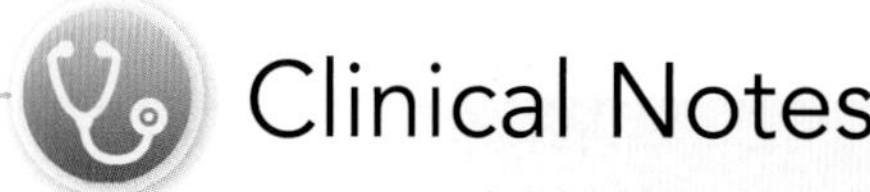

Clinical Notes

Accessory Nerve Injury

The accessory nerve can be injured as the result of penetrating wounds to the neck (eg, stab wounds). Loss of the trapezius muscle was discussed earlier in this chapter in the context of the shoulder joint.

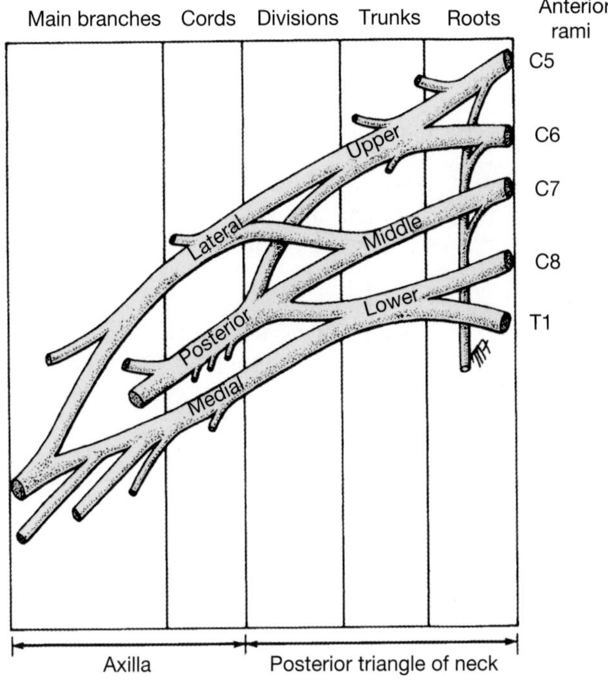

Figure 3.74 Formation of the main parts of the brachial plexus. Note the locations of the different parts.

the neck and form a complex nerve network termed the **brachial plexus** (Figs. 3.74 and 3.75). Individual nerves branch off the brachial plexus and distribute through the upper limb. Thus, nerve fibers that originate in single segments of the spinal cord contribute to the composition of multiple individual nerves. Therefore, each nerve that branches off the brachial plexus carries fibers from multiple segments of the spinal cord.

The brachial plexus is divided schematically into subparts termed **roots**, **trunks**, **divisions**, **cords**, and **(terminal) branches** (see Fig. 3.74). To help remember these parts, think: "Robert (roots) Taylor (trunks) drinks (divisions) cold (cords) beer (branches)."

The roots are the anterior rami of spinal nerves C5 to T1. The roots of C5 and C6 unite to form the **upper trunk**, the root of C7 continues as the **middle trunk**, and the roots of C8 and T1 unite to form the **lower trunk**. Each trunk then divides into **anterior** and **posterior divisions**. The anterior divisions of the upper and middle trunks unite to form the **lateral cord**, the anterior division of the lower trunk continues as the **medial cord**, and the posterior divisions of all three trunks join to form the **posterior cord**.

The plexus occupies a cervicobrachial position (ie, it lies within the neck and the upper limb). The clavicle overlies the plexus in such a way that it effectively divides the plexus into upper supraclavicular and lower infraclavicular parts. The roots, trunks, and divisions of the brachial plexus reside in the upper portion, in the lower part of the posterior triangle of the neck. These are fully described in Chapter 9 (Head and Neck). The three cords are in the infraclavicular region, in the axilla, where they are arranged around the axillary artery (Fig. 3.76; see also Fig. 3.34). Here, the brachial plexus and the axillary artery and vein are enclosed together in a connective tissue wrapping termed the **axillary sheath**.

All three cords of the brachial plexus lie above and lateral to the first part of the axillary artery (see Figs. 3.34 and 3.76). The medial cord crosses behind the artery to reach the medial side of the second part of the artery (see Fig. 3.76). The posterior cord lies behind the second part of the artery, and the lateral cord lies on the lateral side of the second part of the artery. Thus, the cords of the plexus are named according to

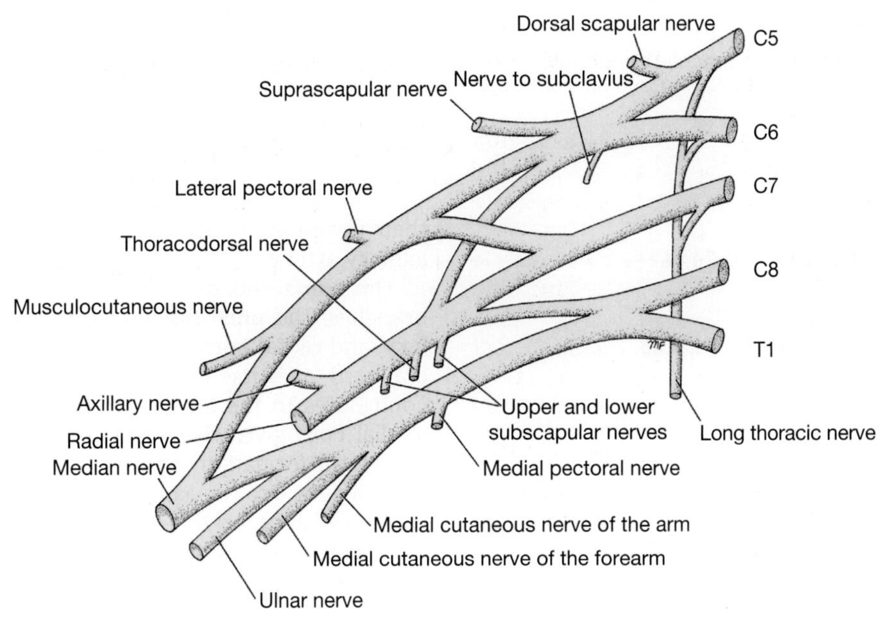

Figure 3.75 Roots, trunks, divisions, cords, and terminal branches of the brachial plexus.

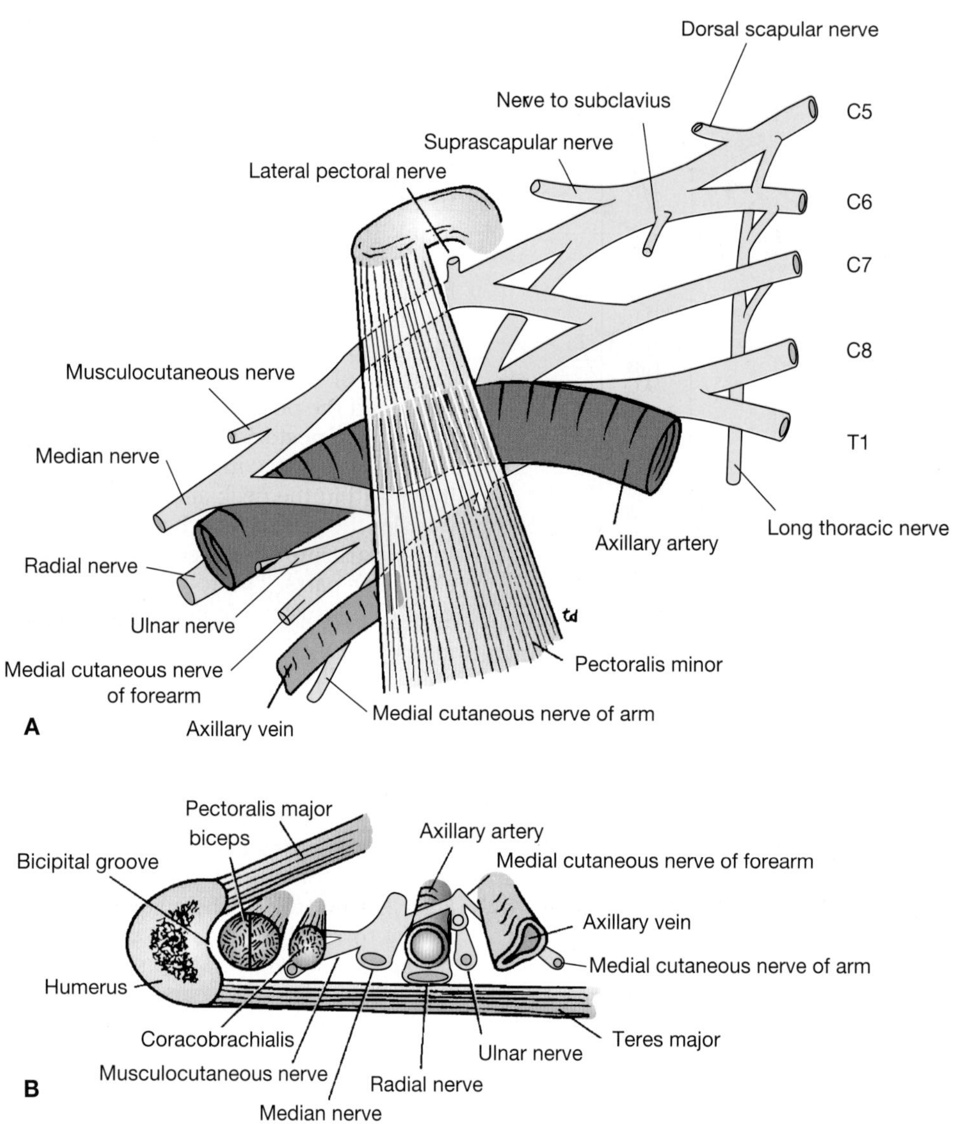

Figure 3.76 **A.** Relations of the brachial plexus and its branches to the axillary artery and vein. **B.** Section through the axilla at the level of the teres major muscle.

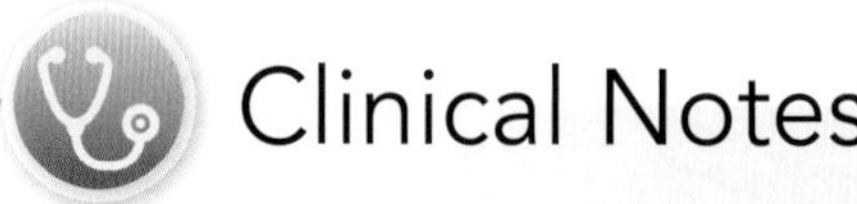

Clinical Notes

Axillary Sheath and Brachial Plexus Nerve Block

Because the axillary sheath encloses the axillary vessels and the brachial plexus, a brachial plexus nerve block can easily be obtained. The distal part of the sheath is closed with finger pressure, and a syringe is inserted into the proximal part of the sheath. The anesthetic solution is then injected into the sheath, and the solution is massaged along the sheath to produce the nerve block. The position of the sheath can be verified by feeling the pulsations of the third part of the axillary artery.

their positional relationship to the second part of the axillary artery.

The cords end by dividing into five terminal nerve branches: the **musculocutaneous**, **median**, **ulnar**, **axillary**, and **radial nerves** (see Figs. 3.75 and 3.76). The lateral cord gives rise to the musculocutaneous nerve and contributes to the formation of the median nerve. The medial cord gives rise to the ulnar nerve and contributes to the formation of the median nerve. The posterior cord divides into the axillary and radial nerves. The axillary nerve supplies the shoulder region. The other four nerves are the main branches that distribute through the osseofascial compartments of the upper limb (Fig. 3.77).

The branches of the different parts of the brachial plexus are as follows. The branches and their distributions are summarized in Table 3.13. The distributions of the

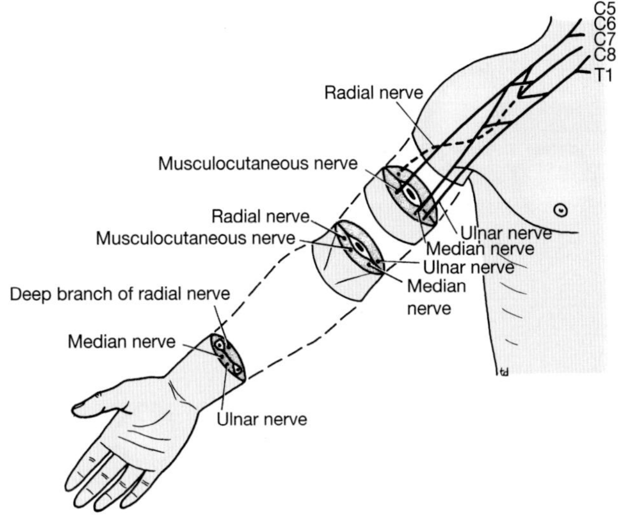

Figure 3.77 Distribution of the main branches of the brachial plexus to different osseofascial compartments of the arm and forearm.

five terminal branches are summarized in Figures 3.78 through 3.81.

- **Roots**
  Dorsal scapular nerve (C5)
  Long thoracic nerve (C5 to C7)
- **Upper trunk**
  Nerve to subclavius (C5, C6)
  Suprascapular nerve (C5, C6)
- **Lateral cord**
  Lateral pectoral nerve
  Musculocutaneous nerve
  Lateral root of median nerve
- **Medial cord**
  Medial pectoral nerve
  Medial cutaneous nerve of arm and medial cutaneous nerve of forearm
  Ulnar nerve
  Medial root of median nerve
- **Posterior cord**
  Upper and lower subscapular nerves
  Thoracodorsal nerve (middle subscapular nerve)
  Axillary nerve
  Radial nerve

Table 3.13 Summary of Brachial Plexus Branches and Distribution

BRANCHES	DISTRIBUTION
Roots	
Dorsal scapular nerve (C5)	Rhomboid minor, rhomboid major, levator scapulae muscles
Long thoracic nerve (C5 to C7)	Serratus anterior muscle
Upper Trunk	
Suprascapular nerve (C5, C6)	Supraspinatus and infraspinatus muscles
Nerve to subclavius (C5, C6)	Subclavius
Lateral Cord	
Lateral pectoral nerve (C5 to C7)	Pectoralis major muscle
Musculocutaneous nerve (C5 to C7)	Coracobrachialis, biceps brachii, most of brachialis muscles; supplies skin along lateral border of forearm when it becomes the lateral cutaneous nerve of forearm
Lateral root of median nerve (C5 to C7)	See medial root of median nerve
Posterior Cord	
Upper subscapular nerve (C5, C6)	Subscapularis muscle
Thoracodorsal nerve (C6 to C8)	Latissimus dorsi muscle
Lower subscapular nerve (C5, C6)	Subscapularis and teres major muscles
Axillary nerve (C5, C6)	Deltoid and teres minor muscles; upper lateral cutaneous nerve of arm supplies skin over lower half of deltoid muscle
Radial nerve (C5 to C8; T1)	Triceps, anconeus, small part of brachialis, extensor carpi radialis longus; via deep radial nerve branch supplies extensor muscles of forearm: supinator, extensor carpi radialis brevis, extensor carpi ulnaris, extensor digitorum, extensor digiti minimi, extensor indicis, abductor pollicis longus, extensor pollicis longus, extensor pollicis brevis; skin, lower lateral cutaneous nerve of arm, posterior cutaneous nerve of arm, and posterior cutaneous nerve of forearm; skin on lateral side of dorsum of hand and dorsal surface of lateral three and a half fingers; articular branches to elbow, wrist, and hand

(continued)

Table 3.13 Summary of Brachial Plexus Branches and Distribution *(Continued)*

BRANCHES	DISTRIBUTION
Medial Cord	
Medial pectoral nerve (C8; T1)	Pectoralis major and minor muscles
Medial cutaneous nerve of arm joined by intercostal brachial nerve from second intercostal nerve (C8; T1, T2)	Skin of medial side of arm
Medial cutaneous nerve of forearm (C8; T1)	Skin of medial side of forearm
Ulnar nerve (C8; T1)	Flexor carpi ulnaris and medial half of flexor digitorum profundus, flexor digiti minimi, opponens digiti minimi, abductor digiti minimi, adductor pollicis, third and fourth lumbricals, interossei, palmaris brevis, skin of medial half of dorsum of hand and palm, skin of palmar and dorsal surfaces of medial one and a half fingers
Medial root of median nerve (with lateral root) forms median nerve (C5 to C8; T1)	Pronator teres, flexor carpi radialis, palmaris longus, flexor digitorum superficialis, abductor pollicis brevis, flexor pollicis brevis, opponens pollicis, first two lumbricals (by way of anterior interosseous branch), flexor pollicis longus, flexor digitorum profundus (lateral half), pronator quadratus; palmar cutaneous branch to lateral half of the palm and digital branches to palmar surface of lateral three and a half fingers; articular branches to the elbow, wrist, and carpal joints

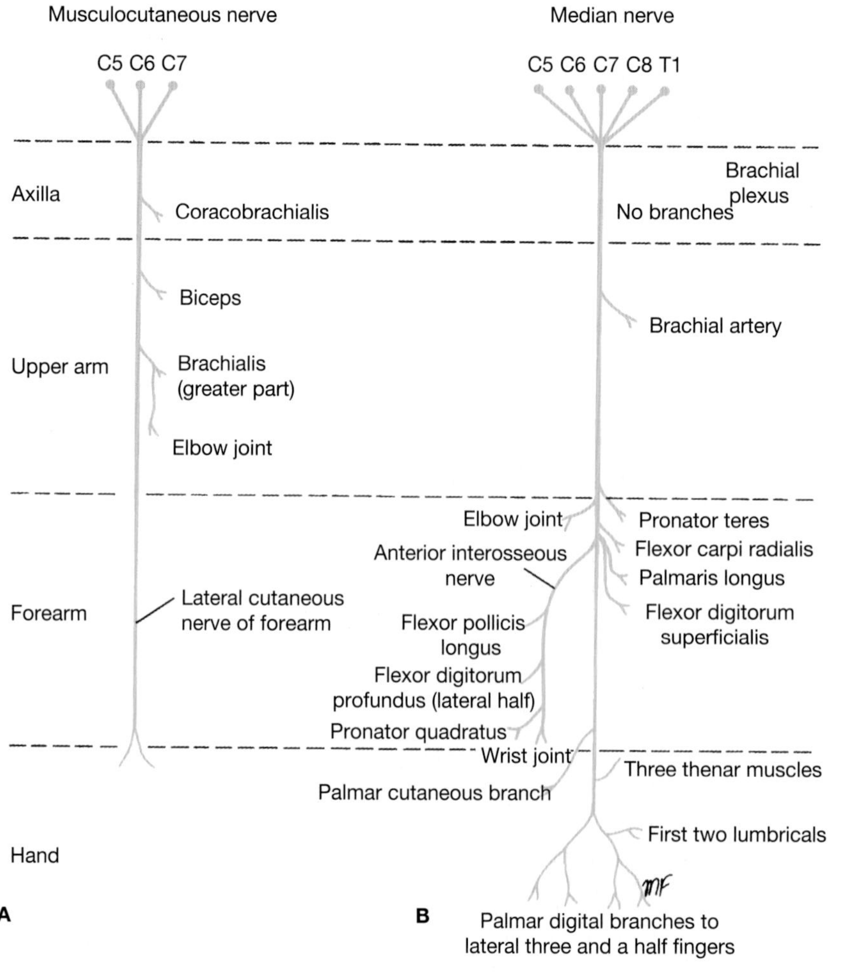

Figure 3.78 Summary of the main branches of the musculocutaneous **(A)** and median **(B)** nerves.

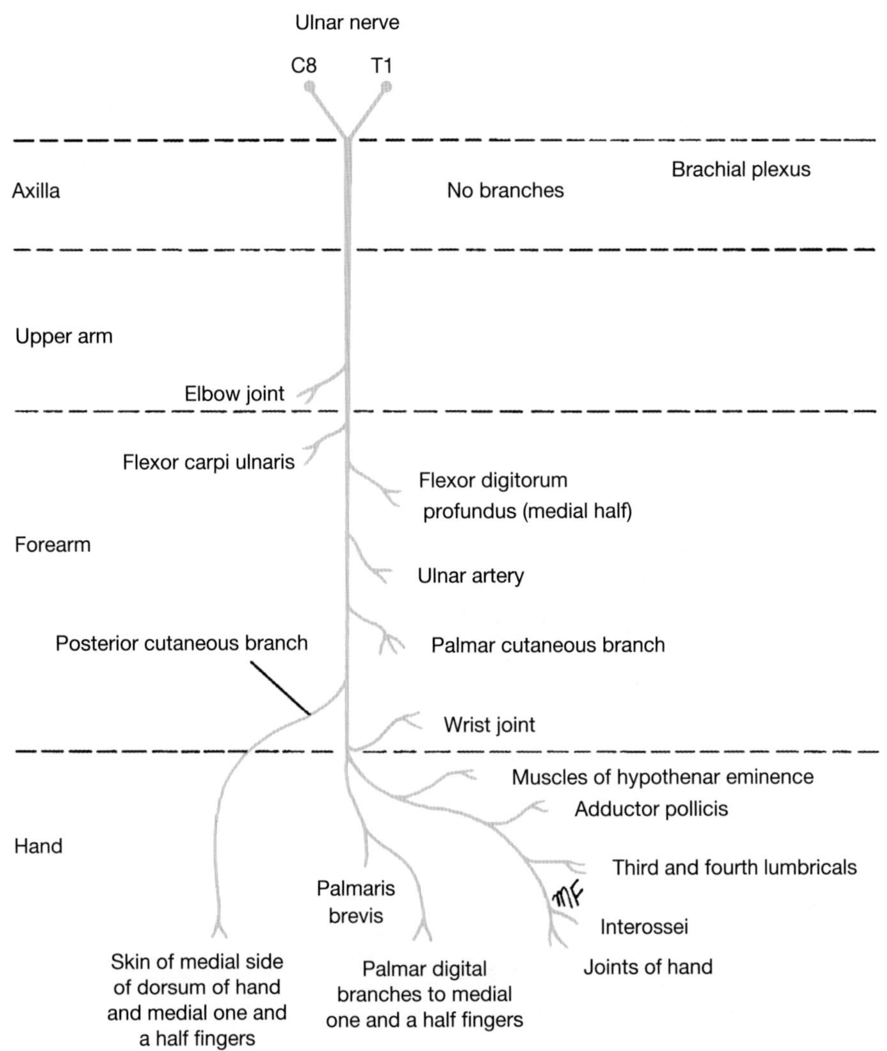

Figure 3.79 Summary of the main branches of the ulnar nerve.

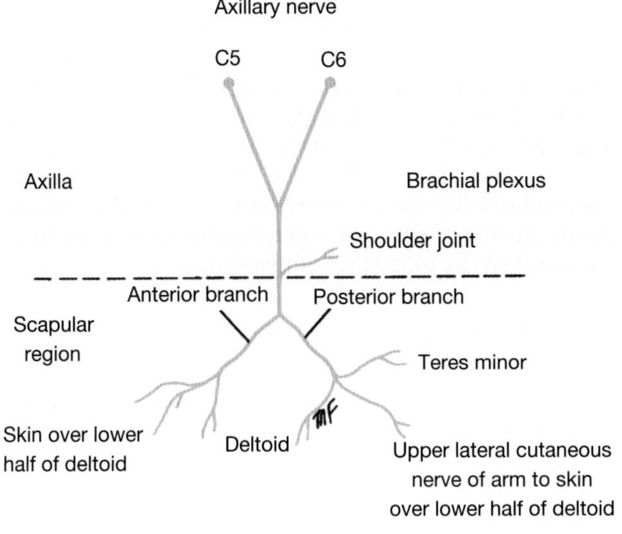

Figure 3.80 Summary of the main branches of the axillary nerve.

Skin

Several cutaneous nerves from multiple sources carry afferent neurons from the skin of the upper limb (Fig. 3.82). The **posterior (dorsal) rami of the spinal nerves** (see Chapter 1, Introduction) supply the skin of the scapular region. However, the C1 and C8 posterior rami do not supply the skin. The **supraclavicular nerves** (C3, C4 from the cervical plexus) provide the sensory nerve supply to the skin over the point of the shoulder to halfway down the deltoid muscle. The **medial cutaneous nerve of the arm** (T1) and the **intercostobrachial nerve** (branch of the T2 intercostal nerve) supply the skin of the armpit and the medial side of the arm. Cutaneous branches of the cords of the brachial plexus and its terminal branches innervate the remainder of the skin of the upper limb.

Branches from Brachial Plexus Roots

The **dorsal scapular nerve** branches from the C5 root of the brachial plexus (see Fig. 3.75) to supply the levator scapulae and rhomboid muscles.

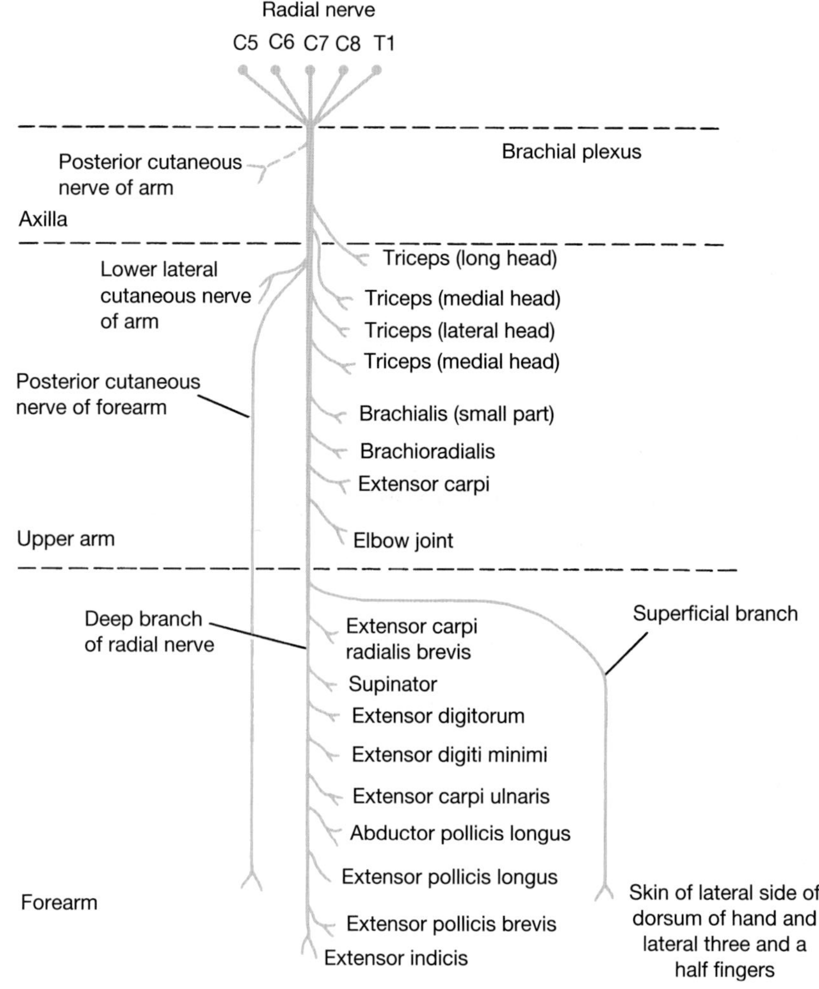

Figure 3.81 Summary of the main branches of the radial nerve.

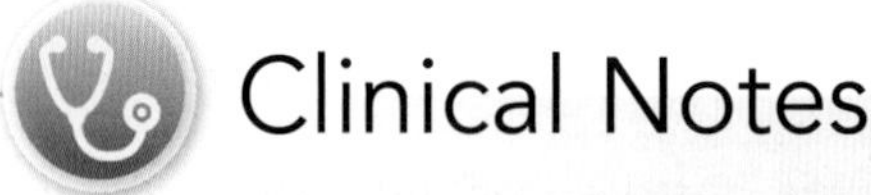

Clinical Notes

Dermatomes and Cutaneous Nerves

Testing the integrity of the C3 to T1 segments of the spinal cord may become necessary. The dermatomes for the upper cervical segments (C3 to C6) are located along the lateral margin of the upper limb; the C7 dermatome is situated on the middle finger; and the dermatomes for C8, T1, and T2 are along the medial margin of the limb. The nerve fibers from a particular segment of the spinal cord, although they exit from the cord in a spinal nerve of the same segment, pass to the skin in two or more different cutaneous nerves.

The supraclavicular nerves innervate the skin over the point of the shoulder and halfway down the lateral surface of the deltoid muscle. Pain may be referred to this region because of inflammatory lesions involving the diaphragmatic pleura or peritoneum. The afferent stimuli reach the spinal cord via the phrenic nerves (C3 to C5). Pleurisy, peritonitis, subphrenic abscess, or gallbladder disease may therefore be responsible for shoulder pain.

The **long thoracic nerve** (C5 to C7) arises from the roots of the brachial plexus in the neck and enters the axilla by passing down over the lateral border of rib 1 deep to the axillary vessels and brachial plexus (see Figs. 3.34 and 3.75). It descends over the superficial surface of the serratus anterior muscle, which it supplies (see Fig. 3.45). The long thoracic nerve is unusual in that it is a motor nerve that enters its target muscle on the muscle's superficial side rather than the more typical deep side of the muscle belly. This relationship places the nerve in a position of greater potential danger from trauma (see the following Clinical Notes).

Branches from Brachial Plexus Trunks and Divisions

The middle and lower trunks of the brachial plexus do not have branches. The following nerves are branches of the upper trunk. The **nerve to the subclavius** (C5 to C6) supplies the subclavius muscle (see Figs. 3.34, 3.75, and 3.76). It is important clinically because it may give a contribution (C5) to the phrenic nerve. This branch, when present, is referred to as the **accessory phrenic nerve**.

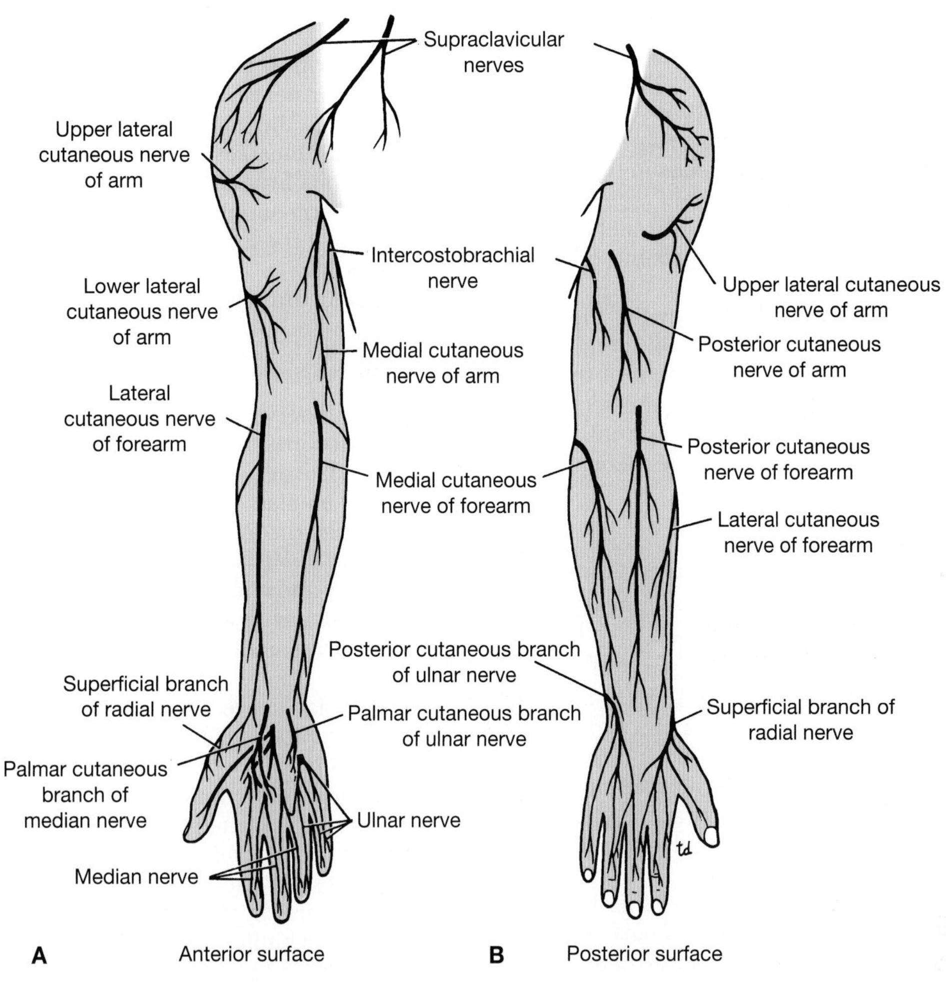

Figure 3.82 Cutaneous innervation of the upper limb. **A.** Anterior surface. **B.** Posterior surface.

The **suprascapular nerve** (C5 to C6) arises in the posterior triangle in the neck and runs downward and laterally to reach the upper edge of the scapula. There, it passes through the suprascapular notch, beneath the suprascapular ligament, to reach the supraspinous fossa (see Fig. 3.41). It supplies the supraspinatus muscle and then continues through the spinoglenoid notch into the infraspinous fossa where it innervates the infraspinatus muscle. The suprascapular nerve also supplies the glenohumeral (shoulder) joint.

The divisions of the brachial plexus give off no branches.

Branches from Brachial Plexus Lateral Cord

The lateral and medial pectoral nerves are so named owing to their origins from the lateral and medial cords of the brachial plexus, respectively. The **lateral pectoral nerve** supplies the pectoralis major muscle, primarily its clavicular head (see Figs. 3.33 and 3.76).

The **musculocutaneous nerve** supplies the coracobrachialis muscle and leaves the axilla by piercing that muscle (see Figs. 3.33 and 3.76). A summary of the complete distribution of the musculocutaneous nerve is given in Figure 3.78A.

The **lateral root of the median nerve** is the direct continuation of the lateral cord of the brachial plexus (see Figs. 3.75 and 3.76). It joins with the medial root to form the median nerve trunk, which passes downward on the lateral side of the axillary artery. The median nerve gives off no branches in the axilla. A summary of the complete distribution of the median nerve is given in Figure 3.78B.

Branches from Brachial Plexus Medial Cord

The **medial pectoral nerve** arises from the medial cord of the brachial plexus; supplies and pierces the pectoralis minor muscle; and next supplies the pectoralis major muscle, primarily its sternocostal head (see Fig. 3.75).

The **medial cutaneous nerve of the arm** (T1) arises from the medial cord of the brachial plexus (see Figs. 3.75 and 3.76) and is joined by the **intercostobrachial nerve** (lateral cutaneous branch of the second intercostal nerve). It supplies the skin on the medial side of the arm (see Fig. 3.82).

The **medial cutaneous nerve of the forearm** arises from the medial cord of the brachial plexus and descends in front of the axillary artery. It supplies the skin on the medial side of the forearm (see Fig. 3.82).

The **ulnar nerve** (C8, T1) arises from the medial cord of the brachial plexus and descends in the interval between the axillary artery and the vein (see Figs. 3.75 and 3.76). The ulnar nerve gives off no branches in the axilla. A summary of the complete distribution of the ulnar nerve is given in Figure 3.79.

The **medial root of the median nerve** is the direct continuation of the medial cord of the brachial plexus (see Figs. 3.75 and 3.76). It crosses in front of the third part of the axillary artery to join the lateral root of the median nerve and form the median nerve trunk. A summary of the complete distribution of the median nerve is given in Figure 3.78B.

Branches from Brachial Plexus Posterior Cord

The **upper and lower subscapular nerves** arise from the posterior cord of the brachial plexus, descend into the axilla, and supply the upper and lower parts of the subscapularis muscle (see Figs. 3.34 and 3.75). In addition, the lower subscapular nerve supplies the teres major muscle.

The **thoracodorsal nerve** (middle subscapular nerve) arises from the posterior cord of the brachial plexus and runs downward into the axilla to supply the latissimus dorsi muscle (see Figs. 3.34 and 3.75).

The **axillary nerve** is one of the terminal branches of the posterior cord of the brachial plexus (see Figs. 3.34 and 3.75). It turns deep and backward and passes through the quadrangular space of the scapular region (see Fig. 3.41 and the earlier description of the quadrangular space). A summary of the complete distribution of the axillary nerve is given in Figure 3.80.

The **radial nerve** is the largest branch of the brachial plexus and lies deep in the axilla, behind the axillary artery (see Figs. 3.34, 3.75, and 3.76). It gives off branches to the heads of the triceps muscle and gives rise to the posterior cutaneous nerve of the arm (see Fig. 3.33). The latter branch is distributed to the skin on the middle of the back of the arm. A summary of the complete distribution of the radial nerve is given in Figure 3.81.

Musculocutaneous Nerve

The musculocutaneous nerve (C5 to C7) originates from the lateral cord of the brachial plexus in the axilla (see Figs. 3.75 and 3.78). It runs downward and laterally, pierces the coracobrachialis muscle (see Fig. 3.34), and then passes downward between the biceps and brachialis muscles (see Fig. 3.48). It appears at the lateral margin of the biceps tendon, pierces the deep fascia just above the elbow, and moves into a superficial position. It then runs down the lateral aspect of the forearm as the **lateral cutaneous nerve of the forearm** (see Fig. 3.82). The name of this nerve makes sense because it is first muscular in its distribution and then cutaneous.

Branches

- **Muscular branches:** The musculocutaneous nerve is the motor nerve to the anterior compartment of the arm (ie, to the coracobrachialis, biceps brachii, and brachialis muscles; see Fig. 3.78).
- **Cutaneous branches:** The lateral cutaneous nerve of the forearm supplies the skin of the front and lateral aspects of the forearm down as far as the root of the thumb.
- **Articular branches** supply the elbow joint.

Median Nerve

The median nerve (C5 to T1) originates from the medial and lateral cords of the brachial plexus in the axilla (see Fig. 3.75). The nerve is so named because it mainly runs along the median axis of the upper limb. It first runs through the arm on the lateral side of the brachial artery (see Fig. 3.48). Halfway down the arm, it crosses the brachial artery and continues downward on its medial side. The median nerve has no branches in the arm, except for a small vasomotor nerve to the brachial artery (see Fig. 3.78).

The median nerve lies deep to the bicipital aponeurosis in the cubital fossa (see Fig. 3.52). The nerve leaves the cubital fossa by passing between the two heads of the pronator teres muscle (see Fig. 3.56). It continues downward sandwiched in the plane between the flexor digitorum superficialis and the flexor digitorum profundus muscles. At the wrist, the median nerve emerges from the lateral border of the flexor digitorum superficialis and lies behind the tendon of the palmaris longus (see Figs. 3.55 and 3.56).

Forearm Branches

- **Muscular branches:** The median nerve is the major motor nerve to the anterior compartment of the forearm. It supplies all the muscles therein, except for the flexor carpi ulnaris and the medial half of the flexor digitorum profundus (see Figs. 3.78 and 3.79). It gives off muscular branches in the cubital fossa to the pronator teres, flexor carpi radialis, palmaris longus, and flexor digitorum superficialis (see Fig. 3.78).
- **Articular branches** supply the elbow joint.
- **Anterior interosseous nerve**.
- **Palmar cutaneous branch** arises in the lower part of the forearm, crosses the superficial side of the flexor retinaculum, and distributes to the skin over the lateral part of the palm (see Fig. 3.82).

Anterior Interosseous Nerve

This nerve arises from the median nerve as the median nerve emerges from between the two heads of the pronator teres muscle. It passes downward on the anterior surface of the interosseous membrane, between the flexor pollicis longus and the flexor digitorum profundus (see Fig. 3.57). It ends on the anterior surface of the carpus.

ANTERIOR INTEROSSEOUS NERVE BRANCHES

- **Muscular branches** supply the flexor pollicis longus, pronator quadratus, and lateral half of the flexor digitorum profundus (see Fig. 3.78).
- **Articular branches** supply the wrist and distal radio-ulnar joints; they also supply the joints of the hand.

The median nerve enters the palm of the hand by passing deep to the flexor retinaculum and through the carpal tunnel (see Fig. 3.65). It is the minor motor nerve to the intrinsic muscles of the hand and supplies the three muscles of the thenar compartment plus the first two lumbricals. The ulnar nerve innervates all the other intrinsic muscles.

Hand Branches

- The **recurrent branch** curves back around the distal border of the flexor retinaculum and lies about one fingerbreadth distal to the tubercle of the scaphoid. It supplies the muscles of the thenar compartment (abductor pollicis brevis, flexor pollicis brevis, and opponens pollicis) and the first lumbrical muscle (see Fig. 3.65).
- The **palmar digital branches** supply the palmar aspect of the lateral three and a half fingers and the distal half of the dorsal aspect of each of those fingers (see Figs. 3.65 and 3.78). One of these branches also supplies the second lumbrical muscle.

Ulnar Nerve

The ulnar nerve (C8, T1) originates from the medial cord of the brachial plexus in the axilla (see Figs. 3.75 and 3.76). It is named for its pathway along the ulnar (medial) side of the upper limb. The ulnar nerve runs downward on the medial side of the brachial artery as far as the middle of the arm (see Fig. 3.48). Here, at the insertion of the coracobrachialis, the nerve pierces the medial intermuscular fascial septum, accompanied by the superior ulnar collateral vessels, and enters the medial aspect of the posterior compartment of the arm. The nerve and vessels descend behind the septum, covered posteriorly by the medial head of the triceps, and then pass behind the medial epicondyle of the humerus (see Fig. 3.50). The ulnar nerve has no branches in the arm except for an articular branch to the elbow joint (see Fig. 3.79).

The ulnar nerve emerges from behind the medial epicondyle of the humerus, crosses the medial collateral ligament of the elbow joint, and enters the medial aspect of the anterior compartment of the forearm by passing between the two heads of the flexor carpi ulnaris (see Figs. 3.56 and 3.57). It then runs down the forearm between the flexor carpi ulnaris and the flexor digitorum profundus muscles. In the distal two thirds of the forearm, the ulnar nerve lies on the medial side of the ulnar artery (see Fig. 3.57). At the wrist, the ulnar nerve becomes superficial and lies between the tendons of the flexor carpi ulnaris and flexor digitorum superficialis muscles (see Figs. 3.55, 3.56, and 3.62).

Forearm Branches

- **Muscular branches:** The ulnar nerve is the minor motor nerve to the anterior compartment of the forearm. It supplies one and a half muscles in the medial aspect of this compartment, the flexor carpi ulnaris and the medial (ulnar) half of the flexor digitorum profundus (see Fig. 3.79). The median nerve and its branches innervate all the other muscles in the anterior compartment of the forearm.
- **Articular branches** supply the elbow joint.
- The **palmar cutaneous branch** is a small branch that arises in the middle of the forearm. It crosses the superficial side of the flexor retinaculum and supplies the skin over the medial part of the palm (see Figs. 3.79 and 3.82).
- The **posterior (dorsal) cutaneous branch** is a large branch that arises in the distal third of the forearm. It winds around the ulna deep to the flexor carpi ulnaris tendon, descends superficial to the extensor retinaculum, and supplies the medial third of the dorsum of the hand (see Figs. 3.58, 3.79, and 3.82). It divides into several **dorsal digital nerves** that supply the medial side of the ring finger and both sides of the little finger.

The ulnar nerve enters the medial part of the palm of the hand by passing superficial to the flexor retinaculum and lateral to the pisiform bone. Here, the nerve lies medial to the ulnar artery (see Figs. 3.55, 3.56, 3.62, and 3.65). The nerve divides into a superficial and a deep branch as it crosses the retinaculum (see Figs. 3.65, 3.68, and 3.79).

Superficial Branch of the Ulnar Nerve

The superficial branch of the ulnar nerve is primarily a cutaneous nerve in the hand. It descends into the palm, lying in the subcutaneous tissue between the pisiform bone and the hook of the hamate (see Figs. 3.61 and 3.65). The nerve lies medial to the ulnar artery. Here, the nerve and artery may lie in a fibro-osseous tunnel (**tunnel of Guyon**) created by fibrous tissue derived from the superficial part of the flexor retinaculum. The nerve may be compressed at this site, giving rise to clinical signs and symptoms.

Branches

- A **muscular branch** supplies the palmaris brevis muscle.
- **Palmar cutaneous branches (common palmar digital and proper palmar digital nerves)** supply the palmar aspect of the medial side of the little finger and the adjacent sides of the little and ring fingers (see Fig. 3.65). They also supply the distal half of the dorsal aspect of each finger.

Deep Branch of the Ulnar Nerve

The deep branch of the ulnar nerve is the primary motor nerve to the intrinsic muscles of the hand. It supplies all the intrinsic muscles except for the three muscles in the thenar compartment and the first two lumbricals, which are innervated by the median nerve. The deep branch curves deeply between the abductor digiti minimi and the flexor digiti minimi (see Figs. 3.68 and 3.69). It pierces the opponens digiti minimi, winds around the lower border of the hook of the hamate, and passes laterally within the concavity of the deep palmar arterial arch. The nerve lies deep down to the long flexor tendons and superficial to the metacarpal bones and interosseous muscles.

Branches

- **Muscular branches** supply the three muscles of the hypothenar eminence (abductor digiti minimi, flexor digiti minimi, and opponens digiti minimi), all the palmar and dorsal interossei, the third and fourth lumbrical muscles, and both heads of the adductor pollicis.

Axillary Nerve

The axillary nerve (C5 to C6) arises from the termination of the posterior cord of the brachial plexus in the axilla (Figs. 3.34 and 3.51). It curves deeply into the axilla and enters the quadrangular space with the posterior circumflex humeral artery (see Fig. 3.41). As the nerve passes through the space, it comes into close relationship with the inferior aspect of the capsule of the shoulder joint and with the medial side of the surgical neck of the humerus. It terminates by dividing into anterior and posterior branches (see Figs. 3.41 and 3.80).

Branches

- An **articular branch** supplies the shoulder joint.
- An **anterior terminal branch** winds around the surgical neck of the humerus deep to the deltoid muscle; it supplies the deltoid and the skin that covers its lower part.
- A **posterior terminal branch** gives off a branch to the teres minor muscle and a few branches to the deltoid and then emerges from the posterior border of the deltoid as the **upper lateral cutaneous nerve of the arm** (see Figs. 3.41 and 3.80).

Radial Nerve

The radial nerve (C5 to T1) originates from the posterior cord of the brachial plexus in the axilla (see Figs. 3.34, 3.75, and 3.76). It is named for its pathway along the radial (lateral) side of the upper limb. The radial nerve is the sole motor nerve to the muscles in the posterior compartments of the arm and forearm (see Fig. 3.81). It also provides extensive cutaneous innervation along the posterior aspect of the entire limb (see Fig. 3.82).

Axillary Branches

- **Muscular branches** supply the long and medial heads of the triceps (see Figs. 3.50 and 3.81).
- The **posterior cutaneous nerve of the arm** supplies the skin of the back of the arm (see Fig. 3.82).

The radial nerve descends out of the axilla and immediately enters the posterior compartment of the arm (see Fig. 3.50). It winds around the back of the arm in the radial groove of the humerus between the heads of the triceps, where it lies in direct contact with the shaft of the humerus (see Fig. 3.50). The profunda brachii vessels accompany the nerve in the radial groove. The nerve then pierces the lateral intermuscular septum above the lateral epicondyle of the humerus, enters the anterior compartment of the arm between the brachialis and brachioradialis muscles, and continues into the cubital fossa (see Fig. 3.52).

Arm Branches

- **Muscular branches** in the spiral groove supply the lateral and medial heads of the triceps and the anconeus. Additional muscular branches in the anterior compartment of the arm, after the nerve has pierced the lateral intermuscular septum, supply the brachialis (a very small branch), brachioradialis, and extensor carpi radialis longus muscles (see Figs. 3.52 and 3.81).
- The **lower lateral cutaneous nerve of the arm** supplies the skin over the lateral and anterior aspects of the lower part of the arm (see Figs. 3.81 and 3.82).
- The **posterior cutaneous nerve of the forearm** runs down the middle of the back of the forearm as far as the wrist (see Figs. 3.81 and 3.82).
- **Articular branches** supply the elbow joint (see Fig. 3.81).

The radial nerve passes downward in the cubital fossa in front of the lateral epicondyle of the humerus, lying between the brachialis muscle on the medial side and the brachioradialis and extensor carpi radialis longus muscles on the lateral side (see Figs. 3.52 and 3.56). The nerve divides into superficial and deep branches at the level of the lateral epicondyle (see Figs. 3.52 and 3.57).

Cubital Fossa Branches

- **Articular branches** supply the elbow joint.
- **Superficial branch of the radial nerve**.
- **Deep branch of the radial nerve** winds around the neck of the radius, within the supinator muscle, and enters the posterior compartment of the forearm (see Fig. 3.57).

Superficial Branch of the Radial Nerve

The superficial branch of the radial nerve is a cutaneous nerve to the wrist and hand. It is the direct continuation of the radial nerve after its main stem has given off its deep branch in front of the lateral epicondyle of the humerus (see Figs. 3.52 and 3.56). It runs down under cover of the brachioradialis muscle on the lateral side of the radial artery. The nerve leaves the artery in the distal part of the forearm, winds around the radius deep to the brachioradialis tendon, descends superficial to the extensor retinaculum, and divides into several **dorsal digital nerves**. These terminal branches supply the lateral two thirds of the dorsum of the hand and the posterior surface over the proximal phalanges of the lateral three and a half fingers (see Fig. 3.82).

The sensory nerve supply to the skin on the dorsum of the hand is derived from the superficial branch of the radial nerve and the posterior cutaneous branch of the ulnar nerve. These nerve territories vary. Commonly, a dorsal digital nerve, a branch of the ulnar nerve, also supplies the lateral side of the ring finger. The dorsal digital branches of the radial and ulnar nerves do not extend far beyond the proximal phalanx. The remainder of the dorsum of each finger receives its nerve supply from palmar digital nerves (branches of the median and ulnar nerves).

Deep Branch of the Radial Nerve

The deep branch arises from the radial nerve in front of the lateral epicondyle of the humerus in the cubital fossa (see Fig. 3.52). It pierces the supinator muscle and winds around the lateral aspect of the neck of the radius in the substance of the muscle to reach the posterior compartment of the forearm (see Figs. 3.52 and 3.57 to 3.59). When the nerve emerges from the supinator muscle in the posterior compartment, it is commonly referred to as the **posterior interosseous nerve**. The nerve descends in the interval between the superficial and deep groups of muscles and eventually reaches the posterior surface of the wrist joint.

BRANCHES

- **Muscular branches** supply the extensor carpi radialis brevis, supinator, extensor digitorum, extensor digiti minimi, extensor carpi ulnaris, abductor pollicis longus, extensor pollicis brevis, extensor pollicis longus, and extensor indicis muscles.
- **Articular branches** supply the wrist and carpal joints.

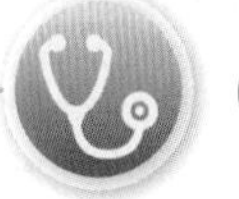

Clinical Notes

Tendon Reflexes and Segmental Innervation of Muscles

Skeletal muscles receive a segmental innervation. Most muscles are innervated by several spinal nerves and therefore by several segments of the spinal cord. A clinician should know the segmental innervation of the following muscles because it is possible to test them by eliciting simple muscle reflexes in the patient:

Biceps brachii tendon reflex: C5 and C6 (flexion of the elbow joint by tapping the biceps tendon)

Triceps tendon reflex: C6 to C8 (extension of the elbow joint by tapping the triceps tendon)

Brachioradialis tendon reflex: C5 to C7 (supination of the radioulnar joints by tapping the insertion of the brachioradialis tendon)

Brachial Plexus Injuries

The roots, trunks, and divisions of the brachial plexus reside in the lower part of the posterior triangle of the neck, whereas the cords and most of the branches of the plexus lie in the axilla. Complete lesions involving all the roots of the plexus are rare. Incomplete injuries are common and are usually caused by traction or pressure; stab wounds can divide individual nerves.

Upper Lesions of Brachial Plexus (Erb–Duchenne Palsy)

Upper lesions of the brachial plexus are injuries resulting from excessive displacement of the head to the opposite side and depression of the shoulder on the same side. This causes excessive traction or even tearing of the C5 and C6 roots of the plexus. It may occur in infants during a difficult delivery or in adults after a blow to or fall on the shoulder. The suprascapular nerve, nerve to the subclavius, and musculocutaneous and axillary nerves all possess nerve fibers derived from the C5 and C6 roots and are therefore functionless. The following muscles are consequently paralyzed: supraspinatus (abductor of the shoulder) and infraspinatus (lateral rotator of the shoulder) because of the suprascapular nerve; subclavius (depresses the clavicle) because of its nerve; coracobrachialis (flexes the shoulder), biceps brachii (supinator of the forearm, flexor of the elbow, weak flexor of the shoulder), and greater part of the brachialis (flexor of the elbow) because of the musculocutaneous nerve; and deltoid (abductor of the shoulder) and teres minor (lateral rotator of the shoulder) because of the axillary nerve. As a result, the limb characteristically hangs limply by the side, medially rotated by the unopposed sternocostal part of the pectoralis major; adducted because of loss of the supraspinatus and deltoid; the forearm is pronated because of loss of the action of the biceps (Fig. 3.83). The position of the upper limb in this condition has been likened to that of a porter or waiter hinting for a tip and so is often referred to as **"waiter's tip posture"** (Fig. 3.84). In addition, sensation is lost over the lower half of the deltoid and down the lateral side of the forearm.

Lower Lesions of Brachial Plexus (Klumpke Palsy)

Lower lesions of the brachial plexus are usually traction injuries caused by excessive abduction of the arm, as occurs in the case of a person falling from a height clutching at an object to save themself. The T1 anterior ramus is usually torn. The nerve fibers from this segment run in the ulnar and median nerves to supply all the small muscles of the hand. The hand has a clawed appearance caused by hyperextension of the metacarpophalangeal joints and flexion of the interphalangeal joints. The extensor digitorum is unopposed by the lumbricals and interossei and extends the metacarpophalangeal joints; the flexor digitorum superficialis and profundus are unopposed by the

(continued)

lumbricals and interossei and flex the middle and terminal phalanges, respectively. In addition, loss of sensation occurs along the medial side of the arm. If the C8 anterior ramus is also damaged, the extent of anesthesia is greater and involves the medial side of the forearm, hand, and medial two fingers.

Lower lesions of the brachial plexus can also be produced by the presence of a cervical rib or malignant metastases from the lungs in the lower deep cervical lymph nodes.

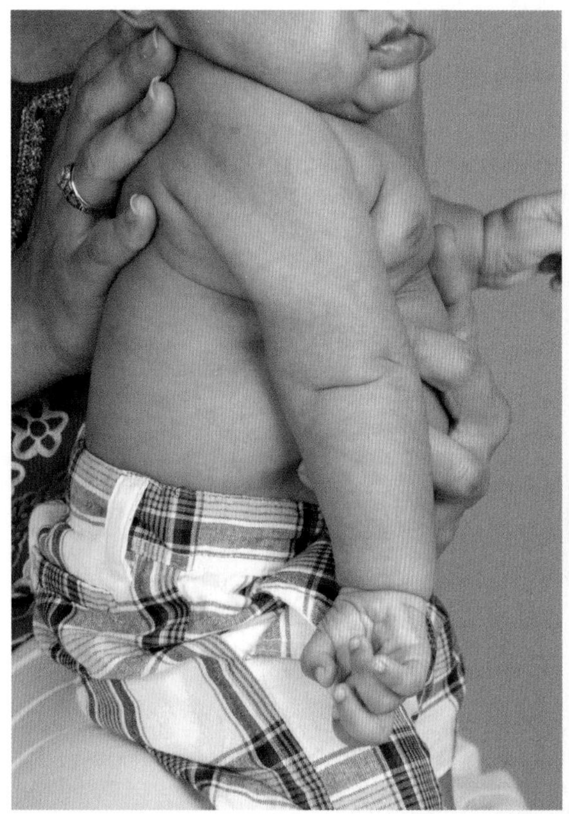

Figure 3.83 A 5-month-old male with right C5/C6 brachial plexus palsy. Note the typical "waiter's tip posture" of shoulder adduction and medial rotation, elbow extension, and forearm pronation.

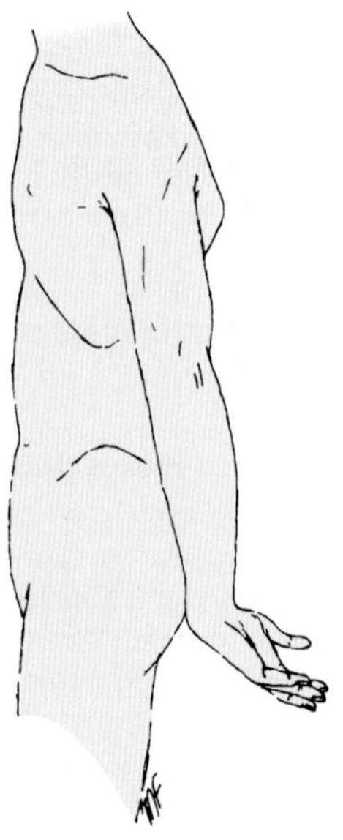

Figure 3.84 Adult with Erb–Duchenne palsy (waiter's tip posture).

Long Thoracic Nerve Injury

Certain neurologic conditions, blows to or pressure on the posterior triangle of the neck, or trauma to the upper lateral chest wall (eg, during the surgical procedure of radical mastectomy) may injure the long thoracic nerve, which arises from the anterior rami of C5 to C7 and supplies the serratus anterior muscle. Paralysis of the serratus anterior results in the inability to rotate the scapula during abduction of the arm above a right angle. Therefore, the patient has trouble raising their arm above their head. The vertebral border and inferior angle of the scapula are no longer kept closely applied to the chest wall and protrude posteriorly in a condition known as "**winged scapula**" (Fig. 3.85).

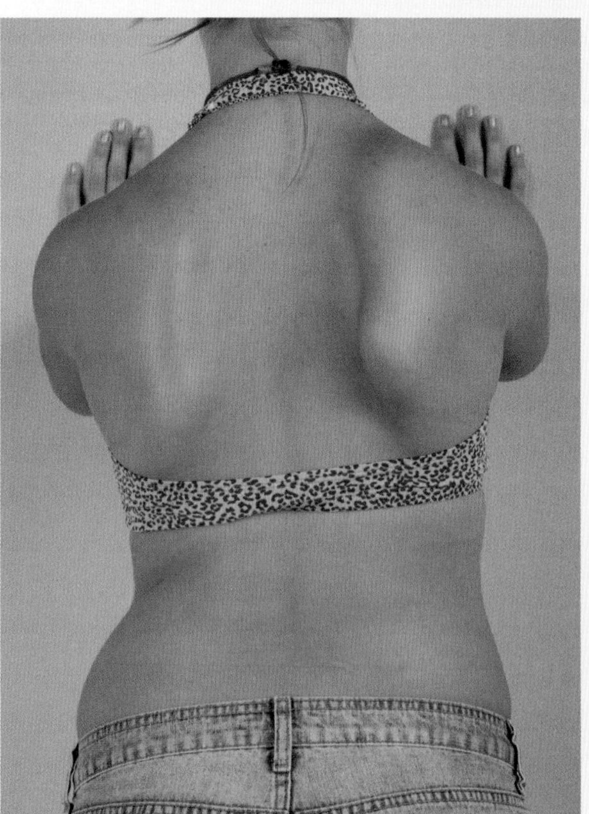

Figure 3.85 A 14-year-old female with neuralgic amyotrophy affecting the right long thoracic nerve. Note the right scapular winging exacerbated by pushing against the wall.

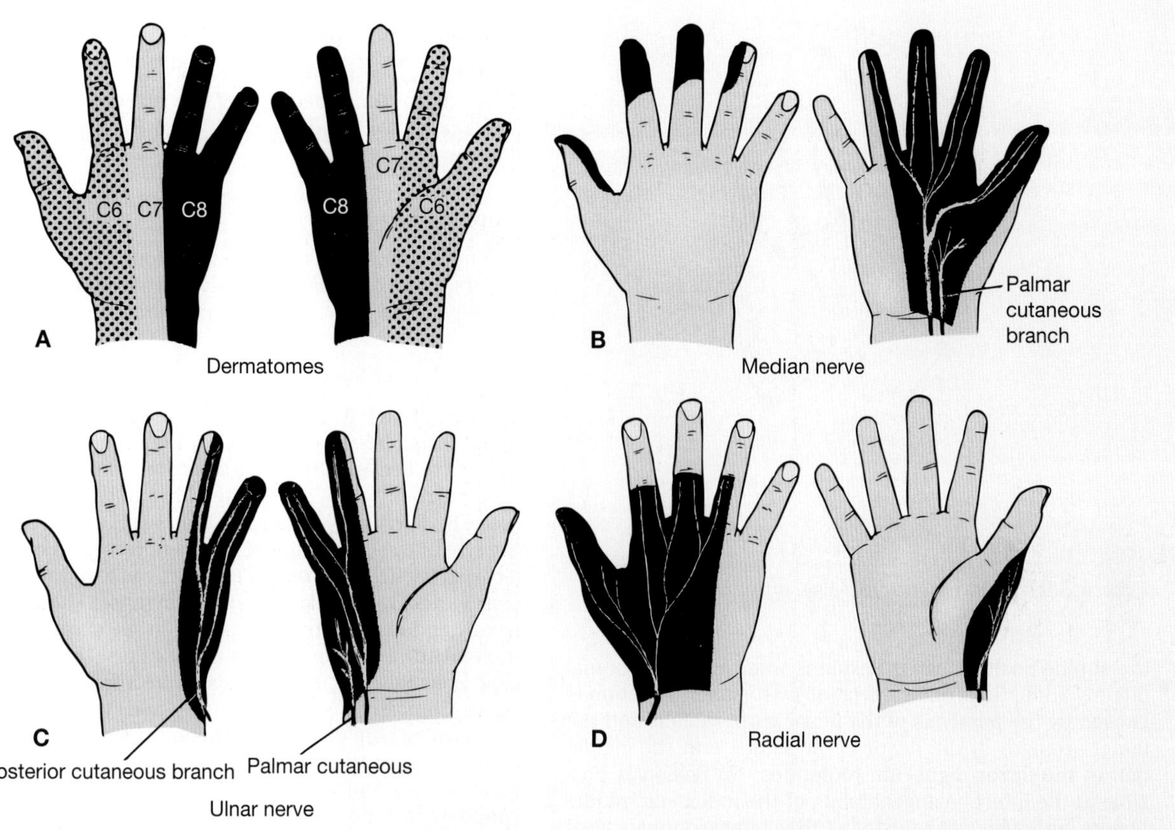

Figure 3.86 Sensory innervation of the skin of the volar (palmar) and dorsal aspects of the hand. **A.** The arrangement of the dermatomes. **B.** Cutaneous territory of the median nerve. **C.** Cutaneous territory of the ulnar nerve. **D.** Cutaneous territory of the radial nerve.

Musculocutaneous Nerve

The musculocutaneous nerve (see Fig. 3.78A) is rarely injured because of its protected position deep to the biceps brachii muscle (see Fig. 3.48). If it is injured high up in the arm, the biceps and coracobrachialis are paralyzed, and the brachialis muscle is greatly weakened (the latter muscle is also supplied partly by the radial nerve). The remainder of the brachialis muscle and the flexors of the forearm then produce flexion of the forearm at the elbow joint. When the forearm is in the prone position, the extensor carpi radialis longus and the brachioradialis muscles assist in flexion of the forearm. There is also sensory loss along the lateral side of the forearm because the musculocutaneous nerve continues as the lateral cutaneous nerve of the forearm (see Fig. 3.82). Wounds or cuts of the forearm can sever the lateral cutaneous nerve of the forearm, resulting in sensory loss along the lateral side of the forearm but not the loss of the muscles in the anterior compartment.

Median Nerve

The median nerve does not give off cutaneous or motor branches in the axilla or in the arm (see Fig. 3.78B). It begins branching in the proximal third of the anterior forearm via unnamed branches and its anterior interosseous branch. It supplies all the muscles of the anterior compartment of the forearm except the flexor carpi ulnaris and the medial half of the flexor digitorum profundus, which are supplied by the ulnar nerve (see Figs. 3.78B and 3.79). In the distal third of the forearm, it gives rise to a palmar cutaneous branch, which crosses superficial to the flexor retinaculum and supplies the skin on the lateral half of the palm (Fig. 3.86B; see also Fig. 3.82). In the palm, the median nerve supplies the muscles of the thenar compartment and the first two lumbricals and gives sensory innervation to the skin of the palmar aspect of the lateral three and a half fingers, including the nail beds on the dorsum (see Figs. 3.78B and 3.86B).

Supracondylar fractures of the humerus occasionally cause injury to the median nerve in the elbow region. Damage here influences the entire functional territory of the nerve. However, penetrating wounds (eg, stab wounds or broken glass wounds) just proximal to the flexor retinaculum are more common causes of injury. Here, the nerve lies in the interval between the tendons of the flexor carpi radialis and flexor digitorum superficialis, overlapped by the palmaris longus. Lesions at the wrist affect only the distal territory of the nerve in the hand.

Median Nerve Lesion: Motor Effects

The pronator muscles of the forearm and the long flexor muscles of the wrist and fingers (except for the flexor carpi ulnaris and the medial half of the flexor digitorum profundus) are paralyzed. As a result, the forearm rests in

(continued)

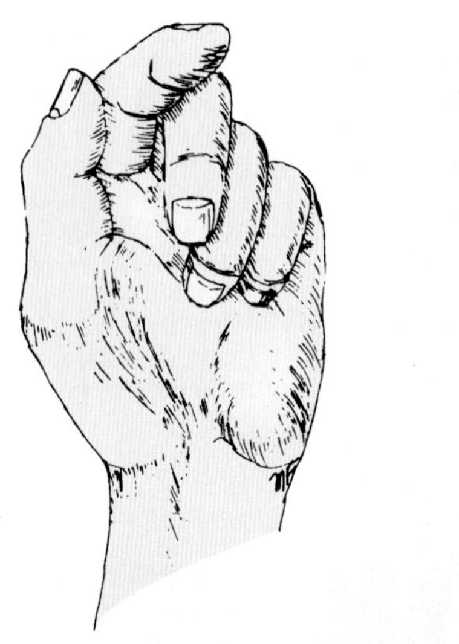

Figure 3.87 Median nerve palsy, anterior view.

the supine position; wrist flexion is weak and is accompanied by adduction (ulnar deviation). The ulnar deviation is caused by the paralysis of the flexor carpi radialis and the intact strength of the flexor carpi ulnaris and the medial half of the flexor digitorum profundus. No flexion is possible at the interphalangeal joints of the index and middle fingers, although weak flexion of the metacarpophalangeal joints of these fingers is attempted by the interossei. When the patient tries to make a fist, the index and, to a lesser extent, the middle fingers tend to remain straight, whereas the ring and little fingers flex (Fig. 3.87). However, the latter two fingers are weakened by the loss of the flexor digitorum superficialis.

The terminal phalanx of the thumb is extended because of paralysis of the flexor pollicis longus. The muscles of the thenar eminence are paralyzed and wasted so that the eminence is flattened. Opposition of the thumb is impossible. The thumb is laterally rotated and adducted. The first two lumbricals are paralyzed, which can be recognized clinically when the patient is asked to make a fist slowly, and the index and middle fingers tend to lag behind the ring and little fingers. Overall, the hand looks flattened and similar to that of a great ape, with the deformity most pronounced on the lateral (radial) aspect of the hand. Thus, the upper limb posture resulting from a median nerve lesion is often referred to as **"ape hand"** (see Fig. 3.87).

Median Nerve Lesion: Sensory Effects

Skin sensation is lost on the lateral half or less of the palm of the hand and the palmar aspect of the lateral three and a half fingers (see Fig. 3.86B). Sensory loss also occurs on the skin of the distal part of the dorsal surfaces of the lateral three and a half fingers. The area of total anesthesia is considerably less because of the overlap of adjacent nerves. Perhaps the most serious disability in median nerve injuries is the loss of the ability to oppose the thumb to the other fingers combined with the loss of sensation over the lateral fingers. In this situation, the delicate pincer-like action of the hand is no longer possible.

Vasomotor Changes

The skin areas involved in sensory loss are warmer and drier than normal because of the arteriolar dilation and absence of sweating resulting from loss of sympathetic control.

Trophic Changes

In longstanding cases, changes are found in the hand and fingers. The skin is dry and scaly, the nails crack easily, and atrophy of the pulp of the fingers is present.

Carpal Tunnel Syndrome

The carpal tunnel, formed by the concave anterior surface of the carpal bones and closed by the flexor retinaculum, is tightly packed with the long flexor tendons of the fingers, their surrounding synovial sheaths, and the median nerve (see Fig. 3.60). Any condition that significantly decreases the size of the carpal tunnel and compresses its contents is a carpal tunnel syndrome. The exact cause of the compression varies, but thickening of the synovial sheaths of the flexor tendons or arthritic changes in the carpal bones are thought to be responsible in many cases. One major possible consequence is compression necrosis of the median nerve. Clinically, the nerve compression syndrome consists of a burning pain or "pins and needles" sensation along the distribution of the median nerve to the lateral three and a half fingers and weakness of the thenar muscles. As you would expect, no paresthesia occurs over the thenar eminence because the palmar cutaneous branch of the median nerve, which passes superficial to the flexor retinaculum, supplies this area of skin. Decompressing the tunnel by making a longitudinal incision through the flexor retinaculum dramatically relieves the condition.

Ulnar Nerve

The ulnar nerve does not give off cutaneous or motor branches in the axilla or in the arm (see Fig. 3.79). It provides motor branches to the flexor carpi ulnaris and the medial half of the flexor digitorum profundus as it enters the forearm from behind the medial epicondyle. Next, it gives off its palmar and posterior cutaneous branches in the distal third of the forearm. The palmar cutaneous branch supplies the skin over the hypothenar eminence; the posterior cutaneous branch supplies the skin over the medial third of the dorsum of the hand and the medial one and a half fingers (see Fig. 3.86C). Not uncommonly, the posterior cutaneous branch supplies two and a half instead of one and a half fingers. It does not supply the skin over the distal part of the dorsum of these fingers.

Having entered the palm by passing superficial to the flexor retinaculum, the **superficial branch of the ulnar nerve** supplies the skin of the palmar surface of the medial one and a half fingers, including their nail beds. It also supplies the palmaris brevis muscle. The **deep branch of the ulnar nerve** supplies all the small muscles of the hand except the muscles of the thenar compartment and the first two lumbricals, which are supplied by the median nerve.

The ulnar nerve is most injured at the elbow, where it lies behind the medial epicondyle, and at the wrist, where it lies with the ulnar artery superficial to the flexor retinaculum. The injuries at the elbow are usually associated with fractures of the medial epicondyle. The superficial position of the nerve at the wrist makes it vulnerable to damage from cuts and stab wounds. Trauma at the elbow can affect the entire functional territory of the nerve, whereas injury at the wrist affects only the distal territory of the nerve in the hand.

Ulnar Nerve Lesion: Motor Effects

The flexor carpi ulnaris and the medial half of the flexor digitorum profundus muscles are paralyzed. The paralysis of the flexor carpi ulnaris can be observed by asking the patient to make a tightly clenched fist. Normally, the synergistic action of the flexor carpi ulnaris tendon can be observed as it passes to the pisiform bone; the tightening of the tendon is absent if the muscle is paralyzed. The profundus tendons to the ring and little fingers are functionless, and the terminal phalanges of these fingers are therefore not capable of being markedly flexed. Flexion of the wrist joint results in abduction, owing to paralysis of the flexor carpi ulnaris. The medial border of the front of the forearm shows flattening owing to the wasting of the underlying ulnaris and profundus muscles.

The small muscles of the hand are paralyzed, except the muscles of the thenar compartment and the first two lumbricals. The patient is unable to adduct and abduct their fingers and consequently is unable to grip a piece of paper placed between the fingers. Remember that the extensor digitorum can abduct the fingers to a small extent but only when the metacarpophalangeal joints are hyperextended.

Adducting the thumb is impossible because the adductor pollicis muscle is paralyzed. If the patient is asked to grip a piece of paper between the thumb and the index finger, they do so by strongly contracting the flexor pollicis longus and flexing the terminal phalanx (**Froment's sign**).

The metacarpophalangeal joints become hyperextended because of the paralysis of the lumbrical and interosseous muscles, which normally flex these joints. The hyperextension of the metacarpophalangeal joints is most prominent in the fourth and fifth fingers because the first and second lumbricals are not paralyzed (they are supplied by the median nerve). The interphalangeal joints are flexed, owing again to the paralysis of the lumbrical and interosseous muscles, which normally extend these joints through the extensor expansion. The flexion deformity at the interphalangeal joints of the fourth and fifth fingers is obvious because the first and second lumbrical muscles of the index and middle fingers are not paralyzed.

In longstanding cases, the hand assumes a characteristic claw-like deformity, with the clawing most pronounced on the medial (ulnar) aspect of the hand (Fig. 3.88). This appearance is often referred to as "**claw hand**" (**main en griffe**; **papal hand**). The claw hand is much more obvious in wrist lesions because the flexor digitorum profundus muscle is not paralyzed, and marked flexion of the terminal phalanges occurs. Wasting of the paralyzed muscles results in flattening of the hypothenar eminence and loss of the convex curve to the medial border of the hand. The dorsum of the hand shows hollowing between the metacarpal bones caused by wasting of the dorsal interosseous muscles.

Ulnar Nerve Lesion: Sensory Effects

In injuries at the elbow, loss of skin sensation occurs over the anterior and posterior surfaces of the medial third of the hand and the medial one and a half fingers (see Fig. 3.86C). In injuries at the wrist, the main ulnar nerve and its palmar cutaneous branch are usually severed; the posterior cutaneous branch, which arises from the ulnar nerve trunk

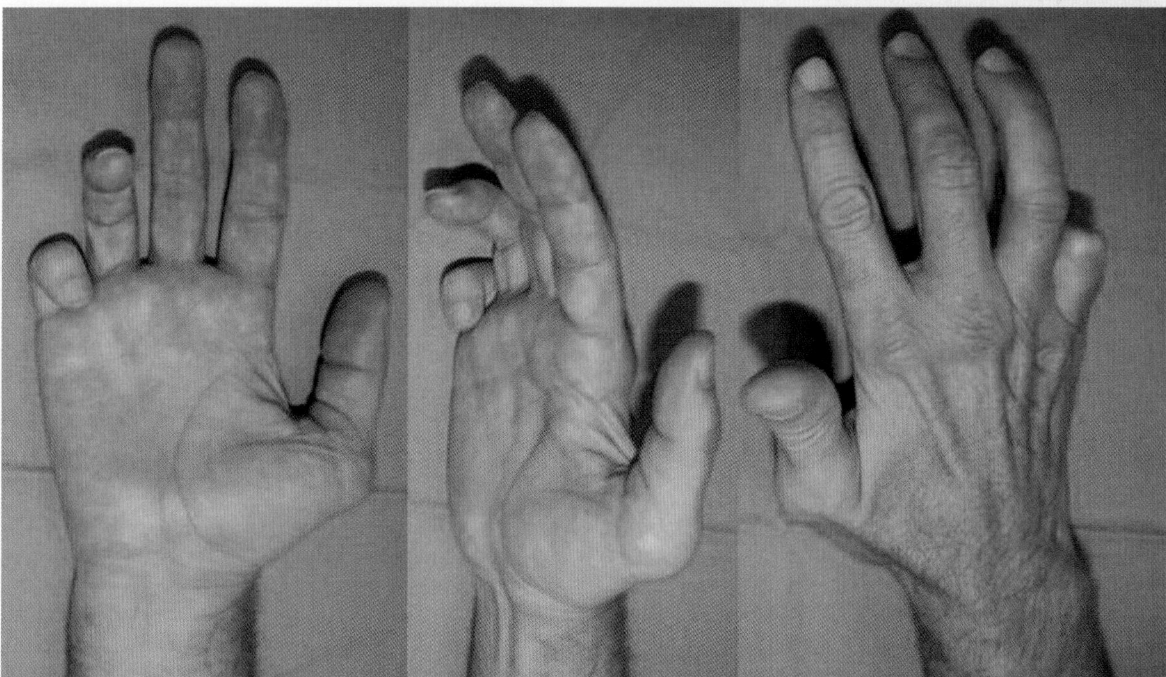

Figure 3.88 Ulnar nerve palsy (claw hand). Note the abnormal posture of the ring and little fingers, the flattening of the hypothenar eminence, and the atrophy over the web of the adductor pollicis.

(continued)

about 2.5 in. (6.25 cm) above the pisiform bone, is usually unaffected. The sensory loss will therefore be confined to the palmar surface of the medial third of the hand and the medial one and a half fingers and to the dorsal aspects of the middle and distal phalanges of the same fingers.

Unlike median nerve injuries, lesions of the ulnar nerve leave a relatively efficient hand. The sensation over the lateral part of the hand is intact, and the pincer-like action of the thumb and index finger is reasonably good, although there is some weakness owing to loss of the adductor pollicis.

Vasomotor Changes

The skin areas involved in sensory loss are warmer and drier than normal because of the arteriolar dilation and absence of sweating resulting from loss of sympathetic control.

Axillary Nerve

The axillary nerve can be injured in dislocations of the glenohumeral (shoulder) joint, by compression of the quadrangular space, or by the pressure of a badly adjusted crutch pressing upward into the armpit. As the nerve passes deeply from the axilla through the quadrangular space, it is particularly vulnerable to trauma from downward displacement of the humeral head in shoulder dislocations or fractures of the surgical neck of the humerus. The deltoid and teres minor muscles are paralyzed as a result (see Fig. 3.80). The paralyzed deltoid wastes rapidly, and the underlying greater tuberosity can be readily palpated. Because the supraspinatus is the only other abductor of the shoulder, this movement is much impaired. Paralysis of the teres minor is not recognizable clinically. The cutaneous branches of the axillary nerve, including the upper lateral cutaneous nerve of the arm, are functionless; consequently, there is a loss of skin sensation over the lower half of the deltoid muscle (see Fig. 3.82).

Radial Nerve

The radial nerve characteristically gives off its branches some distance proximal to the part to be innervated (see Fig. 3.81).

It gives off three branches in the axilla: the posterior cutaneous nerve of the arm, which supplies the skin on the back of the arm down to the elbow; nerve to the long head of the triceps; and the nerve to the medial head of the triceps.

It gives off four branches in the radial groove of the humerus: the lower lateral cutaneous nerve of the arm, which supplies the lateral surface of the arm down to the elbow; posterior cutaneous nerve of the forearm, which supplies the skin down the middle of the back of the forearm as far as the wrist; nerve to the lateral head of the triceps; and the nerve to the medial head of the triceps and the anconeus.

It gives off three branches in the anterior compartment of the arm above the lateral epicondyle: the nerve to a small part of the brachialis, nerve to the brachioradialis, and the nerve to the extensor carpi radialis longus.

In the cubital fossa, it gives off the deep branch of the radial nerve and continues as the superficial radial nerve. The deep branch supplies the extensor carpi radialis brevis and the supinator in the cubital fossa and all the extensor muscles in the posterior compartment of the forearm. The superficial radial nerve is sensory and supplies the skin over the lateral part of the dorsum of the hand and the dorsal surface of the lateral three and a half fingers proximal to the nail beds (see Fig. 3.86D). The ulnar nerve supplies most of the rest of the dorsum of the hand and the dorsal surface of the medial one and a half fingers. The exact cutaneous areas innervated by the radial and ulnar nerves on the hand vary.

The radial nerve is commonly damaged in the axilla and in the radial groove.

Radial Nerve Lesion: Motor Effects

The radial nerve can be injured in the axilla, for example, by the pressure of the upper end of a badly fitting crutch pressing up into the armpit and compressing the nerve or by falling asleep with one arm over the back of a chair. It can also be badly damaged in the axilla by fractures and dislocations of the proximal end of the humerus. When the humerus is displaced downward in inferior dislocations of the glenohumeral joint, the radial nerve, which is wrapped around the back of the shaft of the humerus, is pulled downward, stretching the nerve excessively.

Recall that the radial nerve supplies all the muscles in the posterior compartments of the arm and forearm. The triceps, anconeus, and long extensors of the wrist are paralyzed. The patient is unable to extend their elbow joint, wrist joint, and fingers. **Wristdrop** (flexion of the wrist; Fig. 3.89) occurs because of the action of the unopposed flexor muscles of the wrist and the inability to hold the wrist in extension against gravity. Wristdrop is very disabling because the individual is unable to flex their fingers strongly for the purpose of firmly gripping an object with the wrist fully flexed. (Try it on yourself.) However, if the

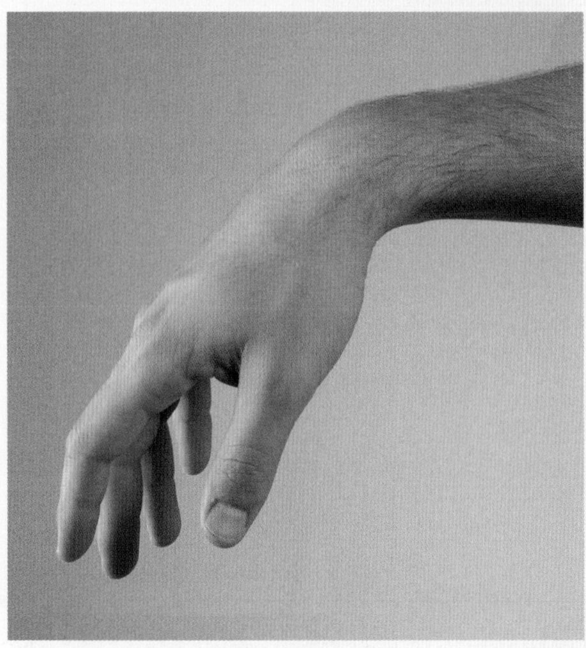

Figure 3.89 Wristdrop, lateral view.

wrist and proximal phalanges are passively extended by holding them in position with the opposite hand, the middle and distal phalanges of the fingers can be extended by the action of the lumbricals and interossei, which are inserted into the extensor expansions. The brachioradialis and supinator muscles are also paralyzed, but supination is still performed well by the biceps brachii.

The radial nerve can be injured in the radial groove of the humerus at the time of fracture of the shaft of the humerus or subsequently involved during the formation of the callus. The pressure of the back of the arm on the edge of the operating table in an unconscious patient has also been known to injure the nerve at this site. The prolonged application of a tourniquet to the arm in a person with a slender triceps muscle is often followed by temporary radial palsy. The injury to the radial nerve occurs most commonly in the distal part of the radial groove, beyond the origin of the nerves to the triceps and the anconeus and beyond the origin of the cutaneous nerves. In this case, the patient can extend the shoulder and elbow but is unable to extend the wrist and the fingers, and wristdrop occurs.

The deep branch of the radial nerve is the motor nerve to the extensor muscles in the posterior compartment of the forearm. It can be damaged in fractures of the proximal end of the radius or during dislocation of the radial head. The nerve supply to the supinator and the extensor carpi radialis longus will be undamaged, and because the latter muscle is powerful, it will keep the wrist joint extended, and wristdrop will not occur.

Radial Nerve Lesion: Sensory Effects

With an axillary lesion of the radial nerve, a small loss of skin sensation occurs down the posterior surface of the lower part of the arm and down a narrow strip on the back of the forearm. A variable area of sensory loss is present on the lateral part of the dorsum of the hand and on the dorsal surface of the roots of the lateral three and a half fingers (see Fig. 3.86D). The area of total anesthesia is relatively small because of the overlap of sensory innervation by adjacent nerves.

If the radial nerve is damaged in the radial groove, a variable small area of anesthesia occurs over the dorsal surface of the hand and the dorsal surface of the roots of the lateral three and a half fingers.

No cutaneous loss occurs following lesion of the deep branch of the radial nerve because this is a motor nerve. Division of the superficial radial nerve, which is sensory, as in a stab wound, results in a variable small area of anesthesia over the dorsum of the hand and the dorsal surface of the roots of the lateral three and a half fingers.

Trophic Changes

Trophic changes are slight.

VASCULATURE

Arteries

The **subclavian artery**, located in the root of the neck, continues as the **axillary artery**, which supplies the upper limb (Fig. 3.90).

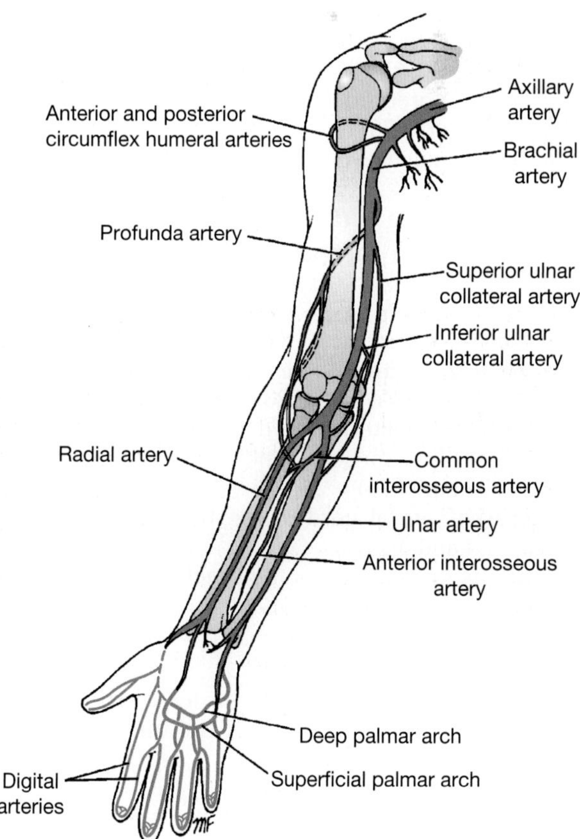

Figure 3.90 Main arteries of the upper limb.

Axillary Artery

The axillary artery (Fig. 3.91; see also Fig. 3.34) begins at the lateral border of rib 1 and ends at the lower border of the teres major muscle, where it continues as the **brachial artery** (see Fig. 3.91). Throughout its course, the artery is closely related to the cords of the brachial plexus and their branches and is enclosed with them in a connective tissue sheath called the **axillary sheath**. This sheath is continuous with the prevertebral fascia in the root of the neck. The pectoralis minor muscle crosses in front of the axillary artery and divides it into three parts (see Figs. 3.76 and 3.91).

First Part of the Axillary Artery

This extends from the lateral border of rib 1 to the upper border of the pectoralis minor (see Fig. 3.91).

RELATIONS

- **Anteriorly:** Pectoralis major and the skin; cephalic vein crosses the artery (see Fig. 3.32)
- **Posteriorly:** Long thoracic nerve (nerve to the serratus anterior; see Fig. 3.34)

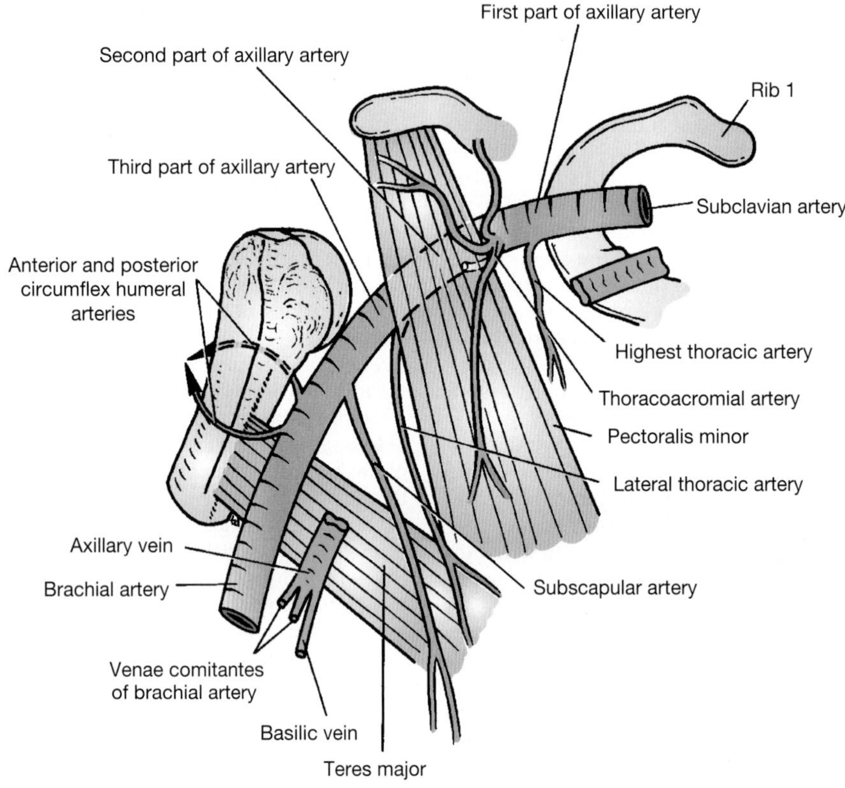

Figure 3.91 Parts of the axillary artery and its branches. Note the formation of the axillary vein at the lower border of the teres major muscle.

- **Laterally:** Three cords of the brachial plexus (see Figs. 3.34 and 3.76)
- **Medially:** Axillary vein (see Fig. 3.34)

Second Part of the Axillary Artery

This lies deep to the pectoralis minor muscle (see Fig. 3.91).

RELATIONS

- **Anteriorly:** Pectoralis minor, pectoralis major, and the skin (see Figs. 3.32, 3.33, 3.76, and 3.91)
- **Posteriorly:** Posterior cord of the brachial plexus, subscapularis muscle, and shoulder joint (see Figs. 3.34 and 3.76)
- **Laterally:** Lateral cord of the brachial plexus (see Figs. 3.34 and 3.76)
- **Medially:** Medial cord of the brachial plexus and the axillary vein (see Figs. 3.34 and 3.76)

Third Part of the Axillary Artery

This extends from the lower border of the pectoralis minor to the lower border of the teres major (see Fig. 3.91).

RELATIONS

- **Anteriorly:** Pectoralis major for a short distance; more distally, the medial root of the median nerve crosses the artery (see Figs. 3.33 and 3.76)
- **Posteriorly:** Subscapularis, latissimus dorsi, and teres major; axillary and radial nerves also lie behind the artery (see Figs. 3.34 and 3.46)
- **Laterally:** Coracobrachialis, biceps, and humerus; lateral root of the median nerve and the musculocutaneous nerve also lie on the lateral side (see Figs. 3.33, 3.34 and 3.76)
- **Medially:** Ulnar nerve, axillary vein, and medial cutaneous nerve of the arm (see Figs. 3.33 and 3.76)

Axillary Artery Branches

Typically, the axillary artery has six branches (see Fig. 3.91). Conveniently for memory, one branch comes from the first part of the artery, two branches from the second part, and three branches from the third part. However, the branching pattern varies extensively, and it is important to recognize the target territories of the branches to verify the identities of the branches.

BRANCH FROM THE FIRST PART

- The **highest thoracic artery** is small and extremely variable. It runs along the upper border of the pectoralis minor to reach the area of ribs 1 and 2.

BRANCHES FROM THE SECOND PART

- The **thoracoacromial artery** is a short trunk that immediately divides into four terminal branches that supply the pectoral muscles and the acromioclavicular region.

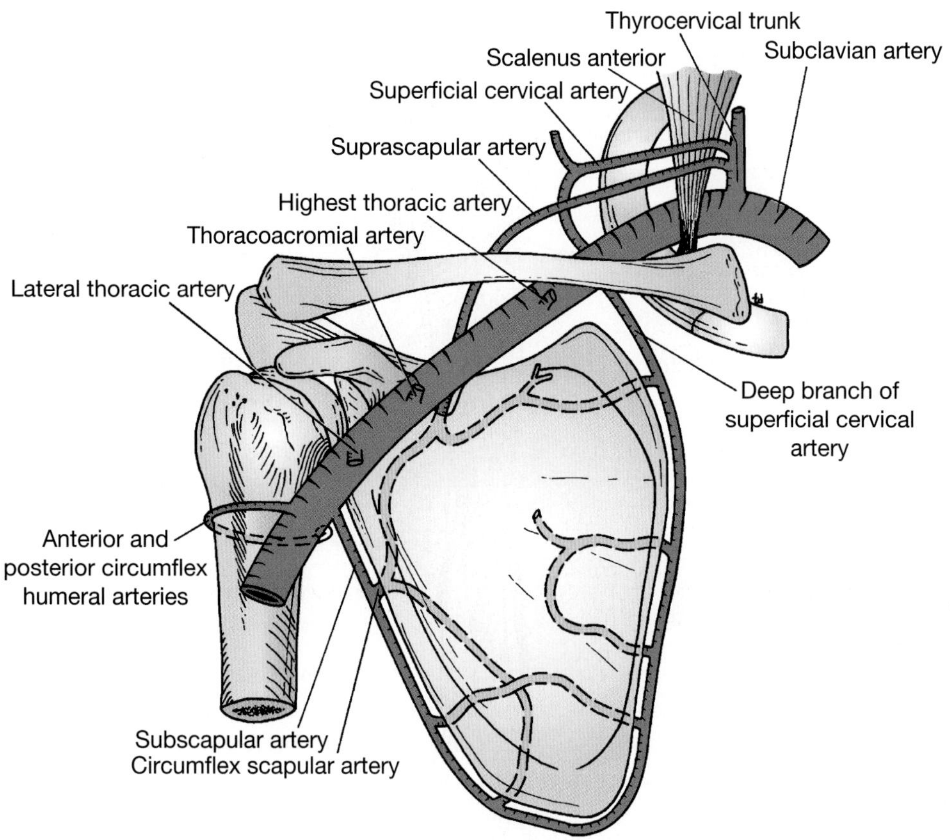

Figure 3.92 Arteries that take part in anastomosis around the shoulder joint.

- The **lateral thoracic artery** runs along the lower (lateral) border of the pectoralis minor along the lateral chest wall.

BRANCHES FROM THE THIRD PART

- The **subscapular artery** is a large vessel that descends along the lower (axillary) border of the scapula. It divides into the circumflex scapular and thoracodorsal arteries. The **circumflex scapular artery** curls around the axillary border of the scapula to reach the infraspinous fossa (Fig. 3.92; see also Fig. 3.41). The **thoracodorsal artery** descends along the latissimus dorsi muscle to reach the lateral thoracic wall.
- The **anterior and posterior circumflex humeral arteries** wind around the front and the back of the surgical neck of the humerus, respectively, and form an anastomosing circle. The posterior artery is the larger of the two and passes through the quadrangular space with the axillary nerve to reach the scapular region (see Fig. 3.41).

Arterial Anastomosis around the Shoulder Joint

The extreme mobility of the shoulder joint may result in kinking of the axillary artery and temporary occlusion of its lumen. To compensate, an important arterial anastomosis exists between certain branches of the subclavian artery and the axillary artery, thus ensuring that an adequate blood flow supplies the upper limb irrespective of the position of the arm (see Fig. 3.92).

Branches from the Subclavian Artery

- The **suprascapular artery** is distributed to the supraspinous and infraspinous fossae of the scapula.
- The **superficial cervical artery** gives off a deep branch that runs down the medial border of the scapula.

Branches from the Axillary Artery

- The **subscapular artery** and its **circumflex scapular branch** supply the subscapular and infraspinous fossae of the scapula, respectively.
- **Anterior circumflex humeral artery**.
- **Posterior circumflex humeral artery**.

Brachial Artery

The brachial artery (Fig. 3.93; see also Figs. 3.48, 3.52, and 3.90) begins at the lower border of the teres major muscle as a continuation of the axillary artery. It travels through the anterior compartment of the arm. However, its branches supply both the anterior and posterior compartments of the arm, and thus, the brachial artery supplies the entire arm. It terminates opposite the neck of the radius by dividing into the radial and ulnar arteries.

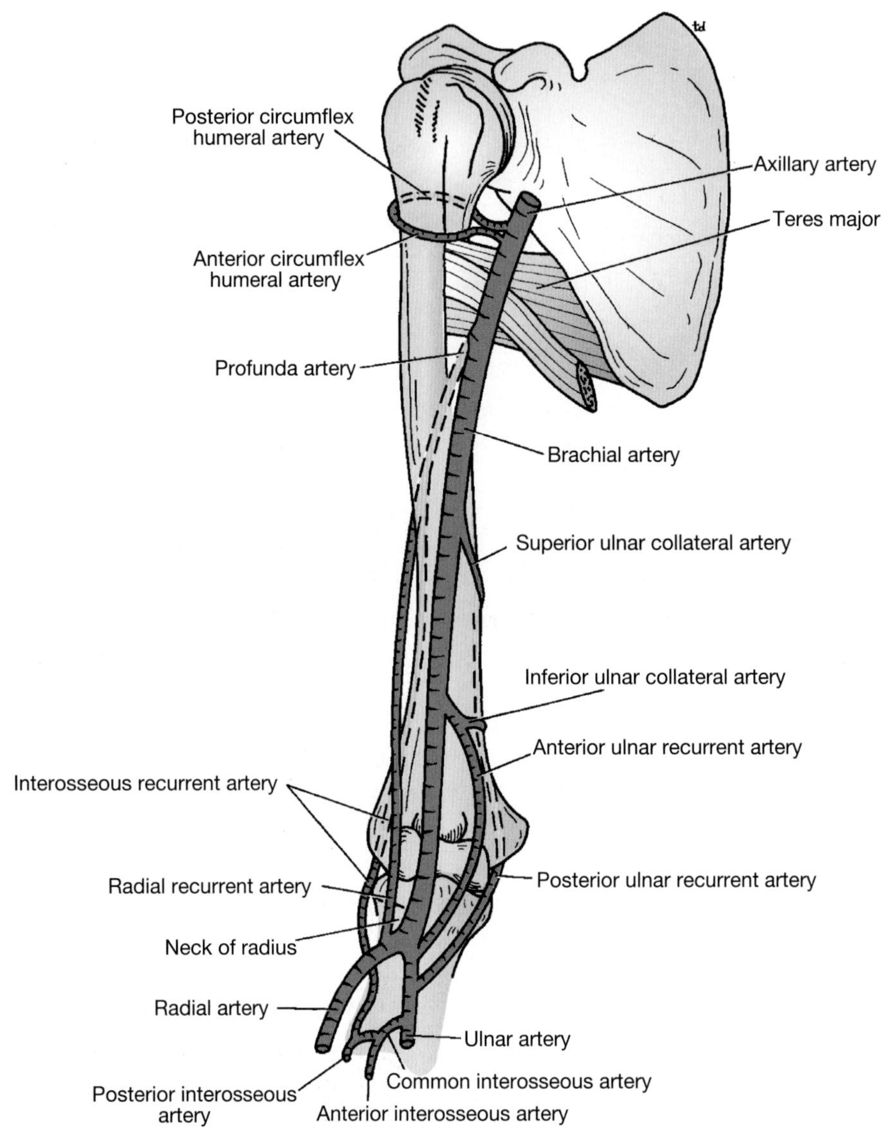

Figure 3.93 Main arteries of the upper arm. Note the arterial anastomosis around the elbow joint.

Relations

Refer to Figure 3.48.

- **Anteriorly:** The vessel is superficial and is overlapped from the lateral side by the coracobrachialis and biceps muscles. The medial cutaneous nerve of the forearm lies in front of the upper part, the median nerve crosses its middle part, and the bicipital aponeurosis crosses its lower part.
- **Posteriorly:** The artery lies on the triceps, coracobrachialis insertion, and brachialis.
- **Medially:** In the upper part of the arm, the ulnar nerve and the basilic vein lie medial to the artery. In the lower part of the arm, the median nerve lies on its medial side.
- **Laterally:** More proximally, the median nerve and the coracobrachialis and biceps muscles. More distally, the tendon of the biceps lies lateral to the artery.

BRANCHES

- **Muscular branches** to the anterior compartment of the arm.
- **Nutrient artery** to the humerus.
- The **profunda brachii (deep brachial) artery** arises near the origin of the brachial artery, accompanies the radial nerve through the radial (spiral) groove of the humerus, and supplies the triceps muscle. It anastomoses with the **radial recurrent artery** (branch of the radial artery) to form part of the collateral circulation around the elbow joint (see Fig. 3.93).
- The **superior ulnar collateral artery** arises near the middle of the arm and follows the ulnar nerve posterior to the medial epicondyle (see Fig. 3.93). It anastomoses with the **posterior ulnar recurrent artery** (branch of the ulnar artery) to form part of the collateral circulation around the elbow joint (see Figs. 3.57 and 3.93).

- The **inferior ulnar collateral artery** arises near the termination of the brachial artery and passes anterior to the medial epicondyle. It anastomoses with the **anterior ulnar recurrent artery** (branch of the ulnar artery) to form part of the collateral circulation around the elbow joint (see Figs. 3.57 and 3.93).

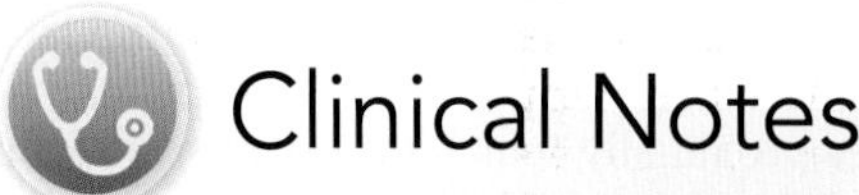

Clinical Notes

Arterial Anastomosis and Axillary Artery Ligation

The existence of the anastomosis around the shoulder joint is vital to preserving the upper limb should it be necessary to ligate the axillary artery. Notice that it is critical to ligate the axillary artery proximal to the subscapular artery to maintain adequate collateral flow to the upper limb (see Fig. 3.92).

Ulnar Artery

The ulnar artery is the larger of the two terminal branches of the brachial artery (see Figs. 3.52 and 3.90). It begins in the cubital fossa at the level of the neck of the radius (see Fig. 3.52). It descends through the medial (ulnar) aspect of the anterior compartment of the forearm (see Fig. 3.57) and enters the palm superficial to the flexor retinaculum in company with the ulnar nerve (see Figs. 3.60 to 3.62). It ends by forming the superficial palmar arch, often anastomosing with the superficial palmar branch of the radial artery (see Figs. 3.62 and 3.65).

Ulnar Artery in the Forearm

In the proximal forearm, the ulnar artery lies deep to most of the flexor muscles (see Fig. 3.57). More distally, it becomes superficial and lies between the tendons of the flexor carpi ulnaris and the tendons of the flexor digitorum superficialis (see Fig. 3.56). As the artery crosses over the flexor retinaculum, it lies just lateral to the pisiform bone and is covered only by skin and fascia, making this a good site for taking the ulnar pulse.

FOREARM BRANCHES

- **Muscular branches** to neighboring muscles.
- **Anterior and posterior ulnar recurrent branches** that take part in the arterial anastomoses around the elbow joint. (See the above descriptions of the ulnar collateral arteries; Figs. 3.57 and 3.93.)
- Branches that take part in the arterial **anastomosis around the wrist joint**.
- The **common interosseous artery** arises from the upper part of the ulnar artery and, after a brief course, divides into the **anterior and posterior interosseous arteries** (see Figs. 3.57 and 3.90). The interosseous arteries pass distally on the anterior and posterior surfaces of the interosseous membrane, respectively. They provide **nutrient arteries to the radius and ulna**, supply adjacent muscles in the anterior and posterior compartments, and end by taking part in the anastomosis around the wrist joint.

Ulnar Artery in the Hand

The ulnar artery enters the hand superficial to the flexor retinaculum on the lateral side of the ulnar nerve and the pisiform bone (see Figs. 3.62 and 3.65). The artery gives off a **deep palmar branch** and then continues into the palm as the **superficial palmar arch**. On entering the palm, the superficial palmar arch curves laterally deep to the palmar aponeurosis and superficial to the long flexor tendons. The arch is completed on the lateral side by anastomosing with the **superficial palmar branch of the radial artery**. The curve of the arch lies across the palm, level with the distal border of the fully extended thumb.

The superficial arch gives rise to three **common palmar digital arteries** (see Figs. 3.62 and 3.65). Each common artery divides into two **proper palmar digital arteries** that supply adjacent sides of two digits.

The **deep palmar branch** of the ulnar artery arises superficial to the flexor retinaculum, passes deep between the abductor digiti minimi and the flexor digiti minimi, and joins the radial artery to complete the deep palmar arch (see Figs. 3.65, 3.68, and 3.69).

Radial Artery

The radial artery is the smaller of the two terminal branches of the brachial artery (see Figs. 3.52 and 3.90). It begins in the cubital fossa at the level of the neck of the radius (see Fig. 3.52) and descends through the lateral (radial) aspect of the anterior compartment of the forearm (see Figs. 3.55 and 3.56). It ends by forming the deep palmar arch in the hand, often anastomosing with the deep palmar branch of the ulnar artery (see Figs. 3.68 and 3.69).

Radial Artery in the Forearm

In the proximal forearm, the radial artery lies deep to the brachioradialis muscle (see Fig. 3.55). In the middle third of its course, it runs medial to the superficial branch of the radial nerve. In the distal forearm, the radial artery lies on the anterior surface of the radius, between the tendons of the brachioradialis and flexor carpi radialis muscles and is covered only by skin and fascia (see Figs. 3.55 and 3.62). This is the ideal site for taking the radial pulse.

FOREARM BRANCHES

- **Muscular branches** to neighboring muscles.
- The **radial recurrent artery** takes part in the arterial anastomosis around the elbow joint. (See the above description of the profunda brachii artery; Figs. 3.56 and 3.93.)
- The **superficial palmar branch** arises just proximal to the wrist (see Fig. 3.65), enters the palm of the hand, and joins the ulnar artery to complete the superficial palmar arch.

Radial Artery in the Hand

The radial artery leaves the forearm by winding around the lateral aspect of the wrist to reach the posterolateral surface of the hand (see Figs. 3.56 and 3.59). The artery enters the floor of the anatomic snuffbox, lying on the lateral ligament of the wrist joint and passing deep to the tendons of the abductor pollicis longus and extensor pollicis brevis muscles (see Fig. 3.59). The vessel continues under the tendon of the extensor pollicis longus to reach the interval between the two heads of the first dorsal interosseous muscle. Here, the artery dives between the muscle heads to enter the deep aspect of the palm of the hand (see Figs. 3.59 and 3.69).

On entering the palm, the radial artery curves medially between the oblique and transverse heads of the adductor pollicis and continues as the **deep palmar arch** (see Figs. 3.68 and 3.69). The deep palmar arch curves medially deep to the long flexor tendons and superficial to the metacarpal bones and the interosseous muscles. The arch is completed on the medial side by the deep palmar branch of the ulnar artery. The curve of the arch lies at a level with the proximal border of the extended thumb.

Immediately on entering the palm, the radial artery gives off the arteria radialis indicis, which supplies the lateral side of the index finger, and the arteria princeps pollicis, which divides into two and supplies the lateral and medial sides of the thumb. The deep palmar arch sends branches proximally, which take part in anastomoses around the wrist joint, and distally, to join the digital branches of the superficial palmar arch.

Before it dives to form the deep palmar arch, the radial artery gives rise to the **dorsal carpal arch** on the dorsum of the hand. Branches of the dorsal carpal arch take part in anastomoses around the wrist joint and supply the digits (see Fig. 3.59).

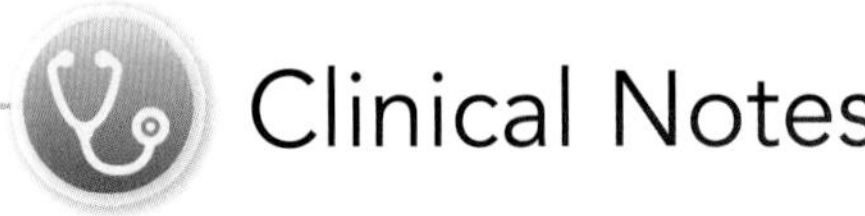

Arterial Injury

The arteries of the upper limb can be damaged by penetrating wounds or may require ligation in amputation operations. Because of the existence of an adequate collateral circulation around the shoulder, elbow, and wrist joints, ligation of the main arteries of the upper limb is not followed by tissue necrosis or gangrene, provided that the arteries forming the collateral circulation are not diseased, and the patient's general circulation is satisfactory. Nevertheless, days or weeks may be required for the collateral vessels to open sufficiently to provide the distal part of the limb with the same volume of blood as previously supplied by the main artery.

Arterial Palpation and Compression

A clinician must know where the arteries of the upper limb can be palpated or compressed in an emergency. The subclavian artery, as it crosses rib 1 to become the axillary artery, can be palpated in the root of the posterior triangle of the neck (see Fig. 3.92). The artery can be compressed here against rib 1 to stop a catastrophic hemorrhage. The third part of the axillary artery can be felt in the axilla as it lies in front of the teres major muscle (see Figs. 3.33 and 3.91). The brachial artery can be palpated in the arm as it lies on the brachialis and is overlapped from the lateral side by the biceps brachii (see Fig. 3.48).

The radial artery lies superficially in front of the distal end of the radius, between the tendons of the brachioradialis and flexor carpi radialis (see Fig. 3.55). This is where the clinician takes the radial pulse. If the pulse cannot be felt, try finding the radial artery on the other wrist. Occasionally, a congenitally abnormal radial artery can be difficult to feel. The radial artery can be less easily felt as it crosses the anatomic snuffbox (see Fig. 3.105).

The ulnar artery can be palpated as it crosses superficial to the flexor retinaculum in company with the ulnar nerve. The artery lies lateral to the pisiform bone, separated from it by the ulnar nerve. The artery is commonly damaged here in laceration wounds in front of the wrist.

Allen's Test

The Allen's test is used to determine the patency of the ulnar and radial arteries. With the patient's hands resting in their lap, compress the radial arteries against the anterior surface of each radius and ask the patient to tightly clench their fists, which closes off the superficial and deep palmar arterial arches. When the patient is asked to open their hands, the skin of the palms is at first white, and then normally the blood quickly flows into the arches through the ulnar arteries, causing the palms to promptly turn pink. This establishes that the ulnar arteries are patent. The patency of the radial arteries can be established by repeating the test but this time compressing the ulnar arteries where they lie lateral to the pisiform bones.

Arterial Innervation and Raynaud Disease

Sympathetic nerves innervate the arteries of the upper limb. The preganglionic fibers originate from cell bodies in the T2 to T8 segments of the spinal cord. They ascend in the sympathetic trunk and synapse in the middle cervical, inferior cervical, first thoracic, or stellate ganglia. The postganglionic fibers join the nerves that form the brachial plexus and are distributed to the arteries within the branches of the plexus. For example, the digital arteries of the fingers are supplied by postganglionic sympathetic fibers that run in the digital nerves. Vasospastic diseases involving digital arterioles, such as Raynaud disease, may require a cervicodorsal preganglionic sympathectomy to prevent necrosis of the fingers. The operation is followed by arterial vasodilation, with consequent increased blood flow to the upper limb.

Veins

The veins of the upper limb can be divided into two groups: **superficial and deep**. The deep veins comprise the **venae comitantes** and the **axillary vein**. The venae comitantes are usually paired and accompany the large and medium-sized arteries (see Chapter 1: Introduction).

Superficial Veins

The superficial veins of the upper limb lie in the superficial fascia (Fig. 3.94). The superficial venous network begins with the **dorsal venous arch** in the dorsum of the hand. This arch lies proximal to the metacarpophalangeal joints. The greater part of the blood from the whole hand drains into the arch, which receives digital veins and freely communicates with the deep veins of the palm through the interosseous spaces. The dorsal venous arch drains into the **cephalic** and **basilic veins** at its lateral and medial ends, respectively.

Cephalic Vein

The cephalic vein arises from the lateral side of the dorsal venous arch on the back of the hand and winds around the lateral border of the forearm. It then ascends into the cubital fossa and up the front of the arm in the superficial fascia on the lateral side of the biceps. It dives into the deltopectoral triangle, pierces the clavipectoral fascia, and terminates by draining into the axillary vein. As the cephalic vein passes up the upper limb, it receives a variable number of tributaries from the lateral and posterior surfaces of the limb (see Fig. 3.94A). The **median cubital vein**, a branch of the cephalic vein in the cubital fossa, runs upward and medially and joins the basilic vein. The median cubital vein is normally present, but the form in which it connects the cephalic and basilic veins varies (see Fig. 3.94B). In the cubital fossa, the median cubital vein crosses over the brachial artery and the median nerve, but it is separated from them by the bicipital aponeurosis.

Basilic Vein

The basilic vein arises from the medial side of the dorsal venous arch on the back of the hand and winds around the medial border of the forearm. It then ascends into the cubital fossa and up the front of the arm in the superficial fascia on the medial side of the biceps (see Fig. 3.94A). Halfway up the arm, it pierces the deep fascia and at the lower border of the teres major joins the venae comitantes of the brachial artery to form the axillary vein on the medial side of the biceps. In its course, the basilic vein receives the median cubital vein and a variable number of tributaries from the medial and posterior surfaces of the upper limb.

Axillary Vein

The axillary vein (see Fig. 3.32) is formed at the lower border of the teres major muscle by the union of the venae comitantes of the brachial artery and the basilic vein (see Fig. 3.91). It runs upward on the medial side of the axillary artery and ends at the lateral border of rib 1 by becoming the subclavian vein. The axillary vein receives tributaries that correspond to the branches of the axillary artery and the cephalic vein.

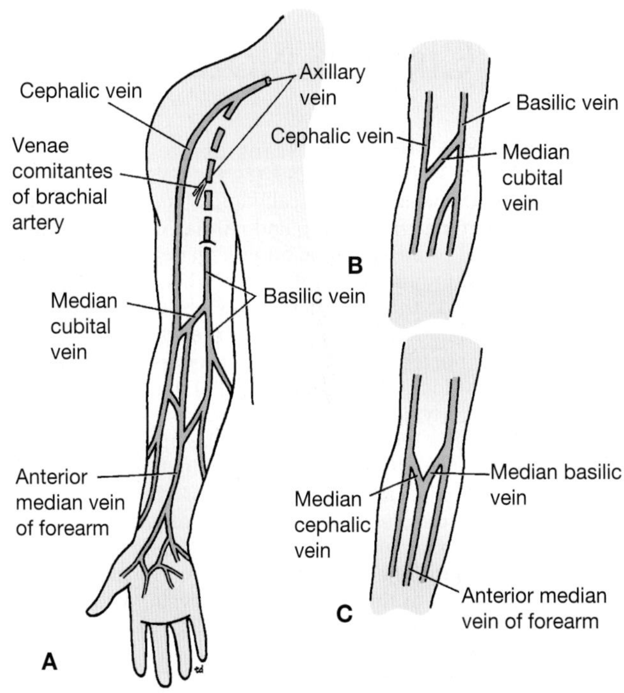

Figure 3.94 Superficial veins of the upper limb. **A.** Main venous channels. **B, C.** Common variations seen in the region of the elbow.

Nerve Supply of Veins

Like the arteries, the smooth muscle in the wall of the veins is innervated by sympathetic postganglionic nerve fibers that provide vasomotor tone. The origin of these fibers is like those of the arteries.

LYMPH

The lymph vessels in the upper limb ultimately drain into an extensive network of axillary lymph nodes.

Axillary Lymph Nodes

The axillary lymph nodes (20 to 30) collect lymph from a large territory. These nodes drain lymph vessels from the lateral quadrants of the breast, the superficial lymph vessels from the thoracoabdominal walls above the level of the umbilicus, the skin of the back above the level of the iliac crests, and the vessels from the upper limb. The lymph nodes are arranged in six groups (Fig. 3.95).

- **Anterior (pectoral) group:** Lying along the lower (lateral) border of the pectoralis minor, deep to the pectoralis major, these nodes receive lymph vessels from the lateral quadrants of the breast and superficial vessels from the anterolateral abdominal wall above the level of the umbilicus.

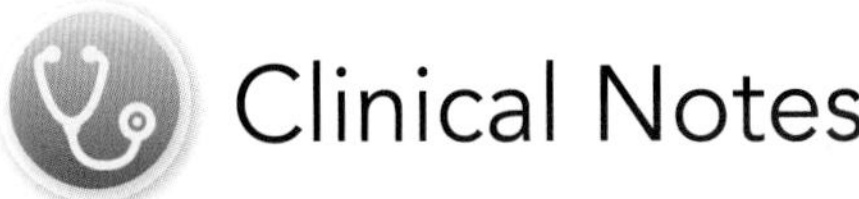

Clinical Notes

Venipuncture and Blood Transfusion

The superficial veins are clinically important and are used for venipuncture, transfusion, and cardiac catheterization. Every clinical professional, in an emergency, should know where to obtain blood from the arm. When a patient is in a state of shock, the superficial veins are not always visible. The cephalic vein usually lies in the superficial fascia, immediately posterior to the styloid process of the radius. In the cubital fossa, the median cubital vein is separated from the underlying brachial artery by the bicipital aponeurosis. This is important because the aponeurosis protects the artery from the mistaken introduction of irritating drugs that should have been injected into the vein. In the deltopectoral triangle, the cephalic vein frequently communicates with the external jugular vein by a small vein that crosses in front of the clavicle. Fracture of the clavicle can result in rupture of this communicating vein, with the formation of a large hematoma.

Intravenous Transfusion and Hypovolemic Shock

In extreme hypovolemic shock, excessive venous tone may inhibit venous blood flow and thus delay the introduction of intravenous blood into the vascular system.

Anatomy of Basilic and Cephalic Vein Catheterization

The median cubital or basilic veins are the veins of choice for central venous catheterization, because from the cubital fossa until the basilic vein reaches the axillary vein, the basilic vein increases in diameter and is in direct line with the axillary vein (see Fig. 3.94). The valves in the axillary vein may be troublesome, but abduction of the shoulder joint may permit the catheter to move past the obstruction.

The cephalic vein does not increase in size as it ascends the arm, and it frequently divides into small branches as it lies within the deltopectoral triangle. One or more of these branches may ascend over the clavicle and join the external jugular vein. In its usual method of termination, the cephalic vein joins the axillary vein at a right angle. It may be difficult to maneuver the catheter around this angle.

Spontaneous Thrombosis of Axillary Vein

Spontaneous thrombosis of the axillary vein occasionally occurs after excessive and unaccustomed movements of the arm at the shoulder joint.

- **Posterior (subscapular) group:** Lying in front of the subscapularis muscle, these nodes receive superficial lymph vessels from the back, down as far as the level of the iliac crests.
- **Lateral group:** Lying along the medial side of the axillary vein, these nodes receive most of the lymph vessels of the upper limb (except those superficial vessels draining the lateral side—see infraclavicular nodes, below).
- **Central group:** Lying in the center of the axilla, in the axillary fat deep to the pectoralis minor, these nodes receive lymph from the above three groups.
- **Infraclavicular (deltopectoral) group:** These nodes are not strictly axillary nodes because they are located outside the axilla. They lie in the deltopectoral groove between the deltoid and pectoralis major muscles and receive superficial lymph vessels from the lateral side of the hand, the forearm, and the arm.
- **Apical group:** Lying at the apex of the axilla at the lateral border of rib 1, these nodes receive the primary lymph drainage from all the other axillary nodes.

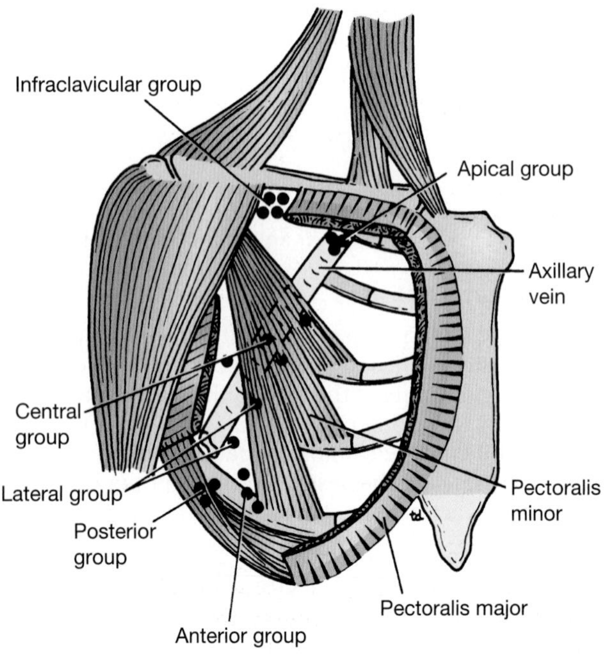

Figure 3.95 Different groups of lymph nodes in the axilla.

The apical nodes drain into the **subclavian lymph trunk.** On the left side, this trunk drains into the thoracic duct. On the right side, it drains into the right lymph trunk. Alternatively, the subclavian lymph trunks may drain directly into one of the large veins at the root of the neck.

Superficial and Deep Lymph Vessels

The superficial lymph vessels draining the superficial tissues of the upper limb pass upward to the axilla (Fig. 3.96).

The lymph vessels of the fingers pass along their borders to reach the webs. From here, the vessels ascend onto the dorsum of the hand. Lymph vessels on the palm form a plexus drained by vessels that ascend in the front of the forearm or pass around the medial and lateral

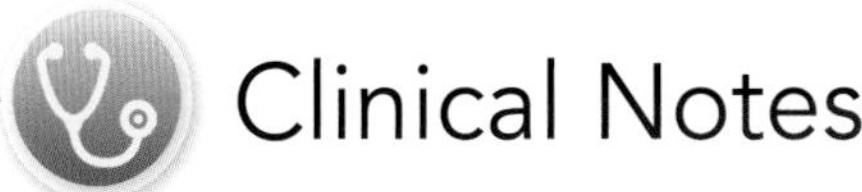

Axillary Lymph Node Examination

Examination of the axillary lymph nodes always forms part of the clinical examination of the breast. With the patient standing or sitting, they are asked to place their hand of the side to be examined on their hip and push hard medially. This action of adduction of the shoulder joint causes the pectoralis major muscle to contract maximally so that it becomes hard like a board. The examiner then palpates the axillary nodes (see Fig. 3.95) as follows:

- The anterior (pectoral) nodes may be palpated by pressing forward against the posterior surface of the pectoralis major muscle on the anterior wall of the axilla.
- The posterior (subscapular) nodes may be palpated by pressing backward against the anterior surface of the subscapularis muscle on the posterior wall of the axilla.
- The lateral nodes may be palpated against the medial side of the axillary vein. The examiner's fingers are pressed laterally against the axillary vein and the pulsating axillary artery.
- The central nodes may be palpated in the center of the axilla between the pectoralis major (anterior wall) and the subscapularis (posterior wall).
- For the apical nodes, the patient is asked to relax their shoulder muscles and let their upper limb hang down at the side. The examiner then gently places the tips of the fingers of the examining hand high up in the axilla to the outer border of rib 1. The nodes can be felt if they are enlarged.

borders to join vessels on the dorsum of the hand. Lymph vessels from the thumb and lateral fingers and the lateral areas of the hand, forearm, and arm follow the cephalic vein to the infraclavicular group of nodes.

The superficial vessels from the medial fingers and the medial areas of the hand and forearm follow the basilic vein to the cubital fossa. Here, some of the vessels drain into the **supratrochlear lymph node**, whereas others bypass the node and accompany the basilic vein to the axilla, where they drain into the lateral group of axillary nodes. The supratrochlear lymph node lies in the superficial fascia over the upper part of the cubital fossa, above the trochlea. The efferent vessels from the supratrochlear node also drain into the lateral axillary nodes.

The deep lymphatic vessels draining the muscles and deep structures of the arm drain into the lateral group of axillary nodes.

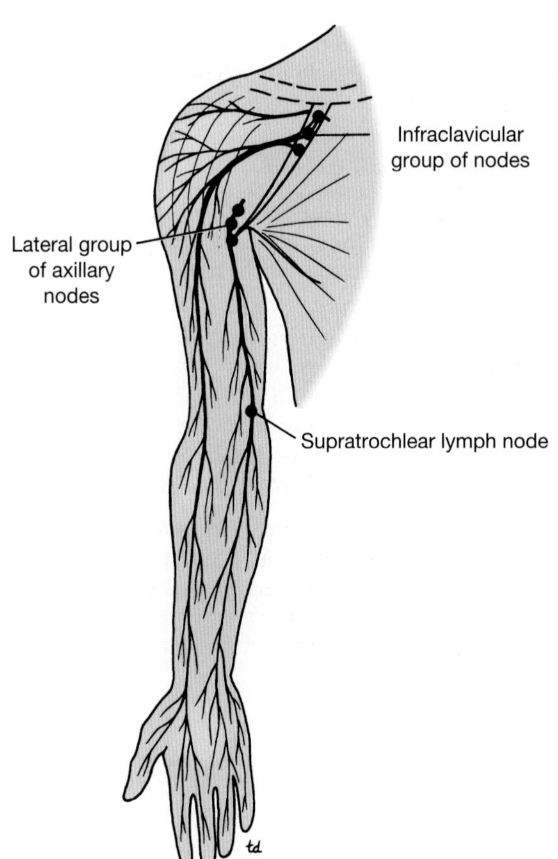

Figure 3.96 Superficial lymphatics of the upper limb. Note the positions of the lymph nodes.

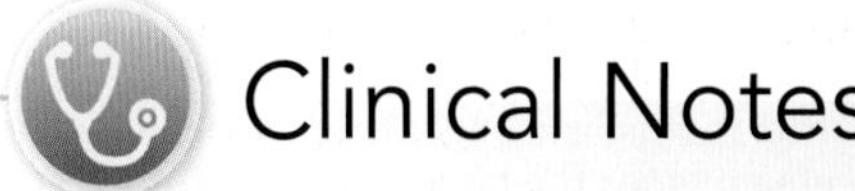

Lymphangitis

Infection of the lymph vessels (lymphangitis) of the arm is common. Red streaks along the course of the lymph vessels are characteristic of the condition. The lymph vessels from the thumb and index finger and the lateral part of the hand follow the cephalic vein to the infraclavicular group of axillary nodes; those from the middle, ring, and little fingers and from the medial part of the hand follow the basilic vein to the supratrochlear node, which lies in the superficial fascia just above the medial epicondyle of the humerus and from there to the lateral group of axillary nodes.

Lymphadenitis

Once the infection reaches the lymph nodes, they become enlarged and tender, a condition known as lymphadenitis. Most of the lymph vessels from the fingers and palm pass to the dorsum of the hand before passing up into the forearm. This explains the frequency of inflammatory edema, or even abscess formation, which may occur on the dorsum of the hand after infection of the fingers or palm.

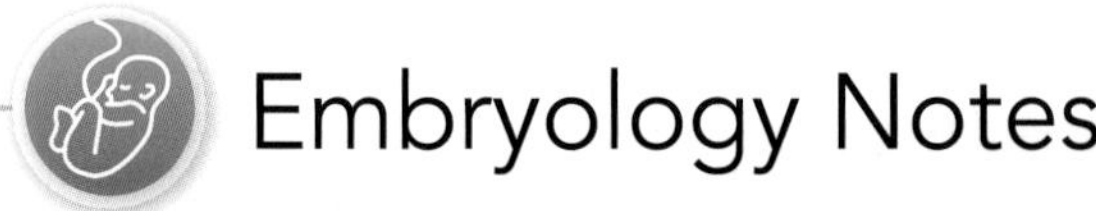

Embryology Notes

Upper Limb Development

The limb buds appear during week 6 of development as the result of a localized proliferation of somatopleuric mesenchyme. This causes the overlying ectoderm to bulge from the trunk as two pairs of flattened paddles (Fig. 3.97). The arm buds develop before the leg buds and lay at the level of the C3 to T2 segments. The flattened limb buds have a cephalic preaxial border and a caudal postaxial border. As the limb buds elongate, the anterior rami of the spinal nerves situated opposite the bases of the limb buds start to grow into the limbs. The mesenchyme situated along the preaxial border becomes associated and innervated with the C4 to C8 nerves, whereas the mesenchyme of the postaxial border becomes associated with the C8 and T1 nerves.

Later, the mesenchymal masses divide into anterior and posterior groups, and the nerve trunks entering the base of each limb also divide into anterior and posterior divisions. The mesenchyme within the limbs differentiates into individual muscles that migrate within each limb. Because of these two factors, the anterior rami of the spinal nerves become arranged in complicated plexuses found near the base of each limb so that the brachial plexus is formed.

Amelia

Congenital absence of one or more limbs (**amelia**) or partial absence (**ectromelia**) may occur. A defective limb may possess a rudimentary hand at the extremity of the limb, or a well-developed hand may spring from the shoulder with absence of the intermediate portion of the limb (**phocomelia**) (Fig. 3.98).

Congenital Absence of the Radius

Occasionally, the radius is congenitally absent, and the growth of the ulna pushes the hand laterally (Fig. 3.99).

Syndactyly

Syndactyly is webbing of the fingers. It is usually bilateral and often familial (Fig. 3.100). Plastic repair of the fingers is carried out at age 5 years. "Lobster hand" is a form of syndactyly associated with a central cleft dividing the hand into two parts. It is a heredofamilial disorder, for which plastic surgery is indicated when possible.

Brachydactyly

In brachydactyly, one or more phalanges are absent in several fingers. If the thumb is functioning normally, surgery is not indicated (Fig. 3.101).

Floating Thumb

A floating thumb results if the metacarpal bone of the thumb is absent but the phalanges are present. Plastic surgery is indicated, when possible, to improve the functional capabilities of the hand (Fig. 3.102).

Polydactyly

In polydactyly, one or more extra digits develop. It tends to run in families. The additional digits are removed surgically.

Macrodactyly (Local Gigantism)

Macrodactyly affects one or more digits; these may be of adult size at birth, but the size usually diminishes with age (Fig. 3.103). Surgical removal may be necessary.

Spinal cord
Posterior vertebral muscles
Posterior ramus
Prevertebral muscles
Anterior ramus
Scalenus medius
Scalenus anterior
Posterior muscles of girdle
Extensor muscles of arm
Esophagus
Trachea
Thyroid gland
Flexor muscles of arm
Arm bud
Anterior muscles of girdle
Infrahyoid muscles

Figure 3.97 Section through the lower cervical region and the formation of the upper limb bud. Note the presence of the developing bones and muscles from the mesenchyme.

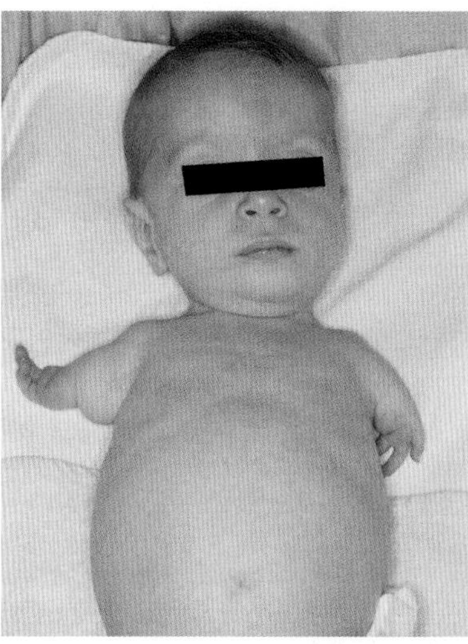

Figure 3.98 Ectromelia. (Courtesy of G. Avery.)

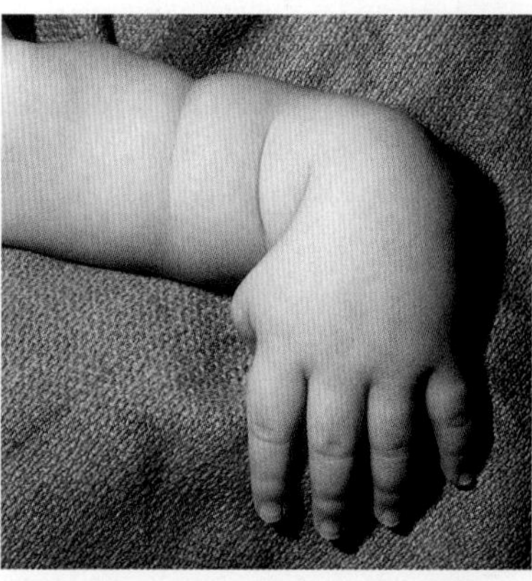

Figure 3.99 Congenital absence of the radius.

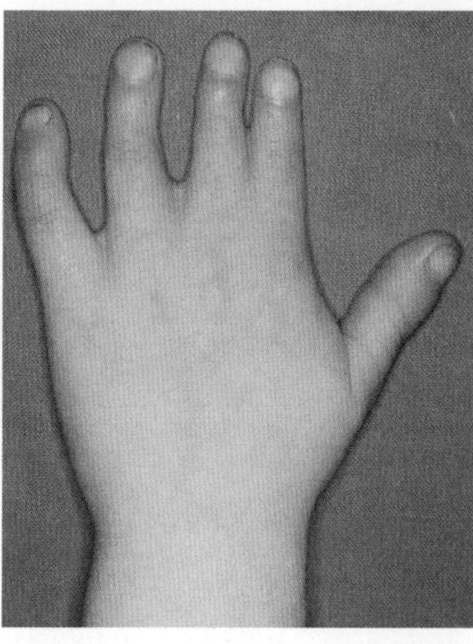

Figure 3.100 Partial syndactyly. (Courtesy of L. Thompson.)

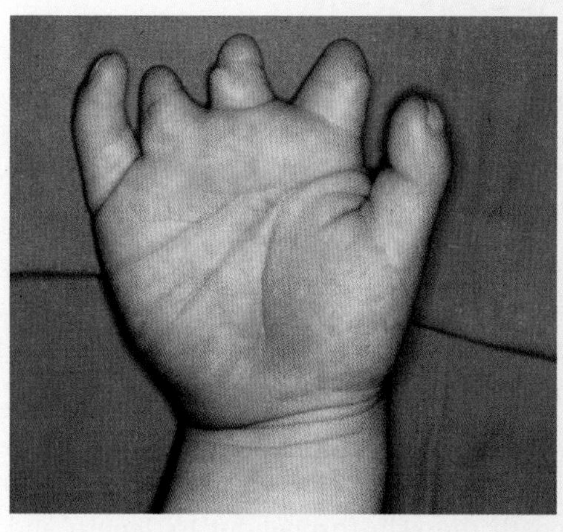

Figure 3.101 Brachydactyly due to defects of the phalanges. (Courtesy of L. Thompson.)

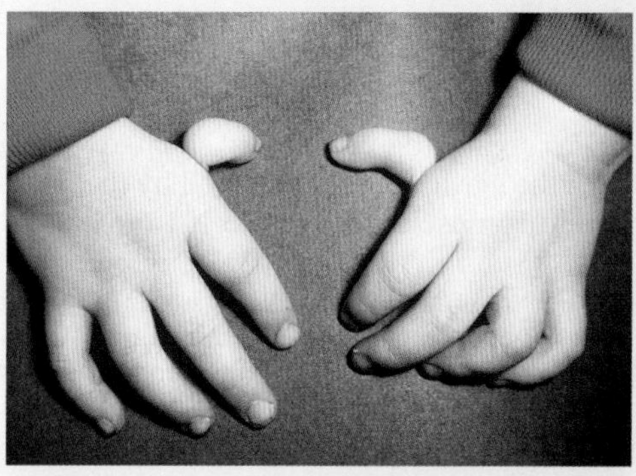

Figure 3.102 Floating thumb. The metacarpal bone of the thumb is absent, but the phalanges are present. (Courtesy of R. Chase.)

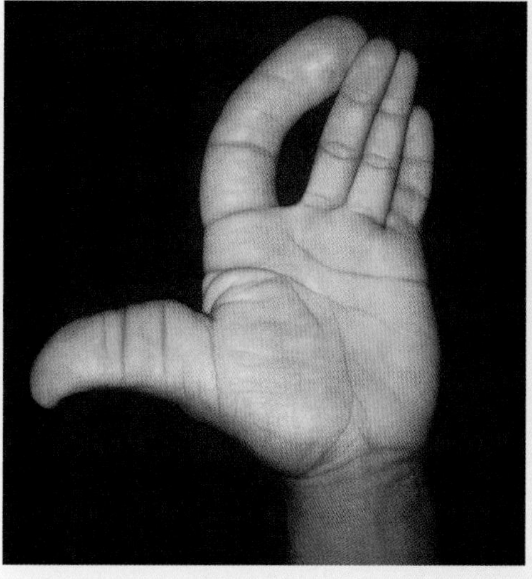

Figure 3.103 Macrodactyly affecting the thumb and index finger. (Courtesy of R. Neviaser.)

SURFACE ANATOMY

Anterior Surface of Chest

The features included here are mainly those related to the upper limb. A more comprehensive list of surface anatomy features is included in Chapter 4 (Thorax).

Suprasternal Notch

The suprasternal notch is the superior margin of the manubrium sterni and is easily palpated between the prominent medial ends of the clavicles in the midline (Figs. 3.104 and 3.105).

Clavicle

The clavicle is situated at the root of the neck. It lies just beneath the skin throughout its length and can be easily palpated (Fig. 3.106; see also Figs. 3.104 and 3.105). The positions of the sternoclavicular and acromioclavicular joints can be easily identified. Note that the medial end of the clavicle projects above the margin of the manubrium sterni.

Deltopectoral Triangle

This small, triangular depression is situated below the outer third of the clavicle and is bounded by the pectoralis major and deltoid muscles (see Figs. 3.104 and 3.105).

Axillary Folds

The **anterior axillary fold** is formed by the lower margin of the pectoralis major muscle and can be palpated between the finger and thumb (see Figs. 3.104 through 3.106). This can be made to stand out by asking the patient to press their hand against their ipsilateral hip. The **posterior axillary fold** is formed by the tendon of latissimus dorsi as it passes around the lower border of the teres major muscle. It can be easily palpated between the finger and thumb (Figs. 3.107 and 3.108).

Axilla

The axilla should be examined with the forearm supported and the pectoral muscles relaxed. With the arm by the side, the inferior part of the head of the humerus can be easily palpated through the floor of the axilla. The pulsations of the axillary artery can be felt high up in the axilla, and, around the artery, the cords of the brachial plexus can be palpated. The upper ribs, covered by the serratus anterior muscle, form the medial wall of the axilla. The serrations of the **serratus anterior** can be seen and felt in a muscular person (see Fig. 3.105B). The coracobrachialis and biceps brachii muscles and the bicipital groove of the humerus form the lateral wall.

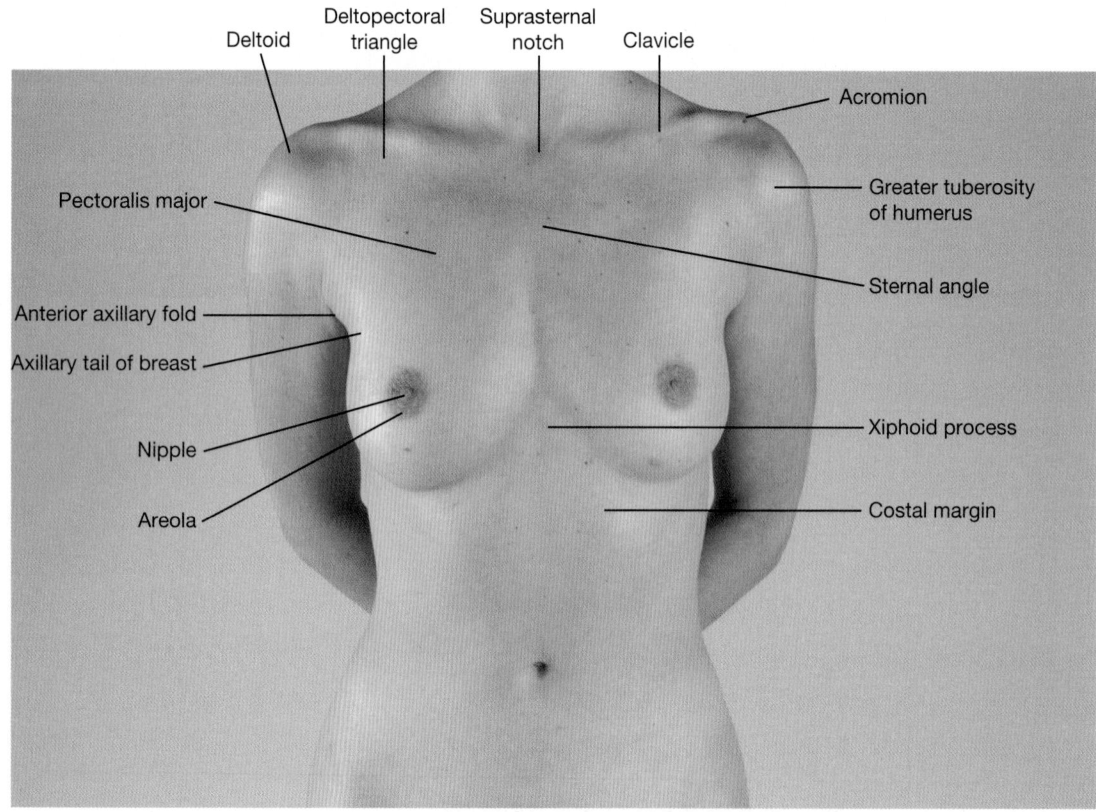

Figure 3.104 Anterior view of the pectoral region in a young woman with her arms held behind her back, showing the surface anatomy of the chest.

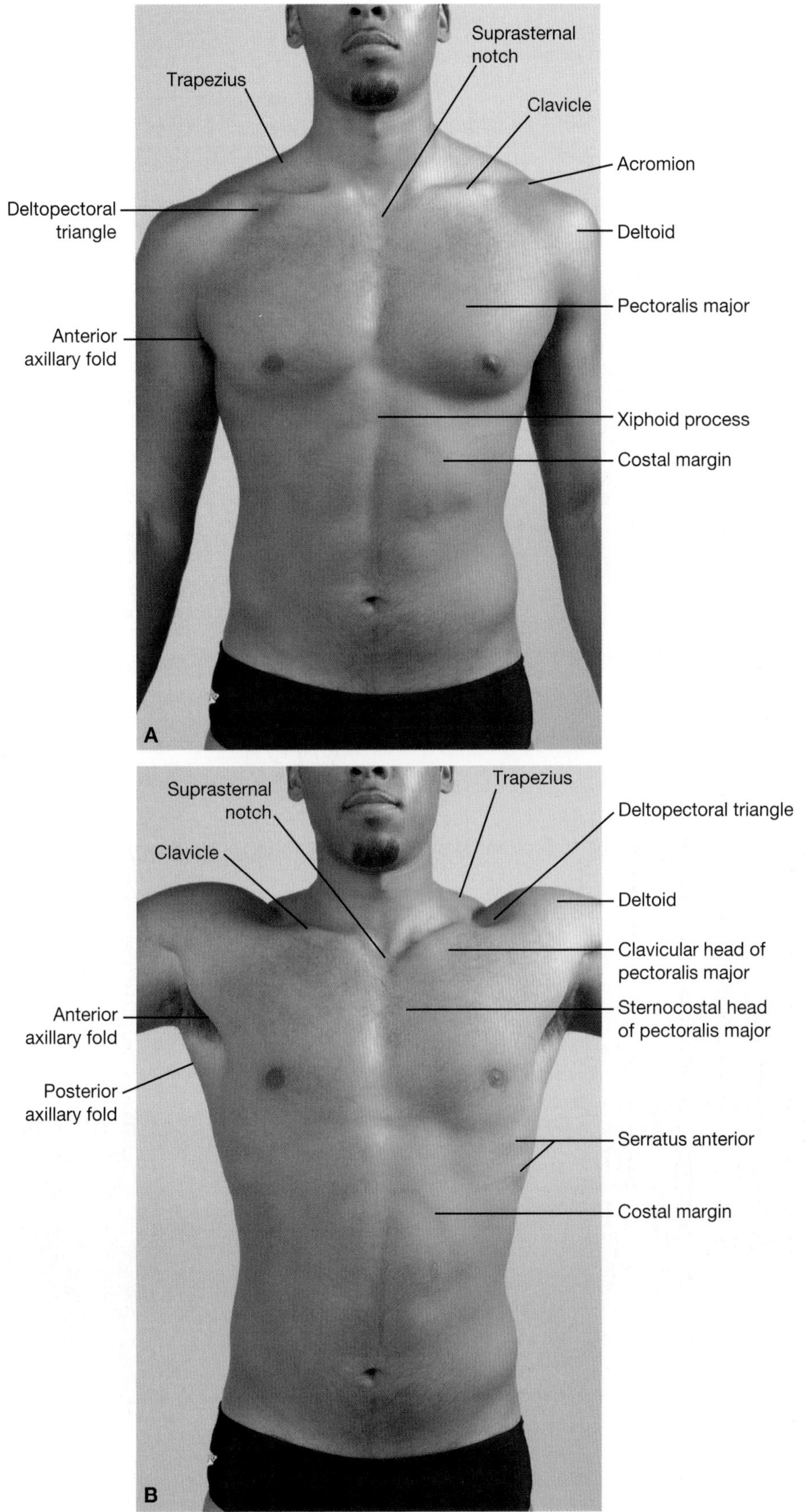

Figure 3.105 Anterior views of the pectoral region in a young man showing the surface anatomy of the chest. **A.** With the arms by the sides. **B.** With the arms abducted.

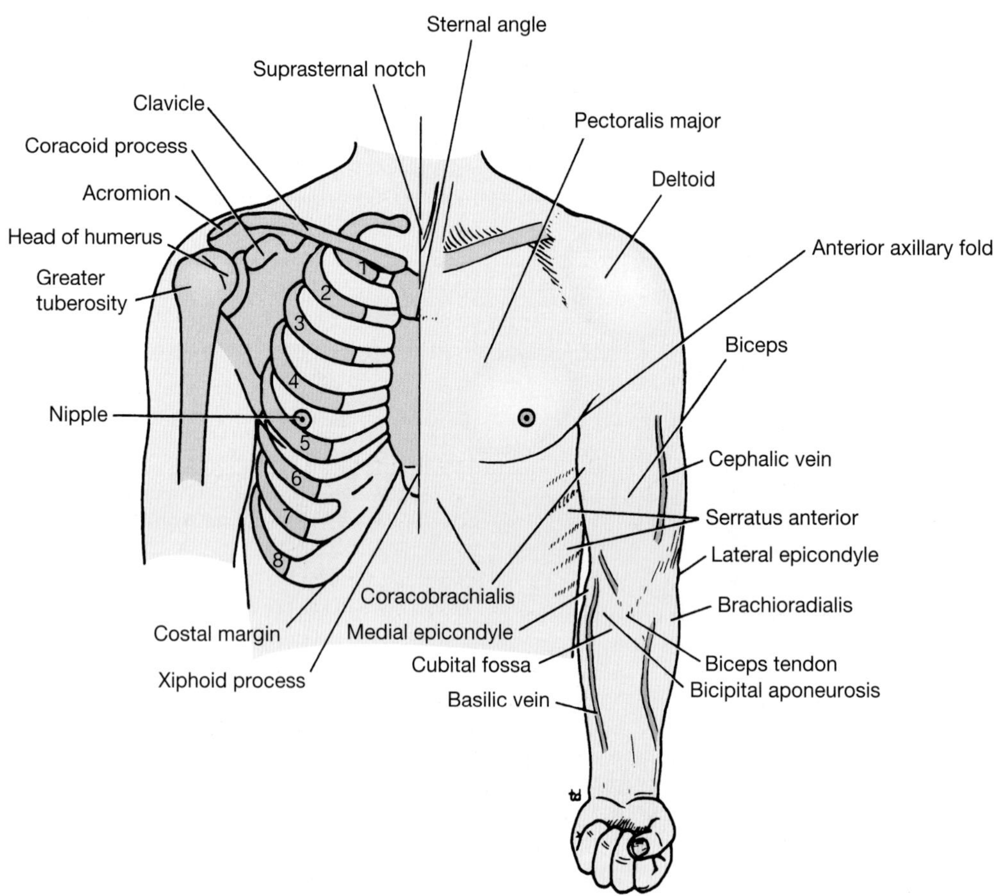

Figure 3.106 Anterior view showing the surface anatomy of the chest, shoulder, and upper limb.

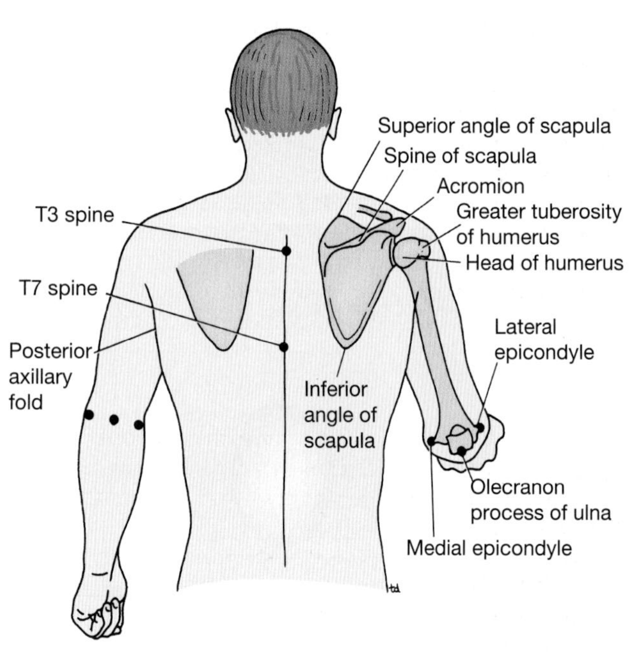

Figure 3.107 Posterior view showing the surface anatomy of the scapula, shoulder, and elbow regions.

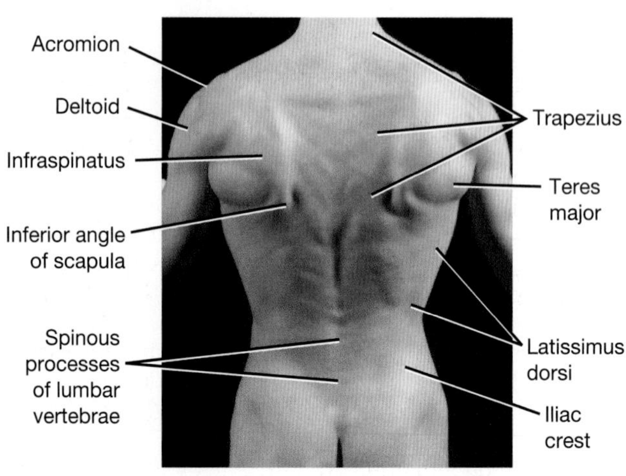

Figure 3.108 Posterior view showing the surface anatomy of the back in a young man.

Posterior Surface of Shoulder

The features included here are mainly related to the upper limb. More comprehensive lists of surface anatomy features are included in Chapters 2 (Back) and 4 (Thorax).

Cervical and Thoracic Vertebrae Spinous Processes

The spinous processes can be palpated in the posterior midline (see Figs. 3.107 and 3.108). The index finger should be placed on the skin in the midline on the posterior surface of the neck and drawn downward in the nuchal groove. The spinous process of the C7 vertebra (vertebra prominens) is the first to be felt. The overlapping spines of the thoracic vertebrae are below this level. The large ligament called the **ligamentum nuchae** covers the spines of the C1 to C6 vertebrae.

Scapula

The tip of the **coracoid process** of the scapula (see Fig. 3.106) can be felt on deep palpation in the lateral part of the deltopectoral triangle; it is covered by the anterior fibers of the deltoid muscle. The **acromion** forms the lateral extremity of the spine of the scapula. It is subcutaneous and easily located (see Figs. 3.104 through 3.108).

Immediately below the lateral edge of the acromion is the smooth, rounded curve of the shoulder produced by the **deltoid muscle**, which covers the **greater tuberosity of the humerus** (see Figs. 3.104 through 3.108).

The **crest of the spine of the scapula** can be palpated and traced medially to the **medial border of the scapula**, which it joins at the level of the T3 spine (see Fig. 3.107).

The **superior angle of the scapula** can be felt through the trapezius muscle and lies opposite the T2 spine.

The **inferior angle of the scapula** can be palpated opposite the T7 spine (see Figs. 3.107 and 3.108).

Breast

In children and men, the breast anatomy is rudimentary, and the glandular tissue is confined to a small area beneath the pigmented areola. In young women, it is usually hemispherical and slightly pendulous, overlaps ribs 2 to 6 and their costal cartilages, and extends from the lateral margin of the sternum to the midaxillary line. The greater part of the breast lies in the superficial fascia and can be moved freely in all directions. Its upper lateral edge (**axillary tail**) extends around the lower border of the pectoralis major and enters the axilla, where it comes into close relationship with the axillary vessels (see Fig. 3.104). In middle-age multiparous women, the breast may be large and pendulous; in older women, the breast may be smaller.

In the living individual, the breast is soft because the fat contained within it is fluid. On careful palpation with the open hand, the breast has a firm, overall lobulated consistency, produced by its glandular tissue.

The **nipple** projects from the lower half of the breast, but its position in relation to the chest wall varies greatly and depends on the development of the gland. In males and immature females, the nipples are small and usually lie over the fourth intercostal spaces about 4 in. (10 cm) from the midline. A circular area of pigmented skin (the **areola**) surrounds the base of the nipple (see Fig. 3.104). Pink in color in the young girl, the areola becomes darker in color in the second month of the first pregnancy and never regains its former tint. The underlying areolar glands produce tiny tubercles on the areola.

Elbow Region

The **medial and lateral epicondyles of the humerus** and the **olecranon process of the ulna** can be palpated (see Figs. 3.106 and 3.107). When the elbow joint is extended, these bony points lie on the same straight line; when the elbow is flexed, these three points form the boundaries of an equilateral triangle.

The **head of the radius** can be palpated in a depression on the posterolateral aspect of the extended elbow, distal to the lateral epicondyle. The head of the radius can be felt to rotate during pronation and supination of the forearm.

The **cubital fossa** is a skin depression in front of the elbow (see Figs. 3.51 and 3.106), and the boundaries can be seen and felt; the brachioradialis muscle forms the lateral boundary, and the pronator teres forms the medial boundary. The **tendon of the biceps** muscle can be palpated as it passes downward into the fossa, and the **bicipital aponeurosis** can be felt as it leaves the tendon to join the deep fascia on the medial side of the forearm. The tendon and aponeurosis are most easily felt if the elbow joint is flexed against resistance.

The **ulnar nerve** can be palpated where it lies behind the medial epicondyle of the humerus. It feels like a rounded cord; when it is compressed, a "pins and needles" sensation is felt along the medial part of the hand.

The **brachial artery** can be felt to pulsate as it passes down the arm, overlapped by the medial border of the biceps muscle. In the cubital fossa, it lies deep to the bicipital aponeurosis. At a level just below the head of the radius, it divides into the radial and ulnar arteries.

The **posterior border of the ulna** bone is subcutaneous and can be palpated along its entire length.

Wrist and Hand

At the wrist, the **styloid processes of the radius** (Fig. 3.109B) and ulna can be palpated. The styloid process of the radius lies about 0.75 in. (1.9 cm) distal to that of the ulna.

The dorsal tubercle of the radius is palpable on the posterior surface of the distal end of the radius.

The **head of the ulna** is most easily felt with the forearm pronated; the head then stands out prominently on the lateral side of the wrist (see Fig. 3.22). The rounded head can be distinguished from the more distal pointed styloid process.

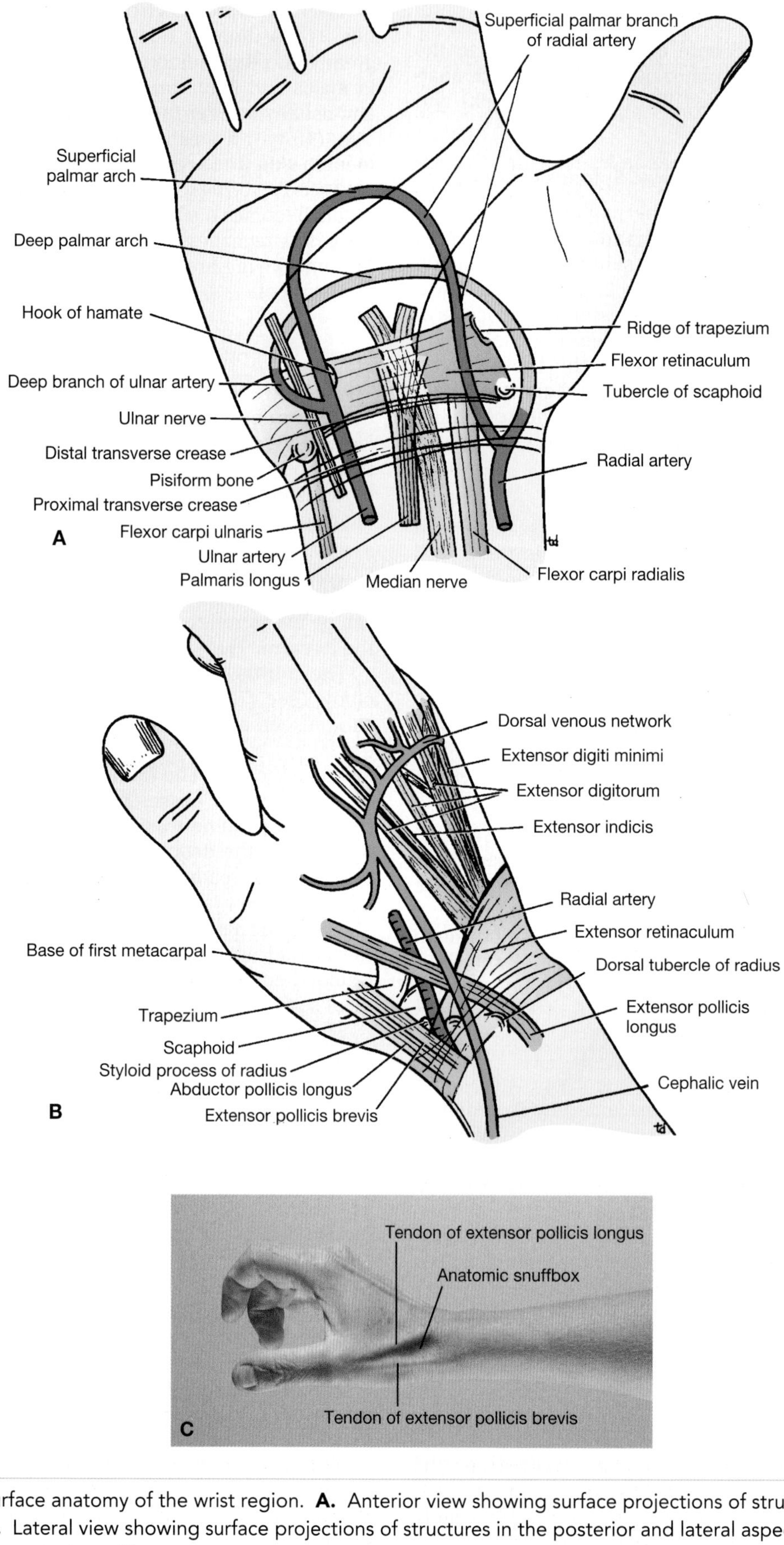

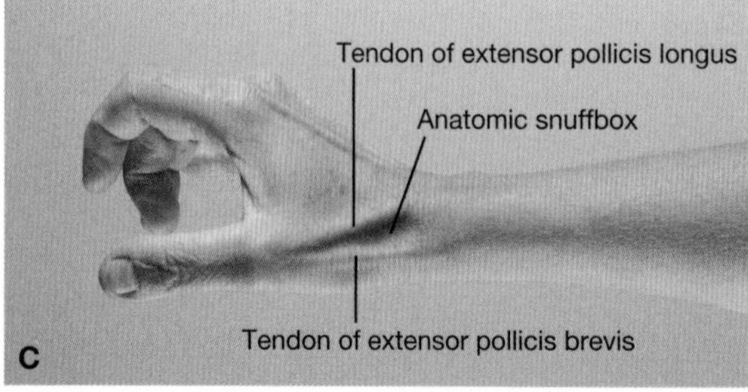

Figure 3.109 Surface anatomy of the wrist region. **A.** Anterior view showing surface projections of structures in the palmar aspect. **B.** Lateral view showing surface projections of structures in the posterior and lateral aspects. **C.** Lateral view showing the anatomic snuffbox.

The **pisiform bone** can be felt on the medial side of the anterior aspect of the wrist between the two transverse creases (see Figs. 3.51 and 3.109A). The **hook of the hamate bone** can be felt on deep palpation of the hypothenar eminence, a fingerbreadth distal and lateral to the pisiform bone.

The transverse creases seen in front of the wrist are important landmarks (see Fig. 3.109A). The **proximal transverse crease** lies at the level of the wrist joint. The **distal transverse crease** corresponds to the proximal border of the flexor retinaculum.

Important Structures Lying in Front of the Wrist

Radial Artery

The pulsations of the radial artery can easily be felt anterior to the distal third of the radius (see Figs. 3.55 and 3.109A). Here, it lies just beneath the skin and fascia lateral to the tendon of flexor carpi radialis muscle.

Tendon of Flexor Carpi Radialis

The tendon of the flexor carpi radialis lies medial to the pulsating radial artery (see Figs. 3.51 and 3.109A).

Tendon of Palmaris Longus

If present, the tendon of the palmaris longus lies medial to the tendon of flexor carpi radialis and overlies the median nerve (see Figs. 3.51 and 3.109A).

Tendons of Flexor Digitorum Superficialis

The tendons of the flexor digitorum superficialis are a group of four that lie medial to the tendon of palmaris longus and can be seen moving beneath the skin when the fingers are flexed and extended.

Tendon of Flexor Carpi Ulnaris

The tendon of the flexor carpi ulnaris is the most medially placed tendon on the front of the wrist and can be followed distally to its insertion on the pisiform bone (see Figs. 3.51 and 3.109A). The tendon can be made prominent by asking the patient to clench their fist (the muscle contracts to assist in fixing and stabilizing the wrist joint).

Ulnar Artery

The pulsations of the ulnar artery can be felt lateral to the tendon of flexor carpi ulnaris (see Fig. 3.109A).

Ulnar Nerve

The ulnar nerve lies immediately medial to the ulnar artery (see Fig. 3.109A).

Important Structures Lying on the Lateral Side of the Wrist

Anatomic Snuffbox

The anatomic snuffbox is a skin depression that lies distal to the styloid process of the radius. It is bounded medially by the **tendon of extensor pollicis longus** and laterally by the **tendons of abductor pollicis longus** and **extensor pollicis brevis** (see Fig. 3.109B,C). In its floor can be palpated the **styloid process of the radius** (proximally) and the **base of the first metacarpal bone** of the thumb (distally); between these bones beneath the floor lie the **scaphoid** and the **trapezium** (felt but not identifiable). The **radial artery** can be palpated within the snuffbox as the artery winds around the lateral margin of the wrist to reach the dorsum of the hand. The **cephalic vein** can also sometimes be recognized crossing the snuffbox as it ascends the forearm.

Important Structures Lying on the Back of the Wrist

Lunate

The lunate lies in the proximal row of carpal bones. It can be palpated just distal to the dorsal tubercle of the radius when the wrist joint is flexed.

Important Structures Lying in the Palm

Recurrent Branch of the Median Nerve

The recurrent branch to the muscles of the thenar eminence curves around the lower border of the flexor retinaculum and lies about one fingerbreadth distal to the tubercle of the scaphoid (see Fig. 3.65).

Superficial Palmar Arterial Arch

The superficial palmar arterial arch is in the central part of the palm (see Fig. 3.109A) and lies on a line drawn across the palm at the level of the distal border of the fully extended thumb.

Deep Palmar Arterial Arch

The deep palmar arterial arch is also located in the central part of the palm (see Fig. 3.109A) and lies on a line drawn across the palm at the level of the proximal border of the fully extended thumb.

Metacarpophalangeal Joints

The metacarpophalangeal joints lie approximately at the level of the distal transverse palmar crease. The **interphalangeal joints** lie at the level of the middle and distal finger creases.

Important Structures Lying on the Dorsum of the Hand

The **tendons of extensor digitorum**, the **extensor indicis**, and the **extensor digiti minimi** can be seen and felt as they pass distally to the bases of the fingers (see Fig. 3.109B).

Dorsal Venous Network

The network of superficial veins can be seen on the dorsum of the hand (see Fig. 3.109B). The network drains upward into the lateral cephalic vein and a medial basilic vein.

The **cephalic vein** crosses the anatomic snuffbox and winds around onto the anterior aspect of the forearm. It then ascends into the arm and runs along the lateral border of the biceps (see Fig. 3.94). It ends by piercing the deep fascia in the deltopectoral triangle and enters the axillary vein.

The **basilic vein** can be traced from the dorsum of the hand around the medial side of the forearm and reaches the anterior aspect just below the elbow. It pierces the deep fascia at about the middle of the arm. The **median cubital vein** (or median cephalic and median basilic veins) links the cephalic and basilic veins in the cubital fossa (see Fig. 3.94).

To identify these veins easily, apply firm pressure around your upper arm and repeatedly clench and relax your fist. By this means, the veins become distended with blood.

Clinical Case Discussion

A diagnosis of subcoracoid dislocation of the right shoulder joint was made, complicated by damage to the axillary and radial nerves. The head of the humerus was displaced downward to below the coracoid process of the scapula by the initial trauma and was displaced further by the pull of the muscles (subscapularis, pectoralis major). The loss of shoulder curvature was caused by the displacement of the humerus (greater tuberosity) medially so that it no longer pushed the overlying muscle (deltoid) laterally. The extensive loss of skin sensation to the right upper limb was the result of damage to the axillary and radial nerves.

For a clinician to be able to make a diagnosis in this case and to be able to interpret the clinical findings, they must have considerable knowledge of the anatomy of the shoulder joint (Fig. 3.110). Furthermore, the clinician must know the relationship of the axillary and radial nerves to the joint and the distribution of these nerves to the parts of the upper limb.

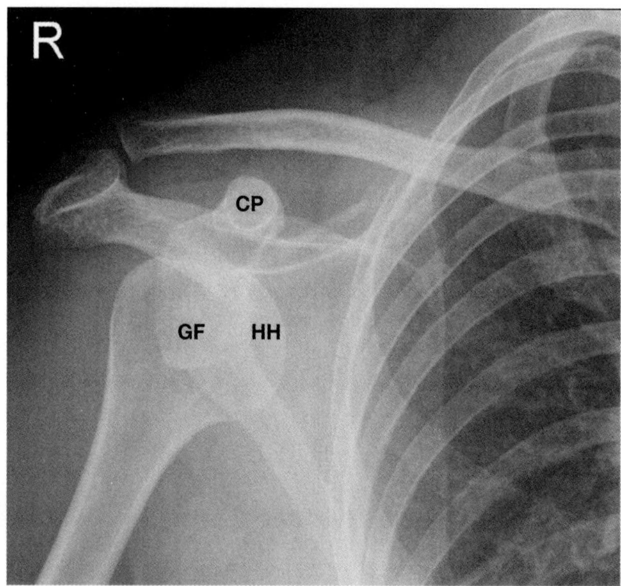

Figure 3.110 Anterior dislocation of the right shoulder (glenohumeral) joint. Note the displacement of the humeral head into a subcoracoid position. CP, coracoid process; GF, glenoid fossa; HH, humeral head.

Key Concepts

Osteology

- A bony framework forms the core of each region of the upper limb.
- The clavicle and scapula form the shoulder girdle, the humerus forms the arm (brachium), and the radius and ulna form the forearm (antebrachium). The eight carpal bones (scaphoid, lunate, triquetrum, pisiform, trapezium, trapezoid, capitate, hamate) form the wrist (carpus). The metacarpal bones and the phalanges form the hand (manus) and digits.
- Bony features are functionally significant in the context of muscle/ligament attachments and movement deficits resulting from fracture (eg, most of the rotator cuff muscles attach to the greater tubercle of the humerus, the triceps attaches to the olecranon process of the ulna, and the biceps brachii is detached following an avulsion fracture of the radial tuberosity).
- Several bony features have significant relations with key neurovascular structures that must be considered in case of bone fractures (eg, surgical neck of the humerus with the axillary nerve and posterior humeral circumflex vessels, midshaft of the humerus with the radial nerve and profunda brachii vessels, and medial epicondyle of the humerus with the ulnar nerve).

Joints

- Numerous, mostly synovial, joints allow the great mobility of the upper limb. The shoulder and elbow regions each contain three individual joints. Likewise, the wrist and hand contain multiple joints.
- The shoulder region contains the sternoclavicular, acromioclavicular, and glenohumeral ("shoulder") joints.
- The elbow contains the humeroulnar, humeroradial, and proximal radioulnar joints.
- The proximal and distal radioulnar joints are the primary joints that allow pronation and supination.
- The wrist complex includes the radiocarpal, intercarpal, and carpometacarpal joints.

Breast

- Breasts are specialized integumentary glands that secrete milk.
- The lymph drainage of the breast is clinically important because of its role in metastasis of cancer. Much of the lymph drainage of the breast runs through the network of axillary lymph nodes.
- The axillary tail is an extension of the upper lateral quadrant of the breast into the axilla that must be recognized in breast examination.

Axilla

- The axilla (armpit) is a pyramid-shaped space between the arm and side of the chest.
- It conveys major blood vessels (axillary artery and vein and their branches), nerves (brachial plexus), and lymph channels (axillary nodes).
- The pectoralis minor muscle divides the axilla into three subregions that are useful in describing the pathways of the arteries and lymph drainage.

Cubital Fossa

- The cubital fossa is a triangular depression in the anterior aspect of the elbow. It contains several neurovascular structures that pass between the arm and forearm.

Carpal Tunnel

- The carpal tunnel is an osseofascial passage through the wrist.
- The carpal bones and the overlying flexor retinaculum form the carpal tunnel.
- Several muscle tendons and the median nerve pass through the carpal tunnel. Abnormal compression of these may result in carpal tunnel syndrome.

Palm

- The palm contains fascial spaces, and the distal palmar side of each finger contains a pulp space. These spaces can dictate the direction and extent of infections in the hand and fingers.

Back and Shoulder Muscles

- Several muscles in the chest and back are developmentally and functionally upper limb muscles.
- The pectoralis major and minor and the serratus anterior connect the upper limb to the thoracic wall.
- The superficial group of muscles of the back connects the vertebral column with the upper limb.
- Muscles in the scapular region connect the scapula with the humerus.
- The rotator cuff is a group of four scapular muscles that act on the shoulder (glenohumeral) joint and assist in stabilizing that joint.

Arm

- The arm (brachium) contains two osseofascial compartments, anterior and posterior.
- The muscles in the anterior compartment contribute to flexion of the shoulder and elbow and to power supination.
- The muscle in the posterior compartment acts in extension of the shoulder and elbow.

Forearm

- The forearm (antebrachium) contains three osseofascial compartments: anterior, posterior, and lateral.
- The muscles in the anterior compartment contribute largely to flexion of the wrist and digits and to pronation.
- The muscles in the posterior compartment contribute largely to extension of the wrist and digits and to supination.
- The muscles in the lateral compartment contribute mainly to flexion of the elbow and extension of the wrist.

Hand

- The hand contains five osseofascial compartments, four (thenar, hypothenar, central, interosseous) on the anterior (palmar) aspect and one (dorsal/extensor) on the posterior side.
- The anterior compartments house many small muscles that produce complex fine movements of the digits, including opposition of the thumb.
- The dorsal compartment contains the long tendons of extrinsic muscles of the hand.

Nerves

- The spinal accessory nerve (cranial nerve XI) supplies one muscle (trapezius) of the upper limb. The brachial plexus supplies all other motor and sensory aspects of the upper limb.
- Several nerves (eg, suprascapular, long thoracic, thoracodorsal) supply the shoulder region.
- Five terminal branches of the brachial plexus (musculocutaneous, median, ulnar, radial, and axillary nerves) supply the shoulder and the upper limb proper.
- The musculocutaneous nerve supplies the muscles in the anterior compartment of the arm and the skin on the lateral border of the forearm. Lesion of this nerve results in part of the "waiter's tip" presentation.

- The median nerve supplies most of the muscles in the anterior compartment of the forearm and a small number of intrinsic hand muscles, including the entire thenar compartment. Lesion of the median nerve results in an "ape hand" presentation.
- The ulnar nerve supplies one and a half muscles in the anterior compartment of the forearm plus most of the intrinsic muscles of the hand. Lesion of this nerve results in a "claw hand" presentation.
- The radial nerve supplies all the muscles in the posterior compartments of the arm and forearm, plus the lateral compartment of the forearm. Lesion of the radial nerve results in a "wristdrop" presentation.
- The axillary nerve supplies two muscles in the shoulder (including the deltoid) and the skin on the lower lateral side of the shoulder. Lesion of the axillary nerve contributes to the "waiter's tip" posture.
- The median, radial, and ulnar nerves provide the cutaneous innervation of the hand.

Arterial Supply

- The subclavian artery continues as the axillary artery, which supplies the upper limb.
- The axillary artery travels through the axilla. The pectoralis minor divides this vessel into three parts. The second part defines the cords of the brachial plexus.
- The brachial artery is the continuation of the axillary artery through the arm. The brachial artery terminates in the cubital fossa by dividing into the radial and ulnar arteries.
- The radial and ulnar arteries supply the forearm and hand. The ulnar artery provides the main blood flow into the superficial palmar arch. The radial artery is the main feeder into the deep palmar arch.

Venous Supply

- The superficial venous drainage of the upper limb begins with the dorsal venous arch in the hand. This arch drains into the cephalic and basilic veins at its lateral and medial ends.
- The median cubital vein connects the cephalic and basilic veins in the cubital fossa.
- The cephalic and basilic veins drain into the axillary vein.

Lymphatic Drainage

- Lymph drainage of the upper limb mainly parallels the cephalic and basilic veins up into the axilla.
- An extensive complex of axillary lymph nodes collects lymph from the upper limb, much of the breast, and a large area of the thoracoabdominal walls and the back.

Surface Anatomy and Medical Imaging

- Numerous features of the upper limb are readily visible and palpable in standard modes of medical imaging and in surface anatomy examination.

4 Thorax

CLINICAL CASE 1

A 20-year-old innocent female bystander was shot during an exchange of gunfire. On examination in the emergency department, she showed signs of severe hemorrhage and was in a state of shock. Her pulse was rapid, and her blood pressure was dangerously low. A small entrance wound was noted about 1 cm wide in the fourth left intercostal space about 3 cm from the lateral margin of the sternum but no exit wound. The left side of her chest was dull on percussion, and breath sounds were absent on that side of the chest. A chest tube was immediately inserted through the chest wall. Because of the massive amount of blood pouring out of the tube, the attending physician decided to enter the chest (thoracotomy). The physician carefully counted the ribs to find the fourth intercostal space and cut the layers of tissue to enter the pleural space (cavity). She was very careful to avoid important anatomic structures.

CLINICAL CASE 2

A 54-year-old female visited the emergency department with a complaint of a sudden excruciating knifelike pain in the front of her chest. During the examination, she said that she could also feel the pain in her back between the shoulder blades. On questioning, she said that she felt no pain down the arms or in the neck. Her blood pressure was 200/110 mm Hg in the right arm and 120/80 mm Hg in the left arm.

See the Clinical Case Discussions at the end of this chapter for further insights.

CHAPTER OUTLINE

LEARNING OBJECTIVES

The purpose of this chapter is to review the basic anatomy of the thorax to understand normal functional relationships and the basis for common injuries, pain, motor deficits, congenital defects, medical imaging, and general surface examination.

1. Identify the bones of the thoracic cage and their major features. Describe the functional aspects of these structures.
2. Identify the bony components, major supporting ligaments, and movements permitted at the joints of the thoracic cage.
3. Describe the structure of the thoracic wall, including its layers and the contents of a typical intercostal space. Note the arrangement of the intercostal muscles and neurovascular elements. Note collateral routes and major anastomoses of arteries.
4. Describe the development, structure, position, and actions of the diaphragm. Identify its innervation and indicate the segmental sources and pathways taken by these nerves to reach the diaphragm. Describe the mechanics of respiration, including a comparison of the roles of the diaphragm, thoracic cage, and thoracoabdominal muscles in normal respiration.
5. Trace the course of motor and sensory innervation of the thoracic wall. Predict the functional consequences of lesions of individual peripheral nerves.
6. Trace the flow of blood to and through the thoracic wall by describing the courses and branching patterns of the major arteries and veins. Identify the territories supplied and drained by the major vessels. Note the main collateral routes and describe the composition of significant anastomoses.
7. Describe the pattern of lymphatic drainage of the thoracic wall, including the relationship of this drainage to that of the axilla and breast.
8. Identify the major subdivisions of the thoracic cavity and describe their contents. Identify the subdivisions of the mediastinum and describe their contents.
9. Identify the major longitudinal structures (eg, trachea, esophagus, vagus nerves, phrenic nerves, aorta, sympathetic networks, azygous system, and thoracic duct) running through the thoracic cavity and describe their courses and relationships.
10. Identify the parietal and visceral pleurae, their different components, the pleural recesses, and the boundaries of the pleura in projection onto the body surface.
11. Identify and differentiate the right and left lungs, including their lobes and fissures. Identify the impressions made on the surfaces of each lung by the major surrounding structures.
12. Identify the primary, secondary, and tertiary branches of the bronchial tree. Identify the bronchi and the pulmonary arteries and veins at the hilar surface of each lung. Define a bronchopulmonary segment and relate such segmentation to the organization of the bronchial and vascular trees.

13. Identify the parietal and visceral pericardia, their relationship to the parietal pleurae and diaphragm, and their projections onto the body surface.
14. Describe the gross structure of the heart, including the fibrous cardiac skeleton.
15. Trace the course of blood flow through the right and left sides of the heart. Identify the internal structures of each chamber and the location and structure of each of the valves.
16. Identify the sounds of the normal heart. Relate these to the flow of blood through the heart and the actions of the cardiac valves.
17. Identify the anatomical and auscultation projections of each of the cardiac valves onto the body surface.
18. Trace the flow of blood through each of the major coronary vessels. Identify which vessels supply the main flow to and drainage from each of the chambers and the interventricular septum as well as possible anastomoses and collateral vascular pathways.
19. Describe the conducting system and extrinsic innervation of the heart.
20. Trace the flow of blood from the thoracic walls and cavity to the heart by describing the formation and courses of the caval and azygos venous tracts. Indicate anastomoses and collateral connections between these and other tracts and discuss the clinical significance of such connections.
21. Trace the primary drainage routes of lymph from the organs and walls of the thoracic cavity to the points of venous connection.
22. Identify the major structures of the thorax in standard medical imaging.
23. Locate the surface projections and palpation points of the major thoracic structures in a basic surface examination.

OVERVIEW

The chest, or thorax (*thora* is Greek for "breastplate"; "chest"), is the region of the body between the neck and the abdomen. It is flattened in front and behind but rounded at the sides. Skin and muscles of the shoulder girdle cover the exterior of the thoracic wall, whereas parietal pleura lines its inner surface. The skeletal framework of the thoracic walls is the **thoracic cage**. This is formed by the thoracic part of the vertebral column posteriorly, the ribs and intercostal spaces laterally on either side, and the sternum and costal cartilages anteriorly (Fig. 4.1). Superiorly, the thorax communicates with the neck; inferiorly, it is separated from the abdomen by the diaphragm. The thoracic cage protects the lungs and heart and provides attachment for the muscles of the thorax, upper extremity, abdomen, and back.

The thoracic cavity can be divided into a median portion, the **mediastinum**, and the laterally placed pleurae and lungs. The lungs are covered by a thin, serous membrane called the **visceral pleura**, which passes from each lung at its root (ie, where the main air passages and blood vessels enter) to the inner surface of the chest wall, where it is called the **parietal pleura**. This arrangement of the pleura forms two independent membranous sacs called the **pleural cavities**, one on each side of the thorax, between the lungs and the thoracic walls.

The thoracic cage and the diaphragm bound the thoracic cavity. However, the thoracic cavity is much smaller than the limits of the thoracic cage because the diaphragm deeply invaginates the lower margins of the thoracic cage. Also, the cavity extends upward into the root of the neck about one fingerbreadth above the clavicle on each side. The diaphragm is the only structure (apart from the pleura and the peritoneum) that separates the thoracic from abdominal viscera.

OSTEOLOGY

The thoracic skeleton forms an osseocartilaginous, cagelike unit that surrounds and protects the heart, lungs, and adnexa. It also covers all or parts of certain upper abdominal organs (eg, liver, stomach, spleen, kidneys). The thoracic cage is a component of the axial skeleton and is formed by the sternum, ribs, costal cartilages, and thoracic vertebrae.

Sternum

The sternum (*stern* is Greek for "breast"; "breastbone") is the elongate, flat bone that lies in the midline of the anterior chest wall. The adult sternum consists of three parts: **manubrium**, **body**, and **xiphoid process** (see Fig. 4.1).

The **manubrium** (*manubri* is Latin for "handle") is the upper part of the sternum. It articulates with the body of the sternum at the **manubriosternal joint**, and it also articulates with the clavicles and with the costal cartilage 1 and the upper part of the costal cartilage 2 on each side. It lies opposite the T3 and T4 vertebrae

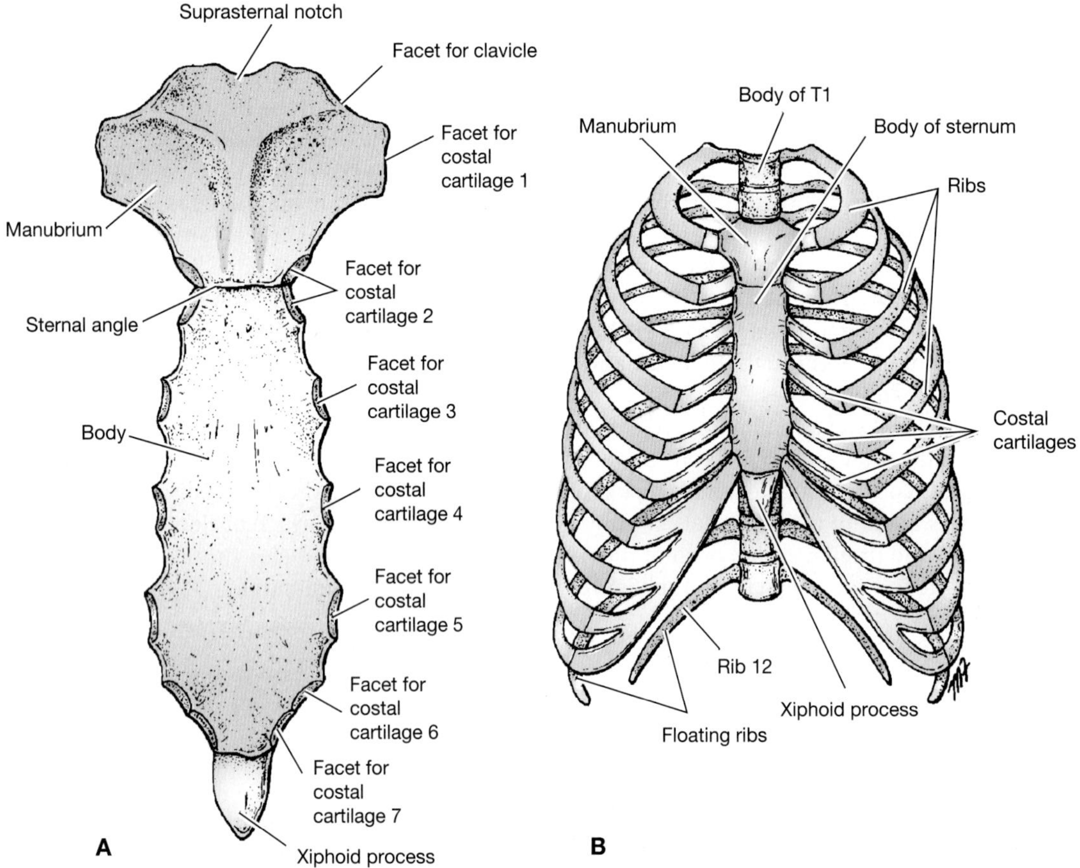

Figure 4.1 **A.** Anterior view of the sternum. **B.** Sternum, ribs, and costal cartilages forming the thoracic skeleton.

(Fig. 4.2). The **suprasternal (jugular) notch** is the easily palpable, concave notch on the superior border of the manubrium. The **clavicular notch** is an ovoid articular surface at each superolateral corner of the manubrium, on each side of the jugular notch. Each holds the sternal end of a clavicle.

The **body** is the relatively long, middle part of the sternum. It articulates above with the manubrium at the manubriosternal joint and below with the xiphoid process at the **xiphisternal joint**. It articulates with costal cartilages 2 to 7 on each side (see Fig. 4.1).

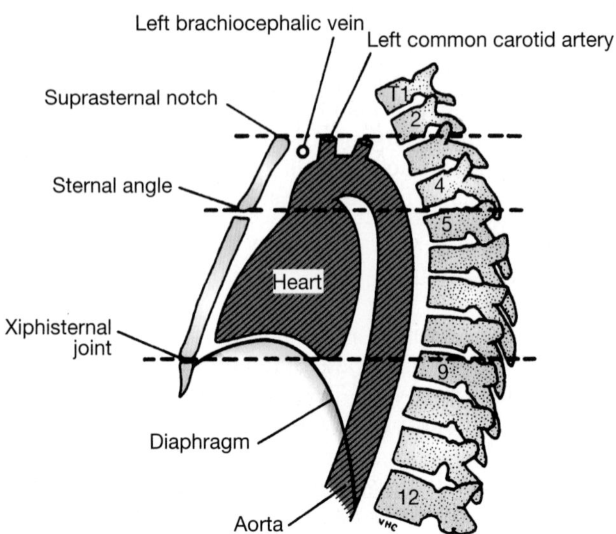

Figure 4.2 Lateral view of the thorax showing the relationship of the surface markings to the vertebral levels.

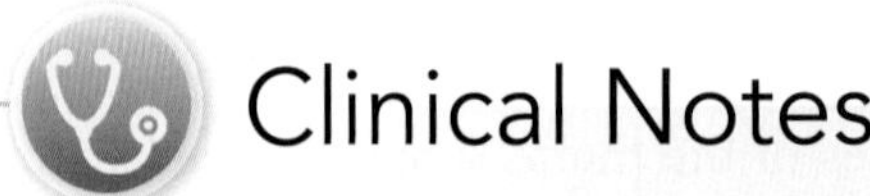

Sternum and Marrow Biopsy

The sternum is subcutaneous and readily palpable along its entire length. Like the ribs, it consists largely of highly vascular cancellous bone enclosed by a thin shell of compact bone. It possesses red hematopoietic marrow throughout life. Because of its morphology and shallow depth in the chest, the sternum can be punctured readily in a needle biopsy procedure (sternal puncture) for aspiration of red marrow. Under a local anesthetic, a wide-bore needle is inserted into the marrow cavity through the anterior surface of the bone. The sternum may also be split in surgery to allow the surgeon to gain easy access to the heart, great vessels, and thymus.

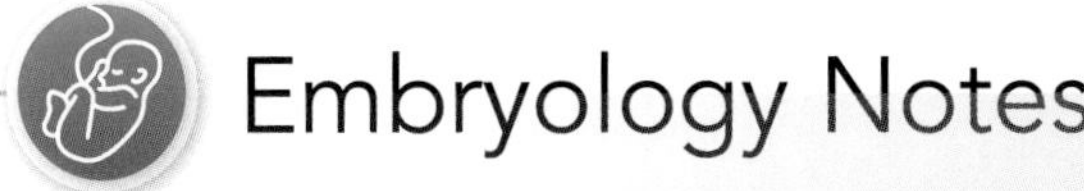

Embryology Notes

Sternum Development

The adult sternum consists of three parts: **manubrium**, **body**, and **xiphoid process** (see Fig. 4.1). Prenatally, it consists of six main parts. The first and last parts remain distinguishable as the manubrium and xiphoid process, respectively. The middle four parts (**sternebrae**) fuse to form the body. The three main parts were named after the resemblance of the sternum to the short sword favored by Roman troops and gladiators—thus, the manubrium (= handle), the body (in older terminology = gladiolus = small sword), and the xiphoid process (= sword point).

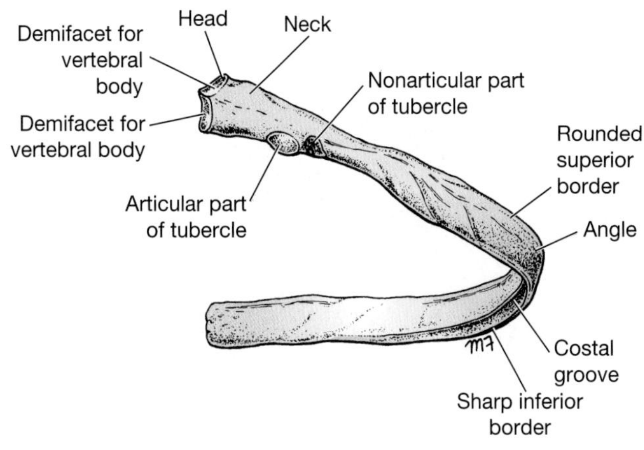

Figure 4.3 Right rib 5, as seen from the posterior aspect.

The **xiphoid process** (*xiph* is Greek for "sword") is the small, "pointed" (at its inferior end), most inferior part of the sternum. It is a thin plate of cartilage that becomes ossified at its proximal end during adult life. However, it is highly variable in size, shape, and degree of ossification. No ribs or costal cartilages attach to it. However, costal cartilage 7 may have a shared attachment with the xiphoid process and the body. The xiphisternal joint lies opposite the body of the T9 vertebra (see Fig. 4.2). The inferior end of the xiphoid provides attachment for the linea alba of the abdominal wall.

The articulation of the manubrium with the body forms the **sternal angle** (angle of Louis), which can be recognized by the presence of a transverse ridge on the anterior aspect of the sternum (see Figs. 4.1 and 4.2). The sternal angle is an important landmark for thoracic anatomy because it marks (1) the manubriosternal joint (a symphyseal joint), (2) the attachment points of the second costal cartilages (thus, these attach to both manubrium and body), (3) a horizontal line that typically projects posteriorly onto the T4 intervertebral disc, and (4) the plane of separation between the superior and inferior mediastina.

Ribs

Ribs (*cost* is Latin for "rib") are the elongate, flattened, arched bones that form a large part of the thoracic wall (see Fig. 4.1). They consist largely of highly vascular cancellous bone enclosed by a thin shell of compact bone. Normally, both males and females have 12 pairs of ribs. The posterior (dorsal; vertebral) end of each rib articulates with one or two thoracic vertebrae. The anterior (ventral; sternal) ends have variable relations that allow the ribs to be categorized as "true," "false," or "floating." **True ribs** (pairs 1 to 7) are connected directly to the sternum via individual costal cartilages. **False ribs** (pairs 8 to 10) are connected to the sternum via individual costal cartilages that join and attach collectively to the seventh costal cartilages. **Floating ribs** (pairs 11 to 12) do not attach to the sternum.

Typical Ribs

All ribs share a common structural floor plan. A typical rib is a long, twisted, flat bone having a rounded, smooth superior border and a sharp, thin inferior border (Figs. 4.3 and 4.4). The anterior end of each rib is attached to the corresponding costal cartilage (Fig. 4.4).

A rib has a head, neck, tubercle, body, angle, and costal groove. The **head** is the posterior (vertebral) end of the rib and has two facets for articulation with the numerically corresponding vertebral body and that of the vertebra immediately above (see Figs. 4.3 and 4.4). The **neck** is the flattened, slightly constricted portion situated between the head and the tubercle. The **tubercle** is a prominence on the outer posterior surface of the rib at the junction of the neck with the body. It has a facet for articulation with the transverse process of the numerically corresponding vertebra. The **body** (shaft) is the long, thin, flattened, and twisted (on its long axis) part that extends from the tubercle to the anterior (sternal) end. The **costal groove** is the elongate depression along the inferior aspect of the internal surface of the shaft of the rib. This holds the intercostal vessels and nerve. The **angle** is the point (usually slightly distal to the tubercle) at which the body of the rib bends sharply and turns from a lateral to a more anteriorly directed orientation. The **anterior (sternal) end** of the rib is flat and has a depression for the costal cartilage.

First Rib

The rib 1 is important clinically because of its close relationship to the lower nerves of the brachial plexus and the main vessels to the arm, namely, the subclavian artery and vein (Fig. 4.5). This rib is small and flattened from above downward. The scalenus anterior muscle is attached to its upper surface and inner border. Anterior to the scalenus anterior, the subclavian vein crosses the rib; posterior to the muscle attachment, the subclavian artery and the lower trunk of the brachial plexus cross the rib and lie in contact with the bone.

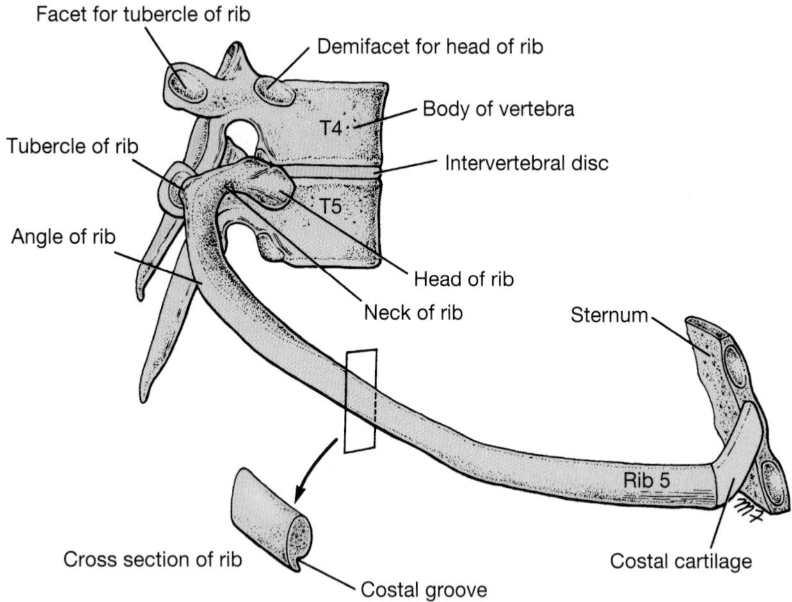

Figure 4.4 Right rib 5 as it articulates with the vertebral column posteriorly and the sternum anteriorly. Note that the rib head articulates with the vertebral body of its own number and that of the vertebra immediately above. Note also the presence of the costal groove along the inferior border of the rib.

Costal Cartilages

Costal cartilages are bars of cartilage connecting ribs 1 to 7 to the lateral edge of the sternum and ribs 8 to 10 to the cartilage immediately above. The cartilages of ribs 11 and 12 end in the abdominal musculature (see Fig. 4.1). The costal cartilages contribute significantly to the elasticity and mobility of the thoracic walls. In old age, the costal cartilages tend to lose some of their flexibility as the result of superficial calcification.

Vertebrae

The basic anatomy of vertebrae is described in Chapter 2. Normally, only the thoracic vertebrae carry ribs, and these vertebrae have unique structures for that purpose.

Costal facets (*facet* is Latin for "little face") are small articular surfaces at approximately the posterolateral aspect of the body, at the junction of the body and the pedicle (Fig. 4.6; see also Fig. 4.4). Typical thoracic vertebrae (T2 to T8) have two on each side. One is located

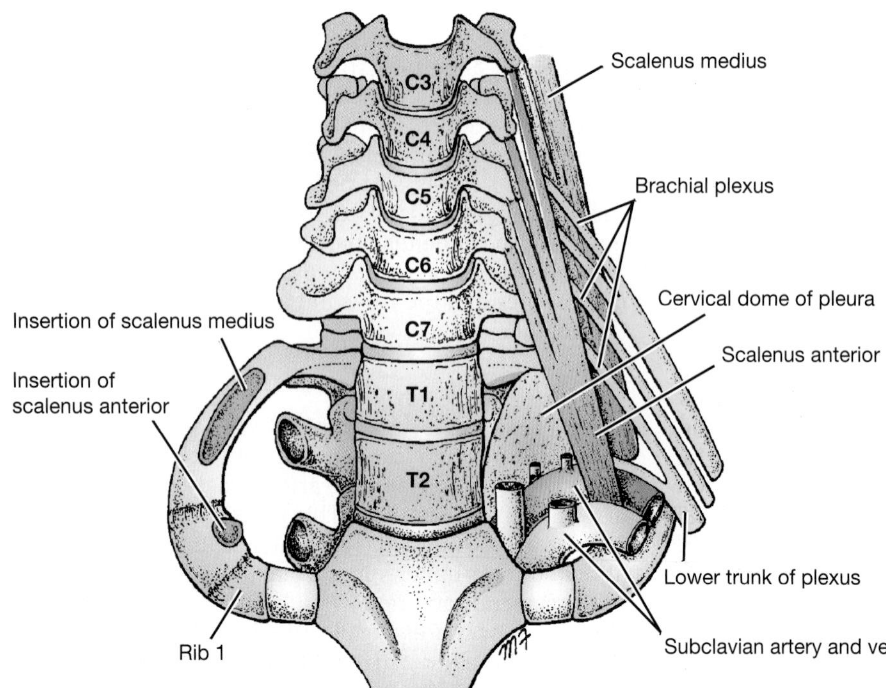

Figure 4.5 Thoracic outlet showing the cervical dome of pleura on the left side of the body and its relationship to the inner border of rib 1. Note also the presence of brachial plexus and subclavian vessels. (Anatomists often refer to the thoracic outlet as the thoracic inlet.)

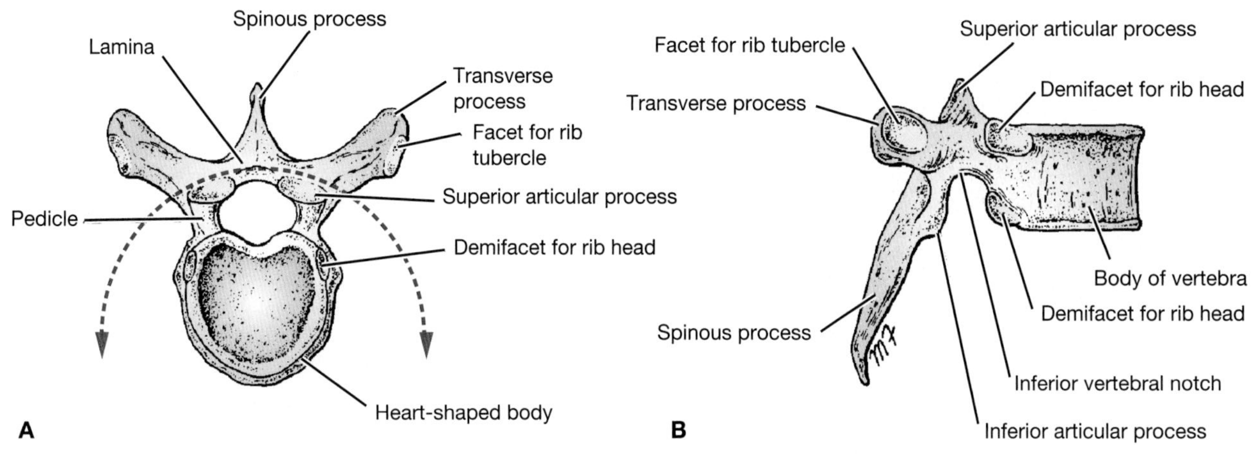

Figure 4.6 Thoracic vertebra. **A.** Superior surface. **B.** Lateral surface.

superiorly (**superior costal facet**). One is located inferiorly (**inferior costal facet**). These are the sites where the heads of the ribs articulate with the body. Adjacent typical thoracic vertebrae share the articulations of ribs. Thus, the head of an individual rib articulates with both the superior costal facet of the numerically corresponding vertebral body and the inferior costal facet of the vertebra immediately above. Because each of these facets carries half of the rib articulation, each is commonly termed a **demifacet** (*demi-* is French for "half"). The T1 vertebra has a full costal facet (instead of a superior demifacet) for the head of rib 1, plus an inferior demifacet for the superior half of the head of rib 2. (Think about these directional terms!) The T11 and T12 vertebrae each have full costal facets (located mainly on the pedicles) instead of demifacets because the heads of ribs 11 and 12 articulate only with their own individual vertebrae.

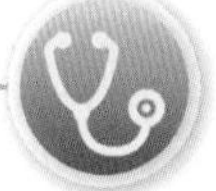

Clinical Notes

Cervical Rib

A cervical rib (ie, a rib arising from the anterior tubercle of the transverse process of the C7 vertebra) occurs in about 0.5% of humans (Fig. 4.7). It may have a free anterior end, may be connected to the first rib by a fibrous band, or may articulate with rib 1. The importance of a cervical rib is that it may apply pressure on the lower trunk of the brachial plexus, causing pain down the medial side of the forearm and hand and wasting of the small muscles of the hand. It can also exert pressure on the overlying subclavian artery and interfere with the circulation of the upper limb.

Rib Excision

To gain entrance to the thoracic cavity, thoracic surgeons commonly perform a rib excision. A longitudinal incision is made through the periosteum on the outer surface of the rib, and a segment of the rib is removed. A second longitudinal incision is then made through the bed of the rib, which is the inner covering of the periosteum. After the operation, the rib regenerates from the osteogenetic layer of the periosteum.

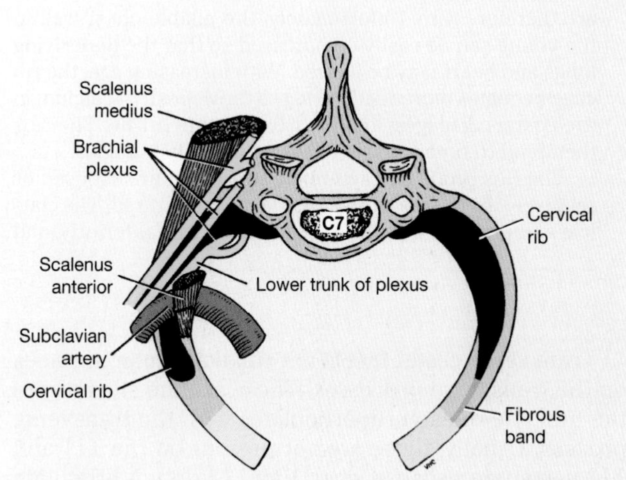

Figure 4.7 Thoracic outlet as seen from above. Note the presence of the cervical ribs (*black*) on both sides. On the right side of the thorax, the rib is almost complete and articulates anteriorly with rib 1. On the left side of the thorax, the rib is rudimentary but is continued forward as a fibrous band attached to costal cartilage 1. Note that the cervical rib may exert pressure on the lower trunk of the brachial plexus and may kink the subclavian artery.

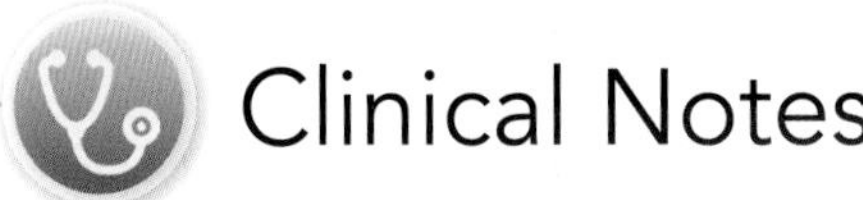

Clinical Notes

Thoracic Cage Distortion

The shape of the thorax can be distorted by congenital anomalies of the vertebral column or by the ribs. Destructive disease of the vertebral column that produces lateral flexion or scoliosis results in marked distortion of the thoracic cage.

Traumatic Injury to Thorax

Traumatic injury to the thorax is common, especially from motor vehicle accidents.

Sternum Fracture

The sternum is a resilient structure held in position by relatively pliable costal cartilages and bendable ribs. For these reasons, fracture of the sternum is not common; however, it does occur in high-speed motor vehicle accidents. Remember that the heart lies posterior to the sternum and may be severely contused by the sternum on impact.

Rib Contusion

Bruising of a rib, secondary to trauma, is the most common rib injury. In this painful condition, a small hemorrhage occurs beneath the periosteum.

Rib Fractures

Fractures of the ribs are common chest injuries. In children, the ribs are highly elastic, and fractures in this age group are therefore rare. Unfortunately, the pliable chest wall in the young can be easily compressed so that the underlying lungs and heart may be injured. With increasing age, the rib cage becomes more rigid, owing to the deposit of calcium in the costal cartilages, and the ribs become brittle. The ribs then tend to break at their weakest part, their angles.

The ribs prone to fracture are those that are exposed or relatively fixed. Ribs 5 to 10 are the most fractured. The clavicle and pectoral muscles protect ribs 1 to 4 anteriorly, and the scapula and its associated muscles do so posteriorly. Ribs 11 and 12 float and move with the force of impact.

Because the rib is sandwiched between the skin externally and the delicate pleura internally, not surprisingly, the jagged ends of a fractured rib may penetrate the lungs and present as a pneumothorax.

Severe localized pain is usually the most important symptom of a fractured rib. The intercostal nerves above and below the rib innervate the periosteum of each rib. To encourage the patient to breathe adequately, performing an intercostal nerve block may be necessary to relieve the pain.

Flail Chest

In severe crush injuries, several ribs may break. If limited to one side, the fractures may occur near the rib angles and anteriorly near the costochondral junctions. This causes flail chest, in which a section of the chest wall is disconnected from the rest of the thoracic wall. If the fractures occur on either side of the sternum, the sternum may be flail. In either case, the stability of the chest wall is lost, and the flail segment is sucked in during inspiration and driven out during expiration, producing paradoxical and ineffective respiratory movements.

Traumatic Injury to Back of Chest

The vertebral column forms the posterior midline wall of the chest. In severe posterior chest injuries, the possibility of a vertebral fracture with associated injury to the spinal cord should be considered. Also remember the presence of the scapula, which overlies the ribs 1 to 7. This bone is covered with muscles and is fractured only in cases of severe trauma.

Traumatic Injury to Abdominal Viscera and Chest

Recognizing that the upper abdominal organs—namely, the liver, stomach, and spleen—may be injured by trauma to the rib cage is important. In fact, any injury to the chest below the level of the nipple line may involve abdominal organs as well as thoracic organs.

Transverse costal facets are small articular surfaces on the transverse processes. These are the sites where the tubercle of each rib articulates with the transverse process. Usually, these are not present on the T11 and T12 vertebrae because ribs 11 and 12 do not articulate with the transverse processes.

JOINTS

Numerous joints link the elements of the thoracic cage and may limit or permit movement, depending on the specific joint. The intervertebral joints are described in Chapter 2. The sternal and costal joints are outlined below.

Sternal Joints

The manubriosternal joint is a cartilaginous joint between the manubrium and the body of the sternum. A small amount of angular movement is possible here during respiration. The xiphisternal joint is a cartilaginous joint between the xiphoid process and the body of the sternum. The xiphoid process usually fuses with the body of the sternum during middle age.

Joints of Heads of Ribs

Rib 1 and ribs 10 to 12 have a single synovial joint with their corresponding vertebral body. For ribs 2 to 9, the head articulates by means of a synovial joint with the corresponding vertebral body and that of the vertebra above it (see Fig. 4.4). A strong intra-articular ligament connects the head to the intervertebral disc.

Joints of Tubercles of Ribs

The tubercle of a rib articulates by means of a synovial joint with the transverse process of the corresponding vertebra (see Fig. 4.4). This joint is absent on ribs 11 and 12.

Joints of Ribs and Costal Cartilages

These joints are cartilaginous joints. No movement is possible here.

Joints of Costal Cartilages with Sternum

The first costal cartilages articulate with the manubrium by cartilaginous joints that do not permit movement (see Fig. 4.1). Costal cartilages 2 to 7 articulate with the lateral border of the sternum by synovial joints. In addition, costal cartilages 6 to 19 articulate with one another along their borders by small synovial joints. The cartilages of ribs 11 and 12 do not articulate with the sternum and are embedded in the abdominal musculature.

Rib and Costal Cartilage Movements

The first ribs and their costal cartilages are fixed to the manubrium and are immobile. Raising and lowering the ribs during respiration is accompanied by movements in both the joints of the head and the tubercle, permitting the neck of each rib to rotate around its own axis.

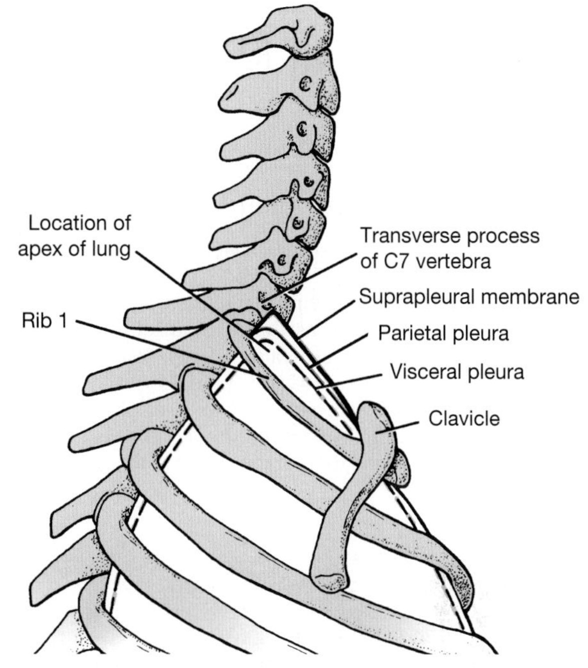

Figure 4.8 Lateral view of the upper opening of the thoracic cage showing how the apex of the lung projects superiorly into the root of the neck. The apex of the lung is covered with visceral and parietal layers of pleura and is protected by the suprapleural membrane, a thickening of the endothoracic fascia.

THORACIC OPENINGS

Numerous gaps connect the thorax with other regions and/or separate the bones of the thoracic cage from one another. Relatively large apertures occur at the upper and lower limits of the thorax, whereas relatively narrow and elongate intercostal spaces separate adjacent ribs.

Thoracic Apertures

The chest cavity communicates with the root of the neck through a narrow opening called the **superior thoracic aperture**, or **thoracic outlet** (see Fig. 4.5). This is called an outlet because important vessels and nerves emerge from the thorax here to enter the neck and upper limbs. The body of the T1 vertebra forms the posterior boundary of the thoracic outlet, the medial edges of the first ribs and their costal cartilages mark the lateral boundaries, and the superior margin of the manubrium sterni forms the anterior border. The outlet is obliquely directed, facing upward and forward, and conveys the esophagus, trachea, and several vessels and nerves. Because of the angled tilt of the opening, the apices of the lungs and pleurae project upward into the neck (Fig. 4.8).

The thoracic cavity communicates with the abdomen through a large opening called the **inferior thoracic aperture** (see Fig. 4.2). The body of the T12 vertebra forms the posterior boundary of this opening, the curving costal margin marks its lateral boundaries, and the xiphisternal joint forms the anterior border. The diaphragm closes the inferior aperture. Structures that pass between the thoracic and abdominal cavities (eg, esophagus, aorta) must either pierce the diaphragm or go around it.

Suprapleural Membrane

The thoracic outlet transmits structures that pass between the thorax and the neck (esophagus, trachea, blood vessels, etc.) and for the most part lie close to the midline. A dense fascial layer called the **suprapleural membrane** closes the thoracic outlet on either side of these structures (see Fig. 4.8). This tent-shaped fibrous sheet attaches laterally to the medial border of rib 1 and costal cartilage; medially to the fascia investing the structures passing from the thorax into the neck; and, at its apex, to the tip of the transverse process of the C7 vertebra. It protects the underlying cervical pleura and resists the changes in intrathoracic pressure occurring during respiratory movements.

Endothoracic Fascia

The endothoracic fascia is a thin layer of loose connective tissue that separates the parietal pleura from the thoracic wall. The suprapleural membrane is a thickening of this fascia.

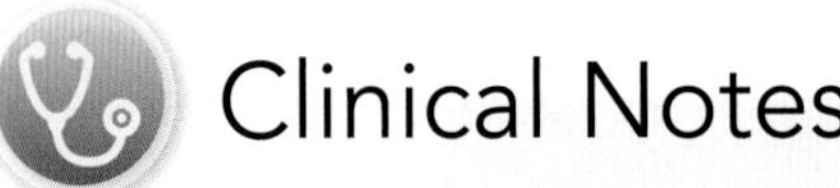

Clinical Notes

Thoracic Outlet Syndrome

The brachial plexus of nerves (C5 to C8 and T1) and the subclavian artery and vein are closely related to the upper surface of rib 1 and the clavicle as they enter the upper limb (see Fig. 4.5). Obstruction of the thoracic outlet may compress these neurovascular structures in this area, a condition known as **thoracic outlet syndrome**. Most of the symptoms are caused by pressure on the lower trunk of the plexus, causing pain down the medial side of the forearm and hand and wasting of the small muscles of the hand. Pressure on the blood vessels may compromise the circulation of the upper limb.

Intercostal Spaces

Intercostal spaces are the gaps between adjacent ribs. A needle passing through the entire depth of an intercostal space must penetrate seven structural layers (Fig. 4.9). These are most pronounced in the lateral aspect of the thoracic wall. In superficial to deep sequence, the layers are the following:

1. Skin
2. Superficial fascia
3. Deep fascia
4. Intercostal muscles
5. Endothoracic fascia
6. Extrapleural fatty layer
7. Parietal pleura

Depending on the specific location on the thoracic wall, an additional layer of muscle, the serratus anterior, may cover the intercostal muscle layer. The three intercostal muscles all act as muscles of respiration. From superficial to deep, these are the external, internal, and innermost intercostal muscles. The innermost intercostal muscle is lined internally by the endothoracic fascia, which is lined internally by a highly variable extrapleural fatty layer and then the parietal pleura. The intercostal nerves and blood vessels run between the intermediate and deepest layers of muscles.

MUSCLES

The muscles of the thoracic walls are summarized in Table 4.1.

Intercostal Muscles

Three intercostal muscles fill the intercostal spaces. The **external intercostal muscle** is the most superficial of the three muscle layers (see Fig. 4.9). Its fibers are directed downward and forward from the inferior border of the rib above to the superior border of the rib below. The muscle extends forward to the costal cartilage where it is replaced by an aponeurosis, the **anterior (external) intercostal membrane** (Fig. 4.10).

The **internal intercostal muscle** forms the intermediate layer (see Fig. 4.9). Its fibers are directed downward and backward from the subcostal groove of the rib above to the upper border of the rib below. The muscle extends backward from the sternum in front to the angles of the ribs behind, where the muscle is replaced

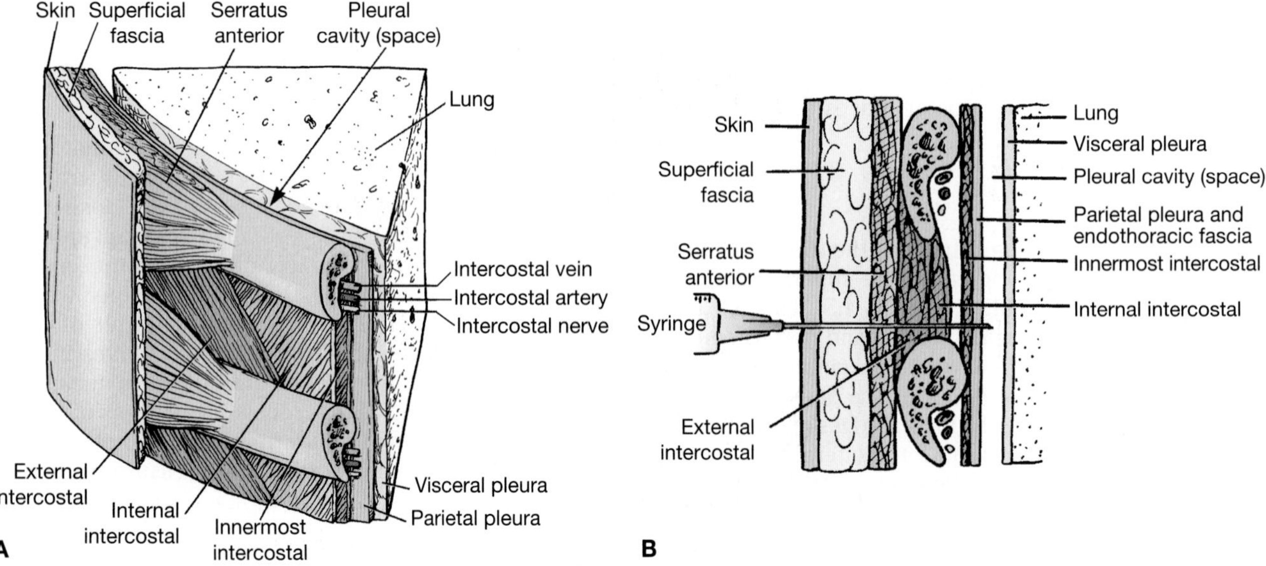

Figure 4.9 **A.** Section through an intercostal space. **B.** Structures penetrated by a needle when it passes from skin surface to pleural cavity. Depending on the site of penetration, the pectoral muscles will be pierced in addition to the serratus anterior muscle.

Table 4.1 Thorax Muscles

NAME OF MUSCLE	ORIGIN	INSERTION	NERVE SUPPLY	ACTION
External intercostal muscle (11) (fibers pass downward and forward)	Inferior border of rib	Superior border of rib below	Intercostal nerves	Stabilize the rib cage: With first rib fixed, they raise ribs during inspiration and thus increase anteroposterior and transverse diameters of thorax
Internal intercostal muscle (11) (fibers pass downward and backward)	Inferior border of rib	Superior border of rib below	Intercostal nerves	Stabilize the rib cage: With last rib fixed by abdominal muscles, they lower ribs during expiration
Innermost intercostal muscle (incomplete layer)	Adjacent ribs	Adjacent ribs	Intercostal nerves	Assists external and internal intercostal muscles
Diaphragm	Xiphoid process; costal cartilages 5 to 10, L1 to L3 vertebrae	Central tendon	Phrenic nerve	Most important muscle of inspiration; increases vertical diameter of thorax by pulling central tendon downward; assists in raising lower ribs; also used in abdominal straining and weightlifting
Levatores costarum (12)	Tip of transverse process of C7 and T1 to T11 vertebrae	Rib below	Posterior rami of thoracic spinal nerves	Elevates ribs; possibly proprioception
Serratus posterior superior	Lower cervical and upper thoracic spines	Upper ribs	Intercostal nerves	Proprioception; possibly raises ribs and therefore an inspiratory muscle
Serratus posterior inferior	Upper lumbar and lower thoracic spines	Lower ribs	Intercostal nerves	Proprioception; possibly depresses ribs and therefore an expiratory muscle

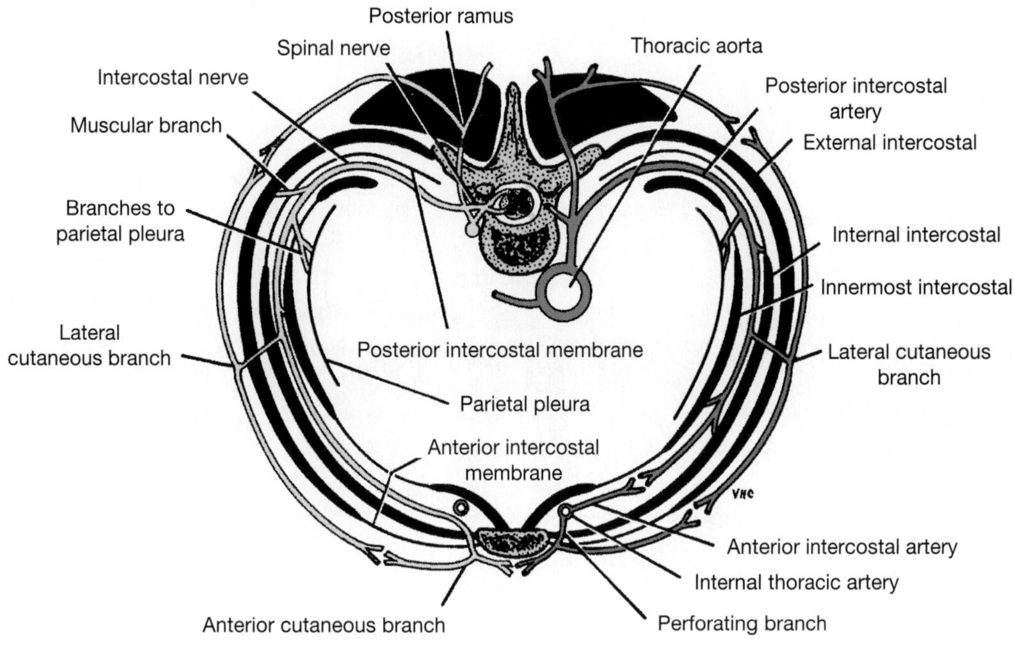

Figure 4.10 Cross section of the thorax showing distribution of a typical intercostal nerve and a posterior and an anterior intercostal artery.

by an aponeurosis, the **posterior (internal) intercostal membrane** (see Fig. 4.10).

The **innermost intercostal muscle** forms the deepest layer (see Fig. 4.9) and corresponds to the transversus abdominis muscle in the anterior abdominal wall. It is an incomplete muscle layer and crosses more than one intercostal space. It is related internally to the endothoracic fascia and parietal pleura and externally to the intercostal nerves and vessels. The innermost intercostal muscle can be divided into three portions, which are more or less separate from one another (see Fig. 4.10). The anterior portion is the **transversus thoracis** muscle, the lateral portion is the **innermost intercostal** muscle, and the posterior portion is the **subcostalis** muscle.

Actions

The primary function of the intercostal muscles during respiration appears to be to stabilize the position of the ribs to maintain the intercostal spaces. Their actions in elevation (external intercostals) and depression (internal intercostals) of the ribs are most likely to occur during forced respiration. In addition, the tone of the intercostal muscles during the different phases of respiration serves to strengthen the tissues of the intercostal spaces, thus preventing the sucking in or the blowing out of the tissues with changes in intrathoracic pressure. For further details concerning the action of these muscles, see Mechanics of Respiration later in this chapter.

Nerve Supply

The corresponding intercostal nerves supply the intercostal muscles. The intercostal nerves and blood vessels (neurovascular bundle), as in the abdominal wall, run between the middle and innermost layers of muscles (see Figs. 4.9A and 4.10). They are arranged in the following order from above downward: intercostal vein, intercostal artery, and intercostal nerve (ie, VAN).

Diaphragm

The diaphragm is a thin muscular and tendinous septum that separates the chest cavity above from the abdominal cavity below (Fig. 4.11). Structures that pass between the thoracic and abdominal cavities (eg, esophagus, aorta) must either pierce the diaphragm or go around it.

The diaphragm is the most important muscle of respiration. It is dome shaped and consists of a peripheral muscular part, which arises from the margins of the thorax, and a centrally placed tendon. The origin of the diaphragm can be divided into three parts: a **sternal part** arising from the posterior surface of the xiphoid process, a **costal part** arising from the deep surfaces of ribs 7 to 12 and their costal cartilages, and a **vertebral part** arising by vertical columns (crura) and from the arcuate ligaments. The **right crus** arises from the sides of the bodies of the L1 to L3 vertebrae and the intervertebral discs. The **left crus** arises from the sides of the bodies of the L1 and L2 vertebrae and the intervertebral disc. Lateral to the crura, the diaphragm arises from the **medial** and **lateral arcuate ligaments**. The medial arcuate ligament extends from the side of the body of the L2 vertebra to the tip of the transverse process of the L1 vertebra. The lateral arcuate ligament extends from the tip of the transverse process of the L1 vertebra to the lower border of rib 12. The **median arcuate ligament**,

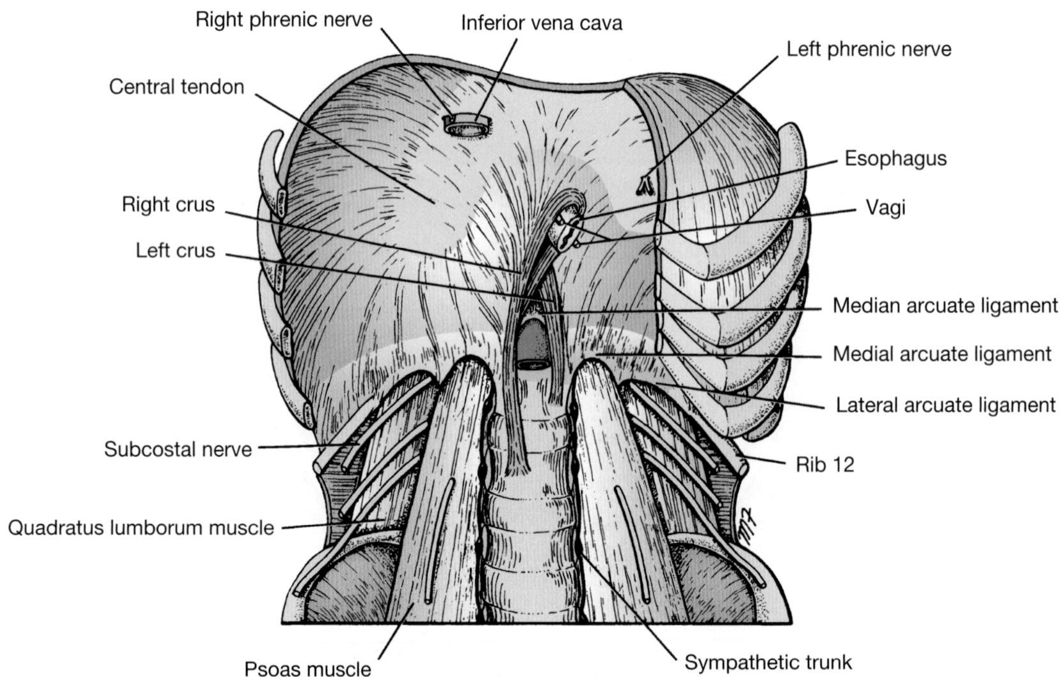

Figure 4.11 Diaphragm as seen from below. The anterior portion of the right side has been removed. Note the sternal, costal, and vertebral origins of the muscle and the important structures that pass through it.

which crosses over the anterior surface of the aorta, connects the medial borders of the two crura.

The diaphragm inserts into a **central tendon**, which is shaped like three leaves. The superior surface of the tendon is partially fused with the inferior surface of the fibrous pericardium. Some of the muscle fibers of the right crus pass up to the left and surround the esophageal orifice in a sling like loop. These fibers appear to act as a sphincter and possibly assist in the prevention of regurgitation of the stomach contents into the thoracic part of the esophagus.

Diaphragm Shape

As seen from in front, the diaphragm curves up into **right** and **left domes** (**cupulae**). The right dome reaches as high as the upper border of rib 5, and the left dome may reach the lower border. The right dome lies at a higher level because of the large size of the right lobe of the liver. The central tendon lies at the level of the xiphisternal joint. The domes support the right and left lungs, whereas the central tendon supports the heart. The levels of the diaphragm vary with the phase of respiration, posture, and the degree of distention of the abdominal viscera. The diaphragm is lower when a person is sitting or standing; it is higher in the supine position and after a large meal.

When seen from the side, the diaphragm has the appearance of an inverted "J," with the long limb extending up from the vertebral column, and the short limb extending forward to the xiphoid process (see Fig. 4.2).

Blood Supply of the Diaphragm

Blood vessels supply and drain the diaphragm on both its superior (thoracic) and inferior (abdominal) sides. The **superior phrenic arteries** (branches of the thoracic aorta) and **pericardiacophrenic** and **musculophrenic arteries** (branches of the internal thoracic arteries) supply the superior aspect. The **inferior phrenic arteries** (usually the first branches of the abdominal aorta) supply the inferior side. The primary veins draining the diaphragm follow the arteries.

Nerve Supply of the Diaphragm

The right and left phrenic nerves (C3 to C5) provide the entire motor supply to the diaphragm. Each phrenic nerve distributes across the inferior side of the diaphragm and supplies approximately the ipsilateral half of the diaphragm. Thus, functionally, the diaphragm operates as two hemidiaphragms.

The phrenic nerves also carry most of the sensation from the parietal pleura and peritoneum covering the central surfaces of the diaphragm. Intercostal nerves 6 to 11 and the subcostal nerves supply the periphery of the diaphragm.

Diaphragmatic Action

On contraction, the diaphragm pulls down its central tendon and increases the vertical diameter of the thorax. Thus, the diaphragm flattens during contraction (inspiration) and elevates during relaxation (expiration).

Diaphragmatic Function

The diaphragm has four main functions:

- **Muscle of inspiration:** On contraction, the diaphragm pulls its central tendon down and increases the vertical diameter of the thorax. The diaphragm is the most important muscle used in inspiration.
- **Muscle of abdominal straining:** The contraction of the diaphragm assists the contraction of the muscles of the anterolateral abdominal wall in raising the intra-abdominal pressure for micturition, defecation, and parturition. Taking a deep breath and closing the glottis of the larynx further aids this mechanism. The diaphragm is unable to rise because of the air trapped in the respiratory tract. Now and again, air is allowed to escape, producing a grunting sound.
- **Weight-lifting muscle:** In a person taking a deep breath and holding it (fixing the diaphragm), the diaphragm assists the muscles of the anterolateral abdominal wall in raising the intra-abdominal pressure to such an extent that it helps support the vertebral column and prevent flexion. This greatly assists the postvertebral muscles in the lifting of heavy weights. Needless to say, adequate sphincteric control of the bladder and anal canal is important under these circumstances.
- **Thoracoabdominal pump:** The descent of the diaphragm decreases the intrathoracic pressure and, at the same time, increases the intra-abdominal pressure. This pressure change compresses the blood in the inferior vena cava and forces it upward into the right atrium of the heart. Lymph within the abdominal lymph vessels is also compressed, and the negative intrathoracic pressure aids its passage upward within the thoracic duct. The presence of valves within the thoracic duct prevents backflow.

Diaphragm Openings

The diaphragm has three main openings (see Fig. 4.11):

- The **aortic opening** lies anterior to the body of the T12 vertebra and between the crura. It transmits the aorta, the thoracic duct, and the azygos vein. Notice that the aortic opening is not a true opening within the diaphragm. Rather, it is a gap behind the posterior margin of the diaphragm.
- The **esophageal opening** lies at the level of the T10 vertebra in a sling of muscle fibers derived from the right crus. It transmits the esophagus, right and left vagus nerves, esophageal branches of the left gastric vessels, and the lymphatics from the lower third of the esophagus.
- The **caval opening** lies at the level of the T8 vertebra, in the central tendon. It transmits the inferior vena cava and terminal branches of the right phrenic nerve.

In addition to these openings, the sympathetic splanchnic nerves pierce the crura, the sympathetic trunks pass posterior to the medial arcuate ligament on each side, and the superior epigastric vessels pass between the sternal and costal origins of the diaphragm on each side.

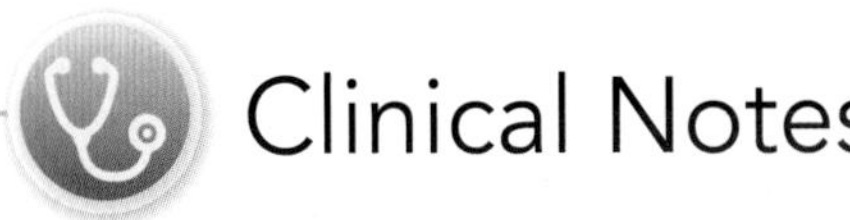

Clinical Notes

Hiccup

Hiccup is the involuntary spasmodic contraction of the diaphragm accompanied by the approximation of the vocal folds and closure of the glottis of the larynx. It is a common condition in normal individuals and occurs after eating or drinking because of gastric irritation of the vagus nerve endings. However, it may be a symptom of disease such as pleurisy, peritonitis, pericarditis, or uremia.

Diaphragm Paralysis

A single dome of the diaphragm (ie, a hemidiaphragm) may be paralyzed by crushing or sectioning of the phrenic nerve in the neck. This may be necessary in the treatment of certain forms of lung tuberculosis when the physician wishes to rest the lower lobe of the lung on one side. Occasionally, the contribution from the C5 spinal nerve joins the phrenic nerve late as a branch from the nerve to the subclavius muscle. This is known as an **accessory phrenic nerve**. To obtain complete paralysis under these circumstances, the nerve to the subclavius muscle must also be sectioned. Recognize that a paralyzed hemidiaphragm assumes a hyperelevated posture rather than a depressed (flattened) posture.

Penetrating Injuries to Diaphragm

Penetrating injuries to the diaphragm can result from stab or bullet wounds to the chest or abdomen. Any penetrating wound to the chest below the level of the nipples should be suspected of causing damage to the diaphragm until proved otherwise. The arching domes of the diaphragm can reach the level of rib 5 (the right dome can reach a higher level).

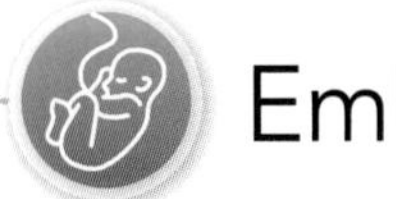

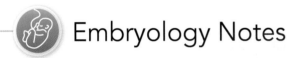

Embryology Notes

Diaphragm Development

The diaphragm is formed from the following structures: (a) **septum transversum**, which forms the muscle and central tendon; (b) two **pleuroperitoneal membranes**, which are largely responsible for the peripheral areas of the diaphragmatic pleura and peritoneum that cover its upper and lower surfaces, respectively; and (c) **dorsal mesentery of the esophagus**, in which the crura develop.

The septum transversum is a mass of mesoderm that is formed in the neck by the fusion of the myotomes of the C3 to C5 cervical segments. With the descent of the heart from the neck to the thorax, the septum is pushed caudally, pulling its nerve supply with it. Thus, cervical nerves C3 to C5 form the phrenic nerve, which supplies the diaphragm.

The pleuroperitoneal membranes grow medially from the body wall on each side until they fuse with the septum transversum anterior to the esophagus and with the dorsal mesentery posterior to the esophagus. During the process of fusion, the mesoderm of the septum transversum extends into the other parts, forming all the musculature of the diaphragm.

The motor nerve supply to the entire muscle of the diaphragm is the phrenic nerve. The central pleura on the upper surface of the diaphragm and the peritoneum on the lower surface are also formed from the septum transversum, which explains their sensory innervation from the phrenic nerve. The sensory innervation of the peripheral parts of the pleura and peritoneum covering the peripheral areas of the upper and lower surfaces of the diaphragm is from the T7 to T12 nerves. This is understandable, because the peripheral pleura and peritoneum from the pleuroperitoneal membranes are derived from the body wall.

Diaphragmatic Hernias

Congenital hernias occur as the result of incomplete fusion of the septum transversum, the dorsal mesentery, and the pleuroperitoneal membranes from the body wall. The hernias occur at the following sites: (a) pleuroperitoneal canal (more common on the left side; caused by failure of fusion of the septum transversum with the pleuroperitoneal membrane), (b) opening between the xiphoid and costal origins of the diaphragm, and (c) esophageal hiatus.

Acquired hernias may occur in middle-age people with weak musculature around the esophageal opening in the diaphragm. These hernias may be either sliding (hiatal) or paraesophageal (Fig. 4.12).

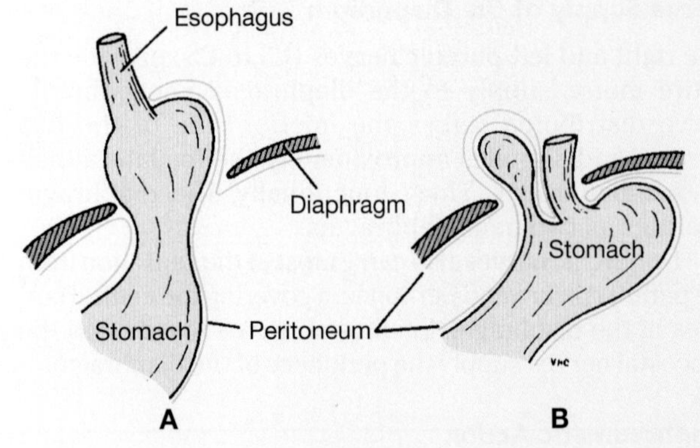

Figure 4.12 **A.** Sliding esophageal hernia. **B.** Paraesophageal hernia.

Levatores Costarum

The levatores costarum muscles comprise 12 pairs. Each is triangular and inserts into the rib below its origin. They elevate the ribs, but their role in respiration is questionable. They may serve as proprioceptive devices.

Serratus Posterior Muscles

The **serratus posterior superior** and **serratus posterior inferior** are thin, flat muscles that comprise the intermediate layer of muscles of the back (see Chapter 2). The superior muscle passes downward and laterally and inserts into the upper ribs. The inferior muscle passes upward and laterally and inserts into the lower ribs. Both are supplied by adjacent intercostal nerves.

Traditionally, these muscles have been described as respiratory muscles because of their alignments, with the superior muscle denoted as acting in inspiration to elevate the ribs, and the inferior muscle acting in expiration to depress the ribs. However, more recent work suggests both muscles may have proprioceptive functions rather than motor actions.

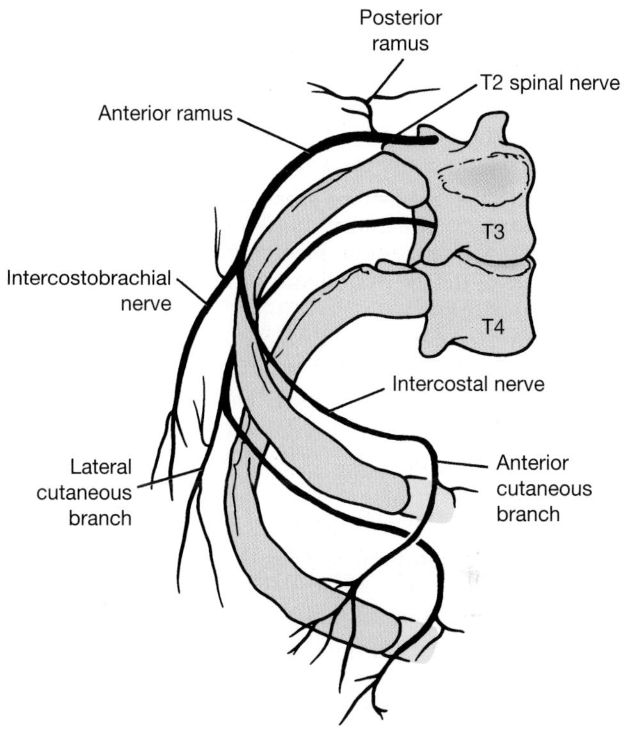

Figure 4.13 The distribution of two intercostal nerves relative to the rib cage.

THORACIC WALL NERVES

The **intercostal nerves** supply the entire thoracic wall. These nerves are the anterior rami of the T1 to T11 spinal nerves (Fig. 4.13; see also Fig. 4.10). The anterior ramus of the T12 nerve lies in the abdomen and runs forward in the abdominal wall as the **subcostal nerve**.

Each intercostal nerve enters an intercostal space between the parietal pleura and the posterior intercostal membrane (see Figs. 4.9 and 4.10). It then runs forward inferiorly to the intercostal vessels in the subcostal groove of the corresponding rib, between the innermost intercostal and internal intercostal muscles (Fig. 4.14; see also Figs. 4.9 and 4.10). Nerves 1 to 6 are distributed within their intercostal spaces. Intercostal nerves 7 to 9 leave the anterior ends of their intercostal spaces by passing deep to the costal cartilages, to enter the anterior abdominal wall. Nerves 10 and 11 pass directly into the abdominal wall.

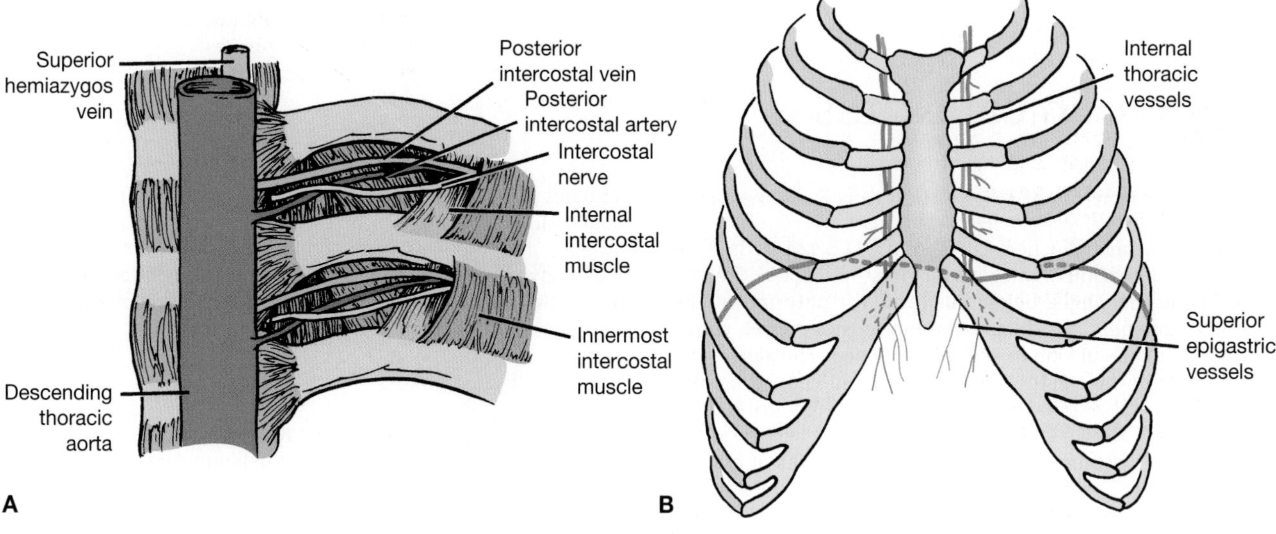

Figure 4.14 **A.** Internal view of the posterior end of two typical intercostal spaces; the posterior intercostal membrane has been removed for clarity. **B.** Anterior view of the chest showing the courses of the internal thoracic vessels. These vessels descend about one fingerbreadth from the lateral margin of the sternum.

Branches

See Figures 4.10 and 4.13.

- **Rami communicantes** connect the intercostal nerve to a ganglion of the sympathetic trunk (see Fig. 1.23). The gray and white rami are adjacent to one another.
- The **collateral branch** runs forward inferiorly to the main nerve on the upper border of the rib below.
- The **lateral cutaneous branch** reaches the skin on the side of the chest. It divides into an anterior and a posterior branch.
- The **anterior cutaneous branch**, which is the terminal portion of the main trunk, reaches the skin near the midline. It divides into a medial and a lateral branch.
- **Muscular branches** run to the intercostal muscles.
- **Pleural sensory branches** go to the parietal pleura.
- **Peritoneal sensory branches** (7th to 11th intercostal nerves only) run to the parietal peritoneum.

The **first intercostal nerve** joins the brachial plexus by a large branch that is equivalent to the lateral cutaneous branch of typical intercostal nerves. The remainder of the first intercostal nerve is small, and an anterior cutaneous branch does not exist.

The **second intercostal nerve** joins the medial cutaneous nerve of the arm by a large branch named the **intercostobrachial nerve** (see Fig. 3.32), which is equivalent to the lateral cutaneous branch of other nerves. Therefore, the second intercostal nerve supplies the skin of the armpit and the upper medial side of the arm. In coronary artery disease, pain is referred along this nerve to the medial side of the arm.

With the exceptions noted, the first six intercostal nerves supply the skin and the parietal pleura covering the outer and inner surfaces of each intercostal space, respectively, plus the intercostal muscles of each intercostal space and the levatores costarum and serratus posterior muscles.

In addition, the 7th to 11th intercostal nerves supply the skin and the parietal peritoneum covering the outer and inner surfaces of the abdominal wall, respectively, plus the anterolateral abdominal wall muscles (which include the external oblique, internal oblique, transversus abdominis, and rectus abdominis muscles).

THORACIC WALL VASCULATURE

The **subclavian artery**, **axillary artery**, and **thoracic aorta** supply the thoracic walls. The subclavian artery provides blood through its **superior intercostal** and **internal thoracic** branches. The axillary artery supplies via its **superior thoracic** and **lateral thoracic** branches. The thoracic aorta gives off **posterior intercostal** and **subcostal** branches.

Internal Thoracic Artery

The internal thoracic artery supplies the anterior wall of the body from the clavicle to the umbilicus. It is a branch of the first part of the subclavian artery in the neck. It descends vertically on the pleura behind the costal cartilages, a fingerbreadth lateral to the sternum, and ends in intercostal space 6 by dividing into the superior epigastric and musculophrenic arteries (see Figs. 4.10 and 4.14B).

Branches

- Two **anterior intercostal arteries** supply intercostal spaces 1 to 6.
- **Perforating arteries** accompany the terminal branches of the corresponding intercostal nerves.
- The **pericardiacophrenic artery** accompanies the phrenic nerve and supplies the pericardium.
- **Mediastinal arteries** supply the contents of the anterior mediastinum (eg, the thymus).
- The **superior epigastric artery** enters the rectus sheath of the anterior abdominal wall and supplies the rectus muscle as far as the umbilicus.
- The **musculophrenic artery** runs around the costal margin of the diaphragm and supplies the lower intercostal spaces and the diaphragm.

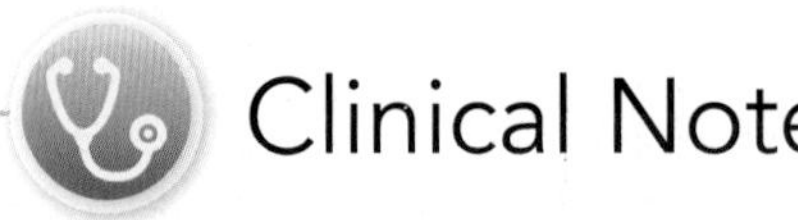

Clinical Notes

Skin Innervation of Chest Wall and Referred Pain

The supraclavicular nerves (C3 and C4) provide the cutaneous innervation of the anterior chest wall above the level of the sternal angle. Below this level, the anterior and lateral cutaneous branches of the intercostal nerves supply oblique bands of skin in regular sequence. The skin on the posterior surface of the chest wall is supplied by the posterior rami of the spinal nerves. The arrangement of the dermatomes is shown in Figures 1.25 and 1.26.

An intercostal nerve not only supplies areas of skin but also supplies the ribs, costal cartilages, intercostal muscles, and parietal pleura lining the intercostal space. Furthermore, intercostal nerves 7 to 11 leave the thoracic wall and enter the anterior abdominal wall to supply dermatomes on the anterior abdominal wall, muscles of the anterior abdominal wall, and parietal peritoneum. This latter fact is of great clinical importance because it means that disease in the thoracic wall may be revealed as pain in a dermatome that extends across the costal margin into the anterior abdominal wall. For example, a pulmonary thromboembolism or pneumonia with pleurisy involving the costal parietal pleura could give rise to abdominal pain and tenderness and rigidity of the abdominal musculature. The abdominal pain in these instances is called **referred pain**.

Herpes Zoster

Herpes zoster, or **shingles**, is a relatively common condition caused by the reactivation of the latent varicella-zoster virus in a patient who has previously had chickenpox. The lesion is seen as an inflammation and degeneration of the sensory neurons in a cranial or spinal nerve with the formation of vesicles and inflammation of the skin. In the thorax, the first symptom is a band of dermatomal pain in the distribution of the sensory neurons in a thoracic spinal nerve, followed in a few days by a skin eruption. The condition occurs most frequently in patients older than age 50 years.

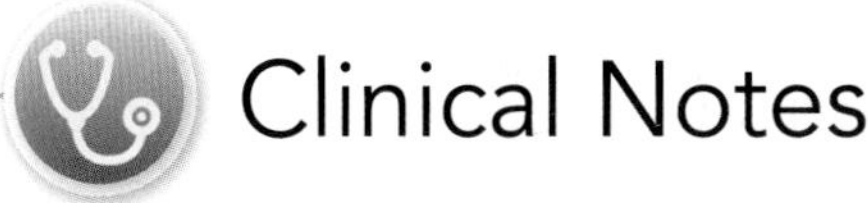

Intercostal Nerve Block

The skin and the parietal pleura cover the outer and inner surfaces of each intercostal space, respectively. Intercostal nerves 7 to 11 supply the skin and the parietal peritoneum covering the outer and inner surfaces of the anterolateral abdominal wall, respectively. Therefore, an intercostal nerve block will also anesthetize these areas. In addition, the periosteum of the adjacent ribs is anesthetized.

Indications

Intercostal nerve block is indicated for repair of lacerations of the thoracic and abdominal walls, for relief of pain in rib fractures, and to allow pain-free respiratory movements.

Procedure

To produce analgesia of the anterior and lateral thoracic and abdominal walls, the intercostal nerve should be blocked before the lateral cutaneous branch arises at the midaxillary line. The ribs may be identified by counting down from rib 2 (opposite the sternal angle) or up from rib 12. The needle is directed toward the rib near the lower border (see Fig. 4.9B), and the tip comes to rest near the subcostal groove, where the local anesthetic is infiltrated around the nerve. Remember that the order of structures lying in the neurovascular bundle from above downward is intercostal vein, artery, and nerve and that these structures are situated between the posterior intercostal membrane of the internal intercostal muscle and the parietal pleura (see Figs. 4.9 and 4.10). Furthermore, laterally, the nerve lies between the internal intercostal muscle and the innermost intercostal muscle (see Fig. 4.14A).

Anatomy of Complications

Pneumothorax can occur if the needlepoint misses the subcostal groove and penetrates too deeply through the parietal pleura. **Hemorrhage** is caused by the puncture of the intercostal blood vessels. This is a common complication, so aspiration should always be performed before injecting the anesthetic. A small hematoma may result.

Internal Thoracic Vein

The internal thoracic vein accompanies the internal thoracic artery and drains into the brachiocephalic vein on each side.

Intercostal Arteries and Veins

Each intercostal space contains a large single posterior intercostal artery and two small anterior intercostal arteries (see Figs. 4.10 and 4.14A).

- The **posterior intercostal arteries** of the first two spaces are branches from the superior intercostal artery, a branch of the costocervical trunk of the subclavian artery. The posterior intercostal arteries of the lower nine spaces are branches of the descending thoracic aorta.
- The **anterior intercostal arteries** of spaces 1 to 6 are branches of the internal thoracic artery, which arises from the first part of the subclavian artery. The anterior intercostal arteries of spaces 7 to 11 are branches of the musculophrenic artery, one of the terminal branches of the internal thoracic artery.

Each intercostal artery gives off branches to the muscles, skin, and parietal pleura. The branches to the superficial structures are particularly large in the breast region in females. The anterior and posterior intercostal arteries typically anastomose with one another at approximately the costochondral junctions.

The corresponding **posterior intercostal veins** drain posteriorly into the **azygos** or **hemiazygos veins** (Fig. 4.15; see also Fig. 4.14A). The **anterior intercostal veins** drain anteriorly into the internal thoracic and musculophrenic veins.

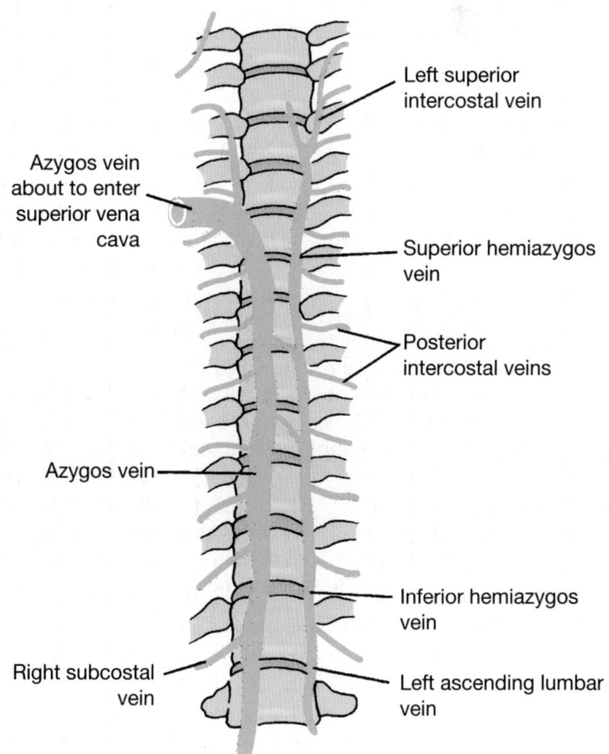

Figure 4.15 Common arrangement of the azygos vein, superior hemiazygos (accessory hemiazygos) vein, and inferior hemiazygos (hemiazygos) vein.

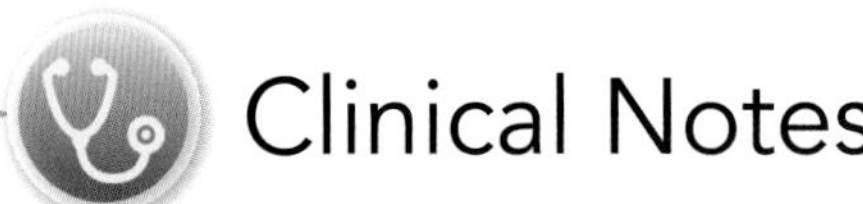

Clinical Notes

Internal Thoracic Artery in Coronary Artery Disease Treatment

In patients with occlusive coronary disease caused by atherosclerosis, the diseased arterial segment can be bypassed by inserting a graft. The graft most used is the great saphenous vein of the leg. However, the myocardium can be revascularized in some patients by surgically mobilizing one of the internal thoracic arteries and joining its distal cut end to a coronary artery.

Arterial Anastomoses

The anterior intercostal arteries (branches of the subclavian artery via the internal thoracic and musculophrenic arteries) and the lower nine posterior intercostal arteries (branches of the thoracic aorta) typically anastomose with one another at approximately the costochondral junctions (see Fig. 4.10). These important connections create collateral circulatory routes that potentially allow blood flow to bypass obstructions in the thoracic aorta or the proximal part of the subclavian artery. These anastomoses are notably prominent in circumventing the constriction present in **postductal coarctation of the aorta**.

Thoracic Wall Lymph Drainage

The lymph drainage of the skin of the anterior chest wall passes to the **anterior axillary lymph nodes**; that from the posterior chest wall passes to the **posterior axillary nodes** (Fig. 4.16). The lymph drainage of the intercostal spaces passes forward to the **internal thoracic nodes**, situated along the internal thoracic artery, and posteriorly to the **posterior intercostal nodes** and the **para-aortic nodes** in the posterior mediastinum. The lymphatic drainage of the breast is described in Chapter 3.

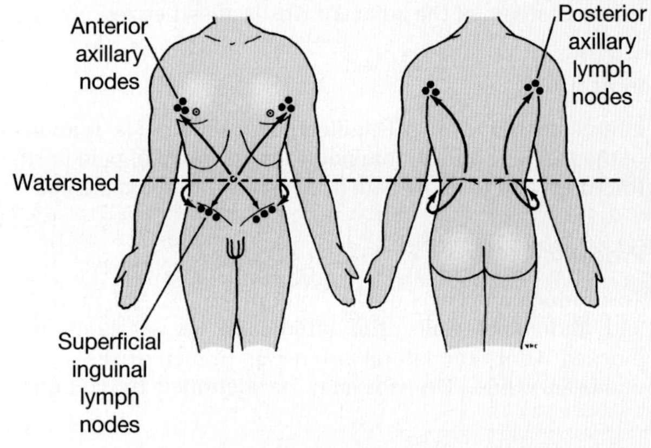

Figure 4.16 Lymph drainage of the skin of the thorax and abdomen. Note that levels of the umbilicus anteriorly and iliac crests posteriorly may be regarded as watersheds for lymph flow.

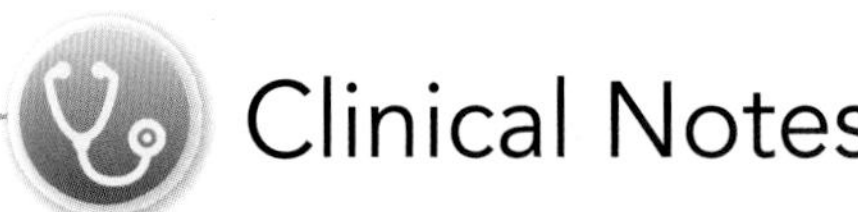

Clinical Notes

Needle Thoracostomy

Needle thoracostomy is creating and maintaining an opening into the thoracic cavity by using a needle. This may be necessary in patients with tension pneumothorax (air in the pleural cavity under pressure) or to drain fluid (blood or pus) away from the pleural cavity to allow the lung to reexpand. It may also be necessary to withdraw a sample of pleural fluid for microbiologic examination.

Anterior Approach

For the anterior approach, the patient is in the supine position. The sternal angle is identified, and costal cartilage 2, rib 2, and intercostal space 2 are found in the midclavicular line.

Lateral Approach

For the lateral approach, the patient is lying on their lateral side. Intercostal space 2 is identified as above, but the anterior axillary line is used.

The skin is prepared in the usual way, and a local anesthetic is introduced along the course of the needle above the upper border of rib 3. The thoracostomy needle pierces the following structures as it passes through the chest wall (see Fig. 4.9B): (a) skin, (b) superficial fascia (in the anterior approach, the pectoral muscles are then penetrated), (c) serratus anterior muscle, (d) external intercostal muscle, (e) internal intercostal muscle, (f) innermost intercostal muscle, (g) endothoracic fascia, and (h) parietal pleura. The needle should be kept close to the upper border of rib 3 to avoid injuring the intercostal vessels and nerve in the subcostal groove.

Tube Thoracostomy

The preferred insertion site for a tube thoracostomy is intercostal space 4 or 5 at the anterior axillary line (Fig. 4.17). The tube is introduced through a small incision. The neurovascular bundle changes its relationship to the ribs as it passes forward in the intercostal space. In the most posterior part of the space, the bundle lies in the middle of the intercostal space. As the bundle passes forward to the rib angle, it becomes closely related to the costal groove on the lower border of the rib above and maintains that position as it courses forward.

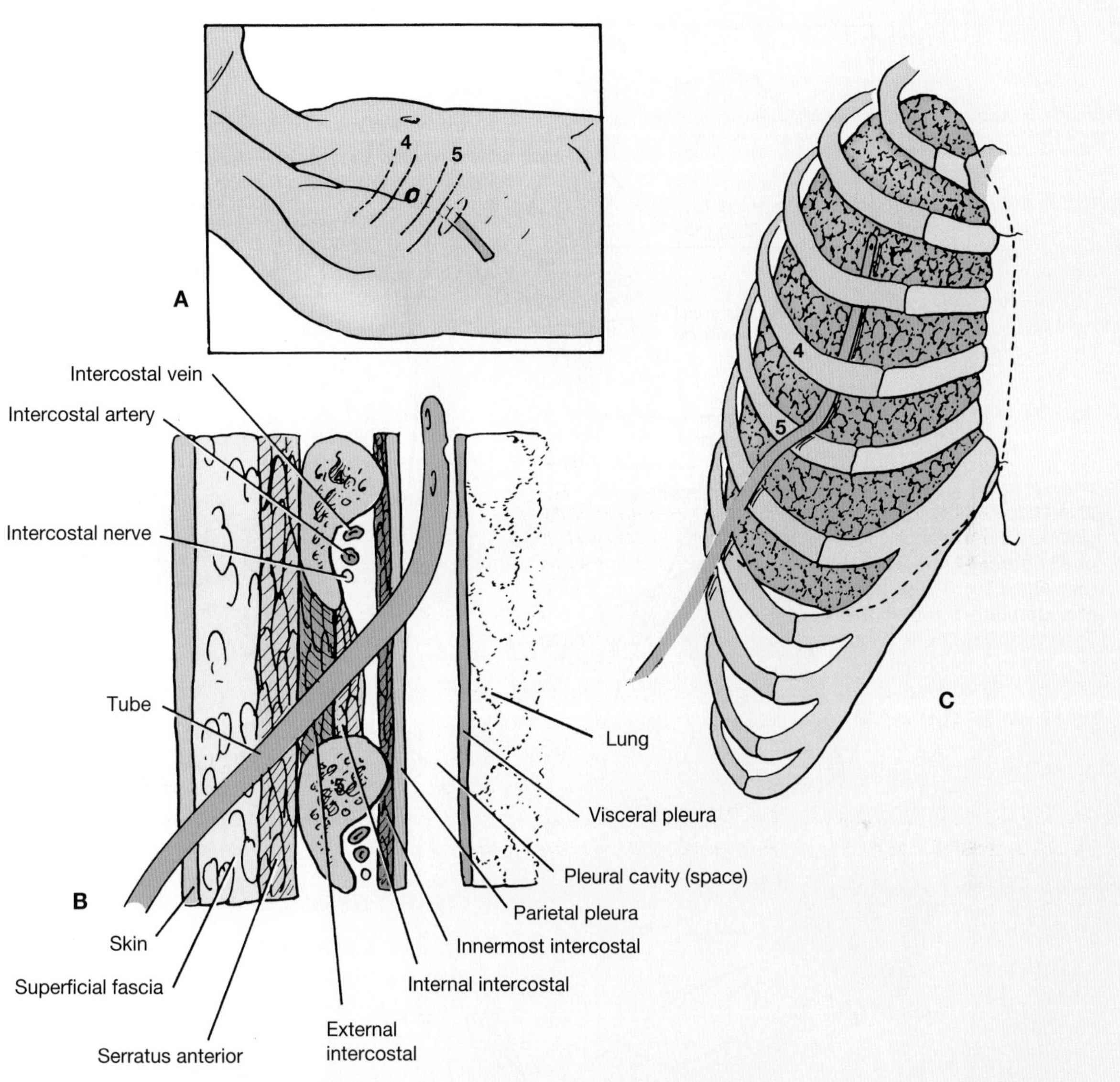

Figure 4.17 Tube thoracostomy. **A.** Site for insertion of the tube at the anterior axillary line. The skin incision is usually made over the intercostal space one below the space to be pierced. **B.** Various layers of tissue penetrated by the scalpel and later the tube as they pass through the chest wall to enter the pleural cavity (space). The incision through the intercostal space is kept close to the upper border of the rib to avoid injuring the intercostal vessels and nerve. **C.** Tube advancing superiorly and posteriorly in the pleural space.

The introduction of a thoracostomy tube or needle through the lower intercostal spaces is possible provided that the presence of the domes of the diaphragm is remembered as they curve upward into the rib cage as far as rib 5 (higher on the right). Avoid damaging the diaphragm and entering the peritoneal cavity and injuring the liver, spleen, or stomach.

Thoracotomy

Thoracotomy is making an incision through the thoracic wall into the pleural space. This may be a lifesaving procedure in patients with penetrating chest wounds and uncontrolled intrathoracic hemorrhage. After preparing the skin in the usual way, the physician makes an incision over intercostal space 4 or 5, extending from the lateral margin of the sternum to the anterior axillary line (Fig. 4.18). Whether to make a right or left incision depends on the site of the injury. The chest should be entered from the left side for access to the heart and aorta. The following tissues are incised (see Fig. 4.17): (a) skin, (b) subcutaneous tissue, (c) serratus anterior and pectoral muscles, (d) external intercostal muscle and anterior intercostal membrane, (e) internal intercostal muscle, (f) innermost intercostal muscle, (g) endothoracic fascia, and (h) parietal pleura. Avoid the internal thoracic artery, which runs vertically downward behind the costal cartilages about a fingerbreadth lateral to the margin of the sternum, and the intercostal vessels and nerve, which extend forward in the subcostal groove in the upper part of the intercostal space.

(continued)

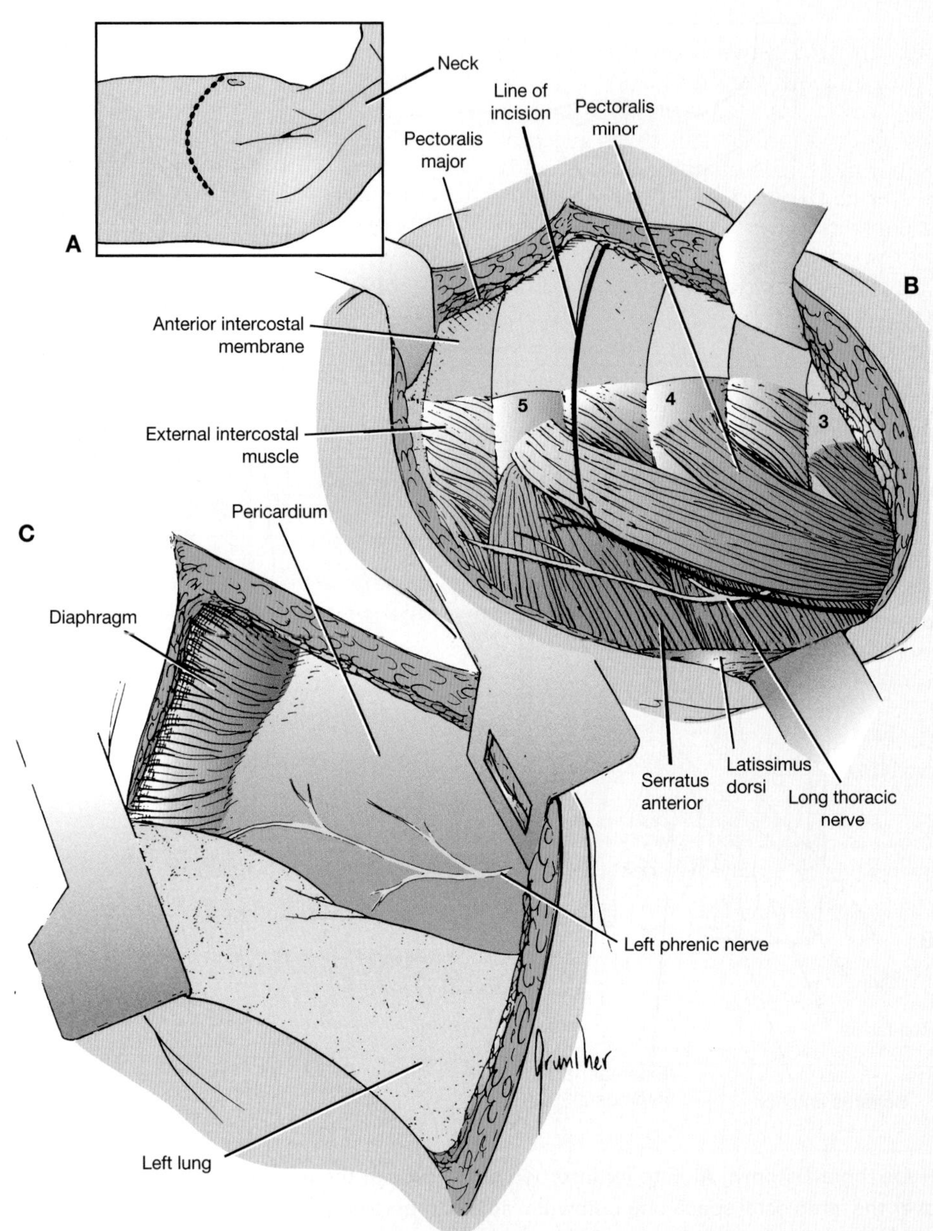

Figure 4.18 Left thoracotomy. **A.** Site of skin incision over intercostal space 4 or 5. **B.** Exposed ribs and associated muscles. The line of incision through the intercostal space should be placed close to the upper border of the rib to avoid injuring the intercostal vessels and nerve. **C.** Pleural space opened, and the left side of the mediastinum exposed. The left phrenic nerve descends over the pericardium beneath the mediastinal pleura. The collapsed left lung must be pushed out of the way to visualize the mediastinum.

Anatomic and Physiologic Thoracic Changes with Aging

Certain anatomic and physiologic changes take place in the thorax with advancing years:

- The rib cage becomes more rigid and loses its elasticity as the result of calcification and even ossification of the costal cartilages. This also alters their usual radiographic appearance.
- The stooped posture (kyphosis), so often seen in older adults because of degeneration of the intervertebral discs and/or bodies, decreases the chest capacity.
- Disuse atrophy of the thoracic and abdominal muscles can result in poor respiratory movements.
- Degeneration of the elastic tissue in the lungs and bronchi results in impairment of the movement of expiration.

These changes, when severe, diminish the efficiency of respiratory movements and impair the individual's ability to withstand respiratory disease.

MEDIASTINUM

The mediastinum is the area between the sternum, the two pleural cavities, and the vertebral column (Figs. 4.19 to 4.21). Though thick, it is a movable partition that extends superiorly to the thoracic outlet and the root of the neck and inferiorly to the diaphragm. It extends anteriorly to the sternum and posteriorly to the vertebral column. It contains the remains of the thymus, the heart and large blood vessels, trachea and esophagus, thoracic duct and lymph nodes, vagus and phrenic nerves, and the sympathetic trunks.

The mediastinum is divided into **superior** and **inferior mediastina** by an imaginary plane passing from the sternal angle anteriorly to the lower border of the body of the T4 vertebra posteriorly (see Fig. 4.20). This plane is a noteworthy landmark in that it marks several key structures. From anterior to posterior, these are the:

- Joint between the manubrium and body of the sternum
- Second costosternal joint
- Demarcation between the ascending aorta and the arch of the aorta
- Demarcation between the arch of the aorta and the descending thoracic aorta
- Bifurcation of the trachea
- Level of the left primary bronchus
- T4 intervertebral disc

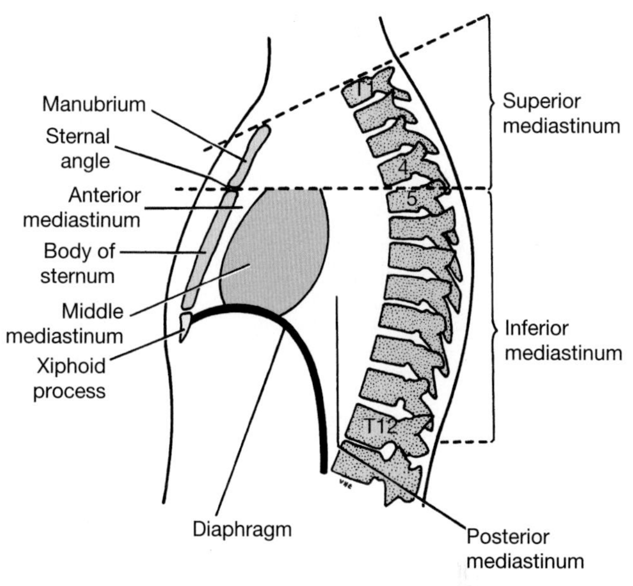

Figure 4.20 Subdivisions of the mediastinum.

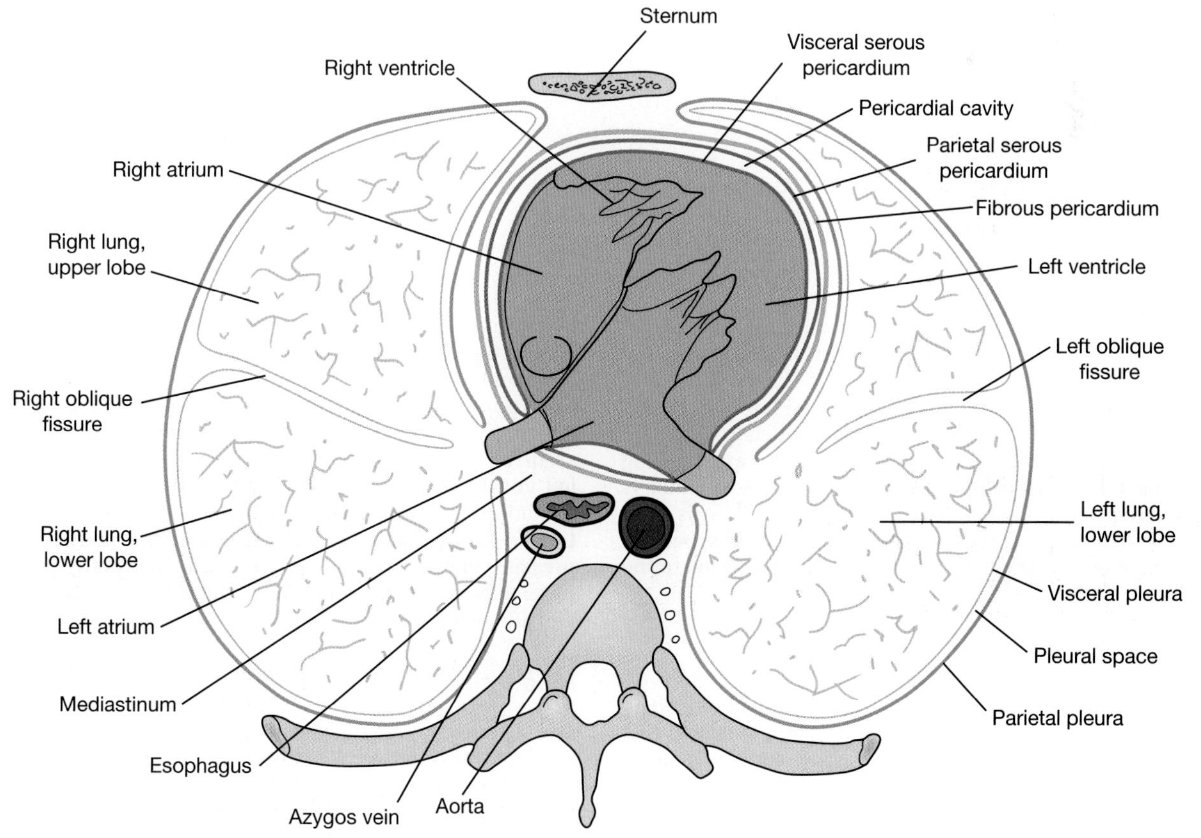

Figure 4.19 Cross section of the thorax at the level of the T8 vertebra. Note the arrangement of the pleura and pleural cavity (*space*) and the fibrous and the serous pericardia. Recall that cross sections are normally viewed from below and that the observer's right is the subject's left.

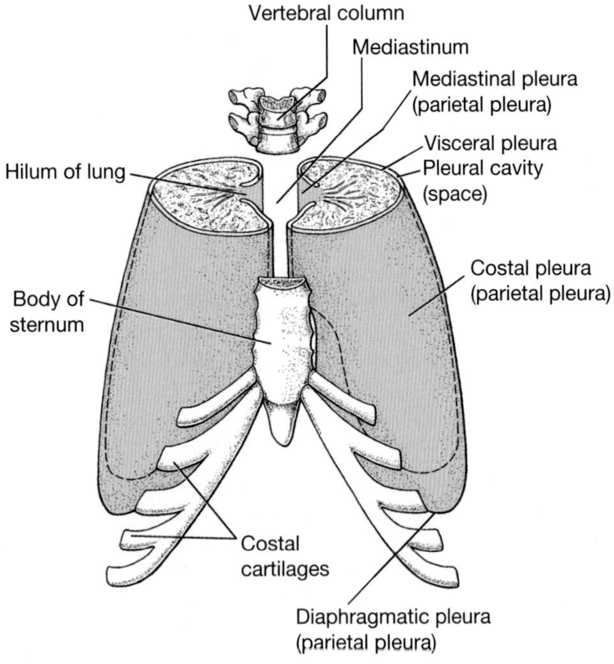

Figure 4.21 Pleurae from above and in front. Note the position of the mediastinum and the hilum of each lung.

The inferior mediastinum is further subdivided into the **middle mediastinum**, which consists of the pericardium and heart; the **anterior mediastinum**, which is a space between the pericardium and the sternum; and the **posterior mediastinum**, which lies between the pericardium and the vertebral column.

Superior Mediastinum

For purposes of orientation, remember that the major superior mediastinal structures are arranged in the following order from anterior to posterior: (1) thymus, (2) large veins, (3) large arteries, (4) trachea, (5) esophagus and thoracic duct, and (6) sympathetic trunks.

The superior mediastinum is bounded in front by the manubrium sterni and behind by the T1 to T4 vertebrae (see Fig. 4.20).

Inferior Mediastinum

For purposes of orientation, remember that the major inferior mediastinal structures are arranged in the following order from anterior to posterior: (1) thymus, (2) heart within the pericardium with the phrenic nerves on each side, (3) esophagus and thoracic duct, (4) descending aorta, and (5) sympathetic trunks.

The inferior mediastinum is bounded in front by the body of the sternum and behind by the T5 to T12 vertebrae (see Fig. 4.20).

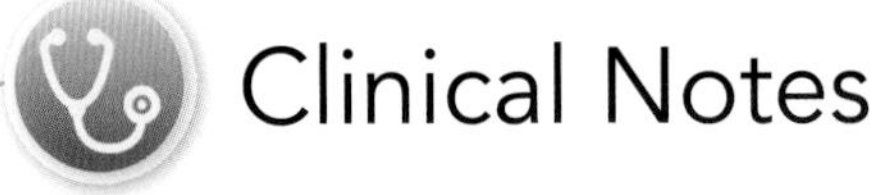

Clinical Notes

Deflection of the Mediastinum

In the cadaver, the mediastinum is an inflexible, fixed structure because of the hardening effect of the preserving fluids. However, in life, it is very mobile; the lungs, heart, and large arteries are in rhythmic pulsation, and the esophagus distends as each bolus of food passes through it.

If air enters the pleural cavity (**pneumothorax**), the lung on that side immediately collapses, and the mediastinum is displaced to the opposite side. This condition reveals itself by the patient being breathless and in a state of shock; on examination, the trachea and the heart are displaced to the opposite side.

Mediastinitis

The structures that make up the mediastinum are embedded in loose connective tissue that is continuous with that of the root of the neck. Thus, it is possible for a deep infection of the neck to spread readily into the thorax, causing mediastinitis. Penetrating wounds of the chest involving the esophagus also may cause mediastinitis. In esophageal perforations, air escapes into the connective tissue spaces and ascends beneath the fascia to the root of the neck, causing **subcutaneous emphysema**.

Mediastinal Tumors or Cysts

Because many vital structures are crowded together within the mediastinum, their functions can be disrupted by an enlarging tumor or organ. A tumor of the left lung can rapidly spread to involve the mediastinal lymph nodes, which, on enlargement, may compress the left recurrent laryngeal nerve, producing paralysis of the left vocal fold. An expanding cyst or tumor can partially occlude the superior vena cava, causing severe congestion of the veins of the upper part of the body. Other pressure effects can be seen on the sympathetic trunks; phrenic nerves; and, sometimes, the trachea; main bronchi; and esophagus.

Mediastinoscopy

Mediastinoscopy is a diagnostic procedure whereby specimens of tracheobronchial lymph nodes are obtained without opening the pleural cavities. A small incision is made in the midline in the neck just above the suprasternal notch, and the superior mediastinum is explored down to the region of the bifurcation of the trachea. The procedure can be used to determine the diagnosis and degree of spread of carcinoma of the bronchus.

PLEURAE

The paired pleurae and lungs lie on either side of the mediastinum within the thoracic cavity. Each pleural membrane has two parts: a **parietal layer** and a **visceral layer** (Fig. 4.22; see also Figs. 4.19 and 4.21). The parietal layer lines the thoracic wall, covers the thoracic surface of the diaphragm and the lateral aspect of the mediastinum, and extends into the root of the neck to line the undersurface of the suprapleural membrane at the thoracic outlet (see Fig. 4.8). The visceral layer completely covers the outer surface of the lung and extends into the depths of the interlobar fissures (Figs. 4.23 and 4.24; see also Fig. 4.19). It is thinner than the parietal layer.

Layers and Cavity

The two layers are continuous with one another via a cuff of pleura that surrounds the structures entering and leaving the lung at the hilum of each lung (see Figs. 4.19 and 4.21 to 4.23). This cuff hangs down as a loose fold called the **pulmonary ligament** and allows for movement of the pulmonary vessels and large bronchi during respiration (see Fig. 4.23).

The parietal and visceral layers of pleura are separated from one another by a slit-like space, the **pleural cavity** (see Figs. 4.19, 4.21, and 4.22). (Clinicians are increasingly using the term **pleural space** instead of the anatomic term pleural cavity. This is probably to avoid the confusion between the pleural cavity [slit-like] space and the larger thoracic cavity.) The pleural cavity normally contains only a small amount of tissue fluid, the **pleural fluid**. Pleural fluid covers the surfaces of the pleura as a thin film, which causes surface tension adhesion of the pleural layers and permits them to move on each other with minimal friction. Thus, the pleural cavity is a potential space under normal conditions and is discernible only under abnormal conditions (eg, when the lung is displaced by air or excess fluid).

For purposes of description, the parietal pleura is divided according to the region in which it lies or the surface that it covers (see Figs. 4.21 to 4.23). The **cervical pleura** (**cupula**) extends up into the neck, lining the undersurface of the suprapleural membrane (see Figs. 4.8 and 4.24). It reaches a level of 1 to 1.5 in. (2.5 to 4 cm) above the medial third of the clavicle. The **costal pleura** lines the inner surfaces of the ribs, costal cartilages, intercostal spaces, sides of the vertebral bodies, and the back of the sternum. The **diaphragmatic pleura** covers the thoracic surface of the diaphragm. In quiet respiration, the costal and diaphragmatic pleurae are in apposition to each other below the lower border of the lung. In deep inspiration, the margins of the base

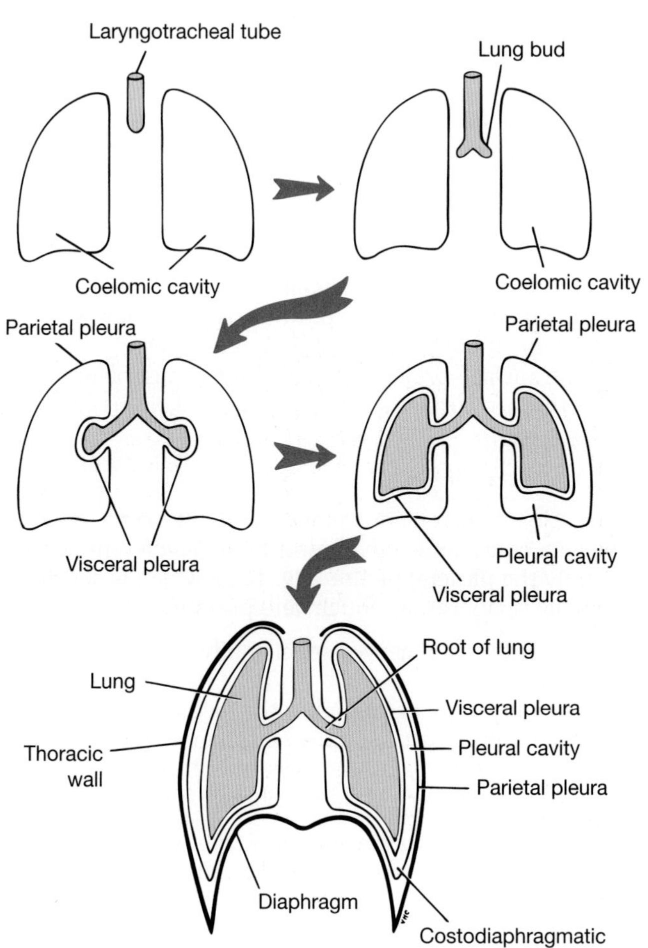

Figure 4.22 Formation of the lungs. Note that each lung bud invaginates the wall of the coelomic cavity and then grows to fill a greater part of the cavity. Note also that the lung is covered with visceral pleura and the thoracic wall is lined with parietal pleura. The original coelomic cavity is reduced to the slit-like pleural cavity because of the growth of the lung.

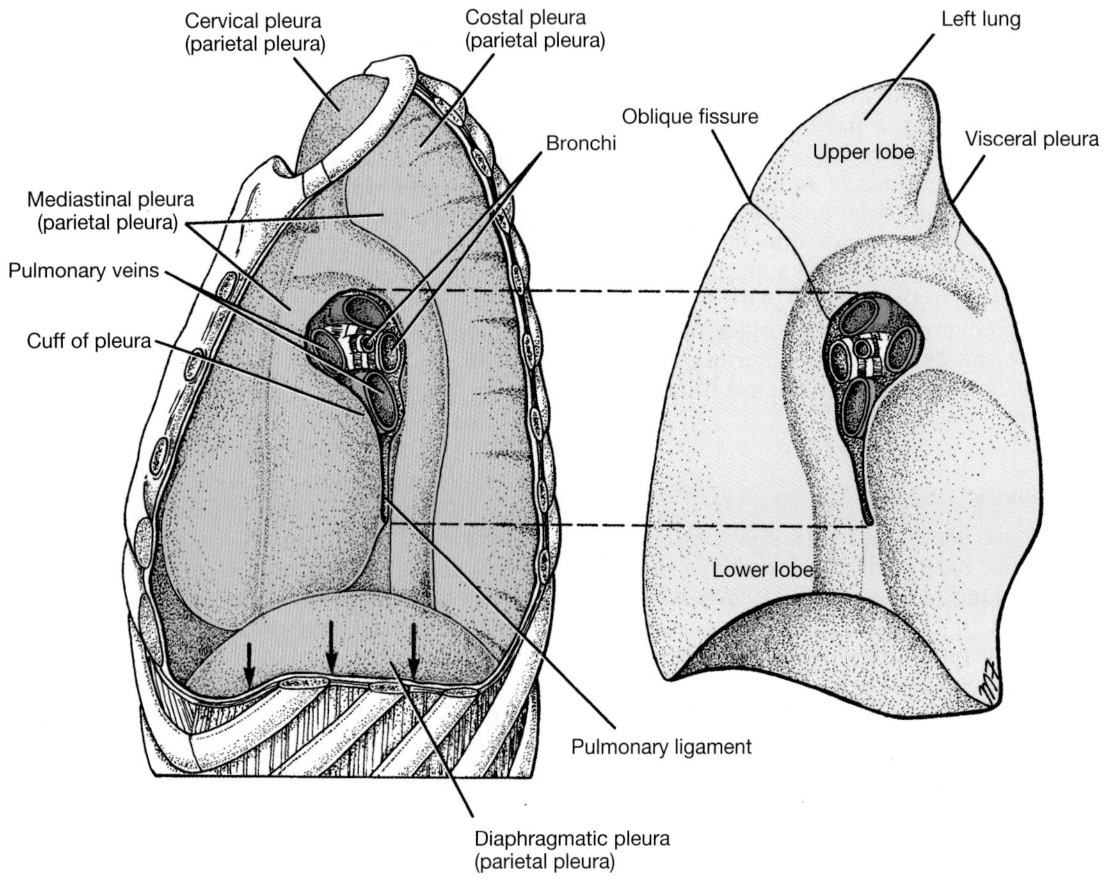

Figure 4.23 Different areas of the parietal pleura. Note the cuff of pleura (*dotted lines*) that surrounds the structures forming the root of the left lung at the hilum. The parietal and visceral layers of pleura become continuous here. *Arrows* indicate the position of the costodiaphragmatic recess.

of the lung descend, and the costal and diaphragmatic pleurae separate. This lower area of the pleural cavity into which the lung expands on inspiration is referred to as the **costodiaphragmatic recess** (see Figs. 4.22 and 4.23). The **mediastinal pleura** covers and forms the lateral boundary of the mediastinum. It reflects as a cuff around the vessels and bronchi at the hilum of the lung and here becomes continuous with the visceral pleura. Thus, each lung lies free except at its hilum, where it is attached to the blood vessels and bronchi that constitute the **lung root**. During full inspiration, the lungs expand and fill the pleural cavities. However, during quiet inspiration, the lungs do not fully occupy the pleural cavities at four sites: the right and left costodiaphragmatic recesses and the right and left costomediastinal recesses.

The **costodiaphragmatic recesses** are slit-like spaces between the costal and diaphragmatic parietal pleurae separated only by a capillary layer of pleural fluid. During inspiration, the lower margins of the lungs descend into the recesses. During expiration, the lower margins of the lungs ascend so that the costal and diaphragmatic pleurae come together again.

The **costomediastinal recesses** are situated along the anterior margins of the pleura. They are slit-like spaces between the costal and mediastinal parietal pleurae, which are separated by a capillary layer of pleural fluid. During inspiration and expiration, the anterior borders of the lungs slide in and out of the recesses.

The surface projections of the lungs and pleurae are described in Surface Anatomy at the end of this chapter.

Nerve Supply

The pleural layers are innervated differently despite being a continuous membrane. Somatic afferent nerves supply the parietal pleura (Fig. 4.25), which is sensitive to pain, temperature, touch, and pressure:

- The intercostal nerves segmentally supply the costal pleura.
- The phrenic nerve supplies the mediastinal pleura.
- The phrenic nerve supplies the diaphragmatic pleura over the dome, and the lower intercostal nerves supply the periphery of the diaphragmatic pleura.

Visceral afferent nerves supply the visceral pleura, which is sensitive to stretch but insensitive to common sensations such as pain and touch. These nerves run in company with autonomic nerves from the pulmonary plexus (see Fig. 4.25).

Infrahyoid muscles
Thymus
Left common carotid artery
Brachiocephalic artery
Left internal jugular vein
Internal thoracic artery
Right phrenic nerve
Left phrenic nerve
Right vagus nerve
Left vagus nerve
Left subclavian artery
Cervical dome of pleura
Left recurrent laryngeal nerve
Trachea
T1
T1 nerve
A
Rib 1
Thoracic duct
Sympathetic trunk
Esophagus

Thymus
Manubrium sterni
Superior vena cava
Arch of aorta
Left phrenic nerve
Right phrenic nerve
Right lung
Left vagus nerve
Left lung
Azygos vein
T4
Left recurrent laryngeal nerve
B
Right vagus nerve
Trachea
Thoracic duct
Sympathetic trunk
Esophagus

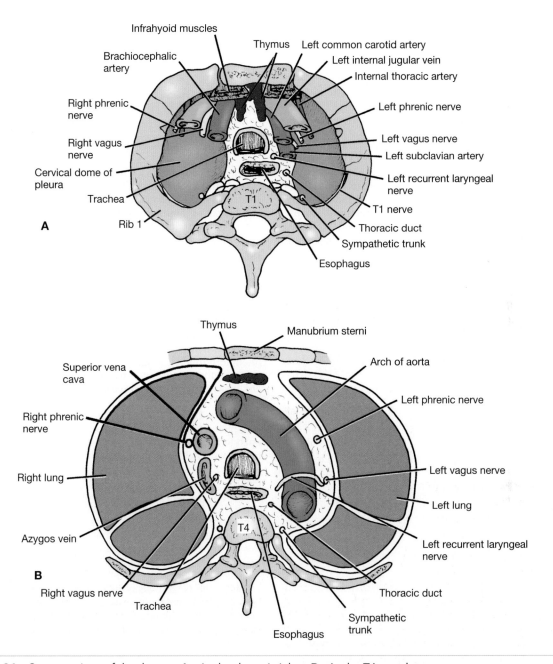

Figure 4.24 Cross sections of the thorax. **A.** At the thoracic inlet. **B.** At the T4 vertebra.

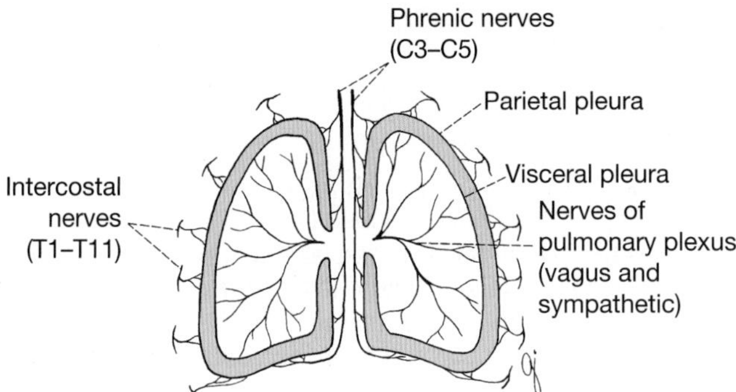

Figure 4.25 Diagram showing the innervation of the parietal and visceral layers of pleura.

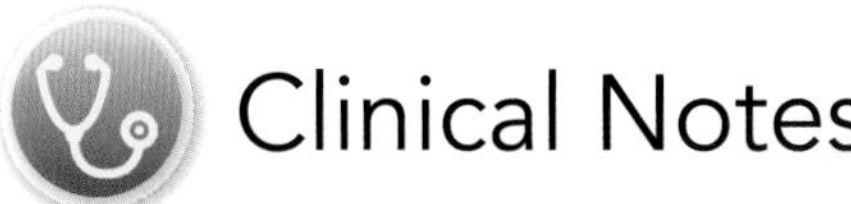

Clinical Notes

Pleural Fluid

The pleural cavity normally contains 5 to 10 mL of clear fluid, which lubricates the apposing surfaces of the visceral and parietal pleurae during respiratory movements. Hydrostatic and osmotic pressures stimulate formation of the fluid. Because the hydrostatic pressures are greater in the capillaries of the parietal pleura than in the capillaries of the visceral pleura (pulmonary circulation), the capillaries of the visceral pleura normally absorb the pleural fluid. Any condition that increases production of the fluid (eg, inflammation, malignancy, congestive heart disease) or impairs drainage (eg, collapsed lung) results in abnormal accumulation of fluid, called a **pleural effusion**. The presence of 300 mL of fluid in the costodiaphragmatic recess in an adult is sufficient for clinical detection. The clinical signs include decreased lung expansion on the side of the effusion, with decreased breath sounds and dullness on percussion over the effusion (Fig. 4.26).

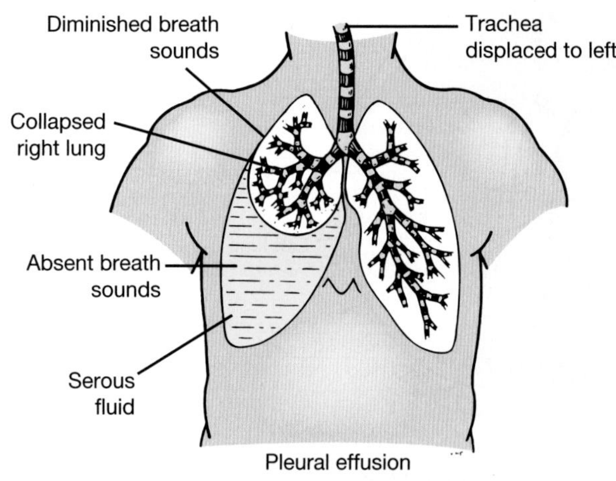

Figure 4.26 Right-sided pleural effusion. The mediastinum is displaced to the left, the right lung is compressed, and the bronchi are narrowed. Auscultation would reveal only faint breath sounds over the compressed lung and absent breath sounds over fluid in the pleural cavity.

Pleurisy

Inflammation of the pleura (**pleuritis** or **pleurisy**), secondary to inflammation of the lung (eg, pneumonia), results in inflammatory exudate coating the pleural surfaces, which causes roughening of the surfaces. This roughening produces friction, which can be heard with the stethoscope as a **pleural rub** on inspiration and expiration. Fibroblasts often invade the exudate, resulting in deposition of collagen and formation of **pleural adhesions** that bind the visceral pleura to the parietal pleura.

Pneumothorax, Empyema, and Pleural Effusion

Air can enter the pleural cavity from the lungs or through the chest wall (**pneumothorax**) as the result of disease or injury (eg, interstitial lung disease, gunshot wounds). In the former treatment of tuberculosis, air was purposely injected into the pleural cavity to collapse and rest the lung. This was known as **artificial pneumothorax**. A **spontaneous pneumothorax** is a condition in which air enters the pleural cavity suddenly without its cause being immediately apparent. Investigation usually reveals that air has entered from a diseased lung and a bulla (bleb) has ruptured.

Wounds that penetrate the thoracic wall (eg, stab wounds) may pierce the parietal pleura so that the pleural cavity is open to the outside air. This condition is called **open pneumothorax**. Each time the patient inspires, it is possible to hear air under atmospheric pressure being sucked into the pleural cavity. Sometimes, the clothing and the layers of the thoracic wall combine to form a valve so that air enters on inspiration but cannot exit through the wound. In these circumstances, the air pressure builds up on the wounded side and pushes the mediastinum toward the opposite side. In this situation, a collapsed lung is on the injured side, and the opposite lung is compressed by the deflected mediastinum. This dangerous condition is called a **tension pneumothorax**.

Air in the pleural cavity associated with serous fluid is known as **hydropneumothorax**, associated with pus as **pyopneumothorax**, and associated with blood as **hemopneumothorax**. In hemopneumothorax, trauma to the chest may result in bleeding from blood vessels in the chest wall, from vessels in the chest cavity, or from a lacerated lung. A collection of pus (without air) in the pleural cavity is called an **empyema**. The presence of excess serous fluid in the pleural cavity is referred to as a **pleural effusion** (see Fig. 4.26). Fluid (serous, blood, or pus) can be drained from the pleural cavity through a wide-bore needle, as described earlier in Needle Thoracostomy.

LOWER RESPIRATORY TRACT

The respiratory tract (respiratory tree) is the network of passageways that supplies air to the lungs. The **upper respiratory tract** includes the nasal passages and sinuses, pharynx, larynx, and upper portion of the trachea. The **lower respiratory tract (tracheobronchial tree)** includes the lower portion of the trachea, the bronchi, and the bronchioles (Fig. 4.27).

Trachea

The trachea is a mobile cartilaginous and membranous tube (Figs. 4.28 to 4.30; see also Fig. 4.27). It begins in the neck as the continuation of the larynx at the lower border of the cricoid cartilage at the level of the C6 vertebra. It descends in the midline of the neck. In the thorax, the trachea runs through the superior mediastinum, in approximately the midline. It ends by dividing into right and left

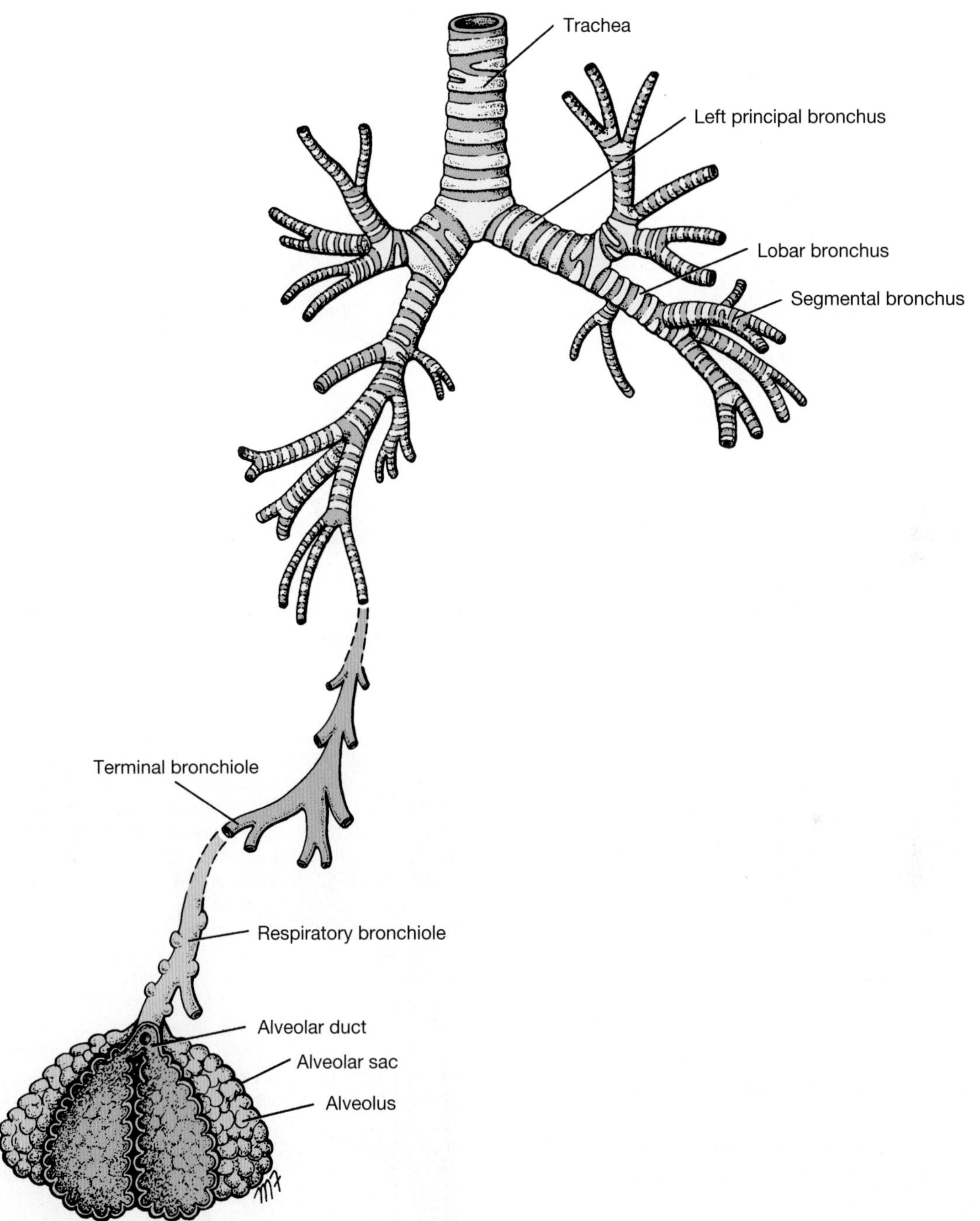

Figure 4.27 Lower respiratory tract, including the trachea, bronchi, bronchioles, alveolar ducts, alveolar sacs, and alveoli. Note the path taken by inspired air from the trachea to the alveoli.

principal (main) bronchi at the level of the sternal angle (opposite the disc between the T4 and T5 vertebrae). During expiration, the bifurcation rises by about one vertebral level and during deep inspiration may lower as far as the T6 vertebra. In adults, the trachea is about 4.5 in. (11.25 cm) long and 1 in. (2.5 cm) in diameter.

U-shaped bars (tracheal rings) of hyaline cartilage embedded in the tracheal wall support and maintain the patency of the trachea (see Figs. 4.27 and 4.29). The **trachealis muscle** (a smooth muscle) connects the posterior free ends of the cartilages. The posterior discontinuity permits the esophagus to expand into the trachea during swallowing.

The relations of the trachea in the neck are described in Chapter 9.

The relations of the trachea in the superior mediastinum of the thorax are as follows:

- **Anteriorly:** The sternum, thymus, left brachiocephalic vein, origins of the brachiocephalic and left common carotid arteries, and the arch of the aorta (see Figs. 4.24A and 4.28)

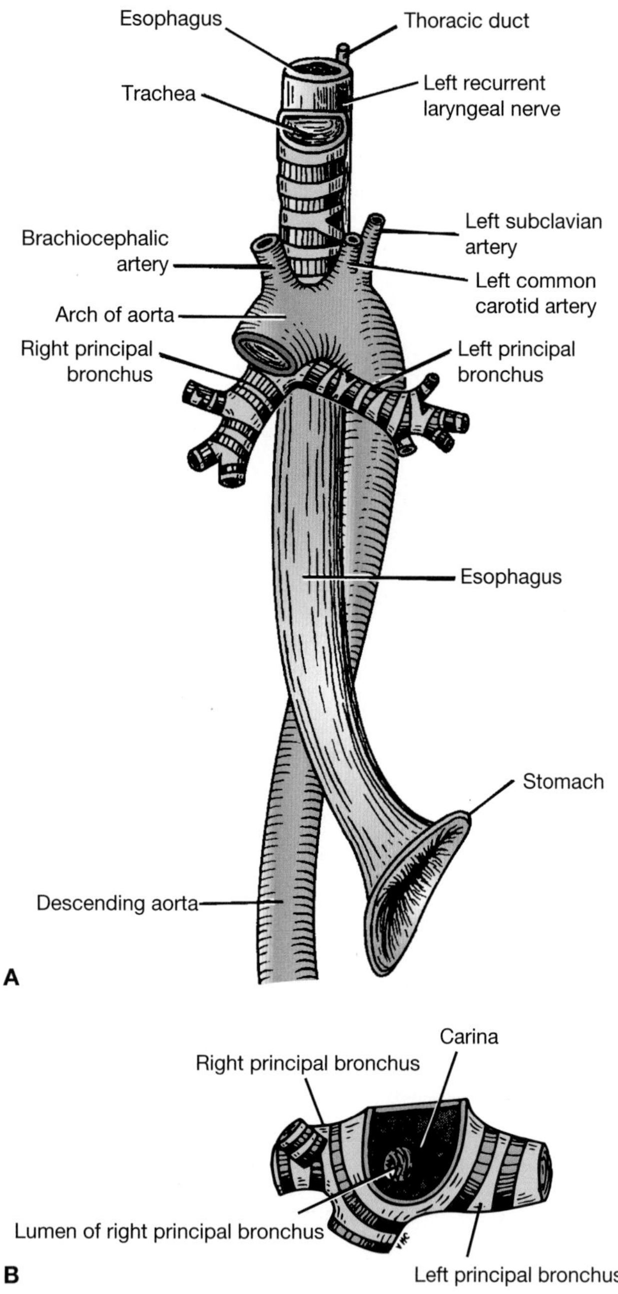

Figure 4.28 Thoracic part of the trachea. **A.** Note that the right principal bronchus is wider and is a more direct continuation of the trachea than the left. **B.** Bifurcation of the trachea as viewed from above.

- **Posteriorly:** The esophagus and the left recurrent laryngeal nerve (see Fig. 4.24)
- **Right side:** The azygos vein, right vagus nerve, and the pleura (Figs. 4.31A and 4.32A; see also Fig. 4.24)
- **Left side:** The arch of the aorta, left common carotid and left subclavian arteries, left vagus and left phrenic nerves, and the pleura (see Figs. 4.24, 4.31B, and 4.32B)

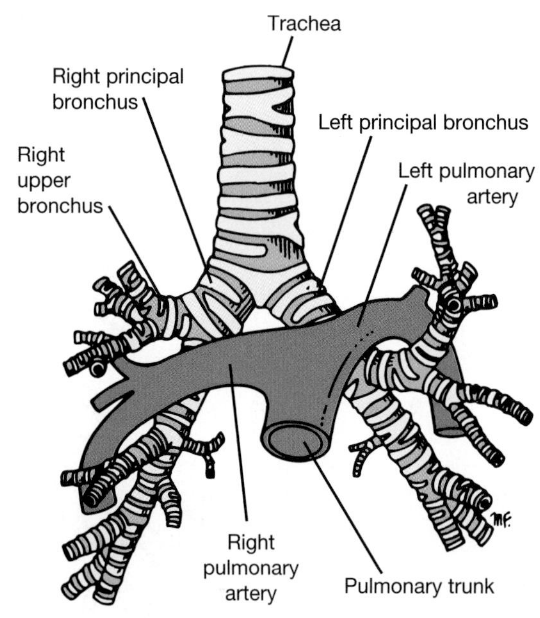

Figure 4.29 Relationship of the pulmonary arteries to the bronchial tree.

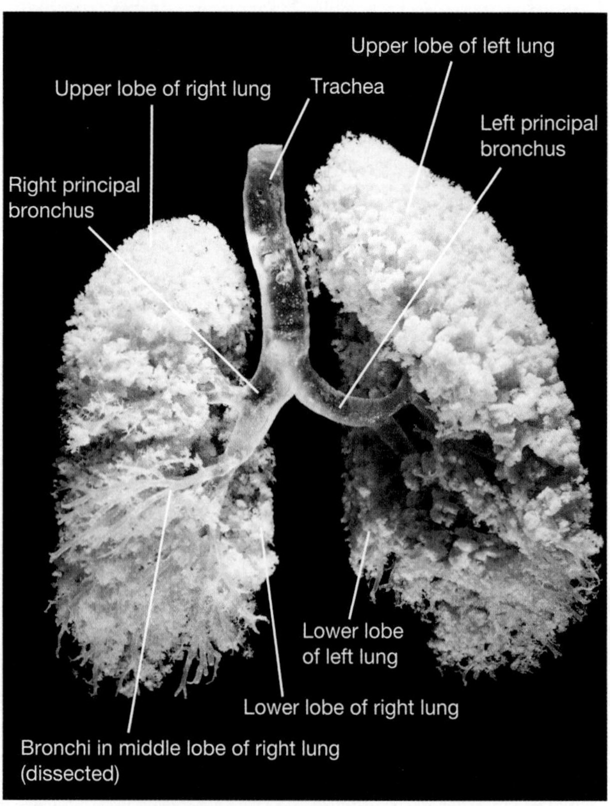

Figure 4.30 Plastinated specimen of an adult trachea, principal bronchi, and lung. Some of the lung tissue has been dissected to reveal the larger bronchi. Note that the right main bronchus is wider and a more direct continuation of the trachea than the left main bronchus.

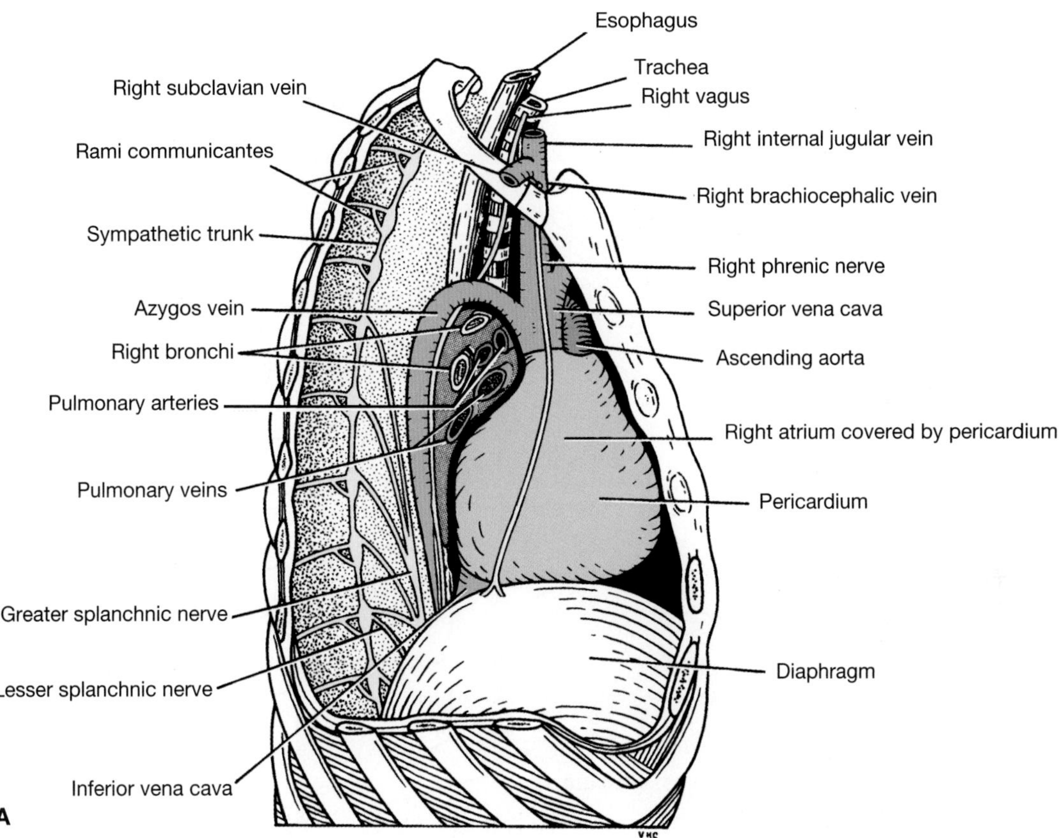
Esophagus
Trachea
Right vagus
Right subclavian vein
Right internal jugular vein
Rami communicantes
Right brachiocephalic vein
Sympathetic trunk
Right phrenic nerve
Azygos vein
Superior vena cava
Right bronchi
Ascending aorta
Pulmonary arteries
Right atrium covered by pericardium
Pulmonary veins
Pericardium
Greater splanchnic nerve
Diaphragm
Lesser splanchnic nerve
Inferior vena cava
A

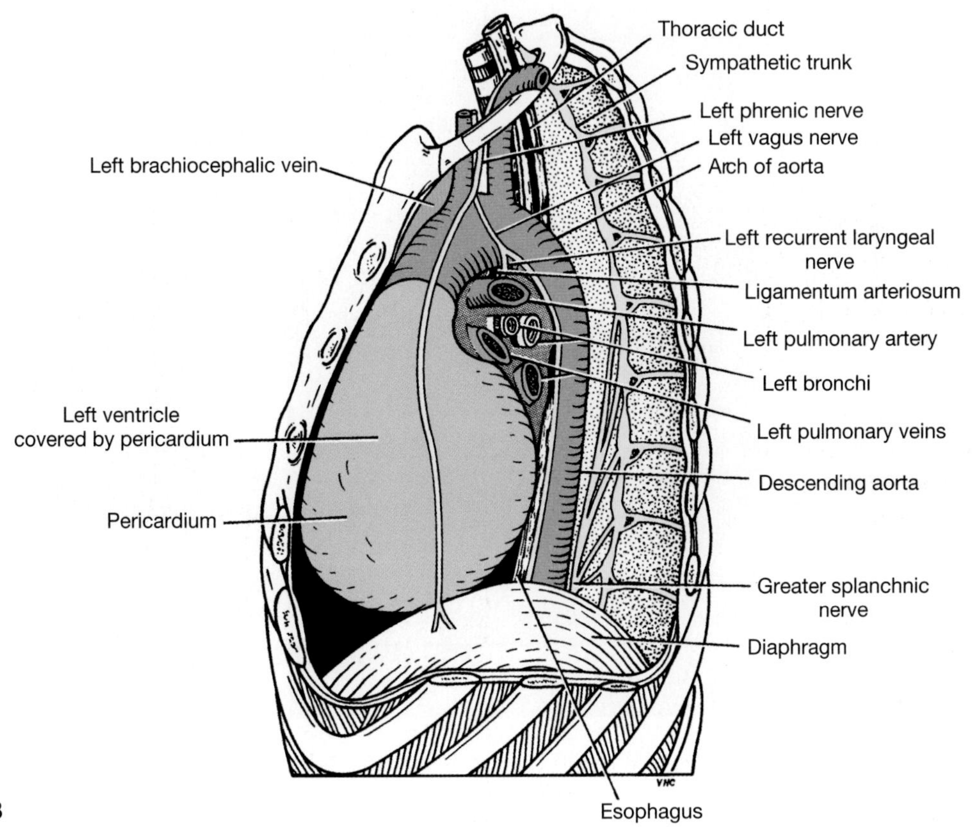
Thoracic duct
Sympathetic trunk
Left phrenic nerve
Left vagus nerve
Left brachiocephalic vein
Arch of aorta
Left recurrent laryngeal nerve
Ligamentum arteriosum
Left pulmonary artery
Left bronchi
Left ventricle covered by pericardium
Left pulmonary veins
Descending aorta
Pericardium
Greater splanchnic nerve
Diaphragm
B
Esophagus

Figure 4.31 Lateral views of the mediastinum. **A.** Right side. **B.** Left side.

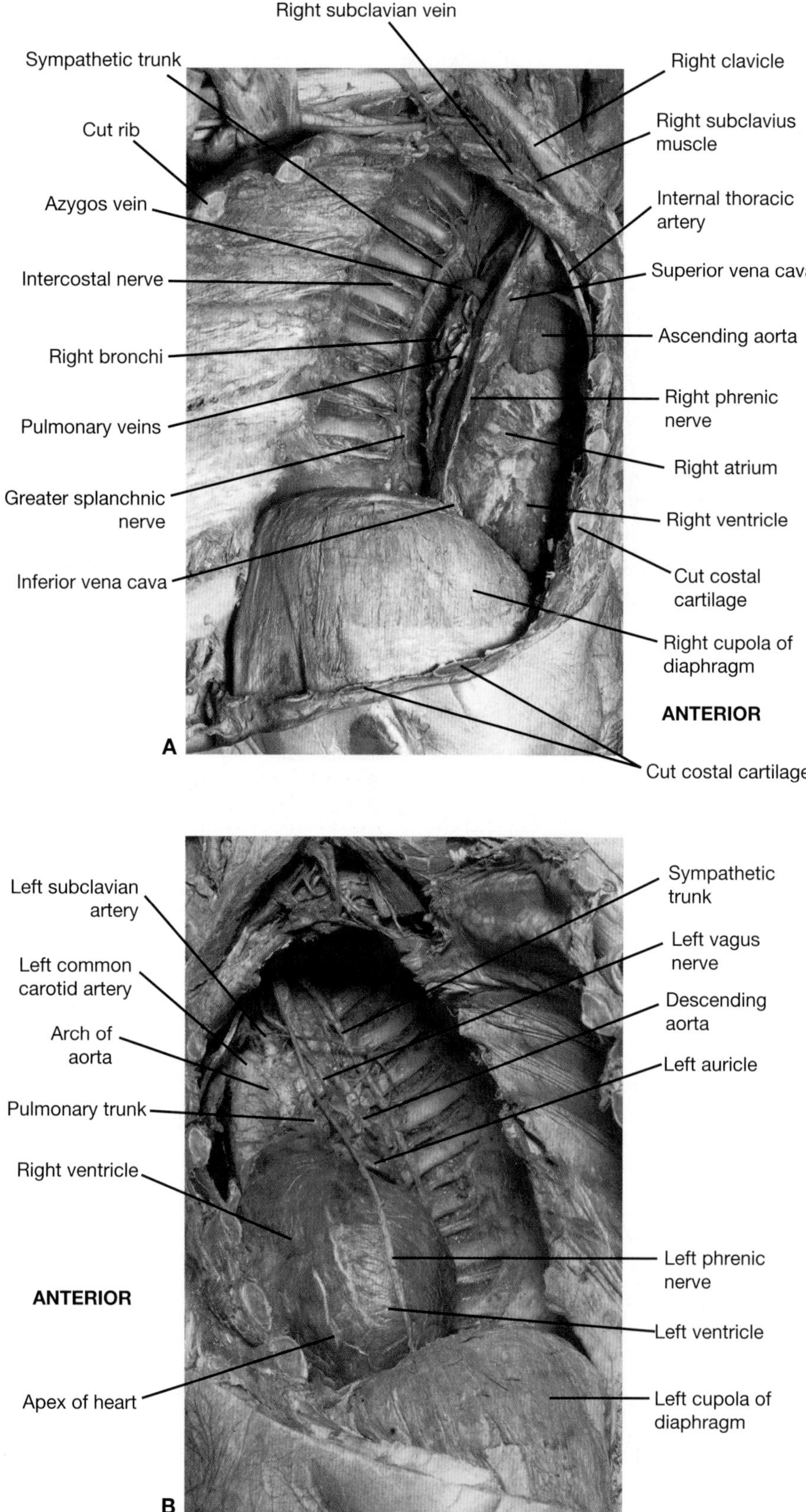

Figure 4.32 Dissection of the mediastinum. The lungs, pericardium, and costal parietal pleura have been removed. **A.** Right side. **B.** Left side.

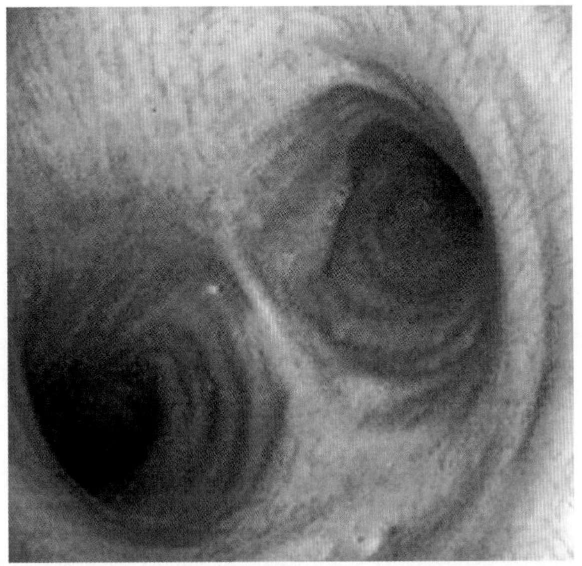

A

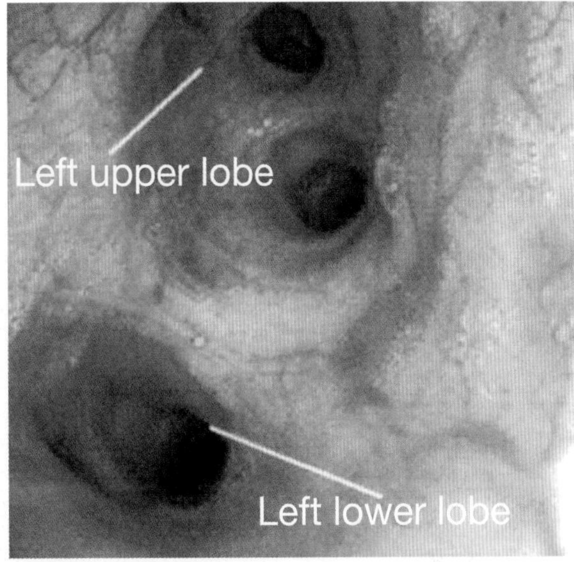

B

Figure 4.33 Interior of the bronchial tree as seen through an operating bronchoscope. **A.** Bifurcation of the trachea. Note the ridge of the carina in the center and the opening into the right main bronchus on the right, which is a more direct continuation of the trachea. **B.** Left main bronchus. The openings into the left upper lobe bronchus and its division and the left lower lobe bronchus are indicated. (Both images are courtesy of E. D. Andersen.)

Blood Supply

The inferior thyroid arteries (branches of the subclavian arteries) supply the upper two thirds of the trachea, and the bronchial arteries (branches of the thoracic aorta) supply the lower third.

Lymph Drainage

The lymph drains into the pretracheal and paratracheal lymph nodes and the deep cervical nodes.

Nerve Supply

The vagus and recurrent laryngeal nerves carry the sensory nerve supply. Sympathetic nerves supply the trachealis muscle.

Bronchi

The trachea bifurcates behind the arch of the aorta into the **right** and **left principal** (**primary** or **main**) **bronchi** (see Figs. 4.27 to 4.30). The **carina** is a small ridge at the inferior end of the junction of the trachea and the principal bronchi that separates the openings of the bronchi (Fig. 4.33A; see also Fig. 4.28B). The bronchi divide dichotomously, eventually giving rise to several million terminal bronchioles that terminate in one or more respiratory bronchioles. Each respiratory bronchiole divides into 2 to 11 alveolar ducts that enter the alveolar sacs. The alveoli arise from the walls of the sacs as diverticula (see Bronchopulmonary Segments, to follow).

Each principal bronchus supplies an entire lung (see Fig. 4.30). The principal bronchi next divide into lobar (secondary) bronchi that supply the individual lobes of the lungs. The right principal (main) bronchus is wider, shorter, and more vertical than the left and is about 1 in. (2.5 cm) long (see Figs. 4.27, 4.28, 4.30, and 4.33). Before entering the hilum of the right lung, the principal bronchus gives off the **superior lobar bronchus**. On entering the hilum, it divides into a **middle** and an **inferior lobar bronchus**.

The left principal (main) bronchus is narrower, longer, and more horizontal than the right and is about 2 in. (5 cm) long. It passes to the left below the arch of the aorta and in front of the esophagus (see Fig. 4.28A). On entering the hilum of the left lung, the principal bronchus divides into a **superior** and an **inferior lobar bronchus**.

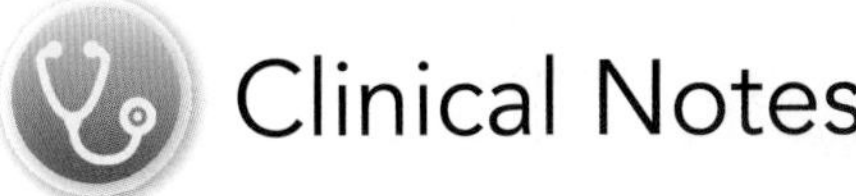

Clinical Notes

Compression of the Trachea

In the neck, a unilateral or bilateral enlargement of the thyroid gland can cause gross displacement or compression of the trachea. A dilatation of the aortic arch (eg, an aneurysm) can compress the trachea. With each cardiac systole, the pulsating aneurysm may tug at the trachea and left bronchus, a clinical sign that can be felt by palpating the trachea in the suprasternal notch.

(continued)

Tracheitis or Bronchitis

The recurrent laryngeal nerves innervate the mucosa lining much of the trachea. **Tracheitis** or **bronchitis** gives rise to a raw, burning sensation felt deep to the sternum instead of actual pain. Many thoracic and abdominal viscera, when diseased, give rise to discomfort that is felt in the midline (see Chapter 5, Abdominal Pain). It seems that organs possessing sensory innervation that is not, under normal conditions, directly relayed to consciousness display this phenomenon. The afferent fibers from these organs traveling to the central nervous system (CNS) accompany autonomic nerves.

Foreign Body Aspiration

Inhalation of foreign bodies into the lower respiratory tract is common, especially in children. Pins, screws, nuts, bolts, peanuts, and parts of chicken bones and toys have all found their way into the bronchi. Parts of the teeth may be inhaled while a patient is under anesthesia during a difficult dental extraction. Because the right principal bronchus is the wider, more vertical, and more direct continuation of the trachea (see Figs. 4.27, 4.30, and 4.33A), foreign bodies tend to enter the right instead of the left main bronchus. From there, they usually pass into the middle or inferior lobar bronchi. Large, aspirated objects commonly lodge in the right main bronchus, whereas small objects tend to stop in the right inferior lobar bronchus.

Bronchoscopy

Bronchoscopy enables examination of the interior of the trachea, its bifurcation, the carina, and the main bronchi (see Fig. 4.33). With experience, it is possible to examine the interior of the lobar bronchi and the beginning of the first segmental bronchi. This procedure also facilitates obtaining biopsy specimens of mucous membrane and removal of inhaled foreign bodies (even an open safety pin).

Lodgment of a foreign body in the larynx or edema of the mucous membrane of the larynx secondary to infection or trauma may require immediate relief to prevent asphyxiation. Tracheostomy is a method commonly used to relieve complete obstruction (see Chapter 9, Clinical Notes on the larynx).

LUNGS

During life, the lungs are soft and spongy and very elastic. If the thoracic cavity were opened, the lungs would immediately shrink to one third or less in volume. In the child, they are pink, but with age, they become dark and mottled because of the inhalation of dust particles that become trapped in the phagocytes of the lung. City dwellers and coal miners show this especially well. One lung lies on each side of the mediastinum. Therefore, the heart and great vessels and other structures in the mediastinum separate them from each other. Each lung is conical, covered with visceral pleura, attached to the mediastinum only by its root, and suspended free in its own pleural cavity (see Fig. 4.22).

Each lung has a blunt **apex**, which projects upward into the neck for about 1 in. (2.5 cm) above the clavicle; a concave **base** that sits on the diaphragm; a convex **costal surface**, which corresponds to the concave chest wall; and a concave **mediastinal surface**, which is molded to the pericardium and other mediastinal structures (Fig. 4.34). At about the middle of this surface is the **hilum**, a depression in which the **root** of the lung attaches (see Fig. 4.21). The structures that enter or leave the lung (ie, the bronchi, pulmonary artery and veins, lymph vessels, bronchial vessels, and nerves)

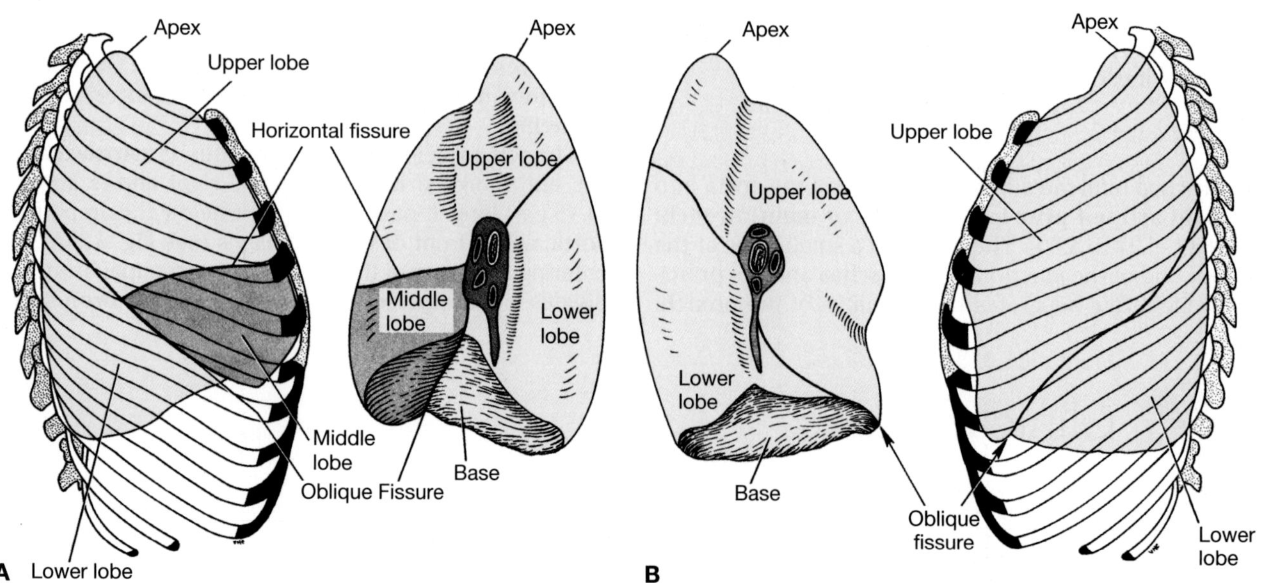

Figure 4.34 Lateral and medial surfaces of the lungs. **A.** Right lung. **B.** Left lung.

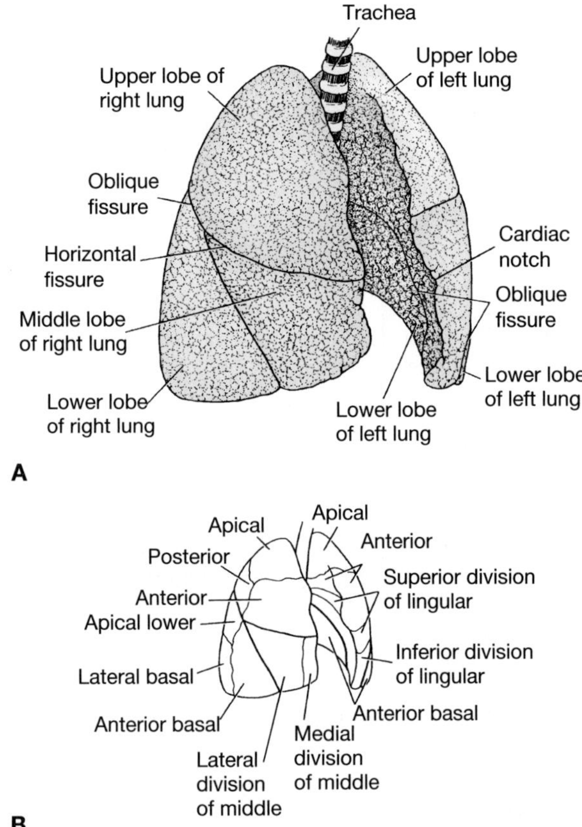

Figure 4.35 Lungs viewed from the right. **A.** Lobes. **B.** Bronchopulmonary segments.

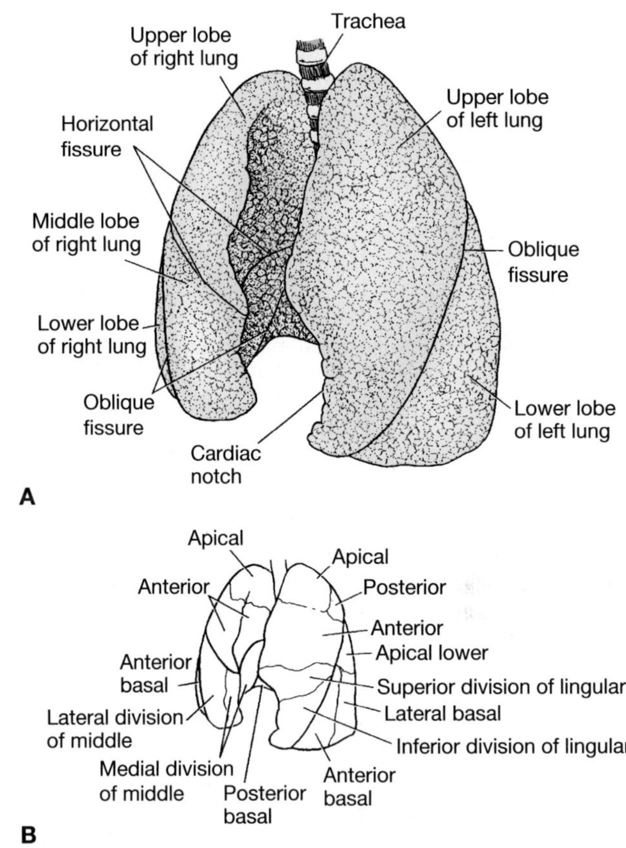

Figure 4.36 Lungs viewed from the left. **A.** Lobes. **B.** Bronchopulmonary segments.

form the root of the lung. The root is surrounded by a tubular sheath of pleura, which joins the mediastinal parietal pleura to the visceral pleura covering the lungs (see Figs. 4.22, 4.23, 4.31, and 4.32).

The anterior lung borders are thin and overlap the heart. The **cardiac notch** is a concave indentation of the anterior margin of the left lung that leaves the anterior surface of the heart relatively exposed (Figs. 4.35 to 4.37). The **lingula** is the tongue-like projection of the anterior margin of the left lung that extends from the inferior end of the cardiac notch. The posterior border of each lung is thick and lies beside the vertebral column.

Lobes and Fissures

Deep fissures divide the right and left lungs into unequal numbers of lobes. The organization of the lobes and fissures is summarized in Table 4.2 and illustrated in Figures 4.34 to 4.36.

Bronchopulmonary Segments

The bronchopulmonary segments are the anatomic, functional, and surgical units of the lungs. Each lobar (secondary) bronchus, which passes to a lobe of the lung, gives off branches called **segmental (tertiary) bronchi** (see Fig. 4.27). Each segmental bronchus passes

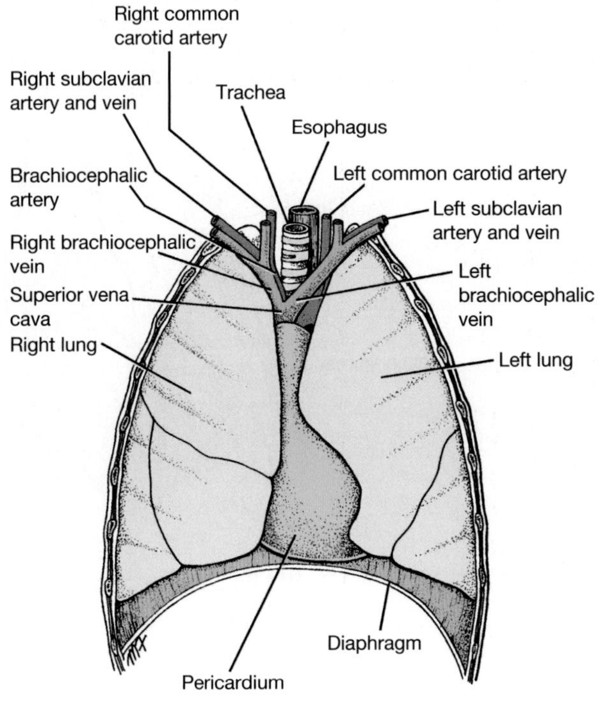

Figure 4.37 Pericardium and the lungs exposed from in front.

Table 4.2 Lung Lobes and Fissures

	FISSURES	LOBES
Right Lung (slightly larger)	1. Horizontal: runs along approximately the horizontal line of costal cartilage 4 to intersect the oblique fissure in the midaxillary line. 2. Oblique: runs at roughly a T2 (posterior) to T6 (anterior) angulation.	1. Upper (superior) 2. Middle 3. Lower (inferior)
Left Lung	1. Oblique: similar course as in the right lung. No horizontal fissure.	1. Upper (superior) 2. Lower (inferior)

Note: In both lungs, the upper lobes lie more anteriorly, whereas the lower lobes lie more posteriorly. The middle lobe is a small triangular lobe that lays anteroinferiorly, between the other two lobes, bounded by the horizontal and oblique fissures.

to a structurally and functionally independent unit of a lung lobe called a **bronchopulmonary segment**, which is bounded by connective tissue walls (Fig. 4.38). A branch of the pulmonary artery accompanies the segmental bronchus, but the tributaries of the pulmonary veins run in the connective tissue between adjacent bronchopulmonary segments. Each segment has its own lymphatic vessels and autonomic nerve supply.

Each segmental bronchus divides repeatedly upon entering a bronchopulmonary segment (see Figs. 4.27

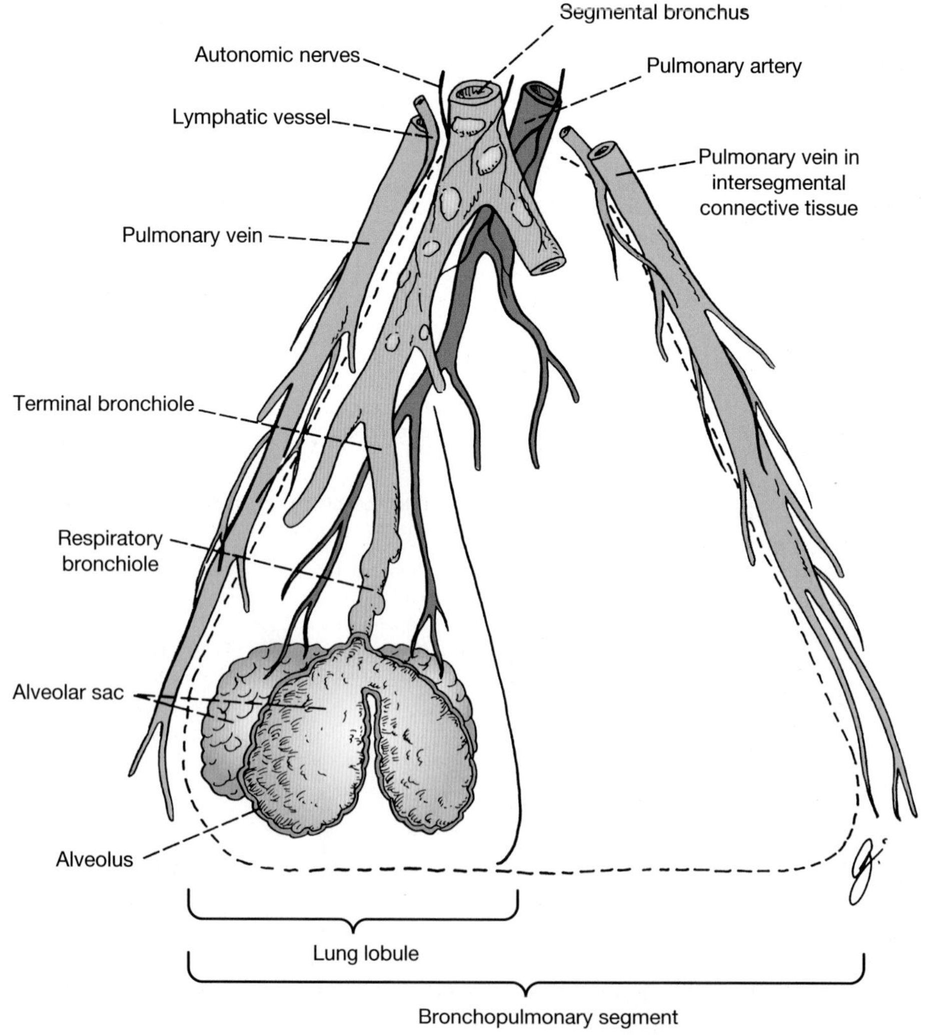

Figure 4.38 Bronchopulmonary segment and a lung lobule. Note that the pulmonary veins lie within the connective tissue septa that separate adjacent segments.

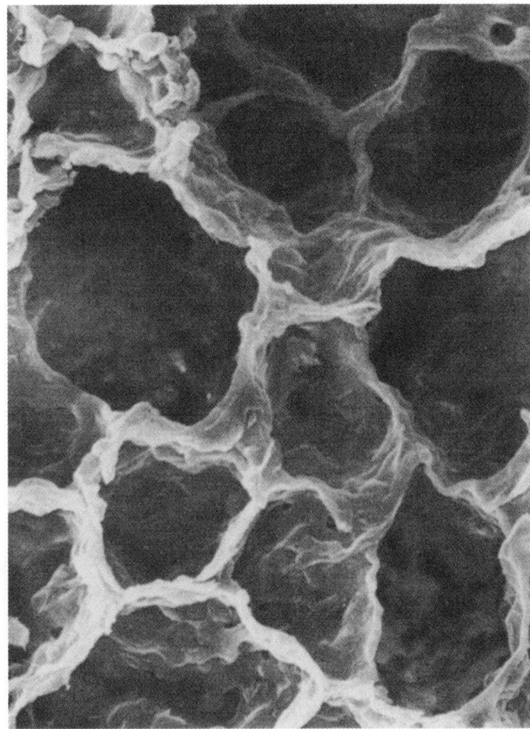

Figure 4.39 Scanning electron micrograph of the lung showing numerous alveolar sacs. The alveoli are the depressions, or alcoves, along the walls of the alveolar sac. (Courtesy of Dr. M. Koering.)

and 4.38). As the bronchi become smaller, irregular plates of cartilage, which become smaller and fewer in number, gradually replace the tracheal rings. The smallest bronchi divide and give rise to **bronchioles**, which are <1 mm in diameter. Bronchioles possess no cartilage in their walls and are lined with columnar ciliated epithelium. The submucosa possesses a complete layer of circularly arranged smooth muscle fibers.

The bronchioles then divide and give rise to **terminal bronchioles**, which show delicate outpouchings from their walls. Gas exchange between blood and air takes place in the walls of these outpouchings, which explains the name **respiratory bronchiole**. The diameter of a respiratory bronchiole is about 0.5 mm. The respiratory bronchioles end by branching into **alveolar ducts**, which lead into tubular passages with numerous thin-walled outpouchings called **alveolar sacs**. The alveolar sacs consist of several **alveoli** opening into a single chamber (Fig. 4.39; see also Figs. 4.27 and 4.38). A rich network of blood capillaries surrounds each alveolus. Gaseous exchange takes place between the air in the alveolar lumen and the alveolar wall into the blood within the surrounding capillaries.

The main characteristics of a bronchopulmonary segment are as follows:

- It is a subdivision of a lung lobe.
- It is pyramid shaped, with its apex directed toward the lung root.
- It is surrounded by connective tissue.
- It has three defining components: a centrally located **segmental (tertiary) bronchus**, a **segmental artery** that accompanies the segmental bronchus, and **intersegmental veins** located in the connective tissue walls between adjacent bronchopulmonary segments.
- It has its own lymph vessels and autonomic nerves.
- Because it is a structural unit, a diseased segment can be removed surgically.

The functional flow pattern within each bronchopulmonary segment is as follows:

- Air enters and leaves the center of each bronchopulmonary segment via the segmental bronchus.
- Deoxygenated blood enters the center of each bronchopulmonary segment via the segmental artery (a branch of the pulmonary artery).
- Oxygenated blood leaves the bronchopulmonary segment via the intersegmental veins located around the periphery of each segment. These veins drain into the pulmonary veins.

Typically, the right lung has 10 bronchopulmonary segments, and the left lung has 8 to 10. Although the general arrangement of the bronchopulmonary segments is clinically important, memorizing the details is not essential for anyone not intending to specialize in pulmonary medicine or surgery.

The main bronchopulmonary segments (see Figs. 4.35 and 4.36) are as follows:

- **Right lung**
  Superior lobe: Apical, posterior, anterior
  Middle lobe: Lateral, medial
  Inferior lobe: Superior (apical), medial basal, anterior basal, lateral basal, posterior basal
- **Left lung**
  Superior lobe: Apical, posterior, anterior, superior lingular, inferior lingular
  Inferior lobe: Superior (apical), medial basal, anterior basal, lateral basal, posterior basal

Blood Supply

Two separate arterial systems supply the lungs. One is the nonrespiratory circuit that supplies the tissues of the respiratory tree and lungs. The second system is the respiratory (pulmonary) circuit, across which gas exchange occurs.

Nonrespiratory Circuit

The **bronchial arteries** (branches of the descending aorta) supply the bronchi, the connective tissue of the lung, and the visceral pleura. The **bronchial veins** (which communicate with the pulmonary veins) drain into the azygos and hemiazygos veins.

Respiratory (Pulmonary) Circuit

The **segmental arteries** (terminal branches of the pulmonary arteries) carry deoxygenated blood into the

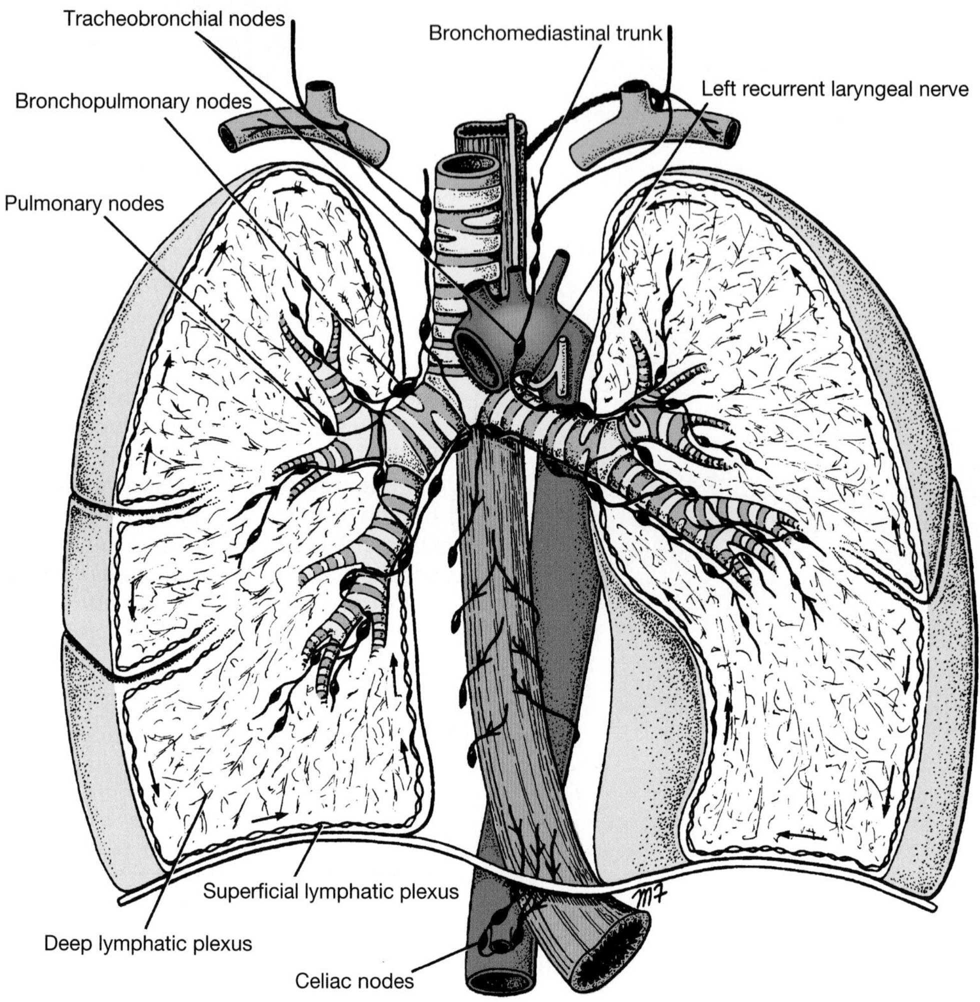

Figure 4.40 Lymph drainage of the lungs and lower end of the esophagus.

bronchopulmonary segments and to the alveoli (see Fig. 4.38). **Intersegmental veins**, carrying oxygenated blood from the alveolar capillaries, follow the connective tissue septa bounding the bronchopulmonary segments to the pulmonary veins and to the lung root (see Fig. 4.38). Two pulmonary veins leave each lung root (see Fig. 4.31) to empty into the left atrium of the heart.

Lymph Drainage

The lymph vessels originate in superficial and deep plexuses (Fig. 4.40); they are not present in the alveolar walls. The **superficial (subpleural) plexus** lies beneath the visceral pleura and drains over the surface of the lung toward the hilum, where the lymph vessels enter the **bronchopulmonary nodes**. The **deep plexus** travels along the bronchi and pulmonary vessels toward the hilum of the lung, passing through **pulmonary nodes** located within the lung substance; the lymph then enters the bronchopulmonary nodes in the hilum of the lung. All the lymph from the lung leaves the hilum and drains into the **tracheobronchial nodes** and then into the **bronchomediastinal lymph trunks**.

Nerve Supply

Sympathetic nerve fibers (derived from the sympathetic chains), parasympathetic nerve fibers (derived from the vagus nerves), and visceral afferent fibers intermingle at the root of each lung and form the **pulmonary plexuses**. Branches of the pulmonary plexuses mainly follow the bronchi into and within the lungs.

Afferent impulses derived from the bronchial mucous membrane and from stretch receptors in the alveolar walls travel with both sympathetic and parasympathetic nerves to the CNS. Table 4.3 summarizes lung autonomic functions.

Mechanics of Respiration

Respiration consists of two alternating phases, **inspiration** and **expiration**, which are accomplished by increasing and decreasing the capacity of the thoracic cavity. The mechanics of each phase differ depending on whether respiration occurs under quiet or forced conditions. The rate of respiration varies between 16 and 20 breaths per minute in normal resting patients and is faster in children and slower in older adults.

Table 4.3 Lung Autonomic Functions

SYMPATHETIC	PARASYMPATHETIC
Bronchodilatation (inhibitory to bronchial smooth muscle)	Bronchoconstriction (motor to bronchial smooth muscle)
Vasoconstriction (motor to pulmonary vessels)	Vasodilatation (inhibitory to pulmonary vessels)
Inhibitory to alveolar glands of the bronchial tree (type II secretory epithelial cells of the alveoli)	Secretomotor to glands of the bronchial tree

Quiet Inspiration

Compare the thoracic cavity to a box with a single entrance at the top, which is a tube called the trachea (Fig. 4.41A). Elongating all its diameters increases the capacity of the box, resulting in air under atmospheric pressure entering the box through the tube.

Now consider the three diameters of the thoracic cavity and how they may be increased (see Fig. 4.41).

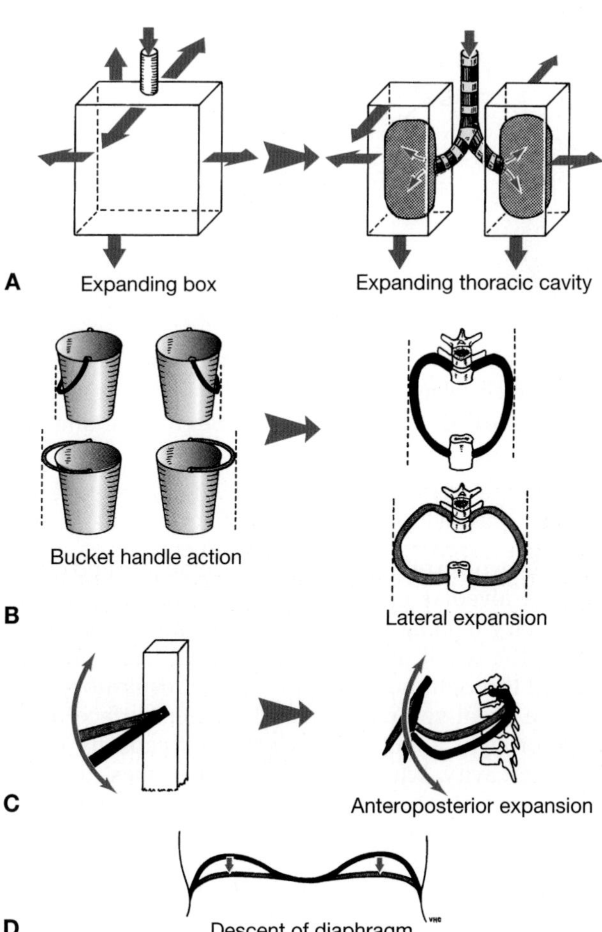

Figure 4.41 How the capacity of the thoracic cavity is increased during inspiration. **A.** All diameter expansion. **B.** Transverse expansion. **C.** Anteroposterior expansion. **D.** Vertical expansion.

Vertical Diameter

Theoretically, the roof could be raised and the floor lowered. The roof is formed by the suprapleural membrane and is fixed. Conversely, the mobile diaphragm forms the floor. When the diaphragm contracts, the domes flatten and the level of the diaphragm lowers, thus increasing the vertical diameter of the thoracic cavity (Fig. 4.41D).

Anteroposterior Diameter

If the downward-sloping ribs were raised at their sternal ends, the anteroposterior diameter of the thoracic cavity would be increased, and the lower end of the sternum would be thrust forward (Fig. 4.41C). This happens when rib 1 is fixed by the contraction of the scalene muscles of the neck and when the intercostal muscles contract (Fig. 4.42). This mechanism stabilizes the sizes of the intercostal spaces and raises the ribs toward rib 1.

Transverse Diameter

The ribs articulate in front with the sternum via their costal cartilages and behind with the vertebral column. Because the ribs curve downward as well as forward around the chest wall, they resemble bucket handles (Fig. 4.41B). It therefore follows that when the ribs are raised (like bucket handles), the transverse diameter of the thoracic cavity increases. As described previously, this occurs by fixing rib 1 and raising the other ribs to it by contracting the intercostal muscles (see Fig. 4.42).

An additional factor that must not be overlooked is the effect of the descent of the diaphragm on the abdominal viscera and the tone of the muscles of the anterior abdominal wall. As the diaphragm descends on inspiration, intra-abdominal pressure rises. This rise in pressure is accommodated by the reciprocal relaxation of the abdominal wall musculature. However, a point is reached when no further abdominal relaxation is possible, and the liver and other upper abdominal viscera act as a platform that resists further diaphragmatic descent. On further contraction, the diaphragm will now have its central tendon supported from below, and its shortening muscle fibers will assist the intercostal muscles in raising the lower ribs (see Fig. 4.42).

Apart from the diaphragm and the intercostals, other less important muscles also contract on inspiration and assist in elevating the ribs, namely, the levatores costarum muscles and (possibly) the serratus posterior superior muscles.

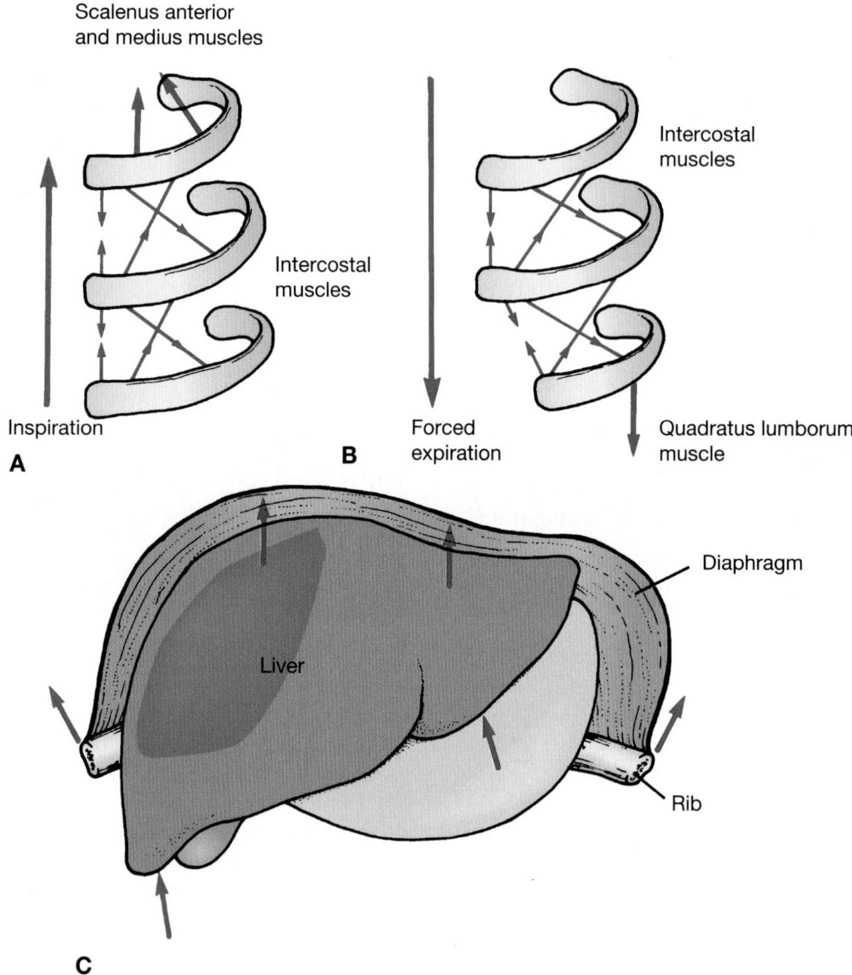

Figure 4.42 Mechanics of respiration. **A.** How the intercostal muscles raise the ribs during inspiration. Note that the scalene muscles fix rib 1 or, in forced inspiration, raise it. **B.** How the intercostal muscles can be used in forced expiration, provided that rib 12 is fixed or is made to descend by the abdominal muscles. **C.** How the liver provides the platform that enables the diaphragm to raise the lower ribs.

Forced Inspiration

Maximum increase in the capacity of the thoracic cavity occurs in forced deep inspiration. Every muscle that can raise the ribs is brought into action, including the scalenus anterior and medius and the sternocleidomastoid. In respiratory distress, the action of all the muscles already engaged becomes more violent, and the scapulae are fixed by the trapezius, levator scapulae, and rhomboid muscles, enabling the serratus anterior and the pectoralis minor to pull up the ribs. Grasping a chair back or table can support the upper limbs, allowing the sternal heads of the pectoralis major muscles to also assist the process.

Lung Changes on Inspiration

In inspiration, the root of the lung descends, and the level of the bifurcation of the trachea may lower by as much as two vertebrae. The bronchi elongate and dilate, and the alveolar capillaries dilate, thus assisting the pulmonary circulation. Air is drawn into the bronchial tree as the result of the positive atmospheric pressure exerted through the upper part of the respiratory tract and the negative pressure on the outer surface of the lungs brought about by the increased capacity of the thoracic cavity. With expansion of the lungs, the elastic tissue in the bronchial walls and connective tissue are stretched. As the diaphragm descends, the costodiaphragmatic recess of the pleural cavity opens, and the expanding sharp lower edges of the lungs descend to a lower level.

Quiet Expiration

Quiet expiration is largely a passive phenomenon caused by the elastic recoil of the lungs, the relaxation of the intercostal muscles and diaphragm, and an increase in the tone of the muscles of the anterior abdominal wall, which forces the relaxing diaphragm upward. The serratus posterior inferior muscles may play a minor role in pulling down the lower ribs.

Forced Expiration

Forced expiration is an active process brought about by the forcible contraction of the musculature of the anterior abdominal wall. The quadratus lumborum also contracts and pulls rib 12 down. Under these circumstances, some of the intercostal muscles may contract, pull the ribs together, and depress them toward the lowered rib 12 (see Fig. 4.42). The serratus posterior inferior and the latissimus dorsi muscles may also play minor roles.

Lung Changes on Expiration

The roots of the lungs and the bifurcation of the trachea ascend during expiration. The bronchi shorten and contract. The elastic tissue recoils, and the lungs become reduced in size. Increasing areas of the diaphragmatic and costal parietal pleura come into apposition with the upward movement of the diaphragm, and the costodiaphragmatic recess reduces in size. The lower margins of the lungs shrink and rise to a higher level.

Types of Respiration

In infants and young children, the ribs are nearly horizontal. Thus, they must rely mainly on the descent of the diaphragm to increase their thoracic capacity on inspiration. Because this is accompanied by a marked inward and outward excursion of the anterior abdominal wall, which is easily seen, respiration at this age is referred to as the **abdominal type of respiration**.

After age 2 years, the ribs become more oblique, and the adult form of respiration is established. A biological sex difference exists in the type of respiratory movements in adults. Females tend to rely mainly on the movements of the ribs rather than on the descent of the diaphragm on inspiration. This is referred to as the **thoracic type of respiration**. Males use both the thoracic and abdominal forms of respiration but mainly the abdominal form.

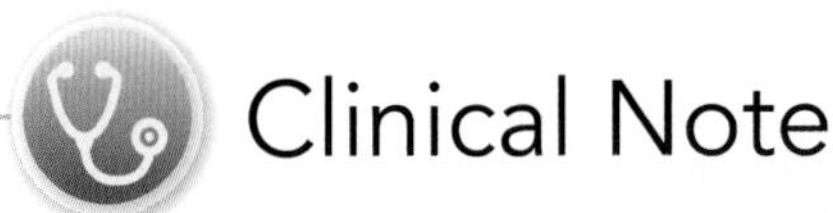

Physical Examination of the Lungs

For physical examination, remember that the upper lobes of the lungs are most easily examined from the front of the chest and the lower lobes from the back. Areas of all lobes can be examined in the axillae.

Lung Trauma

A physician must always remember that the apex of the lung projects up into the neck (1 in. [2.5 cm] above the clavicle) and can be damaged by stab or bullet wounds in this area.

Although the lungs are well protected by the bony thoracic cage, a splinter from a fractured rib can nevertheless penetrate the lung, and air can escape into the pleural cavity, causing a pneumothorax and lung collapse. It can also find its way into the lung connective tissue. From there, the air moves under the visceral pleura until it reaches the lung root. It then passes into the mediastinum and up to the neck. Here, it may distend the subcutaneous tissue, a condition known as **subcutaneous emphysema**.

The changes in the position of the thoracic and upper abdominal viscera and the level of the diaphragm during different phases of respiration relative to the chest wall are of considerable clinical importance. A penetrating wound in the lower part of the chest may or may not damage the abdominal viscera, depending on the phase of respiration at the time of injury.

Pain and Lung Disease

Lung tissue and the visceral pleura are devoid of pain-sensitive nerve endings, so that pain in the chest is always the result of conditions affecting the surrounding structures. In tuberculosis or pneumonia, for example, pain may never be experienced.

Once lung disease crosses the visceral pleura and the pleural cavity to involve the parietal pleura, pain becomes a prominent feature. Lobar pneumonia with pleurisy, for example, produces a severe tearing pain, accentuated by deep inspiration or coughing. Because the lower part of the costal parietal pleura receives its sensory innervation from intercostal nerves 7 to 11, which also innervate the skin of the anterior abdominal wall, pleurisy in this area commonly produces pain that is referred to the abdomen. This could result in a mistaken diagnosis of an acute abdominal lesion.

In a similar manner, pleurisy of the central part of the diaphragmatic pleura, which receives sensory innervation from the phrenic nerves (C3 to C5), can lead to referred pain over the shoulder because the supraclavicular nerves (C3 and C4) supply the skin of this region.

Surgical Access to the Lungs

Surgical access to the lung or mediastinum is commonly undertaken through an intercostal space (see Thoracotomy earlier in this chapter). Special rib retractors allow wide separation of the ribs. The costal cartilages are sufficiently elastic to permit considerable bending. This method permits good exposure of the lungs.

(continued)

Segmental Resection of the Lung (Segmental Pulmonary Resection)

A localized chronic lesion such as that of tuberculosis or a benign neoplasm may require surgical removal. If the disease is restricted to a bronchopulmonary segment, it is possible to dissect out that segment and remove it, leaving the surrounding lung intact. Segmental resection requires that the radiologist and thoracic surgeon have a sound knowledge of the bronchopulmonary segments and that they cooperate fully to localize the lesion accurately before operation.

Bronchogenic Carcinoma

Bronchogenic carcinoma accounts for about one third of all cancer deaths in males and is becoming increasingly common in females. It commences in most patients in the mucous membrane lining the larger bronchi and is therefore situated close to the hilum of the lung. The neoplasm rapidly spreads to the tracheobronchial and bronchomediastinal nodes and may involve the recurrent laryngeal nerves, leading to hoarseness. Lymphatic spread via the bronchomediastinal trunks may result in early involvement in the lower deep cervical nodes just above the level of the clavicle. Hematogenous spread to the bones and the brain commonly occurs.

Bronchial Constriction (Bronchial Asthma)

One of the problems associated with bronchial asthma is the spasm of the smooth muscle in the wall of the bronchioles. This particularly reduces the diameter of the bronchioles during expiration, usually causing the asthmatic patient to experience great difficulty in expiring, although inspiration is accomplished normally. The lungs consequently become greatly distended, and the thoracic cage becomes permanently enlarged, forming the so-called barrel chest. In addition, the airflow through the bronchioles is further impeded by the presence of excess mucus, which the patient is unable to clear because an effective cough cannot be produced.

Loss of Lung Elasticity

Many diseases of the lungs, such as emphysema and pulmonary fibrosis, destroy the elasticity of the lungs, and the lungs are unable to recoil adequately, causing incomplete expiration. The respiratory muscles in these patients must assist in expiration, which no longer is a passive phenomenon.

Loss of Lung Distensibility

Diseases such as silicosis, asbestosis, cancer, and pneumonia interfere with the process of expanding the lung in inspiration. A decrease in lung compliance and the chest wall then occurs, and a greater effort has to be undertaken by the inspiratory muscles to inflate the lungs.

Postural Drainage

Excessive accumulation of bronchial secretions in a lobe or segment of a lung can seriously interfere with the normal flow of air into the alveoli. Furthermore, the stagnation of such secretions is often quickly followed by infection. To aid in the normal drainage of a bronchial segment, a physiotherapist often alters the position of the patient so that gravity assists in the process of drainage. Sound knowledge of the bronchial tree is necessary to determine the optimum position of the patient for good postural drainage.

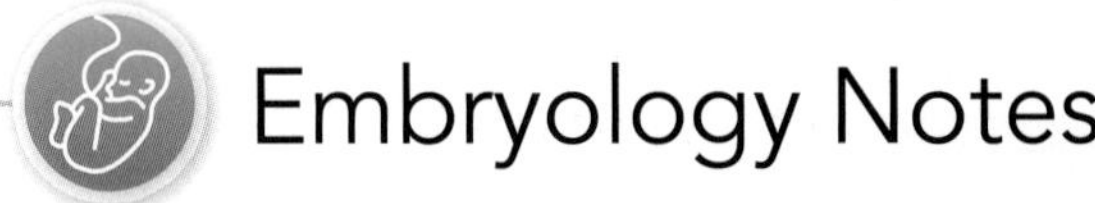

Embryology Notes

Development of the Lungs and Pleura

The lower respiratory tract develops from the embryonic foregut. Initially, a longitudinal groove, the **laryngotracheal groove**, develops in the endodermal lining of the floor of the pharynx. This gives rise to the **laryngotracheal tube** (**respiratory diverticulum**, **lung bud**) (Fig. 4.43; see also Fig. 4.22). A **tracheoesophageal septum** partitions the laryngotracheal tube from the foregut, forming two structures: a more dorsal **esophagus** and a more ventral (anterior) **respiratory primordium**. The laryngotracheal tube grows caudally into the splanchnic mesoderm and divides distally into the **right** and **left lung buds**. Cartilage develops in the mesenchyme surrounding the tube, and the upper part of the tube becomes the larynx, whereas the lower part becomes the trachea.

Each lung bud consists of an endodermal tube surrounded by splanchnic mesoderm; all the tissues of the corresponding lung are derived from this. Each bud grows laterally and projects into the pleural part of the embryonic coelom (see Figs. 4.22 and 4.43). The lung bud divides into two or three lobes, corresponding to the number of main bronchi and lobes found in the fully developed lung. Each main bronchus then divides repeatedly in a dichotomous manner, until the terminal bronchioles and alveoli form. The division of the terminal bronchioles, with the formation of additional bronchioles and alveoli, continues for some time after birth.

Splanchnic mesoderm forms the visceral pleura, whereas somatic mesoderm forms the parietal pleura. By month 7, the capillary loops connected with the pulmonary circulation are sufficiently well developed to support life, should premature birth take place. With the onset of respiration at

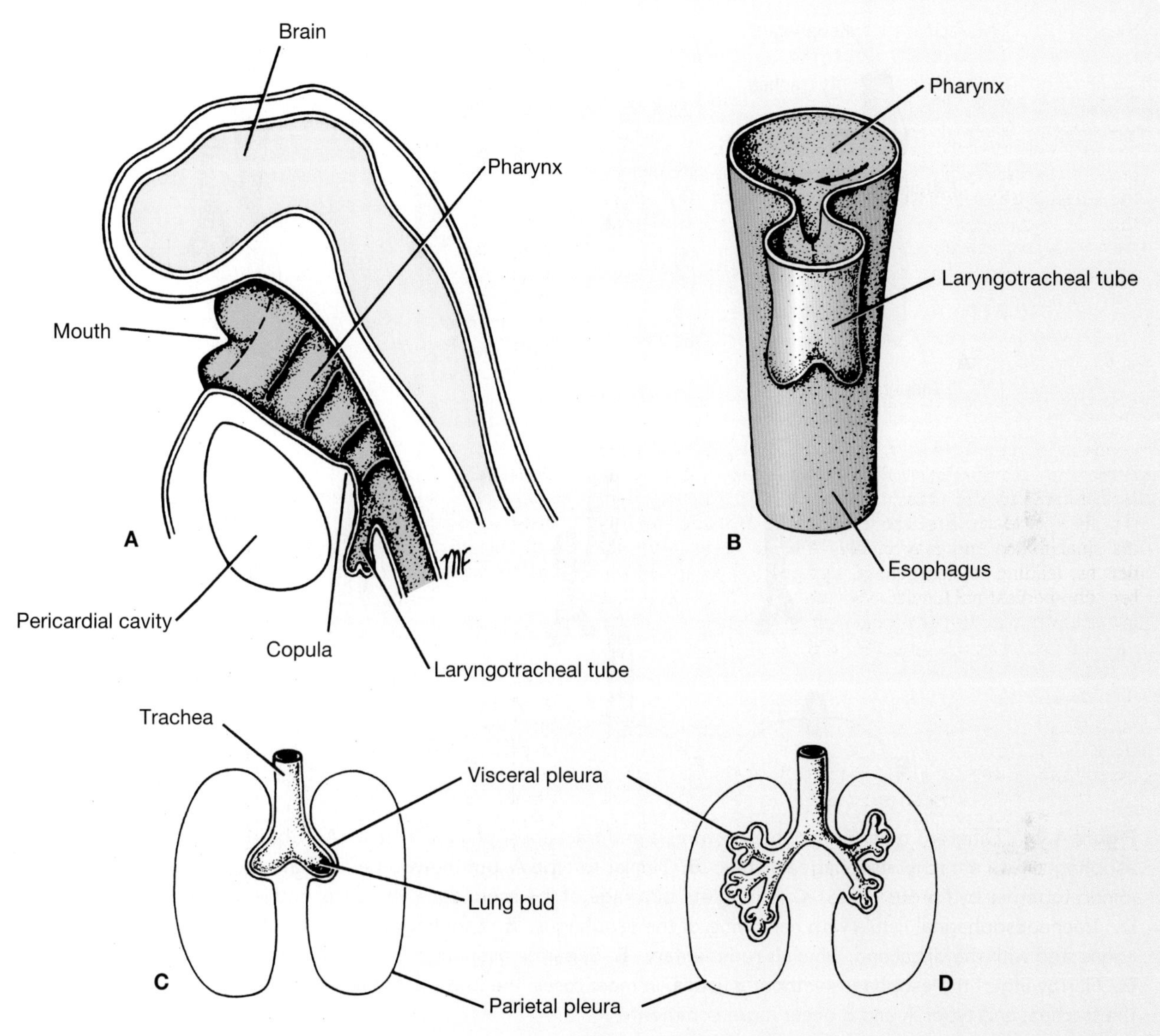

Figure 4.43 Development of the lungs. **A.** Laryngotracheal groove and tube have been formed. **B.** Margins of the laryngotracheal groove fuse to form the laryngotracheal tube. **C.** Lung buds invaginate the wall of the intraembryonic coelom. **D.** Lung buds divide to form the main bronchi.

birth, the lungs expand, and the alveoli dilate. However, the alveoli in the periphery of each lung become fully expanded only after 3 or 4 days of postnatal life.

Congenital Anomalies: Esophageal Atresia and Tracheoesophageal Fistula

If the margins of the laryngotracheal groove fail to fuse properly, an abnormal connection (a fistula) may be left between the laryngotracheal tube and the esophagus. If the tracheoesophageal septum formed by the fusion of the margins of the laryngotracheal groove is deviated posteriorly, the lumen of the esophagus would be much reduced in diameter. The different types of atresia, with and without fistula, are shown in Figure 4.44. Obstruction of the esophagus prevents the child from swallowing saliva and milk, leading to aspiration into the larynx and trachea, which may result in pneumonia.

(continued)

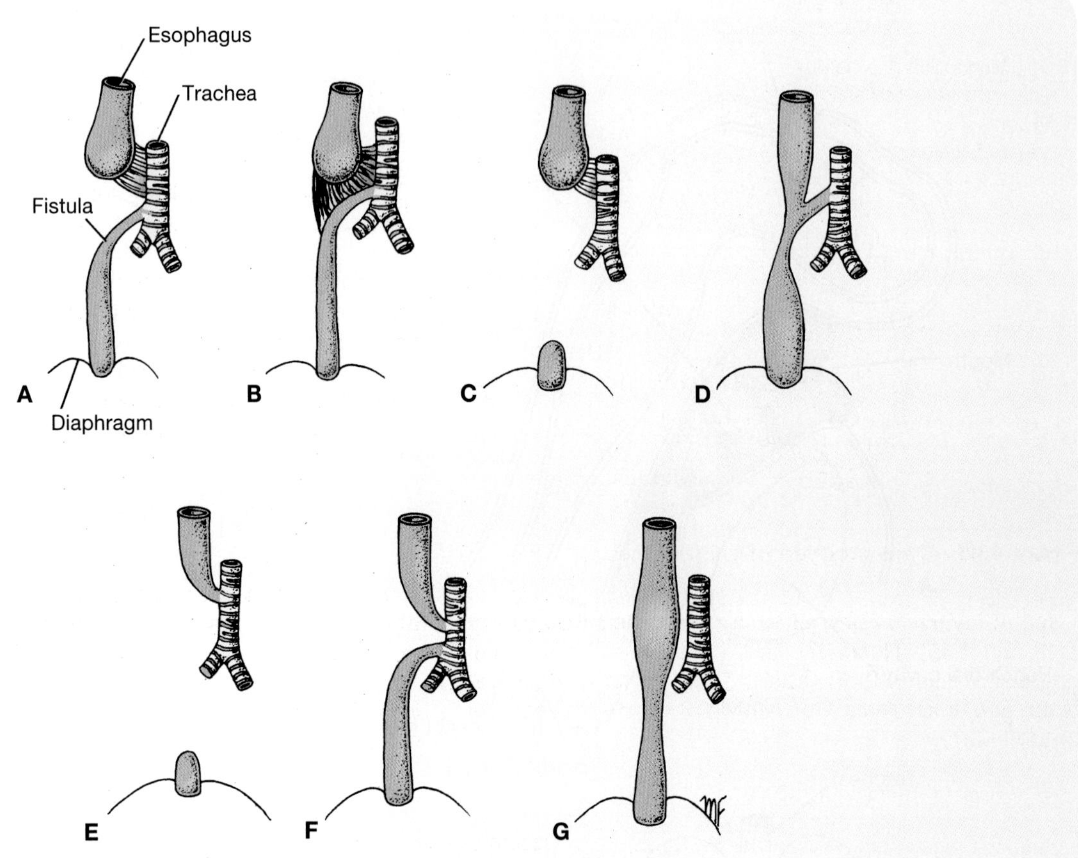

Figure 4.44 Different types of esophageal atresia and tracheoesophageal fistula. **A.** Complete blockage of the esophagus with a tracheoesophageal fistula. **B.** Similar to type A, but the two parts of the esophagus are joined together by fibrous tissue. **C.** Complete blockage of the esophagus; the distal end is rudimentary. **D.** Tracheoesophageal fistula with narrowing of the esophagus. **E.** Esophagotracheal fistula; the esophagus is not connected with the distal end, which is rudimentary. **F.** Separate esophagotracheal and tracheoesophageal fistulas. **G.** Narrowing of the esophagus without a fistula. In most cases, the lower esophageal segment communicates with the trachea, and types A and B occur more commonly.

PERICARDIUM

The pericardium is a fibroserous sac that encloses the heart and the roots of the great vessels (see Fig. 4.37). Its function is to restrict excessive movements of the heart as a whole and to serve as a lubricated container in which the different parts of the heart can contract free of the surrounding structures. The pericardium lies within the middle mediastinum (see Figs. 4.20, 4.31, and 4.37), posterior to the body of the sternum and costal cartilages 2 to 6 and anterior to the T5 to T8 vertebrae.

Fibrous Pericardium

The fibrous pericardium is the strong, fibrous, outer layer of the sac (Fig. 4.45; see also Fig. 4.19). It attaches firmly below to the central tendon of the diaphragm. It fuses with the outer coats of the great blood vessels passing through it—namely, the aorta, the pulmonary trunk, the superior and inferior venae cavae, and the pulmonary veins (Figs. 4.45 and 4.46). The fibrous pericardium attaches in front of the sternum by fibrous bands called the **sternopericardial ligaments**.

Serous Pericardium

The serous pericardium lines the fibrous pericardium and coats the heart. It is divided into parietal and visceral layers (see Figs. 4.19 and 4.45).

The **parietal layer** lines the inner surface of the fibrous pericardium and reflects around the roots of the great vessels to become continuous with the visceral layer of serous pericardium that closely covers the heart (see Figs. 4.45 and 4.46).

The **visceral layer** is closely applied to the superficial surface of the heart and is often called the **epicardium**. The slit-like space between the parietal and

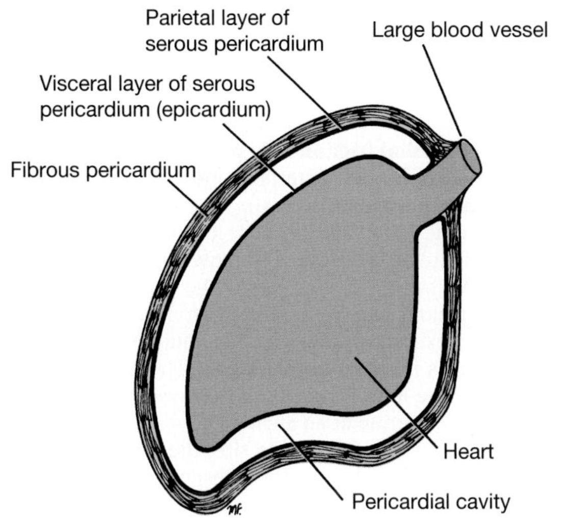

Figure 4.45 Different layers of the pericardium.

visceral layers is referred to as the **pericardial cavity** (see Fig. 4.45). Normally, the cavity contains a small amount of tissue fluid (about 50 mL), the **pericardial fluid**, which acts as a lubricant to facilitate movements of the heart.

Pericardial Sinuses

The pericardial sinuses are spaces posterior to the heart formed by the reflections of the serous pericardium around the great vessels. The reflection around the large veins forms an inverted U-shaped cul-de-sac called the **oblique sinus** (see Fig. 4.46). This runs along the long axis of the heart, from the apex to the ascending aorta. The relatively short horizontal space between the reflection of the serous pericardium around the aorta and pulmonary trunk and the reflection around the large veins is the **transverse sinus**. The pericardial sinuses form because of the way the heart bends during development (see Embryology Notes, below). They are extensions of the pericardial cavity and not separate compartmental spaces.

Nerve Supply

The phrenic nerves carry sensory fibers from the fibrous pericardium and the parietal layer of the serous pericardium (see Figs. 4.31 and 4.46). Visceral afferent fibers travel with branches of the sympathetic trunks and the vagus nerves from the visceral layer of the serous pericardium.

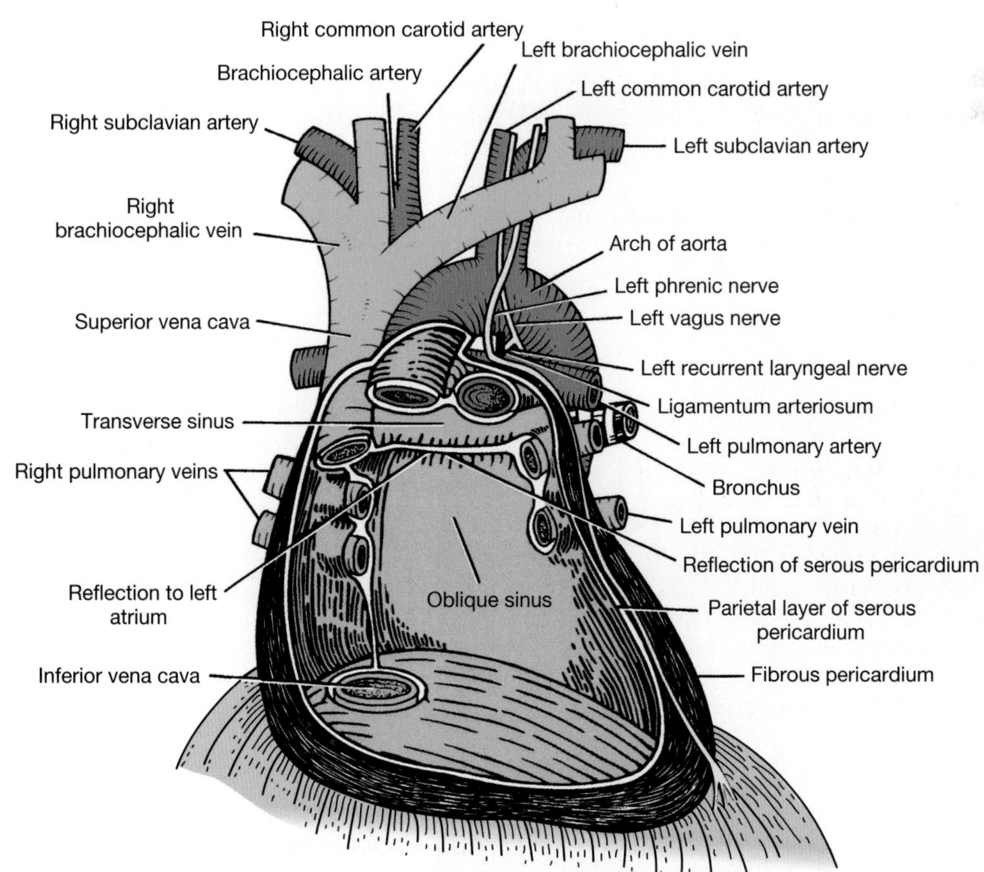

Figure 4.46 Great blood vessels and the interior of the pericardium.

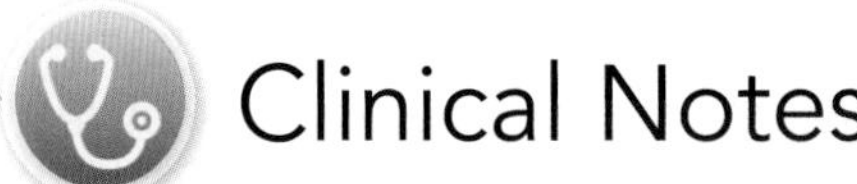

Clinical Notes

Pericarditis

Pericarditis is inflammation of the pericardium. In this condition, excessive pericardial fluid may accumulate in the pericardial cavity, which can compress the thin-walled atria and interfere with the filling of the heart during diastole. Such compression of the heart is called **cardiac tamponade**.

Cardiac tamponade can also occur secondary to stab or gunshot wounds when the chambers of the heart have been penetrated. Blood escapes into the pericardial cavity and can restrict the filling of the heart.

Roughening of the visceral and parietal layers of serous pericardium by inflammatory exudate in acute pericarditis produces **pericardial friction rub**, which can be felt on palpation and heard through a stethoscope.

Constrictive pericarditis occurs when the fibrous pericardium becomes too rigid because of inflammation. This results in heightened resistance to movements of the heart and blood flow.

Pericardial fluid can be aspirated from the pericardial cavity should excessive amounts accumulate in pericarditis. This process is called **paracentesis**. The needle can be introduced to the left of the xiphoid process in an upward and backward direction at an angle of 45° to the skin. When paracentesis is performed at this site, the pleura and lung are not damaged because of the presence of the cardiac notch in this area.

HEART

The heart is an enlarged, internally subdivided blood vessel specialized for pumping. Its major unique and dominant functional feature is a myocardial layer composed largely of cardiac muscle. The heart is somewhat pyramid shaped and lies within the pericardium in the middle mediastinum (Fig. 4.47; see also Figs. 4.20 and 4.46). It is connected at its base to the great blood vessels but otherwise lies free within the pericardium.

The heart contains four chambers, two **atria** and two **ventricles** (Figs. 4.48 to 4.50; see also Fig. 4.47). The atria and ventricles are connected via **atrioventricular valves**. The atria receive venous blood, pump blood

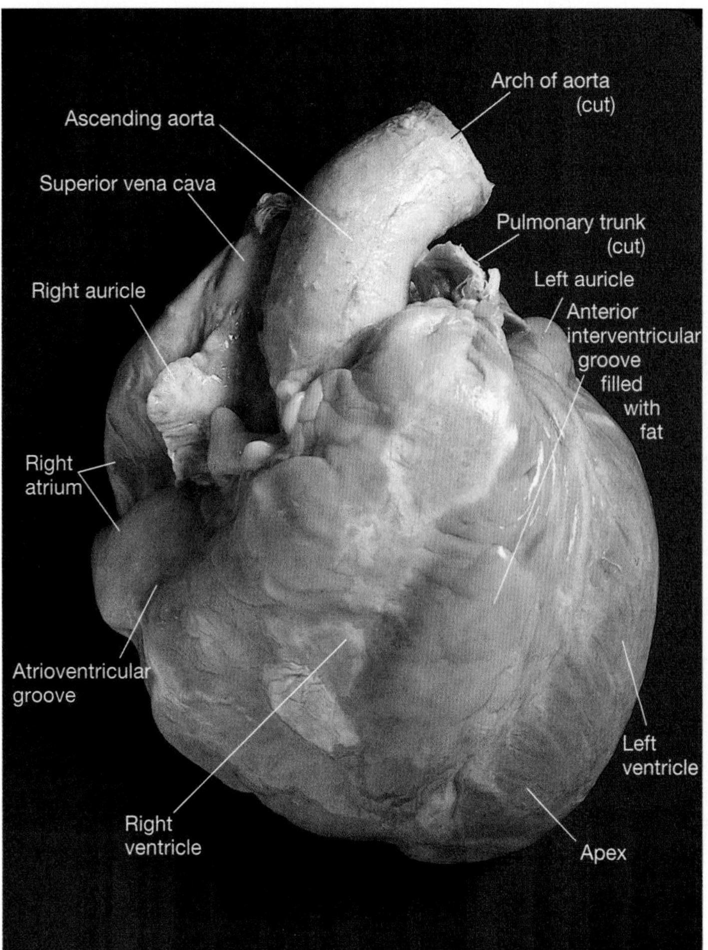

Figure 4.47 Anterior surface of the heart; the fibrous pericardium and the parietal serous pericardium have been removed. Note the presence of fat beneath the visceral serous pericardium in the atrioventricular and interventricular grooves. The coronary arteries are embedded in this fat.

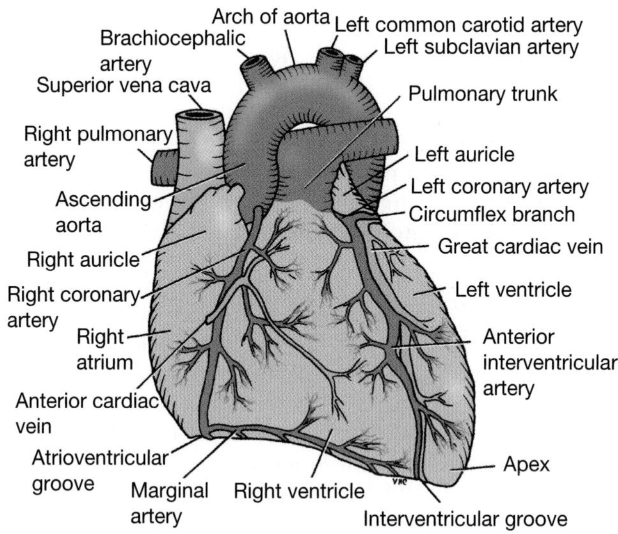

Figure 4.48 Anterior surface of the heart and the great blood vessels. Note the course of the coronary arteries and the cardiac veins.

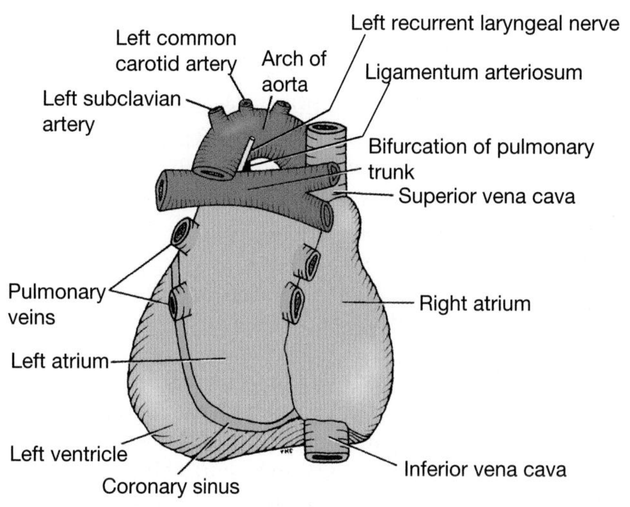

Figure 4.49 Posterior surface, or the base, of the heart.

only to the immediately adjacent ventricles, and therefore are low-pressure chambers. The ventricles pump arterial blood out of the heart, must impart pulmonary and systemic pulses of blood, and therefore are comparatively high-pressure chambers. The ventricles are the major sources of energy for the circulation of blood.

The heart has two functional circuits, the right heart, and the left heart. The **right heart** (right atrium and right ventricle) is the **pulmonary circuit** pump. In this, blood travels a relatively short distance to the lungs and back against low peripheral resistance. The **left heart** (left atrium and left ventricle) is the **systemic circuit** pump. Here, blood travels a long distance through the body against high peripheral resistance.

Orientation

The heart is aligned obliquely within the thorax, with an apex (pointed end) directed downward, forward, and to

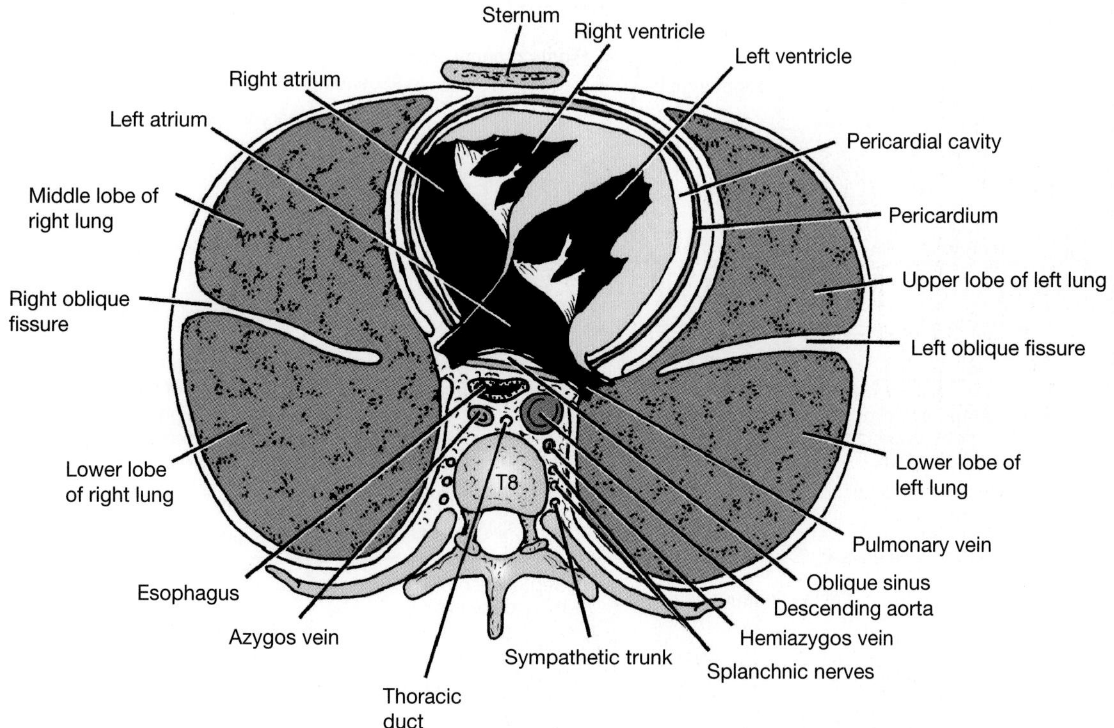

Figure 4.50 Cross section of the thorax at the T8 vertebra.

the left (see Figs. 4.47 and 4.48). About two thirds of the heart lies to the left of the midline and one third to the right of the midline.

The left ventricle forms the **apex** of the heart. It lies at the level of left intercostal space 5, 3.5 in. (9 cm) from the midline. The apex beat can usually be seen and palpated.

Surfaces

The heart has three surfaces: sternocostal (anterior), diaphragmatic (inferior), and base (posterior) (see Figs. 4.47 to 4.49).

The right atrium and the right ventricle are separated from each other by the vertical **atrioventricular groove (coronary sulcus)** and mainly form the **sternocostal (anterior) surface** (see Figs. 4.47 and 4.48). The right ventricle is separated from the left ventricle by the **anterior interventricular groove**.

The right and left ventricles (separated by the posterior interventricular groove) mainly form the **diaphragmatic (inferior) surface** of the heart. The inferior surface of the right atrium, into which the inferior vena cava opens, also forms part of this surface.

The left atrium (which receives the four pulmonary veins) forms the **base** of the heart, or the **posterior surface** (see Fig. 4.49). Note that the base of the heart is called the base because the heart is pyramid shaped and the base lies opposite the apex. The heart does not rest on its base; it rests on its diaphragmatic (inferior) surface.

Borders

The right atrium forms the **right border** of the heart (see Fig. 4.48). The left auricle and left ventricle form the **left border**. The right ventricle mainly forms the **inferior (lower) border (right margin)**, but the right atrium contributes a small portion. These borders are important to recognize when examining a radiograph of the heart (see Radiographic Anatomy later in this chapter).

Heart Structure

The heart wall has three layers. The visceral layer of serous pericardium (**epicardium**) makes up the external layer. Cardiac muscle (**myocardium**) is the primary constituent of the middle layer. A layer of endothelium (**endocardium**) lines the inner surface and forms the internal layer of the heart. The atrial portion of the heart has relatively thin walls, whereas the ventricular portion of the heart has thick walls (see Fig. 4.50).

Two internal septa divide the heart into its four chambers. The **atrial (interatrial) septum** separates the right and left atria. This septum runs from the anterior wall of the heart backward and to the right. The **ventricular (interventricular) septum** separates the right and left ventricles. This septum lies obliquely, with the right surface facing forward and to the right and the left surface facing backward and to the left. The ventricular septum has a lower, thicker **muscular part** and a smaller upper, thinner **membranous part**. The **anterior** and **posterior interventricular grooves** on the surface of the heart mark the position of the ventricular septum (Fig. 4.51; see also Figs. 4.47 and 4.48).

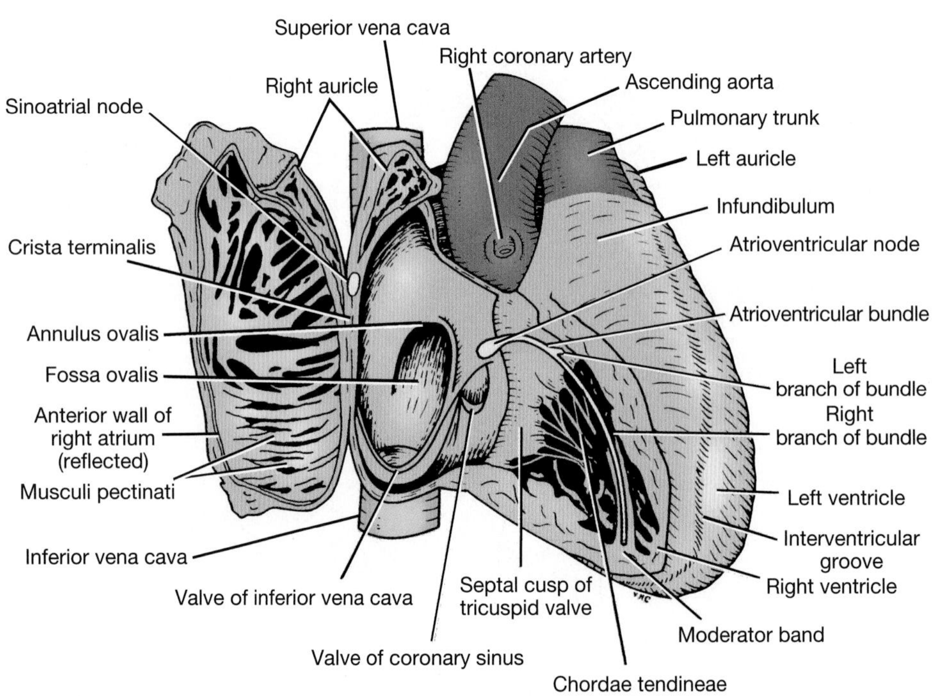

Figure 4.51 Interior of the right atrium and the right ventricle. Note the positions of the sinoatrial node and the atrioventricular node and bundle.

Right Atrium

The right atrium consists of two parts: a **main cavity (atrium proper)** and a small earlike outpouching, the **auricle** (see Figs. 4.48 and 4.51). A vertical groove, the **sulcus terminalis**, runs on the outside of the heart at the junction between the right atrium and the right auricle. It forms a matching ridge, the **crista terminalis** on the inside. The crista marks the boundary between the atrium proper and the auricle. The atrium proper is smooth walled and forms from the embryonic **sinus venosus**. The auricle is roughened or trabeculated by bundles of muscle fibers, the **musculi pectinati (pectinate muscles)**. This area develops from the embryonic primitive atrium.

Openings into the Right Atrium

Blood returns to the heart from the upper half of the body via the **superior vena cava**, which opens into the upper part of the right atrium; it has no valve (see Fig. 4.51). Blood returns to the heart from the lower half of the body through the **inferior vena cava** (larger than the superior vena cava), which opens into the lower part of the right atrium. A rudimentary, nonfunctioning (in the adult) valve, the **valve of the inferior vena cava**, guards the opening of the inferior vena cava.

The **coronary sinus**, which drains most of the blood from the heart wall, opens into the right atrium between the inferior vena cava and the atrioventricular orifice. The **valve of the coronary sinus**, which is rudimentary and nonfunctional in the adult, guards this opening (see Fig. 4.51).

The **right atrioventricular valve (tricuspid valve)** regulates the **right atrioventricular orifice**, which lies anterior to the opening of the inferior vena cava (see Fig. 4.51).

Many small orifices of small veins also drain the wall of the heart and open directly into the right atrium.

Fetal Remnants

The **fossa ovalis** and **annulus ovalis** lie on the **atrial septum**, which separates the right atrium from the left atrium (see Fig. 4.51). The fossa ovalis is a shallow depression that marks the site of the fetal **foramen ovale** (see Embryology Notes to follow). The annulus ovalis forms the upper margin of the fossa. The floor of the fossa represents the **persistent septum primum** of the embryonic heart, and the annulus forms from the lower edge of the **septum secundum**.

The valves of the inferior vena cava and coronary sinus are proportionately larger in the fetal heart and serve to preferentially direct blood flow currents across the right atrium.

Right Ventricle

Blood flows through the **right atrioventricular orifice** passing from the right atrium to the right ventricle. Blood then leaves the ventricle through the **pulmonary orifice** and enters the pulmonary trunk (see Figs. 4.51 and 4.52A,F). The **infundibulum (conus arteriosus)** is the funnel-shaped narrowing of the

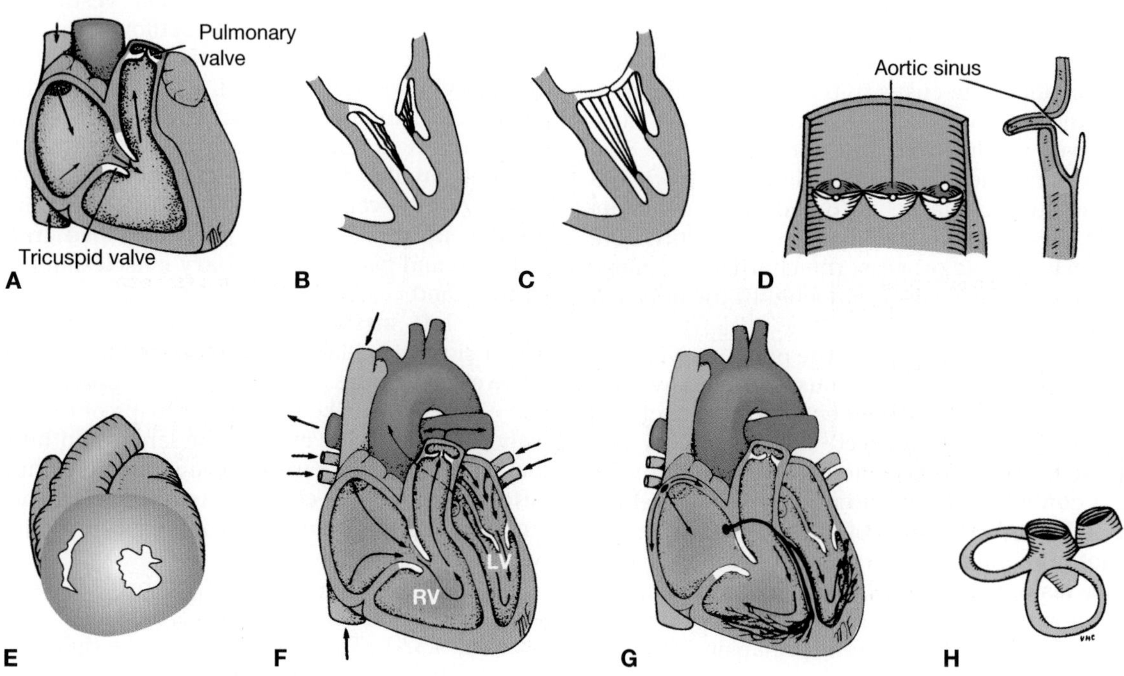

Figure 4.52 **A.** Position of the tricuspid and pulmonary valves. **B.** Mitral cusps with valve open. **C.** Mitral cusps with valve closed. **D.** Semilunar cusps of the aortic valve. **E.** Cross section of the ventricles of the heart. **F.** Path taken by the blood through the heart. **G.** Path taken by the cardiac impulse from the sinoatrial node to the Purkinje network. **H.** Fibrous skeleton of the heart.

ventricular cavity where the cavity approaches the pulmonary orifice. This constitutes the right ventricular outflow tract.

The walls of the right ventricle are much thicker than those of the right atrium and show many internal projecting ridges formed of muscle bundles. These ridges, the **trabeculae carneae**, are characteristic features of the ventricular walls and give the walls a spongelike appearance. There are three forms of trabeculae carneae. The first type comprises the **papillary muscles**, which project inward and attach by their bases to the ventricular wall; their apices connect by fibrous chords (**chordae tendineae**) to the cusps of the tricuspid valve (see Figs. 4.51 and 4.52B,C). The second type attaches at the ends to the ventricular wall and are free in the middle. One of these, the **septomarginal trabecula (moderator band)**, crosses the ventricular cavity from the septal to the anterior wall. It conveys the right branch of the atrioventricular bundle, which is part of the conducting system of the heart, and also resists overdistension of the anterior ventricular wall. The third type is simply composed of prominent ridges.

The **right atrioventricular (tricuspid) valve** guards the right atrioventricular orifice (see Figs. 4.51 and 4.52A,F). The valve consists of **three cusps (leaflets)** formed by a fold of endocardium with some connective tissue enclosed. These are **anterior**, **septal**, and **inferior (posterior) cusps**. The anterior cusp lies anteriorly, the septal cusp lies against the ventricular septum, and the inferior (posterior) cusp lies inferiorly. The bases of the cusps are attached to the fibrous ring of the skeleton of the heart (see below), whereas their free edges and ventricular surfaces are attached to the chordae tendineae (see Fig. 4.52B,C). The chordae tendineae connect the cusps to the papillary muscles. Normally, the right ventricle has three papillary muscles; however, often, there are more. When the ventricle contracts, the papillary muscles contract and prevent the cusps from being forced into the atrium and turning inside out as the intraventricular pressure rises. To assist in this process, the chordae tendineae of one papillary muscle are connected to the adjacent parts of two cusps.

The **pulmonary valve** guards the pulmonary orifice and consists of three **semilunar cusps** formed by folds of endocardium with some connective tissue enclosed (see Fig. 4.52A,D). The curved lower margins and sides of each cusp are attached to the arterial wall, forming a cuplike cavity (a **pulmonary sinus**) behind each cusp. The open mouths of the cusps are directed upward into the pulmonary trunk. No chordae or papillary muscles are associated with these valve cusps; the attachments of the sides of the cusps to the arterial wall prevent the cusps from prolapsing into the ventricle.

The three semilunar cusps are the **anterior**, **right**, and **left cusps**. During ventricular systole, the cusps of the valve are pressed against the wall of the pulmonary trunk by the outrushing blood. During diastole, blood flows back toward the heart and enters the sinuses; the valve cusps fill, come into apposition in the center of the lumen, and close the pulmonary orifice.

Left Atrium

As with the right atrium, the left atrium consists of a **main cavity (atrium proper)** and an **auricle**. The interior of the left atrium proper is smooth, but the left auricle possesses **pectinate muscle** ridges as in the right auricle. However, there is no crista terminalis. The fossa ovalis is not a distinctive structure on the left side of the atrial septum. The left atrium is situated behind the right atrium and forms the greater part of the base (posterior surface) of the heart (see Fig. 4.49). The oblique sinus of the serous pericardium is behind the left atrium, and the fibrous pericardium separates it from the esophagus (see Figs. 4.46 and 4.50).

Openings into the Left Atrium

The four pulmonary veins, two from each lung, open through the posterior wall (see Fig. 5.31) and have no valves. The left atrioventricular orifice is guarded by the mitral valve.

Left Ventricle

Blood enters the left ventricle from the left atrium through the **left atrioventricular orifice** and then leaves the ventricle through the **aortic orifice**, where it passes into the ascending aorta (see Fig. 4.52F). The area just below the aortic orifice is the **aortic vestibule**, which constitutes the left ventricular outflow tract. The walls of the left ventricle are three times thicker than those of the right ventricle (see Fig. 4.52E), and the left intraventricular blood pressure is six times higher than that inside the right ventricle. In cross section, the left ventricle is circular; the right is crescentic because of the bulging of the ventricular septum into the cavity of the right ventricle. There are well-developed **trabeculae carneae** and two large **papillary muscles**, but no moderator band.

The **left atrioventricular (mitral) valve** guards the atrioventricular orifice (see Fig. 4.52). It consists of **two cusps**, **one anterior** and **one posterior**, which have a structure like that of the cusps of the tricuspid valve. The anterior cusp is the larger and intervenes between the atrioventricular and aortic orifices. The attachment of the **chordae tendineae** to the cusps and the papillary muscles is like that of the tricuspid valve.

The **aortic valve** guards the aortic orifice and is almost identical in structure to the pulmonary valve (see Fig. 4.52D). The three cusps are the **right coronary**, **left coronary**, and **posterior (noncoronary)**. Behind each cusp, the aortic wall bulges to form an **aortic sinus**. The aortic walls of the right and left coronary sinuses give origin to the right and left coronary arteries, respectively.

Fibrous Cardiac Skeleton

The skeleton of the heart (see Fig. 4.52H) consists of four interconnected fibrous rings that surround the atrioventricular, pulmonary, and aortic valve orifices and are continuous with the lower part of the atrial septum and the upper membranous part of the ventricular septum. The fibrous rings around the atrioventricular orifices separate the muscular walls of the atria from those of the ventricles but provide attachment for the muscle fibers. The fibrous rings also support and attach the bases of the valve cusps, keeping the valve orifices patent and preventing the valves from overstretching and becoming incompetent. Additionally, the skeleton of the heart forms an electrical insulation between the atria and ventricles, as the electrical impulses of myocardial contractions cannot penetrate the fibrous skeleton. Thus, there is electrical discontinuity between the atria and the ventricles. The net effect of the fibrous skeleton is functional separation of the atrial and ventricular hearts.

Heart Nerve Supply

Extrinsic and intrinsic networks innervate the heart. Both sympathetic and parasympathetic fibers of the autonomic nervous system form the extrinsic nerve supply. The conducting system of the heart forms the intrinsic nerve tract.

Extrinsic Nerve Supply

The **sympathetic supply** originates in upper thoracic spinal cord segments, routes through the cervical and upper thoracic sympathetic chain ganglia, descends through **sympathetic cervical** and **thoracic cardiac nerves**, and enters the **cardiac plexuses** situated below the arch of the aorta around the base of the heart. Postganglionic sympathetic fibers terminate on the sinoatrial and atrioventricular nodes, on cardiac muscle fibers, and on the coronary arteries. Activation of these nerves results in cardiac acceleration, increased force of contraction of the cardiac muscle, and dilatation of the coronary arteries.

The **parasympathetic supply** comes from the vagus nerves. **Vagal cardiac nerve branches** arise in the neck, descend into the thorax, and join into the cardiac plexuses.

Postganglionic parasympathetic fibers terminate on the sinoatrial and atrioventricular nodes and on the coronary arteries. Activation of the parasympathetic nerves results in a reduction in the rate and force of contraction of the heart and constriction of the coronary arteries.

Afferent fibers running with the sympathetic nerves carry nervous impulses that normally do not reach consciousness. However, if the blood supply to the myocardium becomes impaired, pain impulses reach consciousness via this pathway. Afferent fibers running with the vagus nerves take part in cardiovascular reflexes.

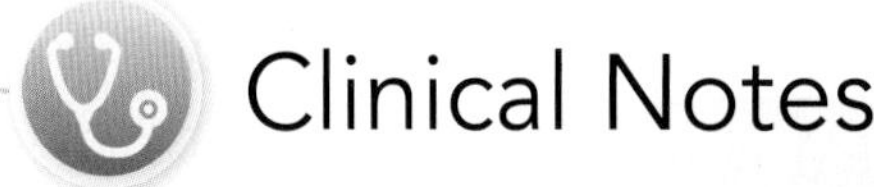

Cardiac Pain

Oxygen deficiency and the accumulation of metabolites, which stimulate the sensory nerve endings in the myocardium, are assumed to cause the pain originating in the heart as the result of acute myocardial ischemia. The afferent nerve fibers ascend to the central nervous system (CNS) through the cardiac branches of the sympathetic trunk and enter the spinal cord through the posterior roots of the T1 to T4 nerves. The nature of the pain varies considerably, from a severe crushing pain to nothing more than a mild discomfort.

The pain is not felt in the heart but is referred to the skin areas supplied by the corresponding spinal nerves. The skin areas supplied by intercostal nerves 1 to 4 and by the intercostobrachial nerve (T2) are therefore affected. The intercostobrachial nerve communicates with the medial cutaneous nerve of the arm and is distributed to the skin on the medial side of the upper part of the arm. A certain amount of spread of nervous information must occur within the CNS, for the pain is sometimes felt in the neck and the jaw.

Myocardial infarction (MI) involving the inferior wall or diaphragmatic surface of the heart often gives rise to discomfort in the epigastrium. Afferent pain fibers from the heart probably ascend in the sympathetic nerves and enter the spinal cord in the posterior roots of the T7 to T9 spinal nerves and give rise to referred pain in the T7 to T9 thoracic dermatomes in the epigastrium.

Because the heart and the thoracic part of the esophagus probably have similar afferent pain pathways, it is not surprising that painful acute esophagitis can mimic the pain of MI.

Intrinsic Nerve Supply (Conducting System)

Cardiac muscle cells have an intrinsic ability to contract spontaneously and to convey the contractile impulse, independent of the extrinsic nervous system. The **conducting system of the heart** is a network of specialized cardiac muscle cells designed to generate rhythmic cardiac impulses and to conduct and coordinate the intrinsic contractions of the myocardium. The normal heart contracts rhythmically at about 70 to 90 beats per minute in the resting adult. The contractile process originates spontaneously in the conducting system, and the impulse travels to different regions of the heart, so the atria contract first and together, followed later by the simultaneous contractions of both ventricles. The functions of the conducting system are as follows:

- Initiate excitation of the atria. This is the "pacemaker function."
- Delay excitation of the ventricles. The slight delay in the passage of the impulse from the atria to the ventricles allows time for the atria to empty their blood into the ventricles before the ventricles contract.
- Penetrate the fibrous cardiac skeleton.
- Spread excitation across the ventricles.

The components of the conducting system are as follows (Fig. 4.53; see also Figs. 4.51 and 4.52G):

- Sinoatrial (SA) node
- Atrioventricular (AV) node
- Atrioventricular bundle (bundle of His)
- Right and left bundle branches
- Subendocardial branches (terminal conducting fibers, Purkinje fibers)

Sinoatrial Node

The SA node is in the wall of the right atrium, at the junction of the crista terminalis and the superior vena cava (see Figs. 4.51 and 4.53). It spontaneously gives origin to rhythmic electrical impulses that spread in all directions through the cardiac muscle of the atria and cause the muscle to contract. Thus, the SA node is referred to as the **"pacemaker" of the heart**. Compared with the terminal conducting fibers, these have a relatively slow conduction velocity, with the atrial excitation wave traveling at ~1 m/s. The SA node is derived from the embryonic **sinus venosus**. Normally, heart rate is determined by the frequency with which the SA node generates impulses. However, autonomic input modulates the activity of the SA node to adjust and balance heart rate as needed.

Atrioventricular Node

The AV node is located on the right, lower side of the atrial septum, between the attachment of the septal cusp of the tricuspid valve and the opening of the coronary sinus (see Figs. 4.51, 4.52G, and 4.53). The atrial excitation wave stimulates the AV node as the wave passes through the atrial myocardium. The slower speed of conduction of the cardiac impulse through the AV node (about 0.1 seconds) delays conduction of impulse from the atria to the ventricles and allows sufficient time for the atria to empty their blood into the ventricles before the ventricles start to contract. The cardiac impulse next travels to the atrioventricular bundle.

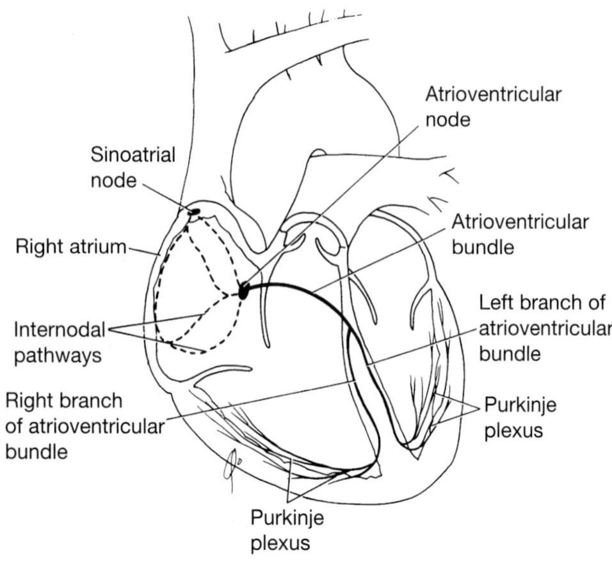

Figure 4.53 Conducting system of the heart. Note the internodal pathways.

Atrioventricular Bundle (Bundle of His)

The AV bundle originates from the AV node, descends behind the septal cusp of the tricuspid valve, and extends into the membranous part of the ventricular septum. The bundle pierces the fibrous skeleton of the heart and is the sole myocardial connection between the atria and the ventricles. Therefore, this is the only route along which the cardiac impulse can travel from the atria to the ventricles (see Fig. 4.53).

Bundle Branches

The AV bundle divides into **right** and **left bundle branches** (one for each ventricle) at the upper border of the muscular part of the ventricular septum. The right bundle branch (RBB) passes down on the right side of the ventricular septum to reach the moderator band, where it crosses to the anterior wall of the right ventricle. Here, it becomes continuous with the fibers of the Purkinje plexus (see Fig. 4.53). The left bundle branch (LBB) pierces the ventricular septum and passes down on its left side beneath the endocardium. It usually divides into two branches (anterior and posterior), which eventually become continuous with the fibers of the Purkinje plexus of the left ventricle.

Subendocardial Branches (Terminal Conducting Fibers, Purkinje Fibers)

The terminal branches of the conducting system ramify throughout the ventricular myocardium in a plexiform fashion. These fibers have the highest conduction velocity (4 to 5 m/s) in the heart.

Internodal Conduction Paths

Impulses from the SA node have been shown to travel to the AV node more rapidly than they can travel by passing along the ordinary myocardium. Some authors explain this phenomenon by describing special internodal pathways in the atrial wall (see Fig. 4.53), which have a structure consisting of a mixture of Purkinje fibers and ordinary cardiac muscle cells. The **anterior internodal pathway** leaves the anterior end of the SA node and passes anterior to the superior vena caval opening. It descends on the atrial septum and ends in the AV node. The **middle internodal pathway** leaves the posterior end of the SA node and passes posterior to the opening of the superior vena cava. It descends on the atrial septum to the AV node. The **posterior internodal pathway** leaves the posterior part of the SA node and descends through the crista terminalis and the valve of the inferior vena cava to the AV node.

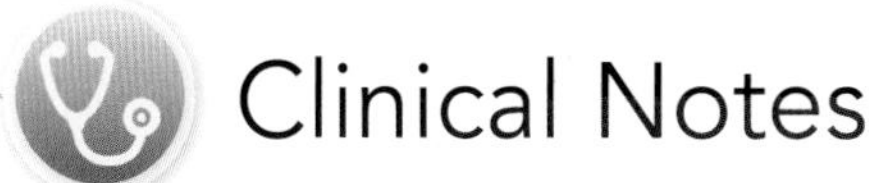

Clinical Notes

Failure of the Conduction System of the Heart

The sinoatrial node is the spontaneous source of the cardiac impulse. The atrioventricular (AV) node is responsible for picking up the cardiac impulse from the atria. The AV bundle is the only route by which the cardiac impulse can spread from the atria to the ventricles. Failure of the bundle to conduct the normal impulses results in alteration in the rhythmic contraction of the ventricles (**arrhythmias**) or, if **complete bundle block** occurs, complete dissociation between the atrial and ventricular rates of contraction. The common cause of defective conduction through the bundle or its branches is atherosclerosis of the coronary arteries, which results in a diminished blood supply to the conducting system.

Commotio Cordis

A blunt nonpenetrating blow to the anterior chest wall over the heart may result in ventricular fibrillation and sudden death. This condition occurs most commonly in the young and adolescents and is often sports related. The sudden blow is frequently produced by a baseball, baseball bat, lacrosse ball, or fist or elbow. The common incidence in the young is most likely due to the compliant chest wall because of the flexible ribs and costal cartilages and the thin undeveloped chest muscles. Apparently, timing of the blow relative to the cardiac cycle is critical; ventricular fibrillation is most likely to occur if the blow occurs during the upstroke of the T wave of the electrical activity of the cardiac muscle.

Heart Arterial Supply

The heart has a small margin for error in its physiology and function. Therefore, it requires a dense vascular system for regulation of blood gases and nutrients. The **right** and **left coronary arteries** provide the arterial supply of the heart. These are the first branches of the aorta. They arise from the ascending aorta immediately above the aortic valve and initially pass around the opposite sides of the pulmonary trunk (Fig. 4.54A; see also Figs. 4.48 and 4.52D). The coronary arteries and their major branches are distributed over the surface of the heart and lie within subepicardial connective tissue. Table 4.4 summarizes the typical pattern of distribution of the coronary arteries in most people.

Right Coronary Artery

The **right coronary artery** arises from the right aortic sinus of the ascending aorta, runs forward between the right side of the pulmonary trunk and the right auricle, and descends almost vertically in the **right atrioventricular groove (coronary sulcus)** (see Figs. 4.48, 4.52D, and 4.54A). At the inferior border of the heart, it continues posteriorly along the atrioventricular groove to anastomose with the left coronary artery in the **posterior interventricular groove**.

Branches

1. The **right conus artery** supplies the anterior surface of the pulmonary conus (infundibulum of the right ventricle) and the upper part of the anterior wall of the right ventricle.
2. Two or three **anterior ventricular branches** supply the anterior surface of the right ventricle. The **right marginal artery** is the largest and runs along the right margin of the anterior surface toward the apex.

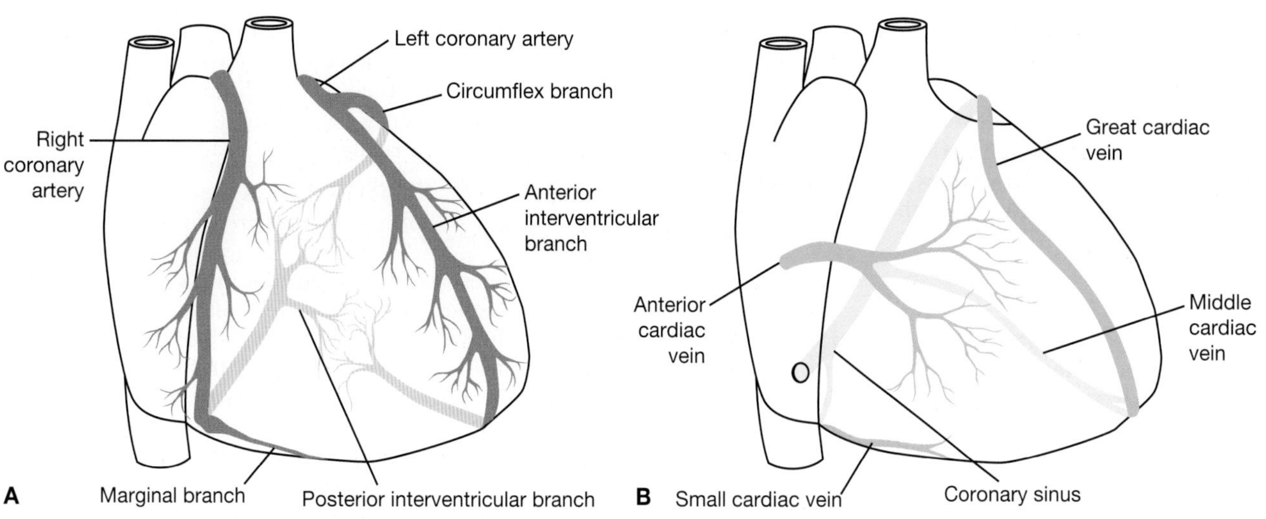

Figure 4.54 Coronary vessels. **A.** Major coronary arteries. **B.** Main coronary veins.

Table 4.4 Typical Distributions of the Coronary Arteries

RIGHT CORONARY ARTERY	LEFT CORONARY ARTERY
Right atrium	Left atrium
Most of the right ventricle	Most of the left ventricle
Left ventricle (diaphragmatic surface)	Small part of right ventricle
Ventricular septum (posterior third)	Ventricular septum (anterior two thirds)
SA node (~60% of people)	SA node (~40% of people)
AV node (~80% of people)	AV bundle + bundle branches

AV, atrioventricular; SA, sinoatrial.

3. Two or three **posterior ventricular branches** supply the diaphragmatic surface of the right ventricle. One of these, the **atrioventricular nodal branch**, supplies the AV node.
4. The **posterior interventricular (posterior descending) artery** runs toward the apex in the **posterior interventricular groove**. It gives off branches to the right and left ventricles, including its inferior wall. It supplies branches to the posterior part of the ventricular septum but not to the apical part, which receives its supply from the anterior interventricular branch of the left coronary artery. The posterior interventricular artery usually is a branch of the right coronary artery. However, it may originate from the circumflex branch of the left coronary artery (see the description of coronary artery dominance below).
5. **Atrial branches** supply the anterior and lateral surfaces of the right atrium. One branch supplies the posterior surface of both the right and left atria. An early branch, the **sinoatrial nodal artery**, supplies the SA node and the right and left atria; in 35% of individuals, it arises from the left coronary artery.

Left Coronary Artery

The **left coronary artery**, which is usually larger than the right coronary artery, supplies the major part of the heart. It arises from the left aortic sinus of the ascending aorta, passes forward between the left side of the pulmonary trunk and the left auricle, enters the AV groove (coronary sulcus), and divides into an anterior interventricular branch and a circumflex branch (see Figs. 4.48, 4.52D, and 4.54A).

Branches

1. The **anterior interventricular artery (left anterior descending artery [LAD])** runs downward along the ventricular septum in the **anterior interventricular groove** to the apex of the heart (see Figs. 4.48 and 4.54A). In most individuals, it then passes around the apex of the heart to enter the posterior interventricular groove and anastomose with the terminal branches of the posterior interventricular branch of the right coronary artery. In about one third of individuals, it ends at the apex of the heart. The anterior interventricular branch supplies the right and left ventricles with numerous branches that also supply the anterior two thirds of the ventricular septum. One larger ventricular branch (**lateral or diagonal artery**) may arise directly from the trunk of the left coronary artery. A small **left conus artery** supplies the pulmonary conus.
2. The **circumflex artery** winds around the **left margin of the heart** in the atrioventricular groove. A **left marginal artery** is a large branch that supplies the left margin of the left ventricle down to the apex. **Anterior** and **posterior ventricular branches** supply the left ventricle. **Atrial branches** supply the left atrium.

Variations in the Coronary Arteries

Variations in the pattern of blood supply to the heart occur commonly, and most affect the blood supply to the diaphragmatic surface of both ventricles. **Coronary artery dominance** refers to the variable origin of the posterior interventricular artery (Fig. 4.55). In **right dominance**, the posterior interventricular artery is a large branch of the right coronary artery (see Fig. 4.55A). Right dominance is present in most individuals (~67%). In **left dominance**, the posterior interventricular artery is a branch of the circumflex branch of the left coronary artery (~15%) (see Fig. 4.55B). In **codominance** (~18%), both the right coronary and circumflex arteries contribute to the formation of the posterior interventricular artery or to multiple branches that substitute for that vessel.

Coronary Artery Anastomoses

Anastomoses (collateral circulation) between the terminal branches of the right and left coronary arteries do exist; however, they are usually not large enough to provide an adequate blood supply to the cardiac muscle should one of the large branches become blocked by disease. Thus, the coronary arteries are generally considered to be **functional end arteries**. A sudden block of one of the larger branches of either coronary artery usually leads to myocardial death (myocardial infarction), although sometimes the collateral circulation is enough to sustain the muscle.

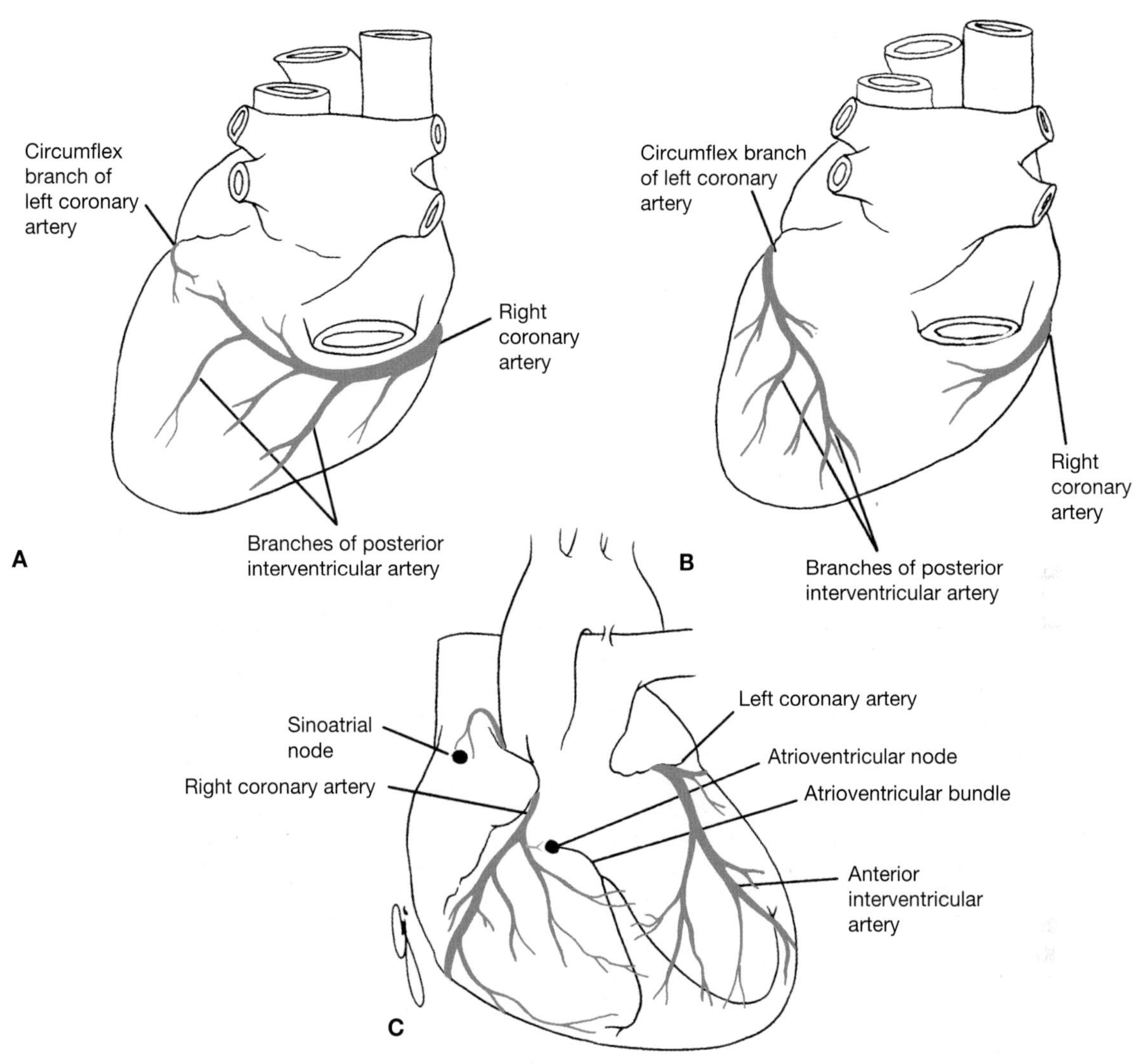

Figure 4.55 **A.** Posterior view of the heart showing the origin and distribution of the posterior interventricular artery in the right dominance. **B.** Posterior view of the heart showing the origin and distribution of the posterior interventricular artery in the left dominance. **C.** Anterior view of the heart showing the relationship of the blood supply to the conducting system.

Heart Venous Drainage

Most blood from the heart wall drains into the right atrium via the **coronary sinus** (see Figs. 4.49 and 4.54B). The coronary sinus is a large, dilated vein that lies in the posterior part of the AV groove (coronary sulcus). It empties into the right atrium just to the left of the inferior vena cava (see Fig. 4.51).

Three main veins drain the heart wall and open into the coronary sinus: the great, middle, and small cardiac veins. Each of these typically accompanies a specific coronary artery (Table 4.5). The **great cardiac vein** drains most of the areas of the heart supplied by the left coronary artery and joins the left end of the coronary sinus (see Fig. 4.54B). The **middle** and **small cardiac veins** drain most of the areas normally supplied by the right coronary artery and drain into the right end of the coronary sinus.

Not all venous blood drains into the coronary sinus. A variable number of small **anterior cardiac veins** drain the anterior surface of the heart and empty directly into the right atrium. Other very small veins may drain directly into the chambers of the heart (usually the atria).

Table 4.5 Major Coronary Veins and Accompanying Coronary Arteries

VEIN	ACCOMPANYING ARTERY
Great cardiac vein	Anterior interventricular artery
Middle cardiac vein	Posterior interventricular artery
Small cardiac vein	Right marginal artery

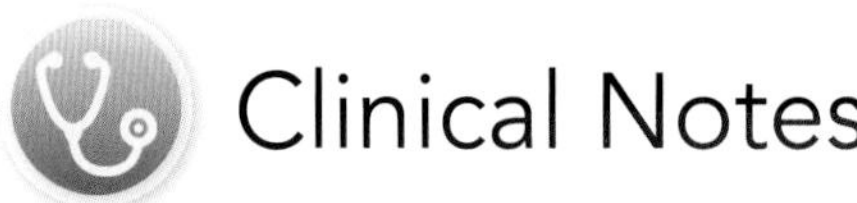

Coronary Artery Disease

The myocardium receives its blood supply through the right and left coronary arteries. Although the coronary arteries have numerous anastomoses at the arteriolar level, they are essentially functional end arteries. A sudden block of one of the large branches of either coronary artery will usually lead to necrosis of the cardiac muscle (**myocardial infarction** [**MI**]) in that vascular area, and often, the patient dies. An acute thrombosis on top of a chronic atherosclerotic narrowing of the lumen causes most cases of coronary artery blockage.

Arteriosclerotic disease of the coronary arteries may present in three ways, depending on the rate of narrowing of the lumina of the arteries: (1) general degeneration and fibrosis of the myocardium occur over many years and are caused by a gradual narrowing of the coronary arteries. (2) **Angina pectoris** is cardiac pain that occurs on exertion and is relieved by rest. In this condition, the coronary arteries are so narrowed that myocardial ischemia occurs on exertion but not at rest. (3) MI occurs when coronary flow is suddenly reduced or stopped, and the cardiac muscle undergoes necrosis. MI is the major cause of death in industrialized nations.

Table 4.6 correlates individual coronary arteries with specific sites of MI and the electrocardiographic signature of each infarct.

Coronary bypass surgery, coronary angioplasty, and coronary artery stenting are now commonly accepted methods of treating coronary artery disease. Coronary bypass surgery involves harvesting a segment of blood vessel and using that to circumvent a blockage in a coronary artery. Many such procedures use the **great saphenous vein** from the lower limb as the donor vessel because of its size and surgical ease of access. Emerging techniques increasingly use the **internal thoracic artery** from the neighboring chest wall to revascularize the heart wall.

Table 4.6 Coronary Artery Lesions, Infarct Location, and ECG Signature

CORONARY ARTERY	INFARCT LOCATION	ECG SIGNATURE
Proximal LAD	Large anterior wall	ST elevation: I, L, V1 to 6
More distal LAD	Anteroapical Inferior wall if wraparound LAD	ST elevation: V2 to 4 ST elevation: II, III, F
Distal LAD	Anteroseptal	ST elevation: V1 to 3
Early obtuse, marginal	High lateral wall	ST elevation: I, L, V4 to 6
More distal marginal branch, circumflex	Small lateral wall	ST elevation: I, L, or V4 to 6 or no abnormality
Circumflex	Posterolateral	ST elevation: V4 to 6; ST depression: V1 to 2
Distal RCA	Small inferior wall	ST elevation: II, III, F; ST depression: I, L
Proximal RCA	Large inferior wall and posterior wall Some lateral wall	ST elevation: II, III, F; ST depression: I, L, V1 to 3 ST elevation: V5 to 6
RCA	Right ventricular Usually inferior	ST elevation: V2R to V4R; some ST elevation: V1; or ST depression V2, V3 ST elevation: II, III, F

ECG, electrocardiographic; LAD, left anterior descending (interventricular); RCA, right coronary artery.

Heart Action

The heart is a muscular pump that normally beats 70 to 90 times per minute in the resting adult and 130 to 150 times per minute in the newborn. The **cardiac cycle** is one complete heartbeat composed of two phases: (1) **systole** (ventricular contraction) and (2) **diastole** (ventricular relaxation). Each phase consists of a series of characteristic changes within the heart as it fills with blood and empties.

The AV valves are closed during ventricular systole (contraction), and the blood is temporarily accommodated in the large veins and atria. The AV valves open once ventricular diastole (relaxation) occurs, and blood passively flows from the atria to the ventricles (see Fig. 4.52F). Atrial systole occurs when the ventricles are nearly full and forces the remainder of the blood in the atria into the ventricles. The SA node initiates the wave of contraction in the atria, which commences around the openings of the large veins and milks the blood toward the ventricles. By this means, blood does not reflux into the veins.

The cardiac impulse, having reached the AV node, is conducted to the papillary muscles by the AV bundle and its branches (see Figs. 4.52G and 4.53). The papillary

Table 4.7 Major Events in the Cardiac Cycle

SYSTOLE	DIASTOLE
Ventricular contraction (shortening and emptying)	Ventricular relaxation (elongation and filling)
First heart sound (lub): closure of the atrioventricular (cuspid) valves (tricuspid and bicuspid)	Second heart sound (dub): closure of the semilunar valves (aortic and pulmonary) and/or blood reflux into the sinuses of the semilunar valves
Tricuspid and bicuspid valves close just after the start of systole	Tricuspid and bicuspid valves open
Aortic and pulmonary valves open during systole	Aortic and pulmonary valves closed

muscles then begin to contract and take up the slack of the chordae tendineae. Meanwhile, the ventricles start contracting, and the AV valves close. The spread of the cardiac impulse along the AV bundle and its terminal branches, including the Purkinje fibers, ensures that myocardial contraction occurs at almost the same time throughout the ventricles.

Once the intraventricular blood pressure exceeds that present in the large arteries (aorta and pulmonary trunk), the semilunar valve cusps are pushed aside, and the blood is ejected from the heart. At the conclusion of ventricular systole, blood begins to move back toward the ventricles and immediately fills the pockets of the semilunar valves. The cusps float into apposition and completely close the aortic and pulmonary orifices.

Classically, two sounds (**lub-dub**) are associated with each heartbeat (cardiac cycle) when listening to the heart with a stethoscope. The first sound (lub) is produced by the contraction of the ventricles and the closure of the tricuspid and mitral valves. The second sound (dub) is produced mainly by the sharp closure of the aortic and pulmonary valves. Table 4.7 summarizes the events related to each phase of the cardiac cycle.

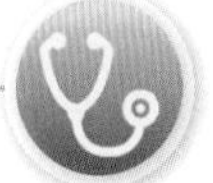

Clinical Notes

Surface Projections and Auscultation of the Heart Valves

The cardiac valves are located deep to the sternum. Each valve has an anatomical projection to a place on the thoracic wall that immediately overlies its position (Fig. 4.56). However, the sounds produced by the valves are projected to auscultation areas that are removed from the anatomic projections and widely separated from each other. This difference is because blood carries sound along the direction of its flow. Thus, each auscultation area is located superficial to the heart chamber or great vessel into which the blood flows after passing each valve. Table 4.8 summarizes the anatomic and auscultation projection areas for each valve.

Valvular Heart Disease

Inflammation of a valve can cause the edges of the valve cusps to stick together. Later, fibrous thickening occurs, followed by loss of flexibility and shrinkage. Narrowing (stenosis) and valvular incompetence (regurgitation) result, and the heart ceases to function as an efficient pump. In rheumatic disease of the mitral valve, not only do the cusps undergo fibrosis and shrink but the chordae tendineae shorten as well, preventing closure of the cusps during ventricular systole.

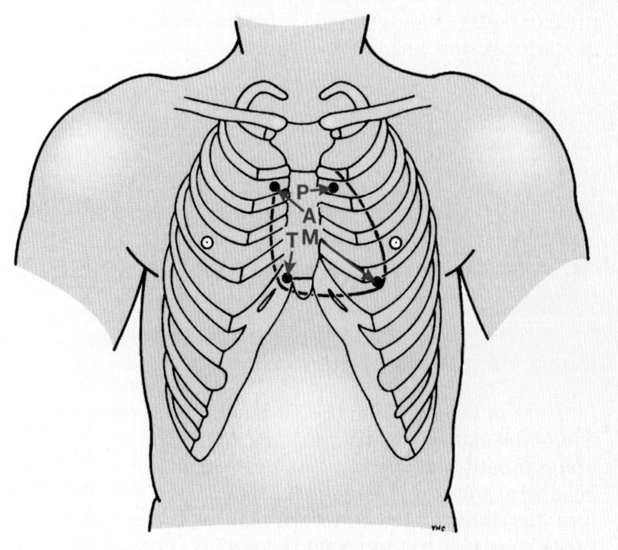

Figure 4.56 Position of the heart valves. *A*, aortic valve; *M*, mitral valve; *P*, pulmonary valve; *T*, tricuspid valve. *Arrows* indicate position where valves may be heard with least interference.

(continued)

Table 4.8 Comparison of Anatomic and Auscultation Areas of the Cardiac Valves[a]

VALVE	ANATOMIC LOCATION	OPTIMAL AUSCULTATION AREA
Tricuspid	Behind the right half of the sternum opposite intercostal space 4	Over the right half of the lower end of the body of the sternum
Bicuspid	Behind the left half of the sternum opposite costal cartilage 4	Over the apex beat, that is, at the level of left intercostal space 5, 3.5 in. (9 cm) from the midline
Pulmonary	Behind the medial end of left costal cartilage 3 and the adjoining part of the sternum	Over the medial end of left intercostal space 2
Aortic	Behind the left half of the sternum opposite intercostal space 3	Over the medial end of right intercostal space 2

[a]See also Figure 4.56.

Valvular Heart Murmurs

Apart from the typical lub-dub sounds of the valves closing, the blood passes through the normal heart silently. However, if the valve orifices become narrowed, or the valve cusps distorted and shrunken by disease, a rippling effect is set up, leading to turbulence and vibrations that are heard as heart murmurs.

Traumatic Asphyxia

The sudden caving in of the anterior chest wall associated with fractures of the sternum and ribs causes a dramatic rise in intrathoracic pressure. Apart from the immediate evidence of respiratory distress, the anatomy of the venous system plays a significant role in the production of the characteristic vascular signs of traumatic asphyxia. The thinness of the walls of the thoracic veins and the right atrium causes their collapse under the raised intrathoracic pressure, and venous blood is dammed back in the veins of the neck and head. This produces venous congestion; bulging of the eyes, which becomes injected; and swelling of the lips and tongue, which becomes cyanotic. The skin of the face, neck, and shoulders becomes purple.

Anatomy of Cardiopulmonary Resuscitation

Cardiopulmonary resuscitation (CPR), achieved by compression of the chest, was originally believed to succeed because of the compression of the heart between the sternum and the vertebral column. However, current evidence indicates that the blood flows in CPR because the whole thoracic cage is the pump; the heart functions merely as a conduit for blood. External chest compressions create an extrathoracic pressure gradient in which the pressure in all chambers and locations within the chest cavity is the same. With compression, blood is forced out of the thoracic cage. The blood preferentially flows out the arterial side of the circulation and back down the venous side because the venous valves in the internal jugular system prevent a useless oscillatory movement. With the release of compression, blood enters the thoracic cage, preferentially down the venous side of the systemic circulation.

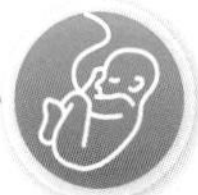

Embryology Notes

Heart Tube Development

Clusters of cells arise in the mesenchyme at the cephalic end of the embryonic disc, cephalic to the site of the developing mouth and the nervous system. These clusters of cells form a plexus of endothelial blood vessels that fuse to form the **right** and **left endocardial heart tubes**. The paired tubes soon fuse to form a single **median endocardial tube** (Fig. 4.57). As the head fold of the embryo develops, the endocardial tube and the pericardial cavity rotate on a transverse axis through almost 180°, so that they come to lie ventral to (in front of) the esophagus and caudal to the developing mouth.

The endocardial tube starts to bulge into the pericardial cavity (see Fig. 4.57) and becomes surrounded by a thick layer of mesenchyme, which differentiates into the **myocardium** and the **visceral layer of the serous pericardium**. This establishes the primitive heart tube, with the cephalic end as the **arterial end** and the caudal end as the **venous end**. The arterial end of the primitive heart is continuous beyond the pericardium with a large vessel, the **aortic sac** (Fig. 4.58). The heart begins to beat during week 3.

The heart tube then undergoes differential expansion, resulting in the formation of four dilatations, separated by grooves (see Fig. 4.58). From the arterial to the venous end, these dilatations are called the **bulbus cordis**, the **ventricle**,

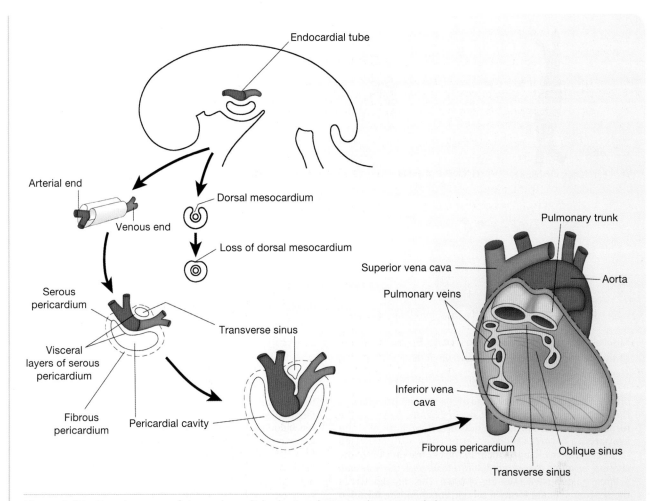

Figure 4.57 Development of the endocardial tube in relation to the pericardial cavity.

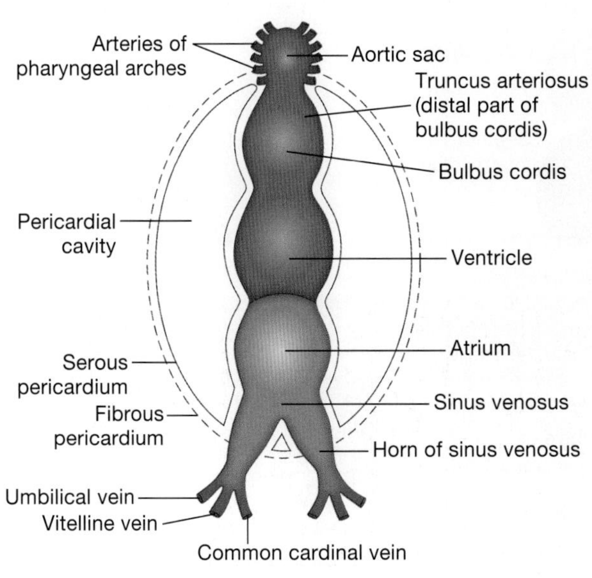

Figure 4.58 Parts of the primitive endocardial heart tube within the pericardium.

the **atrium**, and the **sinus venosus** (including **right** and **left horns**). The bulbus cordis and ventricular parts of the tube elongate more rapidly than the remainder of the tube, and because the arterial and venous ends are fixed by the pericardium, the tube begins to bend (Fig. 4.59). The bend soon becomes U-shaped and then forms a compound S shape, with the atrium lying posterior to the ventricle; thus, the venous and arterial ends are brought close together as they are in the adult. The passage between the atrium and the ventricle narrows to form the **atrioventricular canal**. As these changes occur, the heart tube gradually migrates from the neck region to what will become the thoracic region.

Atria Development

The single primitive atrium divides into two separate right and left atria in the following manner (Fig. 4.60). First, the AV canal widens transversely (see Fig. 4.60A). Then, ventral and dorsal **endocardial (atrioventricular) cushions** form and fuse to form the **septum intermedium**, which divides the canal into right and left halves (see Fig. 4.60A,B). Meanwhile, another septum, the **septum primum**, develops from the roof of the primitive atrium and grows down to fuse with the septum intermedium (see Fig. 4.60A). The

(continued)

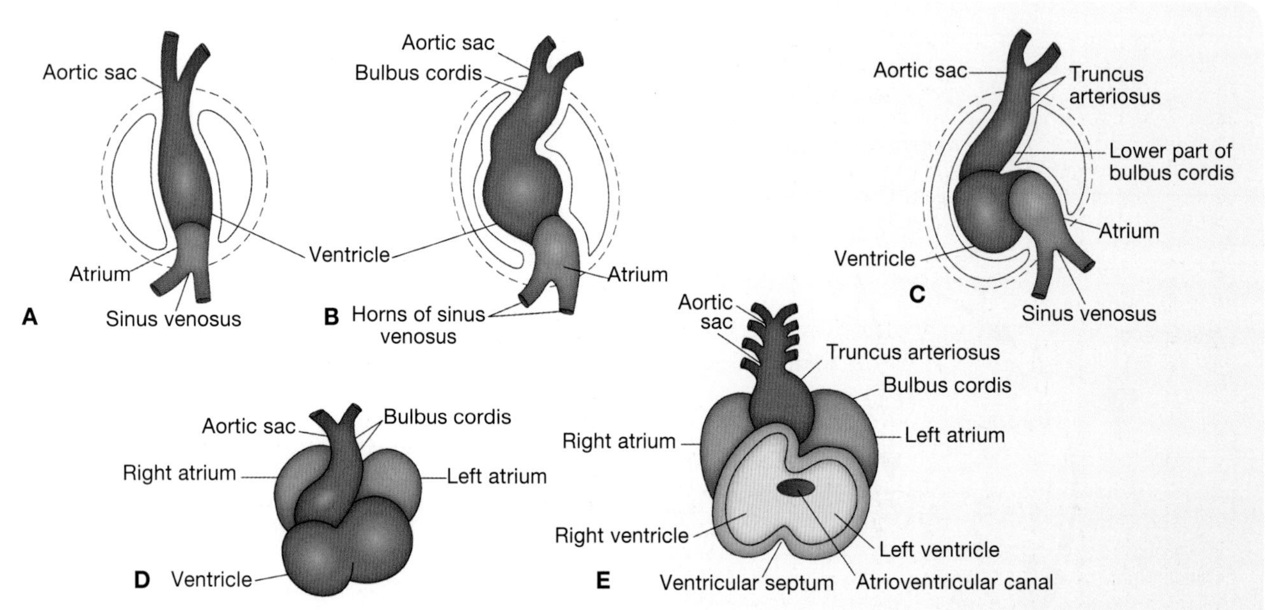

Figure 4.59 Progressive stages **(A to E)** in the bending of the heart tube within the pericardial cavity. The interior of the developing ventricles is shown in **E**.

opening between the lower edge of the septum primum and the septum intermedium that occurs before fusion is the **foramen primum**. The atrium now is divided into right and left parts.

Degenerative changes occur in the central portion of the septum primum before complete closure of the foramen primum takes place (see Fig. 4.60B). This breakdown in the septum primum forms a second foramen, the **foramen secundum**, which allows the right and left atrial chambers to communicate (see Fig. 4.60C). Another, thicker, septum (**septum secundum**) grows down from the atrial roof on the right side of the septum primum (see Fig. 4.60C,D). The lower edge of the septum secundum overlaps the foramen secundum in the septum primum but does not reach the floor of the atrium and does not fuse with the septum intermedium. The space between the free margin of the septum secundum and the septum primum is now known as the **foramen ovale** (see Fig. 4.60D,E).

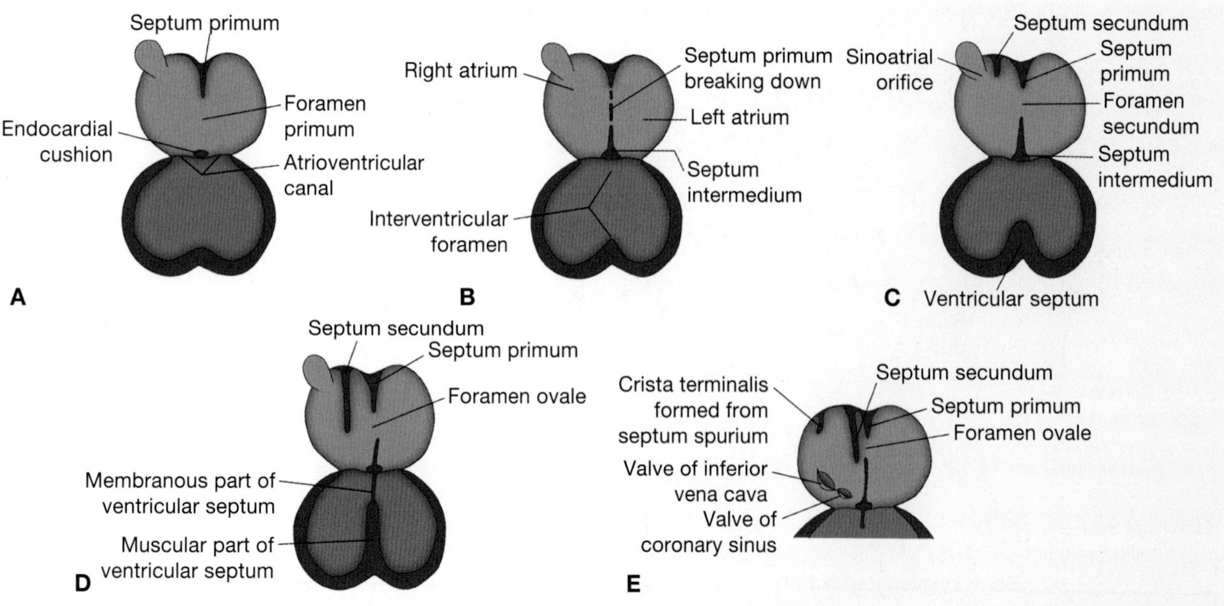

Figure 4.60 Progressive stages **(A to E)** in division of the primitive atrium and ventricle by development of internal septa.

Before birth, the foramen ovale allows oxygenated blood that has entered the right atrium from the inferior vena cava to pass into the left atrium. However, the lower part of the septum primum serves as a flaplike valve to prevent blood from moving from the left atrium to the right atrium. At birth, owing to raised blood pressure in the left atrium, the septum primum is pressed against the septum secundum and fuses with it, and the foramen ovale is closed. Thus, the two atria are separated from each other. The lower edge of the septum secundum seen in the right atrium becomes the **annulus ovalis**, and the depression below this is called the **fossa ovalis**. The right and left **auricular appendages** later develop as small diverticula from the right and left atria, respectively.

Ventricle Development

A muscular partition projects upward from the floor of the primitive ventricle to form the **ventricular septum** (see Fig. 4.60C,D). The space bounded by the crescentic upper edge of the septum and the endocardial cushions forms the **interventricular foramen**. Meanwhile, spiral subendocardial thickenings, the **bulbar ridges**, appear in the distal part of the bulbus cordis. The bulbar ridges then grow and fuse to form a spiral **aorticopulmonary septum** (Fig. 4.61). The interventricular foramen closes as the result of proliferation of the bulbar ridges and the fused endocardial cushions (septum intermedium). This newly formed tissue grows down and fuses with the upper edge of the muscular ventricular septum to form the **membranous part of the septum** (see Fig. 4.60D). The closure of the interventricular foramen not only shuts off the path of communication between the right and left ventricles but also ensures that the right ventricular cavity communicates with the pulmonary trunk and the left ventricular cavity communicates with the aorta. In addition, the right AV opening now connects exclusively with the right ventricular cavity and the left AV opening with the left ventricular cavity.

Development of the Roots and Proximal Portions of the Aorta and the Pulmonary Trunk

The distal part of the bulbus cordis is termed the **truncus arteriosus** (see Fig. 4.58). The spiral aorticopulmonary septum divides the truncus to form the roots and proximal portions of the aorta and pulmonary trunk (see Fig. 4.61). With the establishment of right and left ventricles, the proximal portion of the bulbus cordis becomes incorporated into the right ventricle as the definitive **conus arteriosus** or **infundibulum** and into the left ventricle as the **aortic vestibule**. Just distal to the aortic valves, the two coronary arteries arise as outgrowths from the developing aorta.

Development of the Semilunar Valves of the Aorta and Pulmonary Arteries

After the formation of the aorticopulmonary septum, three swellings appear at the orifices of both the aorta and the pulmonary artery. Each swelling consists of a covering of endothelium over loose connective tissue. Gradually, the swellings become excavated on their upper surfaces to form the semilunar valves.

Atrioventricular Valve Development

After the formation of the septum intermedium, the atrioventricular canal becomes divided into **right** and **left atrioventricular orifices**. Raised folds of the endocardium

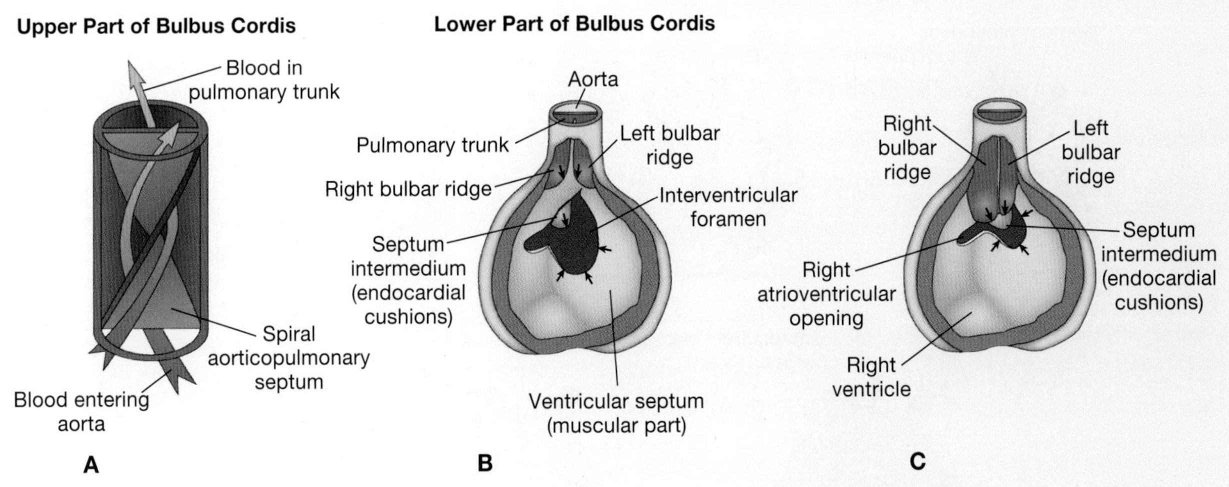

Figure 4.61 Division of the bulbus cordis by the spiral aorticopulmonary septum into the aorta and pulmonary trunk. **A.** Spiral septum in the truncus arteriosus (upper part of the bulbus cordis). **B.** Lower part of the bulbus cordis showing the formation of the spiral septum by fusion of the bulbar ridges (*red*), which then grow down and join the septum intermedium (*blue*) and the muscular part of the ventricular septum. **C.** Area of the ventricular septum that is formed from the fused bulbar ridges (*red*) and the septum intermedium (*blue*) is called the membranous part of the ventricular septum.

(continued)

appear at the margins of these orifices. These folds are invaded by mesenchymal tissue that later becomes hollowed out from the ventricular side. Three valvular cusps are formed about the right AV orifice and constitute the **tricuspid valve**; two cusps are formed about the left AV orifice to become the **bicuspid (mitral) valve**. The newly formed cusps enlarge, and their mesenchymal core becomes differentiated into fibrous tissue. The cusps remain attached at intervals to the ventricular wall by muscular strands. Later, the muscular strands become differentiated into papillary muscles and chordae tendineae.

Atrial Septal Defects

After birth, the foramen ovale closes completely as the result of the fusion of the septum primum with the septum secundum. In 20% to 25% of hearts, a small opening (**probe patency**) persists, but this is usually of such a minor nature that it has no clinical significance. Occasionally, the opening is much larger and results in oxygenated blood from the left atrium passing over into the right atrium (Fig. 4.62B).

Ventricular Septal Defects

Formation of the ventricular septum is complete when the membranous part fuses with the muscular part. Ventricular septal defects (VSDs) are the most common congenital cardiac malformation and may occur in either the membranous or muscular part. They are more common in the muscular part of the septum but are generally more serious defects when occurring in the membranous part. Blood under high pressure passes through the defect from left to right, causing enlargement of the right ventricle. Larger VSDs can shorten life if corrective surgery is not performed.

Tetralogy of Fallot

Normally, the bulbus cordis divides into the aorta and pulmonary trunk because of the formation of the spiral aorticopulmonary septum. This septum forms by the fusion of the bulbar ridges. If the bulbar ridges fail to fuse correctly, unequal division of the bulbus cordis may occur, with consequent narrowing of the pulmonary trunk resulting in interference with the right ventricular outflow (see Fig. 4.62C).

The resulting congenital anomaly, tetralogy of Fallot, is the most common defect in the conotruncal region. The four anatomic abnormalities include stenosis of the pulmonary trunk (narrowing of the right ventricular outflow), a large VSD (mainly in the membranous part), overriding aorta (exit of the aorta immediately above the VSD instead of from the left ventricular cavity only), and severe hypertrophy of the right ventricle (because of the high blood pressure in the right ventricle). The defects, although not necessarily fatal, cause congenital cyanosis and do considerably limit activity. Once the diagnosis has been made, most children can be successfully treated surgically.

Most children find that assuming the squatting position after physical activity relieves their breathlessness. This happens because squatting reduces the venous return by compressing the abdominal veins and increasing the systemic arterial resistance by kinking the femoral and popliteal arteries in the legs; both of these mechanisms tend to decrease the right-to-left shunt through the VSD and improve the pulmonary circulation.

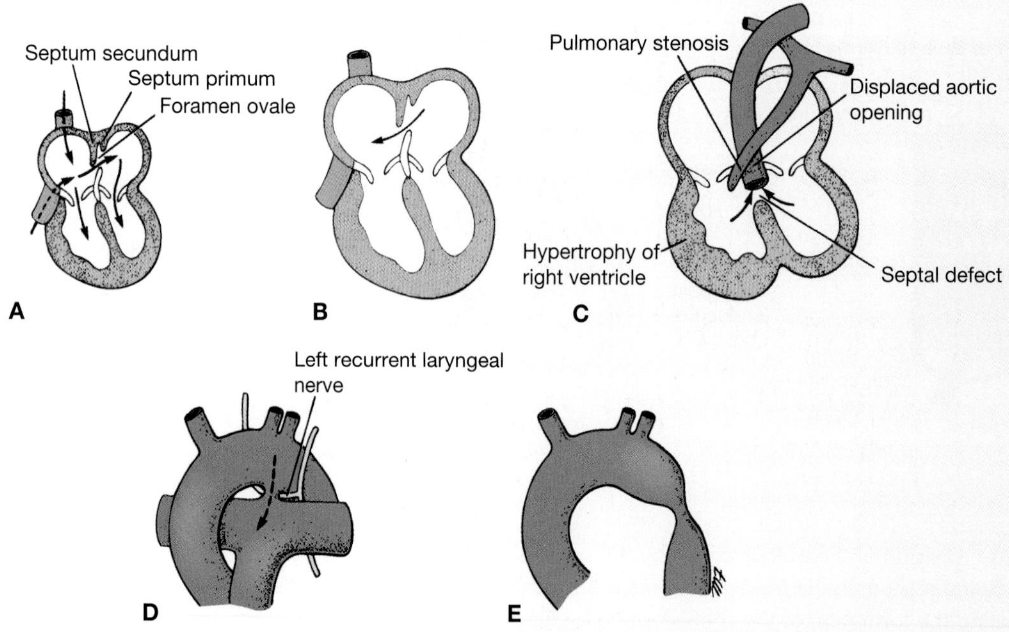

Figure 4.62 **A.** Normal fetal heart. **B.** Atrial septal defect. **C.** Tetralogy of Fallot. **D.** Patent ductus arteriosus (note the close relationship to the left recurrent laryngeal nerve). **E.** Coarctation of the aorta.

LARGE THORACIC ARTERIES

The aorta and pulmonary trunk are the large arteries in the thorax. These two vessels give rise to all arterial flow in the thorax. The aorta provides the systemic circuit flow, and the pulmonary trunk provides the pulmonary circuit flow.

Aorta

The aorta is the main arterial trunk that delivers oxygenated blood from the left ventricle of the heart to the tissues of the body. It consists of four main parts: ascending aorta, arch of the aorta, descending thoracic aorta, and abdominal aorta (Fig. 4.63).

Ascending Aorta

The ascending aorta begins at the base of the left ventricle and runs upward and forward to come to lie behind the right half of the sternum at the level of the sternal angle, where it becomes continuous with the arch of the aorta (see Fig. 4.48). The ascending aorta lies within the fibrous pericardium in the middle mediastinum (see Fig. 4.46) and is enclosed with the pulmonary trunk in a sheath of serous pericardium. At its root, it possesses three bulges, the **sinuses of the aorta**, one behind each aortic valve cusp.

Branches

The coronary arteries are the first branches of the aorta. The right coronary artery arises from the right aortic sinus, and the left coronary artery arises from the left aortic sinus (see Figs. 4.48 and 4.54). The further course of these arteries is described earlier in this chapter (Arterial Supply of the Heart).

Aortic Arch

The arch of the aorta is the continuation of the ascending aorta (see Figs. 4.48 and 4.63). It lies in the superior mediastinum, behind the manubrium sterni, and arches

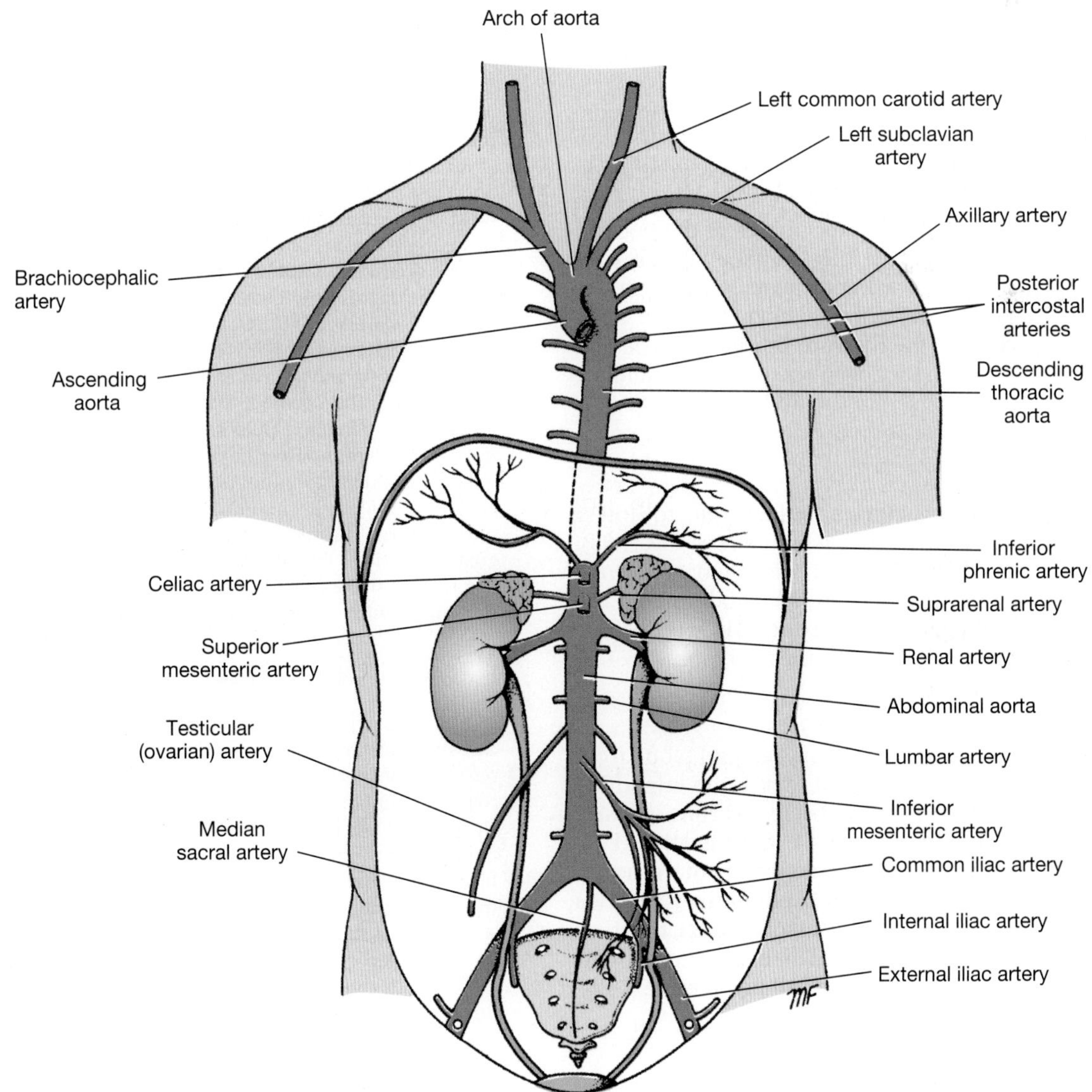

Figure 4.63 Major branches of the aorta.

upward, backward, and to the left in front of the trachea (its main direction is backward). It then passes downward to the left of the trachea and, at the level of the sternal angle, becomes continuous with the descending aorta (see Fig. 4.28A).

Branches

The arch of the aorta gives rise to three major arteries from its superior (convex) surface: brachiocephalic, left common carotid, and left subclavian arteries (see Figs. 4.28A, 4.48, and 4.63). The first branch, the **brachiocephalic artery**, passes upward and to the right of the trachea and divides into the right subclavian and right common carotid arteries behind the right sternoclavicular joint.

The second branch, the **left common carotid artery**, arises on the left side of the brachiocephalic artery. It runs upward and to the left of the trachea and enters the neck behind the left sternoclavicular joint.

The third branch, the **left subclavian artery**, arises from the aortic arch behind the left common carotid artery. It runs upward along the left side of the trachea and the esophagus to enter the root of the neck (see Fig. 4.31B). It arches over the apex of the left lung and continues toward the left upper limb.

Descending Thoracic Aorta

The descending thoracic aorta lies in the posterior mediastinum. It begins as the continuation of the arch of the aorta on the left side of the lower border of the body of the T4 vertebra (ie, opposite the sternal angle). It runs downward, inclining forward and medially to reach the anterior surface of the vertebral column (see Figs. 4.31B and 4.63). At the level of the T12 vertebra, it passes behind the diaphragm (through the aortic opening) in the midline and becomes continuous with the abdominal aorta (see Fig. 4.11). The abdominal aorta is described in Chapter 5.

Branches

Posterior intercostal arteries branch off to lower intercostal spaces 3 to 11 on each side (see Fig. 4.63). **Subcostal arteries** arise on each side and run along the lower border of rib 12 to enter the abdominal wall. **Pericardial**, **esophageal**, and **bronchial arteries** are small branches that distribute to these organs.

Pulmonary Trunk

The pulmonary trunk conveys deoxygenated blood from the right ventricle to the lungs. It leaves the infundibulum (upper part) of the right ventricle and runs upward, backward, and to the left (see Fig. 4.48). It is about 2 in. (5 cm) long and terminates in the concavity of the aortic arch by dividing into **right** and **left pulmonary arteries** (see Fig. 4.29). It lies in the middle mediastinum, together with the ascending aorta, enclosed in the fibrous pericardium and a sheath of serous pericardium (see Fig. 4.46).

Branches

The **right pulmonary artery** runs to the right behind the ascending aorta and superior vena cava to enter the root of the right lung (see Figs. 4.29, 4.31A, and 4.48).

The **left pulmonary artery** runs to the left in front of the descending aorta to enter the root of the left lung (see Figs. 4.29, 4.31B, and 4.48).

The **ligamentum arteriosum** is a fibrous band that connects the bifurcation of the pulmonary trunk to the lower concave surface of the aortic arch (see Figs. 4.31B, 4.46, and 4.49). The ligamentum arteriosum is the remnant of the **ductus arteriosus**, which in the fetus conducts blood from the pulmonary trunk to the aorta, thus bypassing the lungs. The **left recurrent laryngeal nerve** hooks around the lower border of the ductus (see Figs. 4.31B, 4.46, and 4.49), which closes after birth. If it remains patent, aortic blood will enter the pulmonary circulation (see Fig. 4.62D). Surgical ligation of the ductus is then necessary, and the surgeon must take care to preserve the left recurrent laryngeal nerve.

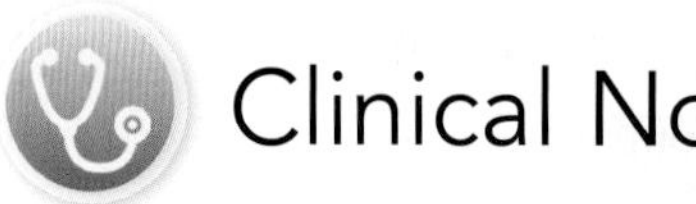

Clinical Notes

Aneurysm and Coarctation of the Aorta

The arch of the aorta lies behind the manubrium sterni. A gross dilatation of the aorta (aneurysm) may show itself as a pulsatile swelling in the suprasternal notch.

Coarctation of the aorta is a congenital narrowing of the aorta just proximal, opposite, or distal to the site of attachment of the ligamentum arteriosum (see Fig. 4.62E). This condition is believed to result from an unusual quantity of ductus arteriosus muscle tissue in the wall of the aorta. When the ductus arteriosus contracts, the ductal muscle in the aortic wall also contracts, and the aortic lumen becomes narrowed. Later, when fibrosis takes place, the aortic wall also is involved, and permanent narrowing occurs.

Clinically, the cardinal sign of aortic coarctation is absent or diminished pulses in the femoral arteries of both lower limbs. To compensate for the diminished volume of blood reaching the lower part of the body, an enormous collateral circulation develops, with dilatation of the internal thoracic, subclavian, and posterior intercostal arteries. The dilated intercostal arteries erode the lower borders of the ribs, producing characteristic notching, which is seen on radiographic examination.

Patent Ductus Arteriosus

The ductus arteriosus represents the distal portion of the sixth left aortic arch and connects the left pulmonary artery (near its origin from the pulmonary trunk) to the beginning of the descending aorta (see Fig. 4.62D). During fetal life, blood passes through it from the pulmonary artery to the aorta, thus bypassing the lungs. After birth, it normally constricts, later closes, and becomes the ligamentum arteriosum.

Failure of the ductus arteriosus to close may occur as an isolated congenital abnormality or may be associated with congenital heart disease. A persistent patent ductus arteriosus (PDA) results in high-pressure aortic blood passing into the pulmonary artery, producing pulmonary hypertension and hypertrophy of the right ventricle. A PDA is life threatening and should be ligated and divided surgically.

LARGE THORACIC VEINS

The brachiocephalic and azygos veins and the superior vena cava are the large veins in the thorax. They receive blood drainage from the head, neck, upper limbs, and thorax. The inferior vena cava receives blood mainly from the body below the diaphragm and has only a brief appearance in the thorax.

Brachiocephalic Veins

The **right** and **left brachiocephalic veins** form at the root of the neck on each side by the union of the respective subclavian and internal jugular veins (Fig. 4.64; see also Figs. 4.31, 4.37, and 4.46). The left brachiocephalic vein passes obliquely downward and to the right behind the manubrium sterni and in front of the large branches of the aortic arch. The right brachiocephalic vein is relatively short and descends almost vertically. The two brachiocephalic veins join to form the superior vena cava (see Fig. 4.64).

Superior Vena Cava

The two brachiocephalic veins join to form the superior vena cava, which conveys all the venous blood from the head and neck and both upper limbs (see Figs. 4.46 and 4.64). It passes downward to end in the right atrium of the heart (see Fig. 4.51). The azygos vein joins the posterior aspect of the superior vena cava just before it enters the pericardium (see Figs. 4.31A and 4.64B).

Azygos Veins

The azygos venous tract consists of the main azygos vein, the inferior hemiazygos vein, and the superior hemiazygos vein (see Figs. 4.15 and 4.64). Collectively,

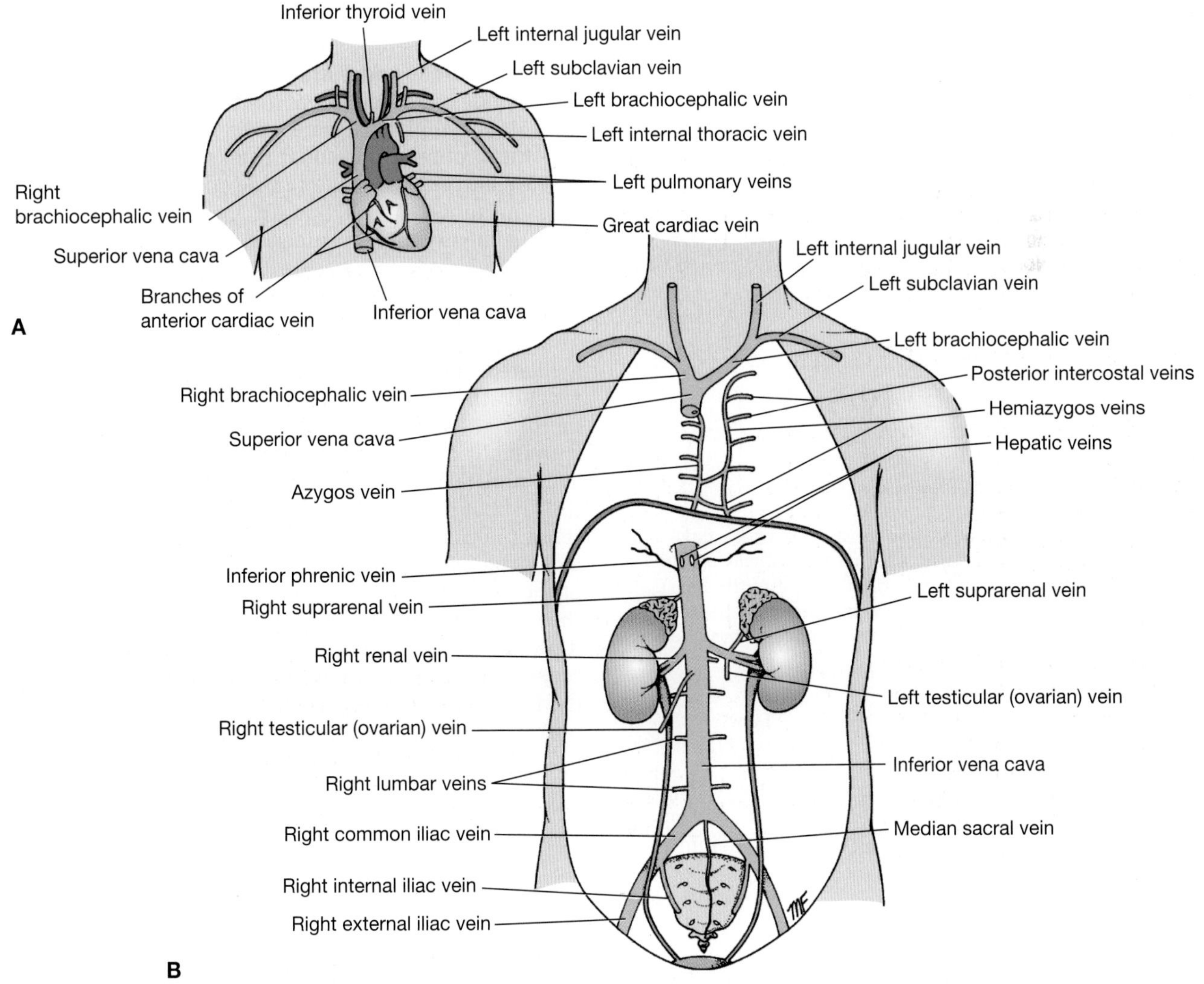

Figure 4.64 **A.** Major veins entering the heart. **B.** Major veins draining into the superior and inferior venae cavae.

they drain blood from the posterior parts of the intercostal spaces, posterior abdominal wall, pericardium, diaphragm, bronchi, and esophagus.

Azygos Vein

The origin of the azygos vein is variable. The union of the **right ascending lumbar vein** and the **right subcostal vein** in the abdomen often forms it (see Fig. 4.15). It ascends through the aortic opening in the diaphragm on the right side of the aorta up to the level of the T5 vertebra (see Fig. 4.64). Here, it arches forward above the root of the right lung to empty into the posterior surface of the superior vena cava (see Fig. 4.31A).

The azygos vein has numerous tributaries, including the **eight lower right intercostal veins**, **right superior intercostal vein**, **superior** and **inferior hemiazygos veins**, and numerous **mediastinal veins**.

Inferior Hemiazygos Vein

The union of the **left ascending lumbar vein** and the **left subcostal vein** in the abdomen often forms the inferior hemiazygos vein. It ascends through the left crus of diaphragm and, at about the level of the T8 vertebra, turns to the right and joins the azygos vein (see Fig. 4.15). It receives as tributaries some **lower left intercostal veins** and **mediastinal veins**.

Superior Hemiazygos Vein

The union of the **left superior intercostal vein** and the **fourth to the eighth intercostal veins** forms the superior hemiazygos vein (see Fig. 4.15). It joins the azygos vein at the level of the T7 vertebra.

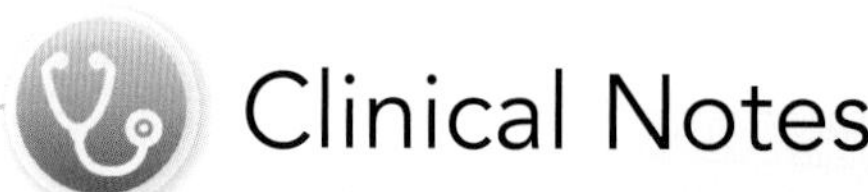

Clinical Notes

Azygos Veins and Caval Obstruction

In obstruction of the superior or inferior venae cavae, the azygos veins provide an alternative pathway for the return of venous blood to the right atrium of the heart. This is possible because these veins and their tributaries connect the superior and inferior venae cavae.

Inferior Vena Cava

The inferior vena cava pierces the central tendon of the diaphragm opposite the T8 vertebra and almost immediately enters the lowest part of the right atrium (see Figs. 4.11, 4.31A, 4.51, and 4.64A).

Pulmonary Veins

Two pulmonary veins leave each lung carrying oxygenated blood to the left atrium of the heart (see Figs. 4.31, 4.49, and 4.50).

THORACIC LYMPHATICS

The lymph vessels in the thorax collect lymph from virtually all parts of the body below the neck and upper limbs. Further, the upper ends of these vessels (located in the root of the neck) typically collect the drainage from the head, neck, and upper limbs.

Thoracic Wall

The lymph vessels of the skin of the anterior thoracic wall drain to the **anterior axillary nodes**, whereas the lymph vessels of the skin of the posterior thoracic wall drain to the **posterior axillary nodes** (see Fig. 4.16). The deep lymph vessels of the anterior parts of the intercostal spaces drain forward to the **internal thoracic nodes** along the internal thoracic blood vessels. From here, the lymph passes to the thoracic duct on the left side and the bronchomediastinal trunk on the right side. The deep lymph vessels of the posterior parts of the intercostal spaces drain backward to the **posterior intercostal nodes** lying near the heads of the ribs. From here, the lymph enters the thoracic duct.

Mediastinum

In addition to the nodes draining the lungs (see Fig. 4.40), other nodes are scattered through the mediastinum. They drain lymph from mediastinal structures and empty into the bronchomediastinal trunks and thoracic duct. Disease and enlargement of these nodes may exert pressure on important neighboring mediastinal structures, such as the trachea and superior vena cava.

Thoracic Duct

The thoracic duct begins below in the abdomen as a dilated sac, the **cisterna chyli** (see Fig. 1.30A). It ascends through the aortic opening of the diaphragm, on the right side of the descending aorta (see Fig. 4.50). It gradually crosses the median plane behind the esophagus and reaches the left border of the esophagus at the level of the lower border of the body of the T4 vertebra (sternal angle) (Fig. 4.24B). It then runs upward along the left edge of the esophagus to enter the root of the neck (Fig. 4.24A). Here, it bends laterally behind the carotid sheath and in front of the vertebral vessels. It turns downward in front of the left phrenic nerve and crosses the subclavian artery to enter the beginning of the left brachiocephalic vein.

At the root of the neck, the thoracic duct receives the **left jugular**, **subclavian**, and **bronchomediastinal lymph trunks**, although they may drain directly into the adjacent large veins. Thus, the thoracic duct conveys all lymph from the lower limbs, pelvic cavity, abdominal cavity, left side of the thorax, and left side of the head, neck, and arm (see Fig. 1.29A,B).

Right Lymphatic Duct

The **right jugular**, **subclavian**, and **bronchomediastinal trunks**, which drain the right side of the head and neck, the right upper limb, and the right side of the thorax, respectively, may join to form the right lymphatic duct (see Fig. 1.29A). This common duct, if present, is about 0.5 in. (1.3 cm) long and opens into the beginning of the right brachiocephalic vein. Alternatively, the trunks may open independently into the great veins at the root of the neck.

THORACIC NERVES

The vagus and phrenic nerves are the major nerves that run through the thoracic cavity. Other nerves (eg, the intercostal nerves) are associated with the thoracic walls and were reviewed earlier in this chapter. The thoracic parts of the sympathetic chains are associated with the thoracic walls and give rise to branches that pass into the thoracic and abdominal cavities. These are reviewed below.

Vagus Nerves

The vagus nerves carry **preganglionic parasympathetic fibers** (and other components) into the thoracic and abdominal cavities. Both give off **cardiac branches** in the neck that descend into the chest. These branches contribute to the pulmonary, esophageal, and cardiac plexuses and supply the lungs, esophagus, and heart, respectively.

The **right vagus nerve** crosses the right subclavian artery and descends into the thorax, first lying posterolateral to the brachiocephalic artery (see Fig. 4.24A), then lateral to the trachea, and medial to the terminal part of the azygos vein (see Fig. 4.31A). It passes behind the root of the right lung and assists in the formation of the **pulmonary plexus**. On leaving the plexus, the vagus passes onto the posterior surface of the esophagus and takes part in the formation of the **esophageal plexus**. It then passes through the esophageal opening of the diaphragm behind the esophagus to reach the posterior surface of the stomach (see Fig. 4.11).

The **left vagus nerve** descends in the thorax between the left common carotid and the left subclavian arteries (see Figs. 4.24A and 4.31B). It then crosses the left side of the aortic arch, where it passes under the left phrenic nerve. The vagus then turns backward behind the root of the left lung and assists in the formation of the **pulmonary plexus**. On leaving the plexus, the vagus passes onto the anterior surface of the esophagus and takes part in the formation of the **esophageal plexus**. It then passes through the esophageal opening in the diaphragm in front of the esophagus to reach the anterior surface of the stomach (see Fig. 4.11).

Branches

Each vagus gives origin to a recurrent laryngeal nerve. The right and left recurrent laryngeal nerves have significantly different relations in the thorax. The **right recurrent laryngeal nerve** arises from the right vagus in the neck, hooks under the right subclavian artery and ascends between the trachea and esophagus. The **left recurrent laryngeal nerve** arises from the left vagus trunk as the nerve crosses the arch of the aorta (see Figs. 4.31B and 4.46). It hooks around the ligamentum arteriosum and ascends in the groove between the trachea and the esophagus on the left side (see Fig. 4.24A). Thus, the left recurrent laryngeal has a much lower origin in the chest and close relations to the arch of the aorta and the ligamentum arteriosum (and prenatally to the ductus arteriosus; see Fig. 4.62D). The recurrent laryngeal nerves supply the trachea and esophagus as they ascend in the neck and ultimately provide the major motor and sensory supply to the larynx.

Phrenic Nerves

The phrenic nerves arise in the neck from the anterior rami of the C3 to C5 nerves (see Chapter 9: Main Nerves in the Neck). The right phrenic nerve descends in the thorax along the right side of the right brachiocephalic vein and the superior vena cava (see Figs. 4.24A,B and 4.31A). It passes in front of the root of the right lung and runs along the right side of the pericardium, which separates the nerve from the right atrium. It then descends on the right side of the inferior vena cava to the diaphragm. Its terminal branches pass through the caval opening in the diaphragm to supply the central part of the peritoneum on its abdominal aspect (see Fig. 4.11).

The **left phrenic nerve** descends in the thorax along the left side of the left subclavian artery. It crosses the left side of the aortic arch (see Fig. 4.31B) and here crosses over the left vagus nerve. It passes in front of the root of the left lung and then descends over the left surface of the pericardium, which separates the nerve from the left ventricle. On reaching the diaphragm, the terminal branches pierce the muscle and supply the central part of the peritoneum on its abdominal aspect (see Fig. 4.11).

The phrenic nerves possess both efferent and afferent fibers. The **efferent fibers** are the sole motor supply to the muscle of the diaphragm. The **afferent fibers** carry sensation to the CNS from the peritoneum covering the central region of the undersurface of the diaphragm, the pleura covering the central region of the upper surface of the diaphragm, and the pericardium and mediastinal parietal pleura.

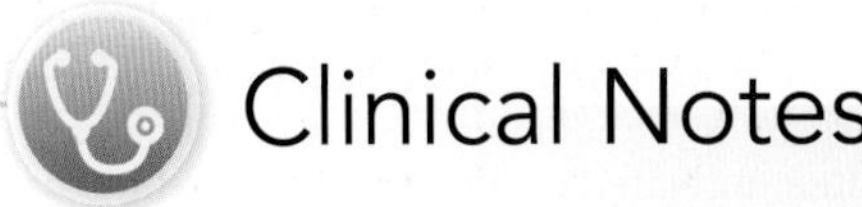

Clinical Notes

Diaphragm Paralysis

The phrenic nerve may be paralyzed because of pressure from malignant tumors in the mediastinum. Surgical crushing or sectioning of the phrenic nerve in the neck, producing paralysis of the diaphragm on one side, was once used as part of the treatment of lung tuberculosis, especially of the lower lobes. In such cases, the immobile dome of the elevated diaphragm rests the lung.

Sympathetic Trunks

The thoracic part of the sympathetic trunk is continuous above with the cervical and below with the lumbar parts of the sympathetic trunk. It is the most laterally placed structure in the mediastinum and runs downward on the heads of the ribs (see Figs. 4.31 and 4.32). It leaves the thorax on the side of the body of the T12 vertebra by passing behind the medial arcuate ligament of the diaphragm.

The thoracic sympathetic trunk has 12 (often only 11) segmentally arranged ganglia, each with a **white** and **gray ramus communicans** passing to the corresponding spinal nerve. The first ganglion is often fused with the inferior cervical ganglion to form the **stellate ganglion**.

Branches

1. **White rami communicantes** connect individual thoracic spinal nerves with the sympathetic chain. These convey preganglionic fibers from the spinal nerves into the sympathetic chain.
2. **Gray rami communicantes** connect sympathetic chain ganglia to their matching thoracic spinal nerves. These rami carry postganglionic fibers that are distributed through the branches of the spinal nerves to the blood vessels, sweat glands, and arrector pili muscles of the skin of the body wall and limbs.
3. **Thoracic splanchnic (visceral) branches** arise from the T1 to T4 or T5 chain ganglia. These carry postganglionic fibers to the pulmonary, cardiac, and esophageal plexuses and on to the lungs, heart, aorta, and esophagus.
4. **Abdominal splanchnic (visceral) nerves** arise from the T5 to T12 chain ganglia (see Fig. 4.31). These carry mainly preganglionic fibers to the abdominal viscera. Three abdominal splanchnic nerves arise from the thoracic part of the sympathetic chain: The **greater splanchnic nerve** arises from ganglia T5 to T9, the **lesser splanchnic nerve** arises from ganglia T10 and T11, and the **lowest (least) splanchnic nerve** arises from ganglion T12. They all enter the abdomen by piercing the crura of the diaphragm. See Chapter 5 for details of the distribution of these nerves in the abdomen.

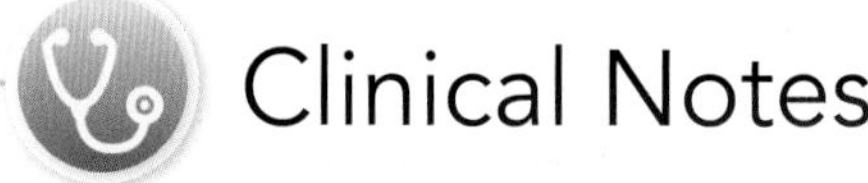

Clinical Notes

Sympathetic Trunk in the Treatment of Raynaud Disease

Preganglionic sympathectomy of the T2 and T3 ganglia can be performed to increase the blood flow to the fingers for such conditions as Raynaud disease. The sympathectomy causes vasodilatation of the arterioles in the upper limb.

Spinal Anesthesia and the Sympathetic Nervous System

A high spinal anesthetic may block the preganglionic sympathetic fibers passing out from the lower thoracic segments of the spinal cord. This produces temporary vasodilatation below this level, with a consequent fall in blood pressure.

Chest Pain

The presenting symptom of chest pain is a common problem in clinical practice. Unfortunately, chest pain is a symptom common to many conditions and may be caused by disease in the thoracic and abdominal walls or in many different thoracic and abdominal viscera. The severity of the pain is often unrelated to the seriousness of the cause. Myocardial pain may mimic esophagitis, musculoskeletal chest wall pain, and other non–life-threatening causes. Unless the physician is astute, a patient may be discharged with a more serious condition than the symptoms indicate. It is not good enough to have a correct diagnosis only 99% of the time with chest pain. An understanding of chest pain helps the physician in the systematic consideration of the differential diagnosis.

Somatic Chest Pain

Pain arising from the chest or abdominal walls is intense and discretely localized. Somatic pain arises in general somatic afferent nerve endings in these structures and is conducted to the central nervous system by segmental spinal nerves.

Visceral Chest Pain

Visceral pain is diffuse and poorly localized. It is conducted to the central nervous system along general visceral afferent nerves that accompany autonomic nerves. Most visceral pain fibers ascend to the spinal cord along sympathetic nerves and enter the cord through the posterior nerve roots of segmental spinal nerves. Some pain fibers from the pharynx and upper part of the esophagus and the trachea enter the central nervous system through parasympathetic nerves via the glossopharyngeal and vagus nerves.

Referred Chest Pain

Referred chest pain is the feeling of pain at a location other than the site of origin of the stimulus but in an area supplied by the same or adjacent segments of the spinal cord. Referred pain can be related to both somatic and visceral structures, for example, myocardial pain referred to the upper limb. A working knowledge of the thoracic dermatomes is essential to understanding chest pain (see Figs. 1.25 and 1.26). See the earlier Clinical Notes (Pain and Lung Disease; Cardiac Pain) in this chapter for a more complete consideration of referred chest pain.

ESOPHAGUS

The esophagus is a tubular structure about 10 in. (25 cm) long that is continuous above with the laryngeal part of the pharynx opposite the C6 vertebra. It passes through the esophageal hiatus of the diaphragm at the level of the T10 vertebra to join the stomach (see Figs. 4.11 and 4.28A).

In the neck, the esophagus lies in front of the vertebral column; laterally, it is related to the lobes of the thyroid gland; anteriorly, it is in contact with the trachea and the recurrent laryngeal nerves (see Chapter 9).

In the thorax, it passes downward and to the left through the superior and then the posterior mediastinum. At the level of the sternal angle, the aortic arch pushes the esophagus to the midline (see Fig. 4.24).

The relations of the thoracic part of the esophagus from above downward are as follows:

- **Anteriorly:** The trachea and the left recurrent laryngeal nerve; the left principal bronchus, which constricts it; and the pericardium, which separates the esophagus from the left atrium (see Figs. 4.24 and 4.50)
- **Posteriorly:** The bodies of the thoracic vertebrae; the thoracic duct; azygos veins; right posterior intercostal arteries; and, at its lower end, the descending thoracic aorta (see Figs. 4.24 and 4.50)
- **Right side:** The mediastinal pleura and the terminal part of the azygos vein (see Fig. 4.31A)
- **Left side:** The left subclavian artery, the aortic arch, the thoracic duct, and the mediastinal pleura (see Fig. 4.31B)

Inferior to the level of the roots of the lungs, the vagus nerves leave the pulmonary plexus and join with sympathetic nerves to form the **esophageal plexus**. The **left vagus** lies anterior to the esophagus, and the **right vagus** lies posterior. At its opening in the diaphragm, the esophagus is accompanied by the two vagi (see Fig. 4.11), branches of the left gastric blood vessels, and lymphatic vessels. Fibers from the right crus of diaphragm pass around the esophagus in the form of a sling.

In the abdomen, the esophagus descends for about 0.5 in. (1.3 cm) and then enters the stomach. It is related to the left lobe of the liver anteriorly and to the left crus of diaphragm posteriorly.

Blood Supply

The upper third of the esophagus is supplied by the **inferior thyroid artery**, the middle third by **esophageal branches from the descending thoracic aorta**, and the lower third by branches from the **left gastric artery**. The veins from the upper third drain into the **inferior thyroid veins**, from the middle third into the **azygos veins**, and from the lower third into the **left gastric vein**, a tributary of the portal vein.

Lymph Drainage

Lymph vessels from the upper third of the esophagus drain into the **deep cervical nodes**, from the middle third into the **superior and posterior mediastinal nodes**, and from the lower third into **nodes along the left gastric blood vessels** and the **celiac nodes** (see Fig. 4.40).

Nerve Supply

The esophagus is supplied by parasympathetic and sympathetic fibers via the **vagi** and **sympathetic trunks**, respectively. In the lower part of its thoracic course, the esophagus is surrounded by the **esophageal nerve plexus**.

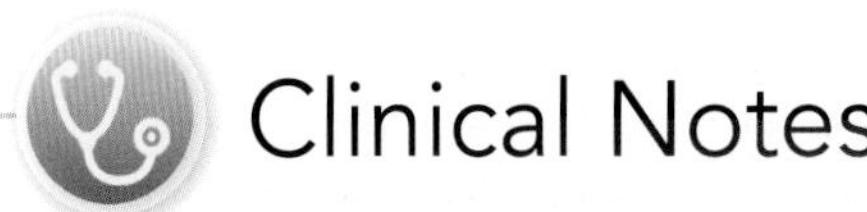

Clinical Notes

Esophageal Constrictions

The esophagus has **three anatomic** and **physiologic constrictions** (Fig. 4.65). The first is where the pharynx joins the upper end, the second is where the aortic arch and the left primary bronchus cross its anterior surface, and the third occurs where the esophagus passes through the diaphragm into the stomach. These constrictions are of considerable clinical importance because they are sites where swallowed foreign bodies can lodge or through which it may be difficult to pass an esophagoscope. Because a slight delay in the passage of food or fluid occurs at these levels, strictures (narrowings) may develop here after drinking caustic fluids. These constrictions are also the common sites of carcinoma of the esophagus. Their respective distances from the upper incisor teeth are 6 in. (15 cm), 10 in. (25 cm), and 16 in. (41 cm), respectively.

Portal-Systemic Venous Anastomosis

An important portal-systemic venous anastomosis occurs at the lower third of the esophagus. (See Chapter 5, Clinical Notes, Portal-Systemic Anastomoses, for other portal-systemic anastomoses.) Here, the **esophageal tributaries of the azygos veins** (systemic veins) anastomose with the **esophageal tributaries of the left gastric vein** (components of the hepatic portal system). Should the portal vein become obstructed (eg, in cirrhosis of the liver), **portal hypertension** develops, resulting in dilatation and varicosity of the portal-systemic anastomoses. Varicose esophageal veins

(continued)

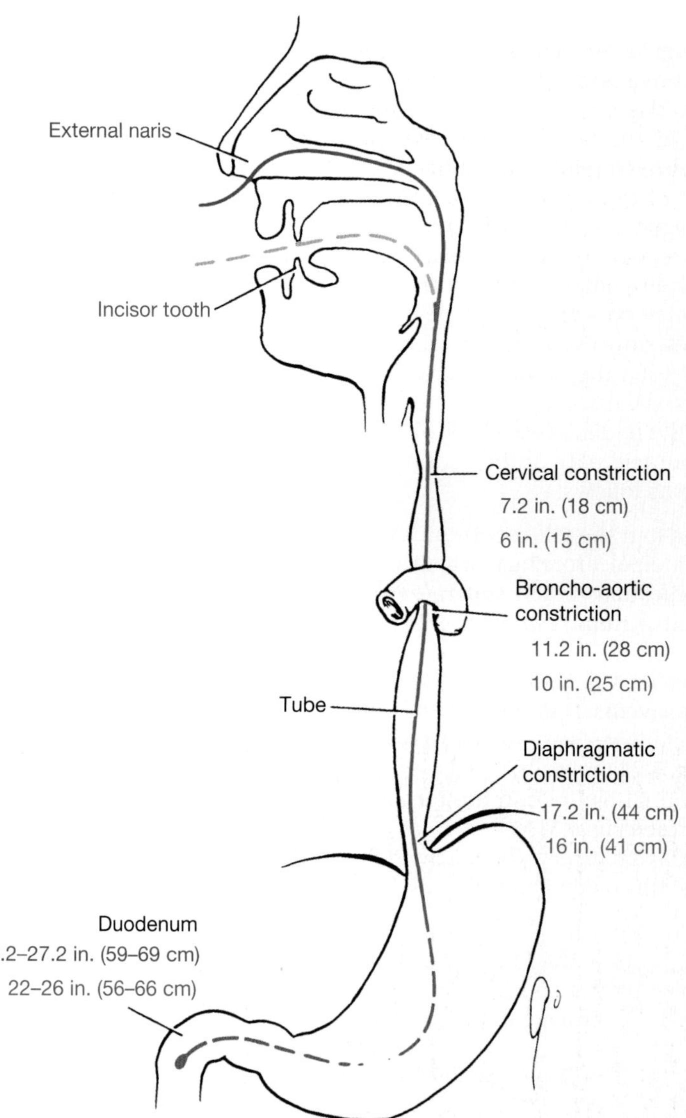

Figure 4.65 Approximate respective distances from the incisor teeth (*blue*) and the nostrils (*red*) to the normal three constrictions of the esophagus. To assist in the passage of a tube to the duodenum, the distances to the first part of the duodenum are also included.

may rupture during the passage of food, causing **hematemesis** (vomiting of blood), which may be fatal.

Carcinoma of Lower Third of the Esophagus

The lymph drainage of the lower third of the esophagus descends through the esophageal opening in the diaphragm and ends in the **celiac nodes** around the celiac artery (see Fig. 4.40). A malignant tumor of this area of the esophagus would therefore tend to spread below the diaphragm along this route. Consequently, surgical removal of the lesion would include not only the primary lesion but also the celiac lymph nodes and all regions that drain into these nodes, namely, the stomach, the upper half of the duodenum, the spleen, and the omenta. Restoration of continuity of the gut is accomplished by performing an esophagojejunostomy.

Esophagus and Left Atrium of the Heart

The anterior wall of the esophagus is closely related to the posterior wall of the left atrium (see Fig. 4.19). A barium swallow may help assess the size of the left atrium in cases of left-sided heart failure, in which the left atrium becomes distended because of backpressure of venous blood.

THYMUS

The thymus is a flattened, bilobed structure (see Fig. 4.24A) lying between the sternum and the pericardium in the anterior mediastinum. It reaches its largest size relative to the size of the body in the newborn infant, at which time it may extend up through the superior mediastinum in front of the great vessels into the root of the neck. The thymus continues to grow until puberty but thereafter undergoes involution. It has a pink, lobulated appearance and is the site for development of T (thymic) lymphocytes.

Blood Supply

The inferior thyroid and internal thoracic arteries supply blood to the thymus.

RADIOGRAPHIC ANATOMY

Only the major features seen on standard posteroanterior and oblique lateral radiographs of the chest are discussed here.

Posteroanterior Radiograph

A **posteroanterior (PA)** radiograph is taken with the anterior wall of the patient's chest touching the cassette holder and with the x-rays traversing the thorax from the posterior to the anterior aspect (Figs. 4.66 and 4.67). First, check to make sure that the radiograph is a true PA radiograph and is not slightly oblique. Look at the sternal ends of both clavicles; they should be equidistant from the vertebral spines.

Now, examine the following in a systematic order:

1. **Superficial soft tissues:** The nipples in both sexes and the breasts in the female may be seen superimposed on the lung fields. The pectoralis major may also cast a soft shadow.
2. **Bones:** The thoracic vertebrae are imperfectly seen. The costotransverse joints and each rib should be examined in order from above downward and compared to the fellows of the opposite side (see Fig. 4.66). The costal cartilages are not usually seen, but if calcified, they will be visible. The clavicles are clearly seen crossing the upper part of each lung field. The medial borders of the

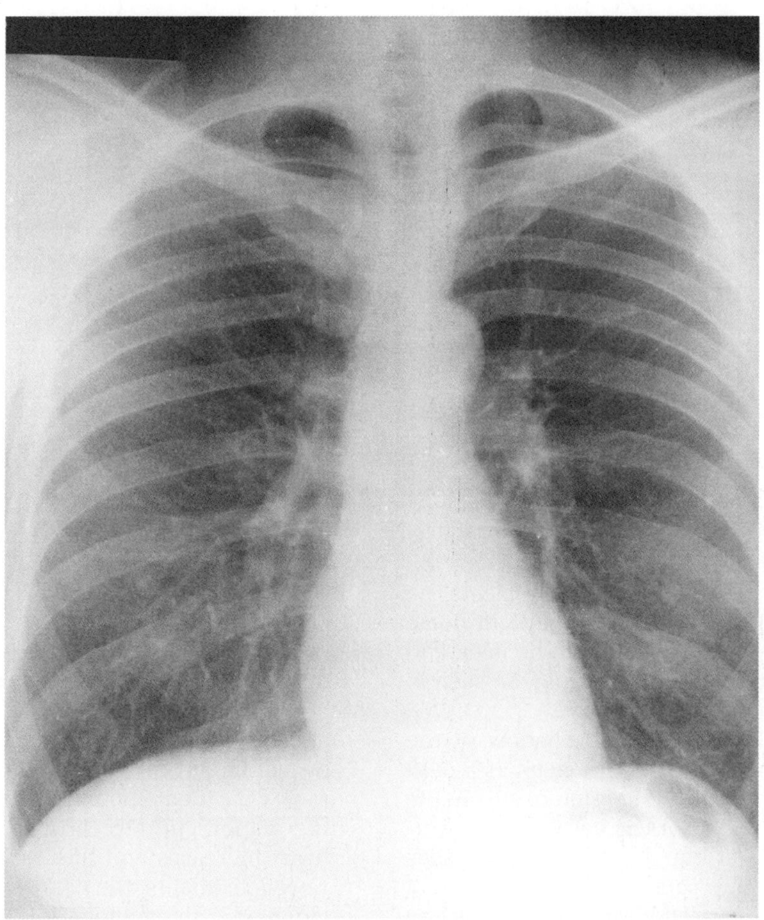

Figure 4.66 Posteroanterior (PA) radiograph of the chest of a healthy adult male.

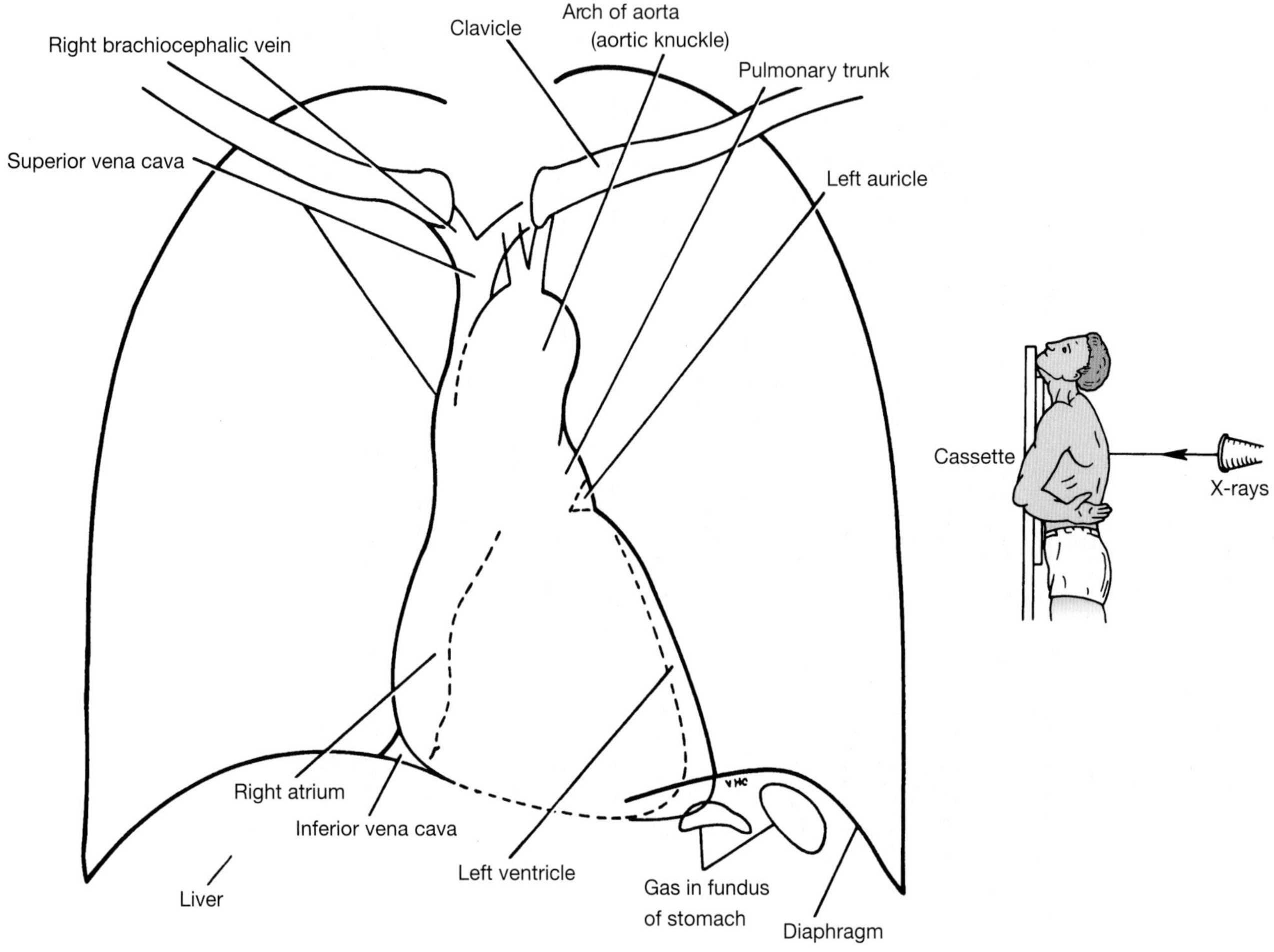

Figure 4.67 Main features observable in the PA radiograph of the chest shown in Figure 4.66. Note the position of the patient in relation to the x-ray source and the cassette holder.

scapulae may overlap the periphery of each lung field.

3. **Diaphragm:** The diaphragm casts dome-shaped shadows on each side; the one on the right is slightly higher than the one on the left. Note the costophrenic angle, where the diaphragm meets the thoracic wall (see Fig. 4.66). Beneath the right dome is the homogeneous, dense shadow of the liver, and beneath the left dome, a gas bubble may be seen in the fundus of the stomach.
4. **Trachea:** The radiolucent, air-filled shadow of the trachea is seen in the midline of the neck as a dark area (see Fig. 4.66). This is superimposed on the lower cervical and upper thoracic vertebrae.
5. **Lungs:** Looking first at the lung roots, one sees relatively dense shadows caused by the presence of the blood-filled pulmonary and bronchial vessels, the large bronchi, and the lymph nodes (see Fig. 4.66). The lung fields, by virtue of the air they contain, readily permit the passage of x-rays. For this reason, the lungs are more translucent on full inspiration than on expiration. The pulmonary blood vessels are seen as a series of shadows radiating from the lung root. When seen end on, they appear as small, round, white shadows. The large bronchi, if seen end on, also cast similar round shadows. The smaller bronchi are not seen.
6. **Mediastinum:** The various structures within the mediastinum, superimposed one on the other, produce a distinctive mediastinal shadow in PA radiographs (see Fig. 4.66). Note the outline of the heart and great vessels. The transverse diameter of the heart should not exceed half the width of the thoracic cage. Remember that on deep inspiration, when the diaphragm descends, the vertical length of the heart increases and the transverse diameter is narrowed. In infants, the heart is always wider and more globular in shape than in adults.

The **right border of the mediastinal shadow** from above downward consists of the right brachiocephalic vein, superior vena cava, right atrium, and (sometimes)

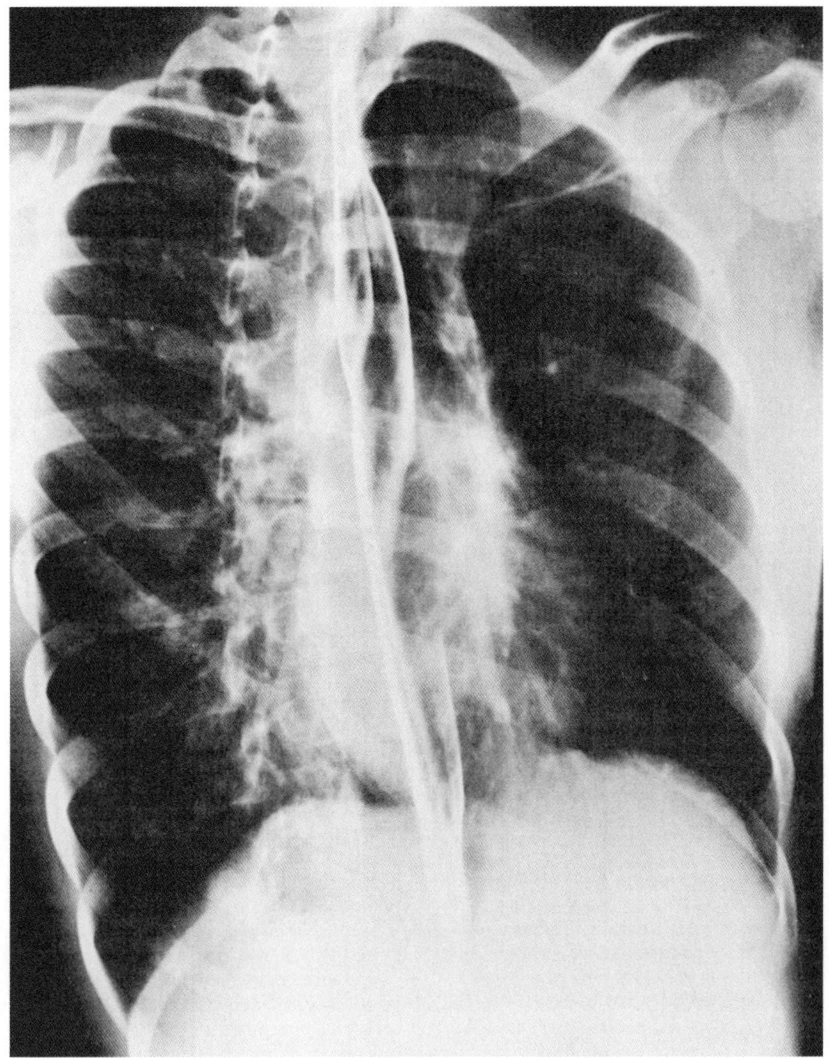

Figure 4.68 Right oblique radiograph of the chest of a healthy adult male after a barium swallow.

the inferior vena cava (see Figs. 4.66 and 4.67). The **left border** consists of a prominence, the **aortic knuckle**, caused by the aortic arch; below this are the left margin of the pulmonary trunk, the left auricle, and the left ventricle. The inferior border of the mediastinal shadow (lower border of the heart) blends with the diaphragm and liver. Note the cardiophrenic angles.

Right Oblique Radiograph

A right oblique radiograph is obtained by rotating the patient so that the right anterior chest wall is touching the cassette holder and the x-rays traverse the thorax from left posterior to right anterior in an oblique direction (Figs. 4.68 and 4.69). The right ventricle largely makes up the heart shadow. A small part of the posterior border is formed by the right atrium. For further details of structures seen on this view, see Figures 4.68 and 4.69.

Left Oblique Radiograph

A left oblique radiograph is obtained by rotation of the patient so that the left anterior chest wall is touching the cassette holder and the x-rays traverse the thorax from right posterior to left anterior in an oblique direction. The heart shadow is largely made up of the right ventricle anteriorly and the left ventricle posteriorly. The aortic arch and the pulmonary trunk may be seen above the heart.

An example of a left lateral radiograph of the chest is shown in Figures 4.70 and 4.71.

Bronchography and Contrast Visualization of the Esophagus

Bronchography is a special study of the bronchial tree by means of the introduction of iodized oil or other contrast medium into a particular bronchus or bronchi,

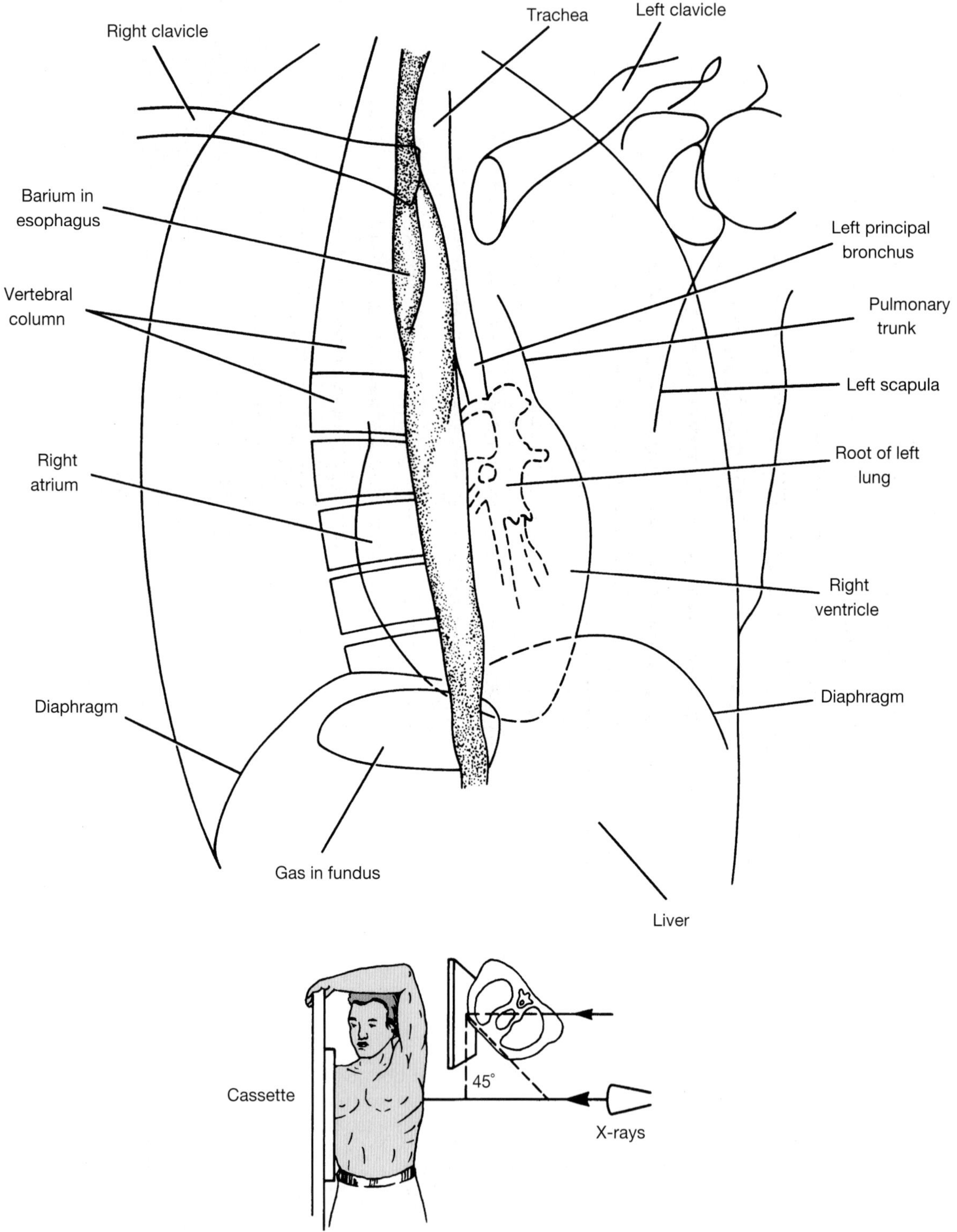

Figure 4.69 Main features observable in the right oblique radiograph of the chest shown in Figure 4.68. Note the position of the patient in relation to the x-ray source and the cassette holder.

usually under fluoroscopic control. The contrast media are nonirritating and sufficiently radiopaque to allow good visualization of the bronchi (Fig. 4.72). After the radiographic examination is completed, the patient is asked to cough and expectorate the contrast medium.

Contrast visualization of the esophagus (see Figs. 4.68 and 4.70) is accomplished by giving the patient a creamy paste of barium sulfate and water to swallow. The aortic arch and the left bronchus cause a smooth indentation on the anterior border of the barium-filled esophagus.

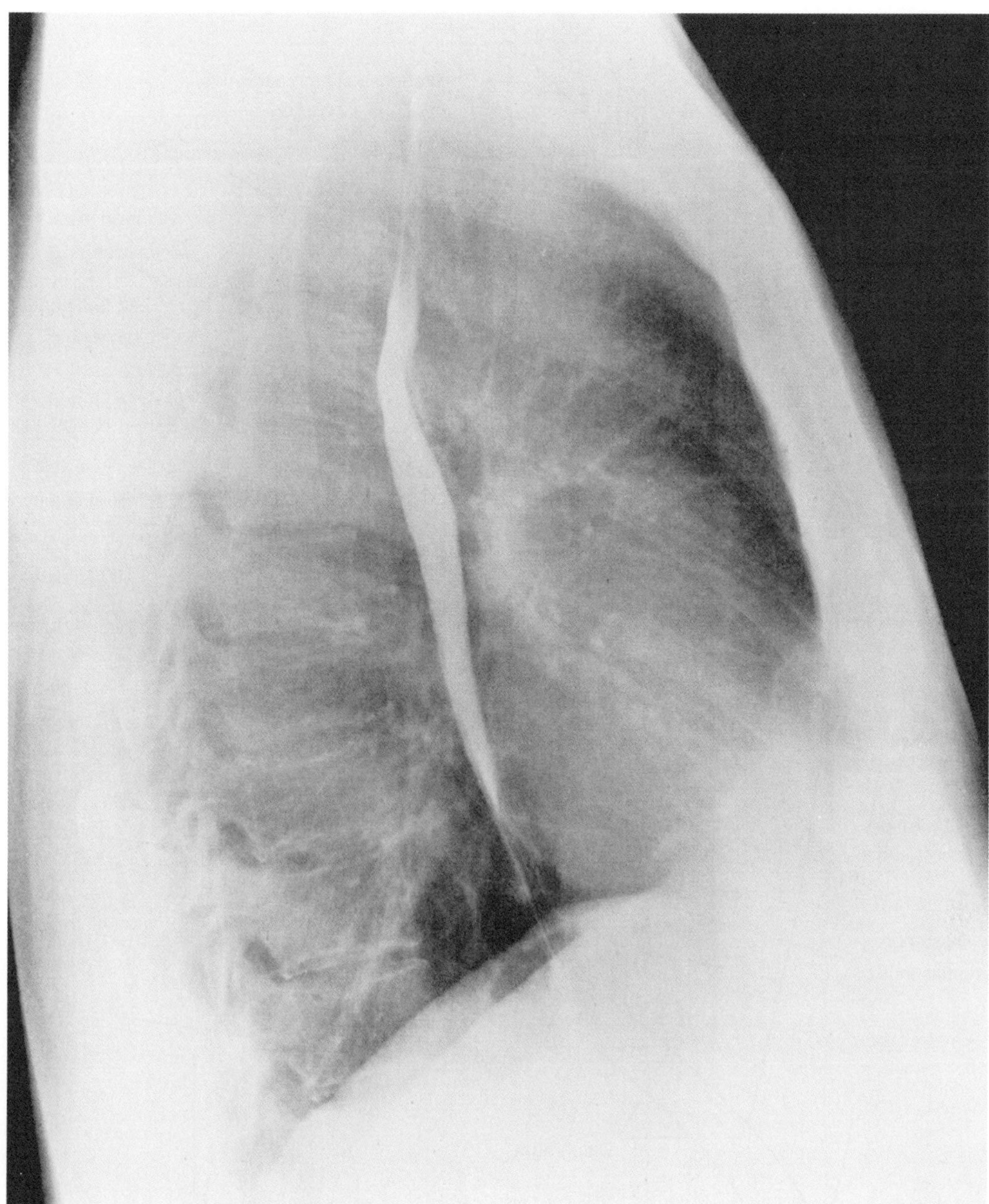

Figure 4.70 Left lateral radiograph of the chest of a healthy adult male after a barium swallow.

This procedure can also be used to outline the posterior border of the left atrium in a left lateral view. An enlarged left atrium causes a smooth indentation of the anterior border of the barium-filled esophagus.

Coronary Angiography

The coronary arteries can be visualized by the introduction of radiopaque material into their lumen. Under fluoroscopic control, a long narrow catheter is passed into the ascending aorta via the femoral artery in the thigh or the radial artery in the forearm. The tip of the catheter is carefully guided into the orifice of a coronary artery, and a small amount of radiopaque material is injected to reveal the lumen of the artery and its branches. The information can be recorded on radiographs (Fig. 4.73) or by cineradiography. Pathologic narrowing or blockage of a coronary artery can be identified using this technique.

Computed Tomography Scanning

Cross-sectional images, such as seen in axial computed tomography (CTs), are critical tools in evaluating the condition of the thorax. Review the cross-sections shown in Figures 4.24, 4.50, and 4.74 as aids in understanding standard CTs of the thorax such as shown in Figures 4.75 and 4.76. Remember, CT scanning relies on the same physics as conventional x-rays (see Chapter 1, Medical Imaging).

(text continue on page 278)

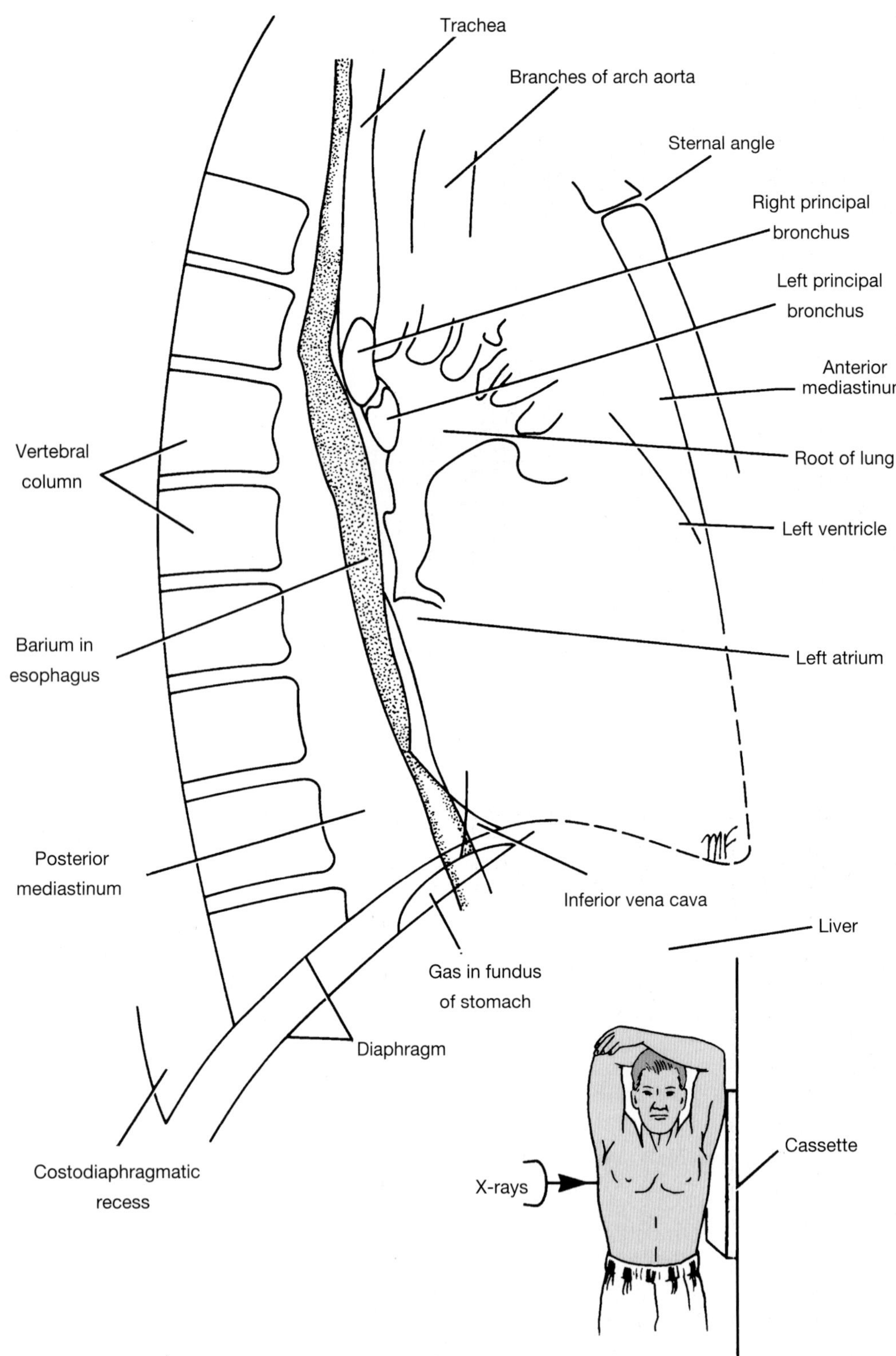

Figure 4.71 Main features observable in a left lateral radiograph of the chest shown in Figure 4.70. Note the position of the patient in relation to the x-ray source and the cassette holder. Also note the relation of the esophagus to the left atrium.

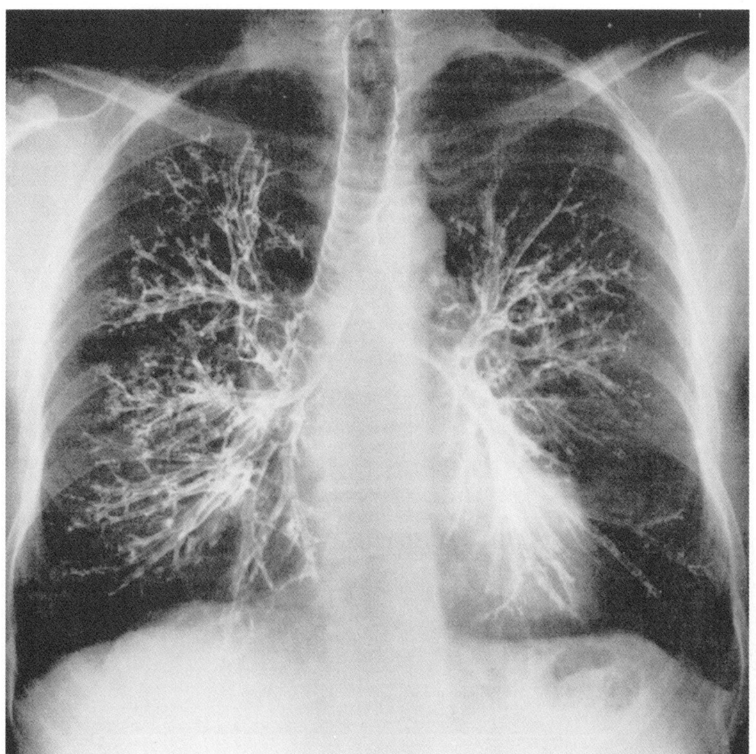

Figure 4.72 Posteroanterior bronchogram of the chest.

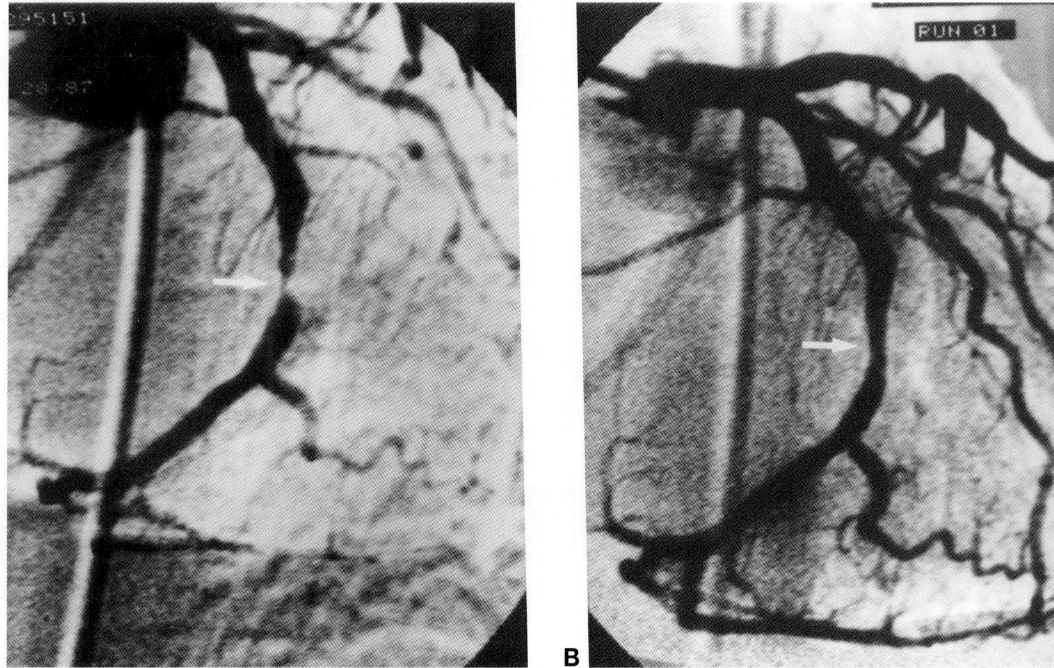

Figure 4.73 Coronary angiograms. **A.** Area of extreme narrowing of the circumflex branch of the left coronary artery (*white arrow*). **B.** Same artery after percutaneous transluminal coronary angioplasty. Inflation of the luminal balloon has dramatically improved the area of stenosis (*white arrow*).

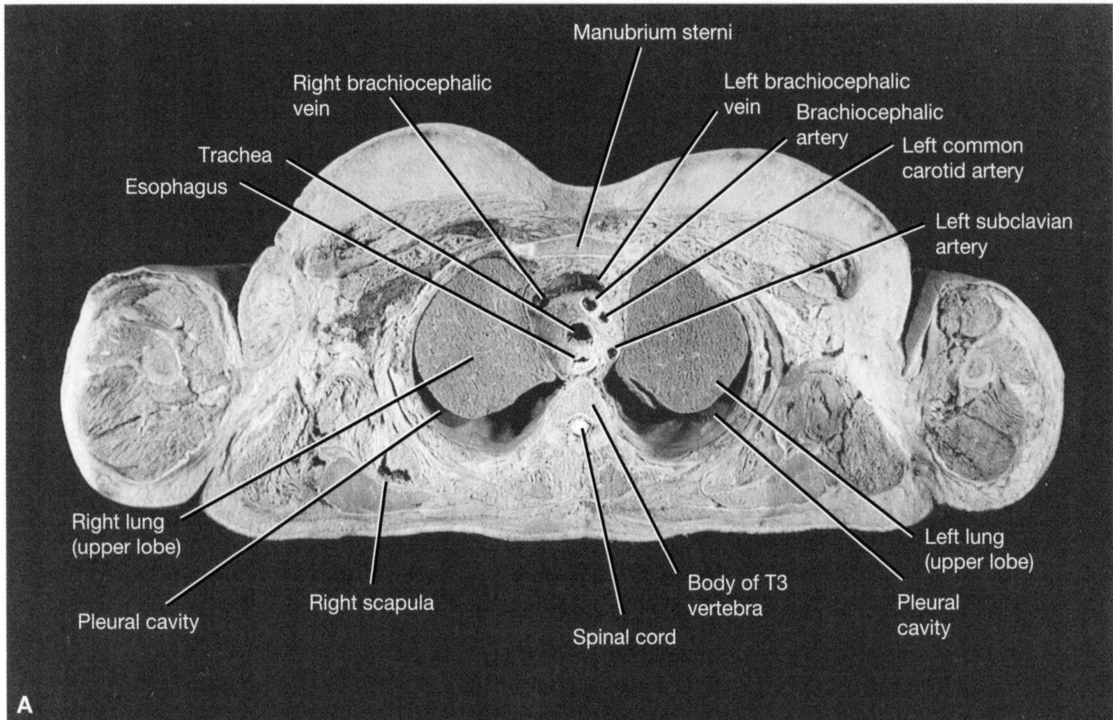

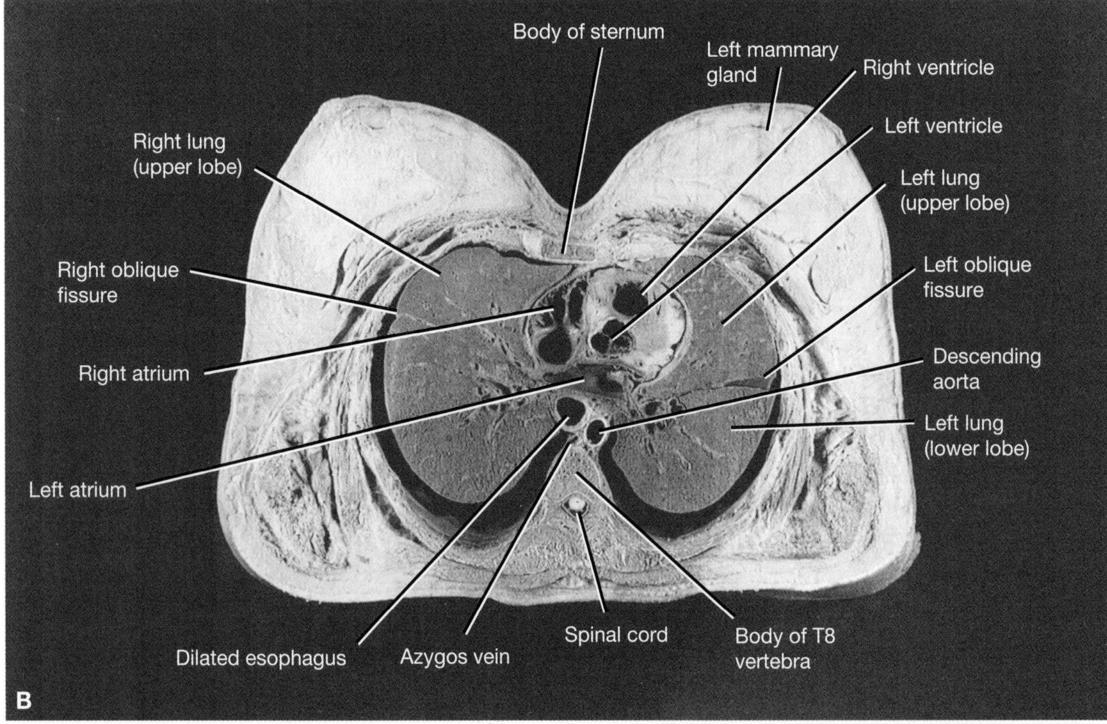

Figure 4.74 Cross sections of the thorax. **A.** At the level of the body of the T3 vertebra. **B.** At the level of the T8 vertebra. Note that in the living, the pleural cavity is only a potential space. The large space seen here is an artifact resulting from the embalming process.

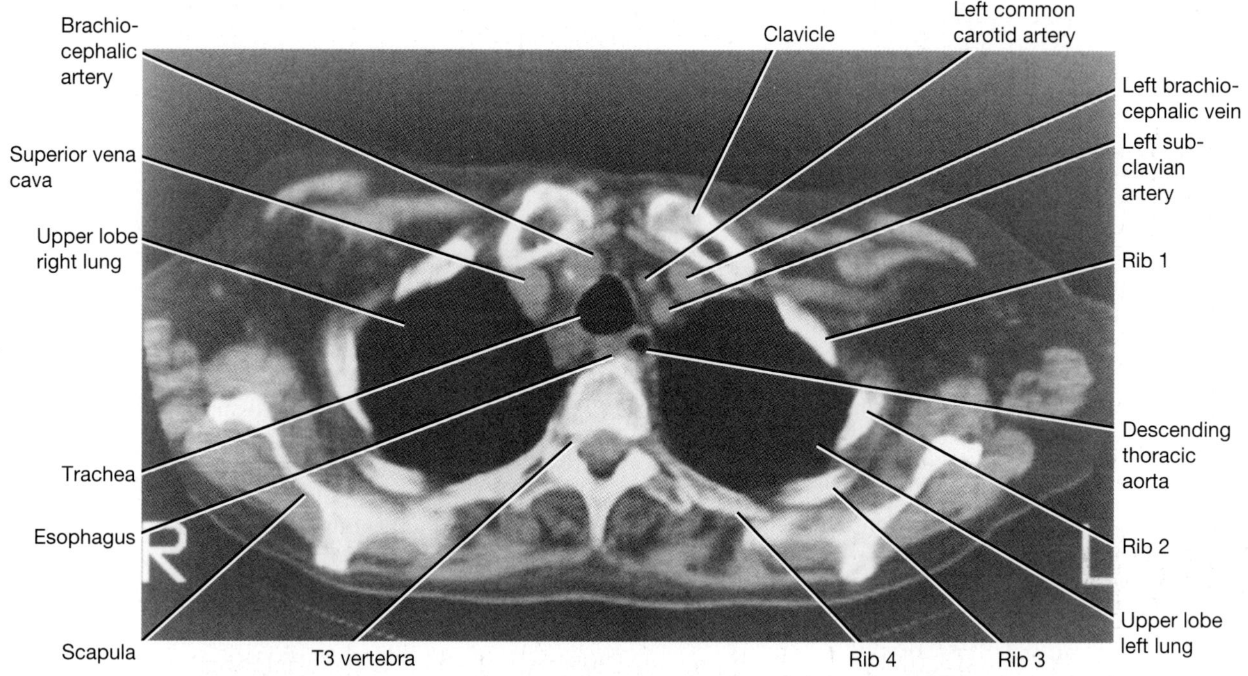

Figure 4.75 Computed tomography scan of the upper part of the thorax at the level of the T3 vertebra.

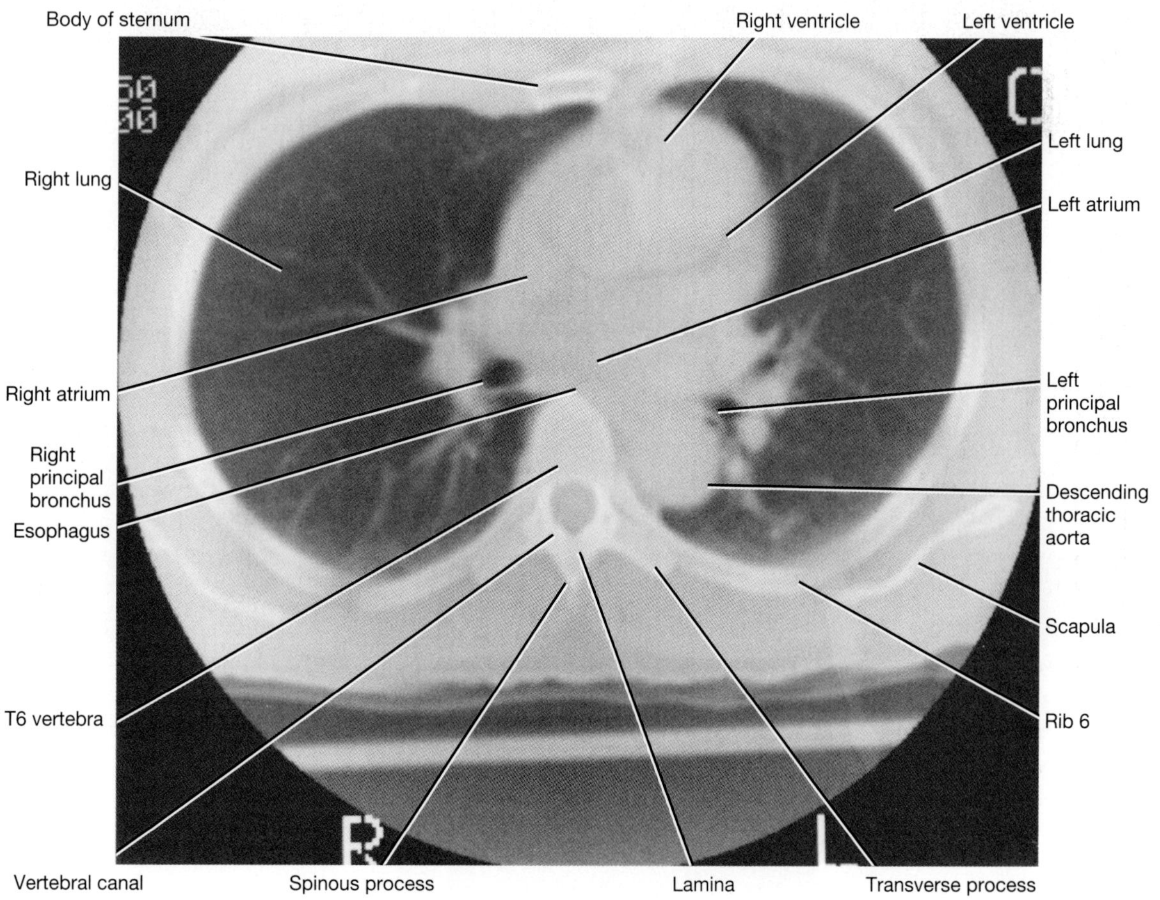

Figure 4.76 Computed tomography scan of the middle part of the thorax at the level of the T6 vertebra.

SURFACE ANATOMY

Refer to Figures 4.77 through 4.84.

Anterior Chest Wall

The **suprasternal notch** is the superior margin of the manubrium sterni and is easily felt between the prominent medial ends of the clavicles in the midline (Figs. 4.77 to 4.79). It lies opposite the lower border of the body of the T2 vertebra (see Fig. 4.2).

The **sternal angle** (angle of Louis) is the angle made between the manubrium and the body of the sternum (see Figs. 4.77 to 4.79). It lies opposite the intervertebral disc between the T4 and T5 vertebrae (see Fig. 4.2). The position of the sternal angle can easily be felt and is often seen as a transverse ridge. The finger moved to the right or to the left will pass directly onto costal cartilage 2 and then rib 2. All ribs may be counted from this point. Occasionally in a very muscular male, large pectoral muscles may obscure the ribs and intercostal spaces. In these cases, it may be easier to count up from rib 12. The **xiphisternal joint** is the joint between the xiphoid process of the sternum and the body of the sternum (see Fig. 4.79). It lies opposite the body of the T9 vertebra (see Fig. 4.2).

The **subcostal angle** is situated at the inferior end of the sternum, between the sternal attachments of the seventh costal cartilages (see Fig. 4.79).

The **costal margin** is the lower boundary of the thorax and is formed by the cartilages of ribs 7 to 10 and the ends of cartilages 11 and 12 (see Figs. 4.77 to 4.79). The lowest part of the costal margin is formed by rib 10 and lies at the level of the L3 vertebra.

The **clavicle** is subcutaneous throughout its entire length and can be easily palpated. It articulates at its lateral extremity with the acromion process of the scapula.

Ribs

Rib 1 lies deep to the clavicle and cannot be palpated. Pressing the fingers upward into the axilla and drawing them downward over the lateral surface of the chest wall can allow feeling the lateral surfaces of the remaining ribs. Rib 12 can be used to identify a particular rib by counting from below. However, in some individuals, rib 12 is very short and difficult to feel. For this reason, an alternative method may be used to identify ribs by first palpating the sternal angle and costal cartilage 2.

Diaphragm

The central tendon of the diaphragm lies directly behind the xiphisternal joint. In the midrespiratory position, the summit of the right dome of the diaphragm arches upward as far as the upper border of rib in the midclavicular line, but the left dome only reaches as far as the lower border.

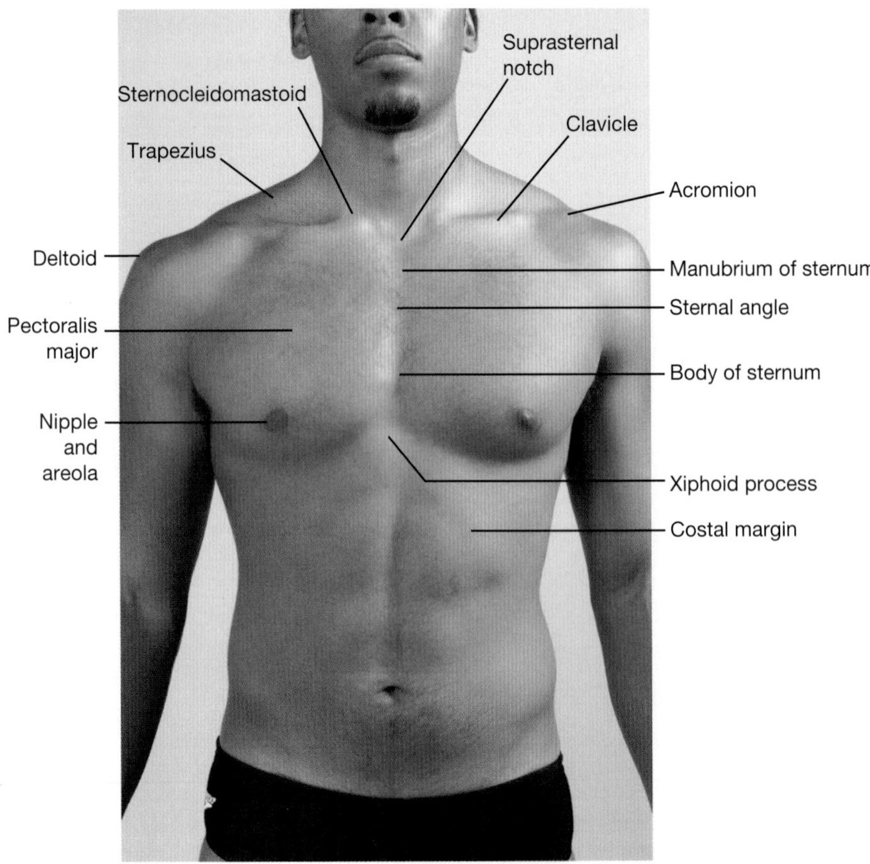

Figure 4.77 Anterior view of the thorax of a young adult male.

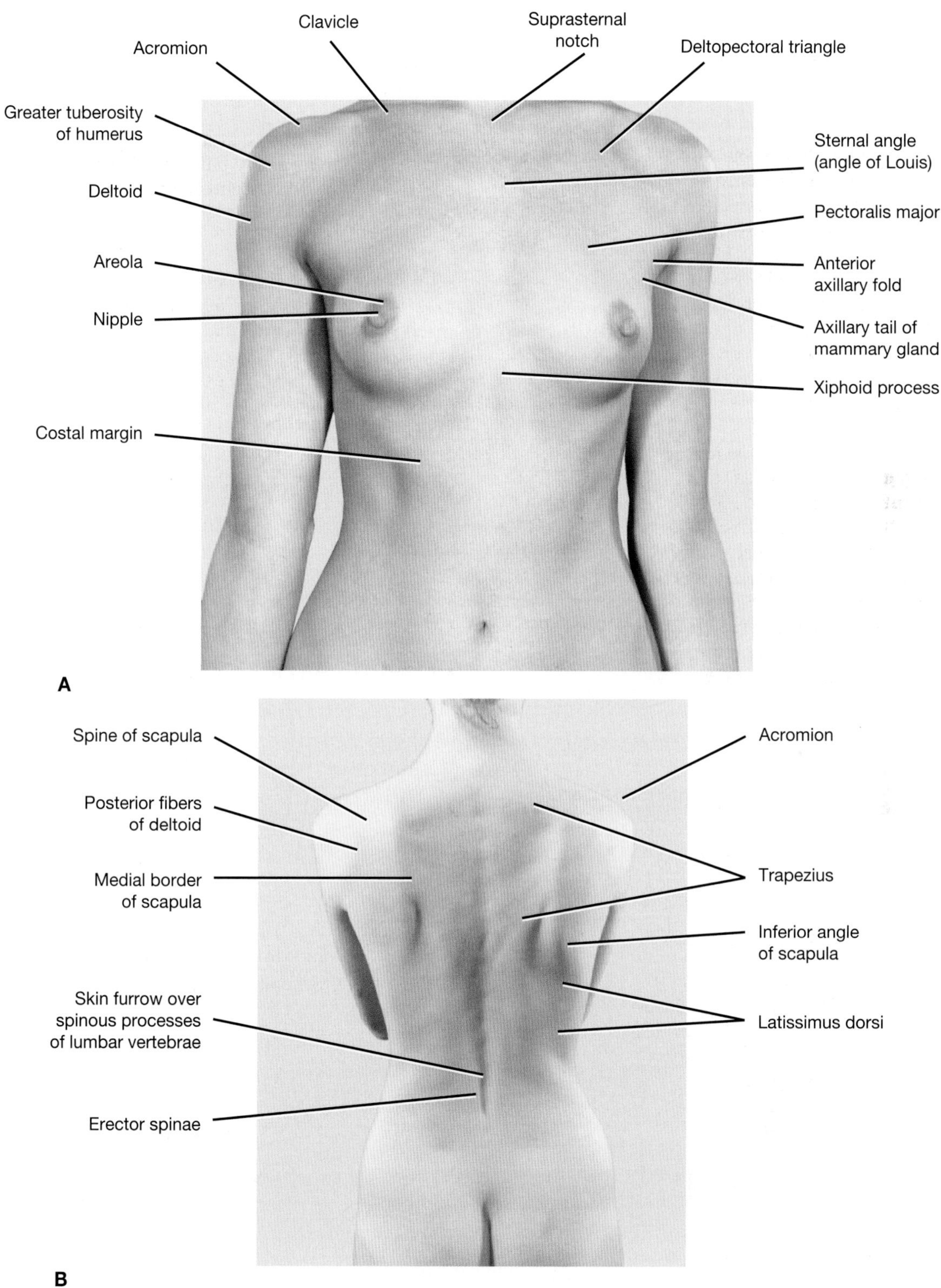

Figure 4.78 Anterior **(A)** and posterior **(B)** views of the thorax of a young adult female.

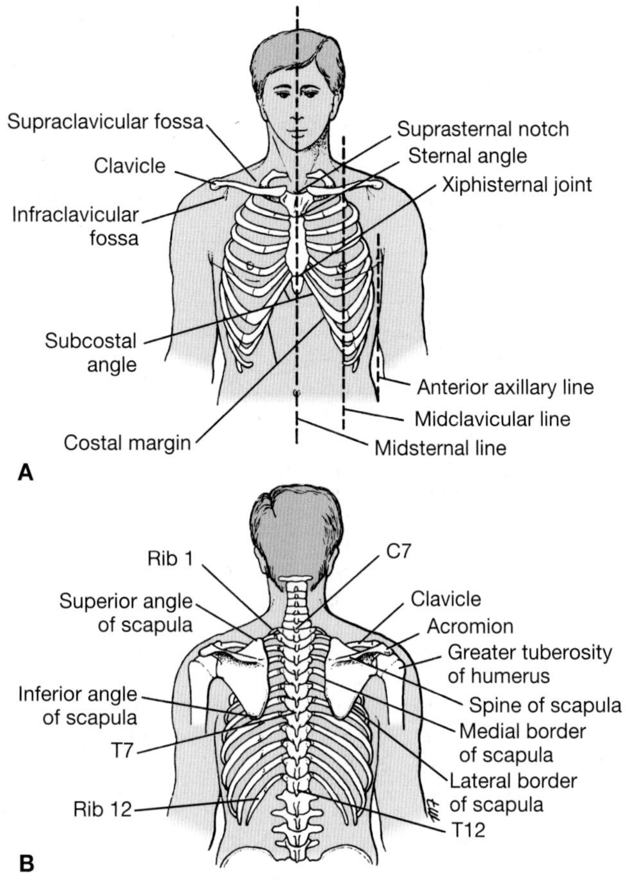

Figure 4.79 Surface landmarks of anterior **(A)** and posterior **(B)** thoracic walls.

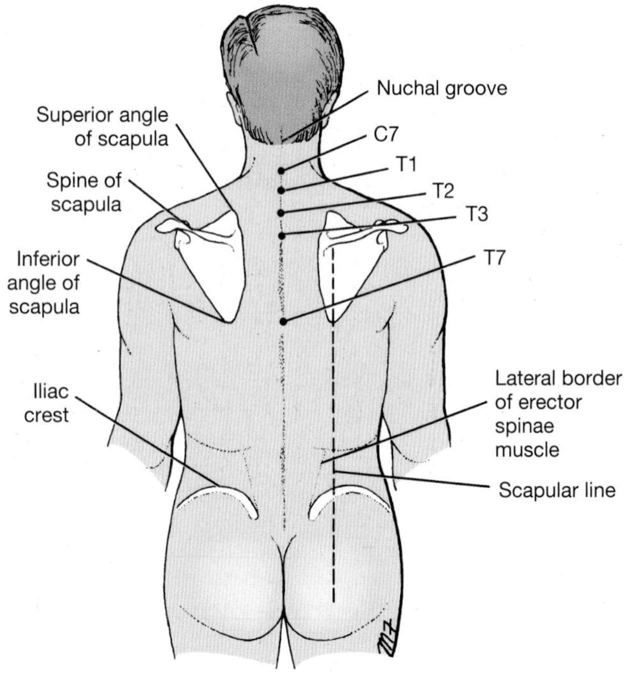

Figure 4.80 Surface landmarks of the posterior thoracic wall.

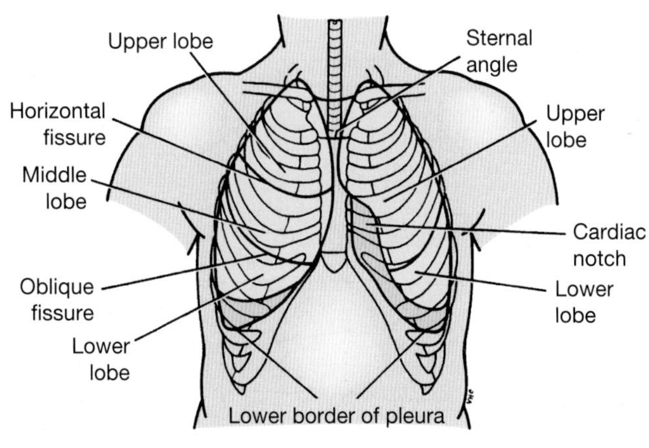

Figure 4.81 Surface markings of the lungs and parietal pleura on the anterior thoracic wall.

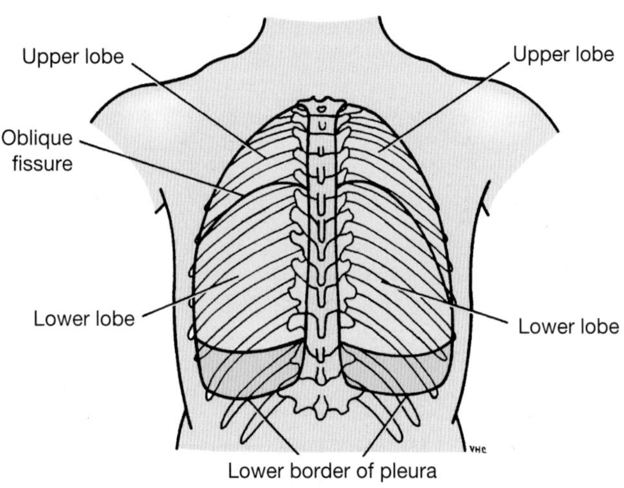

Figure 4.82 Surface markings of the lungs and parietal pleura on the posterior thoracic wall.

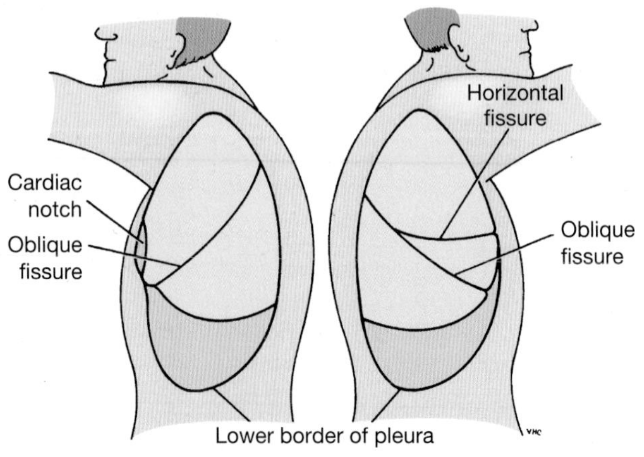

Figure 4.83 Surface markings of the lungs and parietal pleura on the lateral thoracic walls.

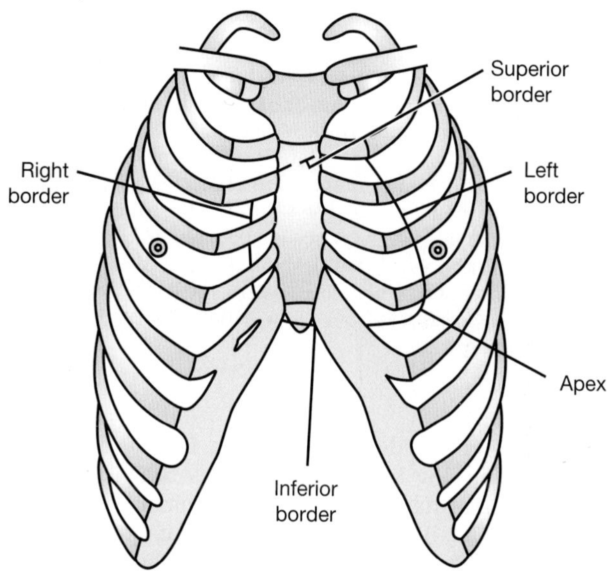

Figure 4.84 Surface markings of the heart.

Nipple

In the male, the nipple usually lies in intercostal space 4 about 4 in. (10 cm) from the midline. In the female, its position is not constant. However, the T4 dermatome always crosses the nipple in both sexes regardless of the form of the breast.

Apex Beat of Heart

The lower portion of the left ventricle forms the apex of the heart. The apex of the heart being thrust forward against the thoracic wall as the heart contracts causes the apex beat. (The heart is thrust forward with each ventricular contraction because of the ejection of blood from the left ventricle into the aorta; the force of the blood in the aorta tends to cause the curved aorta to straighten slightly, thus pushing the heart forward.) The apex beat can usually be felt by placing the flat of the hand on the chest wall over the heart. After the area of cardiac pulsation has been determined, the apex beat is accurately localized by placing two fingers over the intercostal spaces and moving them until the point of maximum pulsation is found. The apex beat is normally found in left intercostal space 5, 3.5 in. (9 cm) from the midline. If you have difficulty in finding the apex beat, have the patient lean forward in the sitting position.

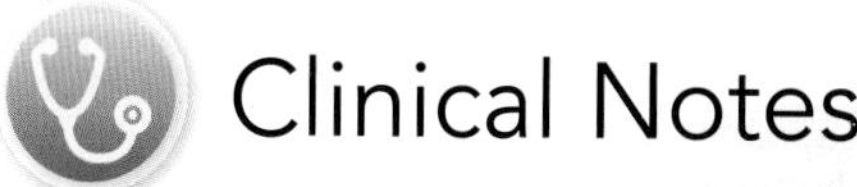

Clinical Notes

Rib and Costal Cartilage Identification

When examining the chest from in front, the sternal angle is an important landmark. Its position can easily be felt and often is seen by the presence of a transverse ridge. The finger moved to the right or to the left passes directly onto costal cartilage 2 and then rib 2. All other ribs can be counted from this point. Rib 12 can usually be felt from behind, but in some obese persons, this may prove difficult.

In a female with pendulous breasts, the examining fingers should gently raise the left breast from below as the intercostal spaces are palpated.

Axillary Folds

The lower border of the pectoralis major muscle forms the **anterior axillary fold** (see Figs. 4.77 and 4.78A). This can be made to stand out by asking the patient to press their hand hard against their hip. The tendon of the latissimus dorsi muscle as it passes around the lower border of the teres major muscle forms the **posterior axillary fold** (see Fig. 4.78B).

Posterior Chest Wall

The **spinous processes** of the thoracic vertebrae can be palpated in the posterior midline (Fig. 4.80; see also Figs. 4.78B and 4.79B). The index finger should be placed on the skin in the midline on the posterior surface of the neck and drawn downward in the nuchal groove. The first spinous process to be felt is that of the C7 vertebrae (**vertebra prominens**). The overlapping spines of the thoracic vertebrae are below this level. A large ligament, the **ligamentum nuchae**, covers the spines of the C1 to C6 vertebrae. It should be noted that the tip of a spinous process of a thoracic vertebra lies posterior to the body of the next vertebra below.

The **scapula** (shoulder blade) is flat and triangular and is located on the upper part of the posterior surface of the thorax. The **superior angle** lies opposite the spine of the T2 vertebra. The **spine** of the scapula is subcutaneous, and the root of the spine lies on a level with the spine of the T3 vertebra. The **inferior angle** lies on a level with the spine of the T7 vertebra.

Clinical Notes

Clinical Examination of Chest

As medical personnel, you will be examining the chest to detect evidence of disease. Your examination consists of inspection, palpation, percussion, and auscultation. **Inspection** shows the configuration of the chest, the range of respiratory movement, and any inequalities on the two sides. The type and rate of respiration are also noted.

Palpation enables the clinician to confirm the impressions gained by inspection, especially of the respiratory movements of the chest wall. Abnormal protuberances or recession of part of the chest wall is noted. Abnormal pulsations are felt, and tender areas detected.

Percussion is a sharp tapping of the chest wall with the fingers. This produces vibrations that extend through the tissues of the thorax. Air-containing organs such as the lungs

(continued)

produce a resonant note; conversely, a more solid viscus such as the heart produces a dull note. With practice, distinguishing the lungs from the heart or liver by percussion is possible.

Auscultation enables the clinician to listen to the breath sounds as air enters and leaves the respiratory passages. If the alveoli or bronchi are diseased and filled with fluid, the nature of the breath sounds will be altered. The rate and rhythm of the heart can be confirmed by auscultation, and the various sounds produced by the heart and its valves during the different phases of the cardiac cycle can be heard. Detecting friction sounds produced by the rubbing together of diseased layers of pleura or pericardium may be possible.

To make these examinations, the clinician must be familiar with the normal structure of the thorax and must have a mental image of the normal position of the lungs and heart in relation to identifiable surface landmarks. Furthermore, the clinician must be able to relate any abnormal findings to easily identifiable bony landmarks to accurately record and communicate them to colleagues. Because the thoracic wall actively participates in the movements of respiration, many bony landmarks change their levels with each phase of respiration. In practice, to simplify matters, the levels given are those usually found at about midway between full inspiration and full expiration.

Orientation Lines

Several imaginary lines are sometimes used to describe surface locations on the anterior and posterior chest walls. Refer to Figures 4.79 and 4.80.

- The **midsternal line** lies in the median plane over the sternum.
- The **midclavicular line** runs vertically downward from the midpoint of the clavicle.
- The **anterior axillary line** runs vertically downward from the anterior axillary fold.
- The **posterior axillary line** runs vertically downward from the posterior axillary fold.
- The **midaxillary line** runs vertically downward from a point situated midway between the anterior and posterior axillary folds.
- The **scapular line** runs vertically downward on the posterior wall of the thorax, passing through the inferior angle of the scapula (arms at the sides)

Trachea

The trachea extends from the lower border of the cricoid cartilage (opposite the body of the C6 vertebra) in the neck to the level of the sternal angle in the thorax (Fig. 4.81). It commences in the midline and ends just to the right of the midline by dividing into the right and the left principal bronchi. At the root of the neck, it may be palpated in the midline in the suprasternal notch.

Lungs

The **apex** of the lung projects into the neck. It can be mapped out on the anterior surface of the body by drawing a curved line, convex upward, from the sternoclavicular joint to a point 1 in. (2.5 cm) above the junction of the medial and intermediate thirds of the clavicle (see Fig. 4.81).

The **anterior border of the right lung** begins behind the sternoclavicular joint and runs downward, almost reaching the midline behind the sternal angle. It then continues downward until it reaches the xiphisternal joint. The **anterior border of the left lung** has a similar course, but at the level of costal cartilage 4, it deviates laterally and extends for a variable distance beyond the lateral margin of the sternum to form the **cardiac notch**. The heart displacing the lung to the left produces this notch. The anterior border then turns sharply downward to the level of the xiphisternal joint.

The **lower border of the lung** in midinspiration follows a curving line, which crosses the rib 6 in the midclavicular line and rib 8 in the midaxillary line and reaches rib 10 adjacent to the vertebral column posteriorly (Figs. 4.82 and 4.83; see also Fig. 4.81). Understand that the level of the inferior border of the lung changes during inspiration and expiration.

The **posterior border of the lung** extends downward from the spinous process of the C7 vertebra to the level of the T10 vertebra and lies about 1.5 in. (4 cm) from the midline.

The **oblique fissure** of the lung can be indicated on the surface by a line drawn from the root of the spine of the scapula obliquely downward, laterally and anteriorly, following the course of rib 6 to costochondral junction 6. In the left lung, the upper lobe lies above and anterior to this line, whereas the lower lobe lies below and posterior to it (see Figs. 4.81 to 4.83).

The **horizontal fissure** is an additional fissure in the right lung only. This fissure may be represented by a line drawn horizontally along costal cartilage 4 to meet the oblique fissure in the midaxillary line (see Figs. 4.81 and 4.83). The upper lobe lies above the horizontal fissure, and the middle lobe lies below it. The lower lobe lies below and posterior to the oblique fissure.

Pleura

The boundaries of the pleural sac can be marked out as lines on the surface of the body. The lines, which indicate the limits of the parietal pleura where it lies close to the body surface, are referred to as the **lines of pleural reflection**.

The **cervical pleura** bulges upward into the neck and has a surface marking identical to that of the apex of the lung. A curved line may be drawn, convex upward, from the sternoclavicular joint to a point 1 in. (2.5 cm) above the junction of the medial and intermediate thirds of the clavicle (see Fig. 4.81).

The **anterior border of the right pleura** runs down behind the sternoclavicular joint, almost reaching the midline behind the sternal angle. It then continues downward until it reaches the xiphisternal joint. The **anterior border of the left pleura** has a similar course, but at the level of costal cartilage 4, it deviates laterally and extends to the lateral margin of the sternum to form the cardiac notch. (Note that the pleural cardiac notch is not as large as the cardiac notch of the lung.) It then turns sharply downward to the xiphisternal joint (see Fig. 4.81).

The **lower border of the pleura** on both sides follows a curved line, which crosses the eighth rib in the midclavicular line and rib 10 in the midaxillary line and reaches rib 12 rib adjacent to the vertebral column—that is, at the lateral border of the erector spinae muscle (see Figs. 4.81 to 4.83). Note that the lower margins of the lungs cross ribs 6, 8, and 10 at the midclavicular lines, the midaxillary lines, and the sides of the vertebral column, respectively. The lower margins of the pleura cross, at the same points, ribs 8, 10, and 12, respectively. The distance between the two borders corresponds to the **costodiaphragmatic recess**.

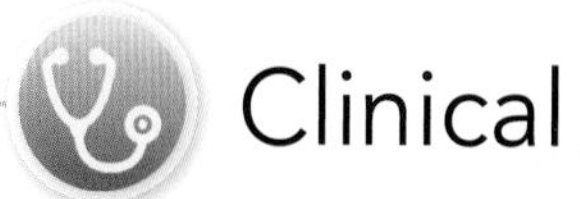

Clinical Notes

Pleural Reflections

Recognizing the surface markings of the pleural reflections and the lobes of the lungs is important. The clinician should have a mental image of the structures that lie beneath the stethoscope when listening to the breath sounds of the respiratory tract.

The **cervical dome of the pleura** and the **apex of the lungs** extend up into the neck so that at their highest point, they lie about 1 in. (2.5 cm) above the clavicle (see Figs. 4.5, 4.8, and 4.81). Consequently, they are vulnerable to stab wounds in the root of the neck or to damage by an anesthetist's needle during nerve block of the lower trunk of the brachial plexus.

Remember also that the **lower limit of the pleural reflection**, as seen from the back, may be damaged during a nephrectomy. The pleura crosses rib 12 and may be damaged during removal of the kidney through an incision in the loin.

Heart

For practical purposes, the heart may be considered to have both an apex and four borders. The **apex**, formed by the left ventricle, corresponds to the apex beat and is found in left intercostal space 5, 3.5 in. (9 cm) from the midline (Fig. 4.84).

The **superior border**, formed by the roots of the great blood vessels, extends from a point on left costal cartilage 2 (remember the sternal angle) 0.5 in. (1.3 cm) from the edge of the sternum to a point on right costal cartilage 3, 0.5 in. (1.3 cm) from the edge of the sternum.

The **right border**, formed by the right atrium, extends from a point on right costal cartilage 3, 0.5 in. (1.3 cm) from the edge of the sternum downward to a point on right costal cartilage 6, 0.5 in. (1.3 cm) from the edge of the sternum.

The **left border**, formed by the left ventricle, extends from a point on left costal cartilage 2, 0.5 in. (1.3 cm) from the edge of the sternum to the apex beat of the heart. The **inferior border**, formed by the right ventricle and the apical part of the left ventricle, extends from right costal cartilage 6 0.5 in. (1.3 cm) from the sternum to the apex beat.

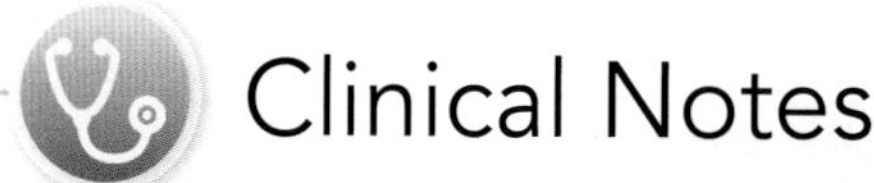

Clinical Notes

Position and Enlargement of Heart

The surface markings of the heart and the position of the apex beat help determine whether the heart has shifted its position in relation to the chest wall or whether the heart is enlarged by disease. The apex beat can often be seen and almost always can be felt. Percussion can determine the position of the margins of the heart.

Thoracic Blood Vessels

The **arch of the aorta** and the roots of the **brachiocephalic** and **left common carotid arteries** lie behind the manubrium sterni (see Fig. 4.2).

The **superior vena cava** and the terminal parts of the **right** and **left brachiocephalic veins** also lie behind the manubrium sterni.

The **internal thoracic vessels** run vertically downward, posterior to the costal cartilages, 0.5 in. (1.3 cm) lateral to the edge of the sternum (see Figs. 4.10 and 4.14B), as far as intercostal space 6.

The **intercostal vessels and nerve** ("vein, artery, nerve"—VAN—is the order from above downward) are situated immediately below their corresponding ribs (see Fig. 4.9).

Mammary Gland

The mammary gland is fully described in Chapter 3 because it is closely related to the pectoral muscles and its main lymph drainage is into the axillary lymph nodes. To summarize, the mammary gland lies in the superficial fascia covering the anterior chest wall (see Fig. 4.78A). It is rudimentary in children and in males. It enlarges and assumes its hemispherical shape in females after puberty. The breast overlies ribs 2 to 6 and their costal cartilages and extends from the lateral margin of the sternum to the midaxillary line in young adult females. Its upper lateral edge extends around the lower border of the pectoralis major and enters the axilla. The breasts may be large and pendulous in middle-aged multiparous females. In females past menopause, the adipose tissue of the breast may diminish, and the hemispherical shape lost; the breasts then become smaller, and the overlying skin is wrinkled.

Clinical Case 1 Discussion

The incision was made in the fourth left intercostal space along a line that extended from the lateral margin of the sternum to the anterior axillary line. The following structures were incised: skin, subcutaneous tissue, pectoral muscles and serratus anterior muscle, external intercostal muscle and anterior intercostal membrane, internal intercostal muscle, innermost intercostal muscle, endothoracic fascia, and parietal pleura. The internal thoracic artery, which descends just lateral to the sternum and the intercostal vessels and nerve, must be avoided as the knife cuts through the layers of tissue to enter the chest. The cause of the hemorrhage was perforation of the left atrium of the heart by the bullet. A clinician must have knowledge of chest wall anatomy to make a reasoned diagnosis and institute treatment.

Clinical Case 2 Discussion

The evaluation of chest pain is one of the most common problems facing an emergency physician. The cause can vary from the simple to one of life-threatening proportions. The severe nature of the pain and its radiation to the back made a preliminary diagnosis of aortic dissection a strong possibility. Myocardial infarction commonly results in referred pain down the inner side of the arm or up into the neck.

Pain impulses originating in a diseased descending thoracic aorta pass to the central nervous system along the path of sympathetic nerves and are then referred along the somatic spinal nerves to the skin of the anterior and posterior chest walls. In this patient, the aortic dissection had partially blocked the origin of the left subclavian artery, which would explain the lower blood pressure recorded in the left arm.

Key Concepts

Thoracic Cage

The thoracic cage consists of the thoracic vertebrae, ribs, costal cartilages, and sternum.

- Most of the thoracic cage is readily palpable in surface anatomy.
- The thoracic cage covers the thoracic organs and also the upper abdominal organs.
- Synovial joints occur between the ribs and the bodies and transverse processes of the thoracic vertebrae and between most costal cartilages and their anterior attachments.
- The ribs act as a unit in respiration. They elevate during inspiration and depress during expiration.
- The thoracic cage has a smaller superior aperture (thoracic outlet) and a larger inferior aperture. The superior aperture transmits structures between the thoracic cavity and the neck and upper limb. The inferior aperture connects the thoracic and abdominal cavities.
- The intercostal spaces are the gaps between the ribs. These contain the intercostal muscles and neurovascular bundles of intercostal veins, arteries, and nerves.

Musculature

Three main groups of muscles act on the thoracic cage: intercostal muscles, the diaphragm, and small thoracic muscles.

- The intercostal muscles are the external intercostal, internal intercostal, and innermost intercostal. These act to stabilize the position of the ribs and move the ribs during forced respiration. The intercostal nerves innervate the intercostal muscles.
- The diaphragm is the major muscle of respiration. It is dome shaped and consists of a peripheral muscular part, which arises from the margins of the thorax, and a centrally placed tendon.
- The phrenic nerves supply each half of the diaphragmatic muscle, resulting in two functional hemidiaphragms.
- The diaphragm contracts (depresses; flattens) during inspiration. This increases the vertical diameter of the thorax, lowers intrathoracic pressure, and elevates intra-abdominal pressure. The diaphragm relaxes (elevates) during expiration. This decreases the vertical diameter of the thorax, increases intrathoracic pressure, and lowers intra-abdominal pressure. A paralyzed diaphragm is abnormally elevated.
- Structures that pass between the thoracic and abdominal cavities must either pierce the diaphragm or go around the edge of the diaphragm.
- The small thoracic muscles include the levatores costarum, serratus posterior superior, and serratus posterior inferior. The role of these muscles in respiration is uncertain. All three muscles may have proprioceptive functions.

Nerve Supply

The intercostal and phrenic nerves supply the thoracic wall and diaphragm, respectively.

- The intercostal nerves are the anterior rami of T1 to T11 spinal nerves.
- The intercostal nerves provide both motor and sensory supplies to the thoracic walls.
- The intercostal nerves extend beyond the costal margins and supply the abdominal wall.
- The phrenic nerves are the sole motor nerves to the diaphragm. They also carry sensory fibers from the pericardial sac and both the pleural and peritoneal surfaces of the diaphragm.

Vasculature

The subclavian artery, axillary artery, and thoracic aorta supply the thoracic walls.

- The subclavian artery provides blood through its superior intercostal and internal thoracic branches.
- The axillary artery supplies via its superior thoracic and lateral thoracic branches.
- The thoracic aorta gives off posterior intercostal and subcostal branches.
- The anterior and posterior intercostal arteries form important anastomoses that connect the subclavian artery and thoracic aorta.

Lymph Drainage

Lymph drainage of the thoracic wall passes to both external and internal nodes.

- Drainage from the skin of the anterior chest wall passes to the anterior axillary nodes.
- Drainage from the posterior chest wall passes to the posterior axillary nodes.
- Drainage of the intercostal spaces passes forward to the internal thoracic nodes and posteriorly to the posterior intercostal nodes and the para-aortic nodes.

Mediastinum

The mediastinum is the area between the sternum, the two pleural cavities, and the vertebral column.

- The mediastinum is divided into superior and inferior mediastina by an imaginary plane passing from the sternal angle anteriorly to the lower border of the body of the T4 vertebra posteriorly.
- The inferior mediastinum is further subdivided into the middle mediastinum, which consists of the pericardium and heart; the anterior mediastinum, which is a space between the pericardium and the sternum; and the posterior mediastinum, which lies between the pericardium and the vertebral column.

Pleurae

- The paired pleurae and lungs lie on either side of the mediastinum within the thoracic cavity.
- Each pleural membrane has two parts: a parietal layer and a visceral layer. The parietal layer lines the thoracic wall, covers the thoracic surface of the diaphragm and the lateral aspect of the mediastinum, and extends into the root of the neck. The visceral layer completely covers the outer surface of the lung and extends into the interlobar fissures. The parietal and visceral layers of pleura are separated from one another by a slit-like space, the pleural cavity.
- The pleural layers are innervated differently despite being a continuous membrane. Somatic afferent nerves supply the parietal pleura, which is sensitive to pain, temperature, touch, and pressure. Visceral afferent nerves supply the visceral pleura, which is sensitive to stretch but is insensitive to common sensations such as pain and touch.

Lower Respiratory Tract

The trachea begins in the neck as the continuation of the larynx. It descends into the thorax through the superior mediastinum. It ends by dividing into right and left principal (main) bronchi. Cartilaginous tracheal rings embedded in the tracheal wall support and maintain the patency of the trachea.

- Each principal bronchus supplies an entire lung. The principal bronchi next divide into lobar (secondary) bronchi that supply the individual lobes of the lungs.

Lungs

- Horizontal and oblique fissures divide the right lung into three lobes. A single oblique fissure divides the left lung into two lobes.
- Each lung is conical, covered with visceral pleura, attached to the mediastinum only by its root, and suspended free in its own pleural cavity.
- Each lung has an apex that extends into the neck; a base that sits on the diaphragm; a costal surface, which corresponds to the chest wall; and a mediastinal surface, which is molded to the pericardium and other mediastinal structures. The structures that enter or leave the lung form the root of the lung. The root of the lung attaches to the hilum.
- Each lobar (secondary) bronchus branches into multiple segmental (tertiary) bronchi. Each segmental bronchus passes to a structurally and functionally independent bronchopulmonary segment.
- Two separate arterial systems supply the lungs. One is the nonrespiratory circuit that supplies the tissues of the respiratory tree and lungs. The second is the respiratory (pulmonary) circuit, across which gas exchange occurs.
- Intersegmental veins carry oxygenated blood from the alveolar capillaries, follow the connective tissue septa bounding the bronchopulmonary segments to the pulmonary veins and to the lung root. Two pulmonary veins leave each lung root and empty into the left atrium of the heart.
- All the lymph from the lung leaves the hilum and drains into the tracheobronchial nodes and then into the bronchomediastinal lymph trunks.
- Sympathetic, parasympathetic, and visceral afferent nerve fibers intermingle at the root of each lung in the pulmonary plexuses. Branches of the pulmonary plexuses mainly follow the bronchi into and within the lungs.

Pericardium

- The pericardium is a fibroserous sac that encloses the heart and the roots of the great vessels. It lies within the middle mediastinum.
- The fibrous pericardium is the strong, fibrous, outer layer of the sac. The serous pericardium lines the fibrous pericardium and coats the heart. It is divided into parietal and visceral layers.
- The parietal layer lines the inner surface of the fibrous pericardium and reflects around the roots of the great vessels to become continuous with the visceral layer of serous pericardium that closely covers the heart. The slit-like space between the parietal and visceral layers is the pericardial cavity.
- The phrenic nerves carry somatic sensory fibers from the fibrous pericardium and the parietal layer of the serous pericardium. Visceral afferent fibers travel with branches of the sympathetic trunks and the vagus nerves from the visceral layer of the serous pericardium.

Heart

- The heart lies within the pericardium, in the middle the mediastinum.
- It contains four chambers: two atria and two ventricles. The atria and ventricles are connected via atrioventricular valves. The atria receive venous blood and pump blood only to the immediately adjacent ventricles. The ventricles pump arterial blood out of the heart.
- The heart has two functional circuits, the right heart and the left heart. The right heart (right atrium and right ventricle) is the pulmonary circuit pump. The left heart (left atrium and left ventricle) is the systemic circuit pump.
- The heart has three surfaces (anterior, inferior, posterior) and three borders (right, left, inferior).
- The right atrium consists of the atrium proper and the auricle. The auricle features internal pectinate muscles. The atrium proper receives blood via the superior and inferior venae cavae and the coronary sinus. The fossa ovalis is located in the atrial septum. The right atrioventricular (tricuspid) valve regulates the opening into the right ventricle.
- The right ventricle features trabeculae carneae. The chordae tendineae attach the cusps of the tricuspid valve to papillary muscles. The pulmonary valve guards the outflow channel into the pulmonary trunk.
- The left atrium consists of an atrium proper and an auricle with pectinate muscles. It receives blood via four pulmonary veins. The left atrioventricular (bicuspid) valve regulates the opening into the left ventricle.
- The left ventricle possesses trabeculae carneae. Chordae tendineae attach the cusps of the bicuspid valve to papillary muscles. The aortic valve regulates the outflow channel into the ascending aorta.
- The heart possesses a fibrous internal skeleton that surrounds the valve orifices.
- Autonomic nerves from the sympathetic trunks and the vagi provide an external nerve supply. The conducting system of the heart forms an internal nerve supply.
- Right and left coronary arteries provide the arterial supply to the heart. Each has multiple branches. However, the left coronary is usually the larger vessel. Most venous blood from the heart drains into the right atrium via the coronary sinus.
- The cardiac cycle is one complete heartbeat composed of systolic and diastolic phases. The differential closing of the heart valves produces the two classic heartbeat sounds (lub-dub).

Large Blood Vessels

- The aorta and pulmonary trunk are the two large arteries of the thorax.
- The aorta consists of ascending, arch, and descending thoracic parts. It provides the systemic arterial flow. The pulmonary trunk provides arterial flow to the lungs.
- The ligamentum arteriosum connects the pulmonary trunk with the aortic arch. The left recurrent laryngeal nerve is closely related to this ligament.
- The brachiocephalic veins, venae cavae, azygos veins, and pulmonary veins are the large veins of the thorax.

Lymphatics

- The thoracic duct conveys all lymph from the lower limbs, pelvic cavity, abdominal cavity, left side of the thorax, and left side of the head, neck, and upper limb to a drainage point at the beginning of the left brachiocephalic vein.
- The right lymphatic duct collects lymph from the right side of the head and neck, right upper limb, and right side of the thorax and empties into the beginning of the right brachiocephalic vein.

Nerves

- The vagus and phrenic nerves and the sympathetic trunks are the main nerves to the thoracic cavity.
- The vagi mainly carry parasympathetic fibers to the pulmonary, esophageal, and cardiac plexuses and on to the lungs, gut tube, and heart. Each vagus gives rise to a recurrent laryngeal nerve that supplies the esophagus, trachea, and larynx.

- The phrenic nerves arise in the neck from the cervical plexus and descend into the thorax. They are the sole motor supply to the diaphragm and also carry sensory fibers from both sides of the diaphragm, the pericardium, and the mediastinal pleura.
- Each sympathetic trunk connects to thoracic spinal nerves via white and gray rami communicantes. Thoracic splanchnic branches supply thoracic viscera. Abdominal splanchnic branches (greater, lesser, least splanchnic nerves) supply the abdominal viscera.

Esophagus

- The esophagus connects the pharynx with the stomach. It lies in front of the vertebral column and behind the trachea.
- The vagi and sympathetic branches contribute to the esophageal plexus, which supplies the innervation of the esophagus.

Thymus

- The thymus gland lies between the sternum and the pericardium in the anterior mediastinum. It is large in neonates but small and essentially vestigial in adults.

Radiology and Surface Anatomy

- Posteroanterior plain films provide optimal x-ray images of the mediastinal shadow, which includes the profile of the heart. Oblique views are useful for imaging other details.
- Coronary angiography permits imaging of the coronary arteries and their branches.
- Cross-sectional images (eg, CTs) are critical tools in evaluating the condition of the thorax.
- Numerous features of the thorax are directly palpable or can be located by projection in standard surface anatomy examination.

5 Abdomen

CLINICAL CASE 1

A 26-year-old male visited his physician for a painful swelling in the left groin; he had vomited four times in the previous 3 hours. On examination, he was dehydrated, and his abdomen was moderately distended. A large, tense swelling, which was very tender on palpation, was present in the left groin and extended down into the scrotum. An attempt to gently push the contents of the swelling back into the abdomen was impossible. A left complete, irreducible, indirect inguinal hernia was diagnosed. The vomiting and abdominal distention were secondary to the intestinal obstruction caused by the herniation of some bowel loops into the hernial sac.

CLINICAL CASE 2

A 15-year-old male presented to his physician with pain in the lower part of the anterior abdominal wall. On examination, he had a temperature of 101°F (38.3°C), a furred tongue, and extreme tenderness in the lower right quadrant. The abdominal muscles in that area were firm (rigid) on palpation and became more spastic when increased pressure was applied (guarding). Acute appendicitis was diagnosed.

See the Clinical Case Discussions at the end of this chapter for further insight.

CHAPTER OUTLINE

LEARNING OBJECTIVES

The purpose of this chapter is to review the basic anatomy of the abdomen to understand normal topographic and functional relationships and the basis for common injuries, pain, motor deficits, congenital defects, medical imaging, and general surface examination.

1. Identify the bones of the abdominal wall and their major features. Describe the functional aspects of these structures.
2. Identify the layers of the abdominal wall. Compare and contrast the formation of the rectus sheath above and below the arcuate line.
3. Identify the muscles of the abdominal wall, noting their attachments, innervation, and major actions.
4. Trace the distribution of the motor and sensory innervation of the abdominal wall. Predict the functional consequences of lesions of individual peripheral nerves.
5. Trace the flow of blood to and from the abdominal wall by describing the courses and branching patterns of the major arteries and veins. Identify the territories supplied and drained by the major vessels. Note the main collateral routes and describe the composition of significant anastomoses.
6. Describe the pattern of lymphatic drainage of the abdominal wall, including the external genitalia.
7. Describe the inguinal canal, its composition, and its surface projections in males and females. Describe the descent of the gonads and their relations to the development of the inguinal canal. Identify the homologous urogenital structures in the abdominal wall and external genitalia.
8. Identify the spermatic cord and its constituent structures. Describe the relations of the components of the cord with structures in the abdominal wall.
9. Identify the structures comprising the external genitalia and their adnexa in males and females.
10. Identify parietal and visceral peritoneum and the major peritoneal folds, reflections, and spaces in the abdomen. Indicate which abdominopelvic organs are intraperitoneal or retroperitoneal. Describe the functional and clinical significance of these arrangements.
11. Identify the organs of the abdominal cavity. Describe the relations, gross structure, blood supply, innervation, lymphatic drainage, and basic function of each.
12. Describe the features that differentiate the duodenum, jejunum, and ileum of the small intestine. Compare the features that distinguish the small from the large intestine. Describe variability in the location of the vermiform appendix.
13. Trace the course of the extrahepatic biliary system from the liver into and out of the gallbladder, and into the duodenum. Note the relations of the bile tract. Trace the course of exocrine pancreatic secretions from their source to the duodenum. Note the relations of this system to the biliary tract.
14. Identify the kidneys and suprarenal glands. Describe their normal positions, relations, and neurovascular supplies. Trace the flow of urine from the gross collecting structures in the kidney to the urinary bladder. Note the relationships of the ureters to surrounding structures.
15. Describe the structure of the posterior abdominal wall. Identify the muscles of the posterior abdominal wall and their attachments, innervation, and major actions.

16. Differentiate the major forms of hernias related to the abdominal wall.
17. Trace the flow of blood into and from the abdomen by describing the courses, branching patterns, and distributions of the major arteries and veins. Note the relations of these vessels to neighboring organs and mesenteries.
18. Identify the major arterial trees/axes and their territories. Note the anastomoses between arterial trees and their importance in providing collateral circulation. Identify and explain the function of vascular arcades within the abdomen. Define and differentiate anatomic versus functional end arteries. Give examples of each and identify the organs they supply.
19. Trace the flow of blood from the abdomen to the heart by describing the formations and courses of the portal and caval venous tracts. Indicate anastomoses between these tracts and describe the clinical significance of such connections. Note the relations of the major veins along their courses.
20. Trace the primary drainage routes of lymph from the abdominal organs and walls to their primary lymph nodes.
21. Identify and trace the pathways of the main somatic and visceral nerves in the abdomen. Identify the lumbar plexus, its segmental origins, and its major peripheral branches. Identify the sources of autonomic innervation. Describe the specific pathways involved in the autonomic innervation of the abdomen. Describe the clinical relevance of these positional relations. Describe the functional consequences of lesions of the main nerves supplying the pelvis and perineum.
22. Identify the major structures of the abdomen in radiographic and cross-sectional examinations.
23. Identify the surface regions of the abdominal wall. Identify the surface projections and palpation points of major abdominal structures.

OVERVIEW

The abdomen is the region of the trunk that lies between the diaphragm above and the pelvic inlet below. This is a primarily soft tissue region, with little bony framework. Therefore, an intact abdominal wall is essential for the support of the abdominal contents. The abdominopelvic cavity extends from the diaphragm above to the pelvic floor below. The pelvic inlet marks the anatomically arbitrary (but descriptively useful) boundary line that demarcates the upper abdominal cavity from the lower pelvic cavity. In reality, the regions are a single, continuous space.

Common abdominal problems include acute pain, swellings, and blunt and penetrating trauma. These problems are complicated by the fact that the abdomen contains multiple organ systems. Further, the physician can feel many abdominal contents through the flexible abdominal wall. Therefore, understanding the spatial relationships of the organs to one another and to the abdominal wall is essential for accurate and complete diagnosis.

OSTEOLOGY

The thoracic cage covers all or parts of the upper abdominal organs (eg, liver stomach, spleen, and kidneys). The abdominal skeleton consists primarily of the lumbar vertebrae, the margin of the thoracic cage, and the iliac and pubic bone elements of the pelvis (Fig. 5.1). These structures provide attachment sites for the abdominal wall muscles and limited support for abdominal organs, but little direct protection for those organs.

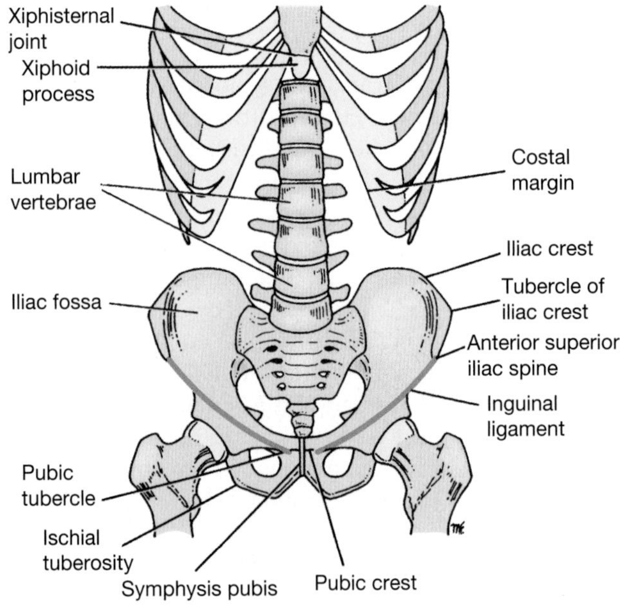

Figure 5.1 Costal margin and bones of the abdomen.

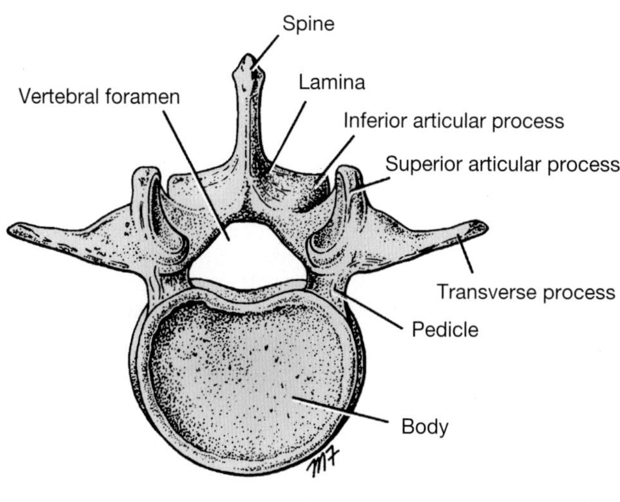

Figure 5.2 L5 vertebra.

Lumbar Vertebrae

The anatomy of the lumbar vertebrae is described in detail in Chapter 2. The **body** of each vertebra (Fig. 5.2) is massive and kidney shaped and bears the greater part of the body weight. The L5 vertebra articulates with the base of the sacrum at the **lumbosacral joint**. The **transverse processes** are long and slender and provide sites of attachment for several abdominal wall muscles.

The **intervertebral discs** (Fig. 5.3) in the lumbar region are thicker than in other regions of the vertebral column. They are wedge shaped and are responsible for the normal posterior concavity (lordosis) in the curvature of the vertebral column in the lumbar region.

Thoracic Cage

The anatomy of the thoracic cage is described in detail in Chapter 4. The components most pertinent to the abdominal wall include the xiphoid process of the sternum, costal margin (costal cartilages 7 to 10), and lower ribs (see Fig. 5.1). The head of rib 12 is different from most others in that it has a single facet for articulation with the body of the T12 vertebra. The anterior end is pointed and has a small costal cartilage, which is embedded in the musculature of the anterior abdominal wall. In many people, it is so short that it fails to protrude beyond the lateral border of the erector spinae muscle on the back.

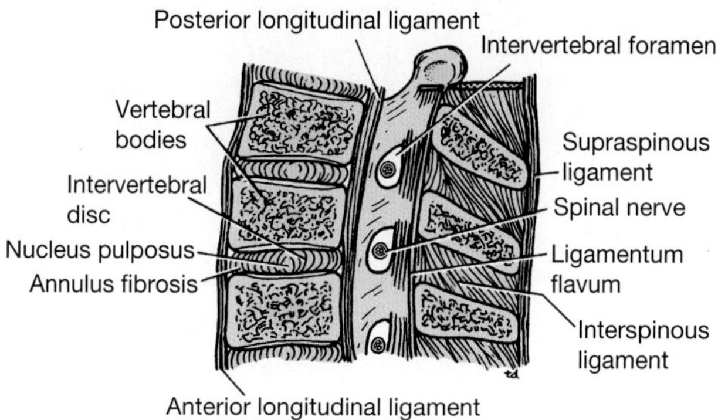

Figure 5.3 Sagittal section of the lumbar part of the vertebral column showing intervertebral discs and ligaments.

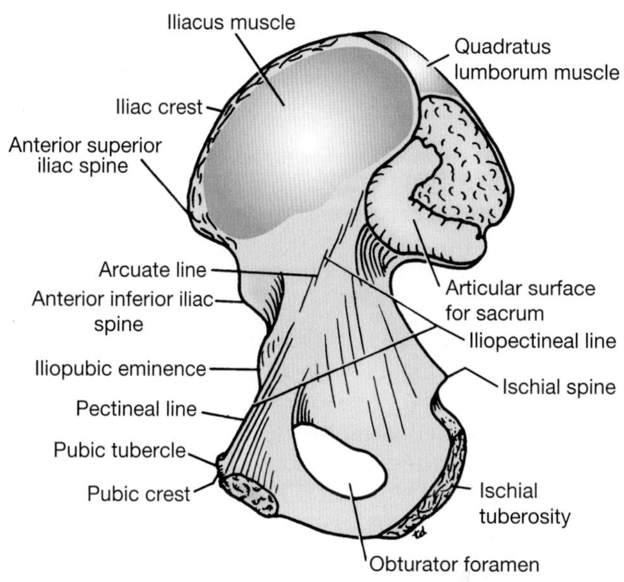

Figure 5.4 Internal aspect of the right hip bone.

Pelvis

The **os coxae** (hip bone) is composed of the ilium, ischium, and pubis (Fig. 5.4; see also Fig. 5.1). The medial surface of the ilium is divided into two parts by the **arcuate line**. The **iliac fossa** is a concave surface above the arcuate line. A flattened surface continuous with the medial surfaces of the pubis and ischium lies below the arcuate line. Note that the arcuate line of the ilium forms the posterior part of the **iliopectineal line**, whereas the **pectineal line** of the pubis forms the anterior part of the iliopectineal line. The iliopectineal line demarcates the false from the true pelvis. See Chapter 6 for further details on the structure of the hip bone.

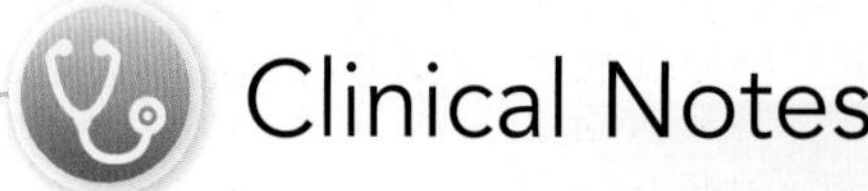

Clinical Notes

General Appearance of the Abdominal Wall

The normal abdominal wall is soft and pliable and moves in and out with respiration. The contour is subject to considerable variation and depends on the tone of its muscles and the amount of fat in the subcutaneous tissue. Well-developed muscles or an abundance of fat can be an obstacle in palpating the abdominal viscera.

ANTEROLATERAL ABDOMINAL WALL

The anterolateral abdominal wall is made up of seven layers:

- Skin
- Superficial fascia
- Deep fascia
- Muscles
- Transversalis fascia
- Extraperitoneal fascia
- Parietal peritoneum

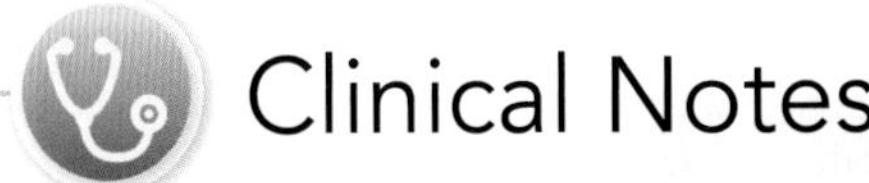

Clinical Notes

Surgical Incisions

If possible, all surgical incisions should be made in the lines of cleavage where the bundles of collagen fibers in the dermis run in parallel rows. An incision along a cleavage line will heal as a narrow scar, whereas one that crosses the lines will heal as wide or heaped-up scars.

Skin

The skin is loosely attached to the underlying structures except at the umbilicus, where it is tethered to the scar tissue. The natural **lines of cleavage** in the skin are constant and run downward and forward almost horizontally around the trunk. The **umbilicus** is a scar representing the site of attachment of the umbilical cord in the fetus; it is situated in the linea alba (see below).

Nerve Supply

The cutaneous nerve supply to the anterolateral abdominal wall is derived from the anterior rami of the T7 to T12 and L1 nerves (Figs. 5.5 and 5.6). The thoracic nerves are the lower five intercostal and the subcostal nerves; the L1 nerve is represented by the iliohypogastric and the ilioinguinal nerves.

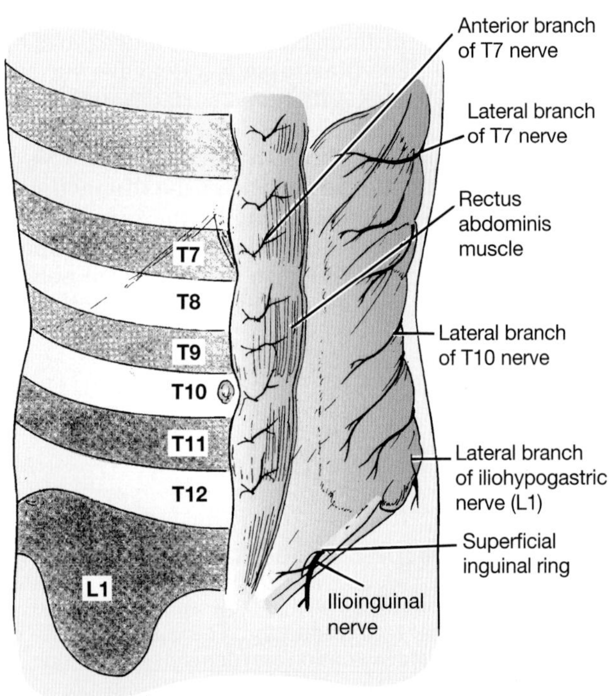

Figure 5.5 Dermatomes and distribution of cutaneous nerves on the anterior abdominal wall.

The dermatome of T7 is in the epigastrium over the xiphoid process (see Fig. 5.5). The dermatome of T10 includes the umbilicus and that of L1 lies just above the inguinal ligament and the symphysis pubis.

Arteries

Branches of the superior and inferior epigastric arteries supply the skin near the midline (see Fig. 5.6). Branches of the intercostal, lumbar, and deep circumflex iliac arteries supply the skin of the flanks. In addition, the superficial epigastric, superficial circumflex iliac, and superficial external pudendal arteries, branches of the femoral artery, supply the skin in the inguinal region.

Veins

Venous drainage from the upper abdominal wall passes mainly into the axillary vein via the lateral thoracic vein (Fig. 5.7). The lower abdominal wall drains into the femoral vein via the superficial epigastric and the great saphenous veins.

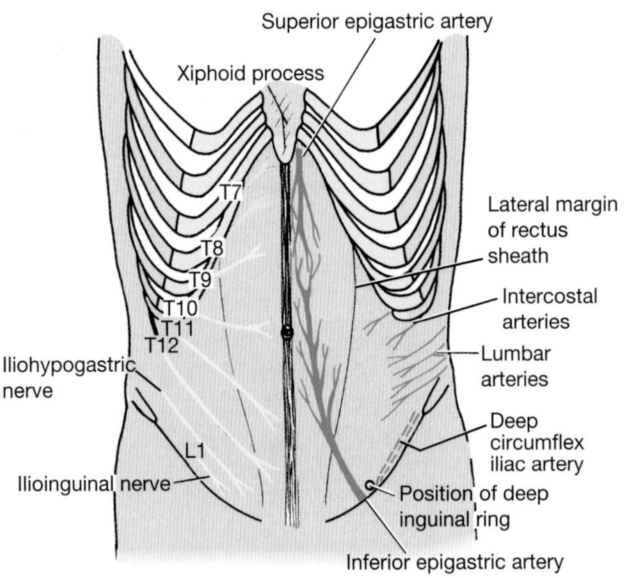

Figure 5.6 Segmental innervation of the anterior abdominal wall (*left*) and arterial supply to the anterior abdominal wall (*right*).

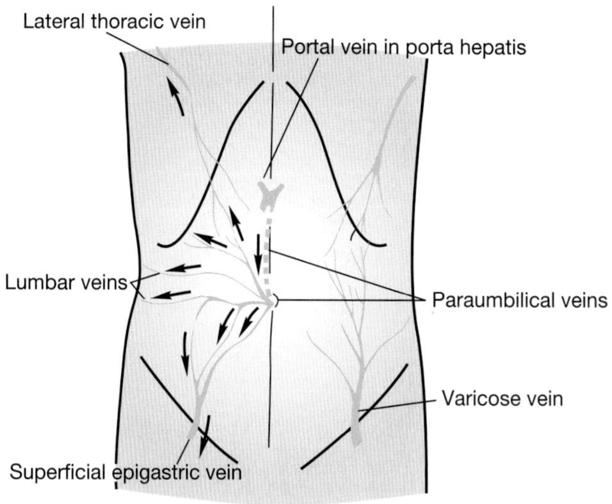

Figure 5.7 Superficial veins of the anterior abdominal wall. On the *left* are anastomoses between systemic veins and the portal vein via paraumbilical veins. *Arrows* indicate the direction taken by venous blood when the portal vein is obstructed. On the *right* is an enlarged anastomosis between the lateral thoracic vein and the superficial epigastric vein. This occurs if either the superior or the inferior vena cava is obstructed.

Superficial Fascia

The superficial fascia is divided into two layers: a more superficial **fatty layer (Camper's fascia)** and a deeper **membranous layer (Scarpa's fascia)** (Fig. 5.8). The fatty layer is continuous with the superficial fat over the rest of the body and may be extremely thick (3 in. [8 cm] or more in obese patients). The membranous layer is thin and fades out laterally and above, where it becomes continuous with the superficial fascia of the back and thorax, respectively. Inferiorly, the membranous layer passes onto the front of the thigh, where it fuses with the deep fascia one fingerbreadth below the inguinal ligament. In the midline inferiorly, the membranous layer of fascia is not attached to the pubis but forms a tubular sheath for the penis (males) or clitoris (females). Below, in the perineum, it enters the wall of the scrotum (males) or labia majora (females). From there, it passes to attachments on each side to the margins of the pubic arch; it is here referred to as **Colles' fascia**. Posteriorly, it fuses with the perineal body and the posterior margin of the perineal membrane (see Fig. 5.8B).

In the scrotum, the fatty layer of the superficial fascia exists as a thin layer of smooth muscle, the **dartos muscle**. The membranous layer of the superficial fascia persists as a separate layer.

Deep Fascia

The deep fascia in the anterolateral abdominal wall is merely a thin layer of connective tissue covering the muscles. It lies immediately deep to the membranous layer of superficial fascia.

Muscles

The anterolateral abdominal wall houses three broad thin sheets of muscle that are most pronounced laterally and become aponeurotic anteriorly. From exterior (superficial) to interior (deep), they are the **external oblique**, **internal oblique**, and **transversus abdominis**

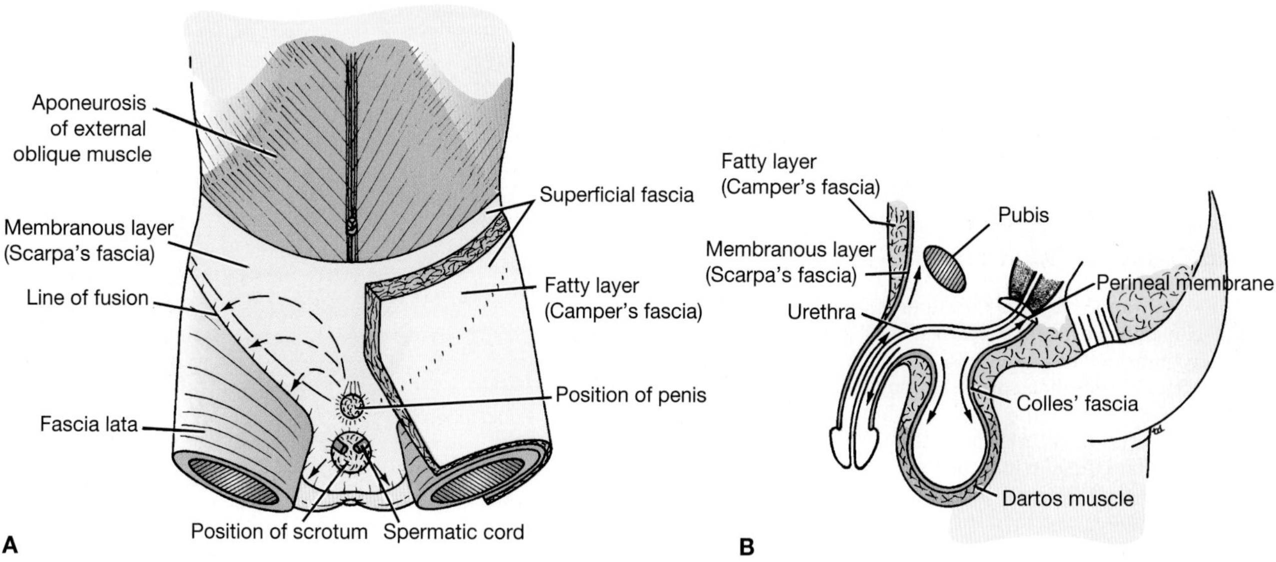

Figure 5.8 Arrangement of the fatty layer and the membranous layer of the superficial fascia in the lower part of the anterior abdominal wall. **A.** Anterior view. Note the line of fusion between the membranous layer and the deep fascia of the thigh (fascia lata). **B.** Sagittal view. Note the attachment of the membranous layer to the posterior margin of the perineal membrane. *Arrows* indicate paths taken by urine in cases of ruptured urethra.

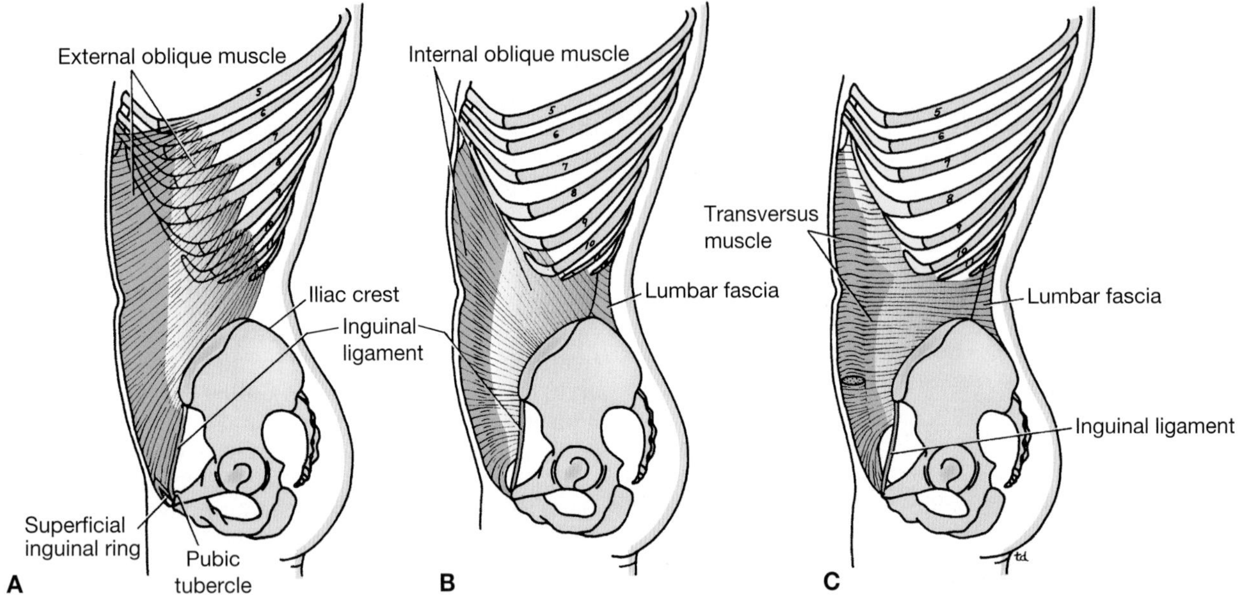

Figure 5.9 Sheet muscles of the anterolateral abdominal wall. **A.** External oblique. **B.** Internal oblique. **C.** Transversus abdominis.

(Fig. 5.9). These are the abdominal equivalents of the intercostal muscles. Additionally, the paired **rectus abdominis** muscles form wide vertical straps on either side of the anterior midline (Fig. 5.10). As the aponeuroses of the three sheets pass forward, they enclose the rectus abdominis to form the **rectus sheath**. The lower part of the rectus sheath might contain a small muscle called the **pyramidalis**. Details of the attachments, innervation, and actions of the anterolateral wall muscles are summarized in Table 5.1.

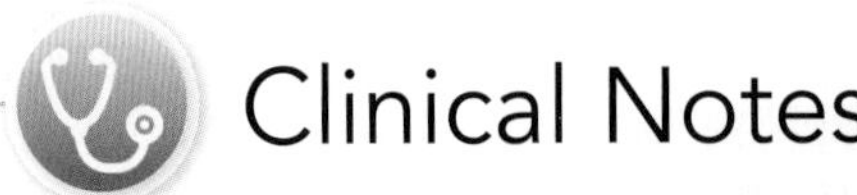

Clinical Notes

Membranous Layer of Superficial Fascia and Extravasation of Urine

The membranous layer of the superficial fascia is important clinically because beneath it is a potential closed space that does not open into the thigh but is continuous with the superficial perineal pouch via the penis and scrotum. Rupture of the penile urethra may be followed by extravasation of urine into the scrotum, perineum, and penis and then up into the lower part of the anterior abdominal wall deep to the membranous layer of fascia. The urine is excluded from the thigh because of the attachment of the fascia to the fascia lata (see Fig. 5.8).

When closing abdominal wounds, a surgeon usually puts in a continuous suture uniting the divided membranous layer of superficial fascia. This strengthens the healing wound, prevents stretching of the skin scar, and makes for a more cosmetically acceptable result.

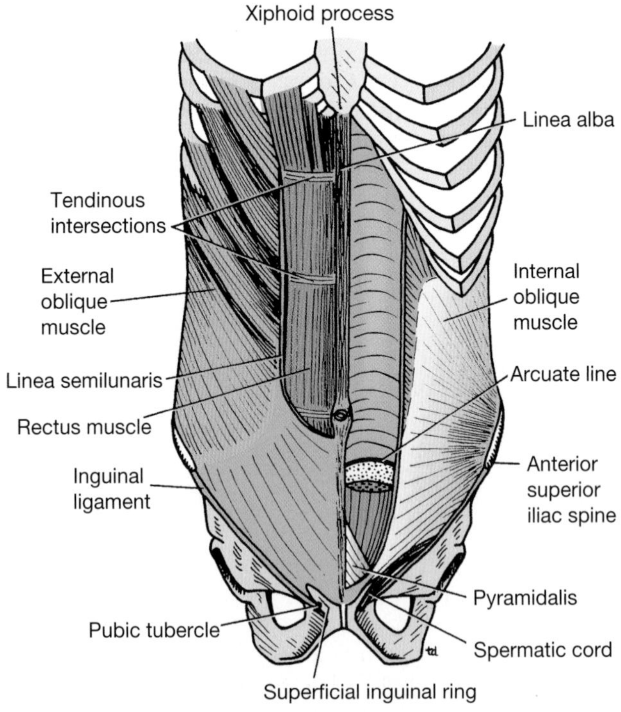

Figure 5.10 Anterior view of the rectus abdominis muscle and the rectus sheath. *Left.* The anterior wall of the sheath has been partly removed, revealing the rectus muscle with its tendinous intersections. *Right.* The posterior wall of the rectus sheath. The edge of the arcuate line is shown at the level of the anterior superior iliac spine.

Table 5.1 Anterior Abdominal Wall Muscles

NAME OF MUSCLE	ORIGIN	INSERTION	NERVE SUPPLY	ACTION
External oblique	Ribs 5 to 12	Xiphoid process, linea alba, pubic crest, pubic tubercle, iliac crest	T7 to T12 nerves and iliohypogastric and ilioinguinal nerves (L1)	Supports abdominal contents; compresses abdominal contents; assists in flexing and rotation of trunk; assists in forced expiration, micturition, defecation, parturition, and vomiting
Internal oblique	Lumbar fascia, iliac crest, lateral two-thirds of inguinal ligament	Ribs 9 to 12 and costal cartilages, xiphoid process, linea alba, symphysis pubis	T7 to T12 nerves and iliohypogastric and ilioinguinal nerves (L1)	As above
Transversus	Lower six costal cartilages, lumbar fascia, iliac crest, lateral third of inguinal ligament	Xiphoid process, linea alba, symphysis pubis	T7 to T12 nerves and iliohypogastric and ilioinguinal nerves (L1)	Compresses abdominal contents
Rectus abdominis	Symphysis pubis and pubic crest	Fifth, sixth, and seventh costal cartilages and xiphoid process	T7 to T12 nerves	Compresses abdominal contents and flexes vertebral column; accessory muscle of expiration
Pyramidalis (if present)	Anterior surface of pubis	Linea alba	T12 nerve	Tenses the linea alba

External Oblique

The external oblique muscle is a broad, thin, muscular sheet, with most of its fibers inserting by means of a wide aponeurosis (see Figs. 5.9 and 5.10). Note that the most posterior fibers passing down to the iliac crest form a posterior free border.

The **superficial inguinal ring**, a triangular defect in the external oblique aponeurosis lies immediately above and medial to the pubic tubercle. The spermatic cord (males) or round ligament of the uterus (females) passes through this opening and carries the **external spermatic fascia** (or the external covering of the round ligament of the uterus) from the margins of the ring (Figs. 5.11 and 5.12).

The lower border of the aponeurosis is folded backward on itself between the anterior superior iliac spine and the pubic tubercle, forming the **inguinal ligament** (Figs. 5.13 and 5.14; see also Fig. 5.9). The **lacunar ligament** extends backward and upward from the medial end of the inguinal ligament to the pectineal line on the superior ramus of the pubis (see Figs. 5.13 and 5.14). Its sharp, free crescentic edge forms the medial margin of the **femoral ring** (see Chapter 8). On reaching the pectineal line, the lacunar ligament becomes continuous with a thickening of the periosteum called the **pectineal ligament**.

The lateral part of the posterior edge of the inguinal ligament gives origin to part of the internal oblique and transversus abdominis muscles (see Figs. 5.9, 5.10, and 5.14). The deep fascia of the thigh, the **fascia lata**, is attached to the inferior rounded border of the inguinal ligament (see Fig. 5.8A).

Internal Oblique

The internal oblique muscle is also a broad, thin, muscular sheet that lies deep to the external oblique. Most of its fibers run at right angles to those of the external oblique and radiate as they pass upward and forward (see Fig. 5.9). The internal oblique has a lower free border that arches over the spermatic cord (males) or round ligament of the uterus (females) and then descends behind it to attach to the pubic crest and the pectineal line (Fig. 5.15; see also Fig. 5.14). Near their insertion, the lowest tendinous fibers are joined by similar fibers from the transversus abdominis to form the **conjoint tendon** (see Figs. 5.14 and 5.15C). The conjoint tendon attaches medially to the **linea alba**, but it has a lateral free border.

As the spermatic cord passes under the lower border of the internal oblique, it carries some muscle fibers that are derived from the internal oblique. These fibers that surround the spermatic cord constitute the **cremaster muscle** (see Figs. 5.14 and 5.15B). The **cremasteric fascia** is the cremaster muscle plus its fascia. The cremaster exerts tension on the spermatic cord and acts to raise or lower the testis.

Transversus Abdominis

The transversus abdominis is a thin sheet of muscle that lies deep to the internal oblique. Its fibers run horizontally forward (see Fig. 5.9). The lowest tendinous fibers join similar fibers from the internal oblique to form the conjoint tendon, which is fixed to the pubic crest and the pectineal line (see Figs. 5.14 and 5.15C).

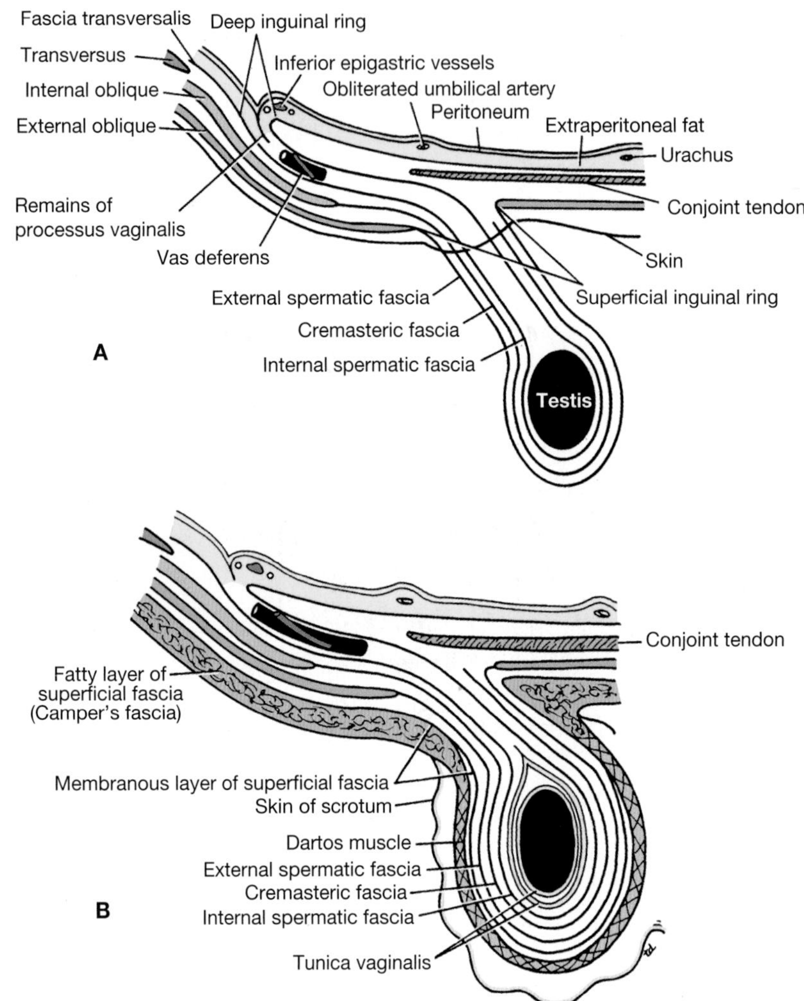

Figure 5.11 **A.** Continuity of the different layers of the anterior abdominal wall with coverings of the spermatic cord. **B.** Skin and superficial fascia of the abdominal wall and scrotum have been included, and the tunica vaginalis is shown.

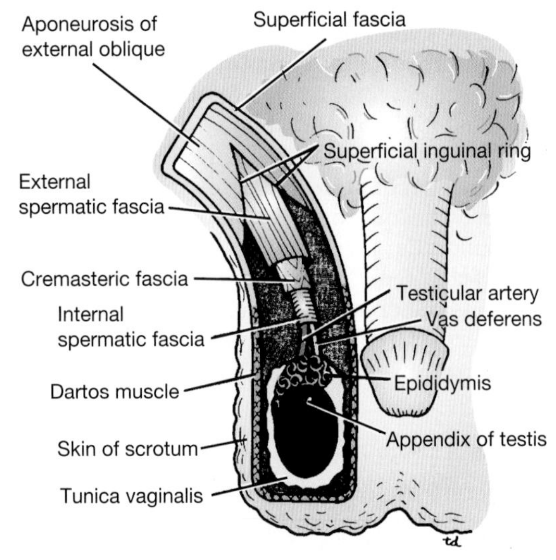

Figure 5.12 Scrotum dissected from in front. Note the spermatic cord and its coverings.

Note that the posterior border of the external oblique muscle is free, whereas the posterior borders of the internal oblique and the transversus muscles are attached to the lumbar vertebrae by the lumbar fascia (see Fig. 5.9).

Rectus Abdominis

The rectus abdominis is a long strap muscle that extends along the whole length of the anterior abdominal wall (Fig. 5.16; see also Fig. 5.10). It is broader above and lies close to the midline, being separated from its fellow by the linea alba.

When the rectus contracts, its lateral margin forms a curved ridge, the **linea semilunaris**, that can be palpated and often seen. This extends from the tip of costal cartilage 9 to the pubic tubercle.

The rectus abdominis muscle is divided into distinct segments by three transverse **tendinous intersections**: one at the level of the xiphoid process, one at the level of the umbilicus, and one halfway between these two. These intersections are strongly attached to the anterior

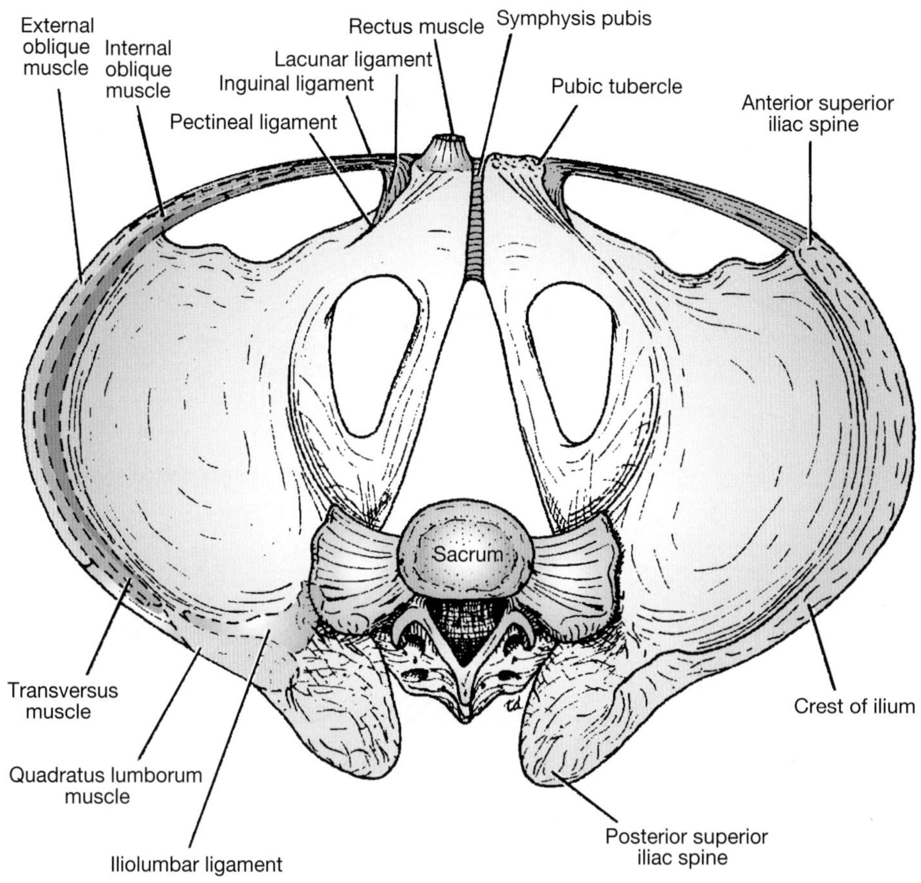

Figure 5.13 Bony pelvis viewed from above. Note the attachments of the inguinal, lacunar, and pectineal ligaments.

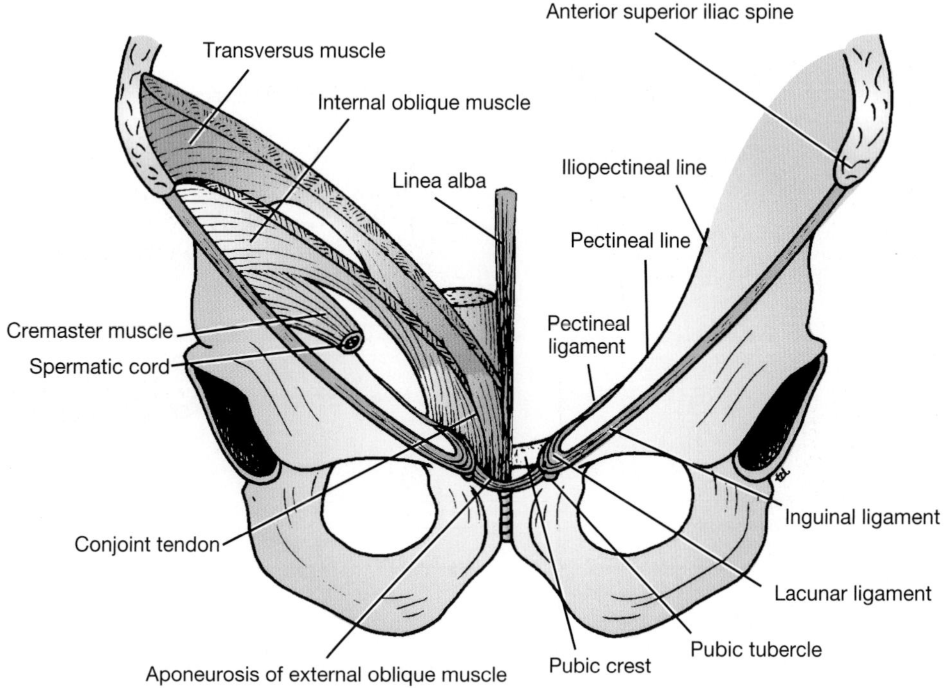

Figure 5.14 Anterior view of the pelvis showing the attachment of the conjoint tendon to the pubic crest and the adjoining part of the pectineal line.

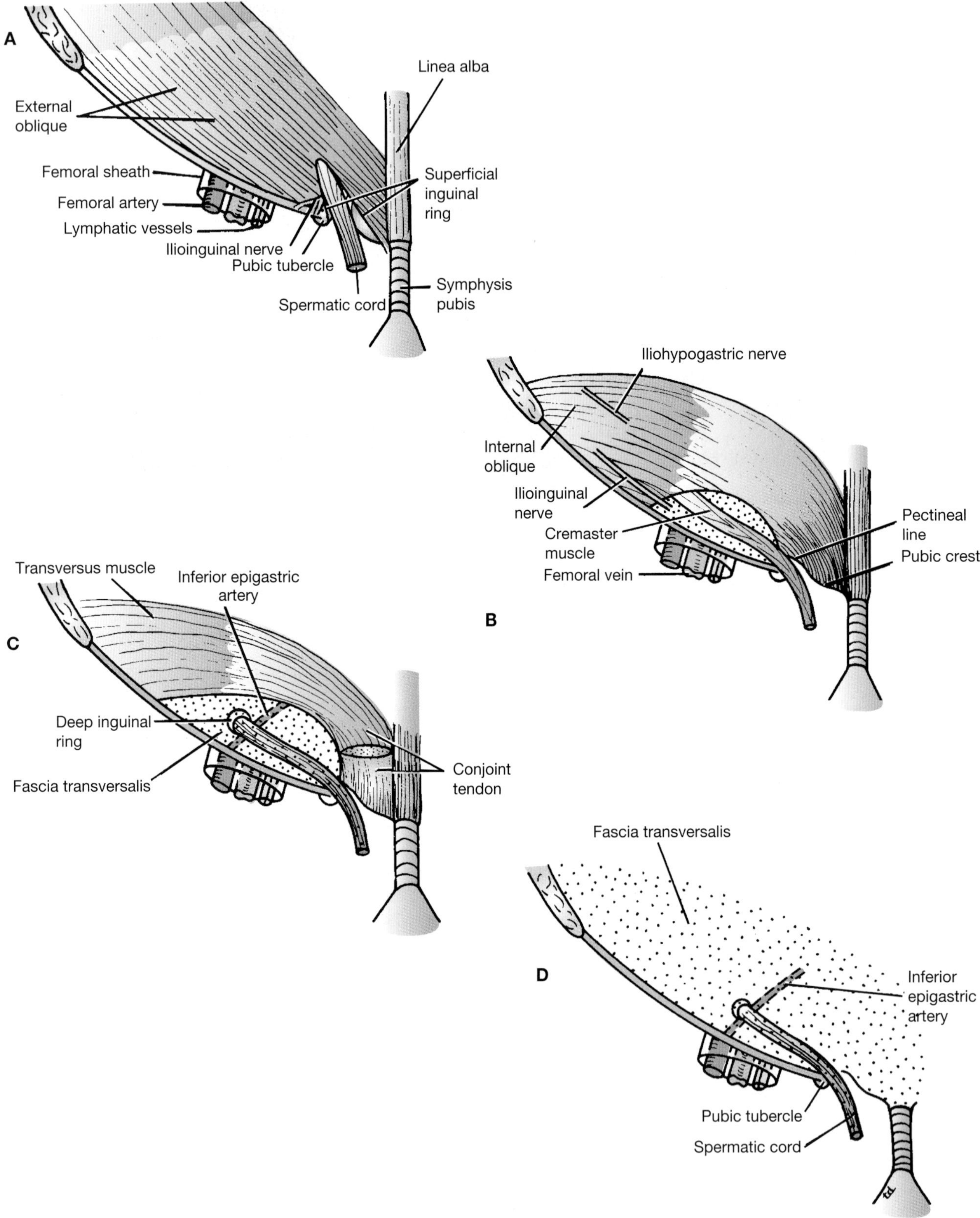

Figure 5.15 Inguinal canal showing the arrangement of the external oblique muscle **(A)**, the internal oblique muscle **(B)**, the transversus abdominis muscle **(C)**, and the transversalis fascia **(D)**. Note that the external oblique and the internal oblique form the anterior wall of the canal, and the transversalis fascia and the conjoint tendon form the posterior wall of the canal. The deep inguinal ring lies lateral to the inferior epigastric artery.

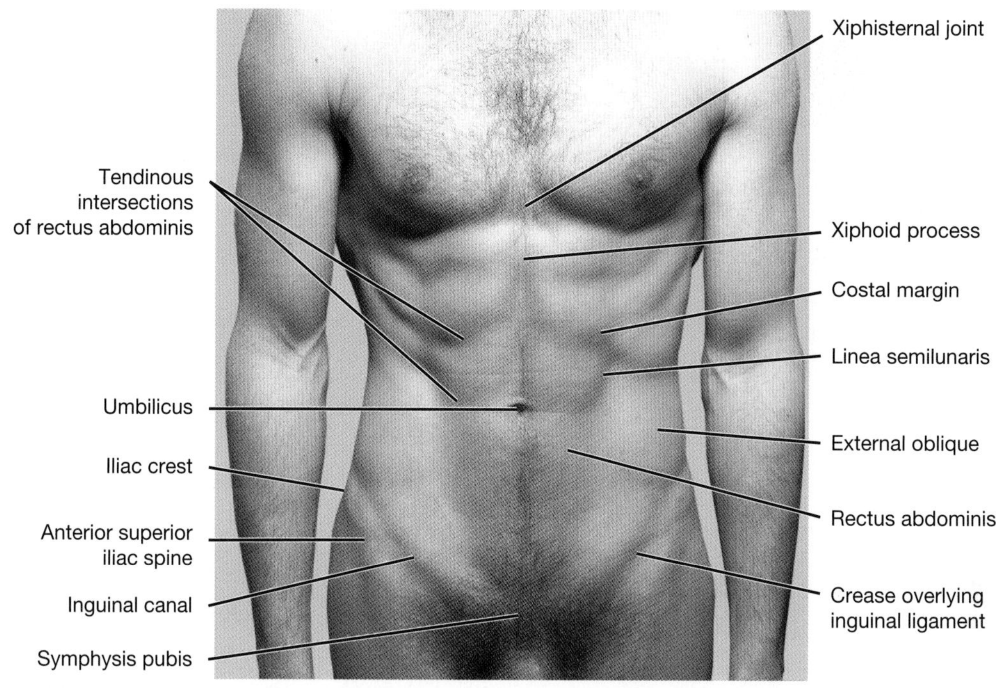

Figure 5.16 Anterior abdominal wall of a young adult male. Note the well-defined rectus abdominis muscles with their pronounced tendinous intersections and linea semilunaris.

wall of the rectus sheath (see below). When the rectus is well developed, the tendinous intersections produce the classic "six-pack abs" appearance (see Fig. 5.16).

The rectus abdominis is enclosed between the aponeuroses of the external oblique, internal oblique, and transversus abdominis, which form the **rectus sheath**.

Pyramidalis

The pyramidalis is a small muscle that lies in front of the lower part of the rectus abdominis (see Fig. 5.10). However, it is often absent.

Rectus Sheath

The rectus sheath is a long fibrous envelope that encloses the rectus abdominis and pyramidalis (if present) muscles. Thus, the sheath has two walls, anterior and posterior. It also contains the anterior rami of the T7 to T12 nerves and the superior and inferior epigastric vessels and lymph vessels. It is formed mainly by the aponeuroses of the three lateral abdominal muscles (Fig. 5.17; see also Fig. 5.10).

The composition of the walls of the rectus sheath changes at different levels. For ease of description, the rectus sheath is generally considered at three levels (Fig. 5.18).

- Above the costal margin, the anterior wall is formed by the aponeurosis of the external oblique. The posterior wall is formed by the thoracic wall (ie, costal cartilages 5 to 7 and the intercostal spaces).
- Between the costal margin and the arcuate line (at about the level of the anterior superior iliac spine), the aponeurosis of the internal oblique splits to enclose the rectus muscle. The external oblique aponeurosis is directed in front of the muscle, and the transversus aponeurosis is directed behind the muscle.
- Between the level of the arcuate line (at about the anterior superior iliac spine) and the pubis, the aponeuroses of all three muscles form the anterior wall. The posterior wall is absent, and the rectus muscle lies in contact with the transversalis fascia.

Note that where the aponeuroses forming the posterior wall pass in front of the rectus at the level of the anterior superior iliac spine, the posterior wall has a free, curved lower border called the **arcuate line** (see Figs. 5.10 and 5.17). At this site, the inferior epigastric vessels enter the rectus sheath and pass upward to anastomose with the superior epigastric vessels.

The rectus sheath is separated from its fellow on the opposite side by a fibrous band called the **linea alba**. This extends from the xiphoid process down to the symphysis pubis and is formed by the fusion of the aponeuroses of the lateral muscles of the two sides. It is wider above the umbilicus and narrows down below the umbilicus to be attached to the symphysis pubis.

The posterior wall of the rectus sheath is not attached to the rectus abdominis muscle. However, the anterior wall is firmly attached to it by the muscle's tendinous intersections.

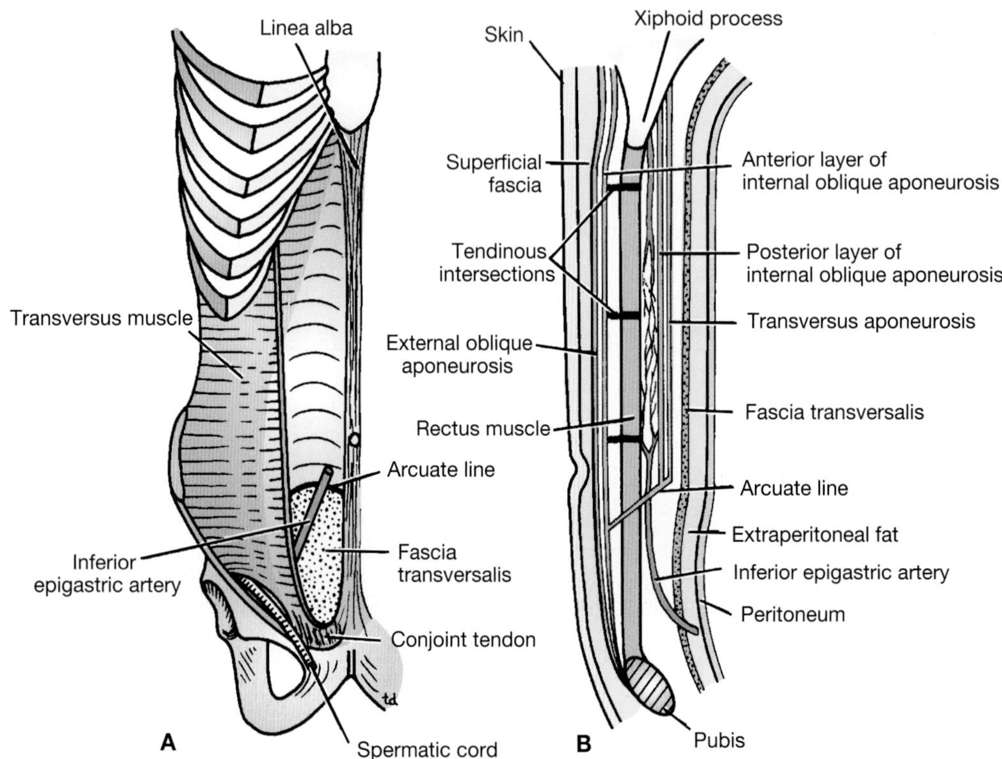

Figure 5.17 Rectus sheath in anterior view **(A)** and in the sagittal section **(B)**. Note the arrangement of the aponeuroses forming the rectus sheath.

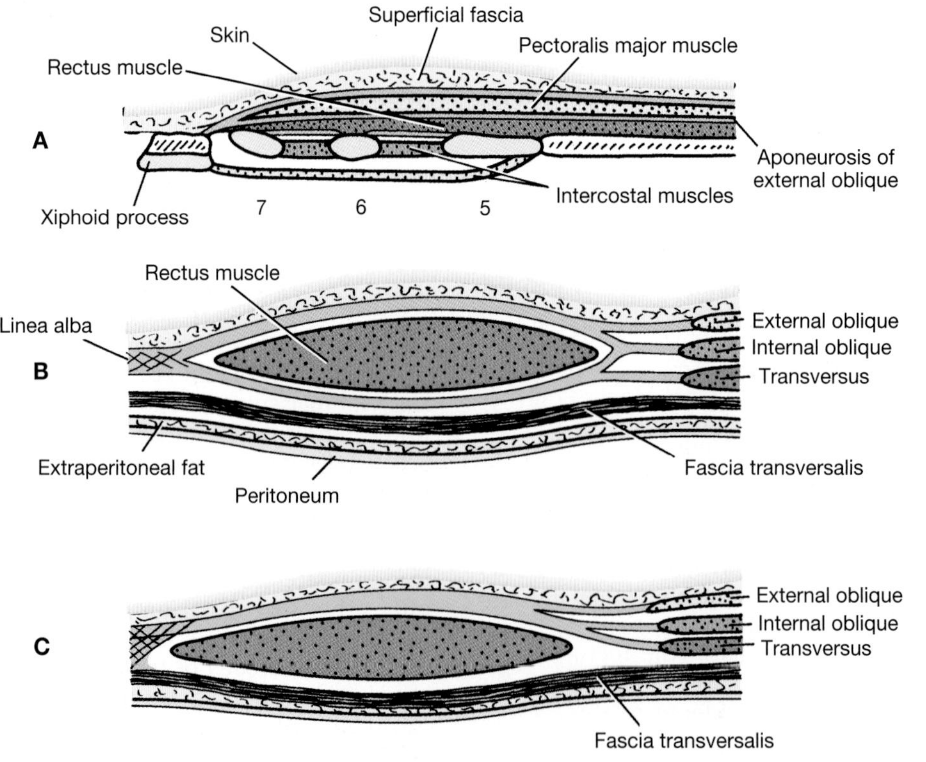

Figure 5.18 Transverse sections of the rectus sheath seen at three levels. **A.** Above the costal margin. **B.** Between the costal margin and the level of the anterior superior iliac spine. **C.** Below the level of the anterior superior iliac spine and above the pubis.

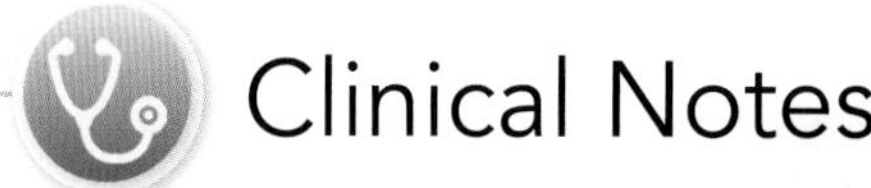

Clinical Notes

Rectus Sheath Hematoma

Hematoma of the rectus sheath is uncommon but important because it is often overlooked. It occurs most often below the level of the umbilicus. The source of the bleeding is the inferior epigastric vein or, more rarely, the inferior epigastric artery. These vessels may be stretched during a severe bout of coughing or in the later months of pregnancy, which may predispose to the condition. The cause is usually blunt trauma to the abdominal wall, such as a fall or a kick. The symptoms that follow the trauma include midline abdominal pain. An acutely tender mass confined to one rectus sheath is diagnostic.

Function

The oblique muscles laterally flex and rotate the trunk (Fig. 5.19). The rectus abdominis flexes the trunk and stabilizes the pelvis, and the pyramidalis keeps the linea alba taut during the process.

The muscles of the anterior and lateral abdominal walls assist the diaphragm during inspiration by relaxing as the diaphragm descends so that the abdominal viscera can be accommodated.

The muscles assist in the act of forced expiration that occurs during coughing and sneezing by pulling down the ribs and sternum. Their tone plays an important part in supporting and protecting the abdominal viscera. By contracting simultaneously with the diaphragm, with the glottis of the larynx closed, they increase intra-abdominal pressure and help in micturition, defecation, vomiting, and parturition.

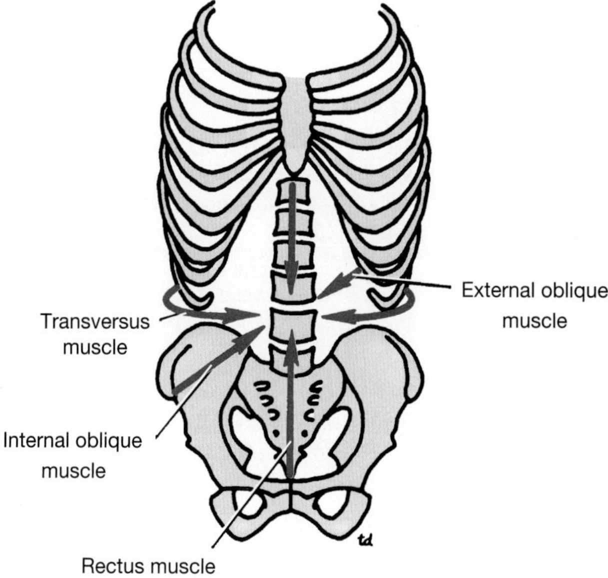

Figure 5.19 Actions of the muscles of the anterior and lateral abdominal walls. *Arrows* indicate the line of pull of different muscles.

Nerve Supply

The T7 to T12 nerves and the iliohypogastric and ilioinguinal nerves (L1) supply the oblique and transversus abdominis muscles (Fig. 5.20; see also Fig. 5.6). The T7 to T12 nerves supply the rectus abdominis. The T12 nerve supplies the pyramidalis.

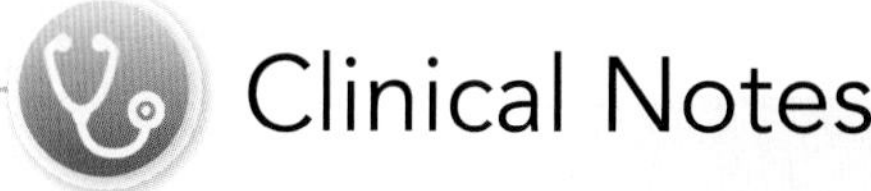

Clinical Notes

Abdominal Muscles, Abdominothoracic Rhythm, and Visceroptosis

The abdominal muscles contract and relax with respiration, and the abdominal wall conforms to the volume of the abdominal viscera. Normally, during inspiration, when the sternum moves forward and the chest expands, the anterior abdominal wall also moves forward—the **abdominothoracic rhythm**. If the anterior abdominal wall remains stationary or contracts inward when the chest expands, the parietal peritoneum is probably inflamed and has caused a reflex contraction of the abdominal muscles.

The shape of the anterolateral abdominal wall depends on the tone of its muscles. A female with poor abdominal muscles and/or who has had multiple pregnancies is often incapable of supporting her abdominal viscera. The lower part of the anterior abdominal wall protrudes forward in a condition known as **visceroptosis**. This should not be confused with an abdominal tumor such as an ovarian cyst or with the excessive accumulation of fat in the fatty layer of the superficial fascia.

Transversalis Fascia

The transversalis fascia is a component of an extensive thin layer of fascia that lies between the muscle layer of the abdominal wall and the parietal peritoneum (Fig. 5.21; see also Fig. 5.17). It is continuous below with a similar fascial layer lining the pelvic walls. Customarily, this fascia is named according to the structure it overlies. For example, the **diaphragmatic fascia** covers the undersurface of the diaphragm, the **transversalis fascia** lines the transversus abdominis, the **psoas fascia** covers the psoas muscle, the **quadratus lumborum fascia** covers the quadratus lumborum, and the **iliac fascia** covers the iliacus muscle.

The abdominal blood and lymph vessels lie within this fascial lining, whereas the principal nerves lie outside the fascia. This fact is important in understanding the **femoral sheath** (see Fig. 5.21). This sheath is simply a downward prolongation of the transversalis and iliac fascial linings around the femoral vessels and lymphatics, for about 1.5 in. (4 cm) into the thigh, behind the inguinal ligament. Because the femoral nerve lies outside the fascial envelope, it has no sheath (see also Chapter 8).

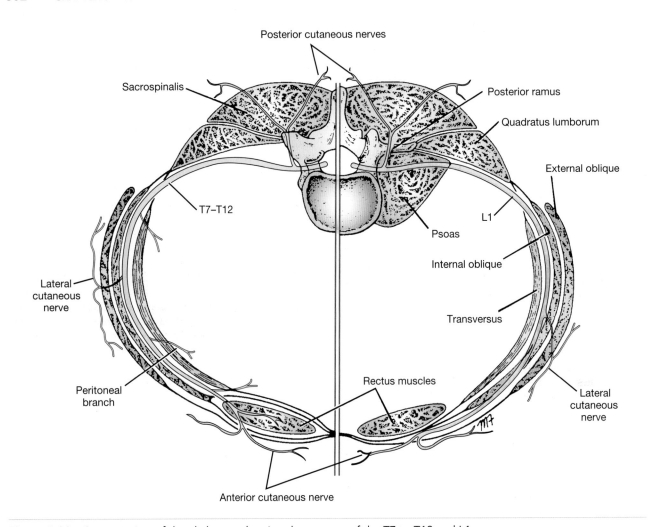

Figure 5.20 Cross section of the abdomen showing the courses of the T7 to T12 and L1 nerves.

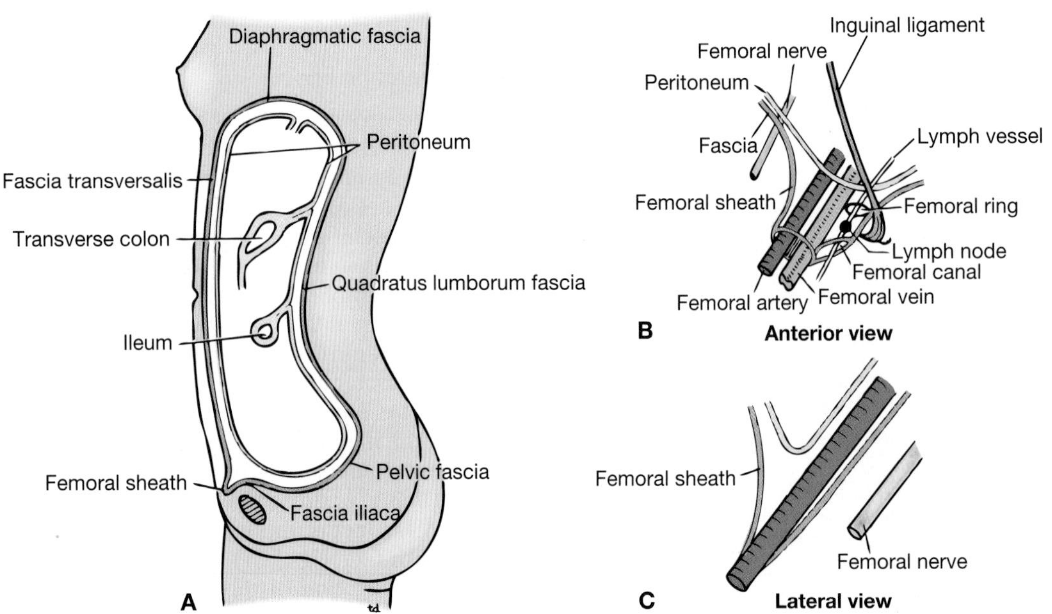

Figure 5.21 **A.** Sagittal section of the abdomen showing the arrangement of the fascial and peritoneal linings of the walls. **B.** Femoral sheath with its contained vessels. **C.** Note that the femoral nerve is devoid of a fascial sheath.

In certain areas of the abdominal wall, the fascial lining performs particularly important functions. Inferior to the level of the arcuate line, the posterior wall of the rectus sheath is devoid of muscular aponeuroses and is formed by the transversalis fascia and parietal peritoneum only (see Figs. 5.17 and 5.18).

At the midpoint between the anterior superior iliac spine and the symphysis pubis, the spermatic cord pierces the transversalis fascia to form the deep inguinal ring (see Fig. 5.15). From the margins of the ring, the fascia continues over the cord as a tubular sheath, the **internal spermatic fascia** (see Fig. 5.11).

Extraperitoneal Fascia

The extraperitoneal fascia is a thin layer of connective tissue that contains a variable amount of fat. It lies between the transversalis fascia and the parietal peritoneum (see Fig. 5.17B).

Parietal Peritoneum

The deep sides of the walls of the abdomen are lined with parietal peritoneum (see Figs. 5.17B and 5.21). This is a thin serous membrane and is continuous below with the parietal peritoneum lining the pelvis (see Chapter 6).

Nerve Supply

The phrenic nerves supply the central part of the diaphragmatic parietal peritoneum, and the lower intercostal nerves supply the peripheral part. The segmental intercostal and lumbar nerves, which also supply the overlying muscles and skin, supply the peritoneum lining the anterior and posterior abdominal walls.

Anterolateral Abdominal Wall Nerves

The anterior rami of the T7 to T12 and L1 nerves supply the anterolateral abdominal wall (see Figs. 5.5, 5.6, and 5.20). The thoracic nerves are the continuations of the lower five intercostal nerves and the subcostal nerves beyond the costal margins (see Fig. 5.6). They pass forward in the interval between the internal oblique and the transversus muscles in the same way the intercostal nerves run forward in the intercostal spaces between the internal intercostal and the innermost intercostal muscles. Collectively, they supply the skin of the anterolateral abdominal wall, the muscles, and the parietal peritoneum. The T7 to T12 nerves pierce the posterior wall of the rectus sheath to supply the rectus muscle and the pyramidalis (T12 only). They terminate by piercing the anterior wall of the sheath and supplying the skin.

The L1 nerve, a branch of the lumbar plexus, has a similar course as the thoracic nerves but does not enter the rectus sheath (see Fig. 5.20). It divides into the iliohypogastric and ilioinguinal nerves (see Figs. 5.5 and 5.6). The **iliohypogastric nerve** pierces the external oblique aponeurosis above the superficial inguinal ring, and the **ilioinguinal nerve** emerges through the ring. They end by supplying the skin just above the inguinal ligament and symphysis pubis.

The dermatomes of the anterolateral abdominal wall are shown in Figure 5.5. Useful landmark references are that the dermatome of T7 is in the epigastrium over the xiphoid process, that of T10 includes the umbilicus, and that of L1 lies just above the inguinal ligament and the symphysis pubis. More simply put:

- Dermatome T7: xiphoid process
- Dermatome T10: umbilicus
- Dermatome L1: pubis

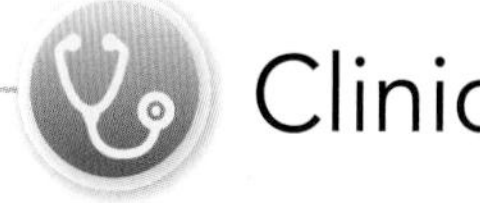

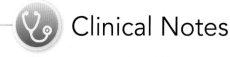

Clinical Notes

Abdominal Pain

Also, see Clinical Notes on Abdominal Pain later in this chapter.

Muscle Rigidity and Referred Pain

Sometimes, a clinician has difficulty in determining whether the muscles of the anterior abdominal wall of a patient are rigid because of underlying inflammation of the parietal peritoneum or whether the patient is voluntarily contracting the muscles because they are conscious of being examined or because the clinician's hand is cold. Asking the patient lying supine on the examination table to rest their arms by their sides and draw up their knees to flex their hip joints usually easily solves this problem. It is practically impossible for a patient to keep their abdominal musculature tensed when the thighs are flexed. Needless to say, the examiner's hand should be warm.

Pleurisy involving the lower costal parietal pleura causes pain in the overlying skin that may radiate down into the abdomen. Although this is unlikely to cause rigidity of the abdominal muscles, it may cause confusion in making a diagnosis.

Anterior Abdominal Nerve Block

An anterior abdominal nerve block is performed to repair lacerations of the anterior abdominal wall.

Area of Anesthesia

The area of anesthesia is the skin of the anterolateral abdominal wall. The relevant nerves are the anterior rami of T7 to T12 nerves and the L1 nerve (ilioinguinal and iliohypogastric nerves).

(continued)

Procedure

The anterior ends of intercostal nerves T7 to T11 enter the abdominal wall by passing posterior to the costal cartilages (see Figs. 5.5 and 5.6). An abdominal field block is most easily carried out along the lower border of the costal margin and then infiltrating the nerves as they emerge between the xiphoid process and rib 10 or 11 along the costal margin (Fig. 5.22).

The ilioinguinal nerve passes forward in the inguinal canal and emerges through the superficial inguinal ring. The iliohypogastric nerve passes forward around the abdominal wall and pierces the external oblique aponeurosis above the superficial inguinal ring. Blocking the two nerves is easily accomplished by inserting the anesthetic needle 1 in. (2.5 cm) above the anterior superior iliac spine on the spinoumbilical line.

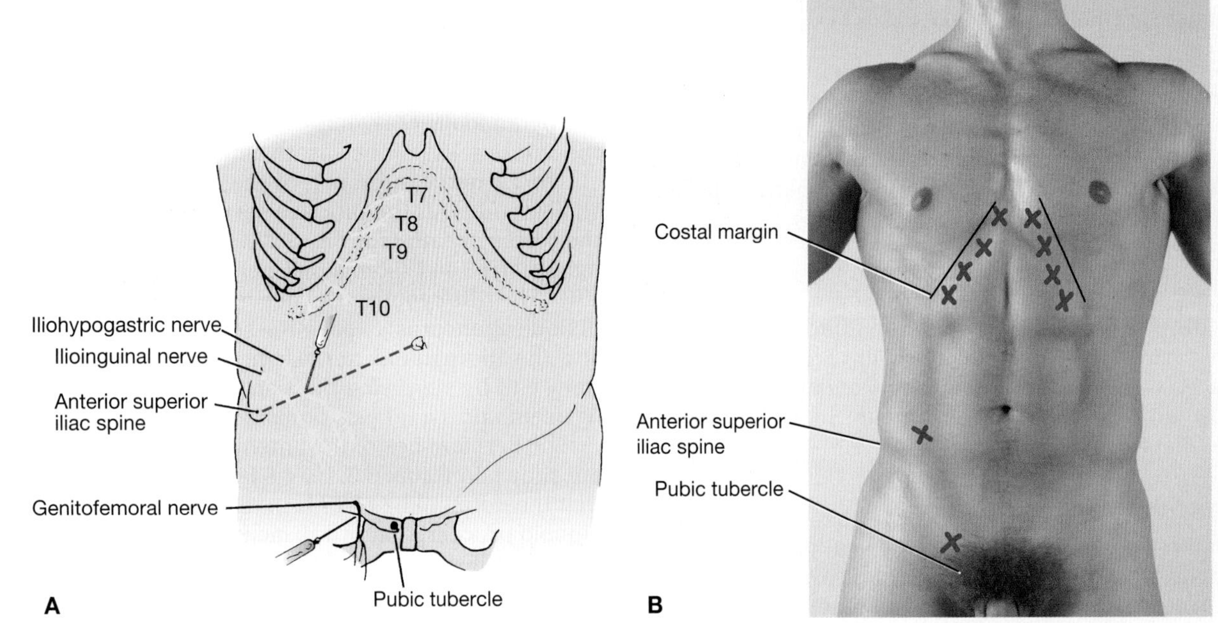

Figure 5.22 Anterior abdominal wall nerve blocks. T7 to T11 **(A)** are blocked (X in **B**) as they emerge from beneath the costal margin. The iliohypogastric and ilioinguinal nerves **(A)** are blocked by inserting the needle about 1 in. (2.5 cm) above the anterior superior iliac spine on the spinoumbilical line (X in **B**). The terminal branches of the genitofemoral nerve **(A)** are blocked by inserting the needle through the skin just lateral to the pubic tubercle and infiltrating the subcutaneous tissue with anesthetic solution (X in **B**).

Anterolateral Abdominal Wall Arteries

The **superior epigastric artery**, one of the terminal branches of the internal thoracic artery, enters the upper part of the rectus sheath between the sternal and costal origins of the diaphragm (see Fig. 5.6). It descends behind the rectus abdominis muscle, supplying the upper central part of the anterior abdominal wall, and anastomoses with the inferior epigastric artery.

The **inferior epigastric artery** is a branch of the external iliac artery just above the inguinal ligament. It runs upward and medially along the medial side of the deep inguinal ring (see Figs. 5.6, 5.11, and 5.15D). It pierces the transversalis fascia to enter the rectus sheath anterior to the arcuate line (see Fig. 5.17). It ascends behind the rectus muscle, supplying the lower central part of the anterior abdominal wall, and anastomoses with the superior epigastric artery.

The **deep circumflex iliac artery** is a branch of the external iliac artery just above the inguinal ligament (see Fig. 5.6). It runs upward and laterally toward the anterosuperior iliac spine and then continues along the iliac crest. It supplies the lower lateral part of the abdominal wall.

The **lower two posterior intercostal arteries**, branches of the descending thoracic aorta, and the **four lumbar arteries**, branches of the abdominal aorta, pass forward between the muscle layers and supply the lateral part of the abdominal wall (see Fig. 5.6).

Anterolateral Abdominal Wall Veins

The superficial veins form a network that radiates out from the umbilicus (see Fig. 5.7). Above, the network drains into the axillary vein via the **lateral thoracic vein** and, below, into the femoral vein via the **superficial epigastric** and **great saphenous veins**. A few small veins, the **paraumbilical veins**, connect the network through the umbilicus and along the ligamentum teres to the portal vein. This forms an important portal–systemic venous anastomosis.

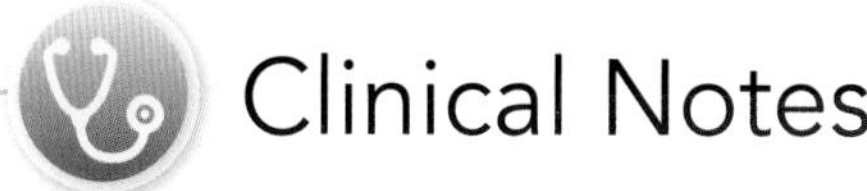

Clinical Notes

Caval Obstruction

If the superior or inferior vena cava is obstructed, the venous blood causes distention of the veins running from the anterior chest wall to the thigh. The lateral thoracic vein anastomoses with the superficial epigastric vein, a tributary of the great saphenous vein of the lower limb. In these circumstances, a tortuous varicose vein may extend from the axilla to the lower abdomen (see Fig. 5.7).

Portal Vein Obstruction

In cases of portal vein obstruction, the superficial veins around the umbilicus and the paraumbilical veins become grossly distended (see Fig. 5.7). The distended subcutaneous veins radiate out from the umbilicus, producing in severe cases the clinical picture referred to as **caput medusae** (Fig. 5.23C).

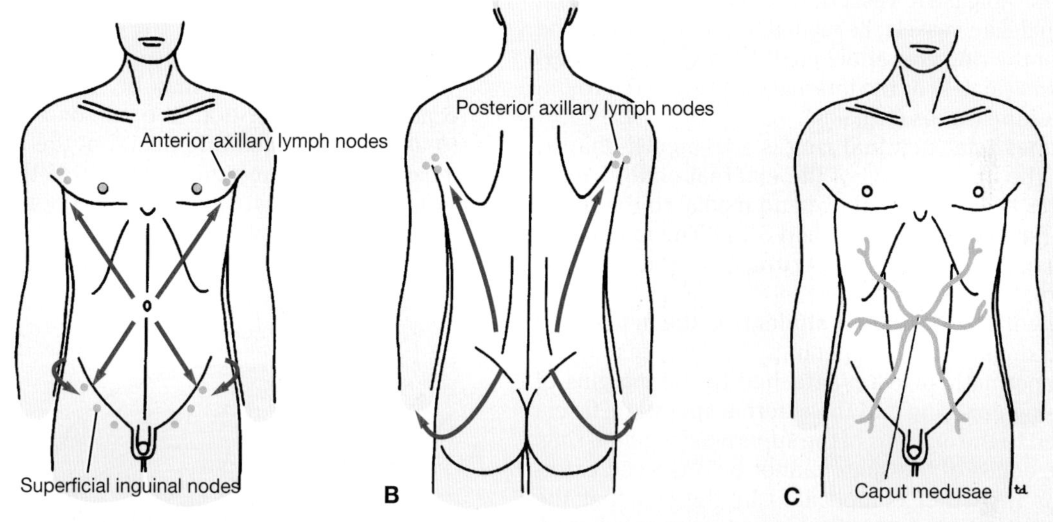

Figure 5.23 **A.** Lymph drainage of the skin of the anterior abdominal wall. **B.** Lymph drainage of the skin of the posterior abdominal wall. **C.** An example of caput medusae in a case of portal obstruction caused by cirrhosis of the liver.

The deep veins of the abdominal wall, the **superior epigastric**, **inferior epigastric**, and **deep circumflex iliac veins**, follow the arteries of the same name and drain into the internal thoracic and external iliac veins. The **posterior intercostal veins** drain into the azygos veins, and the **lumbar veins** drain into the inferior vena cava.

Anterolateral Abdominal Wall Lymphatics

Lymph drainage of the skin of the anterior abdominal wall above the level of the umbilicus is upward to the anterior axillary (pectoral) group of nodes, which can be palpated just beneath the lower border of the pectoralis major muscle (see Fig. 5.23A). Below the level of the umbilicus, the lymph drains downward and laterally to the superficial inguinal nodes. The lymph of the skin of the back above the level of the iliac crests is drained upward to the posterior axillary group of nodes, palpated on the posterior wall of the axilla (see Fig. 5.23B). Below the level of the iliac crests, lymph drains downward to the superficial inguinal nodes.

The deep lymph vessels follow the arteries and drain into the internal thoracic, external iliac, posterior mediastinal, and para-aortic (lumbar) nodes.

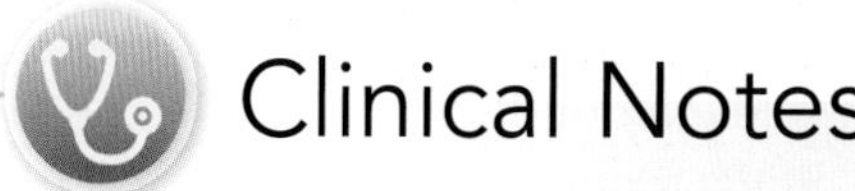

Clinical Notes

Skin and Its Regional Lymph Nodes

Knowledge of the areas of the skin that drain into a particular group of lymph nodes is clinically important in understanding the source of pathology. For example, a swelling in the groin (enlarged superficial inguinal node) could be caused by an infection or malignant tumor of the skin of the lower part of the anterior abdominal wall or that of the buttock.

Inguinal Canal

The inguinal canal is an oblique passage through the lower part of the anterior abdominal wall. In males, it allows structures of the spermatic cord to pass to and from the testis and abdomen. (Normal spermatogenesis takes place only if the testis leaves the abdominal cavity to enter a cooler environment in the scrotum.) In females, the smaller canal allows the round ligament of the uterus to pass from the uterus to the labium majus.

The canal is about 1.5 in. (4 cm) long in the adult and extends from the deep inguinal ring, a hole in the transversalis fascia, downward and medially to the superficial inguinal ring, a hole in the aponeurosis of the external oblique muscle (see Figs. 5.11 and 5.15). It lies parallel to and immediately above the inguinal ligament. In the newborn, the deep ring lies almost directly posterior to the superficial ring so that the canal is considerably shorter at this age. Later, as the result of growth, the deep ring moves laterally.

The **deep inguinal ring**, an oval opening in the transversalis fascia, lies about 0.5 in. (1.3 cm) above the inguinal ligament midway between the anterior superior iliac spine and the symphysis pubis (see Figs. 5.11 and 5.15). The inferior epigastric vessels, which pass upward from the external iliac vessels, lie medial to the deep ring. The margins of the ring give attachment to the **internal spermatic fascia** (males) or the internal covering of the round ligament of the uterus (females).

The **superficial inguinal ring** is a triangular-shaped defect in the aponeurosis of the external oblique muscle and lies immediately above and medial to the pubic tubercle (see Figs. 5.10, 5.12, and 5.15). The margins of the ring, sometimes called the **crura**, give attachment to the **external spermatic fascia**.

A common frustration for students is the inability to see these rings as actual openings. Remember that the internal spermatic fascia is attached to the margins of the deep inguinal ring and the external spermatic fascia is attached to the margins of the superficial inguinal ring. Thus, the edges of the rings cannot be observed externally. This is further complicated by the fact that the superficial ring is not actually a round ring (see above). Compare this arrangement with seeing the openings for the fingers from inside a glove with not seeing the openings when looking at a glove from the outside.

Walls

The inguinal canal has four walls: anterior, posterior, superior (roof), and inferior (floor).

- **Anterior wall:** Formed by the external oblique aponeurosis and reinforced laterally by the origin of the internal oblique from the inguinal ligament (see Figs. 5.10 and 5.15), this wall is strongest where it lies opposite the weakest part of the posterior wall, namely, the deep inguinal ring.
- **Posterior wall:** Formed by the conjoint tendon medially and the transversalis fascia laterally (see Figs. 5.11 and 5.15), this wall is strongest where it lies opposite the weakest part of the anterior wall, namely, the superficial inguinal ring.
- **Superior wall (roof):** This wall is formed by the arching lowest fibers of the internal oblique and transversus abdominis muscles (see Fig. 5.14).
- **Inferior wall (floor):** This wall is formed by the upturned lower edge of the inguinal ligament and, at its medial end, the lacunar ligament (see Fig. 5.14).

Mechanics

The inguinal canal is a site of potential weakness in both sexes. It is interesting to consider how the design of this canal attempts to lessen this weakness.

1. Except in the newborn, the canal is an oblique passage with the weakest areas (superficial and deep rings) lying some distance apart.
2. The fibers of the internal oblique muscle immediately in front of the deep ring reinforce the anterior wall of the canal.
3. The strong conjoint tendon immediately behind the superficial ring reinforces the posterior wall of the canal.
4. On coughing and straining, as in micturition, defecation, and parturition, the arching lowest fibers of the internal oblique and transversus abdominis muscles contract, flattening out the arched roof so that it is lowered toward the floor. The roof may compress the contents of the canal against the floor so that the canal is virtually closed (Fig. 5.24).
5. When straining efforts may be necessary, as in defecation and parturition, the person naturally tends to assume the squatting position; the hip joints are flexed, and the anterior surfaces of the thighs are brought up against the anterior abdominal wall. By this means, the lower part of the anterior abdominal wall is protected by the thighs (see Fig. 5.24).

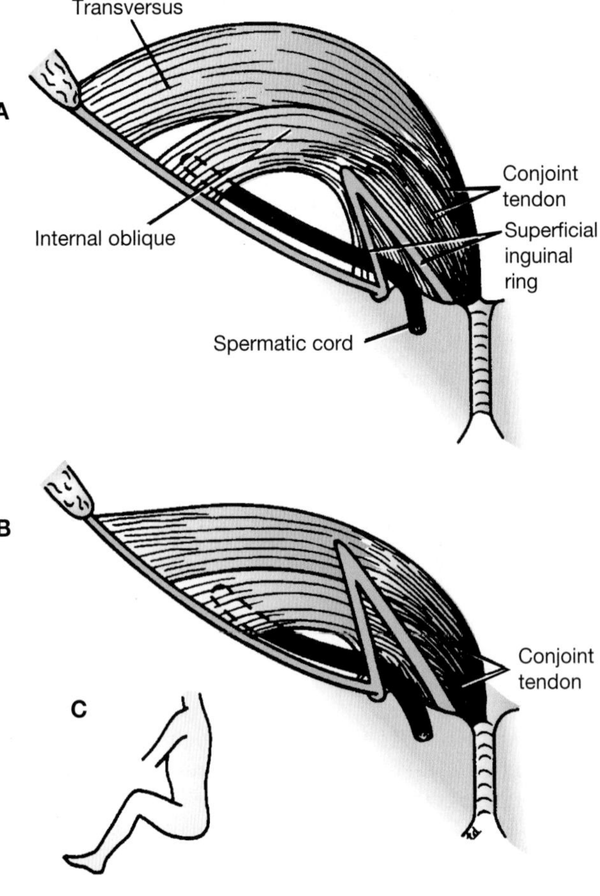

Figure 5.24 Action of the sheet muscles on the inguinal canal. **A.** Muscles relaxed. **B.** Muscles contracted. Note that the canal is "obliterated" when the muscles contract. **C.** Note that the anterior surface of the thigh protects the inguinal region in the squatting position.

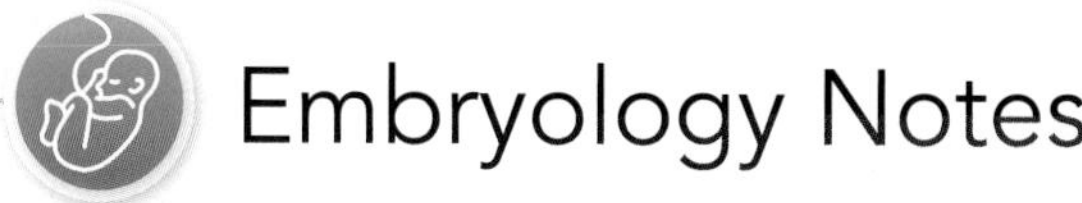

Embryology Notes

Inguinal Canal Development

A peritoneal diverticulum called the **processus vaginalis** forms before the descent of the testis and the ovary from their site of origin high on the posterior abdominal wall (L1) (Fig. 5.25). The processus vaginalis passes through the layers of the lower part of the anterior abdominal wall and acquires a tubular covering from each layer as it does so. It traverses the transversalis fascia at the deep inguinal ring and acquires a tubular covering, the **internal spermatic fascia** (see Fig. 5.11). As it passes through the lower part of the internal oblique muscle, it takes with it some of its lowest fibers, which form the **cremaster muscle**. The muscle fibers are embedded in fascia, and thus the second tubular sheath is known as the **cremasteric fascia**. The processus vaginalis passes under the arching fibers of the transversus abdominis muscle and therefore *does not* acquire a covering from this abdominal layer. On reaching the aponeurosis of the external oblique, it evaginates this to form the superficial inguinal ring and acquires a third tubular fascial coat, the **external spermatic fascia** in males (see Figs. 5.11 and 5.12) and the covering of the round ligament of the uterus in females. The inguinal canal is formed in this manner in both sexes.

Meanwhile, a band of mesenchyme, extending from the lower pole of the developing gonad through the inguinal canal to the labioscrotal swelling, condenses to form the **gubernaculum** (see Fig. 5.25).

In males, the testis descends through the pelvis and inguinal canal during months 7 and 8 of fetal life. The normal stimulus for the descent of the testis is testosterone, which is secreted by the fetal testes. The testis follows the gubernaculum and descends behind the peritoneum on the posterior abdominal wall. The testis then passes behind the processus vaginalis and pulls down its duct, blood vessels, nerves, and lymph vessels. The testis takes up its final position in the developing scrotum by the end of month 8.

Because the testis and its accompanying vessels, ducts, and so on, follow the course previously taken by the processus vaginalis, they acquire the same three coverings as they pass down the inguinal canal. Thus, three concentric layers of fascia cover the spermatic cord: the external spermatic fascia, the cremasteric fascia, and the internal spermatic fascia.

In females, the ovary descends into the pelvis following the gubernaculum (see Fig. 5.25). The gubernaculum attaches to the side of the developing uterus, and the gonad descends no farther. That part of the gubernaculum extending from the uterus into the developing labium majus persists as the round ligament of the uterus. Thus, in females, the only structures that pass through the inguinal canal from the abdominal cavity are the round ligament of the uterus and a few lymph vessels. The lymph vessels convey a small amount of lymph from the body of the uterus to the superficial inguinal nodes.

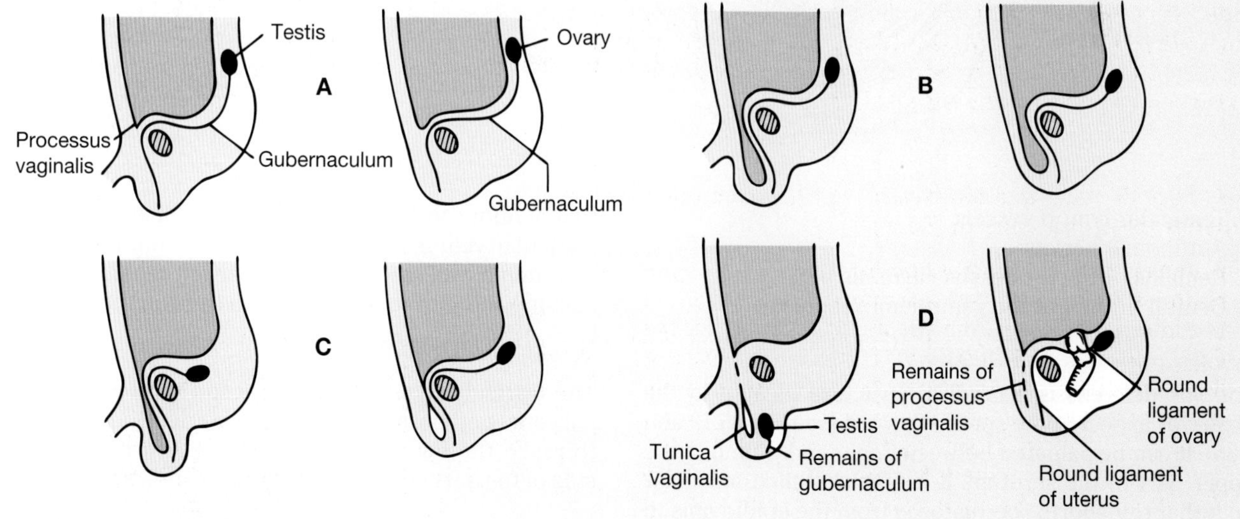

Figure 5.25 Origin **(A)**, development **(B, C)**, and fate **(D)** of the processus vaginalis in the two sexes. Note the descent of the testis into the scrotum and the descent of the ovary into the pelvis.

Spermatic Cord

The spermatic cord is a bundle of structures that pass through the inguinal canal to and from the testis (Fig. 5.26; see also Fig. 5.15). It begins at the deep inguinal ring lateral to the inferior epigastric artery and ends at the testis.

Structures

The structures of the spermatic cord are as follows:

- Vas deferens
- Testicular artery
- Testicular veins (pampiniform plexus)

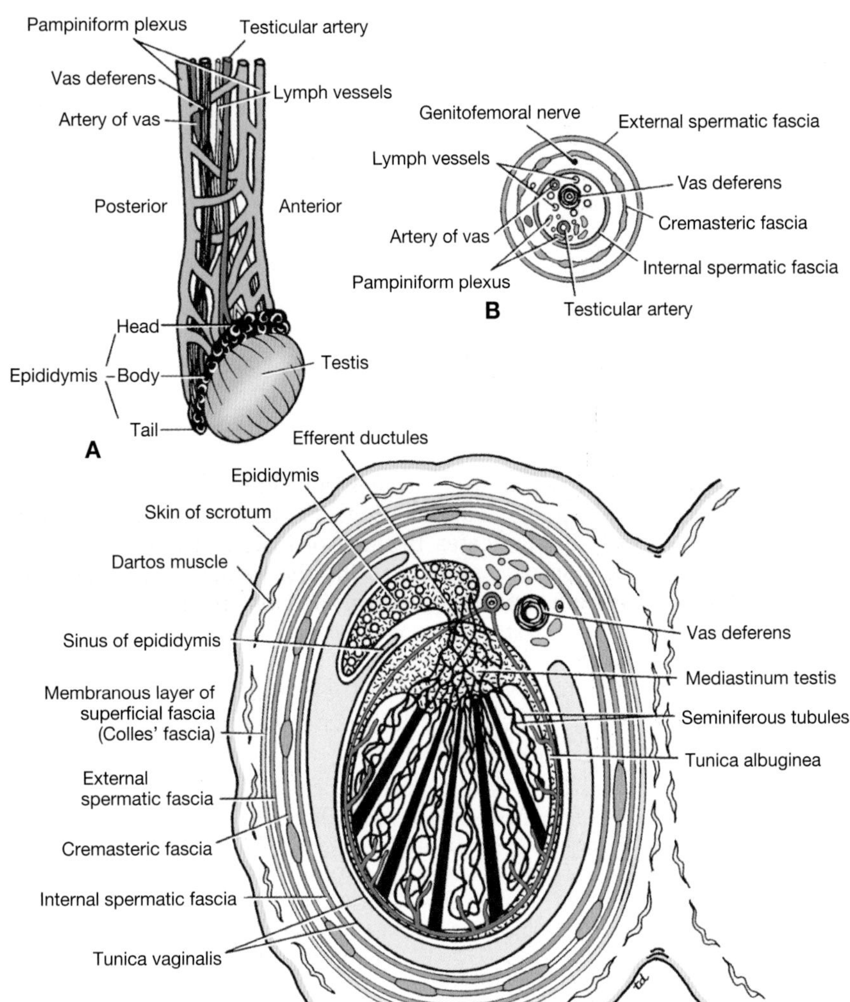

Figure 5.26 Testis, epididymis, spermatic cord, and scrotum. **A.** Spermatic cord and testis. **B.** Transverse section across the spermatic cord and its fasciae. **C.** Testis and epididymis cut across in the horizontal section.

- Testicular lymph vessels
- Autonomic nerves
- Remains of the processus vaginalis
- Genital branch of the genitofemoral nerve

Vas Deferens (Ductus Deferens)

The vas deferens is a cordlike structure located in the posterior aspect of the spermatic cord (see Figs. 5.12 and 5.26). It can be palpated between finger and thumb in the upper part of the scrotum. It is a thick-walled muscular duct that transports spermatozoa from the epididymis to the urethra.

Testicular Artery

A branch of the abdominal aorta (at the level of vertebra L2), the testicular artery is long and slender and descends on the posterior abdominal wall. It traverses the inguinal canal and supplies the testis and the epididymis (see Fig. 5.26).

Testicular Veins

An extensive venous plexus, the **pampiniform plexus**, leaves the posterior border of the testis (see Fig. 5.26). As the plexus ascends, it becomes reduced in size so that at about the level of the deep inguinal ring, a single testicular vein is formed. This runs up on the posterior abdominal wall and drains into the left renal vein on the left side and into the inferior vena cava on the right side.

Lymph Vessels

The testicular lymph vessels ascend through the inguinal canal and pass up over the posterior abdominal wall to reach the lumbar (para-aortic) lymph nodes on the side of the aorta at the level of the L1 vertebra (Fig. 5.27).

Autonomic Nerves

Sympathetic fibers run with the testicular artery from the renal or aortic sympathetic plexuses. Afferent sensory nerves accompany the efferent sympathetic fibers.

Processus Vaginalis

The remains of the processus vaginalis are present within the cord (see below).

Genital Branch of the Genitofemoral Nerve

This nerve supplies the cremaster muscle (see Fig. 5.26; see also Nerves of the Posterior Abdominal Wall later in this chapter).

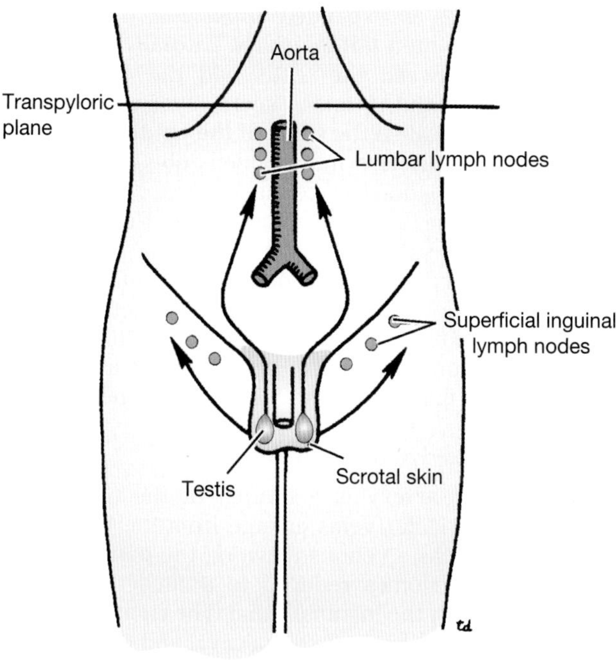

Figure 5.27 Lymph drainage of the testis and the skin of the scrotum.

Spermatic Cord Coverings (Spermatic Fasciae)

The coverings of the spermatic cord are three concentric layers of fascia derived from the layers of the anterior abdominal wall. Each covering is acquired as the processus vaginalis descends into the scrotum through the layers of the abdominal wall (see Fig. 5.25). See the Embryology Notes above (Development of the Inguinal Canal) for an explanation of the formation of the spermatic fasciae.

- **External spermatic fascia** derived from the external oblique aponeurosis and attached to the margins of the superficial inguinal ring
- **Cremasteric fascia** derived from the internal oblique muscle
- **Internal spermatic fascia** derived from the transversalis fascia and attached to the margins of the deep inguinal ring

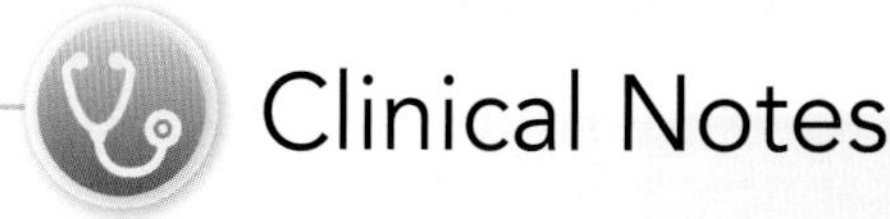

Clinical Notes

Vasectomy

Bilateral vasectomy is a simple operation performed to produce infertility. Under local anesthesia, a small incision is made in the upper part of the scrotal wall, and the vas deferens is divided between ligatures. Spermatozoa may be present in the first few postoperative ejaculations, but that is simply an emptying process. Now only the secretions of the seminal vesicles and prostate constitute the seminal fluid, which can be ejaculated as before.

Scrotum, Testis, and Epididymis

The scrotum is an outpouching of the lower part of the anterior abdominal wall. It contains the testes, the epididymides, and the lower ends of the spermatic cords (see Figs. 5.11, 5.12, and 5.26).

Scrotum

The wall of the scrotum has four layers:

- **Skin**
- **Superficial fascia**
- **Spermatic fasciae**
- **Tunica vaginalis**

Skin

The skin of the scrotum is thin, wrinkled, and pigmented and forms a single pouch. A slightly raised ridge in the midline indicates the line of fusion of the two lateral labioscrotal swellings. (In the female, the swellings remain separate and form the labia majora.)

Superficial Fascia

This is continuous with the fatty and membranous layers of the anterior abdominal wall. However, the fat is replaced by smooth muscle called the **dartos muscle**. This is innervated by sympathetic nerve fibers and is responsible for the wrinkling of the overlying skin. The membranous layer of the superficial fascia (Colles' fascia) is continuous in front with the membranous layer of the anterior abdominal wall (Scarpa's fascia), and behind, it is attached to the perineal body and the posterior edge of the perineal membrane (see Fig. 5.8). At the sides, it is attached to the ischiopubic rami. Both layers of superficial fascia contribute to a median partition that crosses the scrotum and separates the testes from each other.

Spermatic Fasciae

These three layers lie beneath the superficial fascia and are derived from the three layers of the anterior abdominal wall on each side, as previously explained. The external spermatic fascia is derived from the aponeurosis of the external oblique muscle, cremasteric fascia from the internal oblique muscle, and internal spermatic fascia from the transversalis fascia.

The cremaster muscle can be made to contract by stroking the skin on the medial aspect of the thigh. This is called the **cremasteric reflex**. The afferent fibers of this reflex arc travel in the femoral branch of the genitofemoral nerve (L1 and L2), and the efferent motor nerve fibers travel in the genital branch of the genitofemoral nerve. The function of the cremaster muscle is to raise the testis and the scrotum upward for warmth and for protection against injury. For testicular temperature and fertility, see below.

Tunica Vaginalis

This lies within the spermatic fasciae and covers the anterior, medial, and lateral surfaces of each testis (see Figs. 5.11, 5.12, and 5.26). It is the lower expanded part of the processus vaginalis; normally, just before birth, it becomes shut off from the upper part of the processus and the peritoneal cavity. The tunica vaginalis is thus a closed sac, invaginated from behind by the testis.

Scrotal Lymph Drainage

Lymph from the skin and fascia, including the tunica vaginalis, drains into the superficial inguinal lymph nodes (see Fig. 5.27). However, lymph from the testes drains upward to the lumbar nodes, where the testes originated.

Testis

The testis is a firm, mobile organ lying within the scrotum (see Figs. 5.12 and 5.26). The left testis usually lies at a lower level than the right. A tough fibrous capsule, the **tunica albuginea**, surrounds each testis.

A series of **fibrous septa** extend from the inner surface of the capsule and divide the interior of the organ into lobules. One to three coiled **seminiferous tubules** lie within each lobule. The tubules open into a network of channels called the **rete testis**. Small **efferent ductules** connect the rete testis to the upper end of the epididymis (see Fig. 5.26).

Normal spermatogenesis can occur only if the testes are at a temperature lower than that of the abdominal cavity. When they are in the scrotum, they are at a temperature about 3°C lower than the abdominal temperature. The control of testicular temperature in the scrotum is not fully understood, but the surface area of the scrotal skin can be changed reflexively by the contraction of the dartos and cremaster muscles. The testicular veins in the spermatic cord that form the pampiniform plexus—together with the branches of the testicular arteries, which lie close to the veins—probably assist in stabilizing the temperature of the testes by a countercurrent heat exchange mechanism. By this means, the hot blood arriving in the artery from the abdomen loses heat to the blood ascending to the abdomen within the veins.

Epididymis

The epididymis is a firm structure lying posterior to the testis, with the vas deferens lying on its medial side (see Fig. 5.26). It has an expanded upper end, the **head**, a **body**, and a pointed **tail** inferiorly. Laterally, a distinct groove lies between the testis and the epididymis, which is lined with the inner visceral layer of the tunica vaginalis and is called the **sinus of the epididymis**.

The epididymis is a much-coiled tube nearly 20 ft (6 m) long, embedded in connective tissue. The tube emerges from the tail of the epididymis as the vas deferens, which enters the spermatic cord.

The long length of the duct of the epididymis provides storage space for the spermatozoa and allows them to mature. A main function of the epididymis is fluid absorption. Another function may be the addition of substances to the seminal fluid to nourish the maturing sperm.

Testis and Epididymis Blood Supply

The **testicular artery** is a branch of the abdominal aorta. The testicular veins emerge from the testis and the epididymis as a venous network, the **pampiniform plexus**. This becomes reduced to a single vein as it ascends through the inguinal canal. The right testicular vein drains into the inferior vena cava, and the left vein joins the left renal vein.

Testis and Epididymis Lymph Drainage

The lymph vessels (see Fig. 5.27) ascend in the spermatic cord and end in the lymph nodes on the side of the aorta (lumbar or para-aortic nodes) at the level of the L1 vertebra (ie, on the transpyloric plane). This is to be expected because, during development, the testis has migrated from high up on the posterior abdominal wall, down through the inguinal canal, and into the scrotum, dragging its blood supply and lymph vessels after it.

Labia Majora

The labia majora are prominent, hair-bearing folds of skin formed by the enlargement of the genital swellings in the fetus. (In males, the genital swellings fuse in the midline to form the scrotum.) A large amount of adipose tissue and the terminal strands of the round ligaments of the uterus are the contents of the labia.

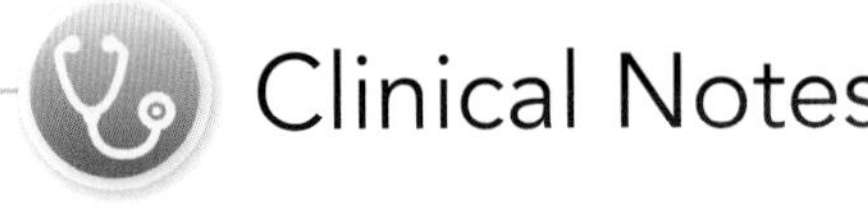

Varicocele

In a varicocele, the veins of the pampiniform plexus are elongated and dilated. It is a common disorder in adolescents and young adults, with most occurring on the left side. This is thought to be because the right testicular vein joins the low-pressure inferior vena cava, whereas the left vein joins the left renal vein, in which the venous pressure is higher. Rarely, malignant disease of the left kidney extends along the renal vein and blocks the exit of the testicular vein. A rapidly developing left-sided varicocele should therefore always lead one to examine the left kidney.

Malignant Tumor of the Testis

A malignant tumor of the testis spreads upward via the lymph vessels to the lumbar (para-aortic) lymph nodes at the level of the L1 vertebra. Later, when the tumor spreads locally to involve the tissues and skin of the scrotum, the superficial inguinal lymph nodes become involved.

Testicular Torsion

Torsion of the testis is a rotation of the testis around the spermatic cord within the scrotum. It is often associated

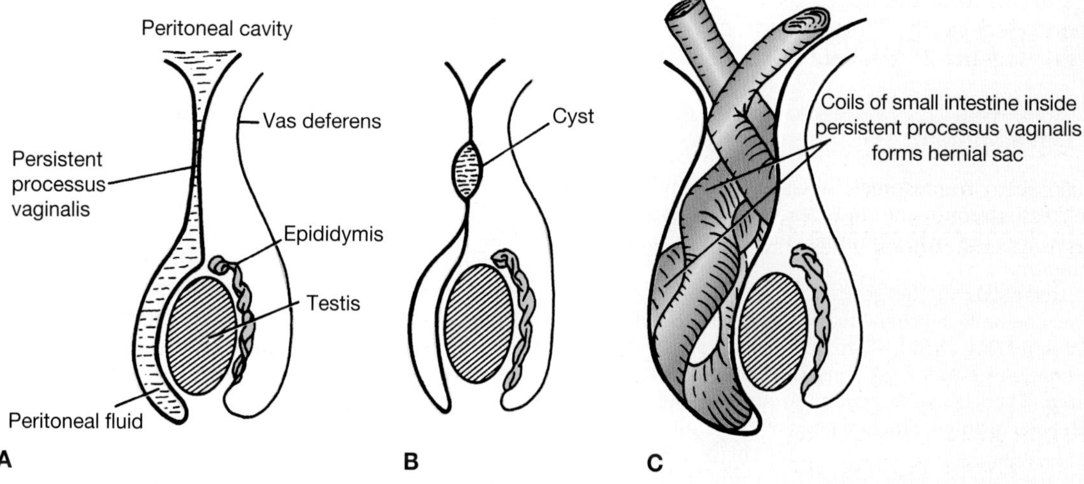

Figure 5.28 Common congenital anomalies of the processus vaginalis. **A.** Congenital hydrocele. **B.** Encysted hydrocele of the cord. **C.** Preformed hernial sac for indirect inguinal hernia.

with an excessively large tunica vaginalis. Torsion commonly occurs in active young men and children and is accompanied by severe pain. If not treated quickly, the testicular artery may be occluded, followed by necrosis of the testis.

Processus Vaginalis

The formation of the processus vaginalis and its passage through the lower part of the anterior abdominal wall with the formation of the inguinal canal in both sexes were described earlier. Normally, the upper part becomes obliterated just before birth, and the lower part remains as the tunica vaginalis.

The processus is subject to the following common congenital anomalies:

1. It may persist partially or in its entirety as a **preformed hernial sac** for an indirect inguinal hernia (Fig. 5.28C).
2. It may become very much narrowed, but its lumen remains in communication with the abdominal cavity. Peritoneal fluid accumulates in it, forming a **congenital hydrocele** (see Fig. 5.28A).
3. The upper and lower ends of the processus may become obliterated, leaving a small intermediate cystic area referred to as an **encysted hydrocele of the cord** (see Fig. 5.28B).

The tunica vaginalis is closely related to the front and sides of the testis. Therefore, it is not surprising to find that inflammation of the testis can cause an accumulation of fluid within the tunica vaginalis. This is referred to as a **hydrocele** (Fig. 5.29A). Most hydroceles are idiopathic.

To remove excess fluid from the tunica vaginalis, a procedure termed **tapping a hydrocele**, a fine trocar and cannula are inserted through the scrotal skin (see Fig. 5.29B). The following anatomic structures are traversed by the cannula: skin, dartos muscle and membranous layer of fascia (Colles' fascia), external spermatic fascia, cremasteric fascia, internal spermatic fascia, and parietal layer of the tunica vaginalis.

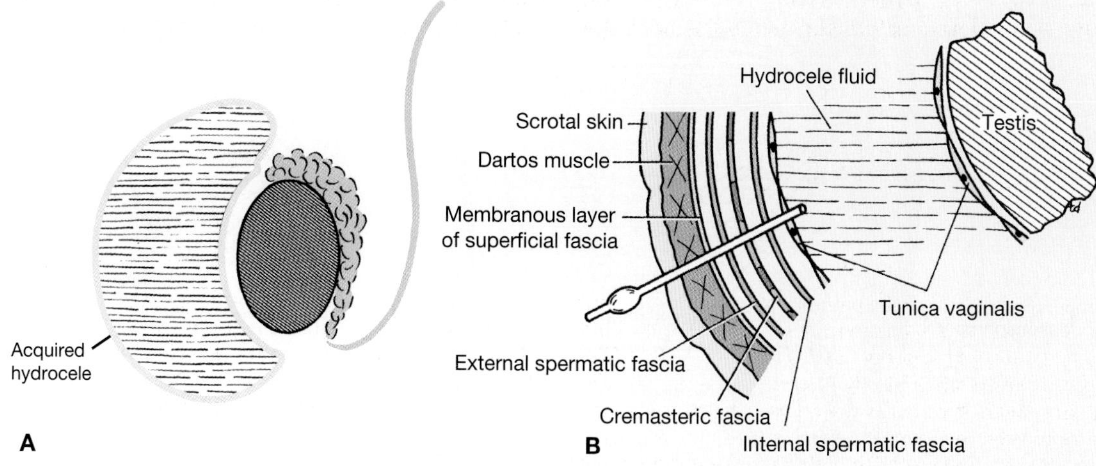

Figure 5.29 Testicular hydrocele. **A.** Tunica vaginalis distended with fluid (hydrocele). **B.** Various anatomic layers traversed by a trocar and a cannula when a hydrocele is tapped.

Embryology Notes

Testis Development

The male sex chromosome causes the genital ridge to secrete testosterone and induces the development of the testis and the other internal and external organs of reproduction.

The **sex cords** of the genital ridge become separated from the coelomic epithelium by the proliferation of the mesenchyme (Fig. 5.30). The outer part of the mesenchyme condenses to form a dense fibrous layer, the **tunica albuginea**. The sex cords become U shaped and form the **seminiferous tubules**. The free ends of the tubules form the **straight tubules**, which join one another in the mediastinum testis to become the **rete testis**. The primordial sex cells in the seminiferous tubules form the **spermatogonia**, and the sex cord cells form the **Sertoli cells**. The mesenchyme in the developing gonad makes up the connective tissue and fibrous septa. The **interstitial cells**, which are already secreting testosterone, are also formed of mesenchyme. The rete testis becomes canalized, and the tubules extend into the mesonephric tissue, where they join the remnants of the mesonephric tubules; the latter tubules become the **efferent ductules** of the testis. The mesonephric duct forms the **duct of the epididymis**, the **vas deferens**, the **seminal vesicle**, and the **ejaculatory duct**.

Testicular Descent

The testis develops high up on the posterior abdominal wall, and in late fetal life, it "descends" behind the

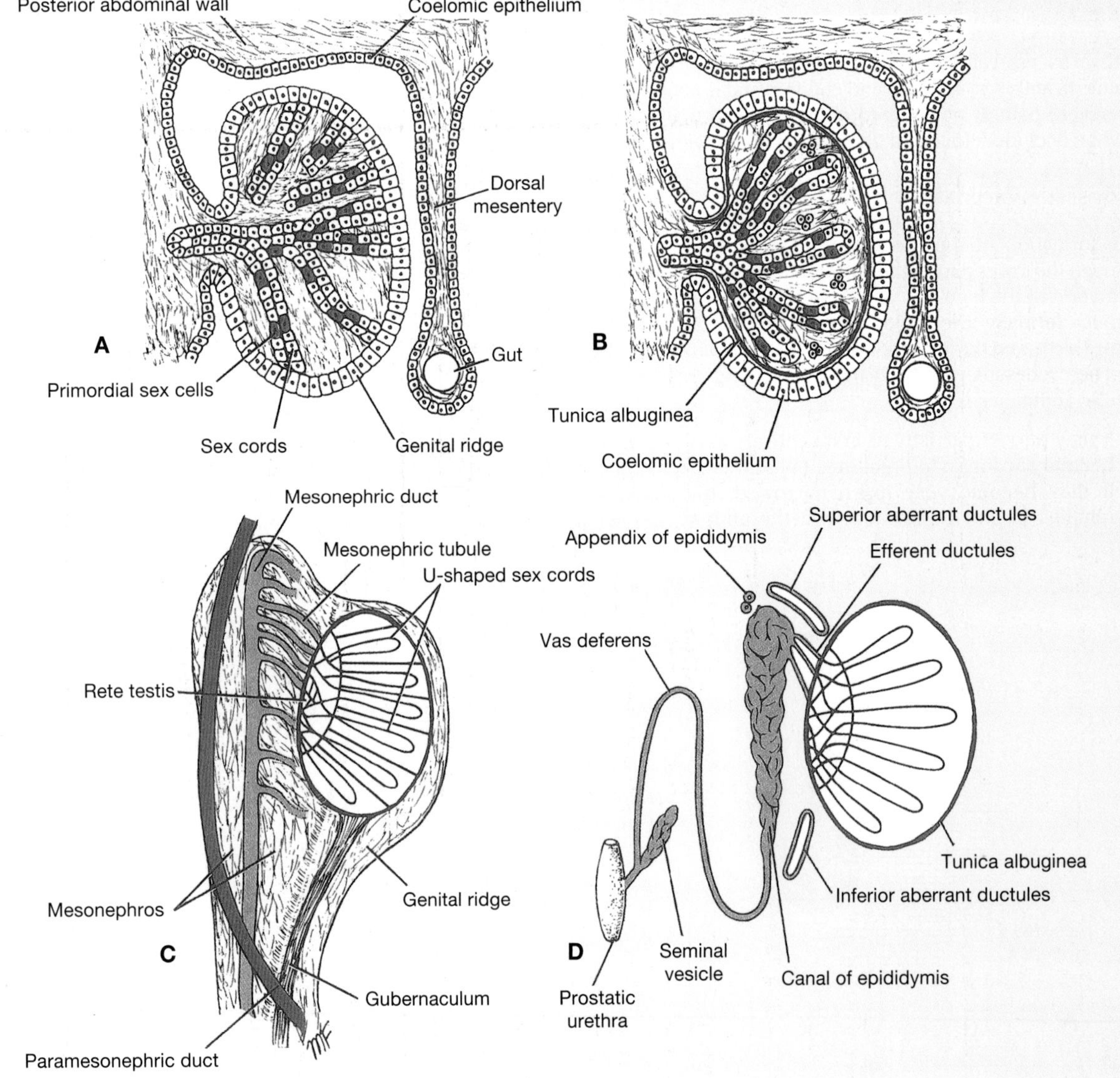

Figure 5.30 Formation **(A)**, development **(B, C)**, and fate **(D)** of the testis and its ducts.

peritoneum, pulling its blood supply, nerve supply, and lymphatic drainage after it. The process of the descent of the testis is shown in Figure 5.25.

Congenital Anomalies

The testis may be subject to the following congenital anomalies.

- **Anterior inversion**, in which the epididymis lies anteriorly and the testis and the tunica vaginalis lie posteriorly.
- **Polar inversion**, in which the testis and epididymis are completely inverted.
- **Imperfect descent (cryptorchidism)**: **Incomplete descent** (Fig. 5.31), in which the testis, although traveling down its normal path, fails to reach the floor of the scrotum may be found within the abdomen, within the inguinal canal, at the superficial inguinal ring, or high up in the scrotum.
- **Maldescent** (Fig. 5.32), in which the testis travels down an abnormal path and fails to reach the scrotum may be found in the superficial fascia of the anterior abdominal wall above the inguinal ligament, in front of the pubis, in the perineum, or in the thigh.

The testes must leave the abdominal cavity because the temperature there retards the normal process of

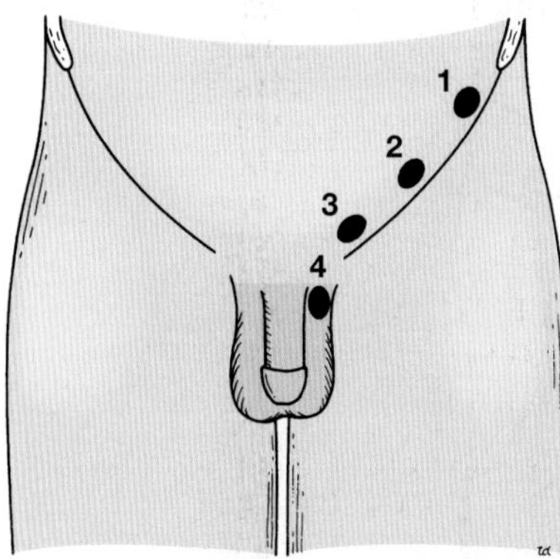

Figure 5.31 Four degrees of incomplete descent of the testis. (1) In the abdominal cavity close to the deep inguinal ring. (2) In the inguinal canal. (3) At the superficial inguinal ring. (4) In the upper part of the scrotum.

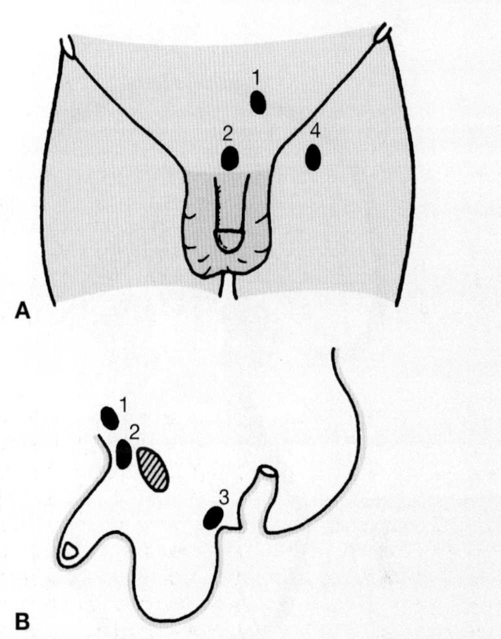

Figure 5.32 Four types of maldescent of the testis. **A.** Anterior view. **B.** Sagittal section. (1) In the superficial fascia of the anterior abdominal wall, above the superficial inguinal ring. (2) At the root of the penis. (3) In the perineum. (4) In the thigh.

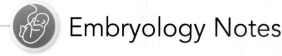

spermatogenesis. If an incompletely descended testis is brought down into the scrotum by surgery before puberty, it will develop and function normally. A maldescended testis, although often developing normally, is susceptible to traumatic injury and, for this reason, should be placed in the scrotum. Many authorities believe that the incidence of tumor formation is greater in testes that have not descended into the scrotum.

The **appendix of the testis** and the **appendix of the epididymis** are embryologic remnants found at the upper poles of these organs that may become cystic. The appendix of the testis is derived from the paramesonephric ducts, and the appendix of the epididymis is a remnant of the mesonephric tubules.

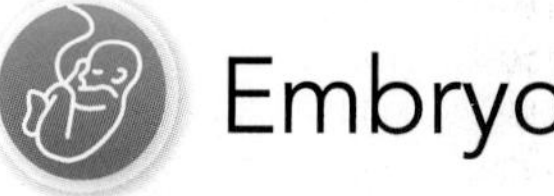

Embryology Notes

Abdominal Wall Development

Following segmentation of the mesoderm, the **lateral mesoderm** (see Chapter 1, Embryology Notes) splits into a **somatic** and a **splanchnic layer** associated with ectoderm and entoderm, respectively (Fig. 5.33). The muscles of the anterior abdominal wall are derived from the somatopleuric mesoderm and retain their segmental innervation from the anterior rami of the spinal nerves. Unlike the thorax, the segmental arrangement becomes lost because of the absence of ribs, and the mesenchyme fuses to form large sheets of muscle. The rectus abdominis retains indications of its segmental origin, as seen by the presence of the tendinous intersections. The somatopleuric mesoderm splits tangentially into three layers, which form the external oblique, internal oblique, and transversus abdominis muscles. The anterior body wall finally closes in the midline during month 3, when the right and left sides meet in the midline and fuse. The line of fusion of the mesenchyme forms the **linea alba**, and on either side of this, the rectus muscles come to lie within their rectus sheaths.

(continued)

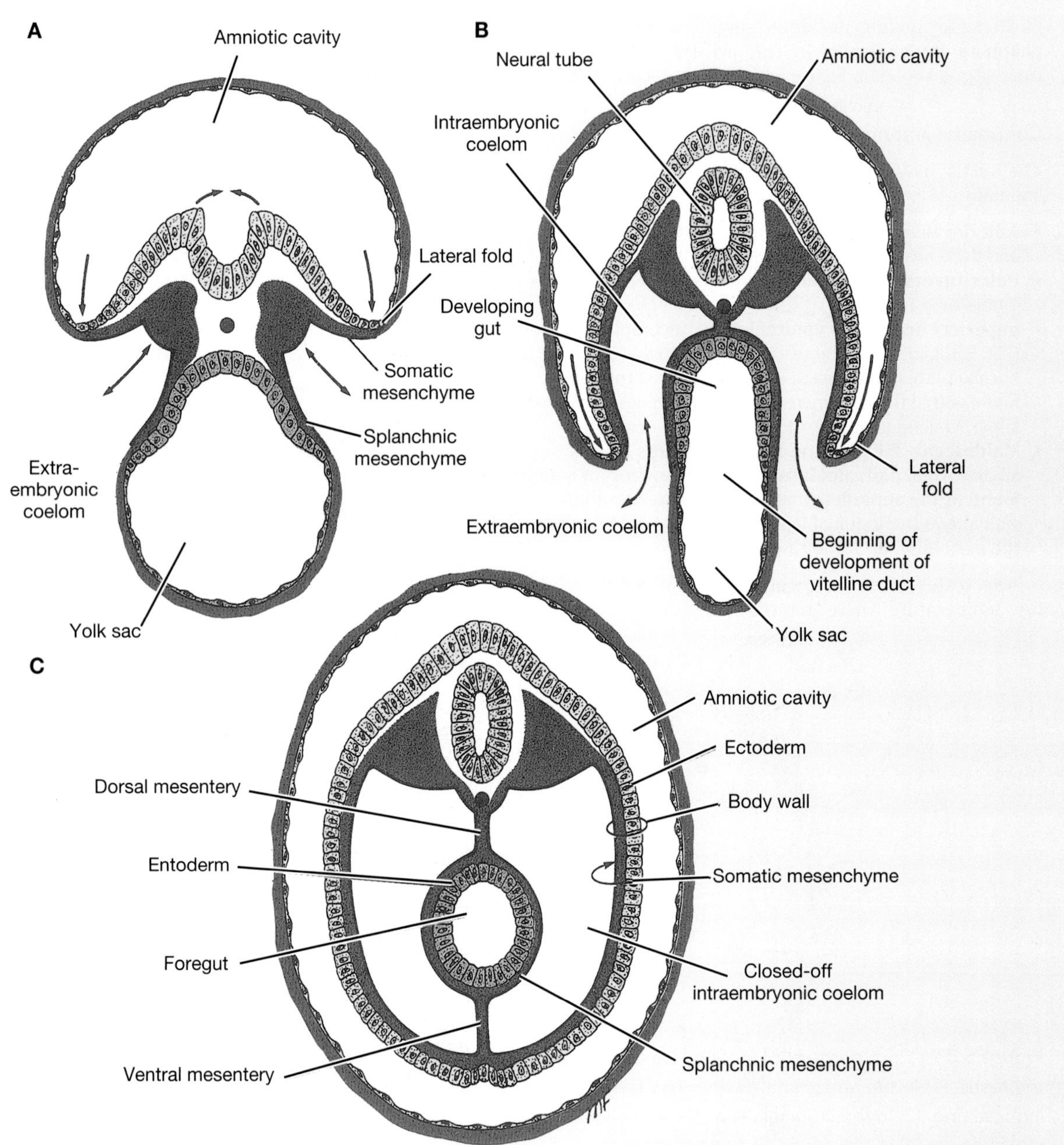

Figure 5.33 Transverse sections through the embryo at different stages of development showing the formation of the abdominal wall and peritoneal cavity. **A.** Intraembryonic coelom in free communication with the extraembryonic coelom (*double-headed arrows*). **B.** Development of the lateral folds of the embryo and the beginning of the closing off of the intraembryonic coelom. **C.** Lateral folds of the embryo finally fused in the midline and closing off the intraembryonic coelom or future peritoneal cavity. Most of the ventral mesentery will break down and disappear.

Umbilical Cord and Umbilicus Development

As the tail fold of the embryo develops, the embryonic attachment of the body stalk to the caudal end of the embryonic disc comes to lie on the anterior surface of the embryo, close to the remains of the yolk sac (Fig. 5.34). The amnion and chorion now fuse, so that the amnion encloses the body stalk and the yolk sac with their blood vessels to form the tubular **umbilical cord**. The mesenchymal core of the cord forms the loose connective tissue called **Wharton's jelly**. The remains of the yolk sac, the vitelline duct, the remains of the allantois, where the umbilical blood vessels are embedded.

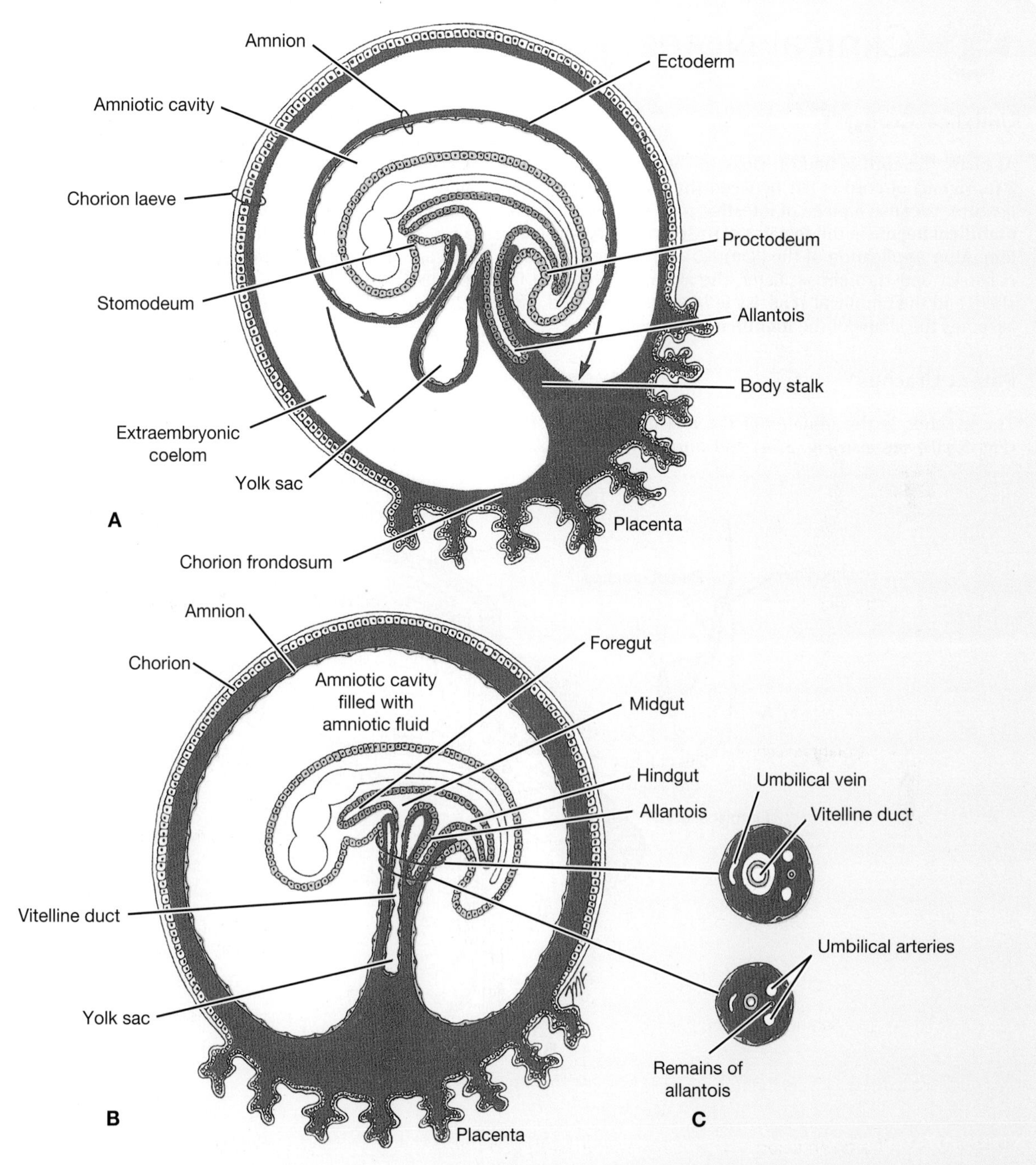

Figure 5.34 Formation of the umbilical cord. **A.** Early formation. **B.** Later formation. Note the expansion of the amniotic cavity (*arrows*) so that the cord becomes covered with amnion. **C.** Note that the umbilical vessels reduce to one vein and two arteries.

The umbilical vessels consist of two arteries that carry deoxygenated blood from the fetus to the chorion (later the placenta). The two umbilical veins convey oxygenated blood from the placenta to the fetus. The right vein soon disappears (see Fig. 5.34).

The umbilical cord is a twisted tortuous structure that measures about 0.75 in. (2 cm) in diameter. It increases in length until, at the end of pregnancy, it is about 20 in. (50 cm) long—that is, about the same length as the infant.

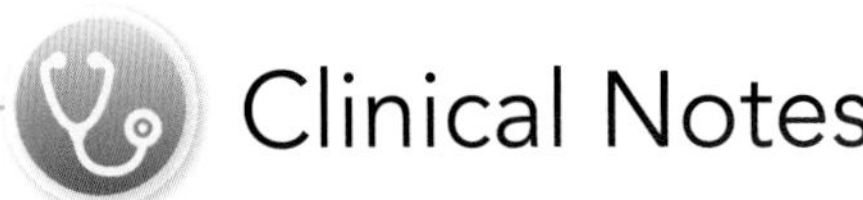

Clinical Notes

Umbilical Cord

At birth, the cord is tied off close to the umbilicus. About 2 in. (5 cm) of cord is left between the umbilicus and the ligature, because a piece of intestine may be present as an **umbilical hernia** in the remains of the extraembryonic coelom. After application of the ligature, the umbilical vessels constrict and thrombose. Later, the stump of the cord is shed, and the umbilical scar tissue becomes retracted and assumes the shape of the **umbilicus**, or **navel**.

Patent Urachus

The urachus is the remains of the **allantois** of the fetus (Fig. 5.35B; see also Fig. 5.34) and normally persists as a fibrous cord that runs from the apex of the bladder to the umbilicus. Occasionally, the cavity of the allantois persists, and urine passes from the bladder through the umbilicus onto the body surface (see Fig. 5.35A). In newborns, it usually reveals itself when a congenital urethral obstruction is present. More often, it remains undiscovered until old age, when enlargement of the prostate may obstruct the urethra.

Vitelline Duct

The vitelline duct connects the developing gut to the yolk sac in the early embryo (see Figs. 5.34 and 5.35B). As normal development proceeds, the duct is obliterated, severs its connection with the small intestine, and disappears.

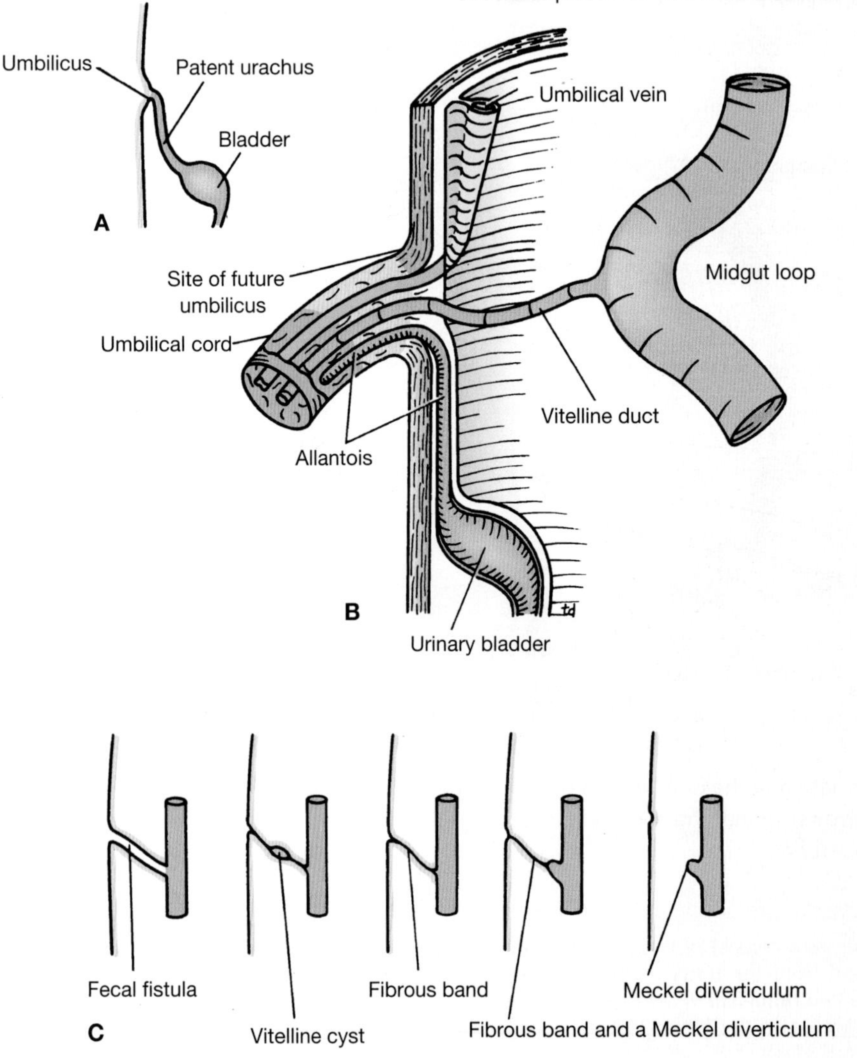

Figure 5.35 Umbilical relations. **A.** Patent urachus. **B.** Normal umbilical relations. **C.** Some common congenital defects.

Persistence of the **vitelline duct** can result in an **umbilical fecal fistula** (see Fig. 5.35C). If the duct remains as a fibrous band, a loop of bowel can become wrapped around it, causing intestinal obstruction.

Meckel's diverticulum is a congenital anomaly representing a persistent portion of the vitelline duct. It occurs in 2% of patients, is located on the antimesenteric side of the small intestine about 2 ft (61 cm) from the ileocolic junction and is about 2 in. (5 cm) long. It can become ulcerated or cause intestinal obstruction.

Umbilical Vessel Catheterization

The umbilical cord is surrounded by the fetal amnion membrane and contains Wharton's jelly. The remains of the vitelline duct and the allantois and the single umbilical vein and the two umbilical arteries are embedded in the jelly (Fig. 5.36). The vein is a larger thin-walled vessel and is located at the 12 o'clock position when facing the umbilicus. The two arteries, which lie adjacent to one another, are smaller and thick-walled and are located at the 4 and 8 o'clock positions when facing the umbilicus.

Indications for Umbilical Artery Catheterization

1. Administration of fluids or blood for resuscitation purposes.
2. Arterial blood gas and blood pressure monitoring. The umbilical arteries may be cannulated most easily during the first few hours after birth, but they may be cannulated up to 6 days after delivery.

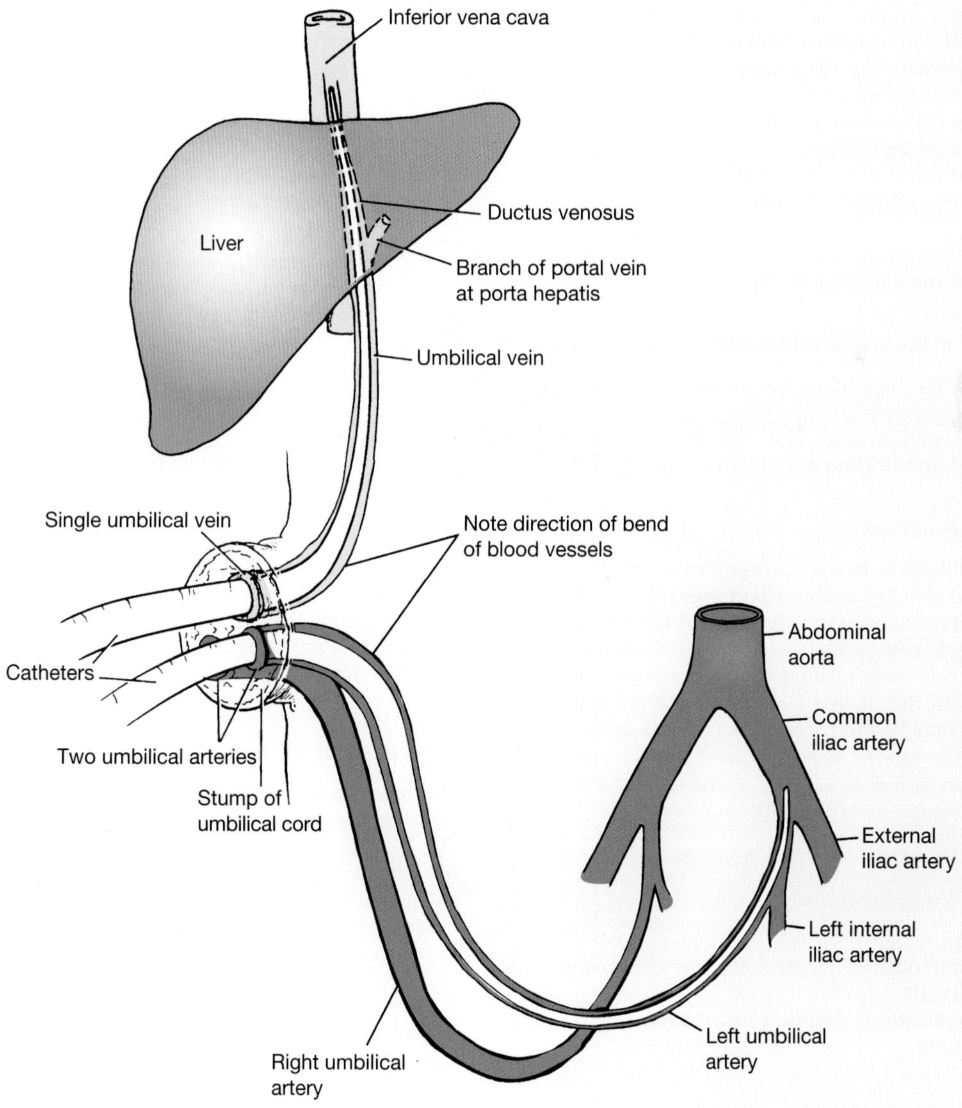

Figure 5.36 Catheterization of the umbilical blood vessels. Arrangement of the single umbilical vein and the two umbilical arteries in the umbilical cord and the paths taken by the catheter in the umbilical vein and the umbilical artery.

(continued)

Anatomy of Procedure

One of the small, thick-walled arteries is identified in Wharton's jelly in the umbilical stump. Because the umbilical arteries are branches of the internal iliac arteries in the pelvis, the catheter is introduced and advanced slowly in the direction of the feet. The catheter can be inserted for about 2.75 in. (7 cm) in a premature infant and 4.75 in. (12 cm) in a full-term infant. The course of the catheter can be confirmed on a radiograph and is as follows: (1) umbilical artery (directed downward into the pelvis), (2) internal iliac artery (acute turn into this artery), (3) common iliac artery, and (4) abdominal aorta.

Anatomy of Complications

- Catheter perforates the arterial wall at a point where the artery turns downward toward the pelvis at the anterior abdominal wall.
- Catheter enters the thin-walled wider umbilical vein instead of the thick-walled smaller artery.
- Catheter enters the thin-walled persistent urachus (urine is returned into catheter).
- Vasospasm of the umbilical and the iliac arteries occurs, causing blanching of the leg.
- Perforation of arteries distal to the umbilical artery occurs, for example, the iliac arteries or even the aorta.
- Other complications include thrombosis, emboli, and infection of the umbilical stump.

Indications for Umbilical Vein Catheterization

1. Administration of fluids or blood for resuscitation purposes.
2. Exchange transfusions. The umbilical vein may be cannulated up to 7 days after birth.

Anatomy of Procedure

The umbilical vein is in the cord stump at the 12 o'clock position (see Fig. 5.36), as described previously, and is easily recognized because of its thin wall and large lumen. The catheter is advanced gently and is directed toward the head because the vein runs in the free margin of the falciform ligament to join the ductus venosus at the porta hepatis. The catheter may be advanced about 2 in. (5 cm) in a full-term infant. The course of the catheter may be confirmed by radiography and is as follows: (1) the umbilical vein, (2) the ductus venosus, and (3) the inferior vena cava (4 to 4.75 in. [10 to 12 cm]).

Anatomy of Complications

- The catheter may perforate the venous wall. This is most likely to occur where the vein turns cranially at the abdominal wall.
- Other complications include liver necrosis, hemorrhage, and infection.

Abdominal Hernias

A hernia is the protrusion of part of the abdominal contents beyond the normal confines of the abdominal wall (Fig. 5.37). It consists of three parts: the **sac**, **contents of the sac**, and **coverings of the sac**. The hernial sac is a pouch (diverticulum) of peritoneum and has a **neck** and a **body**. The hernial contents may consist of any structure found within the abdominal cavity and may vary from a small piece of omentum to a large viscus such as the kidney. The hernial coverings are formed from the layers of the abdominal wall through which the hernial sac passes.

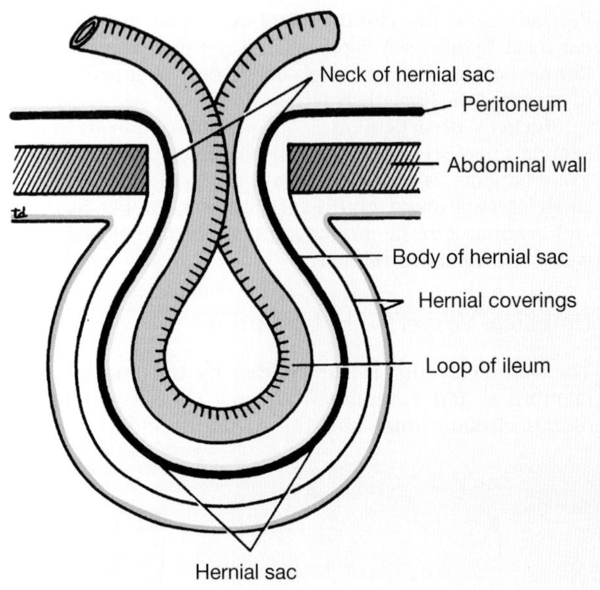

Figure 5.37 Different parts of a hernia.

The common types of abdominal hernias are:

- Inguinal (indirect or direct)
- Femoral
- Umbilical (congenital or acquired)
- Epigastric
- Separation of the recti abdominis
- Incisional
- Hernia of the linea semilunaris (spigelian hernia)
- Lumbar (Petit's triangle hernia)
- Internal

Indirect Inguinal Hernia

The indirect inguinal hernia is the most common form of hernia and is believed to be congenital in origin (Fig. 5.38A). The hernial sac is the remains of the processus vaginalis (an outpouching of peritoneum that in the fetus is responsible for the formation of the inguinal canal [see the earlier description of the development of the inguinal canal]). It follows that the sac enters the inguinal canal through the deep inguinal ring **lateral** to the inferior epigastric vessels. It may extend part of the way along the canal or the full length, as far as the superficial inguinal ring. If the processus vaginalis has not undergone obliteration, the hernia is complete and extends through the superficial inguinal ring down into the scrotum or labium majus. Under these circumstances, the neck of the hernial sac lies at the deep inguinal ring lateral to the inferior epigastric vessels, and the body of the sac resides in the inguinal canal and scrotum (or base of labium majus).

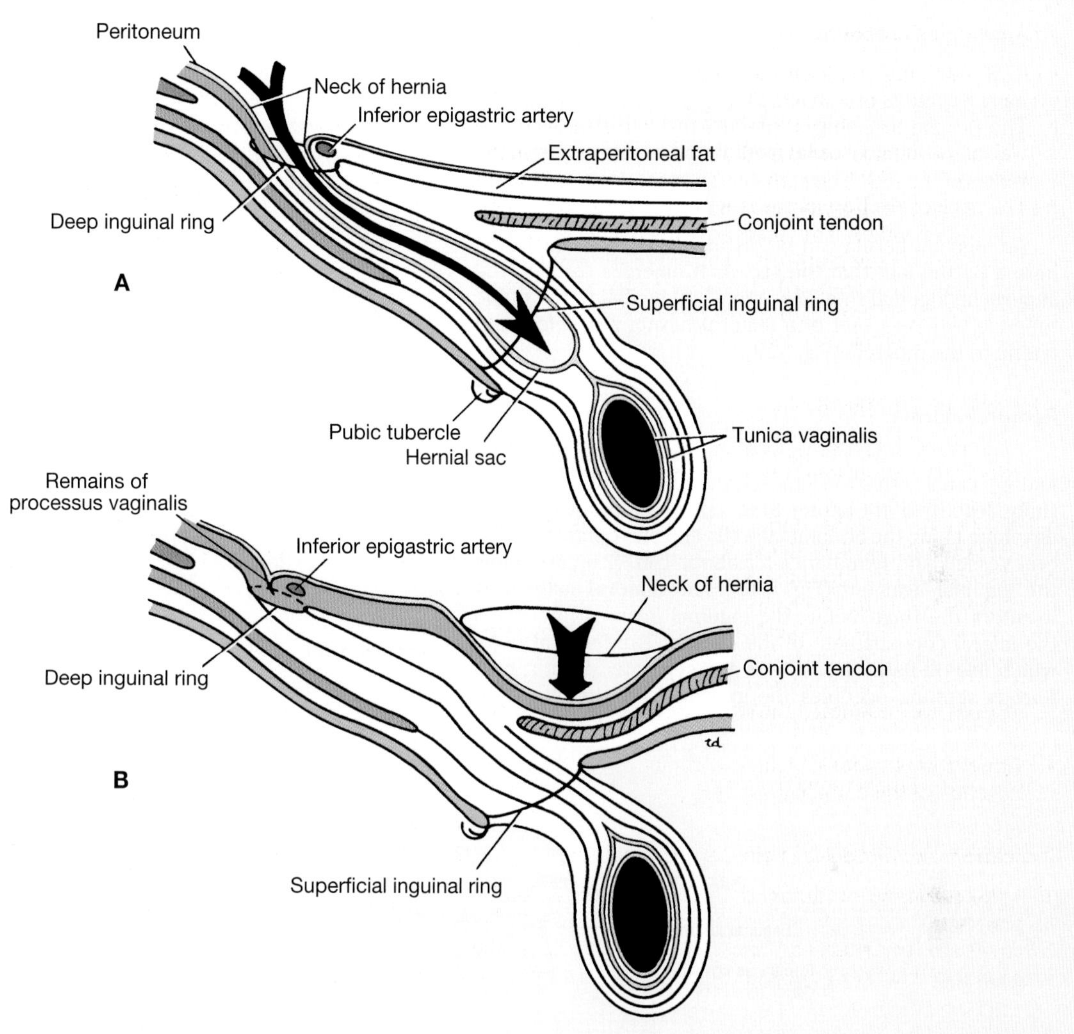

Figure 5.38 Inguinal hernias. **A.** Indirect inguinal hernia. **B.** Direct inguinal hernia. Note that the neck of the indirect inguinal hernia lies lateral to the inferior epigastric artery and the neck of the direct inguinal hernia lies medial to the inferior epigastric artery.

An indirect inguinal hernia is about 20 times more common in males than in females, and nearly one-third are bilateral. It is more common on the right (normally, the right processus vaginalis becomes obliterated after the left; the right testis descends later than the left). It is most common in children and young adults.

The indirect inguinal hernia can be summarized as follows:

- It is the remains of the processus vaginalis and therefore is congenital in origin.
- It is more common than a direct inguinal hernia.
- It is much more common in males than females.
- It is more common on the right side.
- It is most common in children and young adults.
- The hernial sac enters the inguinal canal through the deep inguinal ring and **lateral** to the inferior epigastric vessels. The neck of the sac is narrow.
- The hernial sac may extend through the superficial inguinal ring above and **medial** to the pubic tubercle. (Femoral hernia is located below and lateral to the pubic tubercle.)
- The hernial sac may extend down into the scrotum or labium majus.

Direct Inguinal Hernia

The direct inguinal hernia makes up about 15% of all inguinal hernias. The sac of a direct hernia bulges directly anteriorly through the posterior wall of the inguinal canal **medial** to the inferior epigastric vessels (see Fig. 5.38B). Because of the presence of the strong conjoint tendon (combined tendons of insertion of the internal oblique and transversus muscles), this hernia is usually nothing more than a generalized bulge; therefore, the neck of the hernial sac is wide.

Direct inguinal hernias are rare in females, and most are bilateral. It is a disease of older adult males with weak abdominal muscles.

(continued)

A direct inguinal hernia can be summarized as follows:

- It is common in older males with weak abdominal muscles and is rare in females.
- The hernial sac bulges forward through the posterior wall of the inguinal canal **medial** to the inferior epigastric vessels.
- The neck of the hernial sac is wide.

An inguinal hernia can be distinguished from a femoral hernia by the fact that the sac, as it emerges through the superficial inguinal ring, lies above and medial to the pubic tubercle, whereas that of a femoral hernia lies below and lateral to the tubercle (Fig. 5.39).

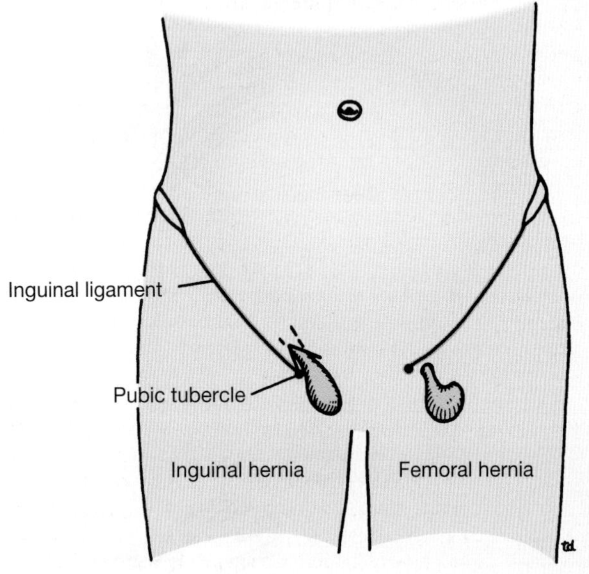

Figure 5.39 Relation of inguinal and femoral hernial sacs to the pubic tubercle.

Femoral Hernia

In a femoral hernia, the hernial sac descends through the femoral canal within the femoral sheath. The femoral sheath (fully described in Chapter 8) is a protrusion of the fascial envelope lining the abdominal walls and surrounds the femoral vessels and lymphatics for about 1 in. (2.5 cm) below the inguinal ligament (Fig. 5.40). The **femoral artery**, as it enters the thigh below the inguinal ligament, occupies the lateral compartment of the sheath. The **femoral vein**, which lies on its medial side and is separated from it by a fibrous septum, occupies the intermediate compartment.

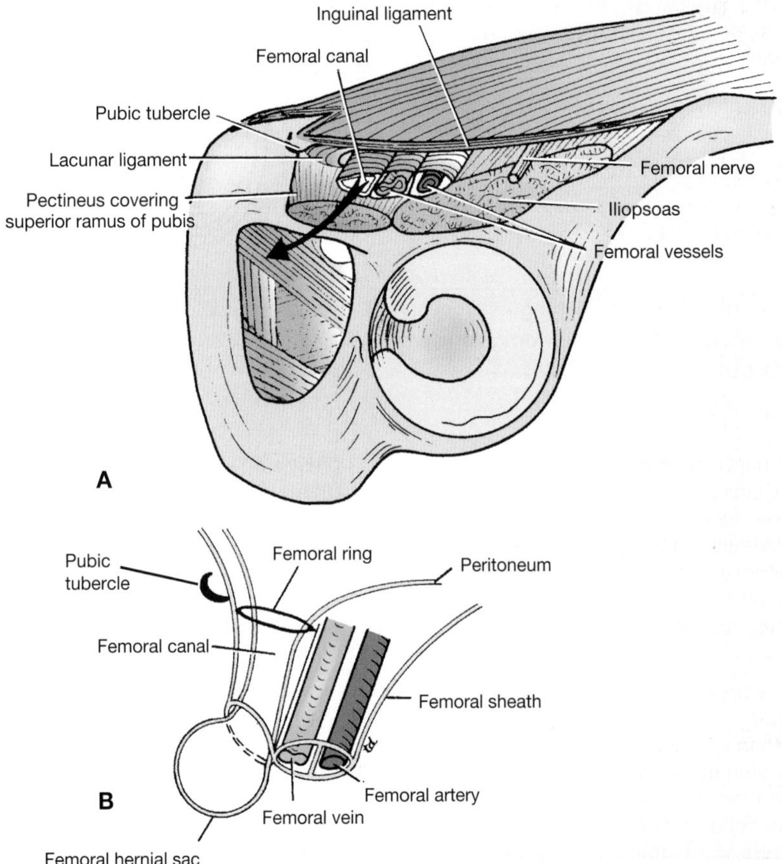

Figure 5.40 Femoral hernia. **A.** The femoral sheath as can be seen from below. *Arrow* emerging from the femoral canal indicates the path taken by the femoral hernial sac. **B.** Note relations of the femoral ring and canal to the hernia.

The **lymph vessels**, which are separated from the vein by a fibrous septum, occupy the most medial compartment. The **femoral canal**, the compartment for the lymphatics, occupies the medial part of the sheath. It is about 0.5 in. (1.3 cm) long, and its upper opening is referred to as the **femoral ring**. The **femoral septum**, which is a condensation of extraperitoneal tissue, plugs the opening of the femoral ring.

A femoral hernia is more common in females than males (possibly because of a wider pelvis and femoral canal). The hernial sac passes down the femoral canal, pushing the femoral septum before it. On escaping through the lower end, it expands to form a swelling in the upper part of the thigh deep to the deep fascia (see Fig. 5.40). With further expansion, the hernial sac may turn upward to cross the anterior surface of the inguinal ligament.

The neck of the sac always lies **below** and **lateral** to the **pubic tubercle** (see Fig. 5.39), which serves to distinguish it from an inguinal hernia. The neck of the sac is narrow and lies at the femoral ring. The ring is related anteriorly to the inguinal ligament, posteriorly to the pectineal ligament and the pubis, medially to the sharp free edge of the lacunar ligament, and laterally to the femoral vein. Because of the presence of these anatomic structures, the neck of the sac is unable to expand. Once an abdominal viscus has passed through the neck into the body of the sac, it may be difficult to push it up and return it to the abdominal cavity (**irreducible hernia**). Furthermore, after straining or coughing, a piece of bowel may be forced through the neck, and the femoral ring may compress its blood vessels, seriously impairing its blood supply (**strangulated hernia**). A femoral hernia is a dangerous disease and should always be treated surgically.

A femoral hernia can be summarized as follows:

- It is a protrusion of abdominal parietal peritoneum down through the femoral canal to form the hernial sac.
- It is more common in females than in males.
- The neck of the hernial sac lies below and lateral to the pubic tubercle.
- The neck of the hernial sac lies at the femoral ring and at that point is related anteriorly to the inguinal ligament, posteriorly to the pectineal ligament and the pubis, laterally to the femoral vein, and medially to the sharp free edge of the lacunar ligament.

Umbilical Hernias

Congenital umbilical hernia, or exomphalos (omphalocele), is caused by a failure of part of the midgut to return to the abdominal cavity from the extraembryonic coelom during fetal life. The hernial sac and its relationship to the umbilical cord are shown in Figure 5.41A.

Acquired infantile umbilical hernia is a small hernia that sometimes occurs in children and is caused by a weakness in the scar of the umbilicus in the linea alba (see Fig. 5.41B). Most become smaller and disappear without treatment as the abdominal cavity enlarges.

Acquired umbilical hernia of adults is more correctly referred to as a **paraumbilical hernia** (see Fig. 5.41C). The hernial sac does not protrude through the umbilical scar, but through the linea alba in the region of the umbilicus. Paraumbilical hernias gradually increase in size and hang downward. The neck of the sac may be narrow, but the body of the sac often contains coils of small and large intestines and omentum. Paraumbilical hernias are much more common in women than in men.

Epigastric Hernia

Epigastric hernia occurs through the widest part of the linea alba, anywhere between the xiphoid process and the umbilicus (see Fig. 5.41D). The hernia is usually small and starts off as a small protrusion of extraperitoneal fat between the fibers of the linea alba. During the following months or years, the fat is forced farther through the linea alba and eventually drags behind it a small peritoneal sac. The body of the sac often contains a small piece of greater omentum. It is common in middle-age manual workers.

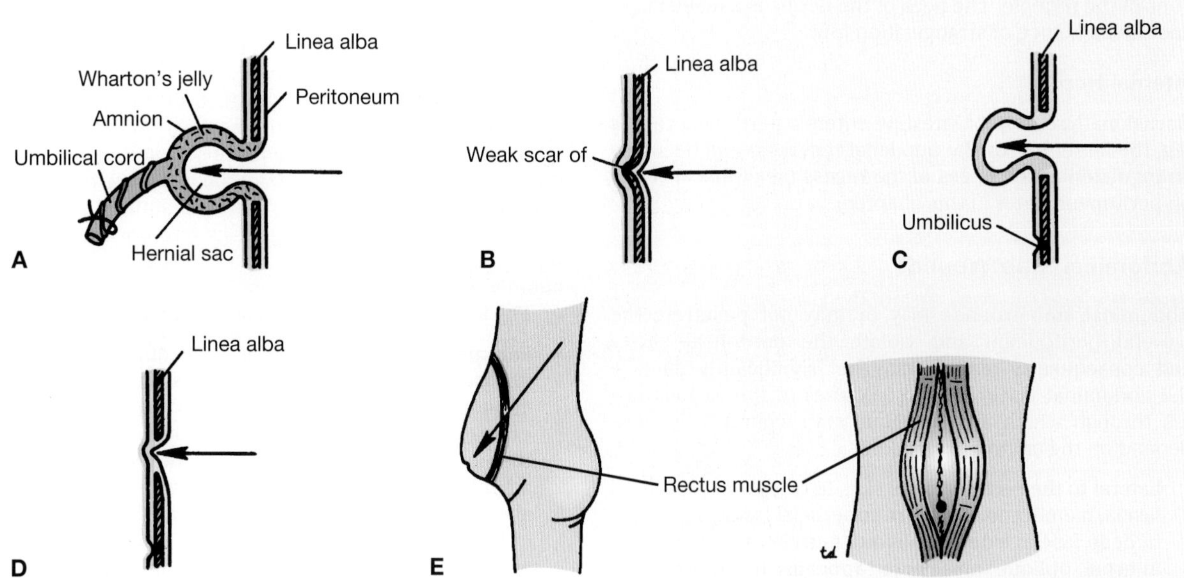

Figure 5.41 Various forms of abdominal hernias. **A.** Congenital umbilical hernia. **B.** Infantile umbilical hernia. **C.** Paraumbilical hernia. **D.** Epigastric hernia. **E.** Lateral and anterior views of separation of the rectus abdominis.

(continued)

Separation of the Recti Abdominis

Separation of the recti abdominis usually occurs in elderly multiparous females with weak abdominal muscles (see Fig. 5.41E). In this condition, the aponeuroses forming the rectus sheath become excessively stretched. When the patient coughs or strains, the recti separate widely, and a large hernial sac, containing abdominal viscera, bulges forward between the medial margins of the recti. This can be corrected by wearing a suitable abdominal belt.

Incisional Hernia

A postoperative incisional hernia is most likely to occur in patients in whom it was necessary to cut one of the segmental nerves supplying the muscles of the anterior abdominal wall. Postoperative wound infection with death (necrosis) of the abdominal musculature is also a common cause. The neck of the sac is usually large, and adhesion and strangulation of its contents are rare complications. In very obese individuals, the extent of the abdominal wall weakness is often difficult to assess.

Linea Semilunaris Hernia (Spigelian Hernia)

The uncommon hernia of the linea semilunaris occurs through the aponeurosis of the transversus abdominis just lateral to the lateral edge of the rectus sheath. It usually occurs just below the level of the umbilicus. The neck of the sac is narrow, so that adhesion and strangulation of its contents are common complications.

Lumbar Hernia

The lumbar hernia occurs through the lumbar triangle and is rare. The lumbar triangle (Petit's triangle) is a weak area in the posterior part of the abdominal wall. It is bounded anteriorly by the posterior margin of the external oblique muscle, posteriorly by the anterior border of the latissimus dorsi muscle, and inferiorly by the iliac crest. The internal oblique and the transversus abdominis muscles form the floor of the triangle. The neck of the hernia is usually large, and the incidence of strangulation low.

Internal Hernia

Occasionally, a loop of intestine enters a peritoneal recess (eg, the lesser sac or the duodenal recesses) and becomes strangulated at the edges of the recess (see Clinical Notes on peritoneum later in this chapter).

Abdominal Stab Wounds

Abdominal stab wounds may or may not penetrate the parietal peritoneum and violate the peritoneal cavity and consequently may or may not significantly damage the abdominal viscera. The structures in the various layers through which an abdominal stab wound penetrates depend on the anatomic location.

- **Lateral to the rectus sheath:** skin, fatty layer of superficial fascia, membranous layer of superficial fascia, thin layer of deep fascia, external oblique muscle or aponeurosis, internal oblique muscle or aponeurosis, transversus abdominis muscle or aponeurosis, transversalis fascia, extraperitoneal connective tissue (often fatty), and parietal peritoneum.
- **Anterior to the rectus sheath:** skin, fatty layer of superficial fascia, membranous layer of superficial fascia, thin layer of deep fascia, anterior wall of rectus sheath, rectus abdominis muscle with segmental nerves and epigastric vessels lying behind the muscle, posterior wall of rectus sheath, transversalis fascia, extraperitoneal connective tissue (often fatty), and parietal peritoneum.
- **In the midline:** skin, fatty layer of superficial fascia, membranous layer of superficial fascia, thin layer of deep fascia, fibrous linea alba, transversalis fascia, extraperitoneal connective tissue (often fatty), and parietal peritoneum.

In an abdominal stab wound, washing out the peritoneal cavity with saline solution (**peritoneal lavage**) can be used to determine whether any damage to viscera or blood vessels has occurred.

Abdominal Gunshot Wounds

Gunshot wounds are much more serious than stab wounds. In most patients, the peritoneal cavity has been penetrated, causing significant visceral damage.

Surgical Incisions

The length and direction of surgical incisions through the anterior abdominal wall to expose the underlying viscera are largely governed by the position and direction of the nerves of the abdominal wall, the direction of the muscle fibers, and the arrangement of the aponeuroses forming the rectus sheath. Ideally, the incision should be made in the direction of the lines of cleavage in the skin so that only a hairline scar is produced. The surgeon sometimes must compromise, placing the safety of the patient first and the cosmetic result second.

Incisions that necessitate the division of one of the main segmental nerves lying within the abdominal wall result in paralysis of part of the anterior abdominal musculature and a segment of the rectus abdominis. The consequent weakness of the abdominal musculature causes the abdominal wall to bulge forward (**visceroptosis**). Extreme cases may require a surgical belt for support.

If the incision can be made in the line of the muscle fibers or aponeurotic fibers as each layer is traversed, on closing the incision the fibers fall back into position and function normally.

Incisions through the rectus sheath are widely used, provided that the rectus abdominis muscle and its nerve supply are kept intact. On closure of the incisions, the anterior and posterior walls of the sheath are sutured separately, and the rectus muscle springs back into position between the suture lines. The result is a very strong repair, with minimum interference with function.

The following incisions are commonly used.

- **Paramedian incision:** This may be supraumbilical, for exposure of the upper part of the abdominal cavity, or infraumbilical, for the lower abdomen and pelvis. In extensive operations in which a large exposure is required, the incision can run the full length of the rectus sheath. The anterior wall of the rectus sheath is exposed and incised about 1 in. (2.5 cm) from the midline. The medial edge of the incision is dissected medially, freeing the anterior wall of the sheath from the tendinous intersections of the rectus muscle. The rectus abdominis muscle is retracted laterally with its nerve supply intact, and the posterior wall of the sheath is exposed. The posterior wall is then incised, together with the transversalis fascia and the peritoneum. The wound is closed in layers.

- **Pararectus incision:** The anterior wall of the rectus sheath is incised medially and parallel to the lateral margin of the rectus muscle. The rectus is freed and retracted medially, exposing the segmental nerves entering its posterior surface. If the opening into the abdominal cavity is to be small, these nerves may be retracted upward and downward. The posterior wall of the sheath is then incised, as in the paramedian incision. The great disadvantage of this incision is that the opening is small, and any longitudinal extension requires that one or more segmental nerves to the rectus abdominis be divided, with resultant postoperative rectus muscle weakness.
- **Midline incision:** This incision is made through the linea alba. The transversalis fascia, the extraperitoneal connective tissue, and the peritoneum are then incised. It is easier to perform above the umbilicus because the linea alba is wider in that region. It is a rapid method of gaining entrance to the abdomen and has the obvious advantage that it does not damage muscles or their nerve and blood supplies. Midline incision has the additional advantage that it may be converted into a T-shaped incision for greater exposure. The anterior and posterior walls of the rectus sheath are then cut across transversely, and the rectus muscle is retracted laterally.
- **Transrectus incision:** The technique of making and closing of this incision is the same as that used in the paramedian incision, except that the rectus abdominis muscle is incised longitudinally and not retracted laterally from the midline. This incision has the great disadvantage of sectioning the nerve supply to that part of the muscle that lies medial to the muscle incision.
- **Transverse incision:** This can be made above or below the umbilicus and can be small or so large that it extends from flank to flank. It can be made through the rectus sheath and the rectus abdominis muscles and through the oblique and transversus abdominis muscles laterally. It is rare to damage more than one segmental nerve so that postoperative abdominal weakness is minimal. The incision gives good exposure and is well tolerated by the patient. Closure of the wound is made in layers. It is unnecessary to suture the cut ends of the rectus muscles, provided that the sheaths are carefully repaired.
- **Muscle splitting (McBurney's incision):** This is chiefly used for cecostomy and appendectomy. It gives limited exposure, and, if any doubt arises about the diagnosis, an infraumbilical right paramedian incision should be used instead. An oblique skin incision is made in the right iliac region about 2 in. (5 cm) above and medial to the anterior superior iliac spine. The external and internal oblique and transversus muscles are incised or split in the line of their fibers and retracted to expose the transversalis fascia and the peritoneum. The latter are now incised, and the abdominal cavity is opened. The incision is closed in layers, with no postoperative weakness.
- **Abdominothoracic incision:** This is used to expose the lower end of the esophagus, as, for example, in esophagogastric resection for carcinoma of this region. An upper oblique or paramedian abdominal incision is extended upward and laterally into the seventh, eighth, or ninth intercostal space, the costal arch is transected, and the diaphragm is incised. Wide exposure of the upper abdomen and thorax is then obtained using a rib-spreading retractor. On completion of the operation, the diaphragm is repaired with nonabsorbable sutures, the costal margin is reconstructed, and the abdominal and thoracic wounds are closed.

Abdominal Paracentesis

Paracentesis of the abdomen may be necessary to withdraw excessive collections of peritoneal fluid, as in ascites secondary to cirrhosis of the liver or malignant ascites secondary to advanced ovarian cancer. Under a local anesthetic, a needle or catheter is inserted through the anterior abdominal wall. The underlying coils of intestine are not damaged because they are mobile and are pushed away by the cannula.

If the cannula is inserted in the midline (Fig. 5.42), it will pass through the following anatomic structures: skin, superficial fascia, deep fascia (very thin), linea alba (virtually bloodless), transversalis fascia, extraperitoneal connective tissue (fatty), and parietal peritoneum.

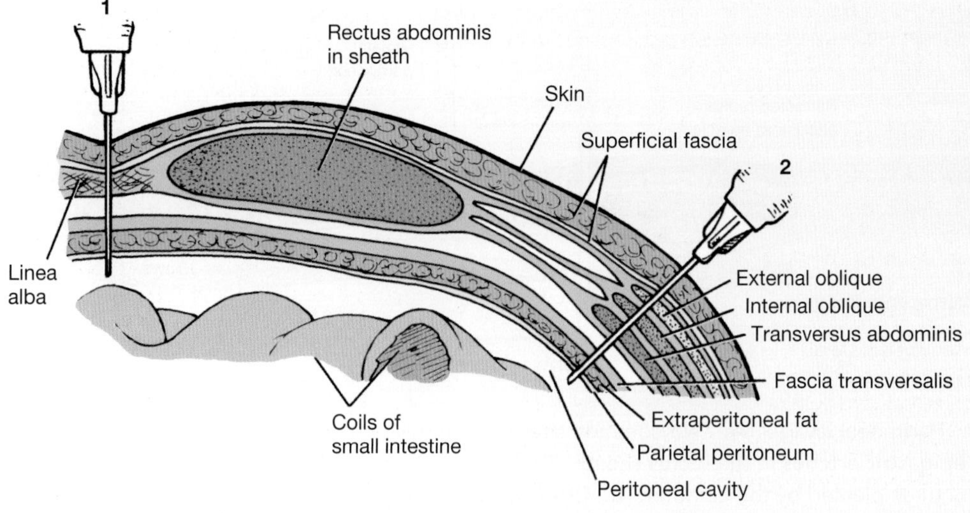

Figure 5.42 Paracentesis of the abdominal cavity in midline (1) and laterally (2).

(continued)

If the cannula is inserted in the flank lateral to the inferior epigastric artery and above the deep circumflex artery, it will pass through the following: skin, superficial fascia, deep fascia (very thin), aponeurosis or muscle of external oblique, internal oblique muscle, transversus abdominis muscle, transversalis fascia, extraperitoneal connective tissue (fatty), and parietal peritoneum.

Anatomy of Peritoneal Lavage

Peritoneal lavage is used to sample the intraperitoneal space for evidence of damage to viscera and blood vessels. It is generally employed as a diagnostic technique in certain cases of blunt abdominal trauma. In nontraumatic situations, peritoneal lavage has been used to confirm the diagnosis of acute pancreatitis and primary peritonitis, to correct hypothermia, and to conduct dialysis.

The patient is placed in the supine position, and the urinary bladder is emptied by catheterization. In small children, the bladder is an abdominal organ (see Chapter 6). In adults, the full bladder may rise out of the pelvis and reach as high as the umbilicus. The stomach is emptied by a nasogastric tube because a distended stomach may extend to the anterior abdominal wall. The skin is anesthetized, and a 2.25 in. (3 cm) vertical incision is made.

Midline Incision Technique

The following anatomic structures are penetrated, in order, to reach the parietal peritoneum (Fig. 5.43B): skin, fatty

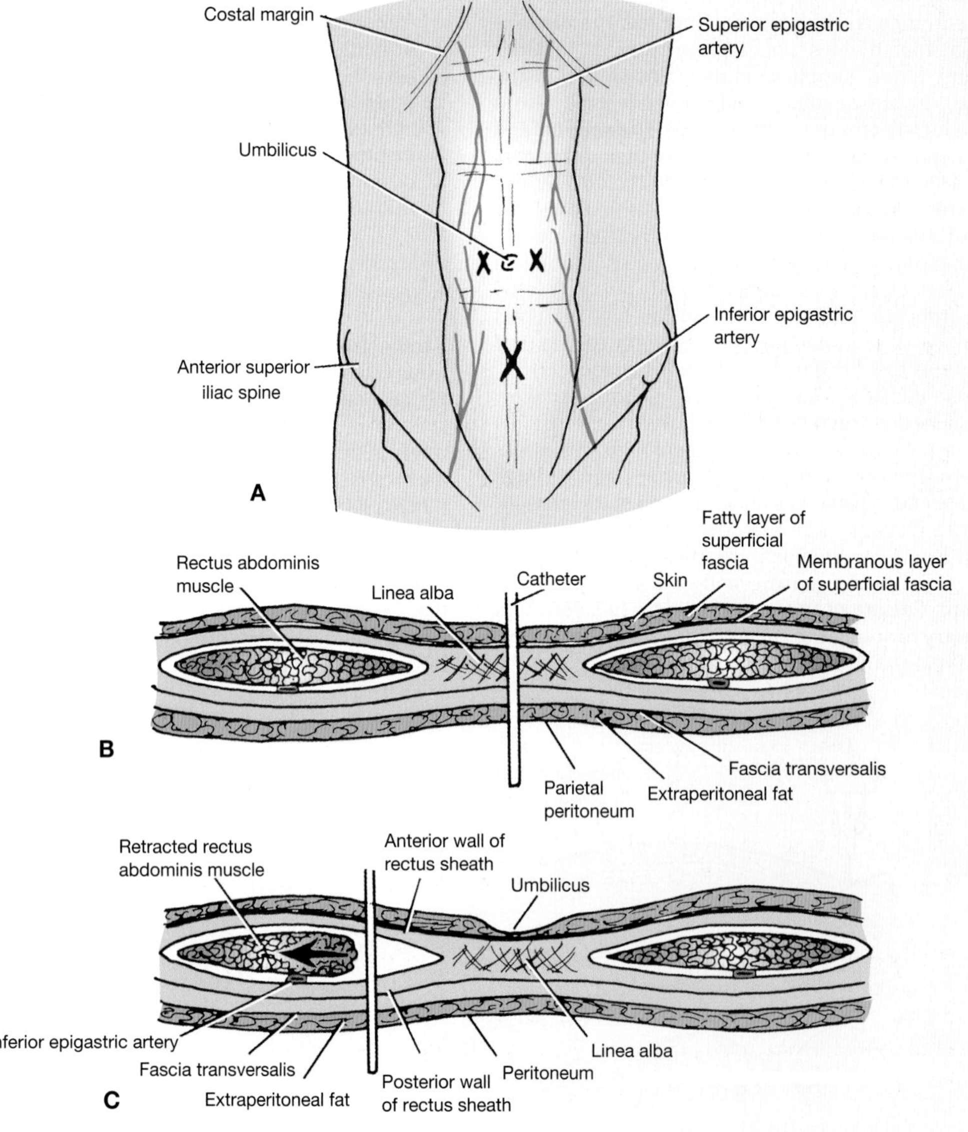

Figure 5.43 Peritoneal lavage. **A.** Two common sites used in this procedure. Note the positions of the superior and inferior epigastric arteries in the rectus sheath. **B.** Cross section of the anterior abdominal wall in the midline. Note the structures pierced by the catheter. **C.** Cross section of the anterior abdominal wall just lateral to the umbilicus. Note the structures pierced by the catheter. The rectus muscle has been retracted laterally.

layer of superficial fascia, membranous layer of superficial fascia, thin layer of deep fascia, linea alba, transversalis fascia, extraperitoneal fat, and parietal peritoneum.

Paraumbilical Incision Technique

The following anatomic structures are penetrated, in order, to reach the parietal peritoneum (see Fig. 5.43C): skin, fatty layer of superficial fascia, membranous layer of superficial fascia, thin layer of deep fascia, anterior wall of rectus sheath, the rectus abdominis muscle (retracted), posterior wall of the rectus sheath, transversalis fascia, extraperitoneal fat, and parietal peritoneum.

It is important that all the small blood vessels in the superficial fascia be secured, because bleeding into the peritoneal cavity might produce a false-positive result. These vessels are the terminal branches of the superficial and deep epigastric arteries and veins.

Anatomy of Complications

- In the midline technique, the incision or trocar may miss the linea alba, enter the rectus sheath, traverse the vascular rectus abdominis muscle, and encounter branches of the epigastric vessels. Bleeding from this source could produce a false-positive result.
- Perforation of the gut by the scalpel or trocar.
- Perforation of the mesenteric blood vessels or vessels on the posterior abdominal wall or pelvic walls.
- Perforation of a full bladder.
- Wound infection.

Endoscopic Surgery

Endoscopic surgery on the gallbladder, bile ducts, and the appendix has become a common procedure. It involves the passage of the endoscope into the peritoneal cavity through small incisions in the anterior abdominal wall. The anatomic structures traversed by the instruments are like those enumerated for peritoneal lavage. Great care must be taken to preserve the integrity of the segmental nerves as they course down from the costal margin to supply the abdominal musculature.

The advantages of this surgical technique are that the anatomic and physiologic features of the anterior abdominal wall are only minimally disrupted, making convalescence brief. The great disadvantages are that the surgical field is small, and the surgeon is limited in the extent of the operation (Fig. 5.44).

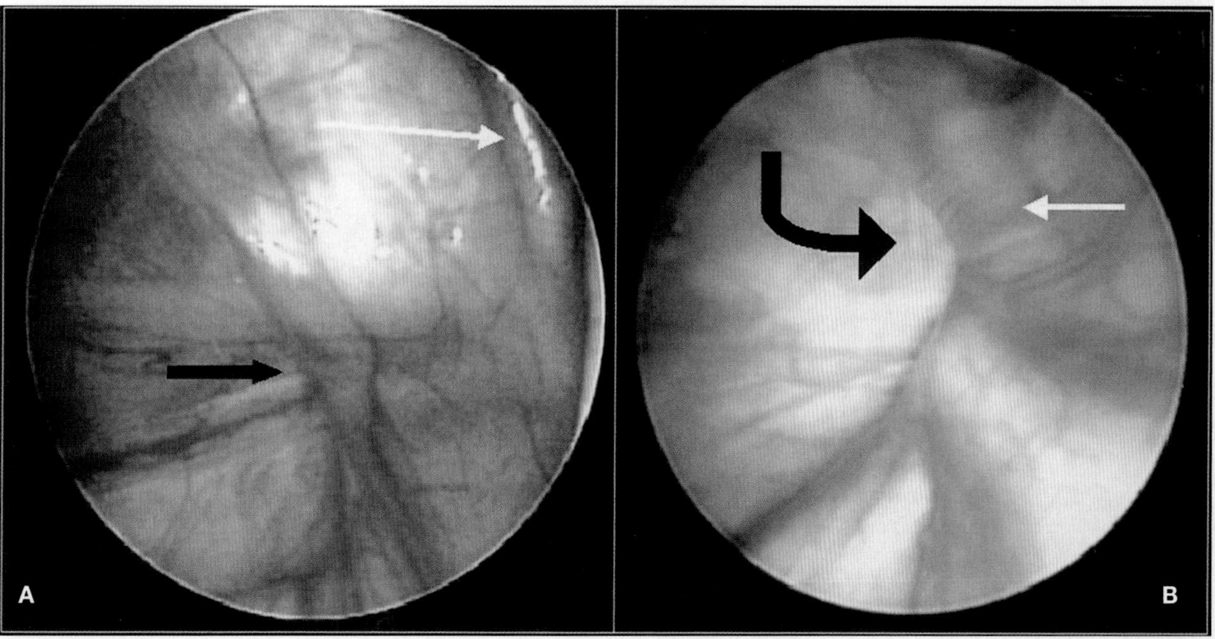

Figure 5.44 Inguinal canal anatomy as viewed during laparoscopic exploration of the peritoneal cavity. **A.** Normal anatomy of the inguinal region from within the peritoneal cavity. *Black arrow* indicates the closed deep inguinal ring; *white arrow* indicates the inferior epigastric vessels. **B.** Indirect inguinal hernia. *Curved black arrow* indicates the mouth of the hernial sac; *white arrow* indicates the inferior epigastric vessels. (Courtesy of N. S. Adzick.)

ABDOMINAL ORGANS OVERVIEW

The abdominal cavity contains many vital organs, including the gastrointestinal (GI) tract, liver, biliary ducts, pancreas, spleen, and parts of the urinary system. These structures are closely packed within the abdominal cavity. Therefore, disease of one can easily involve another. GI tract inflammation and bleeding, malignant disease, and penetrating trauma to the abdomen are just some of the problems facing the clinician. Emergency problems involving the urinary system are common and may present diverse symptoms ranging from excruciating pain to failure to void urine. The aorta and its branches, the inferior vena cava and its tributaries, and the portal vein also lie within the abdomen.

Liver

The liver is a large, highly vascularized organ that occupies the upper part of the abdominal cavity (Figs. 5.45 to 5.47). It lies almost entirely under the cover of the ribs and costal cartilages and extends across the epigastric region.

Gallbladder

The gallbladder is a pear-shaped sac that adheres to the undersurface of the right lobe of the liver. Its blind end, or fundus, projects below the inferior border of the liver (see Figs. 5.45 and 5.46).

Esophagus

The esophagus is a tubular structure that joins the pharynx to the stomach. The esophagus pierces the diaphragm slightly to the left of the midline and after a short course of about 0.5 in. (1.25 cm) enters the stomach on its right side. It is deeply placed, lying behind the left lobe of the liver (see Fig. 5.45).

Stomach

The stomach is a dilated part of the alimentary canal between the esophagus and the small intestine (see Figs. 5.45 and 5.47). It occupies the left upper quadrant, epigastric, and umbilical regions, and much of it lies under cover of the ribs. Its long axis passes downward and forward to the right and then backward and slightly upward.

Small Intestine

The small intestine is termed "small" because of its comparative diameter and not because of its length. It is divided into three regions: duodenum, jejunum, and ileum. The **duodenum** is the first part of the small intestine, and most of it is deeply placed on the posterior abdominal wall. It is situated in the epigastric and umbilical regions. It is a C-shaped tube that extends from the stomach around the head of the pancreas to join the jejunum (see Fig. 5.45). About halfway down its length, the duodenum receives the bile and the pancreatic ducts.

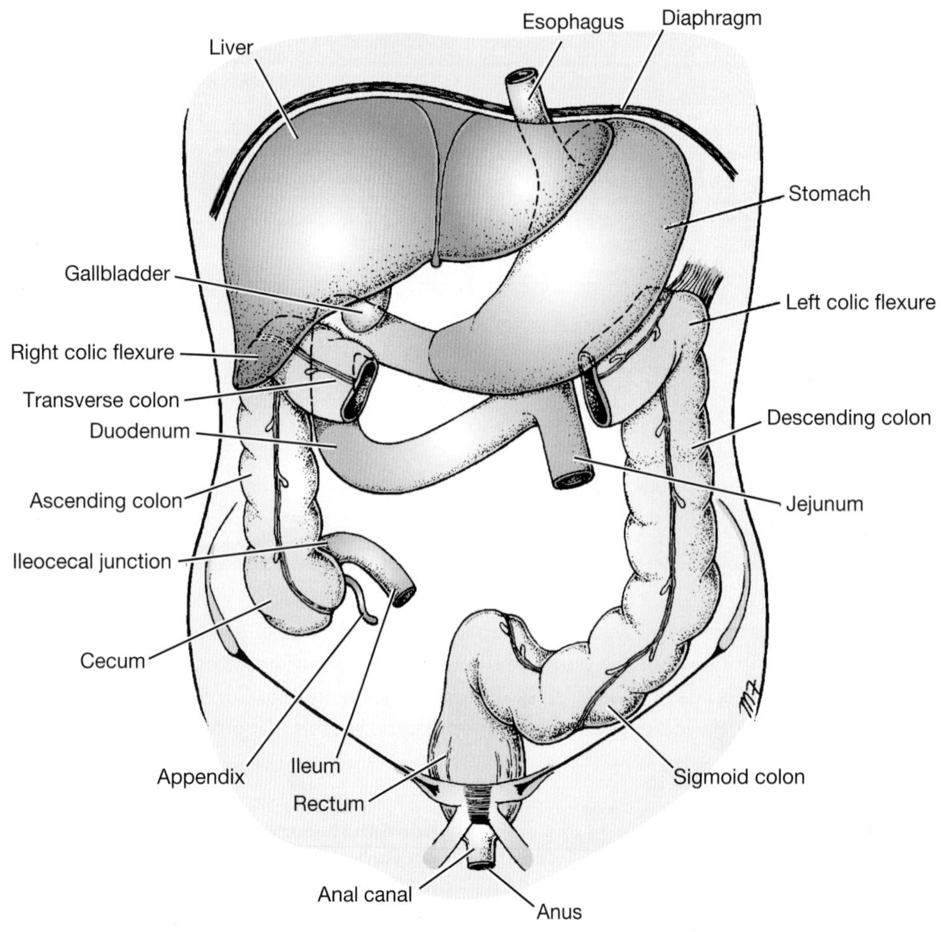

Figure 5.45 General arrangement of abdominal viscera.

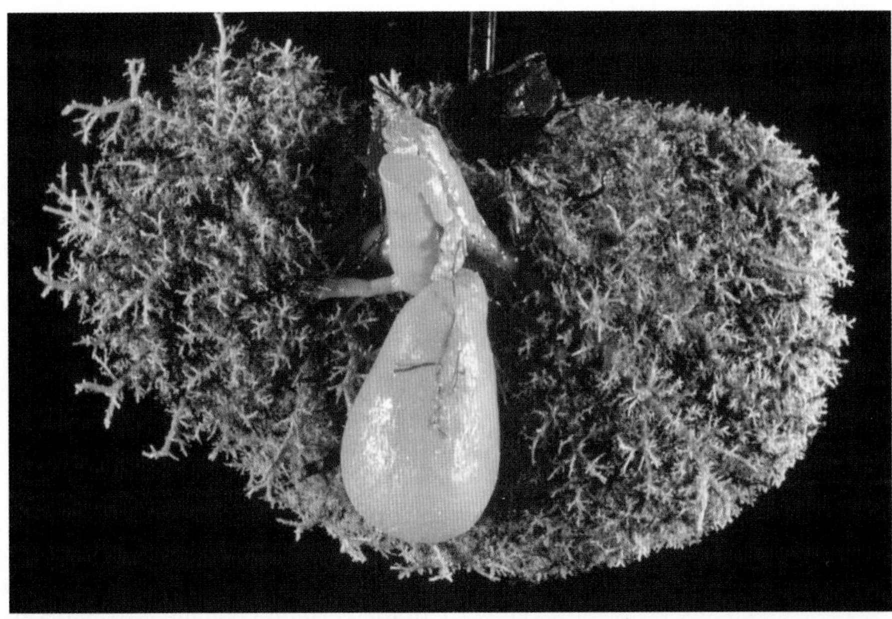

Figure 5.46 Plastinated specimen of the liver as can be seen on its posteroinferior (visceral) surface. The portal vein has been transfused with *white plastic* and the inferior vena cava with *dark blue plastic*. Outside the liver, the distended biliary ducts and gallbladder have been injected with *yellow plastic* and the hepatic artery with *red plastic*. The liver was then immersed in corrosive fluid to remove the liver tissue. Note the profuse branching of the portal vein as its white terminal branches enter the portal canals between the liver lobules; the *dark blue* tributaries of many of the hepatic veins can also be seen.

The jejunum and ileum together measure about 20 ft (6 m) long. The jejunum makes up the upper two fifths of this length. The **jejunum** begins at the duodenojejunal junction, and the **ileum** ends at the ileocecal junction. The coils of jejunum occupy mainly the upper left part of the abdominal cavity, whereas the ileum tends to occupy the lower right part of the abdominal cavity and the pelvic cavity (Fig. 5.48).

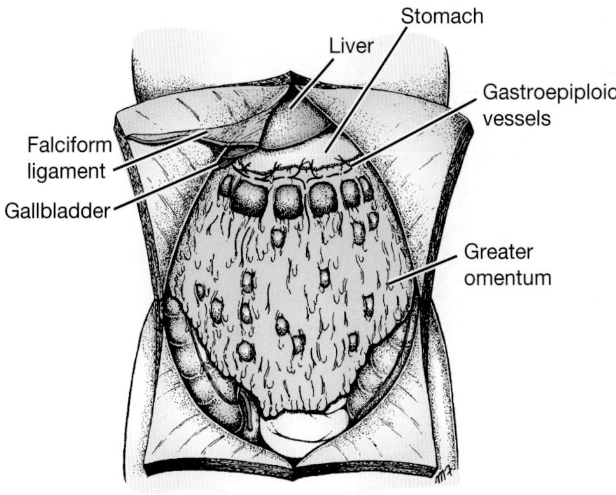

Figure 5.47 Abdominal organs in situ. Note that the greater omentum hangs down in front of the small and large intestines.

Large Intestine

The large intestine is termed "large" because of its comparative diameter and not because of its length. It is divided into the cecum, appendix, ascending colon, transverse colon, descending colon, sigmoid colon,

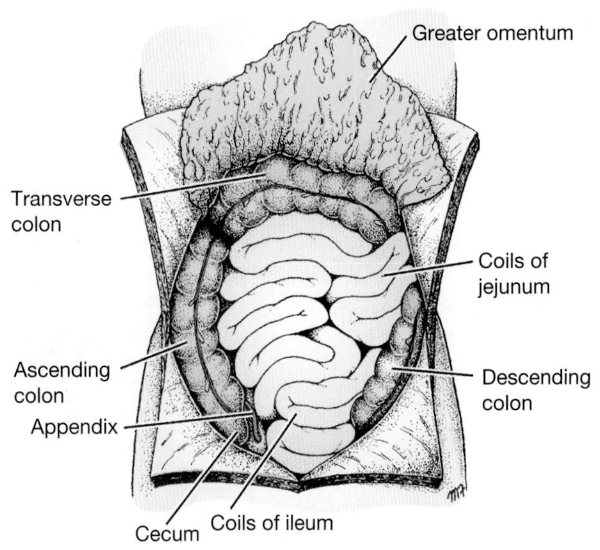

Figure 5.48 Abdominal contents after the greater omentum have been reflected upward. Coils of the small intestine occupy the central part of the abdominal cavity, whereas ascending, transverse, and descending parts of the colon are located at the periphery.

rectum, and anal canal (see Fig. 5.45). The large intestine arches around and encloses the coils of the small intestine (see Fig. 5.48) and tends to be more fixed than the small intestine.

The **cecum** is a blind-ended sac that projects downward in the right iliac region below the ileocecal junction (see Figs. 5.45 and 5.48). The **appendix** (**vermiform appendix**) is a worm-shaped tube that arises from its medial side (see Fig. 5.45).

The **ascending colon** extends upward from the cecum to the inferior surface of the right lobe of the liver, occupying the right lower and upper quadrants (see Figs. 5.45 and 5.48). On reaching the liver, it bends to the left, forming the **right colic (hepatic) flexure**.

The **transverse colon** crosses the abdomen in the umbilical region from the right colic flexure to the left colic flexure. It forms a wide U-shaped curve. In the erect position, the lower part of the U may extend down into the pelvis. The transverse colon, on reaching the region of the spleen, bends downward, forming the **left colic (splenic) flexure** to become the descending colon.

The **descending colon** extends from the left colic flexure to the pelvis below. It occupies the left upper and lower quadrants.

The **sigmoid colon** begins at the pelvic inlet, where it is a continuation of the descending colon (see Fig. 5.45). It hangs down into the pelvic cavity in the form of an S-shaped loop. It joins the rectum in front of the sacrum.

The **rectum** occupies the posterior part of the pelvic cavity. It continuous above with the sigmoid colon and descends in front of the sacrum to leave the pelvis by piercing the pelvic floor. Here, it becomes continuous with the **anal canal** in the perineum.

Pancreas

The pancreas is a soft, lobulated organ that stretches obliquely across the posterior abdominal wall in the epigastric region (Fig. 5.49). It is situated behind the stomach and extends from the duodenum to the spleen.

Spleen

The spleen is a soft mass of lymphatic tissue that occupies the left upper part of the abdomen between the stomach and the diaphragm (see Fig. 5.49). It lies along the long axis of left rib 10.

Kidneys

The kidneys are two reddish brown organs situated high up on the posterior abdominal wall, one on each side of the vertebral column (see Fig. 5.49). The left kidney lies slightly higher than the right (because the left lobe of the liver is smaller than the right). Each kidney gives rise to a **ureter** that runs vertically downward on the psoas muscle.

Suprarenal Glands

The suprarenal glands are two yellowish organs that lie on the upper poles of the kidneys (see Fig. 5.49) on the posterior abdominal wall.

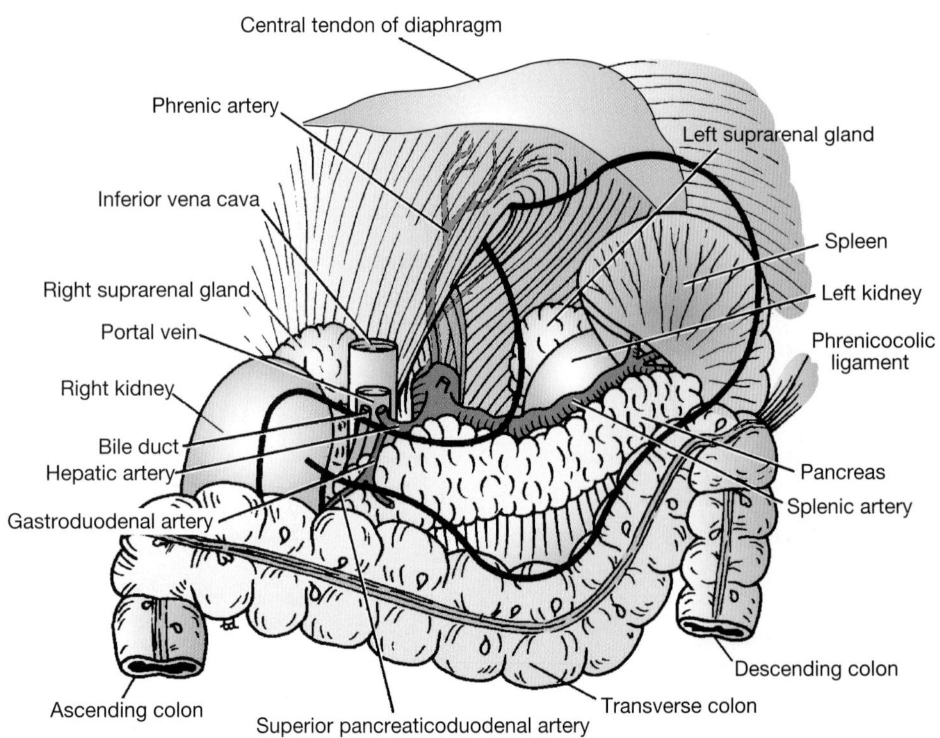

Figure 5.49 Structures situated on the posterior abdominal wall behind the stomach.

PERITONEUM

The peritoneum is a thin serous membrane that lines the walls of the abdominal and pelvic cavities and clothes the viscera (Figs. 5.50 and 5.51). The peritoneum can be regarded as a balloon against which organs are pressed from outside.

General Arrangement

The **parietal peritoneum** lines the walls of the abdominopelvic cavity, and the **visceral peritoneum** covers the organs. The potential space between the parietal and visceral layers, which is in effect the inside space of the balloon, is called the **peritoneal cavity**. In males, this is a closed cavity, but communication with the exterior occurs in females through the uterine tubes, uterus, and vagina.

A layer of connective tissue called the **extraperitoneal tissue** lies between the parietal peritoneum and the fascial lining of the abdominal and pelvic walls. In the area of the kidneys, this tissue contains a large amount of fat, which supports the kidneys.

The peritoneal cavity is the largest cavity in the body and is divided into two parts: greater and lesser sacs (see Figs. 5.50 and 5.51). The **greater sac** is the main compartment and extends from the diaphragm down into the pelvis. The **lesser sac** is smaller and lies behind the stomach. The greater and lesser sacs are in free communication with one another through an oval window called the **opening of the lesser sac**, or the **epiploic foramen** (Fig. 5.52; see also Fig. 5.50B). The peritoneum secretes a small amount of serous fluid, the **peritoneal fluid**, which lubricates the surfaces of the peritoneum and allows free movement between the viscera.

Intraperitoneal and Retroperitoneal Relationships

The terms **intraperitoneal** and **retroperitoneal** describe the relationship of various organs to their peritoneal covering. An organ is intraperitoneal when it is almost totally covered with visceral peritoneum. The stomach, jejunum, ileum, and spleen are good examples of intraperitoneal organs. Retroperitoneal organs lie behind the peritoneum and are only partially covered with visceral

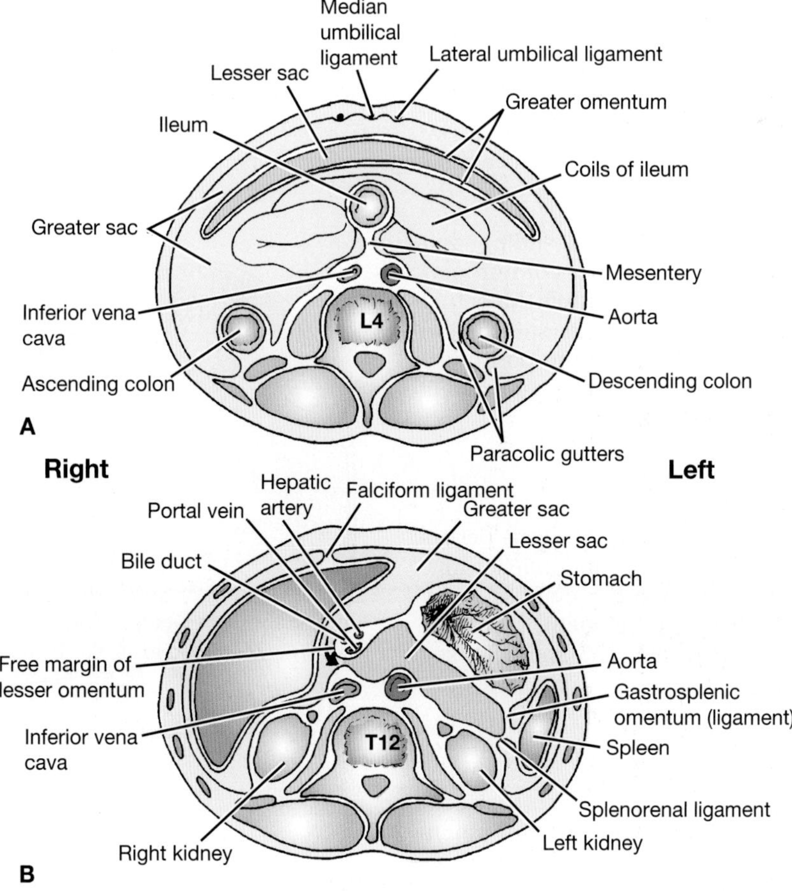

Figure 5.50 Transverse sections of the abdomen showing the arrangement of the peritoneum. **A.** At the level of L4. **B.** At the level of T12. *Arrow* in **(B)** indicates the position of the opening of the lesser sac. These sections are viewed from below.

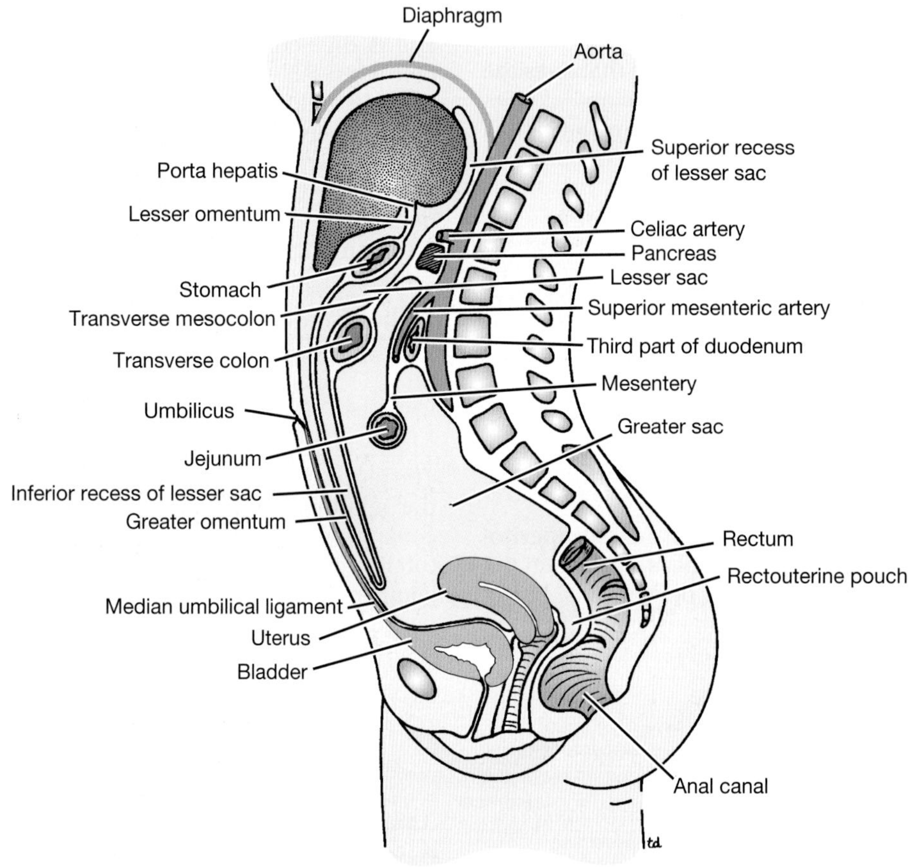

Figure 5.51 Sagittal section of the female abdomen showing the arrangement of the peritoneum.

peritoneum. The pancreas and the ascending and descending parts of the colon are examples of retroperitoneal organs. However, no organ is within the actual peritoneal cavity. An intraperitoneal organ, such as the stomach, appears to be surrounded by the peritoneal cavity, but it is covered with visceral peritoneum and is attached to other organs by omenta.

Peritoneal Ligaments

Peritoneal ligaments are two-layered folds of the peritoneum that connect solid viscera to the abdominal walls. The liver, for example, connects to the diaphragm by the **falciform ligament**, **coronary ligament**, and **right** and **left triangular ligaments** (Figs. 5.53 and 5.54; see also Fig. 5.52).

Omenta

Omenta are two-layered folds of peritoneum that connect the stomach to another viscus. The **greater omentum** connects the greater curvature of the stomach to the transverse colon (see Fig. 5.47). It hangs down like an apron in front of the coils of the small intestine and folds back on itself to attach to the transverse colon (see Fig. 5.51). The **lesser omentum** suspends the lesser curvature of the stomach and the proximal duodenum

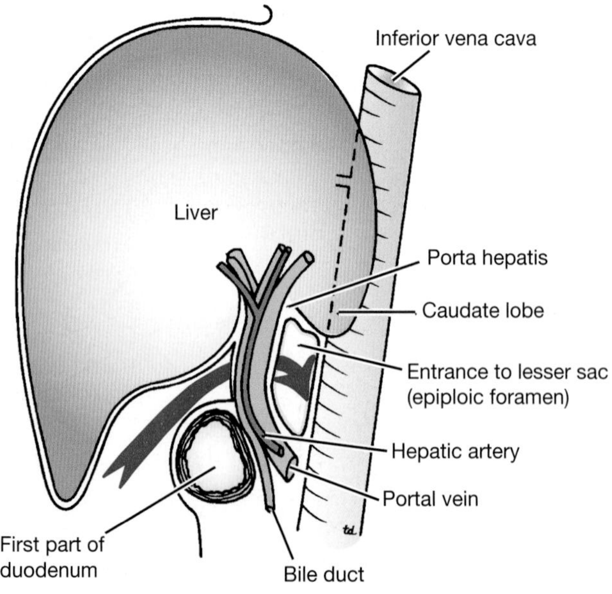

Figure 5.52 Sagittal section through the entrance into the lesser sac showing the important structures that form boundaries to the opening. (Note the *arrow* passing from the greater sac through the epiploic foramen into the lesser sac.)

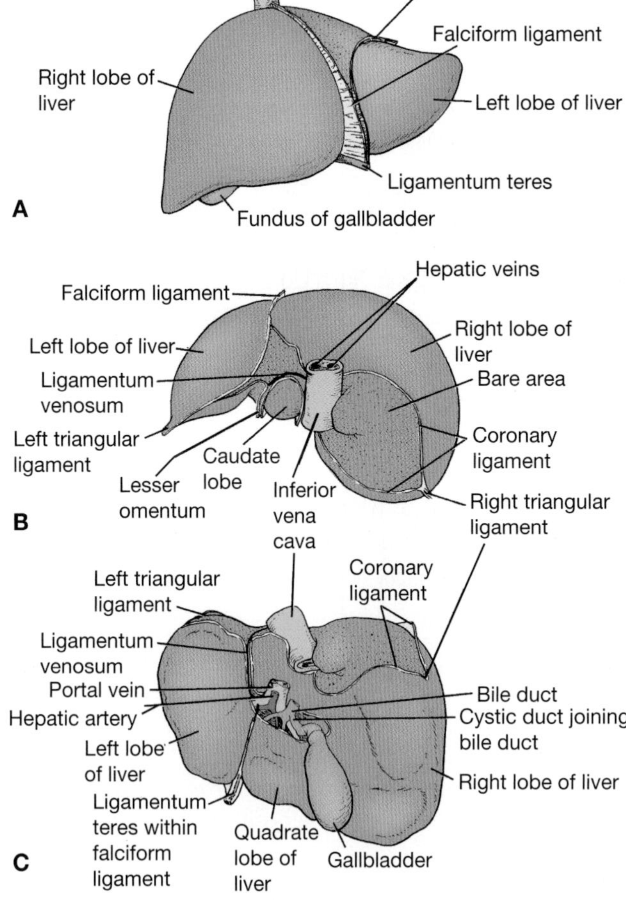

Figure 5.53 The liver as seen from in front **(A)**, from above **(B)**, and from behind **(C)**. Note the position of the peritoneal reflections, bare areas, and peritoneal ligaments.

from the fissure of the ligamentum venosum and the porta hepatis on the undersurface of the liver. The **gastrosplenic omentum (ligament)** connects the stomach to the hilum of the spleen (see Fig. 5.50).

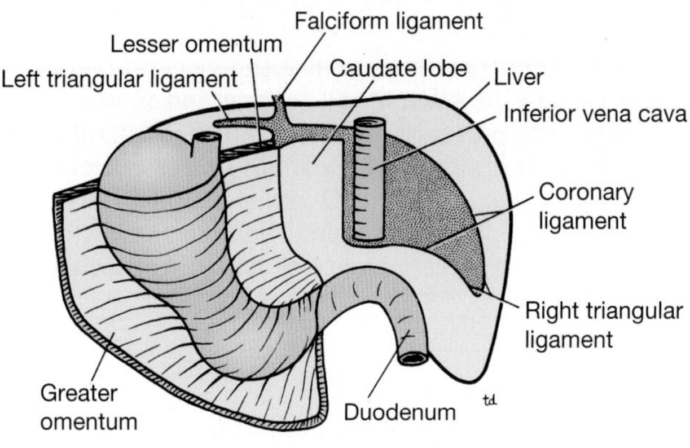

Figure 5.54 Attachment of the lesser omentum to the stomach and the posterior surface of the liver.

Mesenteries

Mesenteries are two-layered folds of the peritoneum connecting parts of the intestines to the posterior abdominal wall, for example, the **mesentery of the small intestine**, the **transverse mesocolon**, and the **sigmoid mesocolon** (see Fig. 5.51).

The peritoneal ligaments, omenta, and mesenteries serve as bridges that permit blood, lymph vessels, and nerves to reach the viscera.

The extent of the peritoneum and the peritoneal cavity should be studied in the transverse and sagittal sections of the abdomen seen in Figures 5.50 and 5.51.

Lesser Sac

The lesser sac lies behind the stomach and the lesser omentum (Fig. 5.55; see also Figs. 5.50 and 5.51). It extends upward as far as the diaphragm and downward between the layers of the greater omentum. The spleen, the gastrosplenic omentum, and the splenorenal ligament form the left margin of the sac (see Fig. 5.55). The right margin opens into the greater sac (the main part of the peritoneal cavity) through the **opening of the lesser sac** or **epiploic foramen** (see Figs. 5.52 and 5.55).

The opening into the lesser sac (epiploic foramen) has the following boundaries:

- **Anteriorly:** Free border of the lesser omentum, the bile duct, the hepatic artery, and the portal vein
- **Posteriorly:** Inferior vena cava
- **Superiorly:** Caudate process of the caudate lobe of the liver
- **Inferiorly:** First part of the duodenum

Duodenal Recesses

Close to the duodenojejunal junction, there may be four small pocket-like pouches of peritoneum called the **superior duodenal**, **inferior duodenal**, **paraduodenal**, and **retroduodenal recesses** (Fig. 5.56).

Cecal Recesses

Folds of peritoneum close to the cecum produce three peritoneal recesses called the **superior ileocecal**, the **inferior ileocecal**, and the **retrocecal recesses** (Fig. 5.57A).

Intersigmoid Recess

The intersigmoid recess is situated at the apex of the inverted, V-shaped root of the **sigmoid mesocolon** (see Fig. 5.57B). Its mouth opens downward.

Subphrenic Spaces

The **right** and **left anterior subphrenic spaces** lie between the diaphragm and the liver, on each side of the falciform ligament (Fig. 5.58). The **right posterior subphrenic space** lies between the right lobe of the liver, the right kidney, and the right colic flexure (Fig. 5.59). The **right extraperitoneal space** lies between the layers of the coronary ligament and is therefore situated between the liver and the diaphragm.

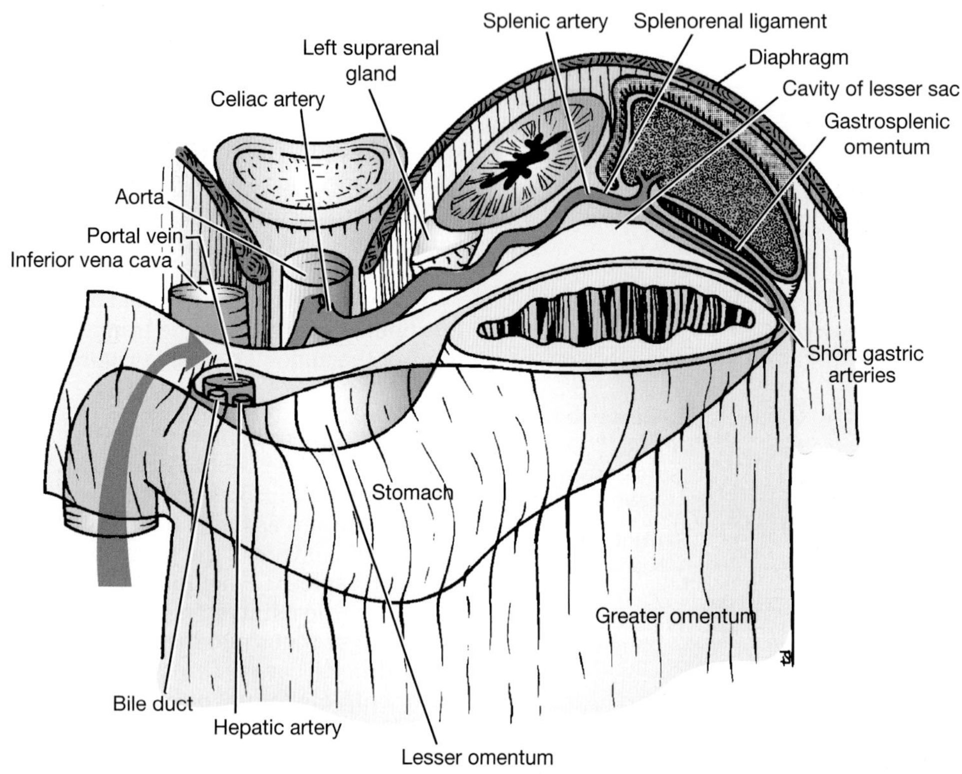

Figure 5.55 Transverse section of the lesser sac showing the arrangement of the peritoneum in the formation of the lesser omentum, the gastrosplenic omentum, and the splenorenal ligament. *Arrow* indicates the position of the opening of the lesser sac.

Paracolic Gutters

The paracolic gutters lie on the lateral and medial sides of the ascending and descending colons, respectively (see Figs. 5.50, 5.58, and 5.59).

The subphrenic spaces and the paracolic gutters are clinically important because they may be sites for the collection and movement of infected peritoneal fluid (see the "Clinical Notes" below).

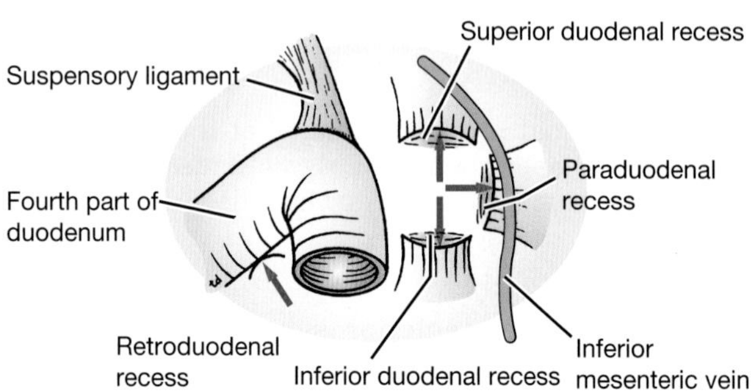

Figure 5.56 Peritoneal recesses, which may be present in the region of the duodenojejunal junction. Note the presence of the inferior mesenteric vein in the peritoneal fold, forming the paraduodenal recess.

Peritoneal Nerve Supply

The **parietal peritoneum**, like the parietal pleura, is sensitive to pain, temperature, touch, and pressure. The parietal peritoneum lining the anterior abdominal wall is supplied by the T7 to T12 and L1 nerves (ie, the same nerves that innervate the overlying muscles and skin). The phrenic nerves supply the central part of the diaphragmatic peritoneum. The T7 to T12 nerves supply the peripheral diaphragmatic peritoneum. The obturator nerve, a branch of the lumbar plexus, mainly supplies the parietal peritoneum in the pelvis.

The **visceral peritoneum**, like the visceral pleura, is sensitive only to stretch and tearing and is not sensitive to touch, pressure, or temperature. Visceral afferent nerves that supply the viscera or are traveling in the mesenteries supply it. Overdistension of a viscus leads to the sensation of pain. The mesenteries of the small and large intestines are sensitive to mechanical stretching.

Peritoneal Functions

The peritoneal fluid, which is pale yellow and somewhat viscid, contains leukocytes. It is secreted by the peritoneum and ensures that the mobile viscera glide easily on one another. As a result of the movements of the

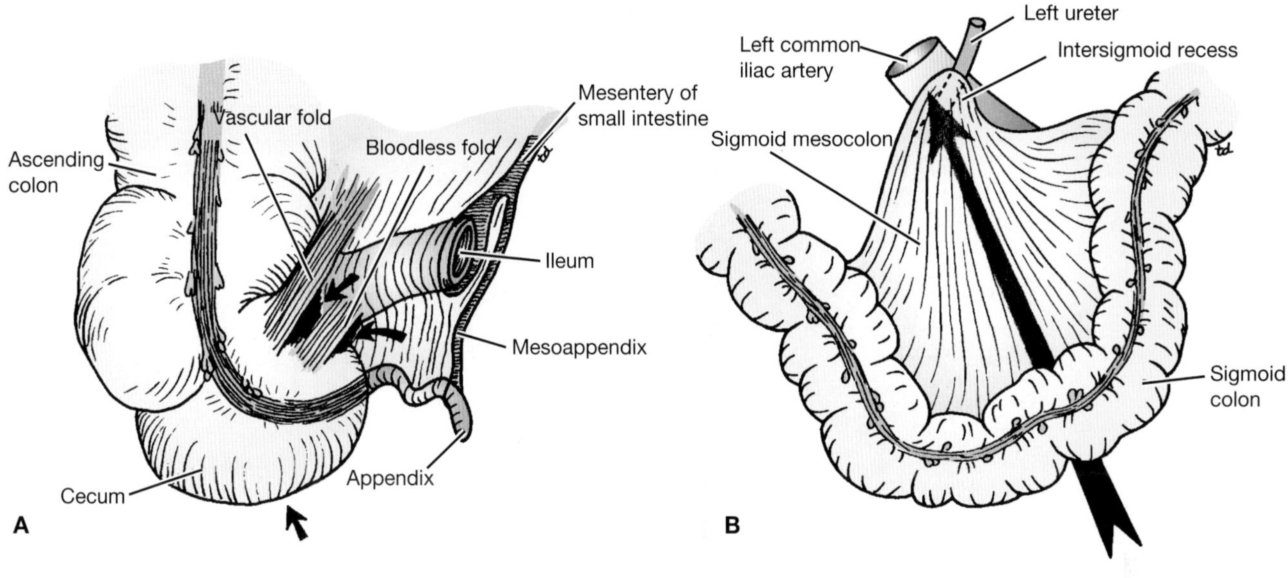

Figure 5.57 Peritoneal recesses (*arrows*) in the region of the cecum **(A)** and the recess related to the sigmoid mesocolon **(B)**.

diaphragm and the abdominal muscles, together with the peristaltic movements of the intestinal tract, the peritoneal fluid is not static. Experimental evidence has shown that particulate matter introduced into the lower part of the peritoneal cavity reaches the subphrenic peritoneal spaces rapidly, whatever the position of the body. Intraperitoneal movement of fluid toward the diaphragm appears to be continuous (see Fig. 5.58), and there it is quickly absorbed into the subperitoneal lymphatic capillaries.

This can be explained on the basis that the area of peritoneum is extensive in the region of the diaphragm and the respiratory movements of the diaphragm aid lymph flow in the lymph vessels.

The peritoneal coverings of the intestine tend to adhere together in the presence of infection. The greater omentum, which is kept constantly mobile by the peristalsis of the neighboring intestinal tract, may cling to other peritoneal surfaces around a focus of infection. In this manner, many intraperitoneal infections are sealed off and remain localized.

The peritoneal folds play an important part in suspending the various organs within the peritoneal cavity and serve as avenues for conveying the blood vessels, lymphatics, and nerves to these organs.

Large amounts of fat are stored in the peritoneal ligaments and mesenteries, and especially large amounts can be found in the greater omentum.

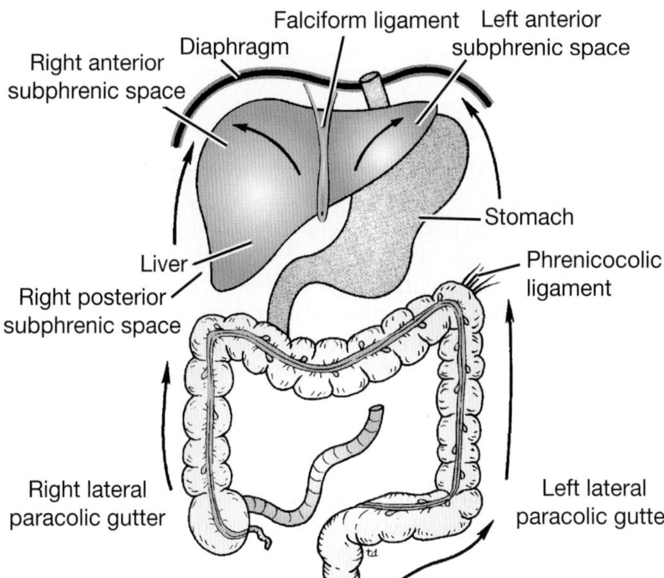

Figure 5.58 Normal direction of flow of the peritoneal fluid from different parts of the peritoneal cavity to the subphrenic spaces.

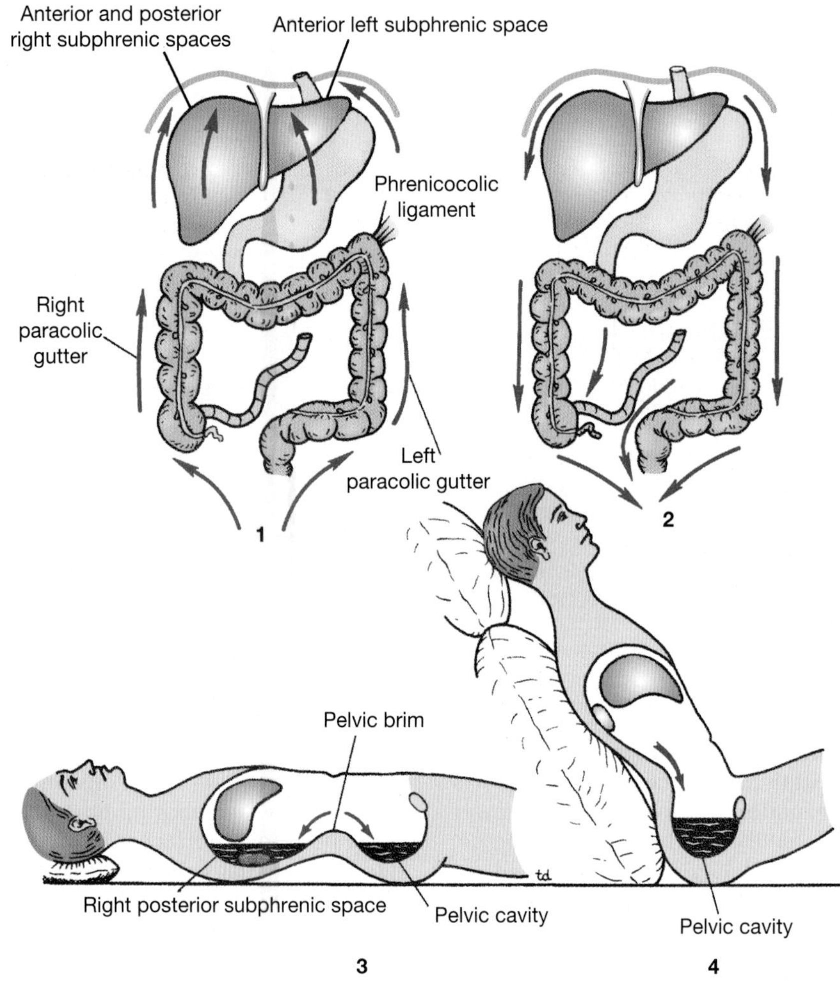

Figure 5.59 Direction of flow of the peritoneal fluid. (1) Normal flow upward to the subphrenic spaces. (2) Flow of inflammatory exudate in peritonitis. (3) The two sites where inflammatory exudate tends to collect when the patient is nursed in the supine position. (4) Accumulation of inflammatory exudate in the pelvis when the patient is nursed in the inclined position.

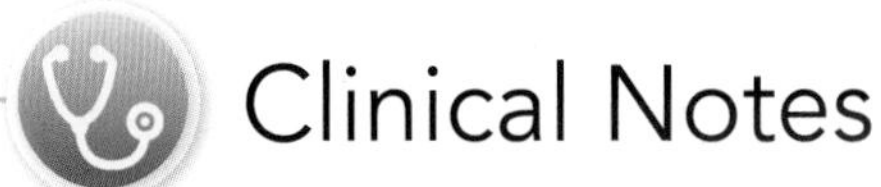

Clinical Notes

Peritoneum and Peritoneal Cavity

The peritoneal cavity is divided into an upper part within the abdomen and a lower part in the pelvis. The abdominal part is further subdivided by the many peritoneal reflections into important recesses and spaces, which, in turn, are continued into the paracolic gutters (see Fig. 5.59).

Peritoneal Fluid Movement

The attachments of the transverse mesocolon and the mesentery of the small intestine to the posterior abdominal wall provide natural peritoneal barriers that may hinder the movement of infected peritoneal fluid from the upper part to the lower part of the peritoneal cavity. Note that when the patient is in the supine position, the right subphrenic peritoneal space and the pelvic cavity are the lowest areas of the peritoneal cavity, and the region of the pelvic brim is the highest area.

Ascites is essentially an excessive accumulation of peritoneal fluid within the peritoneal cavity. Ascites can occur secondary to hepatic cirrhosis (portal venous congestion), malignant disease (eg, cancer of the ovary), or congestive heart failure (systemic venous congestion). In a thin patient, as much as 1,500 mL must accumulate before ascites can be recognized clinically. In obese individuals, a far greater amount must collect before it can be detected. The withdrawal of peritoneal fluid from the peritoneal cavity is described earlier in this chapter in "Clinical Notes, Paracentesis of the Abdomen."

Peritoneal Infection

Infection may enter the peritoneal cavity through several routes: from the interior of the gastrointestinal (GI) tract and gallbladder, through the anterior abdominal wall, via the uterine tubes in females (gonococcal peritonitis in adults and pneumococcal peritonitis in children occur through this route), and from the blood.

Collection of infected peritoneal fluid in one of the **subphrenic spaces** is often accompanied by infection of the pleural cavity. It is common to find localized pus in a pleural space (**empyema**) in a patient with a subphrenic abscess. Infection is thought to spread from the peritoneum to the pleura via the diaphragmatic lymph vessels. A patient with a subphrenic abscess may complain of pain over the shoulder. This also holds true for collections of blood under the diaphragm, which irritate the parietal diaphragmatic peritoneum. The skin of the shoulder is supplied by the supraclavicular nerves (C3 and C4), which have the same segmental origin as the phrenic nerve, which supplies the peritoneum in the center of the undersurface of the diaphragm.

To avoid the accumulation of infected fluid in the subphrenic spaces and to delay the absorption of toxins from intraperitoneal infections, common nursing practice is to sit a patient up in bed with the back at an angle of 45°. In this position, the infected peritoneal fluid tends to gravitate downward into the pelvic cavity, where the rate of toxin absorption is slow (see Fig. 5.59).

Greater Omentum

Surgeons often refer to the greater omentum as the abdominal policeman. The lower and the right and left margins are free, and it moves about the peritoneal cavity in response to the peristaltic movements of the neighboring gut.

Localization of Infection

In the first 2 years of life, the greater omentum is poorly developed and thus is less protective in a young child. Later, however, in an acutely inflamed appendix, for example, the inflammatory exudate causes the omentum to adhere to the appendix and wrap itself around the infected organ (Fig. 5.60). By this means, the infection is often localized to a small area of the peritoneal cavity, thus saving the patient from serious diffuse peritonitis.

Hernial Plug

The greater omentum has been found to plug the neck of a hernial sac and prevent the entrance of coils of small intestine.

Greater Omentum in Surgery

Surgeons sometimes use the omentum to buttress an intestinal anastomosis or in the closure of a perforated gastric or duodenal ulcer.

Torsion

The greater omentum may undergo torsion, and if extensive, the blood supply to a part of it may be cut off, causing necrosis.

Peritoneal Pain

The T7 to T12 and L1 nerves supply the parietal peritoneum lining the anterior abdominal wall. Abdominal pain originating from the parietal peritoneum is therefore of the somatic type and can be precisely localized. It is usually severe (see "Clinical Notes, Abdominal Pain," later in this chapter).

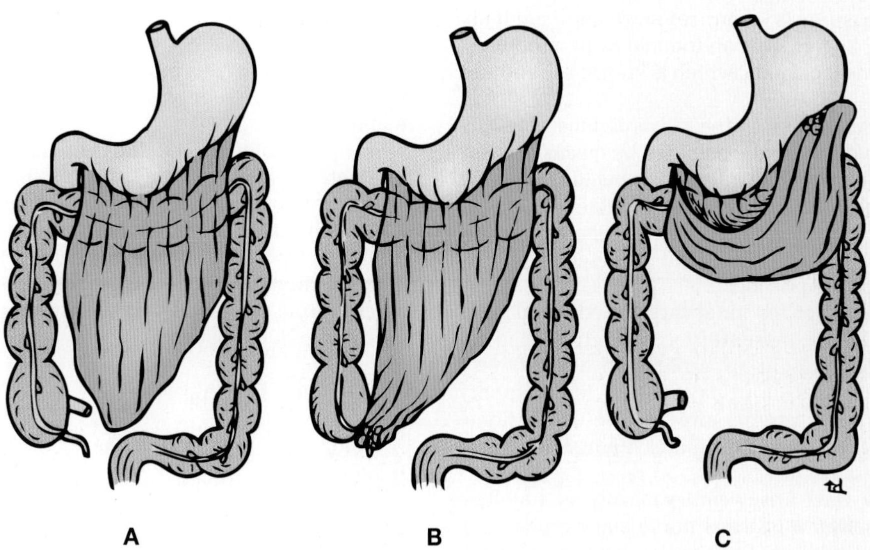

Figure 5.60 Different conditions of the greater omentum. **A.** Normal greater omentum. **B.** Greater omentum wrapped around an inflamed appendix. **C.** Greater omentum adherent to the base of a gastric ulcer. One important function of the greater omentum is to attempt to limit the spread of intraperitoneal infections.

(continued)

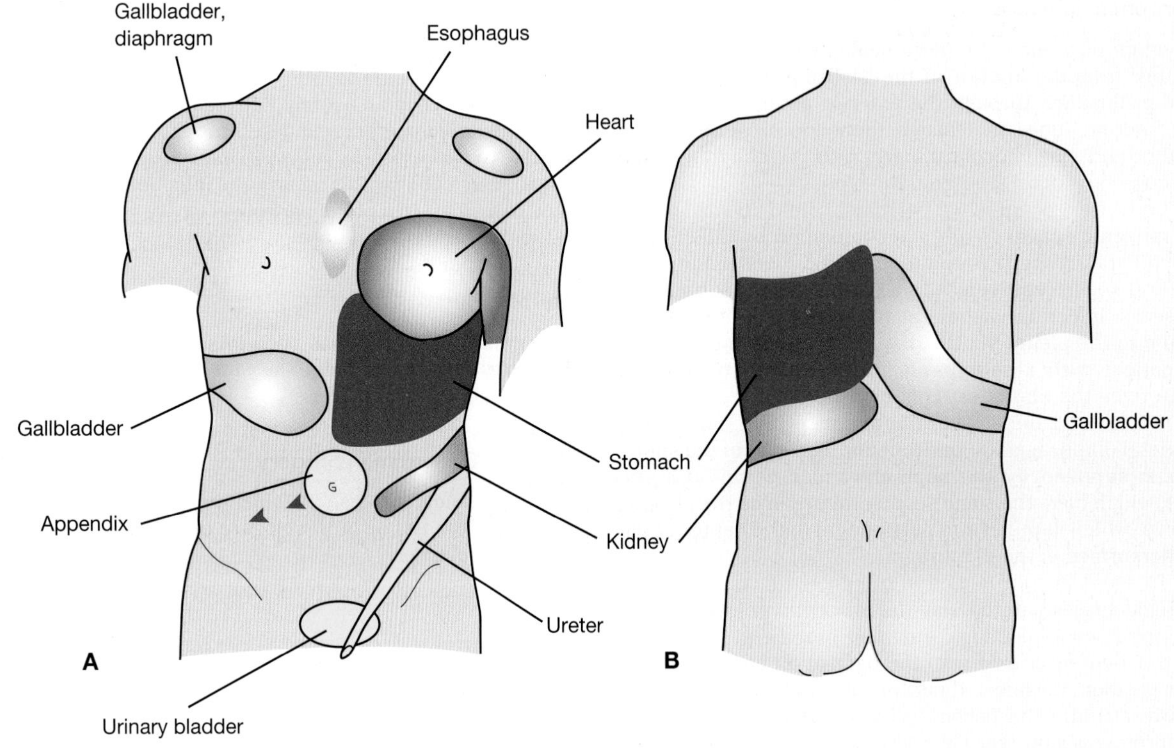

Figure 5.61 Some important skin areas involved in referred visceral pain. **A.** Anterior aspect of trunk. **B.** Posterior trunk.

An inflamed parietal peritoneum is extremely sensitive to stretch. This fact is made use of clinically in diagnosing **peritonitis**. Pressure is applied to the abdominal wall with a single finger over the site of the inflammation. The pressure is then removed by suddenly withdrawing the finger. The abdominal wall rebounds, resulting in extreme local pain, which is known as **rebound tenderness**.

The parietal peritoneum in the pelvis is innervated by the obturator nerve and can be palpated by means of a rectal or vaginal examination. An inflamed appendix may hang down into the pelvis and irritate the parietal peritoneum there. A pelvic examination can detect extreme tenderness of the parietal peritoneum on the right side (see Chapter 6, "Clinical Notes, Pelvic Appendix").

Visceral afferent nerves innervate the visceral peritoneum, including the mesenteries. Stretch caused by overdistension of a viscus or pulling on a mesentery gives rise to the sensation of pain, which is commonly referred to a characteristic site in the skin. Some typical sites of referral of visceral pain are shown in Figure 5.61.

Because the GI tract arises embryonically as a midline structure and receives a bilateral nerve supply, pain may be referred to the midline. Pain arising from an abdominal viscus is dull and poorly localized (see "Clinical Notes, Abdominal Pain," later in this chapter).

Peritoneal Dialysis

Because the peritoneum is a semipermeable membrane, it allows rapid bidirectional transfer of substances across itself. Because the surface area of the peritoneum is enormous, this transfer property has been made use of inpatients with acute renal insufficiency. The efficiency of this method is only a fraction of that achieved by hemodialysis.

A watery solution, the **dialysate**, is introduced through a catheter through a small midline incision through the anterior abdominal wall below the umbilicus. The technique is the same as peritoneal lavage (see "Clinical Notes, Peritoneal Lavage" earlier in this chapter). The products of metabolism, such as urea, diffuse through the peritoneal lining cells from the blood vessels into the dialysate and are removed from the patient.

Internal Abdominal Hernia

Occasionally, a loop of intestine enters a peritoneal pouch or recess (eg, the lesser sac or the duodenal recesses) and becomes strangulated at the edges of the recess. Remember that important structures form the boundaries of the entrance into the lesser sac and that the inferior mesenteric vein often lies in the anterior wall of the paraduodenal recess.

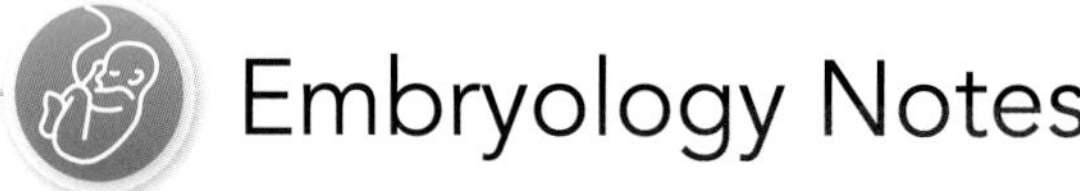

Embryology Notes

Peritoneum and Peritoneal Cavity Development

Once the lateral mesoderm has split into somatic and splanchnic layers, a cavity is formed between the two, called the **intraembryonic coelom**. The peritoneal cavity is derived from that part of the embryonic coelom situated caudal to the septum transversum. In the earliest stages, the peritoneal cavity is in free communication with the extraembryonic coelom on each side (see Fig. 5.33B). Later, with the development of the head, tail, and lateral folds, this wide area of communication becomes restricted to the small area within the umbilical cord.

Early in development, the peritoneal cavity is divided into right and left halves by a central partition formed by the **dorsal mesentery**, the gut, and the small **ventral mesentery** (Fig. 5.62A). However, the ventral mesentery extends only for a short distance along the gut (see below), so that below this level, the right and left halves of the peritoneal cavity are in free communication (see Fig. 5.62B). As a result of the enormous growth of the liver and the enlargement of the developing kidneys, the capacity of the abdominal cavity becomes greatly reduced at about week 6 of development. At this time, the small remaining communication between the peritoneal cavity and extraembryonic coelom becomes important. An intestinal loop is forced out of the abdominal cavity through the umbilicus into the umbilical cord. This **physiologic herniation of the midgut** takes place during week 6.

Peritoneal Ligaments and Mesenteries Formation

The peritoneal ligaments are developed from the ventral and dorsal mesenteries. The **ventral mesentery** is formed from the mesoderm of the septum transversum (derived from the cervical somites, which migrate downward). The ventral mesentery forms the **falciform ligament**, **lesser omentum**, and **coronary** and **triangular ligaments** of the liver (see Fig. 5.62C,D).

The **dorsal mesentery** is formed from the fusion of the splanchnopleuric mesoderm on the two sides of the embryo. It extends from the posterior abdominal wall to

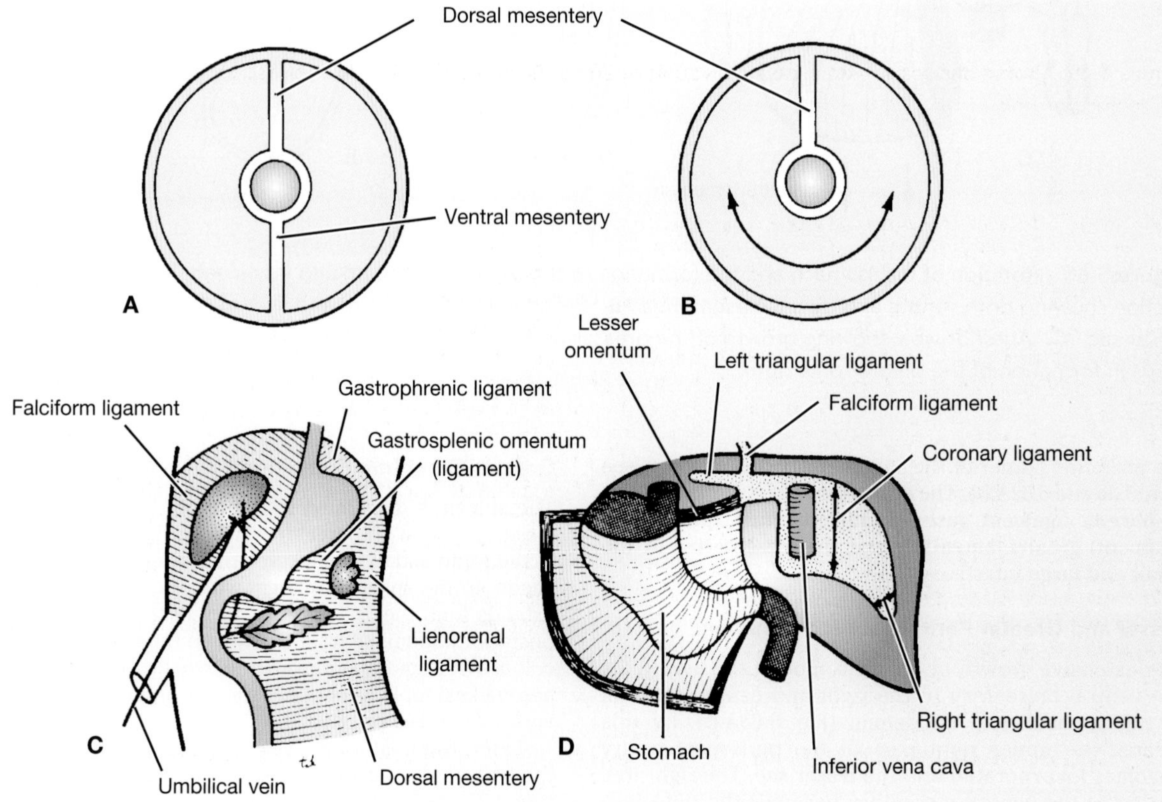

Figure 5.62 Ventral and dorsal mesenteries and the organs that develop within them. **A.** Both ventral and dorsal mesenteries occur in the upper abdomen. **B.** No ventral mesentery in the lower abdomen, thus allowing free communication between both sides of the peritoneal cavity. **C.** Sagittal view showing ventral and dorsal mesenteries. **D.** Posterior view showing derivatives of the ventral mesentery.

(continued)

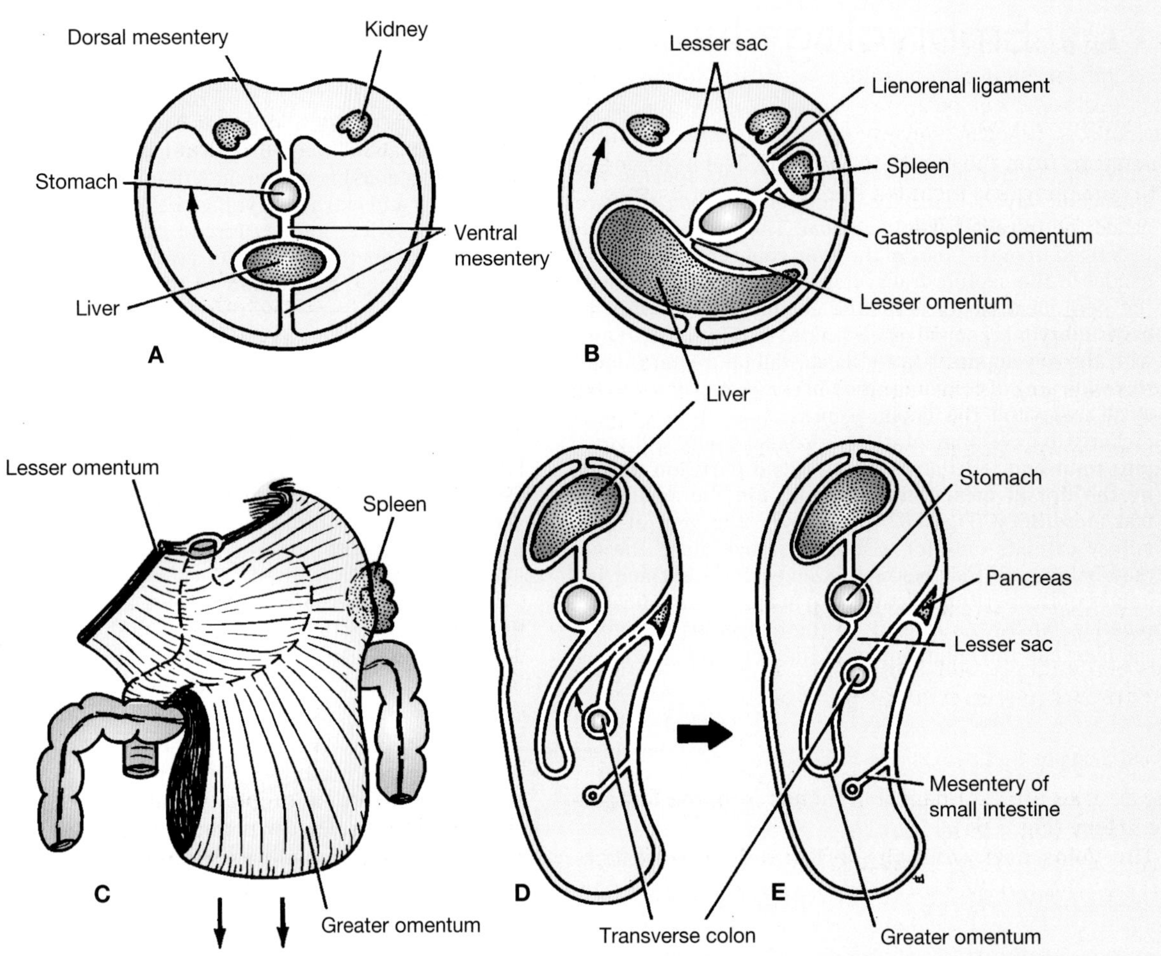

Figure 5.63 Rotation of the stomach and the formation of the greater omentum and lesser sac. **A.** Horizontal section showing both ventral and dorsal mesenteries. **B.** Rotation of the stomach and liver and formation of the lesser sac. **C.** Anterior view showing growth of the greater omentum (*arrows*). **D, E.** Sagittal sections showing final steps in formation of the greater omentum.

the posterior border of the abdominal part of the gut (see Figs. 5.33 and 5.62A,B). The dorsal mesentery forms the **gastrophrenic ligament**, **gastrosplenic omentum**, **splenorenal ligament**, **greater omentum**, and the **mesenteries of the small and large intestines**.

Lesser and Greater Peritoneal Sac Formation

The extensive growth of the right lobe of the liver pulls the ventral mesentery to the right and causes rotation of the stomach and duodenum (Fig. 5.63A,B). By this means, the upper right part of the peritoneal cavity becomes incorporated into the **lesser sac**. The right free border of the ventral mesentery becomes the right border of the lesser omentum and the anterior boundary of the entrance into the lesser sac.

The remaining part of the peritoneal cavity, which is not included in the lesser sac, is called the **greater sac**, and the two sacs are in communication through the **epiploic foramen**.

Greater Omentum Formation

The spleen is developed in the upper part of the dorsal mesentery, and the greater omentum is formed because of the rapid and extensive growth of the dorsal mesentery caudal to the spleen. To begin with, the greater omentum extends from the greater curvature of the stomach to the posterior abdominal wall superior to the transverse mesocolon. With continued growth, it reaches inferiorly as an apron-like double layer of peritoneum anterior to the transverse colon (see Fig. 5.63C).

Later, the posterior layer of the omentum fuses with the transverse mesocolon. As a result, the greater omentum becomes attached to the anterior surface of the transverse colon (see Fig. 5.63D). As development proceeds, the omentum becomes laden with fat. The inferior recess of the lesser sac extends inferiorly between the anterior and the posterior layers of the fold of the greater omentum.

GASTROINTESTINAL TRACT

The gastrointestinal tract includes the stomach, small intestine, large intestine, and the accessory organs that are developmental outgrowths of those organs. Note that this is not the entirety of the digestive system, which runs from the mouth to the anus. The inferior end of the esophagus is included here because of its general relations to the abdomen.

Esophagus (Abdominal Portion)

The esophagus is a muscular, collapsible tube about 10 in. (25 cm) long that joins the pharynx to the stomach. The greater part of the esophagus lies within the thorax (see Chapter 4). The esophagus enters the abdomen through an opening in the right crus of the diaphragm (see Fig. 4.11). After a course of about 0.5 in. (1.25 cm), it enters the stomach on its right side.

Relations

The esophagus is related anteriorly to the posterior surface of the left lobe of the liver and posteriorly to the left crus of the diaphragm. The left and right vagi lie on its anterior and posterior surfaces, respectively.

Blood Supply

The arteries are esophageal branches from the **left gastric artery** (Fig. 5.64).

The veins drain into the **left gastric vein**, a tributary of the portal vein Fig. 5.65) (see also "Clinical Notes: Portal–Systemic Anastomoses," later in this chapter).

Lymph Drainage

The lymph vessels follow the arteries into the **left gastric nodes,** which in turn drain into the celiac lymph nodes (Fig. 5.66).

Nerve Supply

The nerve supply is the **anterior and posterior gastric nerves (vagi)** and **sympathetic branches of the thoracic part of the sympathetic trunk** (Fig. 5.67).

Function

The esophagus conducts food from the pharynx into the stomach. Wavelike contractions of the muscular coat, called **peristalsis**, propel the food onward.

Gastroesophageal Sphincter

No **anatomic sphincter** exists at the lower end of the esophagus. However, the circular layer of smooth muscle in this region serves as a **physiologic sphincter**. As the food descends through the esophagus, relaxation of the muscle at the lower end occurs ahead of the peristaltic wave so that the food enters the stomach. The tonic contraction of this sphincter prevents the stomach contents from regurgitating into the esophagus. The closure of the sphincter is under vagal control, and this can be augmented by the hormone gastrin and reduced in response to secretin, cholecystokinin, and glucagon.

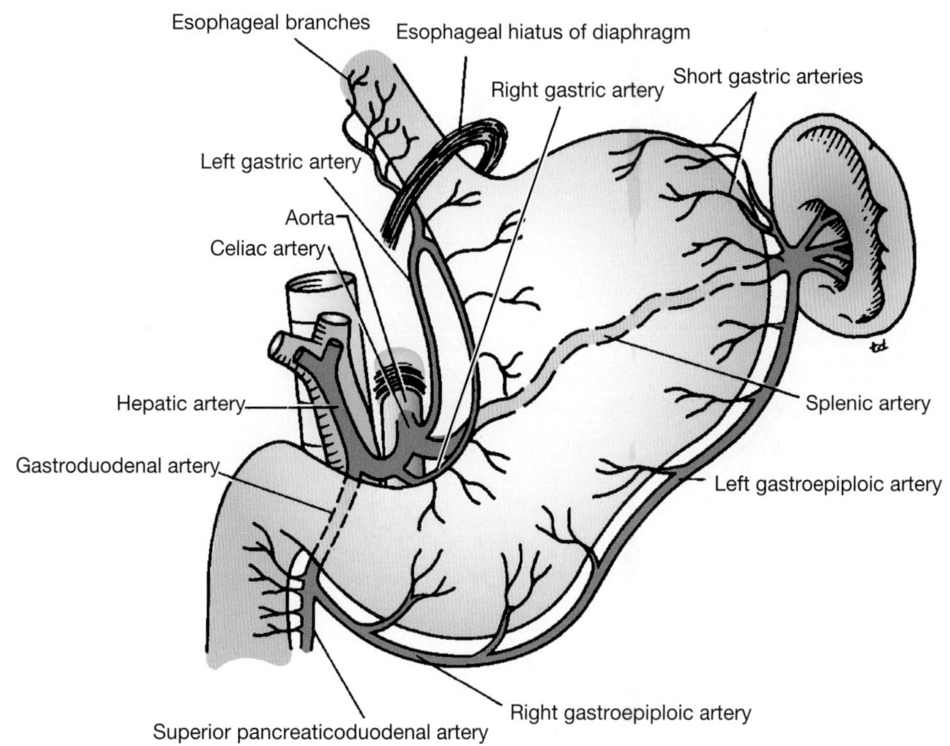

Figure 5.64 Arteries that supply the stomach. Note that all the arteries are derived from branches of the celiac artery.

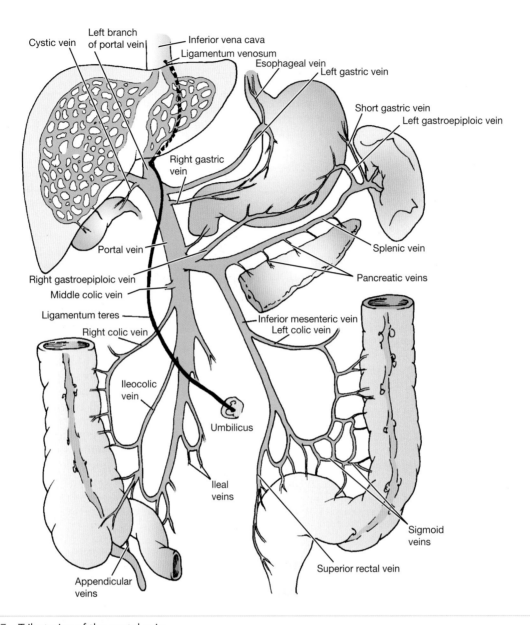

Figure 5.65 Tributaries of the portal vein.

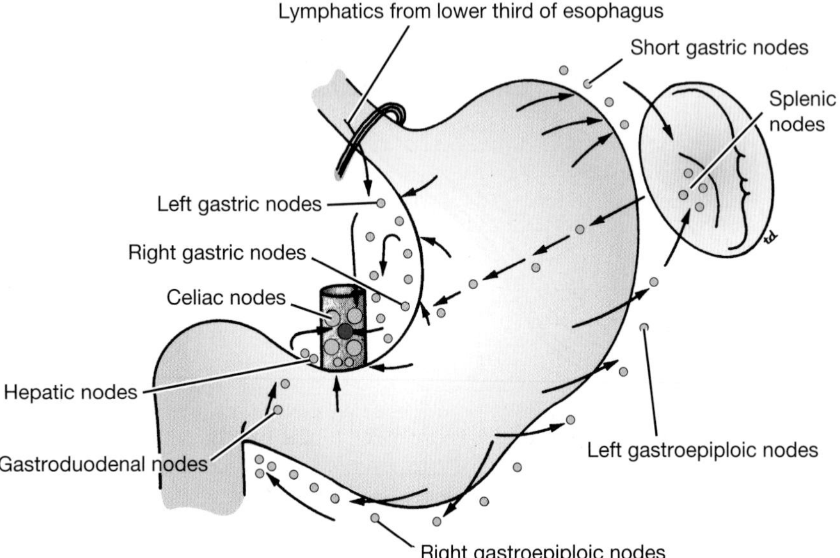

Figure 5.66 Lymph drainage of the stomach. Note that all the lymph eventually passes through the celiac lymph nodes.

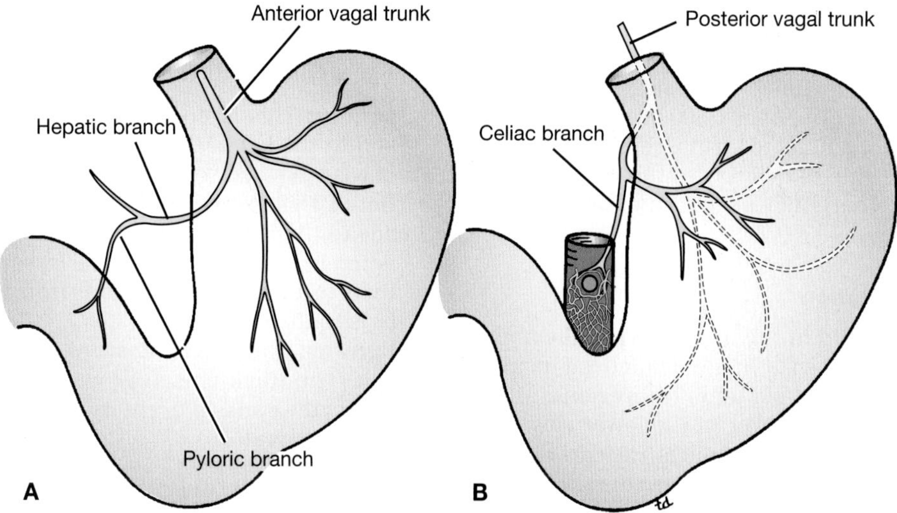

Figure 5.67 Distribution of the vagal trunks within the abdomen. **A.** Anterior vagus distribution. **B.** Posterior vagus distribution. Note that the celiac branch of the posterior vagal trunk is distributed with the sympathetic nerves as far down the intestinal tract as the left colic flexure.

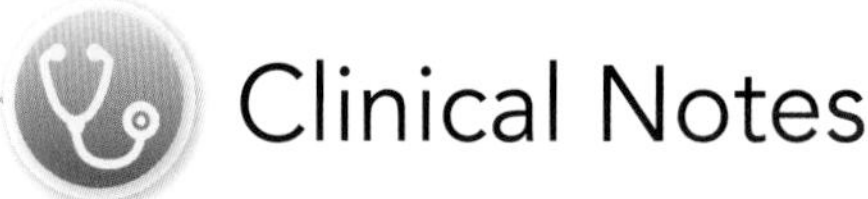

Clinical Notes

Esophagus

The esophagus is narrowed at three sites: (1) at the beginning, behind the cricoid cartilage of the larynx, (2) where the left bronchus and the arch of the aorta cross the front of the esophagus, and (3) where the esophagus enters the stomach (see Fig. 4.65). These three sites may resist the passage of a tube down the esophagus into the stomach.

Achalasia of the Cardia (Esophageal Achalasia)

This condition is a failure of normal relaxation of the gastroesophageal sphincter, resulting in obstruction of flow into the stomach. The cause is unknown, but it is associated with a degeneration of the parasympathetic plexus (Auerbach plexus) in the wall of the esophagus. The primary site of the disorder may be in the innervation of the cardioesophageal sphincter by the vagus nerves. Dysphagia (difficulty in swallowing) and regurgitation are common symptoms that are later accompanied by proximal dilatation and distal narrowing of the esophagus.

Gastroesophageal Reflux Disease

Gastroesophageal reflux disease (GERD) is the most common gastrointestinal disorder seen in outpatient clinics. It consists of a reflux of acid stomach contents into the esophagus producing the symptoms of heartburn on at least two occasions per week. If the reflux continues, the esophageal mucous membrane becomes inflamed. Later, if the condition persists, the lining of the esophagus changes from squamous epithelium to columnar epithelium, causing risk for the development of adenocarcinoma at the lower end of the esophagus. The causes of this disease include failure of the lower esophageal sphincter, hiatus hernia of the diaphragm, and abdominal obesity.

Bleeding Esophageal Varices

The **gastroesophageal anastomosis** is an important **portal–systemic venous anastomosis** that occurs at the lower third of the esophagus (see Fig. 5.65. Also, see "Clinical Notes: Portal–Systemic Anastomoses," later in this chapter). Here, the **esophageal tributaries of the left gastric vein** (which drains into the portal vein) anastomose with the **esophageal tributaries of the azygos veins** (systemic veins). Should the portal vein become obstructed (eg, in cirrhosis of the liver), portal hypertension develops, resulting in dilatation and varicosity of the portal–systemic anastomoses. Varicosed esophageal veins may rupture, causing severe vomiting of blood (**hematemesis**).

The **Sengstaken–Blakemore balloon** is used for the control of massive esophageal hemorrhage from esophageal varices. A gastric balloon anchors the tube against the esophageal–gastric junction. An esophageal balloon occludes the esophageal varices by counterpressure. The tube is inserted through the nose or by using the oral route.

The lubricated tube is passed down into the stomach, and the gastric balloon is inflated. In the average adult, the distance between the external orifices of the nose and the stomach is 17.2 in. (44 cm), and the distance between the incisor teeth and the stomach is 16 in. (41 cm).

Anatomy of Complications

- Difficulty in passing the tube through the nose
- Damage to the esophagus from overinflation of the esophageal tube
- Pressure on neighboring mediastinal structures as the esophagus is expanded by the balloon within its lumen
- Persistent hiccups caused by irritation of the diaphragm by the distended esophagus and irritation of the stomach by the blood

Stomach

The stomach is the dilated portion of the alimentary canal and has three main functions: it stores food (in the adult, it has a capacity of about 1,500 mL), it mixes the food with gastric secretions to form a semifluid **chyme**, and it controls the rate of delivery of the chyme to the small intestine so that efficient digestion and absorption can take place.

Location and Description

The stomach is situated in the upper part of the abdomen, extending from beneath the left costal margin region into the epigastric and umbilical regions. Much of the stomach lies under cover of the lower ribs. It is roughly J shaped and has two openings, the **cardiac** and **pyloric orifices**; two curvatures, the **greater** and **lesser curvatures**; and two surfaces, **anterior** and **posterior surfaces** (Fig. 5.68).

The stomach is relatively fixed at both ends but is very mobile in between. It tends to be high and transversely arranged in the short, obese person (steer-horn stomach) and elongated vertically in the tall, thin person (J-shaped stomach). Its shape undergoes considerable variation in the same person and depends on the volume of its contents, the position of the body, and the phase of respiration.

The stomach is divided into the following parts:

- **Fundus:** This is dome shaped and projects upward and to the left of the cardiac orifice. It is usually full of gas.
- **Body:** This extends from the level of the cardiac orifice to the level of the **incisura angularis**, a constant notch in the lower part of the lesser curvature.
- **Pyloric antrum:** This extends from the incisura angularis to the pylorus.
- **Pylorus:** This is the most tubular part of the stomach. The thick muscular wall is called the **pyloric sphincter**, and the cavity of the pylorus is the **pyloric canal**.

The **lesser curvature** forms the right border of the stomach and extends from the cardiac orifice to the pylorus. It is suspended from the liver by the lesser omentum. The **greater curvature** is much longer than the lesser curvature and extends from the left of the cardiac orifice, over the dome of the fundus, and along the left border of the stomach to the pylorus. The gastrosplenic omentum (ligament) extends from the upper part of the greater curvature to the spleen,

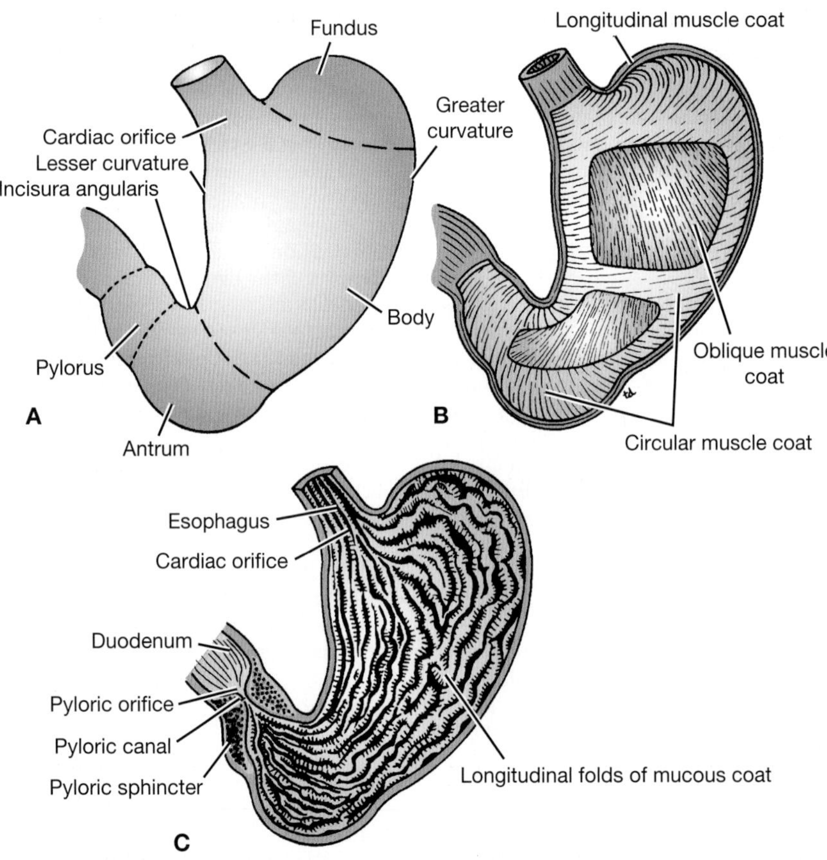

Figure 5.68 Anatomy of the stomach. **A.** Exterior features. **B.** Muscular coats. **C.** Internal structures. Note the increased thickness of the circular muscle forming the pyloric sphincter.

and the greater omentum extends from the lower part of the greater curvature to the transverse colon (see Fig. 5.55).

The **cardiac orifice** is where the esophagus enters the stomach (see Fig. 5.68). Although an anatomic sphincter is not present here, a physiologic mechanism prevents regurgitation of stomach contents into the esophagus (see "Gastroesophageal Sphincter," above).

The **pyloric canal** forms the **pyloric orifice**, which is about 1 in. (2.5 cm) long. The circular muscle coat of the stomach is much thicker here and forms the anatomic and physiologic **pyloric sphincter**. The pylorus lies on the transpyloric plane, and its position can be recognized by a slight constriction on the surface of the stomach.

Pyloric Sphincter Function

The pyloric sphincter controls the outflow of gastric contents into the duodenum. The sphincter receives motor fibers from the sympathetic system and inhibitory fibers from the vagi. In addition, the pylorus is controlled by local nervous and hormonal influences from the stomach and duodenal walls. For example, the stretching of the stomach because of filling will stimulate the myenteric nerve plexus in its wall and reflexively cause relaxation of the sphincter.

The **mucous membrane** of the stomach is thick and vascular and is thrown into numerous folds, or **rugae**, that are mainly longitudinal in direction (see Fig. 5.68C). The folds flatten out when the stomach is distended.

The **muscular wall** of the stomach contains longitudinal fibers, circular fibers, and oblique fibers.

Visceral peritoneum surrounds the stomach. It leaves the lesser curvature as the lesser omentum and the greater curvature as the gastrosplenic omentum and the greater omentum.

Relations

- **Anteriorly:** The anterior abdominal wall, the left costal margin, the left pleura and lung, the diaphragm, and the left lobe of the liver (see Figs. 5.47 and 5.51)
- **Posteriorly:** The lesser sac, the diaphragm, the spleen, the left suprarenal gland, the upper part of the left kidney, the splenic artery, the pancreas, the transverse mesocolon, and the transverse colon (see Figs. 5.49, 5.51, and 5.55)

Arteries

The arteries are derived from the branches of the celiac artery (see Fig. 5.64).

The **left gastric artery** arises from the celiac artery. It passes upward and to the left to reach the esophagus and then descends along the lesser curvature of the stomach. It supplies the lower third of the esophagus and the upper right part of the stomach.

The **right gastric artery** arises from the hepatic artery at the upper border of the pylorus and runs to the left along the lesser curvature. It supplies the lower right part of the stomach.

The **short gastric arteries** arise from the splenic artery at the hilum of the spleen and pass forward in the gastrosplenic omentum (ligament) to supply the fundus.

The **left gastroepiploic artery** arises from the splenic artery at the hilum of the spleen and passes forward in the gastrosplenic omentum (ligament) to supply the stomach along the upper part of the greater curvature.

The **right gastroepiploic artery** arises from the gastroduodenal branch of the hepatic artery. It passes to the left and supplies the stomach along the lower part of the greater curvature.

Veins

The veins drain into the portal circulation (see Fig. 5.65). The **left** and **right gastric veins** drain directly into the portal vein. The **short gastric veins** and the **left gastroepiploic veins** join the splenic vein. The **right gastroepiploic vein** joins the superior mesenteric vein.

Lymph Drainage

The lymph vessels follow the arteries into the left and right gastric nodes, the left and right gastroepiploic nodes, and the short gastric nodes (see Fig. 5.66). All lymph from the stomach eventually passes to the **celiac nodes** located around the root of the celiac artery on the posterior abdominal wall.

Nerve Supply

The nerve supply includes sympathetic fibers derived from the **celiac plexus** and parasympathetic fibers from the right and left vagus nerves (see Fig. 5.67).

The **anterior vagal trunk**, which is formed in the thorax mainly from the left vagus nerve, enters the abdomen on the anterior surface of the esophagus. The trunk, which may be single or multiple, then divides into branches that supply the anterior surface of the stomach. A large hepatic branch passes up to the liver, and from this, a pyloric branch passes down to the pylorus.

The **posterior vagal trunk**, which is formed in the thorax mainly from the right vagus nerve, enters the abdomen on the posterior surface of the esophagus. The trunk then divides into branches that supply mainly the posterior surface of the stomach. A large branch passes to the celiac and superior mesenteric plexuses and is distributed to the intestine as far as the splenic flexure and to the pancreas.

The **sympathetic innervation** of the stomach carries a proportion of pain-transmitting nerve fibers, whereas the parasympathetic vagal fibers are secretomotor to the gastric glands and motor to the muscular wall of the stomach. The pyloric sphincter receives motor fibers from the sympathetic system and inhibitory fibers from the vagi.

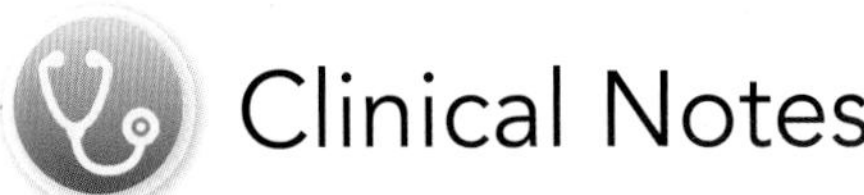

Clinical Notes

Stomach Trauma

Apart from its attachment to the esophagus at the cardiac orifice and its continuity with the duodenum at the pylorus, the stomach is relatively mobile. It is protected on the left by the lower part of the rib cage. These factors greatly protect the stomach from blunt trauma to the abdomen. However, its large size makes it vulnerable to gunshot wounds.

Gastric Ulcer

The mucous membrane of the body of the stomach and, to a lesser extent, that of the fundus produces **acid** and **pepsin**. The secretion of the antrum and pyloric canal is **mucous** and weakly **alkaline** (Fig. 5.69). The secretion of acid and pepsin is controlled by nerves and hormones. The vagus nerves are responsible for nervous control, and the hormone **gastrin**, produced by the antral mucosa, is responsible for hormonal control. In the surgical treatment of chronic gastric and duodenal ulcers, attempts are made to reduce the amount of acid secretion by sectioning the vagus nerves (**vagotomy**) and by removing the gastrin-bearing area of mucosa, the antrum (**partial gastrectomy**).

Gastric ulcers occur in the alkaline-producing mucosa of the stomach, usually on or close to the lesser curvature. A chronic ulcer invades the muscular coats and, in time, involves the peritoneum so that the stomach adheres to neighboring structures. An ulcer situated on the posterior wall of the stomach may perforate into the lesser sac or adhere to the pancreas. Erosion of the pancreas produces pain referred to the back. The splenic artery runs along the upper border of the pancreas, and erosion of this artery may produce fatal hemorrhage. A penetrating ulcer of the anterior stomach wall may result in the escape of stomach contents into the greater sac, producing diffuse peritonitis. The anterior stomach wall may, however, adhere to the liver, and the chronic ulcer may penetrate the liver substance.

Gastric Pain

The sensation of pain in the stomach is caused by the stretching or spasmodic contraction of the smooth muscle in its walls and is referred to the epigastrium. Pain-transmitting **visceral afferent fibers** are believed to leave the stomach in company with the sympathetic nerves. They pass through the celiac ganglia and reach the spinal cord via the **greater splanchnic nerves**.

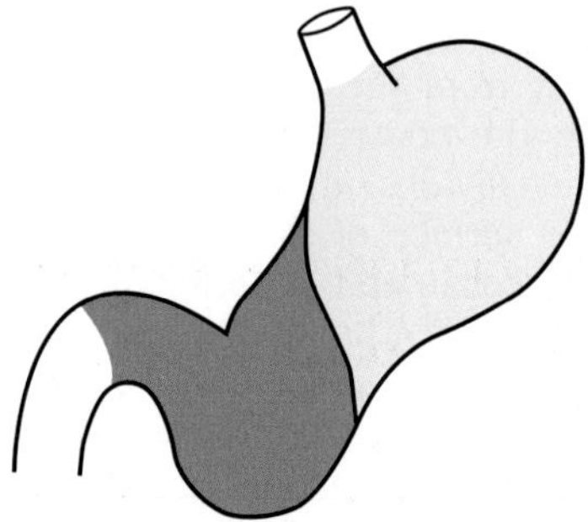

Figure 5.69 Areas of the stomach that produce acid and pepsin (*blue*) and alkali and gastrin (*red*).

Stomach Cancer

Because the lymphatic vessels of the mucous membrane and submucosa of the stomach are in continuity, it is possible for cancer cells to travel to different parts of the stomach, some distance away from the primary site. Cancer cells also often pass through or bypass the local lymph nodes and are held up in the regional nodes. For these reasons, malignant disease of the stomach is treated by **total gastrectomy**, which includes removal of the lower end of the esophagus and the first part of the duodenum, spleen and gastrosplenic and splenorenal ligaments and their associated lymph nodes, splenic vessels, tail and body of the pancreas and their associated nodes, nodes along the lesser curvature of the stomach, and the nodes along the greater curvature, along with the greater omentum. This radical operation is an attempt to remove the stomach en bloc and, with it, its lymphatic field. Anastomosing the esophagus with the jejunum restores the continuity of the gut.

Gastroscopy

Gastroscopy is the viewing of the mucous membrane of the stomach through an illuminated tube fitted with a lens system. The patient is anesthetized, and the **gastroscope** is passed into the stomach, which is then inflated with air. With a flexible fiber-optic instrument, direct visualization of different parts of the gastric mucous membrane is possible. It is also possible to perform a mucosal biopsy through a gastroscope.

Nasogastric Intubation

Nasogastric intubation is a common procedure performed to empty the stomach, to decompress the stomach in cases of intestinal obstruction, or before operations on the gastrointestinal tract. It may also be performed to obtain a sample of gastric juice for biochemical analysis.

1. The patient is placed in the semi upright position or left lateral position to avoid aspiration.
2. The well-lubricated tube is inserted through the wider nostril and is directed backward along the nasal floor.
3. Once the tube has passed the soft palate and entered the oral pharynx, decreased resistance is felt, and the conscious patient will feel like gagging.
4. Some important distances in the adult may be useful. From the nostril (external nares) to the cardiac orifice of the stomach is about 17.2 in. (44 cm), and from the cardiac orifice to the pylorus of the stomach is 4.8 to 5.6 in. (12 to 14 cm). The curved course taken by the tube from the cardiac orifice to the pylorus is usually longer, 6.0 to 10.0 in. (15 to 25 cm) (see Fig. 4.65).

Anatomic Impediments to Nasogastric Tube Passage

- A **deviated nasal septum** makes the passage of the tube difficult on the narrower side.
- **Three sites of esophageal narrowing** may resist the nasogastric tube: (1) at the beginning of the esophagus behind the cricoid cartilage (7.2 in. [18 cm]), (2) where the left bronchus and the arch of the aorta cross the front of the esophagus (11.2 in. [28 cm]), and (3) where the esophagus enters the stomach (17.2 in. [44 cm]) (see Fig. 4.65). Gently grasping the wings of the thyroid cartilage and pulling the larynx forward may overcome the upper esophageal narrowing. This maneuver opens the normally collapsed esophagus and permits the tube to pass down without further delay.

Anatomy of Complications

- The nasogastric tube enters the larynx instead of the esophagus.
- Rough insertion of the tube into the nose will cause nasal bleeding from the mucous membrane.
- Penetration of the wall of the esophagus or stomach. Always aspirate the tube for gastric contents to confirm successful entrance into the stomach.

Small Intestine

The small intestine is the longest part of the alimentary canal and extends from the pylorus of the stomach to the ileocecal junction (see Fig. 5.45). The greater part of digestion and food absorption takes place in the small intestine. It is divided into three parts: **duodenum**, **jejunum**, and **ileum**.

Duodenum

The duodenum is a C-shaped tube, about 10 in. (25 cm) long, which joins the stomach to the jejunum. It receives the openings of the bile and pancreatic ducts. The duodenum curves around the head of the pancreas (Fig. 5.70). The first inch (2.5 cm) of the duodenum resembles the stomach in that it is covered on its anterior and posterior surfaces with peritoneum and has the lesser omentum attached to its upper border and the greater omentum to its lower border. The lesser sac lies behind this short segment. The remainder of the duodenum is retroperitoneal, being only partially covered by peritoneum.

Parts of the Duodenum

The duodenum is situated in the epigastric and umbilical regions and, for purposes of description, is divided into four parts.

FIRST PART OF THE DUODENUM

The first part of the duodenum begins at the pylorus and runs upward and backward on the transpyloric plane at the level of the L1 vertebra (Fig. 5.71; see also Fig. 5.70).

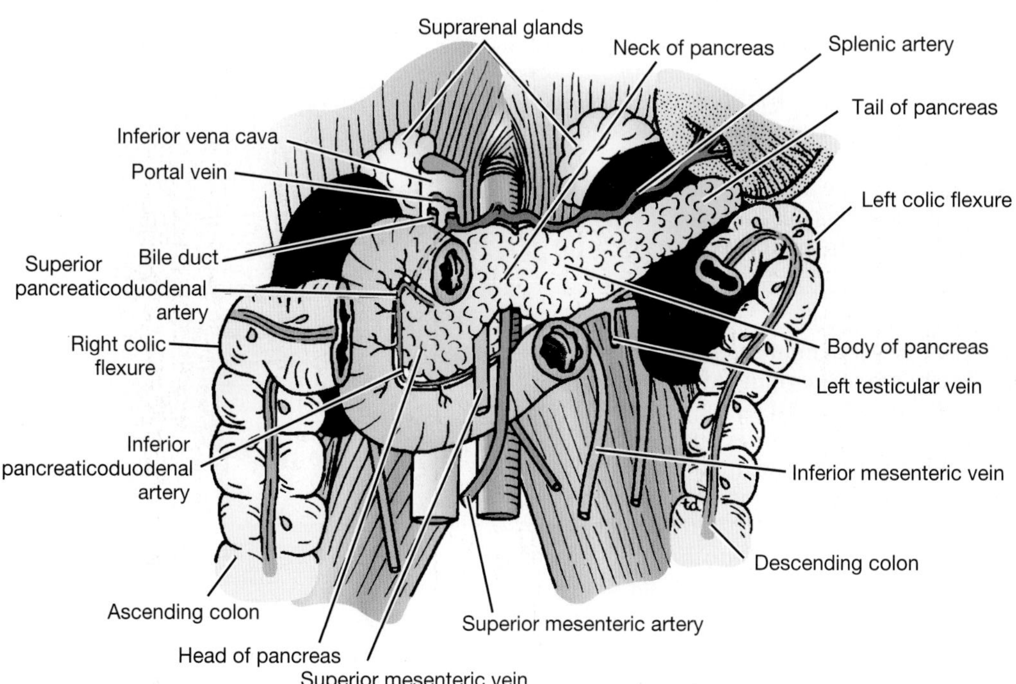

Figure 5.70 Pancreas and anterior relations of the kidneys.

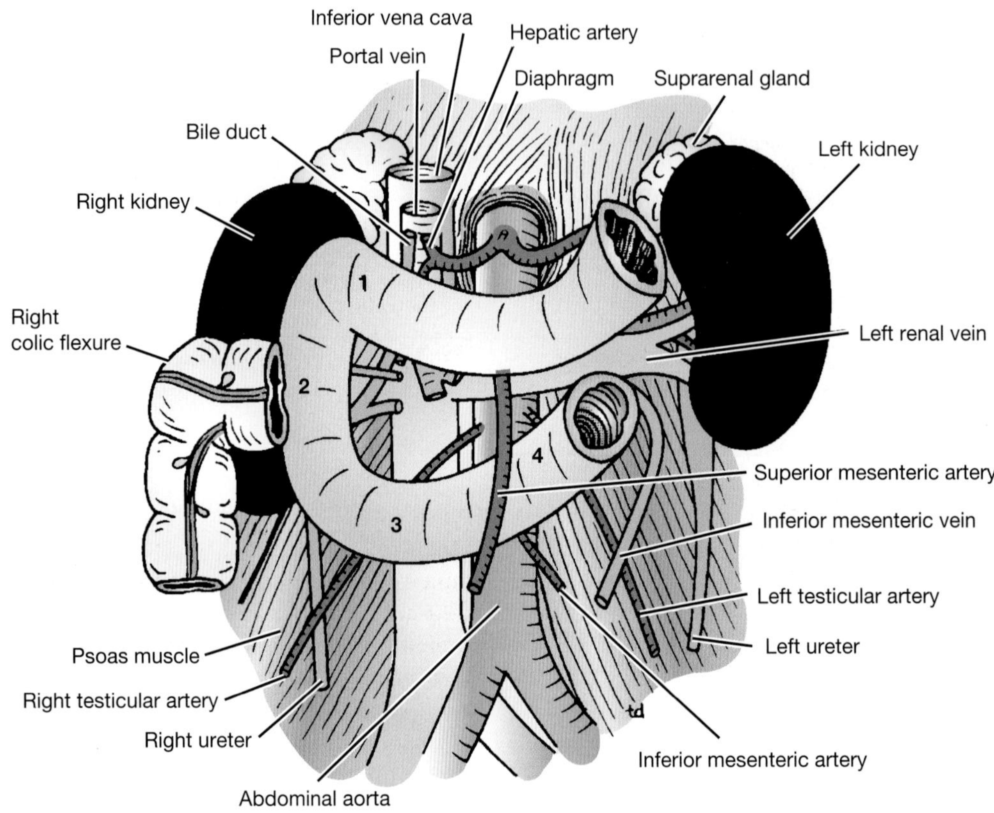

Figure 5.71 Posterior relations of the duodenum and the pancreas. The *numbers* represent the four parts of the duodenum.

The relations of this part are as follows:

- **Anteriorly:** The quadrate lobe of the liver and the gallbladder (see Fig. 5.54)
- **Posteriorly:** The lesser sac (first inch only), gastroduodenal artery, bile duct and portal vein, and the inferior vena cava (see Fig. 5.71)
- **Superiorly:** The entrance into the lesser sac (the epiploic foramen) (see Figs. 5.52 and 5.55)
- **Inferiorly:** The head of the pancreas (see Fig. 5.70)

SECOND PART OF THE DUODENUM

The second part of the duodenum runs vertically downward in front of the hilum of the right kidney on the right side of the L2 and L3 vertebrae (see Figs. 5.70 and 5.71). About halfway down its medial border, the bile duct and the main pancreatic duct pierce the duodenal wall. They unite to form the **ampulla** that opens on the summit of the **major duodenal papilla** (Fig. 5.72). The **accessory pancreatic duct**, if present, opens into the duodenum a little higher up on the **minor duodenal papilla** (see Figs. 5.71 and 5.72).

The relations of this part are as follows:

- **Anteriorly:** The fundus of the gallbladder and the right lobe of the liver, transverse colon, and the coils of the small intestine (Fig. 5.73)

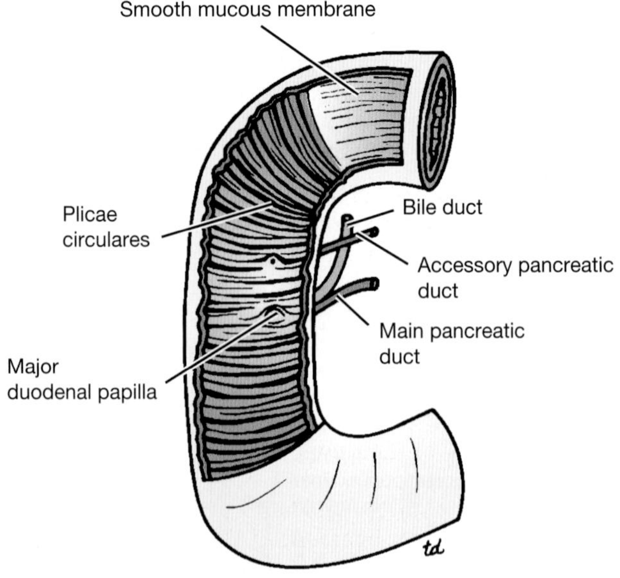

Figure 5.72 Entrance of the bile duct and the main and accessory pancreatic ducts into the second part of the duodenum. Note the smooth lining of the first part of the duodenum, the plicae circulares of the second part, and the major duodenal papilla.

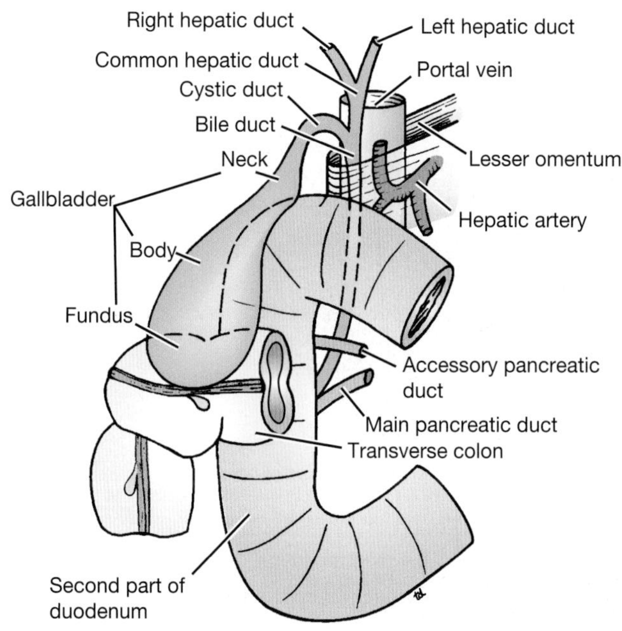

Figure 5.73 Bile ducts and the gallbladder. Note the relation of the gallbladder to the transverse colon and the duodenum.

- **Posteriorly:** The hilum of the right kidney and the right ureter (see Fig. 5.71)
- **Laterally:** The ascending colon, right colic flexure, and right lobe of the liver
- **Medially:** The head of the pancreas, the bile duct, and the main pancreatic duct (see Figs. 5.71 and 5.72)

THIRD PART OF THE DUODENUM

The third part of the duodenum runs horizontally to the left on the subcostal plane, passing in front of the vertebral column and following the lower margin of the head of the pancreas (see Figs. 5.70 and 5.71).

The relations of this part are as follows:

- **Anteriorly:** The root of the mesentery of the small intestine, the superior mesenteric vessels contained within it, and coils of the jejunum (see Figs. 5.70 and 5.71)
- **Posteriorly:** The right ureter, right psoas muscle, inferior vena cava, and the aorta (see Fig. 5.71)
- **Superiorly:** The head of the pancreas (see Fig. 5.70)
- **Inferiorly:** Coils of the jejunum

FOURTH PART OF THE DUODENUM

The fourth part of the duodenum runs upward and to the left to the **duodenojejunal flexure** (see Figs. 5.70 and 5.71). The flexure is held in position by a peritoneal fold, the **suspensory ligament of the duodenum (ligament of Treitz)**, which is attached to the right crus of the diaphragm (see Fig. 5.56).

The relations of this part are as follows:

- **Anteriorly:** The beginning of the root of the mesentery and coils of jejunum (Fig. 5.74)
- **Posteriorly:** The left margin of the aorta and the medial border of the left psoas muscle (see Fig. 5.71)

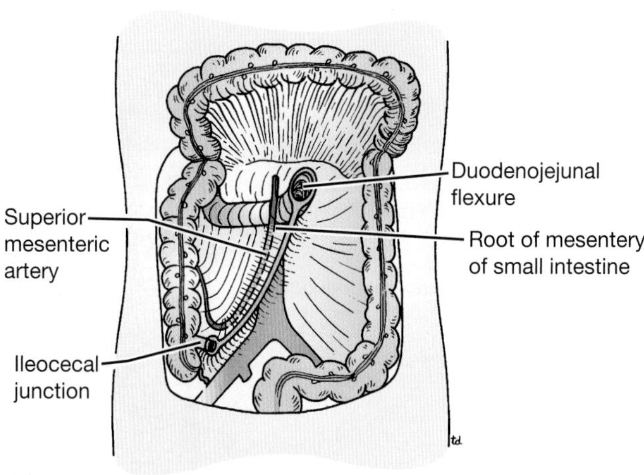

Figure 5.74 Attachment of the root of the mesentery of the small intestine to the posterior abdominal wall. Note that it extends from the duodenojejunal flexure on left of the aorta, downward, and to the right to the ileocecal junction. The superior mesenteric artery lies in the root of the mesentery.

Mucous Membrane and Duodenal Papillae

The mucous membrane of the duodenum is mostly thick. It is smooth in the first part of the duodenum (see Fig. 5.72). However, it is thrown into numerous circular folds called the **plicae circulares** in the remainder of the duodenum. A small, rounded elevation called the **major duodenal papilla** is located at the site where the bile duct and the main pancreatic duct pierce the medial wall of the second part. The accessory pancreatic duct, if present, opens into the duodenum on a smaller papilla about 0.75 in. (1.9 cm) above the major duodenal papilla.

Blood Supply

The **superior pancreaticoduodenal artery**, a branch of the gastroduodenal artery, supplies the upper half (see Figs. 5.64 and 5.70). The **inferior pancreaticoduodenal artery**, a branch of the superior mesenteric artery, supplies the lower half (Fig. 5.75).

The **superior pancreaticoduodenal vein** drains into the portal vein. The inferior vein joins the superior mesenteric vein (see Fig. 5.65).

Lymph Drainage

The lymph vessels follow the arteries. The upper duodenum drains upward via pancreaticoduodenal nodes to the gastroduodenal nodes and then to the **celiac nodes** (see Fig. 5.66). The lower duodenum drains downward via pancreaticoduodenal nodes to the **superior mesenteric nodes** around the origin of the superior mesenteric artery.

Nerve Supply

Sympathetic and parasympathetic (vagus) nerves derived from the celiac and superior mesenteric plexuses supply the duodenum.

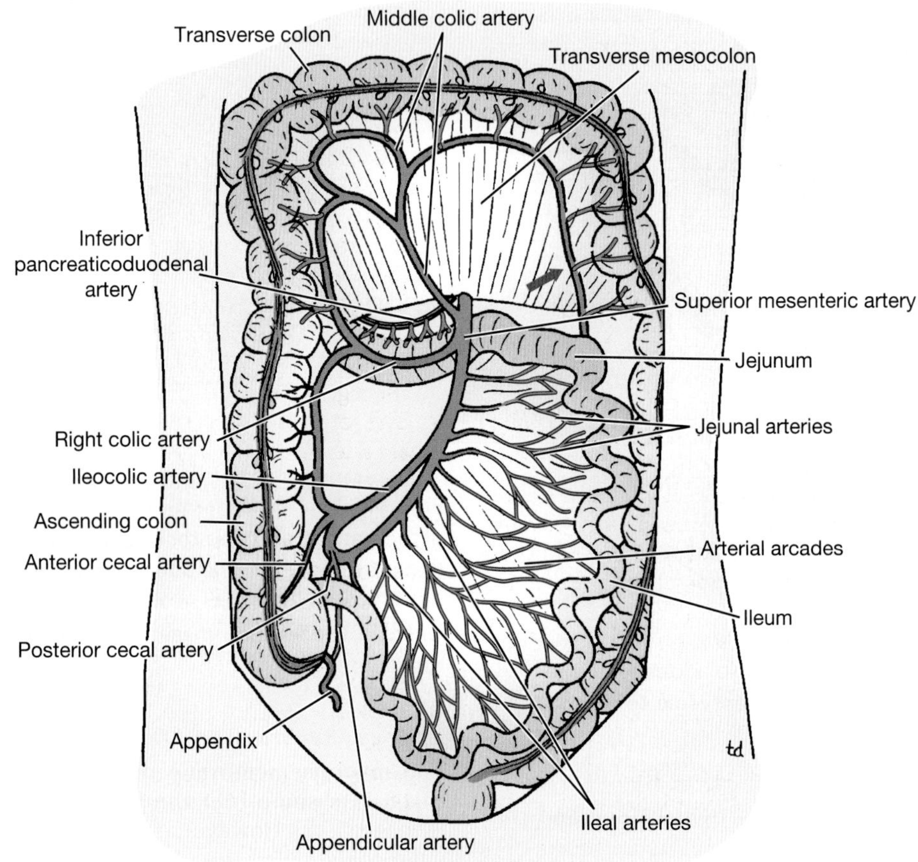

Figure 5.75 Superior mesenteric artery and its branches. Note that this artery supplies blood to the gut from halfway down the second part of the duodenum to the distal third of the transverse colon (*arrow*).

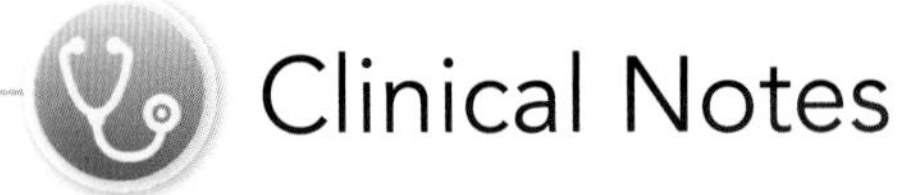

Clinical Notes

Duodenal Trauma

Apart from the first inch, the duodenum is rigidly fixed to the posterior abdominal wall by peritoneum and therefore cannot move away from crush injuries. In severe crush injuries to the anterior abdominal wall, the third part of the duodenum may be severely crushed or torn against the L3 vertebra.

Duodenal Ulcer

As the stomach empties its contents into the duodenum, the acidic **chyme** is squirted against the anterolateral wall of the first part of the duodenum. This is thought to be an important factor in the production of a duodenal ulcer at this site. An ulcer of the anterior wall of the first inch of the duodenum may perforate into the upper part of the greater sac, above the transverse colon. The transverse colon directs the escaping fluid into the right lateral paracolic gutter and thus down to the right iliac fossa. The differential diagnosis between a perforated duodenal ulcer and a perforated appendix may be difficult.

An ulcer of the posterior wall of the first part of the duodenum may penetrate the wall and erode the relatively large **gastroduodenal artery**, causing a severe hemorrhage.

The gastroduodenal artery is a branch of the hepatic artery, which is a branch of the celiac trunk (see Figs. 5.49 and 5.64).

Important Duodenal Relations

The relations to the duodenum of the gallbladder, transverse colon, and right kidney should be remembered. Cases have been reported in which a large gallstone ulcerated through the gallbladder wall into the duodenum. Operations on the colon and right kidney have resulted in damage to the duodenum.

Jejunum and Ileum

The jejunum and ileum together measure about 20 ft (6 m) long. The jejunum makes up the upper two fifths of this length. Each has distinctive features, but there is a gradual change from one to the other. The jejunum begins at the **duodenojejunal flexure**, and the ileum ends at the **ileocecal junction**.

Location and Description

The coils of jejunum and ileum are freely mobile and are attached to the posterior abdominal wall by a fan-shaped fold of the peritoneum known as the **mesentery of the small intestine** (see Fig. 5.74). The long free edge of the fold encloses the mobile intestine. The short root of the fold is continuous with the parietal peritoneum on the posterior abdominal wall along a line that extends downward and to the right from the left side of the L2 vertebra to the region of the right sacroiliac joint. The **root of the mesentery** permits the entrance and exit of the branches of the superior mesenteric artery and vein, lymph vessels, and nerves into the space between the two layers of the peritoneum forming the mesentery.

In the living, the jejunum can be distinguished from the ileum by the following features (Fig. 5.76):

- The jejunum lies coiled in the upper part of the peritoneal cavity below the left side of the transverse mesocolon; the ileum is in the lower part of the cavity and in the pelvis (see Fig. 5.48).
- The jejunum is wider bored, thicker walled, and redder than the ileum. The jejunal wall feels thicker because the permanent infoldings of the mucous membrane, the plicae circulares, are larger, more numerous, and closely set in the jejunum; in the upper part of the ileum, they are smaller and more widely separated, and, in the lower part, they are absent (see Fig. 5.76).
- The jejunal mesentery is attached to the posterior abdominal wall above and to the left of the aorta, whereas the ileal mesentery is attached below and to the right of the aorta.
- The jejunal mesenteric vessels form only one or two **arcades**, with long and infrequent branches (**vasa recta**) passing to the intestinal wall. The ileum receives numerous short terminal vasa recta that arise from a series of three or four or even more arcades.
- At the jejunal end of the mesentery, the fat is deposited near the root and is scanty near the intestinal wall. At the ileal end of the mesentery, the fat is deposited throughout so that it extends from the root to the intestinal wall.
- **Aggregations of lymphoid tissue (Peyer patches)** are present in the mucous membrane of the lower ileum along the antimesenteric border. In the living, these may be visible through the wall of the ileum from the outside.

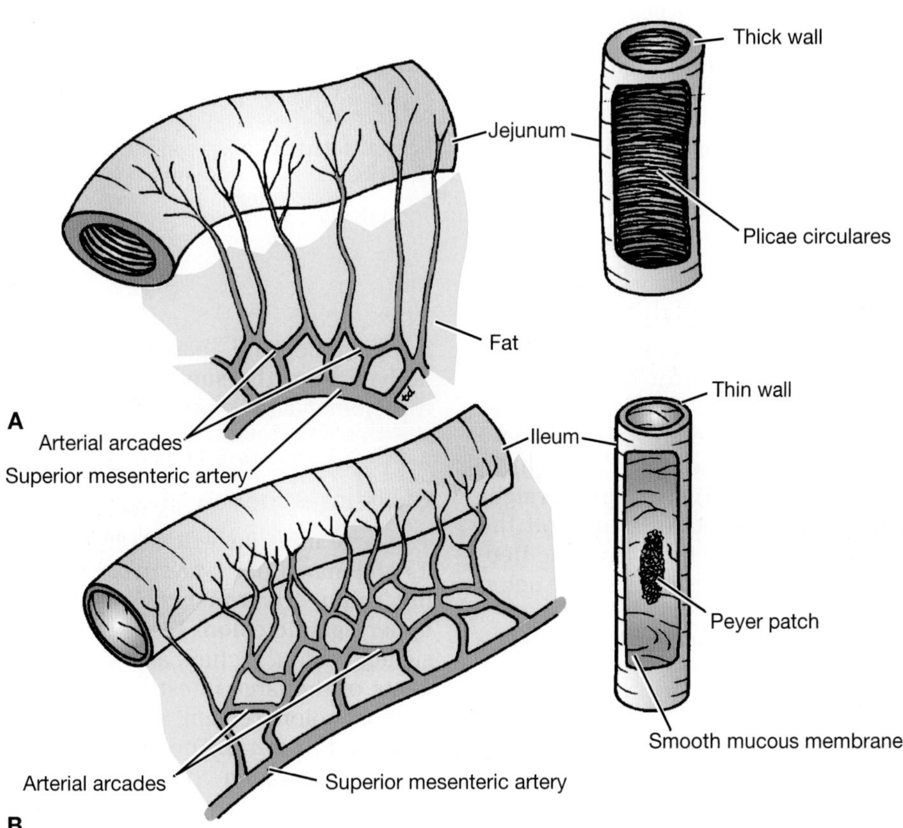

Figure 5.76 Some external and internal differences between the jejunum and the ileum. **A.** Jejunum. **B.** Ileum.

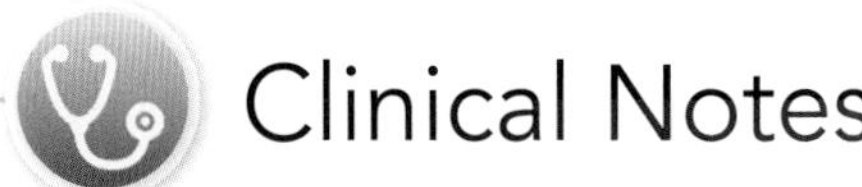

Clinical Notes

Jejunum and Ileum Trauma

Because of its extent and position, the small intestine is commonly damaged by trauma. The extreme mobility and elasticity permit the coils to move freely over one another in instances of blunt trauma. Small, penetrating injuries may self-seal from the mucosa plugging up the hole and the contraction of the smooth muscle wall. Material from large wounds leaks freely into the peritoneal cavity. The presence of the vertebral column and the prominent anterior margin of the S1 vertebra may provide a firm background for intestinal crushing in cases of midline crush injuries. Small-bowel contents have nearly a neutral pH and produce only slight chemical irritation to the peritoneum.

Recognition of the Jejunum and Ileum

Differentiating the jejunum from the ileum may be necessary in cases such as **postoperative burst abdomen**, in which coils of gut are lying free in the patient's bed. The macroscopic differences are described in the previous text above.

Small Intestine Mesenteric Tumors and Cysts

The line of attachment of the mesentery of the small intestine to the posterior abdominal wall extends from a point just to the left of the midline, about 2 in. (5 cm) below the transpyloric plane (L1), coursing downward to the right iliac fossa. A tumor or a cyst of the mesentery, when palpated through the anterior abdominal wall, is more mobile in a direction at right angles to the line of attachment than along the line of attachment.

Pain Fibers from the Jejunum and Ileum

Pain fibers traverse the superior mesenteric sympathetic plexus and pass to the spinal cord via the **splanchnic nerves**. Referred pain from this segment of the gastrointestinal tract is felt in the dermatomes supplied by the T9 to T11 nerves. Strangulation of a coil of the small intestine in an inguinal hernia first gives rise to pain in the region of the umbilicus. Only later, when the parietal peritoneum of the hernial sac becomes inflamed, does the pain become more intense and localized to the inguinal region (see "Clinical Notes, Abdominal Pain," later in this chapter).

Mesenteric Arterial Occlusion

The superior mesenteric artery, a branch of the abdominal aorta, supplies an extensive territory of the gut, from halfway down the second part of the duodenum to the left colic flexure. Occlusion of the artery or one of its branches greatly compromises blood flow to all or part of this segment of the gut. The occlusion may occur as the result of an embolus, a thrombus, an aortic dissection, or an abdominal aneurysm.

Mesenteric Vein Thrombosis

The superior mesenteric vein, which drains the same area of the gut supplied by the superior mesenteric artery, may undergo thrombosis after stasis of the venous bed. Cirrhosis of the liver with portal hypertension may predispose to this condition.

Meckel Diverticulum

Meckel diverticulum, a congenital anomaly of the ileum, is described in the "Embryology Notes" to follow.

Blood Supply

The arterial supply is from branches of the **superior mesenteric artery** (see Fig. 5.75). The **intestinal branches** arise from the left side of the artery and run in the mesentery to reach the gut. They anastomose with one another to form a series of archlike **arcades** (see Figs. 5.75 and 5.76). Multiple straight vessels (**vasa recta**; **arteriae rectae**) branch off the arcades and run to the wall of the intestine. The **ileocolic artery** also supplies the lowest part of the ileum (see Fig. 5.75).

The veins correspond to the branches of the superior mesenteric artery and drain into the **superior mesenteric vein** (see Fig. 5.65).

Lymph Drainage

The lymph vessels pass through many intermediate mesenteric nodes and finally reach the **superior mesenteric nodes**, which are situated around the origin of the superior mesenteric artery.

Nerve Supply

Sympathetic and parasympathetic (vagus) nerves derived from the **superior mesenteric plexus** supply the jejunum and ileum.

Large Intestine

The large intestine extends from the ileum to the anus. Its abdominal parts are the **cecum**, **appendix**, **ascending colon**, **transverse colon**, **descending colon**, and upper **sigmoid colon** (see Figs. 5.45 and 5.75). The lower sigmoid colon, rectum, and **anal canal** are also components of the large intestine and are in the pelvis. The sigmoid colon, rectum, and anal canal are described in detail in Chapter 6. The part of the large intestine identified as the **colon** consists of the cecum through the sigmoid colon. The primary functions of the large intestine are the absorption of water and electrolytes and the storage of undigested material until it can be expelled from the body as feces.

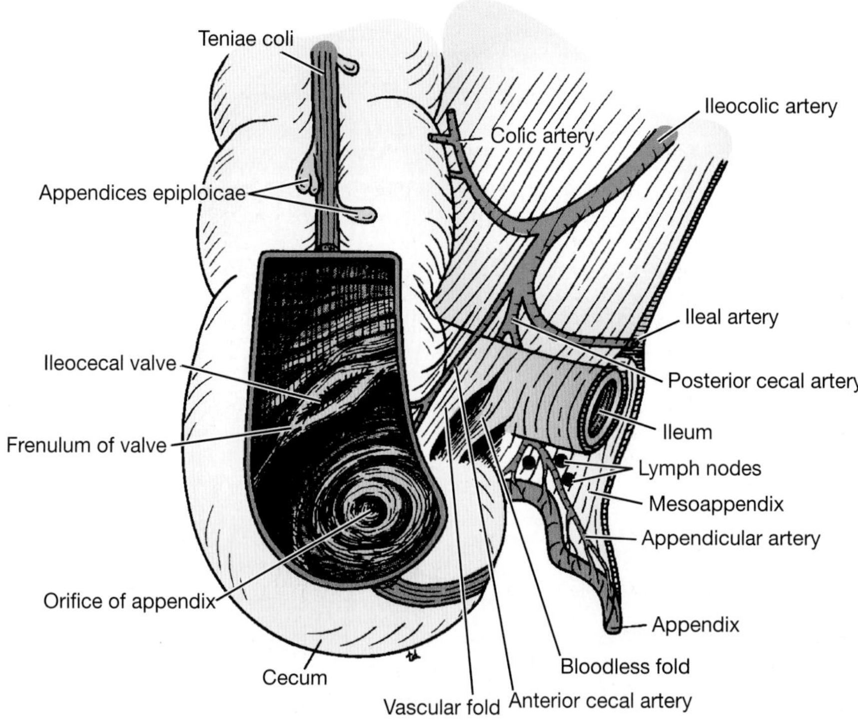

Figure 5.77 Cecum and appendix. Note that the appendicular artery is a branch of the posterior cecal artery. The edge of the mesoappendix has been cut to show the peritoneal layers.

Cecum

The cecum is the part of the large intestine that lies below the level of the junction of the ileum with the large intestine (Fig. 5.77; see also Fig. 5.75). It is a blind-ended pouch that is situated in the right iliac fossa. It is about 2.5 in. (6 cm) long and is completely covered with the peritoneum. It possesses a considerable amount of mobility, although it does not have a mesentery. The appendix is attached to its posteromedial surface. The presence of peritoneal folds in the vicinity of the cecum (see Fig. 5.77) creates the superior ileocecal, the inferior ileocecal, and the retrocecal recesses (see the section on "Peritoneal Pouches, Recesses, Spaces, and Gutters" earlier in this chapter).

As in the colon, the longitudinal muscle is restricted to three flat bands, the **teniae coli**, which converge on the base of the appendix and provide for it a complete longitudinal muscle coat. The cecum is often distended with gas and can then be palpated through the anterior abdominal wall in the living patient.

The terminal part of the ileum enters the large intestine at the junction of the cecum with the ascending colon. The opening is provided with two folds, or lips, which form the so-called ileocecal valve (see below). The appendix communicates with the cavity of the cecum through an opening located below and behind the ileocecal opening.

Relations

- **Anteriorly:** Coils of the small intestine, sometimes part of the greater omentum, and the anterior abdominal wall in the right iliac region.
- **Posteriorly:** The psoas and the iliacus muscles, the femoral nerve, and the lateral cutaneous nerve of the thigh (Fig. 5.78). The appendix is commonly found behind the cecum.
- **Medially:** The appendix arises from the cecum on its medial side (see Fig. 5.77).

Blood Supply

Anterior and **posterior cecal arteries** supply the cecum. These are branches of the ileocolic artery, a branch of the superior mesenteric artery (see Fig. 5.77). The veins correspond to the arteries and drain into the **superior mesenteric vein**.

Lymph Drainage

The lymph vessels pass through several mesenteric nodes and finally reach the **superior mesenteric nodes**.

Nerve Supply

Sympathetic and parasympathetic (vagus) nerves derived from the **superior mesenteric plexus** supply the cecum.

Ileocecal Valve

A rudimentary structure, the ileocecal valve consists of two horizontal folds of mucous membrane that project around the orifice of the ileum (see Fig. 5.77). The valve plays little or no part in the prevention of reflux of cecal contents into the ileum. The circular muscle of the lower end of the ileum (called the **ileocecal sphincter** by physiologists) serves as a sphincter and

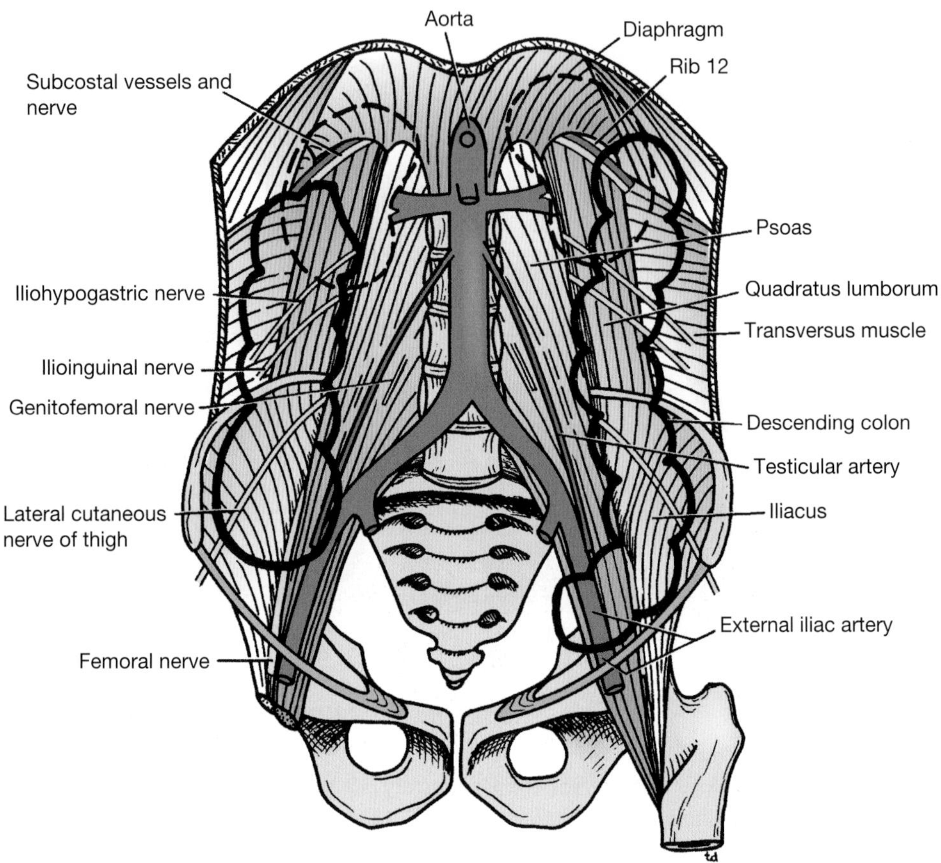

Figure 5.78 Posterior abdominal wall showing posterior relations of the kidneys and the colon.

controls the flow of contents from the ileum into the colon. The smooth muscle tone is reflexively increased when the cecum is distended; the hormone **gastrin**, which is produced by the stomach, causes relaxation of the muscle tone.

Appendix (Vermiform Appendix)

The appendix (see Figs. 5.45 and 5.77) is a narrow, muscular tube containing a large amount of lymphoid tissue. It varies in length from 3 to 5 in. (8 to 13 cm). The base is attached to the posteromedial surface of the cecum about 1 in. (2.5 cm) below the ileocecal junction. The remainder of the appendix is free. It has a complete peritoneal covering, which is attached to the mesentery of the small intestine by a short mesentery of its own, the **mesoappendix**. The mesoappendix contains the appendicular vessels and nerves.

The appendix lies in the right iliac fossa. In relation to the anterior abdominal wall, its base is situated one third of the way up the line joining the right anterior superior iliac spine to the umbilicus (**McBurney's point**). Inside the abdomen, the base of the appendix is easily found by identifying the teniae coli of the cecum and tracing them to the base of the appendix, where they converge to form a continuous longitudinal muscle coat (see Figs. 5.75 and 5.77).

Common Positions of Appendix Tip

The tip of the appendix is subject to a considerable range of movement and may be found in the following positions: (1) hanging down into the pelvis against the right pelvic wall, (2) coiled up behind the cecum, (3) projecting upward along the lateral side of the cecum, and (4) in front of or behind the terminal part of the ileum. The first and second positions are the most common sites.

Blood Supply

The **appendicular artery** is a branch of the posterior cecal artery (see Fig. 5.77). The **appendicular vein** drains into the posterior cecal vein.

Lymph Drainage

The lymph vessels drain into one or two nodes lying in the mesoappendix and then eventually into the **superior mesenteric nodes**.

Nerve Supply

Sympathetic and parasympathetic (vagus) nerves derived from the **superior mesenteric plexus** supply the appendix. Afferent nerve fibers concerned with the conduction of visceral pain from the appendix accompany the sympathetic nerves and enter the spinal cord at the level of the T10 segment.

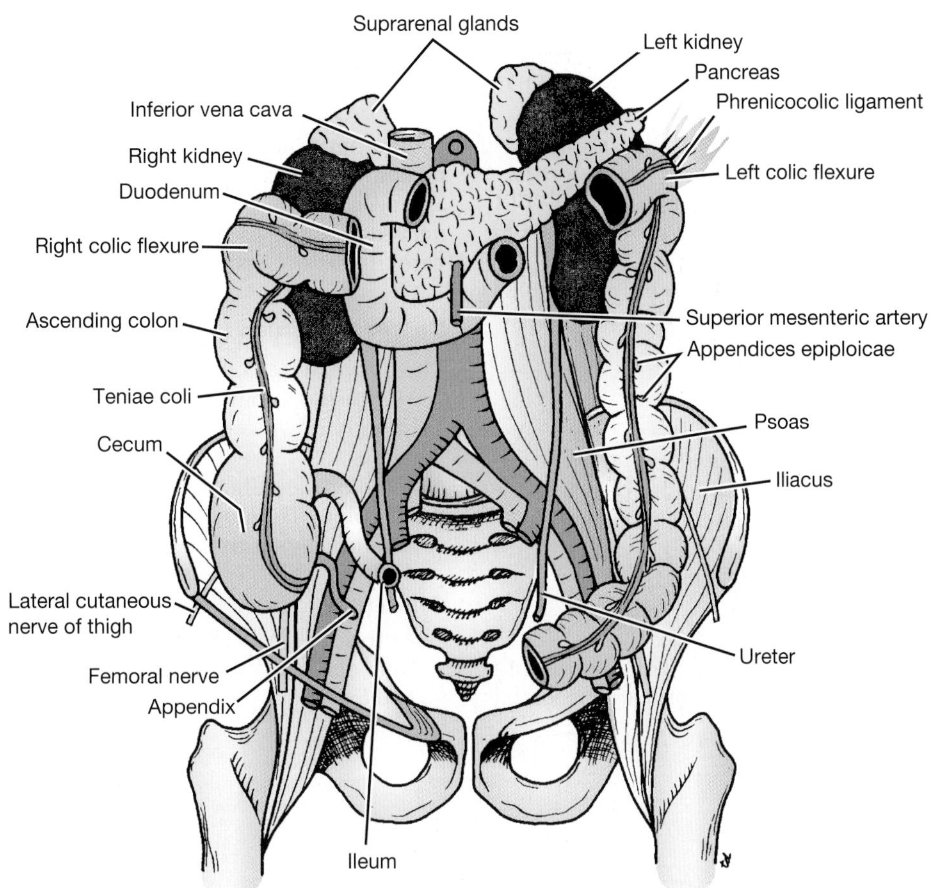

Figure 5.79 Abdominal cavity showing the terminal part of the ileum, the cecum, appendix, ascending colon, right and left colic flexures, and the descending colon. Note the teniae coli and the appendices epiploicae.

Ascending Colon

The ascending colon is about 5 in. (13 cm) long and lies in the right lower quadrant (Fig. 5.79). It extends upward from the cecum to the inferior surface of the right lobe of the liver, where it turns to the left, forming the **right colic (hepatic) flexure**, and becomes continuous with the transverse colon. The peritoneum covers the front and the sides of the ascending colon, binding it to the posterior abdominal wall.

Relations

- **Anteriorly:** Coils of the small intestine, the greater omentum, and the anterior abdominal wall (see Figs. 5.47 and 5.48).
- **Posteriorly:** The iliacus, the iliac crest, the quadratus lumborum, the origin of the transversus abdominis muscle, and the lower pole of the right kidney. The iliohypogastric and the ilioinguinal nerves cross behind it (see Fig. 5.78).

Blood Supply

The **ileocolic** and **right colic** branches of the superior mesenteric artery (see Fig. 5.75) supply this area. The veins correspond to the arteries and drain into the **superior mesenteric vein**.

Lymph Drainage

The lymph vessels drain into lymph nodes lying along the course of the colic blood vessels and ultimately reach the **superior mesenteric nodes**.

Nerve Supply

Sympathetic and parasympathetic (vagus) nerves from the **superior mesenteric plexus** supply this area of the colon.

Transverse Colon

The transverse colon is about 15 in. (38 cm) long and extends across the abdomen, occupying the umbilical region. It begins at the right colic flexure below the right lobe of the liver (see Fig. 5.49) and hangs downward, suspended by the transverse mesocolon from the pancreas (see Fig. 5.51). It then ascends to the **left colic (splenic) flexure** below the spleen. The left colic flexure is higher than the right colic flexure and is suspended from the diaphragm by the **phrenicocolic ligament** (see Fig. 5.79).

The **transverse mesocolon (mesentery of the transverse colon)** suspends the transverse colon from the anterior border of the pancreas (see Fig. 5.51). The mesentery is attached to the superior border of the transverse colon, and the posterior layers of the greater omentum are attached to the inferior border. Because of the length of the transverse mesocolon, the position of the transverse colon is extremely variable and may sometimes reach down as far as the pelvis.

Relations

- **Anteriorly:** The greater omentum and the anterior abdominal wall (umbilical and hypogastric regions) (see Fig. 5.51).
- **Posteriorly:** The second part of the duodenum, head of the pancreas, and the coils of the jejunum and the ileum (see Fig. 5.79).

Blood Supply

The **middle colic artery**, a branch of the superior mesenteric artery, supplies the proximal two-thirds (see Fig. 5.75). The **left colic artery**, a branch of the inferior mesenteric artery, supplies the distal third (Fig. 5.80).

The veins correspond to the arteries and drain into the **superior** and **inferior mesenteric veins**.

Lymph Drainage

The proximal two-thirds drain into the colic nodes and then into the **superior mesenteric nodes**. The distal third drains into the colic nodes and then into the **inferior mesenteric nodes**.

Nerve Supply

Sympathetic and vagal nerves through the **superior mesenteric plexus** innervate the proximal two-thirds. Sympathetic and parasympathetic pelvic splanchnic nerves through the **inferior mesenteric plexus** innervate the distal third.

Descending Colon

The descending colon is about 10 in. (25 cm) long and lies in the left upper and lower quadrants (see Fig. 5.79). It extends downward from the left colic flexure to the pelvic brim, where it becomes continuous with the sigmoid colon. See Chapter 6 for the description of the sigmoid colon. The peritoneum covers the front and the sides and binds it to the posterior abdominal wall.

Relations

- **Anteriorly:** Coils of small intestine, the greater omentum, and the anterior abdominal wall (see Figs. 5.47 and 5.48).

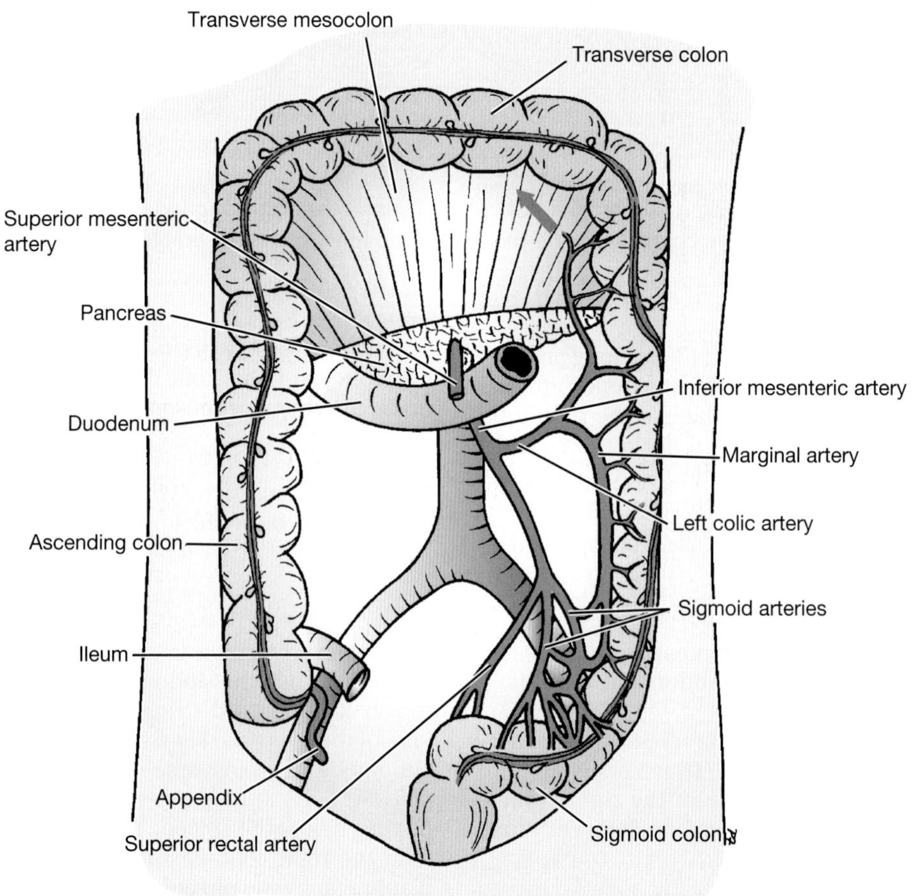

Figure 5.80 Inferior mesenteric artery and its branches. Note that this artery supplies the large bowel from the distal third of the transverse colon to halfway down the anal canal. It anastomoses with the middle colic branch of the superior mesenteric artery (*arrow*).

- **Posteriorly**: The lateral border of the left kidney, origin of the transversus abdominis muscle, quadratus lumborum, iliac crest, iliacus, and the left psoas. The iliohypogastric and ilioinguinal nerves, the lateral cutaneous nerve of the thigh, and the femoral nerve also lie posteriorly (see Fig. 5.78).

Blood Supply

The **left colic** and the **sigmoid branches** of the inferior mesenteric artery supply this area (see Fig. 5.80). The veins correspond to the arteries and drain into the **inferior mesenteric vein**.

Lymph Drainage

Lymph drains into the colic lymph nodes and the **inferior mesenteric nodes** around the origin of the inferior mesenteric artery.

Nerve Supply

The nerve supply is the sympathetic and parasympathetic **pelvic splanchnic nerves** through the inferior mesenteric plexus.

Differences between Small and Large Intestines

External differences between the small and large intestines include the following:

- The small intestine (except the duodenum) is mobile, whereas the ascending and descending parts of the colon are fixed.
- The caliber of the full small intestine is smaller than that of the filled large intestine.
- The small intestine (except the duodenum) has a mesentery that passes downward across the midline into the right iliac fossa.
- The longitudinal muscle of the small intestine forms a continuous layer around the gut. In the large intestine (except for the appendix), the longitudinal muscle is collected into three bands, the **teniae coli** (Fig. 5.81; see also Fig. 5.79).
- The small intestine has no fatty tags attached to its wall. The large intestine has fatty tags, called the **omental appendices** (**appendices epiploicae**; **epiploic appendages**).
- The wall of the small intestine is smooth, whereas that of the large intestine is sacculated in large folds termed **haustra**.

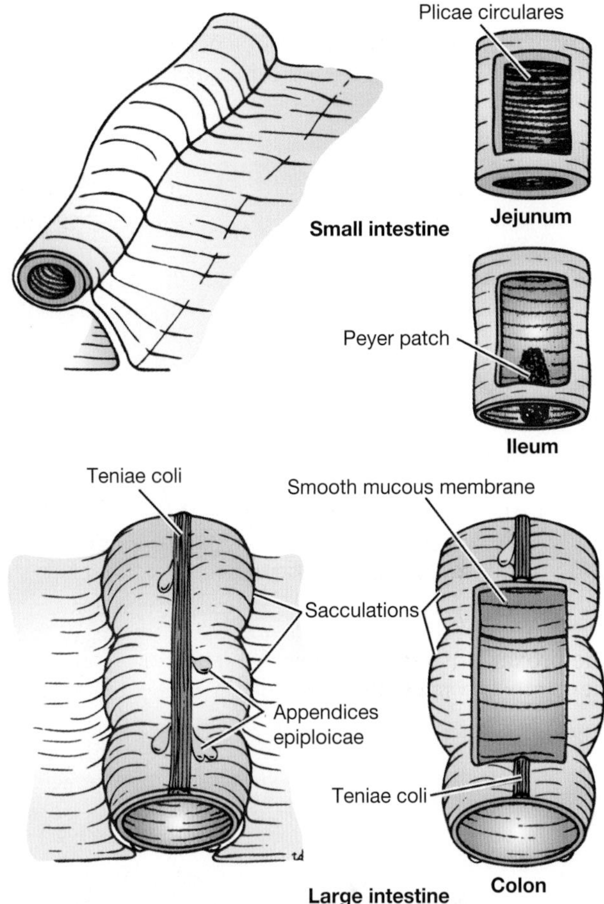

Figure 5.81 Some external and internal differences between the small and large intestines.

Internal differences between the small and large intestines include the following:

- The mucous membrane of the small intestine has permanent folds, called **plicae circulares**, which are absent in the large intestine (see Fig. 5.81).
- The mucous membrane of the small intestine has **villi**, which are absent in the large intestine.
- Aggregations of lymphoid tissue called **Peyer patches** are found in the mucous membrane of the small intestine; these are absent in the large intestine.

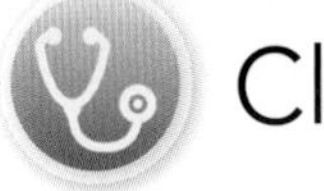

Clinical Notes

Colonoscopy

Because colorectal cancer is a leading cause of death in the Western world, colonoscopy is now being extensively used for early detection of malignant tumors. In this procedure, the mucous membrane of the colon can be directly visualized through an elongated flexible tube, or **endoscope**. Following a thorough washing out of the large bowel, the patient is sedated, and the tube is gently inserted into the anal canal. The interior of the large bowel can be observed from the anus to the cecum (Fig. 5.82). Photographs of suspicious areas, such as polyps, can be taken, and biopsy specimens can be removed for pathologic examination. Although a relatively expensive procedure, it provides a more complete screening examination for colorectal cancer than combined fecal occult blood testing and the examination of the distal colon with **sigmoidoscopy** (see Chapter 6, "Clinical Notes, Sigmoidoscopy").

(continued)

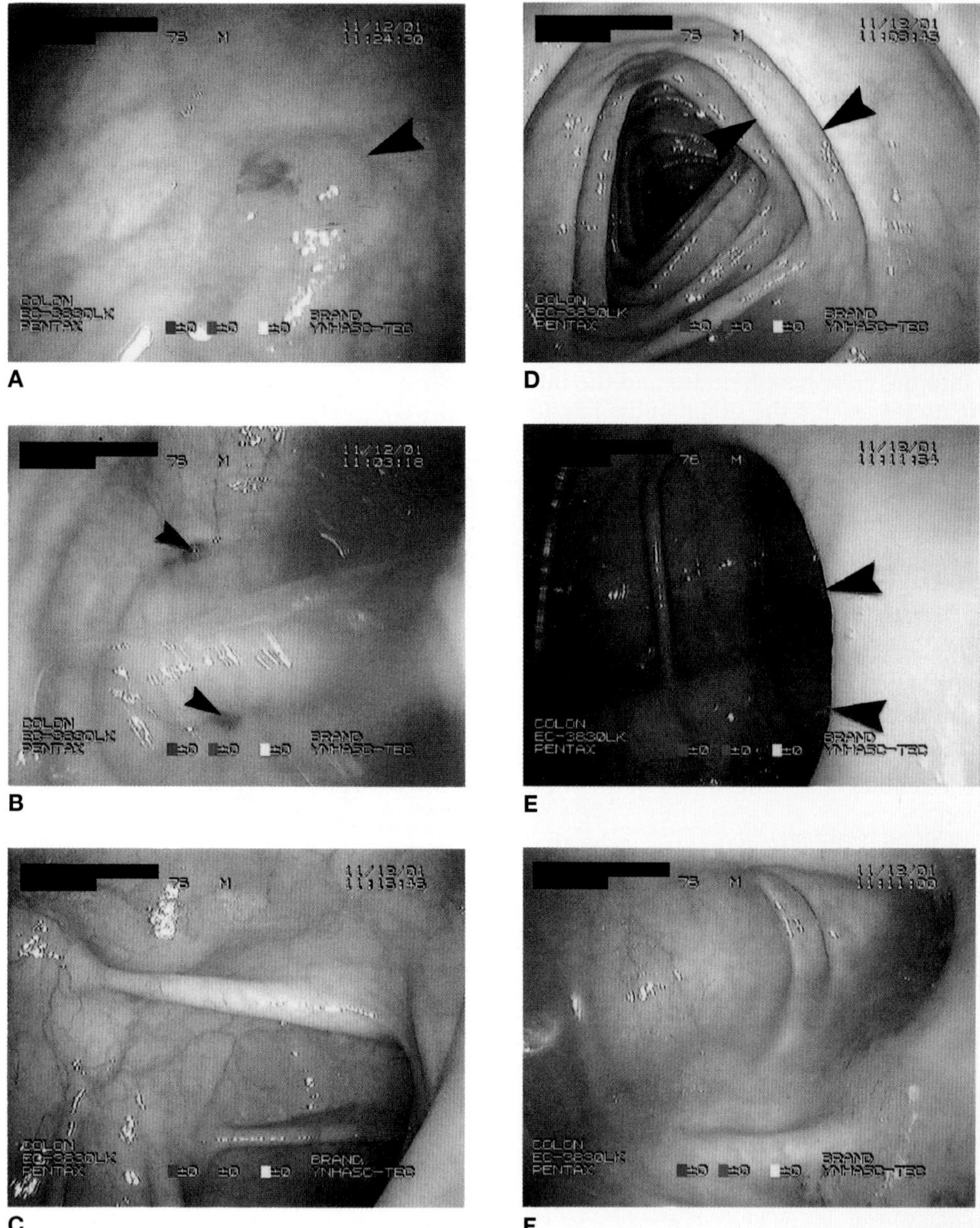

Figure 5.82 Series of the interior of the large bowel taken during a colonoscopy procedure. **A.** Rectal mucosa shows a small benign polyp (*arrowhead*). **B.** Sigmoid mucous membrane shows evidence of a mild diverticulosis. *Arrowheads* indicate the entrances into the mucosal pouches. **C.** Splenic flexure is normal. Note the light reflections from the drops of mucus on the mucous membrane. **D.** Transverse colon shows the characteristic normal folds or ridges (*arrowheads*) between the sacculations of the wall of the colon. **E.** Ileocecal valve shows the upper lip (*arrowheads*) of the valve, which has a normal appearance. **F.** Finally, the mucous membrane lining the inferior wall or floor of the cecum looks normal. (Courtesy of M.H. Brand.)

Appendiceal Position Variability

The inconstancy of the position of the appendix should be recalled when attempting to diagnose appendicitis. A retrocecal appendix, for example, may lie behind a cecum distended with gas, and thus it may be difficult to elicit tenderness on palpation in the right iliac region. Irritation of the psoas muscle, conversely, may cause the patient to keep the right hip joint flexed.

An appendix hanging down in the pelvis may result in absent abdominal tenderness in the right lower quadrant, but deep tenderness may be experienced just above the symphysis pubis. Rectal or vaginal examination may reveal tenderness of the peritoneum in the pelvis on the right side.

Appendiceal Predisposition to Infection

The following factors contribute to the appendix's predilection to infection:

- It is a long, narrow, blind-ended tube, which encourages stasis of large-bowel contents.
- It has a large amount of lymphoid tissue in its wall.
- The lumen has a tendency to become obstructed by hardened intestinal contents (**enteroliths**), which leads to further stagnation of its contents.

Appendiceal Predisposition to Perforation

A long, small artery that does not anastomose with other arteries supplies the appendix. The terminal branches of the appendicular artery supply the blind end of the appendix. Inflammatory edema of the appendicular wall compresses the blood supply to the appendix and often leads to thrombosis of the appendicular artery. These conditions commonly result in necrosis or gangrene of the appendicular wall, with perforation.

Perforation of the appendix or transmigration of bacteria through the inflamed appendicular wall results in infection of the peritoneum of the greater sac. The part that the greater omentum may play in arresting the spread of the peritoneal infection is described in "Clinical Notes (Greater Omentum)" earlier in this chapter.

Appendicitis Pain

Visceral pain in the appendix is produced by distention of its lumen or spasm of its muscle. The afferent pain fibers enter the spinal cord at the level of the T10 segment, and **vague referred pain** is felt in the region of the umbilicus. Later, the pain shifts to where the inflamed appendix irritates the parietal peritoneum. Here the pain is **precise**, **severe**, and **localized** (see "Clinical Notes, Abdominal Pain," later in this chapter).

Cecum and Colon Trauma

Blunt injuries most commonly occur where mobile parts of the colon (transverse and sigmoid) join the fixed parts (ascending and descending). **Penetrating injuries** following stab wounds are common. The multiple anatomic relationships of the different parts of the colon explain why isolated colonic trauma is unusual.

Large Bowel Cancer

Cancer of the large bowel is relatively common in persons older than age 50 years. The growth is restricted to the bowel wall for a considerable time before it spreads via the lymphatics. Bloodstream spread via the portal circulation to the liver occurs late. If a diagnosis is made early and a partial colectomy is performed, accompanied by removal of the lymph vessels and lymph nodes draining the area, a cure can be anticipated.

Diverticulosis

Diverticulosis of the colon is a common clinical condition. It consists of a herniation of the lining mucosa through the circular muscle between the teniae coli and occurs at points where the circular muscle is weakest, that is, where the blood vessels pierce the muscle (Fig. 5.83). The common site for herniation is shown in Figure 5.83B. The term **diverticulitis** refers to the inflammation of a diverticulum or diverticula, and this may result in perforation of the gut wall.

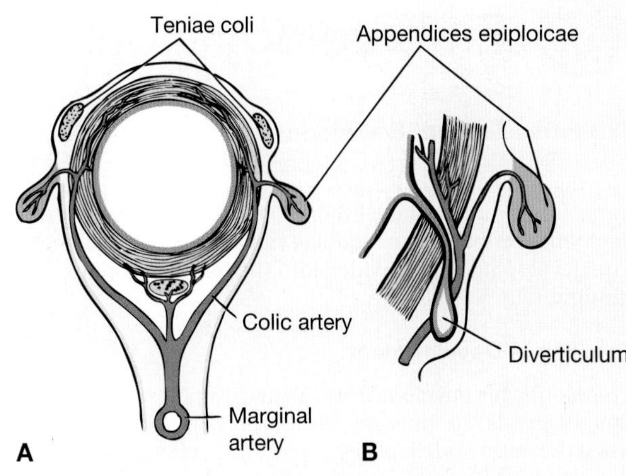

Figure 5.83 Blood supply to the colon **(A)** and formation of the diverticulum **(B)**. Note the passage of the mucosal diverticulum through the muscle coat along the course of the artery.

Cecostomy and Colostomy

Because of their anatomic mobility, the cecum, transverse colon, and sigmoid colon may be brought to the surface through a small opening in the anterior abdominal wall. If the cecum or transverse colon is then opened, the bowel contents may be allowed to drain by this route. These procedures are referred to as cecostomy or colostomy, respectively, and are used to relieve large-bowel obstructions.

Volvulus

Because of its extreme mobility, the sigmoid colon sometimes rotates around its mesentery. This may correct itself spontaneously, or the rotation may continue until the blood supply of the gut is cut off completely.

Intussusception

Intussusception is the telescoping of a proximal segment of the bowel into the lumen of an adjoining distal segment. There is a grave risk of cutting off the blood supply to the gut and developing gangrene. It is common in children. Ileocolic, colocolic, and ileoileal forms do occur, but **ileocolic** is the most common.

The high incidence in children may be caused by the relatively large size of the large bowel compared with the small intestine at this time of life. Another factor may be the possible swelling of Peyer patches secondary to infection. In the latter case, the swollen patch protrudes into the lumen, and violent peristalsis of the ileal wall tries to pass it distally along the gut lumen.

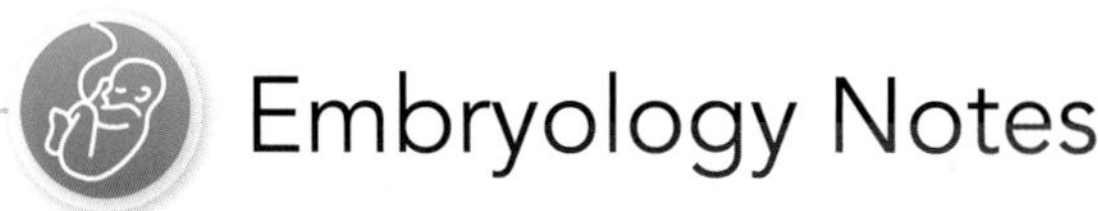

Embryology Notes

Digestive System Development

The digestive tube is formed from the yolk sac. The endoderm forms the epithelial lining, and the splanchnic mesenchyme forms the surrounding muscle and serous coats. The developing gut is divided into the **foregut**, **midgut**, and **hindgut** (Fig. 5.84).

Esophagus Development

The esophagus develops from the narrow part of the foregut that succeeds the pharynx. At first, it is a short tube, but when the heart and diaphragm descend, it elongates rapidly.

Esophageal Atresia

Atresia of the esophagus, with and without fistula, with the trachea is considered in detail in Chapter 4.

Esophageal Stenosis

Esophageal stenosis is a narrowing of the lumen of the esophagus, which commonly occurs in the lower part. It is treated by dilatation.

Congenital Short Esophagus

Abnormal shortness of the esophagus is caused by an **esophageal hiatus hernia** in the diaphragm. Stomach contents flow into the esophagus, resulting in **esophagitis**.

Stomach Development

The stomach develops as a dilatation of the foregut (Fig. 5.85). To begin with, it has a ventral and dorsal mesentery. Very active growth takes place along the dorsal border, which becomes convex and forms the **greater curvature**. The anterior border becomes concave and forms the **lesser curvature**. The **fundus** appears as a dilatation at the upper end of the stomach. At this stage, the stomach has a right and left surface to which the **right and left vagus nerves** are attached, respectively. With the great growth of the right lobe of the liver, the stomach is gradually rotated to the right so that the left surface becomes anterior and the right surface posterior.

The ventral and dorsal mesenteries now change position as a result of rotation of the stomach, and they form the omenta and various peritoneal ligaments. The pouch of the peritoneum behind the stomach is known as the **lesser sac**.

Congenital Hypertrophic Pyloric Stenosis

Hypertrophic pyloric stenosis is a relatively common emergency in infants between ages 3 and 6 weeks. The child ejects the stomach contents with considerable force. The exact cause of the stenosis is unknown, although evidence suggests that the number of autonomic ganglion cells in the stomach wall is fewer than normal. This possibility leads to prenatal neuromuscular incoordination and localized muscular hypertrophy and hyperplasia of the pyloric sphincter. It is much more common in male children.

Duodenum Development

The duodenum is formed from the most caudal portion of the foregut and the most cephalic end of the midgut. This region rapidly grows to form a loop. At this time, the duodenum has a mesentery that extends to the posterior abdominal wall and is part of the dorsal mesentery. A small part of the ventral mesentery is also attached to the ventral border of the first part of the duodenum and the upper half of the second part of the duodenum. When the stomach rotates, the duodenal loop is forced to rotate to the right, where the second, third, and fourth parts adhere to the posterior abdominal wall. Now the peritoneum behind the duodenum disappears. However, some smooth muscle and fibrous tissue that belong to the dorsal mesentery remain as the **suspensory ligament of the duodenum (ligament of Treitz)**, and this fixes the terminal part of the duodenum and prevents it from moving inferiorly (Fig. 5.86). The liver and pancreas arise as endodermal buds from the developing duodenum.

Atresia and Stenosis

During the development of the duodenum, the lining cells proliferate at such a rate that the lumen becomes completely obliterated. Later, as a result of degeneration of

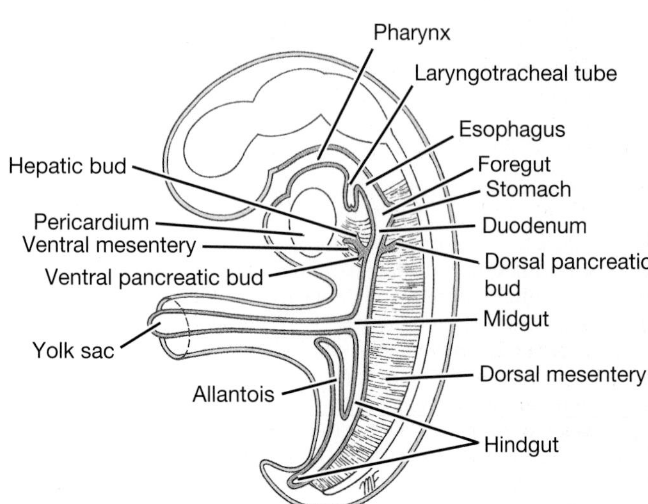

Figure 5.84 Foregut, midgut, and hindgut. The positions of the ventral and dorsal mesenteries, the hepatic bud, and the ventral and dorsal pancreatic buds are also shown.

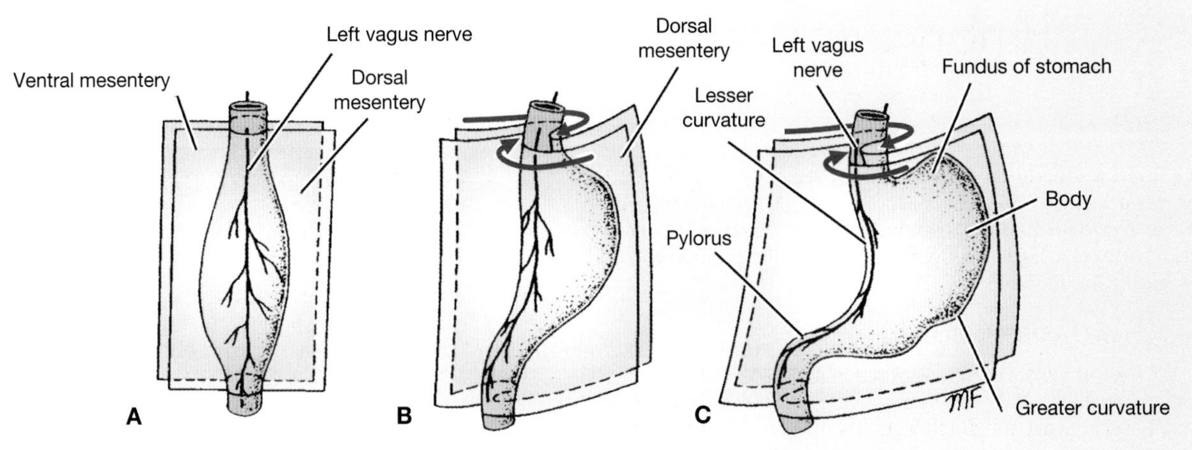

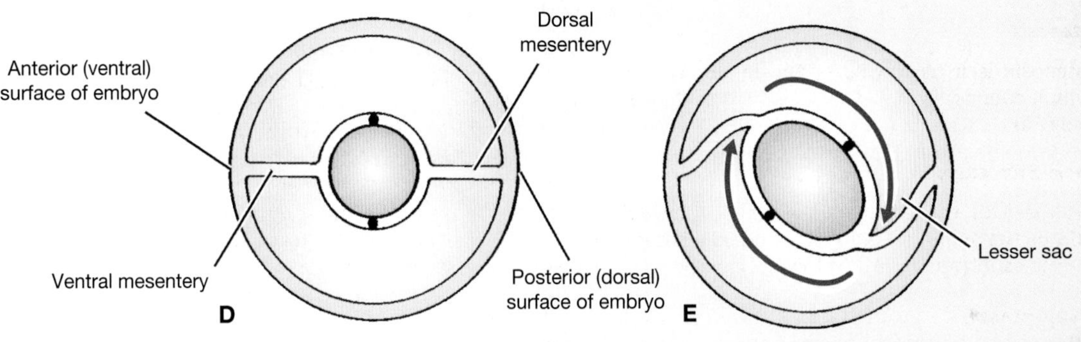

Figure 5.85 Development of the stomach in relation to the ventral and dorsal mesenteries. **A–C.** Lateral views of pre- **(A)**, early **(B)**, and late **(C)** phases of rotation. **D, E.** Cross-sectional views of pre- **(D)** and mid-phases of rotation. Note how the stomach rotates so that the left vagus nerve comes to lie on the anterior surface of the stomach. Note also the position of the lesser sac.

these cells, the gut becomes recanalized. Failure of recanalization could produce atresia or stenosis. Different forms of duodenal atresia and stenosis are shown in Figure 5.87. Vomiting is the most common presenting symptom, and the vomit usually is bile stained. Surgical treatment during the first few days of life is essential.

Midgut Development

The distal duodenum, the jejunum and ileum, and the large intestine as far as the distal third of the transverse colon develop from the midgut. The midgut increases rapidly in length and forms a loop to the apex, on which the **vitelline duct** is attached. This duct passes through the widely open umbilicus (see Fig. 5.84). At the same time, the dorsal mesentery elongates, and passing through it from the aorta to the yolk sac are the **vitelline arteries**. These arteries now fuse to form the superior mesenteric artery, which supplies the midgut and its derivatives. The rapidly growing liver and kidneys now encroach on the abdominal cavity, causing the midgut loop to herniate into the umbilical cord.

A diverticulum appears at the caudal end of the bowel loop, forming the **cecum**. At first, the diverticulum is conical; later, the upper part expands and forms the cecum, whereas the lower part remains rudimentary and forms the **appendix** (Fig. 5.88). After birth, the wall of the cecum grows unequally, and the appendix comes to lie on its medial side.

Although the loop of gut is in the umbilical cord, its **cephalic limb** becomes greatly elongated and coiled and forms the future jejunum and greater part of the ileum. The **caudal limb** of the loop also increases in length, but it remains uncoiled and forms the future distal part of the ileum, the cecum, the appendix, the ascending colon, and the proximal two-thirds of the transverse colon.

Midgut Loop Rotation in the Umbilical Cord and Return to Abdominal Cavity

While in the umbilical cord, the midgut rotates around an axis formed by the superior mesenteric artery and the vitelline duct. Viewing the embryo from the anterior aspect, a **counterclockwise rotation** of ~90° occurs (Fig. 5.89). Later, as the gut returns to the abdominal cavity, the midgut rotates counterclockwise an additional 180°. Thus, a counterclockwise rotation of a total of 270° has occurred (Fig. 5.90).

The rotation of the gut results in part of the large intestine (transverse colon) coming in front of the superior mesenteric artery and the second part of the duodenum;

(continued)

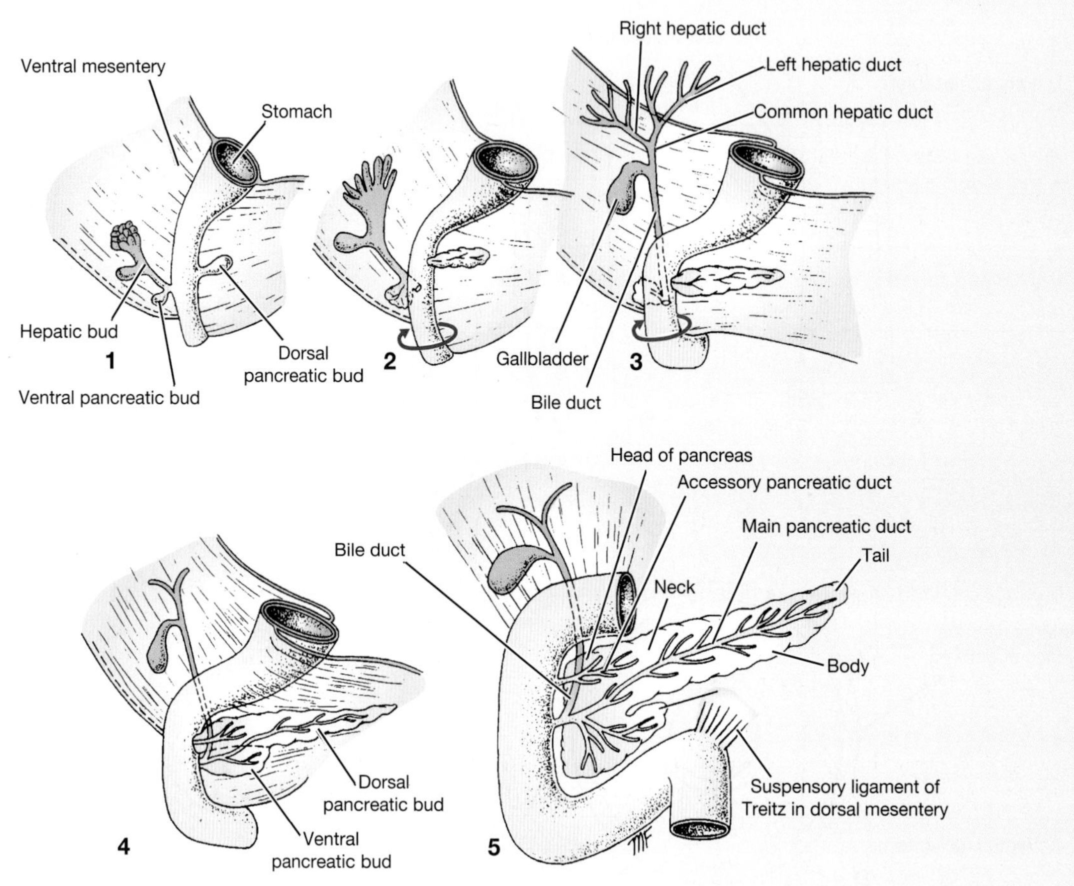

Figure 5.86 Progressive stages (1 to 5) in the development of the pancreas and the extrahepatic biliary apparatus. The *red arrows* indicate the direction of rotation of the duodenum.

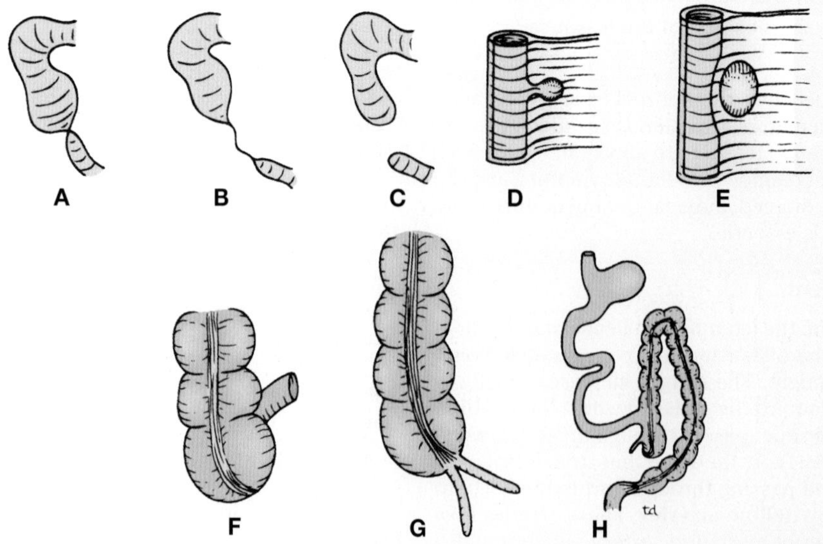

Figure 5.87 Some common congenital anomalies of the intestinal tract. **A–C.** Congenital atresias of the small intestine. **D.** Diverticulum of the duodenum or jejunum. **E.** Mesenteric cyst of the small intestine. **F.** Absence of the appendix. **G.** Double appendix. **H.** Malrotation of the gut, with the appendix lying in the left iliac fossa. For Meckel diverticulum, see Figure 5.35.

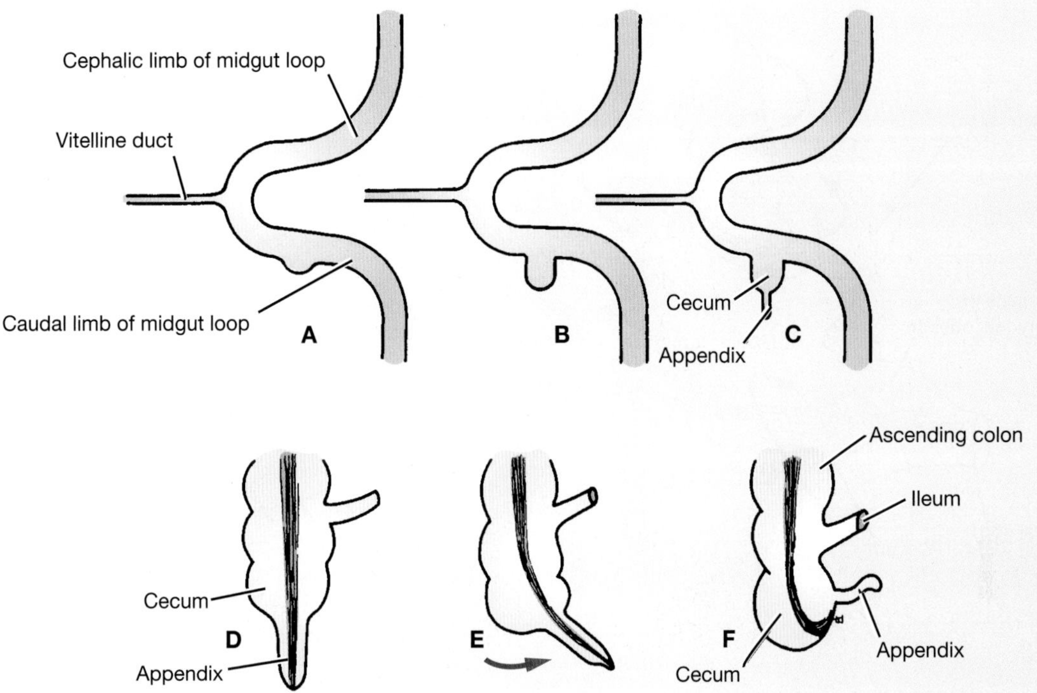

Figure 5.88 Progressive stages **(A–F)** in the development of the cecum and appendix. The *red arrow* indicates the rotation of the appendix. The final stages of development (stages **D–F**) take place after birth.

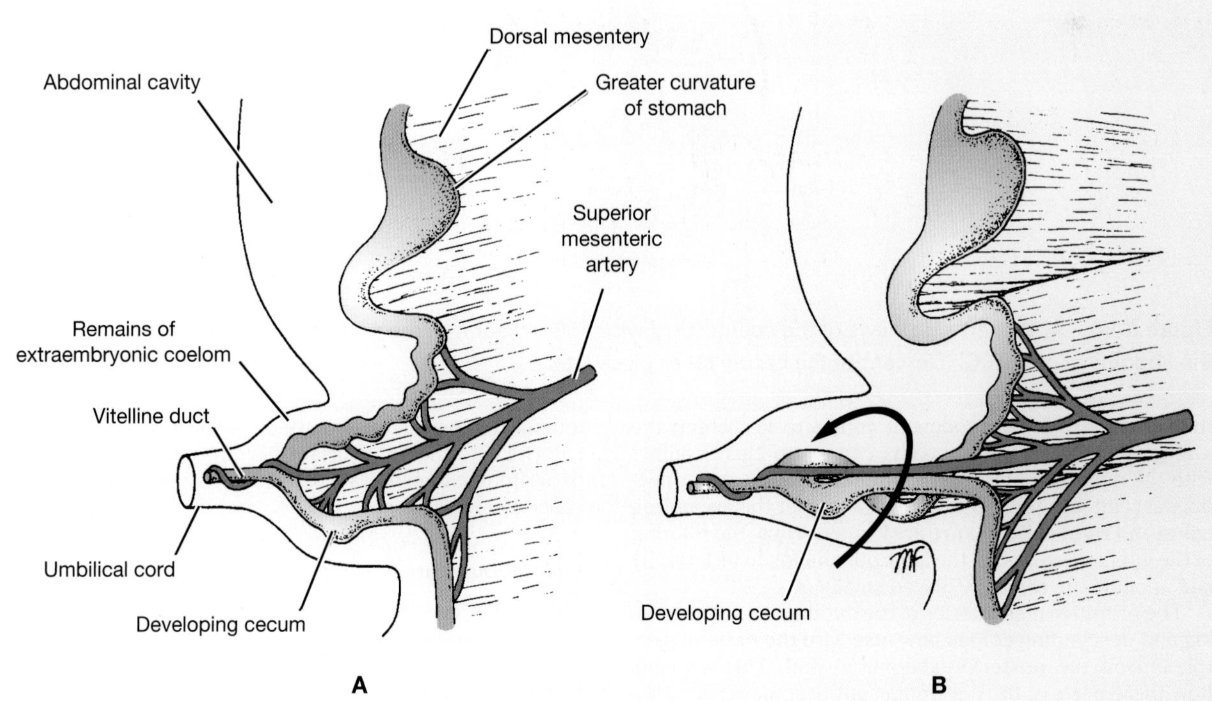

Figure 5.89 Left-side views of the midgut loop before rotation **(A)** and during initial counterclockwise 90° rotation **(B)** while it is in the extraembryonic coelom in the umbilical cord.

(continued)

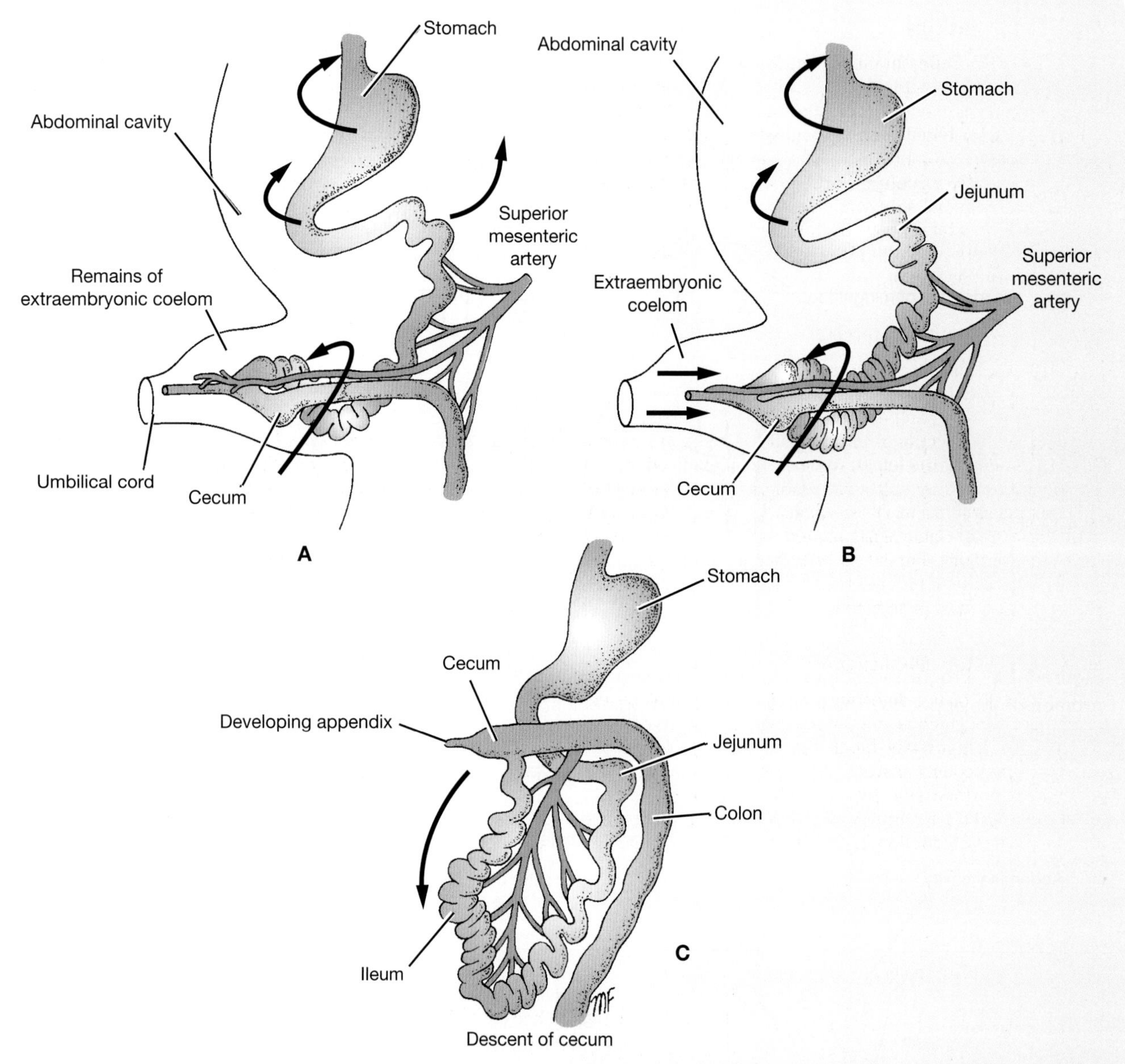

Figure 5.90 **A, B.** Left-side views of the counterclockwise 180° rotation of the midgut loop as it is withdrawn into the abdominal cavity. **C.** Descent of the cecum takes place later.

the third part of the duodenum comes to lie behind the artery. The cecum and appendix come into close contact with the right lobe of the liver. Later, the cecum and appendix descend into the right iliac fossa so that the **ascending colon** and **right colic flexure** are formed. Thus, the rotation of the gut has resulted in the large gut coming to lie laterally and encircle the centrally placed small gut.

The primitive mesenteries of the duodenum and ascending and descending colons now fuse with the parietal peritoneum on the posterior abdominal wall. This explains how these parts of the developing gut become retroperitoneal. The primitive mesenteries of the jejunum and ileum, the transverse colon, and the sigmoid colon persist as the **mesentery of the small intestine**, **transverse mesocolon**, and **sigmoid mesocolon**, respectively.

The rotation of the stomach and duodenum to the right is largely brought about by the great growth of the right lobe of the liver. The left surface of the stomach becomes anterior, and the right surface becomes posterior. A pouch of peritoneum becomes located behind the stomach and is called the **lesser sac**.

Vitelline Duct Fate

The midgut is at first connected with the yolk sac by the vitelline duct. By the time, the gut returns to the abdominal cavity, the duct becomes obliterated and severs its connection with the gut.

Hindgut Development

The left colic flexure, descending colon, sigmoid colon, rectum, and upper half of the anal canal are developed from the hindgut.

Intestinal Diverticula

All coats of the intestinal wall are found in the wall of a **congenital diverticulum**. In the duodenum, diverticula are found on the medial wall of the second and third parts (see Fig. 5.87). Usually, these are symptomless. **Jejunal diverticula** occasionally occur and usually give rise to no symptoms. A **diverticulum of the cecum** is commonly situated on the medial side of the cecum close to the ileocecal valve. It may be subject to acute inflammation and then is confused with appendicitis. Diverticula of the colon are acquired, not congenital.

Intestinal Atresia and Stenosis

The most common site of an atretic or stenotic obstruction is in the duodenum. The next most common sites are the ileum and jejunum, respectively (see Fig. 5.87). Frequently, the obstruction occurs at multiple sites. The cause is possibly the failure of the lumen to become recanalized after it has been blocked by epithelial proliferation of the cells of the mucous membrane. Other causes have been suggested, such as vascular damage associated with twisting or volvulus of the intestine. Persistent bile-stained vomiting occurs from birth. Surgical relief of the obstruction should be carried out as soon as possible.

Digestive System Duplication

In duplication of the digestive system, the normal degeneration of the mucous membrane cells, which have proliferated to temporarily block the lumen, occurs at two sites simultaneously instead of at one. In this way, two lumina are formed side by side. The additional segment of bowel should be removed as soon as possible because it may cause obstruction or be the site of hemorrhage or perforation.

Complete Absence of Rotation or Incomplete Rotation of Midgut Loop

The complete absence of rotation is rare. In cases of incomplete rotation, no further rotation occurs after the initial counterclockwise rotation of 90° in the umbilical cord. Thus, the duodenum, jejunum, and ileum remain on the right side of the abdomen, and the cecum and colon are on the left side (see Fig. 5.87). In other cases, a counterclockwise rotation of 180° occurs, and, although the duodenum may take up its correct position posterior to the superior mesenteric artery, the cecum comes to lie anterior and to the left of the duodenum. Abnormal adhesions form, which run across the anterior surface of the duodenum and cause obstruction to its second part.

Midgut Loop Malrotation

Counterclockwise rotation of 90° followed by clockwise rotation of 90° or 180° may occur. In these cases, the duodenum comes to lie anterior to the superior mesenteric artery, and the colon may come to lie anterior to the mesentery of the small intestine. Repeated vomiting is usually the presenting symptom and is caused by duodenal obstruction. Surgical correction of the incomplete rotation or malrotation of the gut is performed, and all adhesions are divided.

Persistence of the Vitellointestinal Duct

The vitelline duct in the early embryo connects the developing gut to the yolk sac (Fig. 5.91). Normally, as development proceeds, the duct is obliterated, severs its connection with the intestine, and disappears. Persistence of the vitellointestinal duct can result in an **umbilical fistula** (see Fig. 5.35). If the duct remains as a fibrous band, a loop of the small intestine can become wrapped around it, causing intestinal obstruction.

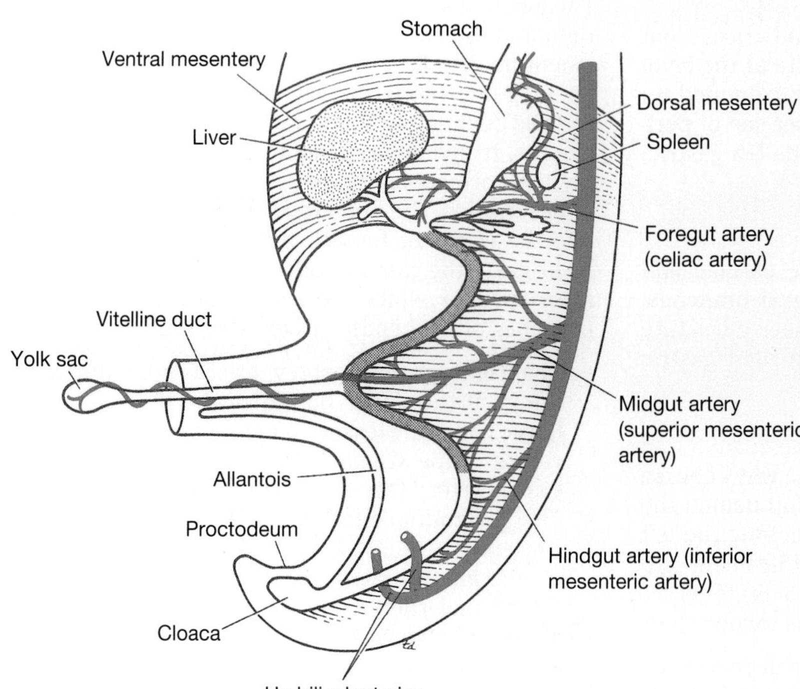

Figure 5.91 Formation of the midgut loop (*shaded*). Note how the superior mesenteric artery and the vitelline duct form an axis for the future rotation of the midgut loop.

(continued)

Meckel Diverticulum

Meckel diverticulum, a congenital anomaly, represents a persistent portion of the **vitellointestinal duct**. The diverticulum is located on the antimesenteric border of the ileum about 2 ft (61 cm) from the ileocecal junction. It is about 2 in. (5 cm) long and occurs in about 2% of individuals. The diverticulum is important clinically, because it may possess a small area of **gastric mucosa**, and bleeding may occur from a "gastric" ulcer in its mucous membrane. Moreover, the pain from this ulcer may be confused with the pain from appendicitis. Should a fibrous band connect the diverticulum to the umbilicus, a loop of small bowel may become wrapped around it, causing intestinal obstruction.

Undescended Cecum and Appendix

In cases of undescended cecum and appendix, an inflammation of the appendix would give rise to tenderness in the right hypochondrium, which may lead to a mistaken diagnosis of inflammation of the gallbladder.

Appendiceal Anomalies

Agenesis of the appendix (failure to develop) is extremely rare; however, a few examples of **double appendix** have been reported (see Fig. 5.87). The possibility of **left-sided appendix** in individuals with transposition of thoracic and abdominal viscera or in cases of arrested rotation of the midgut should always be remembered.

Colon Anomalies

The congenital anomaly of undescended cecum or failure of rotation of the gut so that the cecum lies in the left iliac fossa may give rise to confusion in diagnosis. The pain of appendicitis, for example, although initially starting in the umbilical region, may shift not to the right iliac fossa, but to the right upper quadrant or to the left lower quadrant.

Gastrointestinal Tract Arterial Supply

The arterial supply to the gut is related to the development of the different parts of the gut (see Fig. 5.91). The **celiac artery** is the artery of the foregut and supplies the GI tract from the lower third of the esophagus down as far as the middle of the second part of the duodenum. The **superior mesenteric artery** is the artery of the midgut and supplies the GI tract from the middle of the second part of the duodenum as far as the distal third of the transverse colon. The **inferior mesenteric artery** is the artery of the hindgut and supplies the large intestine from the distal one-third of the transverse colon to halfway down the anal canal.

Celiac Artery

The celiac artery or trunk is very short and arises from the commencement of the abdominal aorta at the level of the T12 vertebra (see Fig. 5.64). It is surrounded by the celiac plexus and lies behind the lesser sac of peritoneum. It has three terminal branches: the left gastric, splenic, and hepatic arteries.

Left Gastric Artery

The small left gastric artery runs to the cardiac end of the stomach, gives off a few esophageal branches, and then turns to the right along the lesser curvature of the stomach. It anastomoses with the right gastric artery (see Fig. 5.64).

Splenic Artery

The large splenic artery runs to the left in a wavy course along the upper border of the pancreas and behind the stomach (see Figs. 5.49 and 5.70). On reaching the left kidney, the artery enters the splenorenal ligament and runs to the hilum of the spleen (see Fig. 5.55). The primary branches of the splenic artery are as follows:

- **Pancreatic branches**: As many as 10 small pancreatic arteries may branch off the splenic artery and supply the pancreas.
- The **left gastro-omental (gastroepiploic) artery** arises near the hilum of the spleen and reaches the greater curvature of the stomach in the gastrosplenic omentum. It passes to the right along the greater curvature of the stomach between the layers of the greater omentum. It anastomoses with the right gastroepiploic artery (see Fig. 5.64).
- The **short gastric arteries**, five or six in number, arise from the end of the splenic artery and reach the fundus of the stomach in the gastrosplenic omentum. They anastomose with the left gastric artery and the left gastro-omental artery (see Fig. 5.64).

Hepatic Artery

The medium-size hepatic artery runs forward and to the right and then ascends between the layers of the lesser omentum (see Figs. 5.51 and 5.55). It lies in front of the opening into the lesser sac and is placed to the left of the bile duct and in front of the portal vein. At the porta hepatis, it divides into right and left branches to supply the corresponding lobes of the liver. For purposes of description, the hepatic artery is sometimes divided into the **common hepatic artery**, which extends from its origin to the gastroduodenal branch, and the **hepatic artery proper**, which is the remainder of the artery. The branches of the hepatic artery are as follows:

- The **right gastric artery** arises from the hepatic artery at the upper border of the pylorus and runs to the left in the lesser omentum along the lesser curvature of the stomach. It anastomoses with the left gastric artery (see Fig. 5.64).
- The **gastroduodenal artery** is a large branch that descends behind the first part of the duodenum. It divides into the **right gastro-omental (gastroepiploic) artery** that runs along the greater curvature of the stomach between the layers of the greater omentum and the **superior pancreaticoduodenal artery** that descends between the second part of the duodenum and the head of the pancreas (see Figs. 5.49 and 5.64).

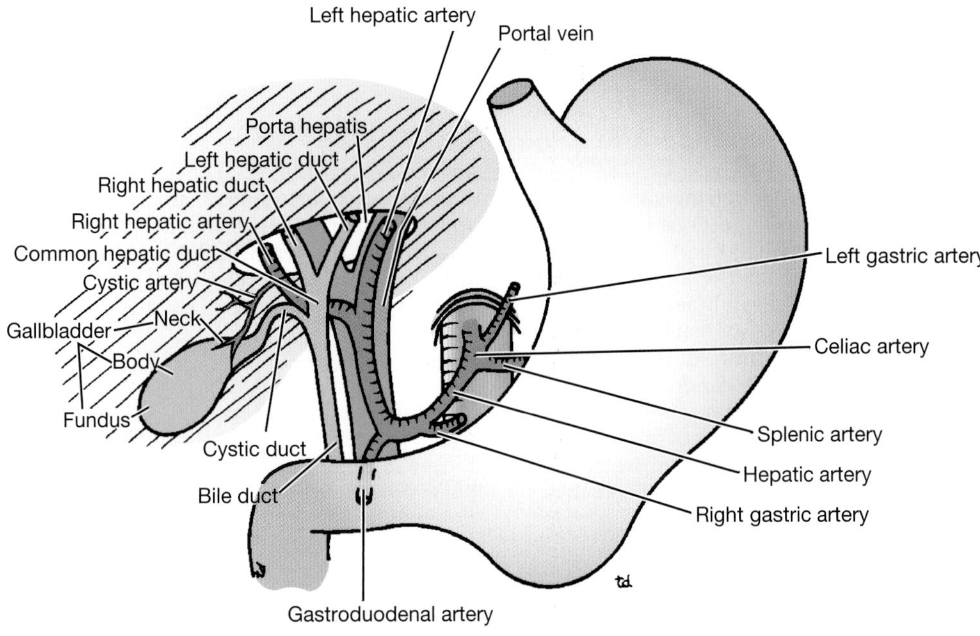

Figure 5.92 Structures entering and leaving the porta hepatis.

- The **right and left hepatic arteries** enter the **porta hepatis**. The right hepatic artery usually gives off the **cystic artery**, which runs to the neck of the gallbladder (Fig. 5.92).

Superior Mesenteric Artery

The superior mesenteric artery supplies the midgut—the distal part of the duodenum, jejunum, ileum, cecum, appendix, ascending colon, and most of the transverse colon (see Fig. 5.75). It arises from the front of the abdominal aorta just below the celiac artery and runs downward and to the right behind the neck of the pancreas and in front of the third part of the duodenum (see Fig. 5.79). It continues downward to the right between the layers of the mesentery of the small intestine and ends by anastomosing with the ileal branch of its own ileocolic branch.

Branches

- The **inferior pancreaticoduodenal artery** passes to the right as a single or double branch along the upper border of the third part of the duodenum and the head of the pancreas. It supplies the pancreas and the adjoining part of the duodenum (see Fig. 5.75).
- The **middle colic artery** runs forward in the transverse mesocolon to supply the transverse colon and divides into right and left branches.
- The **right colic artery** is often a branch of the ileocolic artery. It passes to the right to supply the ascending colon and divides into **ascending and descending branches**.
- The **ileocolic artery** passes downward and to the right. It gives rise to a **superior branch** that anastomoses with the right colic artery and an **inferior branch** that anastomoses with the end of the superior mesenteric artery. The inferior branch gives rise to the **anterior** and **posterior cecal arteries**. The **appendicular artery** is a branch of the posterior cecal artery (see Fig. 5.77).
- The **jejunal** and **ileal branches** are 12 to 15 in number and arise from the left side of the superior mesenteric artery (see Fig. 5.75). Each artery divides into two vessels, which unite with adjacent branches to form a series of **arcades** (see Figs. 5.75 and 5.76). Branches from the arcades divide and unite to form a second, third, and fourth series of arcades. Fewer arcades supply the jejunum than supply the ileum. From the terminal arcades, small straight vessels, the **vasa recta**, supply the intestine.

Inferior Mesenteric Artery

The inferior mesenteric artery supplies the hindgut—the distal third of the transverse colon, left colic flexure, descending colon, sigmoid colon, rectum, and the upper half of the anal canal. It arises from the abdominal aorta about 1.5 in. (3.8 cm) above its bifurcation (see Fig. 5.80). The artery runs downward and to the left and crosses the left common iliac artery. Here, it becomes the **superior rectal artery**.

Branches

- The **left colic artery** runs upward and to the left and supplies the distal third of the transverse colon, left colic flexure, and the upper part of the descending colon. It divides into **ascending** and **descending branches**.
- The **sigmoid arteries** are two or three in number and supply the descending and sigmoid colon.

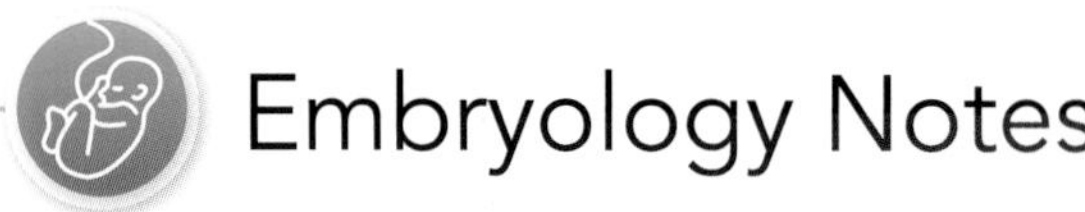

Embryology Notes

Foregut Arteries

The cephalic end of the foregut (which includes the pharynx) and the cervical and thoracic portions of the esophagus are supplied by the ascending pharyngeal arteries, palatine arteries, superior and inferior thyroid arteries, bronchial arteries, and esophageal branches from the aorta. The **celiac artery** supplies the caudal end of the foregut (which includes the distal third of the esophagus, stomach, and proximal half of the duodenum) (see Fig. 5.91). Interestingly, this artery also supplies the liver and pancreas, which are glandular derivatives of this part of the gut. The celiac artery also supplies the spleen, which is not surprising, because this organ develops in the dorsal mesentery of the foregut.

Midgut Artery

The **superior mesenteric artery** supplies the midgut, which extends from halfway along the second part of the duodenum to the left colic flexure. The superior mesenteric artery represents the fused pair of vitelline arteries (see Fig. 5.91).

Hindgut Artery

The **inferior mesenteric artery** supplies the hindgut, which extends from the left colic flexure to halfway down the anal canal (see Fig. 5.91). This represents several ventral branches of the aorta that fuse to form a single artery.

- The **superior rectal artery** is a continuation of the inferior mesenteric artery as it crosses the left common iliac artery. It descends into the pelvis behind the rectum. The artery supplies the rectum and upper half of the anal canal and anastomoses with the middle rectal and inferior rectal arteries.

Marginal Artery

The anastomosis of the colic arteries around the concave margin of the large intestine forms a single arterial line called the marginal artery. This begins at the ileocecal junction, where it anastomoses with the ileal branches of the superior mesenteric artery, and it ends where it anastomoses less freely with the superior rectal artery (see Fig. 5.80).

Gastrointestinal Tract Venous Drainage

The venous blood from the greater part of the GI tract and its accessory organs drains to the liver by the **portal venous system** (see Fig. 5.65). The portal circulation begins as a capillary plexus in the organs it drains and ends by emptying its blood into sinusoids within the liver.

The proximal tributaries drain directly into the portal vein, but the veins forming the distal tributaries correspond to the branches of the celiac artery and the superior and inferior mesenteric arteries.

Portal Vein (Hepatic Portal Vein)

The portal vein (see Fig. 5.65) drains blood from the abdominal part of the GI tract from the lower third of the esophagus to halfway down the anal canal. It also drains blood from the spleen, pancreas, and gallbladder. The portal vein enters the liver and breaks up into sinusoids, from which blood passes into the **hepatic veins** that join the **inferior vena cava**. The portal vein is about 2 in. (5 cm) long and forms behind the neck of the pancreas by the union of the **superior mesenteric** and **splenic veins** (Fig. 5.93). It ascends to the right, behind the first part of the duodenum, and enters the lesser omentum (see Figs. 5.52 and 5.55). It then runs upward in front of the opening into the lesser sac to the porta hepatis, where it lies behind the bile duct and the hepatic artery (see Fig. 5.92). Finally, it divides into **right** and **left terminal branches**.

Tributaries

- **Splenic vein:** This vein leaves the hilum of the spleen and passes to the right in the splenorenal ligament. It unites with the superior mesenteric vein behind the neck of the pancreas to form the portal vein (see Fig. 5.93). It receives the short gastric, left gastro-omental, inferior mesenteric, and pancreatic veins.
- **Inferior mesenteric vein:** This vein ascends on the posterior abdominal wall and joins the splenic vein behind the body of the pancreas. It receives the superior rectal veins, the sigmoid veins, and the left colic vein.
- **Superior mesenteric vein:** This vein ascends in the root of the mesentery of the small intestine. It passes in front of the third part of the duodenum and joins the splenic vein behind the neck of the pancreas. It receives the jejunal, ileal, ileocolic, right colic, middle colic, inferior pancreaticoduodenal, and right gastro-omental veins.
- **Left gastric vein:** This vein drains the left portion of the lesser curvature of the stomach and the distal part of the esophagus. It opens directly into the portal vein (see Fig. 5.65).
- **Right gastric vein:** This vein drains the right portion of the lesser curvature of the stomach and drains directly into the portal vein.
- **Cystic veins:** These veins either drain the gallbladder directly into the liver or join the portal vein.

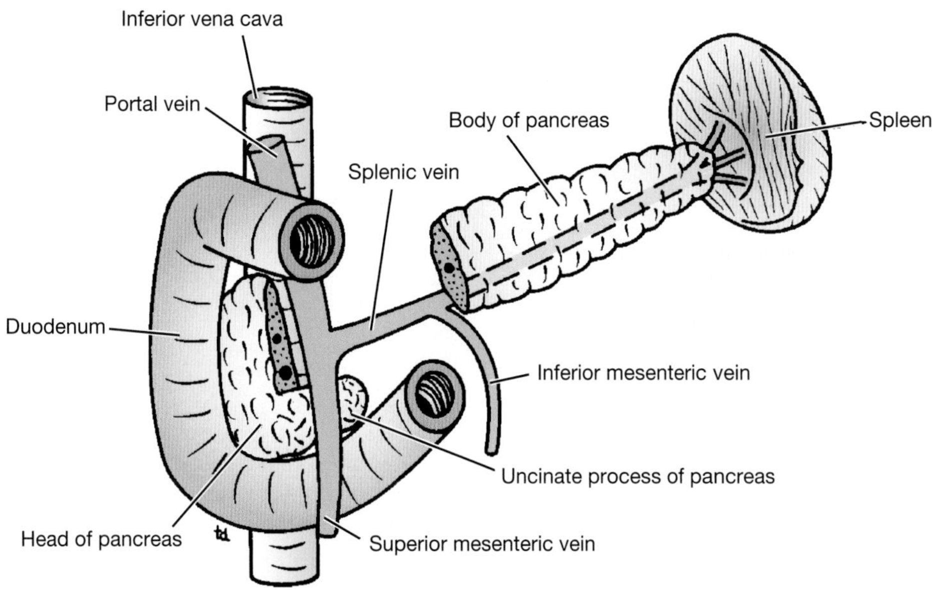

Figure 5.93 Formation of the portal vein behind the neck of the pancreas.

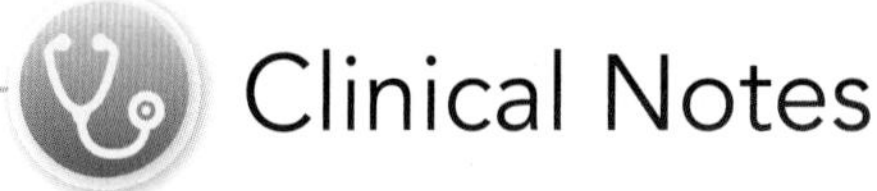

Clinical Notes

Portal–Systemic Anastomoses

Under normal conditions, the portal venous blood traverses the liver and drains into the **inferior vena cava** of the systemic venous circulation by way of the **hepatic veins**. This is the direct route. However, other, smaller communications exist between the portal and systemic systems, and they become important when the direct route becomes blocked (Fig. 5.94).

These communications are as follows:

- **Gastroesophageal anastomosis:** At the lower third of the esophagus, the **esophageal branches of the left gastric vein** (portal tributary) anastomose with the **esophageal veins** draining the middle third of the esophagus into the azygos veins (systemic tributary).
- **Anorectal anastomosis:** Halfway down the anal canal, the **superior rectal veins** (portal tributary) draining the upper half of the anal canal anastomose with the **middle** and **inferior rectal veins** (systemic tributaries), which are tributaries of the internal iliac and internal pudendal veins, respectively.
- **Paraumbilical anastomosis:** The **paraumbilical veins** connect the left branch of the portal vein with the **superficial veins of the anterior abdominal wall** (systemic tributaries). The paraumbilical veins travel in the falciform ligament and accompany the ligamentum teres.
- **Retroperitoneal anastomoses:** The veins of retroperitoneal organs (duodenum, pancreas, ascending colon, and descending colon), plus the liver (portal tributaries), anastomose with the renal, lumbar, and phrenic veins (systemic tributaries).

Portal Hypertension

Portal hypertension is a common clinical condition that influences the portal–systemic anastomoses just described. Enlargement of the portal–systemic connections is frequently accompanied by congestive enlargement of the spleen. **Portacaval shunts** for the treatment of portal hypertension may involve the anastomosis of the portal vein, because it lies within the lesser omentum, to the anterior wall of the inferior vena cava behind the entrance into the lesser sac. The splenic vein may be anastomosed to the left renal vein after removing the spleen.

Portal Vein Blood Flow and Malignant Disease

The portal vein conveys about 70% of the blood that enters the liver. The remaining 30% is oxygenated blood, which passes to the liver via the hepatic artery. The wide angle of union of the splenic vein with the superior mesenteric vein to form the portal vein leads to streaming of the blood flow in the portal vein. The right lobe of the liver receives blood mainly from the intestine, whereas the left lobe plus the quadrate and caudate lobes receive blood from the stomach and the spleen. This distribution of blood may explain the distribution of secondary malignant deposits in the liver.

(continued)

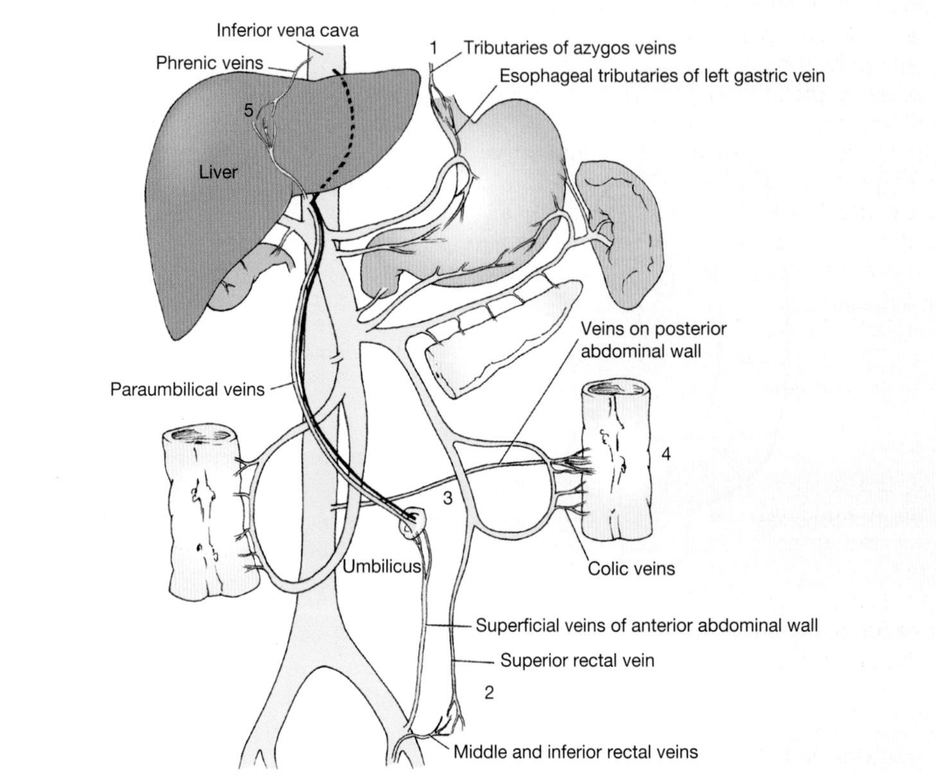

Figure 5.94 Important portal–systemic anastomoses: (1) gastroesophageal, (2) anorectal, (3) paraumbilical, (4) and (5) retroperitoneal.

GASTROINTESTINAL TRACT ACCESSORY ORGANS

The liver, biliary tree, and pancreas develop initially as budlike outgrowths off the GI tract. The spleen is a large lymphoid organ that forms in close association with the GI tract but is not a direct outgrowth of the GI tract.

Liver

The liver is the largest gland in the body and has a wide variety of functions. Three of its basic functions are production and secretion of bile, which is passed into the intestinal tract; involvement in many metabolic activities related to carbohydrate, fat, and protein metabolism; and filtration of the blood, removing bacteria and other foreign particles that have gained entrance to the blood from the lumen of the intestine.

The liver synthesizes heparin, an anticoagulant substance, and has an important detoxicating function. It produces bile pigments from the hemoglobin of worn-out red blood cell corpuscles and secretes bile salts; these together are conveyed to the duodenum by the biliary ducts.

Location and Description

The liver is soft, pliable, and highly vascular and occupies the upper part of the abdominal cavity just beneath the diaphragm (see Figs. 5.45 and 5.46). The greater part of the liver is situated under cover of the right costal margin, and the right hemidiaphragm separates it from the pleura, lungs, pericardium, and heart. The liver extends to the left to reach the left hemidiaphragm. The convex upper surface of the liver is molded to the undersurface of the domes of the diaphragm. The **posteroinferior**, or **visceral surface**, is molded to adjacent viscera and is therefore irregular in shape; it lies in contact with the abdominal part of the esophagus, stomach, duodenum, right colic flexure, right kidney and suprarenal gland, and the gallbladder.

The liver may be divided into a large **right lobe** and a small **left lobe** by the attachment of the peritoneum of the falciform ligament (see Fig. 5.53). The right lobe is further divided into a **quadrate lobe** and a **caudate lobe** by the presence of the gallbladder, the fissure for the ligamentum teres, the inferior vena cava, and the fissure for the ligamentum venosum. Experiments have shown that, in fact, the quadrate and caudate lobes are a functional part of the left lobe of the liver. Thus, the right and left branches of the hepatic artery and portal vein, and the right and left hepatic ducts, are distributed to the right lobe and the left lobe (plus quadrate plus caudate lobes), respectively. Apparently, the two sides overlap very little.

The **porta hepatis**, or **hilum** of the liver, is found on the posteroinferior surface and lies between the caudate and quadrate lobes (see Figs. 5.53 and 5.54). The upper part of the free edge of the lesser omentum is attached to its margins. In it lie the right and left hepatic ducts, right and left branches of the hepatic artery, portal vein, and sympathetic and parasympathetic nerve fibers (see Fig. 5.92). A few hepatic lymph nodes lie here; they drain the liver and gallbladder and send their efferent vessels to the celiac lymph nodes.

The liver is surrounded by a **fibrous capsule** but only partially covered by peritoneum. The liver is made up of **liver lobules**. The **central vein** of each lobule is a tributary of the hepatic veins. In the spaces between the lobules are the **portal canals**, which contain branches of the hepatic artery, portal vein, and a tributary of a bile duct (**portal triad**). The arterial and venous blood passes between the liver cells by means of **sinusoids** and drains into the central vein.

Important Relations

- **Anteriorly:** Diaphragm, right and left costal margins, right and left pleura and lower margins of both lungs, xiphoid process, and anterior abdominal wall in the subcostal angle.
- **Posteriorly:** Diaphragm, right kidney, hepatic flexure of the colon, duodenum, gallbladder, inferior vena cava, and esophagus and fundus of the stomach.

Peritoneal Ligaments

The **falciform ligament**, which is a two-layered fold of the peritoneum, ascends from the umbilicus to the liver (see Fig. 5.53). It has a sickle-shaped free margin that contains the ligamentum teres, the remains of the umbilical vein. The falciform ligament passes on to the anterior and then the superior surfaces of the liver and then splits into two layers. The right layer forms the upper layer of the **coronary ligament**; the left layer forms the upper layer of the **left triangular ligament**. The right extremity of the coronary ligament is known as the **right triangular ligament** of the liver. It should be noted that the peritoneal layers forming the coronary ligament are widely separated, leaving an area of liver devoid of peritoneum. This is the **bare area of the liver**.

The **ligamentum teres** passes into a fissure on the visceral surface of the liver and joins the left branch of the portal vein in the porta hepatis (see Figs. 5.54 and 5.65). The **ligamentum venosum**, a fibrous band that is the remains of the **ductus venosus**, is attached to the left branch of the portal vein and ascends in a fissure on the visceral surface of the liver to attach above to the inferior vena cava (see Figs. 5.53 and 5.65). In the fetus, oxygenated blood is brought to the liver in the **umbilical vein** (ligamentum teres). The greater proportion of the blood bypasses the liver in the ductus venosus (ligamentum venosum) and joins the inferior vena cava. At birth, the umbilical vein and ductus venosus close and become fibrous cords.

The **lesser omentum** arises from the edges of the porta hepatis and the fissure for the ligamentum venosum and passes down to the lesser curvature of the stomach (see Fig. 5.54).

Blood Supply

The **hepatic artery**, a branch of the celiac artery, divides into right and left terminal branches that enter the porta hepatis (see Fig. 5.92). The **portal vein** divides into **right** and **left terminal branches** that enter the porta hepatis behind the arteries. The **hepatic veins** (three or more) emerge from the posterior surface of the liver and drain into the inferior vena cava.

Hepatic Blood Circulation

The blood vessels (see Fig. 5.92) conveying the blood to the liver are the hepatic artery (30%) and portal vein (70%). The hepatic artery brings oxygenated blood to the liver, and the portal vein brings venous blood rich in the products of digestion, which have been absorbed from the GI tract. The arterial and venous blood is conducted to the central vein of each liver lobule by the liver sinusoids. The central veins drain into the right and left hepatic veins, and these leave the posterior surface of the liver and open directly into the inferior vena cava.

Lymph Drainage

The liver produces a large amount of lymph—about one-third to one half of all body lymph. The lymph vessels leave the liver and enter several lymph nodes in the porta hepatis. The efferent vessels pass to the **celiac nodes** (see Fig. 5.66). A few vessels pass from the bare area of the liver through the diaphragm to the **posterior mediastinal lymph nodes**.

Nerve Supply

Sympathetic and parasympathetic nerves form the **celiac plexus**. The anterior vagal trunk gives rise to a large **hepatic branch**, which passes directly to the liver (see Fig. 5.67).

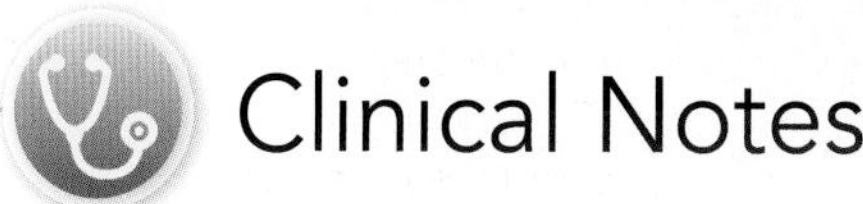

Liver Supports and Surgery

The liver is held in position in the upper part of the abdominal cavity by the attachment of the hepatic veins to the inferior vena cava. The peritoneal ligaments and the tone of the abdominal muscles play a minor role in its support. This fact is important surgically because even if the peritoneal ligaments are cut, the liver can be only slightly rotated.

Liver Trauma

The liver is a soft, friable structure enclosed in a fibrous capsule. Its close relationship to the lower ribs must be emphasized. Fractures of the lower ribs or penetrating wounds of the thorax or upper abdomen are common causes of liver injury. Blunt traumatic injuries from automobile accidents are also common, and severe hemorrhage accompanies tears of this organ.

(continued)

Because anatomic research has shown that the bile ducts, hepatic arteries, and portal vein are distributed in a segmental manner, appropriate ligation of these structures allows the surgeon to remove large portions of the liver in patients with severe traumatic lacerations of the liver or with a liver tumor. Even large, localized carcinomatous metastatic tumors can be successfully removed.

Liver Biopsy

Liver biopsy is a common diagnostic procedure. With the patient holding their breath in full expiration—to reduce the size of the costodiaphragmatic recess and the likelihood of damage to the lung—a needle is inserted through the right eighth or ninth intercostal space in the midaxillary line. The needle passes through the diaphragm into the liver, and a small specimen of liver tissue is removed for microscopic examination.

Subphrenic Spaces

The important subphrenic spaces and their relationship to the liver are described earlier in this chapter. Under normal conditions, these are potential spaces only, and the peritoneal surfaces are in contact. An abnormal accumulation of gas or fluid is necessary for separation of the peritoneal surfaces. The anterior surface of the liver is normally dull on percussion. Perforation of a gastric ulcer is often accompanied by a loss of liver dullness caused by the accumulation of gas over the anterior surface of the liver and in the subphrenic spaces.

Biliary Tree

The biliary tree is the system of ducts that drain and store bile and deliver bile to the small intestine. Bile is secreted by the liver cells at a constant rate of about 40 mL per hour. When digestion is not taking place, the bile is stored and concentrated in the gallbladder; later, it is delivered to the duodenum. The biliary tree consists of the **right** and **left hepatic ducts**, **common hepatic duct**, **bile duct**, **gallbladder**, and the **cystic duct** (see Figs. 5.73 and 5.92).

The smallest interlobular tributaries of the bile ducts are situated in the portal canals of the liver; they receive the bile canaliculi. The interlobular ducts join one another to form progressively larger ducts and, eventually, at the porta hepatis, form the right and left hepatic ducts. The right hepatic duct drains the right lobe of the liver, and the left duct drains the left lobe, caudate lobe, and quadrate lobe.

Hepatic Ducts

The **right** and **left hepatic ducts** emerge from the right and left lobes of the liver in the porta hepatis. After a short course, the hepatic ducts unite to form the common hepatic duct.

The **common hepatic duct** is about 1.5 in. (4 cm) long and descends within the free margin of the lesser omentum. It is joined on the right side by the cystic duct from the gallbladder to form the bile duct.

Bile Duct

The **bile duct** (**common bile duct**) is about 3 in. (8 cm) long. In the first part of its course, it lies in the right free margin of the lesser omentum in front of the opening into the lesser sac. Here, it lies in front of the right margin of the portal vein and on the right of the hepatic artery (see Fig. 5.55). In the second part of its course, it is situated behind the first part of the duodenum (see 5.52) to the right of the gastroduodenal artery (see Fig. 5.49). In the third part of its course, it lies in a groove on the posterior surface of the head of the pancreas (see Fig. 5.73). Here, the bile duct meets the main pancreatic duct.

The bile duct ends below by piercing the medial wall of the second part of the duodenum about halfway down its length (Fig. 5.95). The main pancreatic duct usually joins it, and together, they open into a small ampulla in the duodenal wall called the **hepatopancreatic ampulla** (**ampulla of Vater**). The ampulla opens into the lumen of the duodenum by means of a small papilla, the **major duodenal papilla**. The terminal parts of both ducts and the ampulla are surrounded by circular muscle, known as the **sphincter of the hepatopancreatic ampulla** (**sphincter of Oddi**). Occasionally, the bile and pancreatic ducts open separately into the

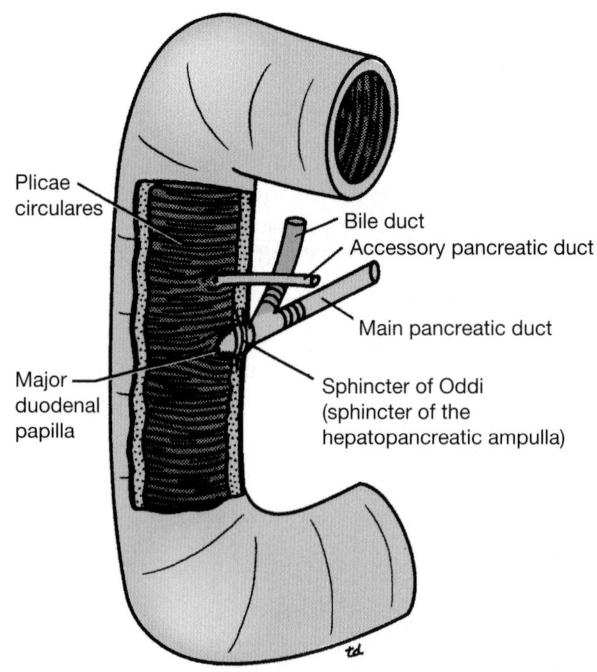

Figure 5.95 Terminal parts of the bile and pancreatic ducts as they enter the second part of the duodenum. Note the sphincter of Oddi and the smooth muscle around the ends of the bile duct and the main pancreatic duct.

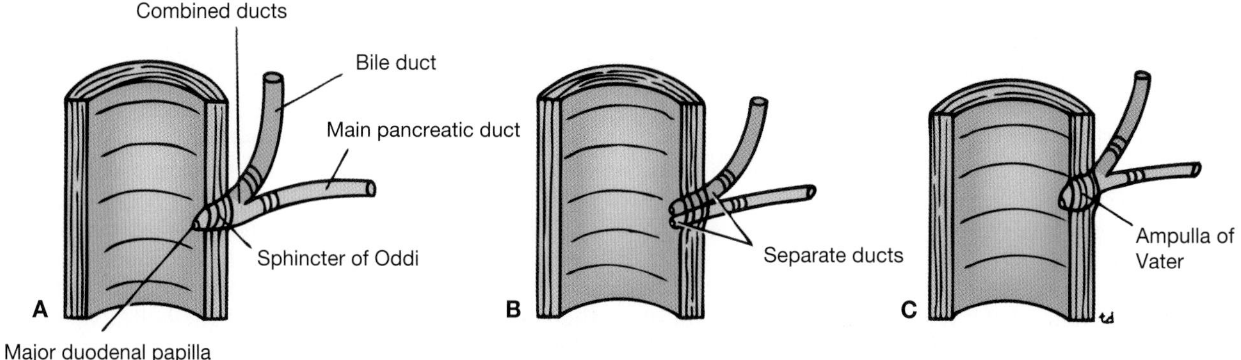

Figure 5.96 Three common variations of terminations of the bile and main pancreatic ducts as they enter the second part of the duodenum. **A.** Both ducts join and drain via the major duodenal papilla, but no ampulla is present. **B.** Each duct opens separately. **C.** Both ducts join and open together into the ampulla at the major papilla.

duodenum. The common variations of this arrangement are shown in Figure 5.96.

Gallbladder

The gallbladder is a pear-shaped sac lying on the undersurface of the liver (Fig. 5.97; see also Figs. 5.46, 5.53, 5.73, and 5.92). It has a capacity of 30 to 50 mL and stores bile, which it concentrates by absorbing water. The gallbladder is divided into the fundus, body, and neck (see Figs. 5.73 and 5.92). The **fundus** is rounded and projects below the inferior margin of the liver, where it meets the anterior abdominal wall at the level of the tip of the ninth right costal cartilage. The **body** lies in contact with the visceral surface of the liver and is directed upward, backward, and to the left. The **neck** becomes continuous with the cystic duct, which runs into the lesser omentum to join the common hepatic duct, to form the bile duct.

The peritoneum surrounds the fundus of the gallbladder and binds the body and neck to the visceral surface of the liver.

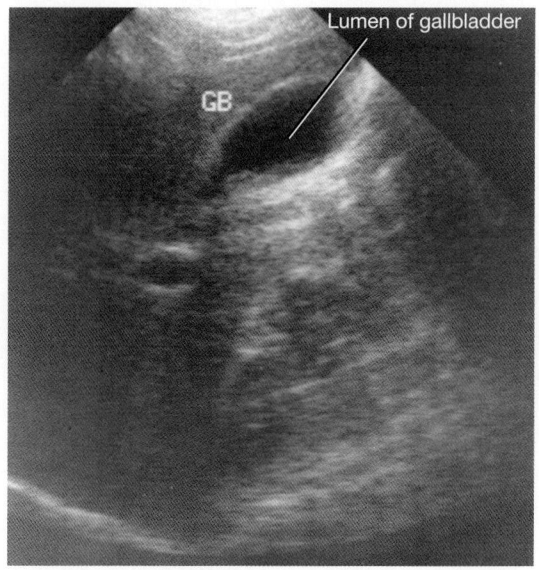

Figure 5.97 Longitudinal sonogram of the upper part of the abdomen showing the lumen of the gallbladder. (Courtesy of Dr. M.C. Hill.)

Relations

- **Anteriorly:** The anterior abdominal wall and the inferior surface of the liver (see Figs. 5.46 and 5.47)
- **Posteriorly:** The transverse colon and the first and second parts of the duodenum (see Fig. 5.73)

Function

When digestion is not taking place, the sphincter of Oddi remains closed, and bile accumulates in the gallbladder. The primary functions of the gallbladder are to store and concentrate bile. When empty or partially filled, the mucous membrane is thrown into convoluted folds that unite with each other, giving the surface a honeycombed appearance. When the gallbladder is distended, the mucosal folds are shorter and more widely spaced.

Bile is delivered to the duodenum as the result of contraction and partial emptying of the gallbladder. The entrance of fatty foods into the duodenum initiates this mechanism. The fat causes release of the hormone **cholecystokinin** from the mucous membrane of the duodenum. The hormone then enters the blood, causing the gallbladder to contract. At the same time, the smooth muscle around the distal end of the bile duct and the ampulla is relaxed, allowing the passage of concentrated bile into the duodenum. Bile salts are important in emulsifying the fat in the intestine and in assisting with its digestion and absorption.

Blood Supply

The **cystic artery**, a branch of the right hepatic artery (see Fig. 5.92), supplies the gallbladder. The **cystic vein** drains directly into the portal vein (see Fig. 5.65). Several very small arteries and veins also run between the liver and gallbladder.

Lymph Drainage

The lymph drains into a cystic lymph node situated near the neck of the gallbladder. From here, the lymph vessels pass to the hepatic nodes along the course of the hepatic artery and then to the **celiac nodes**.

Nerve Supply

Sympathetic and parasympathetic vagal fibers form the celiac plexus. The gallbladder contracts in response to the hormone cholecystokinin, which is produced by the mucous membrane of the duodenum on the arrival of fatty food from the stomach.

Cystic Duct

The cystic duct is about 1.5 in. (3.8 cm) long and connects the neck of the gallbladder to the common hepatic duct to form the bile duct (see Fig. 5.92). It usually is somewhat S shaped and descends for a variable distance in the right free margin of the lesser omentum.

The mucous membrane of the cystic duct is raised to form a spiral fold continuous with a similar fold in the neck of the gallbladder. The fold is commonly known as the **spiral valve**. The function of the spiral valve is to keep the lumen constantly open.

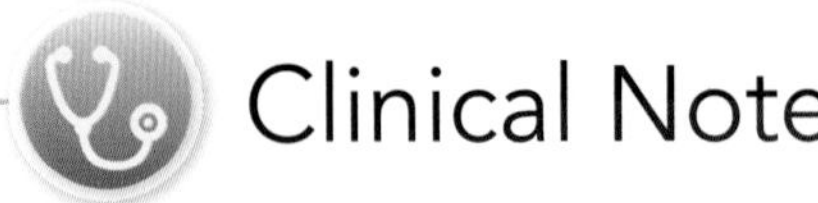

Clinical Notes

Gallstones

Gallstones are usually asymptomatic; however, they can give rise to gallstone colic or produce acute cholecystitis.

Biliary Colic

Biliary colic is usually caused by spasm of the smooth muscle of the wall of the gallbladder to expel a gallstone. Afferent nerve fibers ascend through the celiac plexus and the greater splanchnic nerves to the thoracic segments of the spinal cord. Referred pain is felt in the right upper quadrant or the epigastrium (T7 to T9 dermatomes).

Obstruction of the biliary ducts with a gallstone or by compression by a tumor of the pancreas results in backup of bile in the ducts and development of **jaundice**. The impaction of a stone in the ampulla of Vater may result in the passage of infected bile into the pancreatic duct, producing **pancreatitis**. The anatomic arrangement of the terminal part of the bile duct and the main pancreatic duct is subject to considerable variation (see Fig. 5.96). The type of duct system present determines whether infected bile is likely to enter the pancreatic duct.

Gallstones may ulcerate through the gallbladder wall into the transverse colon or the duodenum. In the former case, they are passed naturally per the rectum, but, in the latter case, they may be held up at the ileocecal junction, producing intestinal obstruction.

Acute Cholecystitis

Acute cholecystitis produces discomfort in the right upper quadrant or epigastrium. Inflammation of the gallbladder may cause irritation of the subdiaphragmatic parietal peritoneum, which is supplied in part by the phrenic nerve (C3 to C5). This may give rise to referred pain over the shoulder, because the supraclavicular nerves (C3 and C4) supply the skin in this area.

Cholecystectomy and Gallbladder Arterial Supply

Before attempting a cholecystectomy operation, the surgeon must be aware of the many variations in the arterial supply to the gallbladder and the relationship of the vessels to the bile ducts (Fig. 5.98). Unfortunately, cases have been reported in which the common hepatic duct or the main bile duct have been included in the arterial ligature with disastrous consequences.

Gallbladder Gangrene

Unlike the appendix, which has a single arterial supply, the gallbladder rarely becomes gangrenous. In addition to the cystic artery, the gallbladder also receives small vessels from the visceral surface of the liver.

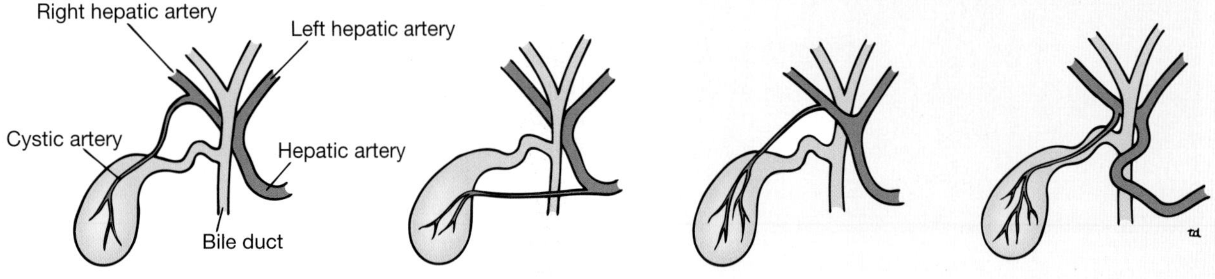

Figure 5.98 Some common variations of blood supply to the gallbladder.

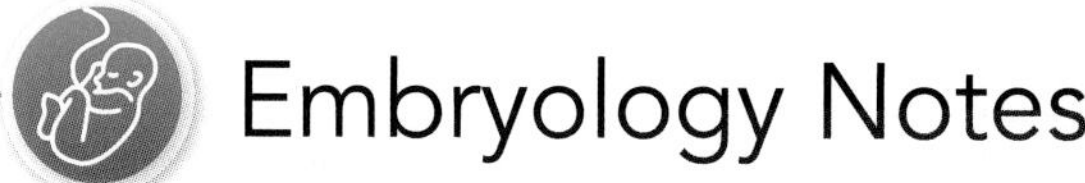

Embryology Notes

Liver and Biliary Tree Development

The liver arises from the distal end of the foregut as a solid bud of endodermal cells (Fig. 5.99; see also Fig. 5.86). The site of origin lies at the apex of the loop of the developing duodenum and corresponds to a point halfway along the second part of the fully formed duodenum. The **hepatic bud** grows anteriorly into the mass of splanchnic mesoderm called the **septum transversum**. The end of the bud now divides into right and left branches, from which columns of endodermal cells grow into the vascular mesoderm. The paired vitelline veins and umbilical veins that course through the septum transversum become broken up by the invading columns of liver cells and form the liver **sinusoids**. The columns of endodermal cells form the **liver cords**. The connective tissue of the liver is formed from the mesenchyme of the septum transversum.

The main hepatic bud and its right and left terminal branches now become canalized to form the **common hepatic duct** and the **right** and **left hepatic ducts**. The liver grows rapidly in size and comes to occupy the greater part of the abdominal cavity; the right lobe becomes much larger than the left lobe.

Gallbladder and Cystic Duct Development

The gallbladder develops from the hepatic bud as a solid outgrowth of cells (see Fig. 5.86). The end of the outgrowth expands to form the **gallbladder**, whereas the narrow stem remains as the **cystic duct**. Later, the gallbladder and cystic duct become canalized. The cystic duct now opens into the **common hepatic duct** to form the **bile duct**.

Biliary Atresia

Failure of the bile ducts to canalize during development causes atresia. Various forms of atresia are shown in Figure 5.100. Jaundice appears soon after birth. Clay-colored stools and very dark urine are also present. Surgical correction of the atresia should be attempted when possible. If the atresia cannot be corrected, the child will die of liver failure.

Absence of Gallbladder

Occasionally, the outgrowth of cells from the hepatic bud fails to develop. In these cases, there is no gallbladder and no cystic duct (Fig. 5.101).

Double Gallbladder

Rarely, the outgrowth of cells from the hepatic bud bifurcates so that two gallbladders are formed (see Fig. 5.101).

Absence of Cystic Duct

In the absence of the cystic duct, the entire outgrowth of cells from the hepatic bud develops into the gallbladder and fails to leave the narrow stem that would normally form the cystic duct. The gallbladder drains directly into the bile duct. The condition may not be recognized when performing a cholecystectomy, and the surgeon may damage the bile duct (see Fig. 5.101).

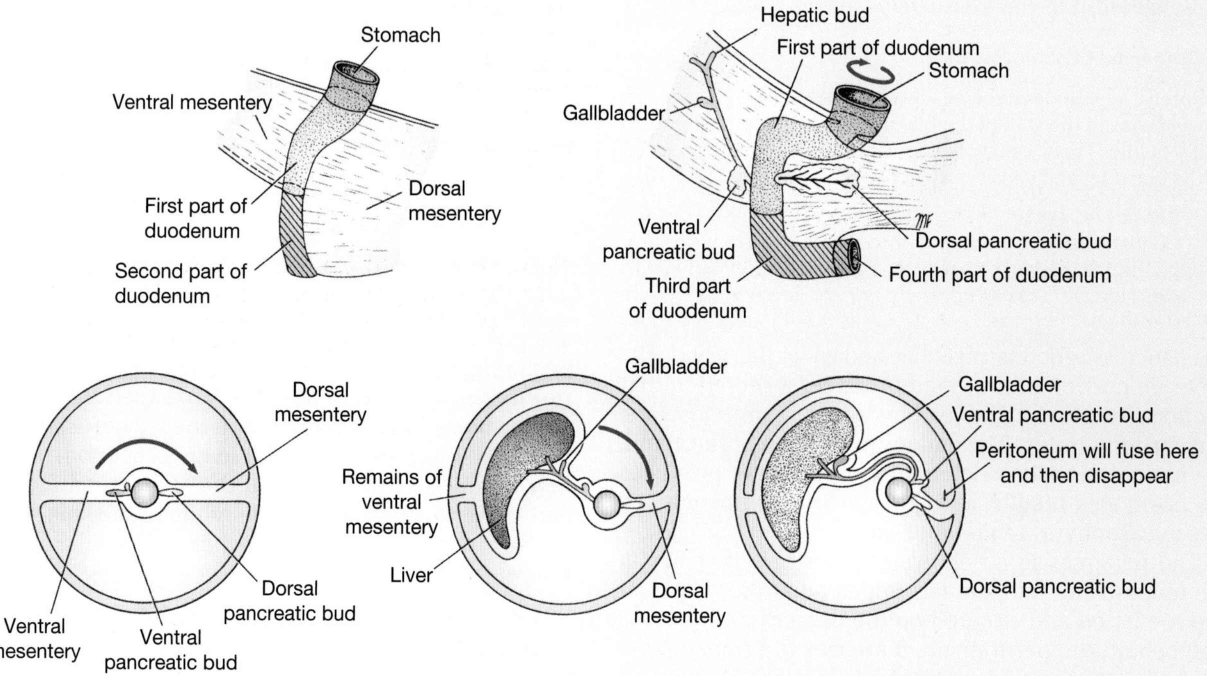

Figure 5.99 Development of the duodenum in relation to the ventral and dorsal mesenteries. *Stippled area*, foregut; *crosshatched area*, midgut. *Red arrows* indicate the direction of rotation of the stomach/upper duodenum.

(continued)

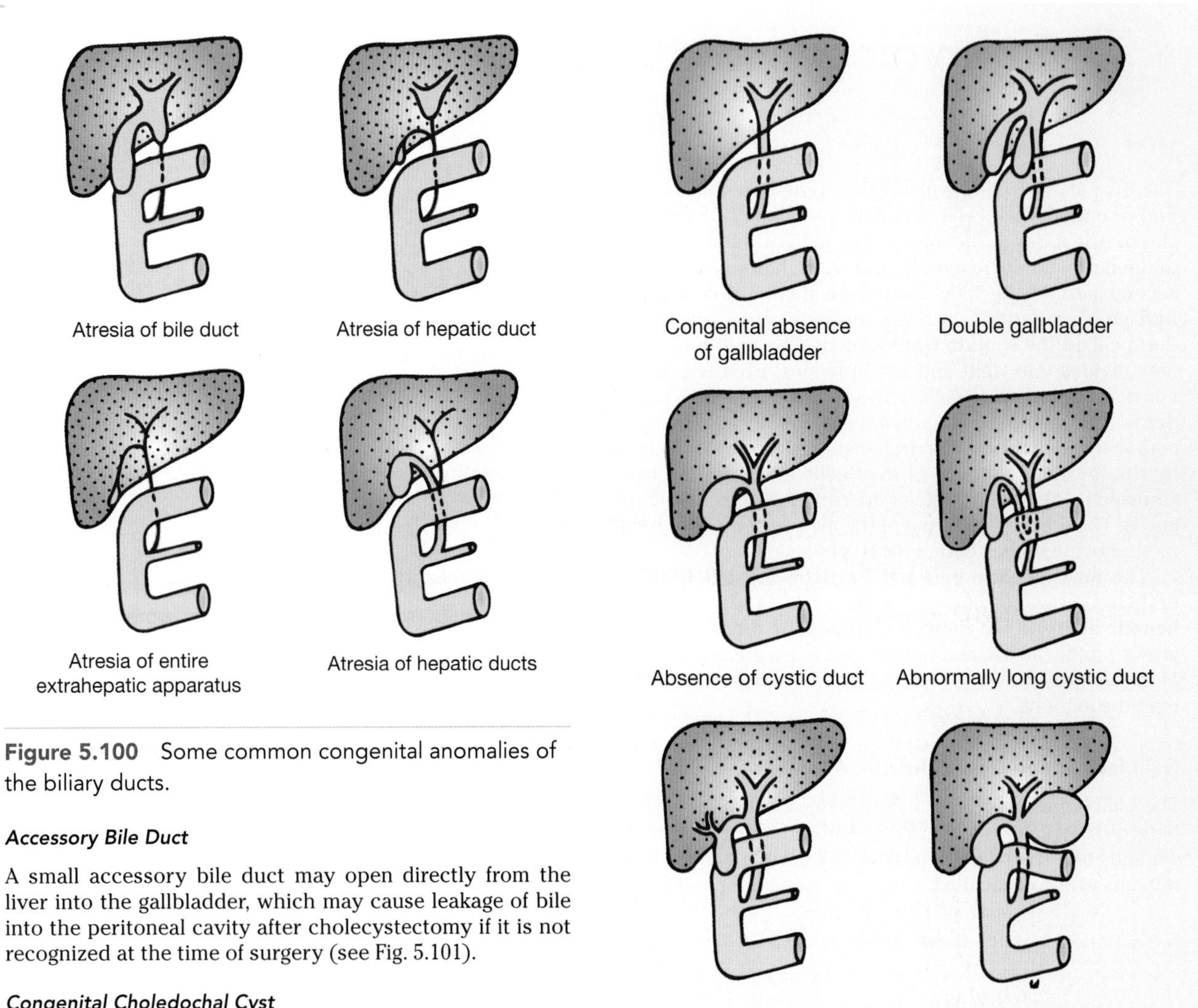

Figure 5.100 Some common congenital anomalies of the biliary ducts.

Accessory Bile Duct

A small accessory bile duct may open directly from the liver into the gallbladder, which may cause leakage of bile into the peritoneal cavity after cholecystectomy if it is not recognized at the time of surgery (see Fig. 5.101).

Congenital Choledochal Cyst

Rarely, a choledochal cyst develops because of an area of weakness in the wall of the bile duct. A cyst can contain 1 to 2 L of bile. The anomaly is important in that it may press on the bile duct and cause obstructive jaundice (see Fig. 5.101).

Figure 5.101 Some common congenital anomalies of the gallbladder.

Pancreas

The pancreas is both an exocrine and endocrine gland. The exocrine portion of the gland produces a secretion that contains enzymes capable of hydrolyzing proteins, fats, and carbohydrates. The endocrine portion of the gland, the **pancreatic islets** (**islets of Langerhans**), produces the hormones **insulin** and **glucagon**, which play a key role in carbohydrate metabolism.

The pancreas is an elongated structure that lies in the epigastrium and the left upper quadrant. It is soft and lobulated and situated on the posterior abdominal wall behind the peritoneum. It crosses the transpyloric plane. The pancreas is divided into a head, neck, body, and tail (Fig. 5.102).

The **head** of the pancreas is disc shaped and lies within the concavity of the duodenum. A part of the head extends to the left behind the superior mesenteric vessels and is called the **uncinate process**.

The **neck** is the constricted portion of the pancreas and connects the head to the body. It lies in front of the beginning of the portal vein and the origin of the superior mesenteric artery from the aorta (see Fig. 5.70).

The **body** runs upward and to the left across the midline. It is somewhat triangular in cross section.

The **tail** passes forward in the splenorenal ligament and comes in contact with the hilum of the spleen.

Relations

- **Anteriorly:** From right to left—the transverse colon and the attachment of the transverse mesocolon, lesser sac, and the stomach (see Figs. 5.49 and 5.51)
- **Posteriorly:** From right to left—the bile duct, portal and splenic veins, inferior vena cava, aorta, origin of the superior mesenteric artery, left psoas muscle, left suprarenal gland, left kidney, and the hilum of the spleen (see Figs. 5.49 and 5.71)

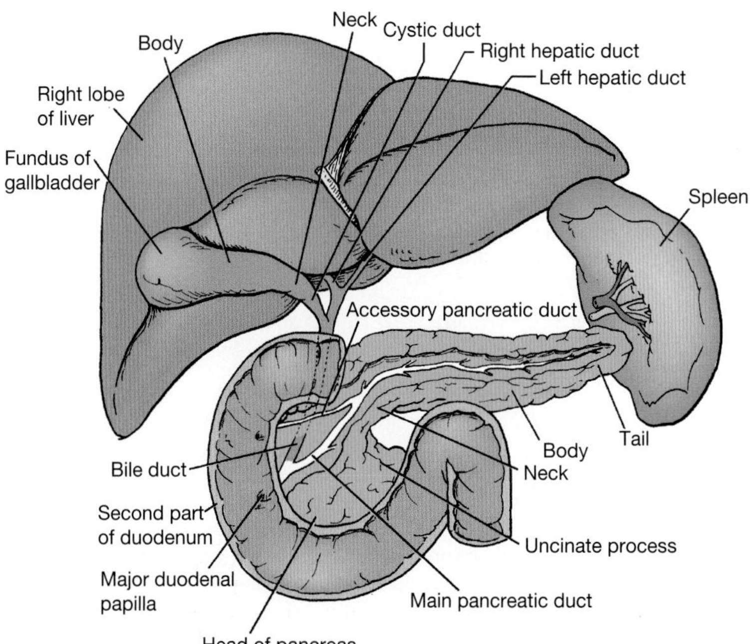

Figure 5.102 Different parts of the pancreas dissected to reveal the duct system.

Pancreatic Ducts

The **main duct of the pancreas** begins in the tail and runs the length of the gland, receiving numerous tributaries on the way (see Fig. 5.102). It opens into the second part of the duodenum at about its middle with the bile duct on the **major duodenal papilla** (see Fig. 5.95). Sometimes, the main duct drains separately into the duodenum.

The **accessory duct of the pancreas**, when present, drains the upper part of the head and then opens into the duodenum a short distance above the main duct on the **minor duodenal papilla** (see Figs. 5.95 and 5.102). The accessory duct frequently communicates with the main duct.

Blood Supply

The **splenic** and the **superior** and **inferior pancreaticoduodenal arteries** (see Fig. 5.70) supply the pancreas. The corresponding veins drain into the portal system.

Lymph Drainage

Lymph nodes are situated along the arteries that supply the gland. The efferent vessels ultimately drain into the **celiac** and **superior mesenteric lymph nodes**.

Nerve Supply

Sympathetic and parasympathetic (vagal) nerve fibers supply the area.

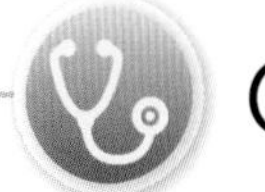

Clinical Notes

Pancreatic Disease Diagnosis

The deep location of the pancreas sometimes gives rise to problems of diagnosis for the following reasons:

- Pain from the pancreas is commonly referred to the back.
- Because the pancreas lies behind the stomach and transverse colon, disease of the gland can be confused with that of the stomach or transverse colon.
- Inflammation of the pancreas can spread to the peritoneum forming the posterior wall of the lesser sac. This in turn can lead to adhesions and the closing off of the lesser sac to form a **pseudocyst**.

Pancreatic Trauma

The pancreas is deeply placed within the abdomen and is well protected by the costal margin and the anterior abdominal wall. However, blunt trauma, such as in a sports injury when a sudden blow to the abdomen occurs, can compress and tear the pancreas against the vertebral column. The pancreas is most commonly damaged by gunshot or stab wounds. Damaged pancreatic tissue releases activated pancreatic enzymes that produce the signs and symptoms of acute peritonitis.

Cancer of the Head of the Pancreas and the Bile Duct

Because of the close relation of the head of the pancreas to the bile duct, cancer of the head of the pancreas often causes obstructive jaundice.

Pancreatic Tail and Splenectomy

The presence of the tail of the pancreas in the splenorenal ligament sometimes results in its damage during splenectomy. The damaged pancreas releases enzymes that start to digest surrounding tissues, with serious consequences.

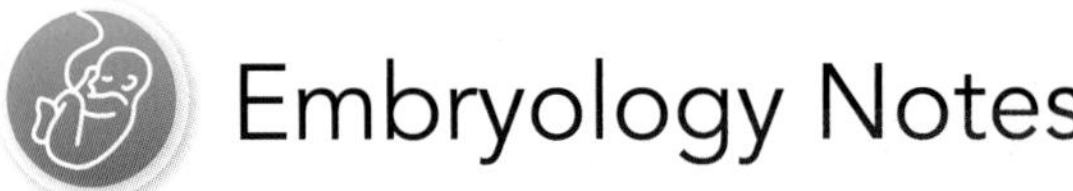

Embryology Notes

Pancreas Development

The pancreas develops from a **dorsal** and **ventral bud** of endodermal cells that arise from the foregut. The dorsal bud originates a short distance above the ventral bud and grows into the dorsal mesentery. The ventral bud arises in common with the hepatic bud, close to the junction of the foregut with the midgut (see Fig. 5.86). A canalized duct system now develops in each bud. The rotation of the stomach and duodenum, together with the rapid growth of the left side of the duodenum, results in the ventral buds coming into contact with the dorsal bud, and fusion occurs (Fig. 5.103).

Fusion also occurs between the ducts, so that the **main pancreatic duct** is derived from the entire ventral pancreatic duct and the distal part of the dorsal pancreatic duct. The main pancreatic duct joins the bile duct and enters the second part of the duodenum. The proximal part of the dorsal pancreatic duct may persist as an **accessory duct**, which may or may not open into the duodenum about 0.75 in. (2 cm) above the opening of the main duct.

Continued growth of the endodermal cells of the now-fused ventral and dorsal pancreatic buds extends into the surrounding mesenchyme as columns of cells. These columns give off side branches, which later become canalized to form **collecting ducts**. Secretory acini appear at the ends of the ducts.

The **pancreatic islets** arise as small buds from the developing ducts. Later, these cells sever their connection with the duct system and form isolated groups of cells that start to secrete **insulin** and **glucagon** at about month 5.

The inferior part of the head and the uncinate process of the pancreas are formed from the ventral pancreatic bud; the superior part of the head, the neck, the body, and the tail of the pancreas are formed from the dorsal pancreatic bud.

Entrance of Bile and Pancreatic Ducts into the Duodenum

As seen from development, the bile duct and the main pancreatic duct are joined to one another. They pass obliquely through the wall of the second part of the duodenum to open on the summit of the **major duodenal papilla**, which is surrounded by the **hepatopancreatic sphincter** (**sphincter of Oddi**) (see Figs. 5.95 and 5.102). In some individuals, they pass separately through the duodenal wall, although in close contact, and open separately on the summit of the duodenal papilla (see Fig. 5.96). In other individuals, the two ducts join and form a common dilatation, the **hepatopancreatic ampulla** (**ampulla of Vater**). This opens on the summit of the duodenal papilla.

Annular Pancreas

In annular pancreas, the ventral pancreatic bud becomes fixed so that, when the stomach and duodenum rotate, the ventral bud is pulled around the right side of the duodenum to fuse with the dorsal bud of the pancreas, thus encircling the duodenum (Fig. 5.104). This may cause obstruction of the duodenum, and vomiting may start a few hours after birth. Early surgical relief of the obstruction is necessary.

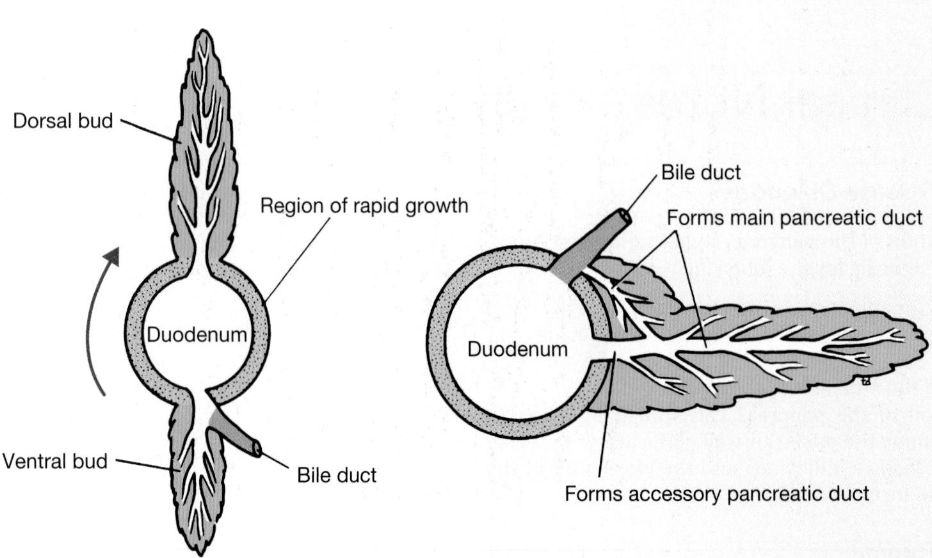

Figure 5.103 Rotation of the duodenum and the unequal growth of the duodenal wall lead to the fusion of the ventral and dorsal pancreatic buds.

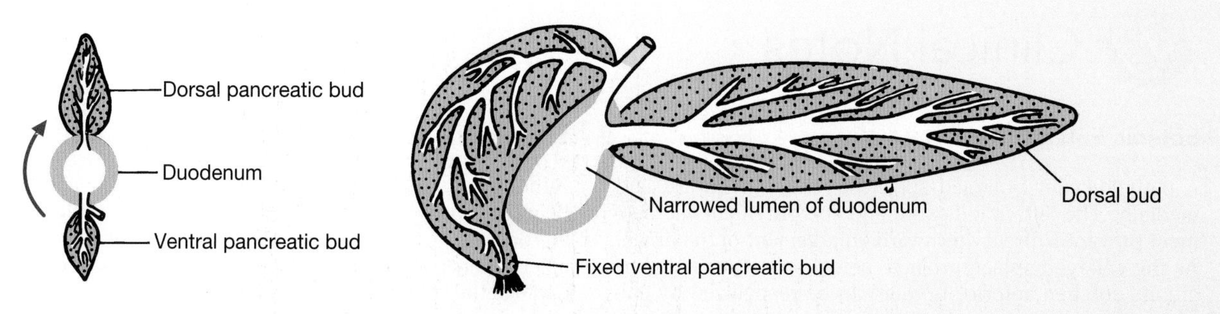

Figure 5.104 Formation of the annular pancreas, producing duodenal obstruction. Note the narrowing of the duodenum.

Ectopic Pancreas

Ectopic pancreatic tissue may be found in the submucosa of the stomach, duodenum, small intestine (including Meckel diverticulum), and gallbladder and in the spleen. It is important in that it may protrude into the lumen of the gut and be responsible for causing intussusception.

Congenital Fibrocystic Disease

Basically, congenital fibrocystic disease in the pancreas is caused by an abnormality in the secretion of mucus. The mucus produced is excessively viscid and obstructs the pancreatic duct, which leads to pancreatitis with subsequent fibrosis. The condition also involves the lungs, kidneys, and liver.

Spleen

The spleen is reddish and is the largest single mass of lymphoid tissue in the body. It is not a component of the GI tract, despite their close relationship. It is oval shaped and has a **notched anterior border**. It lies just beneath the left half of the diaphragm close to ribs 9 to 11. The long axis lies along the shaft of rib 10, and its lower pole extends forward only as far as the midaxillary line and cannot be palpated on clinical examination (Fig. 5.105).

The spleen is surrounded by the peritoneum (see Figs. 5.50 and 5.105), which passes from it at the **hilum** as the gastrosplenic omentum (ligament) to the greater curvature of the stomach (carrying the short gastric and left gastroepiploic vessels). The peritoneum also passes to the left kidney as the splenorenal ligament (carrying the splenic vessels and the tail of the pancreas).

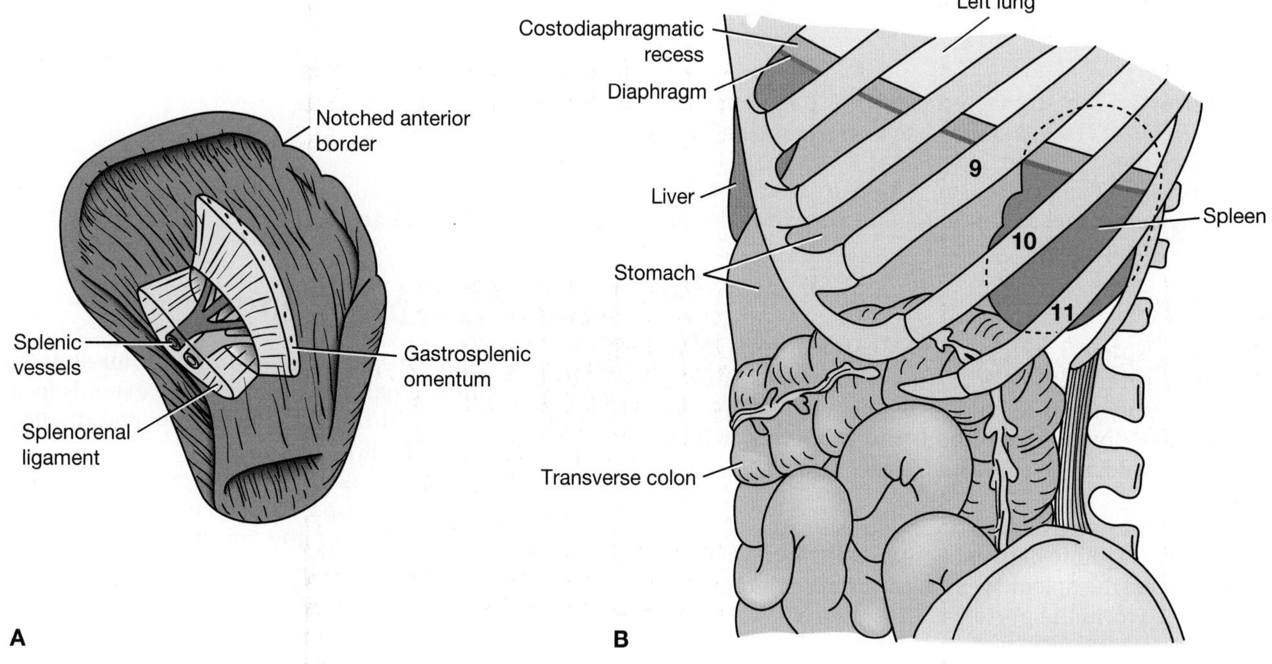

Figure 5.105 Spleen. **A.** It is oval shaped and has a notched anterior border. **B.** Shows the relation of the spleen to adjacent structures.

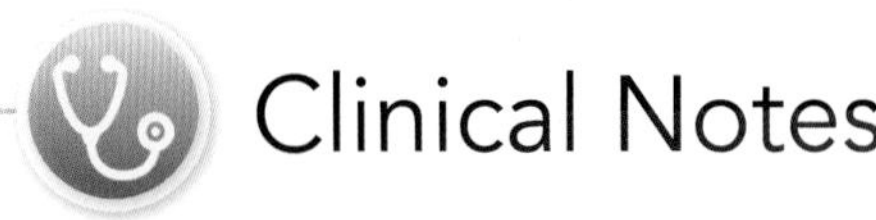

Clinical Notes

Splenic Enlargement

A pathologically enlarged spleen extends downward and medially. The left colic flexure and the phrenicocolic ligament prevent a direct downward enlargement of the organ. As the enlarged spleen projects below the left costal margin, its notched anterior border can be recognized by palpation through the anterior abdominal wall.

The spleen is situated at the beginning of the splenic vein, and in cases of portal hypertension, it often enlarges from venous congestion.

Splenic Trauma

Although anatomically the spleen gives the appearance of being well protected, motor vehicle accidents of the crushing or run-over type commonly produce laceration of the spleen. Penetrating wounds of the lower left thorax can also damage the spleen.

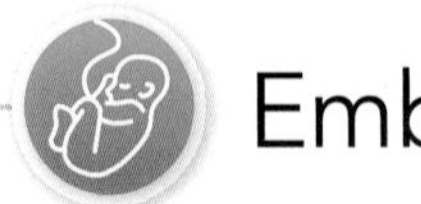

Embryology Notes

Spleen Development

The spleen develops as a thickening of the mesenchyme in the dorsal mesentery (see Fig. 5.91). In the earliest stages, the spleen consists of several mesenchymal masses that later fuse. The notches along its anterior border are permanent and indicate that the mesenchymal masses never completely fuse.

The part of the dorsal mesentery that extends between the hilum of the spleen and the greater curvature of the stomach is called the **gastrosplenic omentum**; the part that extends between the spleen and the left kidney on the posterior abdominal wall is called the **splenorenal ligament**. The **splenic artery**, a branch of the foregut artery (celiac artery), supplies the spleen.

Supernumerary Spleens

In 10% of people, one or more supernumerary spleens may be present, either in the gastrosplenic omentum or in the splenorenal ligament. Their clinical importance is that they may hypertrophy after removal of the major spleen and be responsible for a recurrence of symptoms of the disease for which splenectomy was initially performed.

Relations

- **Anteriorly:** The stomach, tail of the pancreas, left colic flexure. The left kidney lies along its medial border (see Figs. 5.49 and 5.55).
- **Posteriorly:** The diaphragm, left pleura (left costodiaphragmatic recess), left lung, and ribs 9 to 11 (see Figs. 5.55 and 5.105).

Blood Supply

The large **splenic artery** is the largest branch of the celiac artery. It has a tortuous course as it runs along the upper border of the pancreas. The splenic artery then divides into about six branches, which enter the spleen at the hilum (see Figs. 5.49, 5.64, and 5.70).

The **splenic vein** leaves the hilum and runs behind the tail and the body of the pancreas. Behind the neck of the pancreas, the splenic vein joins the superior mesenteric vein to form the portal vein (see Fig. 5.93).

Lymph Drainage

The lymph vessels emerge from the hilum and pass through a few lymph nodes along the course of the splenic artery and then drain into the **celiac nodes**.

Nerve Supply

The nerves accompany the splenic artery and are derived from the **celiac plexus**.

RETROPERITONEAL SPACE

The retroperitoneal space lies on the posterior abdominal wall behind the parietal peritoneum. It extends from the T12 vertebra and rib 12 to the sacrum and the iliac crests below (Fig. 5.106).

The **floor** (**posterior wall**) of the space is formed from medial to lateral by the psoas and quadratus lumborum muscles and the origin of the transversus abdominis muscle. Each of these muscles is covered on the anterior surface by a definite layer of fascia. In front of the fascial layers is a variable amount of fatty connective tissue that forms a bed for the suprarenal glands, the kidneys, ascending and descending parts of the colon, and the duodenum. The retroperitoneal space also contains the ureters and renal and gonadal blood vessels.

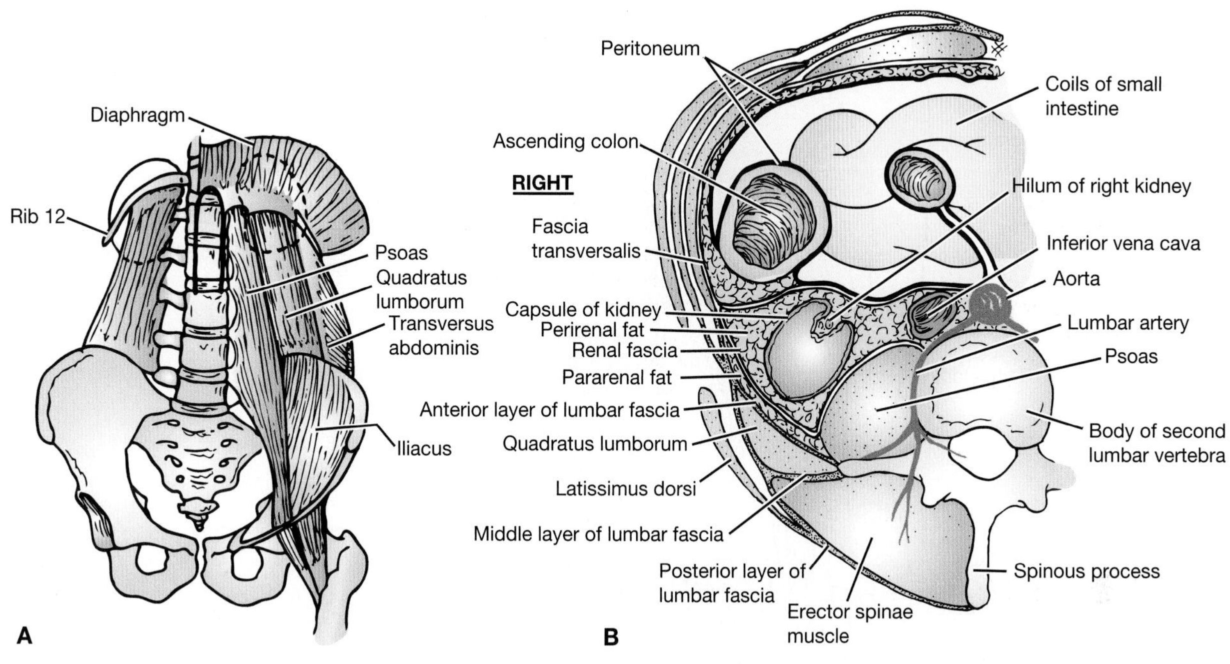

Figure 5.106 Retroperitoneal space. **A.** Structures present on the posterior abdominal wall behind the peritoneum. **B.** Transverse section of the posterior abdominal wall showing structures in the retroperitoneal space as seen from below.

URINARY TRACT

The urinary tract consists of the kidneys, ureters, urinary bladder, and urethra. The bladder and urethra are discussed in Chapter 6.

Kidneys

The two kidneys function to excrete most of the waste products of metabolism. They play a major role in controlling the water and electrolyte balance within the body and in maintaining the acid–base balance of the blood. The waste products leave the kidneys as **urine**, which passes down the **ureters** to the **urinary bladder**, located within the pelvis. The urine leaves the body in the **urethra**.

Location and Description

The kidneys are reddish brown and lie behind the peritoneum high up on the posterior abdominal wall on either side of the vertebral column; they are largely under cover of the costal margin (Fig. 5.107). The right kidney lies slightly lower than the left kidney because of the large size of the right lobe of the liver. With contraction of the diaphragm during respiration, both kidneys move downward in a vertical direction by as much as 1 in. (2.5 cm).

The **hilum** is a vertical slit in the medial concave border of each kidney that is bounded by thick lips of renal substance (Fig. 5.108). The hilum extends into a large cavity called the **renal sinus**. From the front backward, the hilum transmits the renal vein, two branches of the

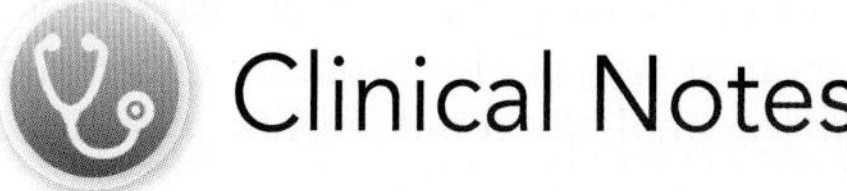

Trauma to Retroperitoneal Space Organs

Palpation of the anterior abdominal wall in the lumbar and iliac regions may give rise to signs indicative of peritoneal irritation (the peritoneum forms the anterior boundary of the space; see Fig. 5.106). In other words, tenderness and muscle spasm (rigidity) may be present. Palpation of the back in the interval between rib 12 and the vertebral column may reveal tenderness suggestive of kidney disease.

Abdominal radiographs may reveal air in the extraperitoneal tissues, indicating perforation of a viscus (eg, ascending or descending colon). Computed tomography (CT) scans can often accurately define the extent of the injury to the extraperitoneal organs.

Abscess Formation

Infection originating in retroperitoneal organs, such as the kidneys, lymph nodes, and retrocecal appendix, may extend widely into the retroperitoneal space.

Leaking Aortic Aneurysm

The blood may first be confined to the retroperitoneal space before rupturing into the peritoneal cavity.

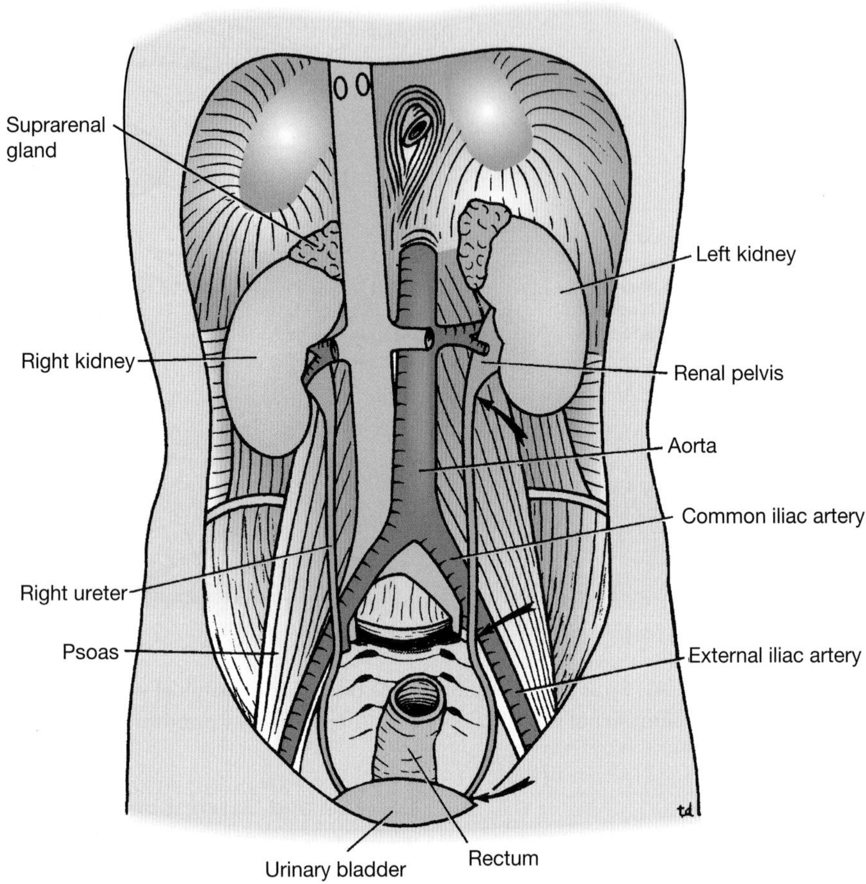

Figure 5.107 Posterior abdominal wall showing the kidneys and the ureters in situ. *Arrows* indicate three sites where the ureter is narrowed.

renal artery, the ureter, and the third branch of the renal artery (VAUA). Lymph vessels and sympathetic fibers also pass through the hilum.

Coverings

The kidneys have the following coverings (see Fig. 5.108B):

- **Fibrous capsule:** This surrounds the kidney and is closely applied to its outer surface.
- **Perirenal fat:** This covers the fibrous capsule.
- **Renal fascia:** This is a condensation of connective tissue that lies outside the perirenal fat and encloses the kidneys and suprarenal glands; it is continuous laterally with the transversalis fascia.
- **Pararenal fat:** This lies external to the renal fascia and is often in large quantity. It forms part of the retroperitoneal fat.

The perirenal fat, renal fascia, and pararenal fat support the kidneys and hold them in position on the posterior abdominal wall.

Renal Structure

Each kidney has a dark brown outer **cortex** and a light brown inner **medulla**. The medulla is composed of about a dozen **renal pyramids**, each having its base oriented toward the cortex and its apex, the **renal papilla**, projecting medially (see Fig. 5.108B). The cortex extends into the medulla between adjacent pyramids as the **renal columns**. Extending from the bases of the renal pyramids into the cortex are striations known as **medullary rays**.

The **renal sinus**, which is the space within the hilum, contains the upper expanded end of the ureter, the **renal pelvis**. This divides into two or three **major calyces**, each of which divides into two or three **minor calyces**. The apex of the renal pyramid, the **renal papilla**, indents each minor calyx.

Important Relations, Right Kidney

Note that many related structures are directly in contact with the kidneys, whereas visceral layers of peritoneum separate others (Fig. 5.109).

- **Anteriorly:** The suprarenal gland, liver, second part of the duodenum, and right colic flexure (see Figs. 5.49 and 5.109).
- **Posteriorly:** The diaphragm; costodiaphragmatic recess of the pleura; rib 12; and the psoas, quadratus lumborum, and transversus abdominis muscles. The subcostal (T12), iliohypogastric, and ilioinguinal nerves (L1) run downward and laterally (see Fig. 5.78).

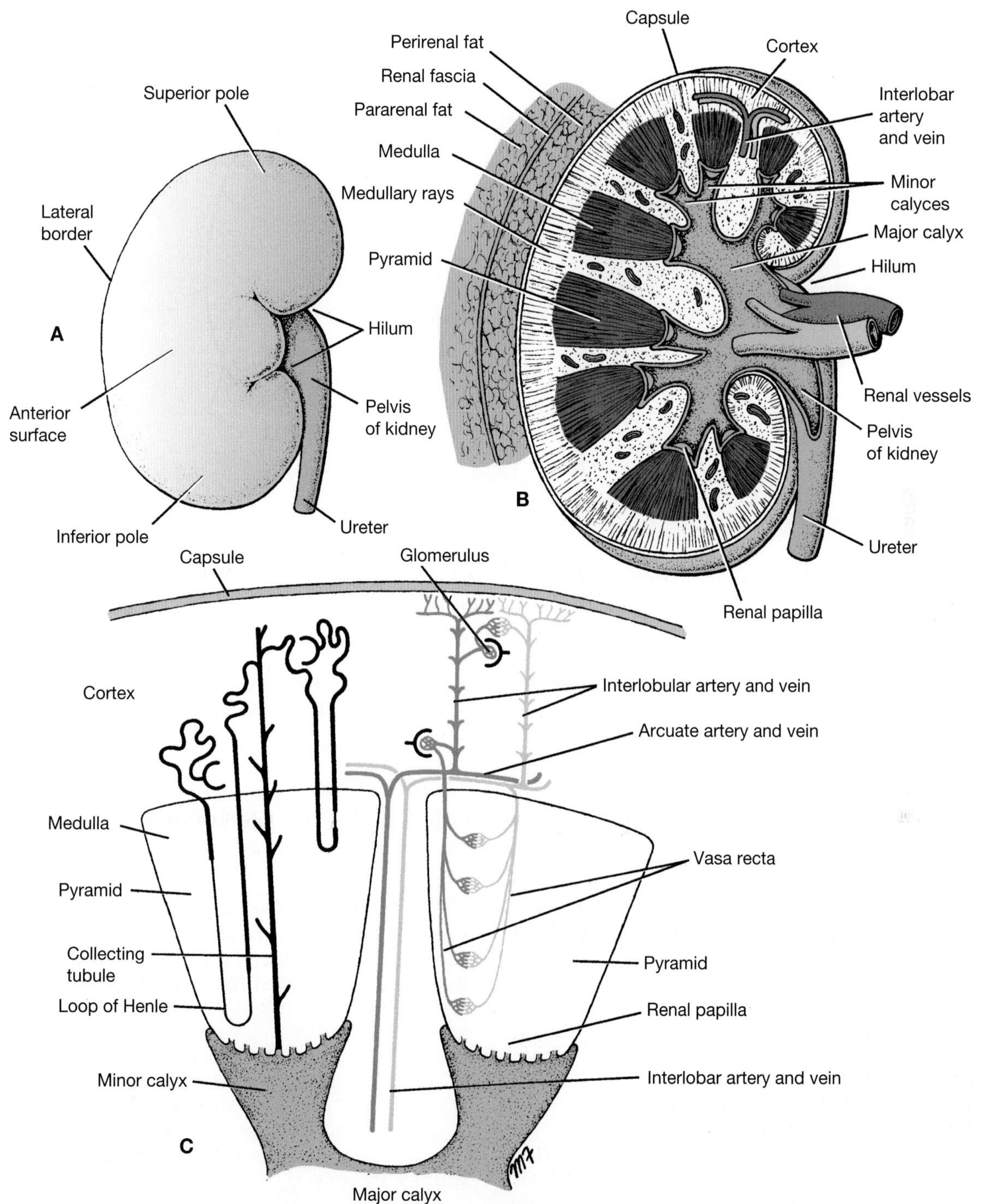

Figure 5.108 **A.** Right kidney, anterior surface. **B.** Right kidney, coronal section showing the cortex, medulla, pyramids, renal papillae, and calyces. **C.** Section of the kidney showing the position of the nephrons and the arrangement of the blood vessels within the kidney.

Important Relations, Left Kidney

- **Anteriorly:** The suprarenal gland, spleen, stomach, pancreas, left colic flexure, and coils of the jejunum (Figs. 5.49 and 5.109).
- **Posteriorly:** The diaphragm; costodiaphragmatic recess of the pleura; ribs 11 (the left kidney is higher) and 12; and the psoas, quadratus lumborum, and transversus abdominis muscles. The subcostal (T12), iliohypogastric, and ilioinguinal nerves (L1) run downward and laterally (see Fig. 5.78).

Blood Supply

The **renal artery** arises from the aorta at the level of the L2 vertebra (see Figs. 5.78 and 5.107). Each renal artery

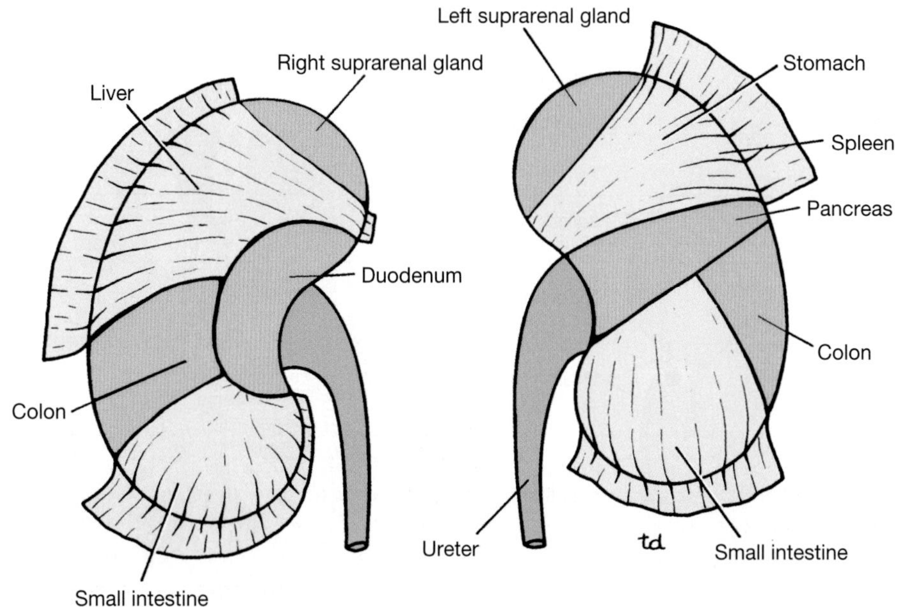

Figure 5.109 Anterior relations of both kidneys. Visceral peritoneum covering the kidneys has been left in position. *Brown* areas indicate where the kidney is in direct contact with the adjacent viscera.

usually divides into five **segmental arteries** that enter the hilum of the kidney. They are distributed to different segments or areas of the kidney. **Lobar arteries** arise from each segmental artery, one for each renal pyramid. Before entering the renal substance, each lobar artery gives off two or three **interlobar arteries** (see Fig. 5.108). The interlobar arteries run toward the cortex on each side of the renal pyramid. At the junction of the cortex and the medulla, the interlobar arteries give off the **arcuate arteries**, which arch over the bases of the pyramids. The arcuate arteries give off several **interlobular arteries** that ascend in the cortex. The **afferent glomerular arterioles** arise as branches of the interlobular arteries.

The **renal vein** emerges from the hilum in front of the renal artery and drains into the inferior vena cava.

Lymph Drainage

Lymph drains to the **lateral aortic lymph nodes** around the origin of the renal artery.

Nerve Supply

The nerve supply is the renal sympathetic plexus. The afferent fibers that travel through the renal plexus enter the spinal cord in the T10 to T12 nerves.

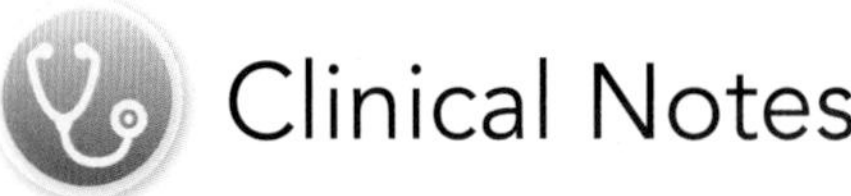

Clinical Notes

Renal Mobility

The kidneys are maintained in their normal position by intra-abdominal pressure and by their connections with the perirenal fat and renal fascia. Each kidney moves slightly with respiration. The right kidney lies at a slightly lower level than the left kidney, and the lower pole may be palpated in the right lumbar region at the end of deep inspiration in a person with poorly developed abdominal musculature. Should the amount of perirenal fat be reduced, the mobility of the kidney may become excessive and produce symptoms of renal colic caused by kinking of the ureter. Excessive mobility of the kidney leaves the suprarenal gland undisturbed because the latter occupies a separate compartment in the renal fascia.

Kidney Trauma

The kidneys are well protected by the lower ribs, the lumbar muscles, and the vertebral column. However, a severe blunt injury applied to the abdomen may crush the kidney against the last rib and the vertebral column. Depending on the severity of the blow, the injury varies from a mild bruising to a complete laceration of the organ. Stab or gunshot wounds usually cause penetrating injuries and often involve other viscera. Because 25% of the cardiac outflow passes through the kidneys, renal injury can result in rapid blood loss. A summary of injuries to the kidneys is shown in Figure 5.110.

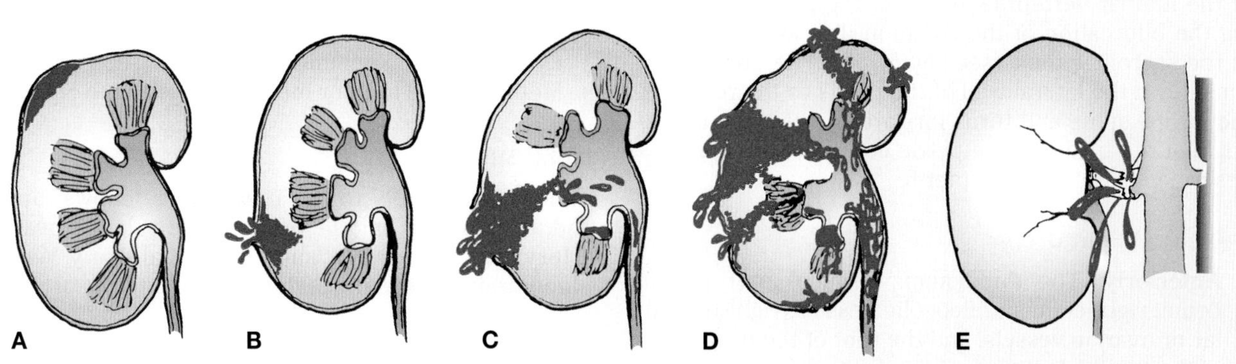

Figure 5.110 Injuries to the kidney. **A.** Contusion with hemorrhage confined to the cortex beneath the intact fibrous capsule. **B.** Tearing of the capsule and the cortex with bleeding occurring into the perirenal fat. **C.** Tearing of the capsule, the cortex, and the medulla. Note the escape of blood into the calyces and therefore the urine. Urine as well as blood may extravasate into the perirenal and pararenal fat and into the peritoneal cavity. **D.** Shattered kidney with extensive hemorrhage and extravasation of blood and urine into the perirenal and pararenal fat; blood also enters the calyces and appears in the urine. **E.** Injury to the renal pedicle involving the renal vessels and possibly the renal pelvis.

Kidney Tumors

Malignant tumors of the kidney have a strong tendency to spread along the renal vein. The left renal vein receives the left testicular vein in the male, and this may rarely become blocked, producing left-sided varicocele (see "Clinical Notes" on scrotum and testes earlier in this chapter).

Renal Pain

Renal pain varies from a dull ache to a severe pain in the flank that may radiate downward into the lower abdomen. Renal pain can result from stretching of the kidney capsule or spasm of the smooth muscle in the renal pelvis. The afferent nerve fibers pass through the **renal plexus** around the renal artery and ascend to the spinal cord through the **lowest splanchnic nerve** in the thorax and the sympathetic trunk. They enter the spinal cord at the level of T12. Pain is commonly referred along the distribution of the subcostal nerve (T12) to the flank and the anterior abdominal wall.

Transplanted Kidneys

The **iliac fossa** on the posterior abdominal wall is the usual site chosen for kidney transplant. The fossa is exposed through an incision in the anterior abdominal wall just above the inguinal ligament. The iliac fossa in front of the iliacus muscle is approached retroperitoneally. The kidney is positioned, and the vascular anastomosis constructed. The **renal artery** is anastomosed end to end to the **internal iliac artery**, and the **renal vein** is anastomosed end to side to the **external iliac vein** (Fig. 5.111).

Anastomosis of the branches of the internal iliac arteries on the two sides is sufficient so that the pelvic viscera on the side of the renal arterial anastomosis are not at risk. **Ureterocystostomy** is then performed by opening the bladder and providing a wide entrance of the ureter through the bladder wall.

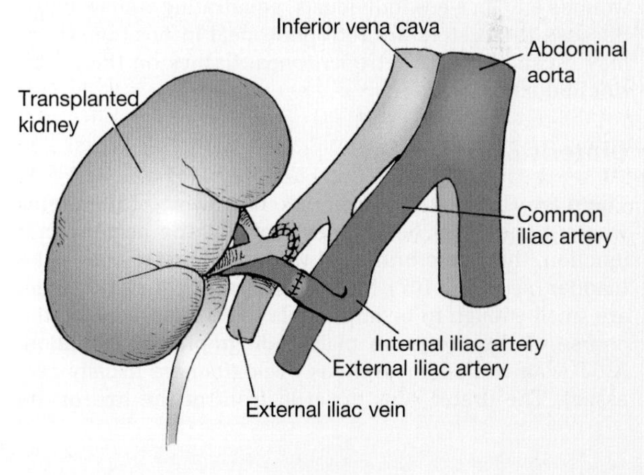

Figure 5.111 Transplanted kidney.

Ureter

The two ureters are muscular tubes that extend from the kidneys to the posterior surface of the urinary bladder (see Fig. 5.107). The urine is propelled along the ureter by peristaltic contractions of the muscle coat, assisted by the filtration pressure of the glomeruli.

Each ureter measures about 10 in. (25 cm) long and resembles the esophagus (also 10 in. long) in having **three constrictions** along its course: (1) where the renal pelvis joins the ureter, (2) where it is kinked as it crosses the pelvic brim, and (3) where it pierces the bladder wall.

The **renal pelvis** is the funnel-shaped expanded upper end of the ureter. It lies within the hilum of the kidney and receives the major calyces (see Fig. 5.110). The ureter emerges from the hilum of the kidney and runs vertically downward behind the parietal peritoneum (adherent to it) on the psoas muscle, which separates it from the tips of the transverse processes of the lumbar vertebrae. It enters the pelvis by crossing the bifurcation of the common iliac artery in front of the sacroiliac joint (see Fig. 5.107). The ureter then runs down the lateral wall of the pelvis to the region of the ischial spine and turns forward to enter the lateral angle of the bladder. The pelvic course of the ureter is described in detail in Chapter 6.

Relations, Right Ureter

- **Anteriorly:** The duodenum, terminal part of the ileum, right colic and ileocolic vessels, right testicular or ovarian vessels, and the root of the mesentery of the small intestine (see Fig. 5.71)
- **Posteriorly:** The right psoas muscle, which separates it from the lumbar transverse processes, and the bifurcation of the right common iliac artery (see Fig. 5.107)

Relations, Left Ureter

- **Anteriorly:** The sigmoid colon and sigmoid mesocolon, left colic vessels, and left testicular or ovarian vessels (see Figs. 5.57 and 5.71)
- **Posteriorly:** The left psoas muscle, which separates it from the lumbar transverse processes, and the bifurcation of the left common iliac artery (see Fig. 5.107)
- **Medially:** The inferior mesenteric vein (see Fig. 5.71)

Blood Supply

The arterial supply to the ureter is as follows: upper end, renal artery; middle portion, testicular or ovarian artery; and, in the pelvis, superior vesical artery. Venous blood drains into veins that correspond to the arteries.

Lymph Drainage

The lymph drains to the **lateral aortic nodes** and the **iliac nodes**.

Nerve Supply

The nerve supply is the renal, testicular (males) or ovarian (females), and hypogastric plexuses (in the pelvis). Afferent fibers travel with the sympathetic nerves and enter the spinal cord in the L1 and L2 segments.

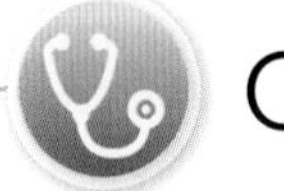

Clinical Notes

Traumatic Ureteral Injuries

Injuries to the ureter are rare because of its protected position and small size. Most injuries are caused by gunshot wounds and, in a few individuals, penetrating stab wounds. Because the ureters are retroperitoneal in position, urine may escape into the retroperitoneal tissues on the posterior abdominal wall.

Ureteric Stones

There are three sites of anatomic narrowing of the ureter where stones may be arrested, namely, the pelviureteral junction, the pelvic brim, and where the ureter enters the bladder (see Fig. 5.107). Most stones, although radiopaque, are small enough to be impossible to see clearly along the course of the ureter on plain radiographic examination. A CT scan and an intravenous pyelogram are usually necessary. The ureter runs down in front of the tips of the transverse processes of the lumbar vertebrae, crosses the region of the sacroiliac joint, swings out to the ischial spine, and then turns medially to the bladder.

The renal pelvis and the ureter send their afferent nerves into the spinal cord at segments T11 to L2. In **renal colic**, strong peristaltic waves of contraction pass down the ureter to pass the stone onward. Spasm of the smooth muscle causes an agonizing colicky pain, which is referred to the skin areas that are supplied by these segments of the spinal cord, namely, the flank, loin, and groin.

When a stone enters the low part of the ureter, the pain is felt at a lower level and is often referred to the testis or the tip of the penis in the male and the labium majus in the female. Sometimes, ureteral pain is referred along the femoral branch of the genitofemoral nerve (L1 and L2) so that pain is experienced in the front of the thigh. The pain is often so severe that afferent pain impulses spread within the central nervous system, giving rise to nausea.

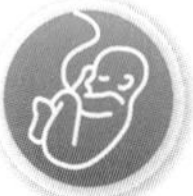

Embryology Notes

Kidney and Ureter Development

Three sets of structures appear in the developing urinary system: **pronephros**, **mesonephros**, and **metanephros**. The metanephros is responsible for the permanent kidney in humans. The metanephros develops from two sources: the **ureteric bud** from the mesonephric duct and the **metanephric cap** from the intermediate cell mass of mesenchyme of the lower lumbar and sacral regions.

Ureteric Bud

The ureteric bud arises as an outgrowth of the **mesonephric duct** (Figs. 5.112 and 5.113). It forms the **ureter**, which dilates at its upper end to form the **pelvis of the ureter**. The pelvis later gives off branches that form the **major calyces**; these, in turn, divide and branch to form the **minor calyces** and the **collecting tubules**.

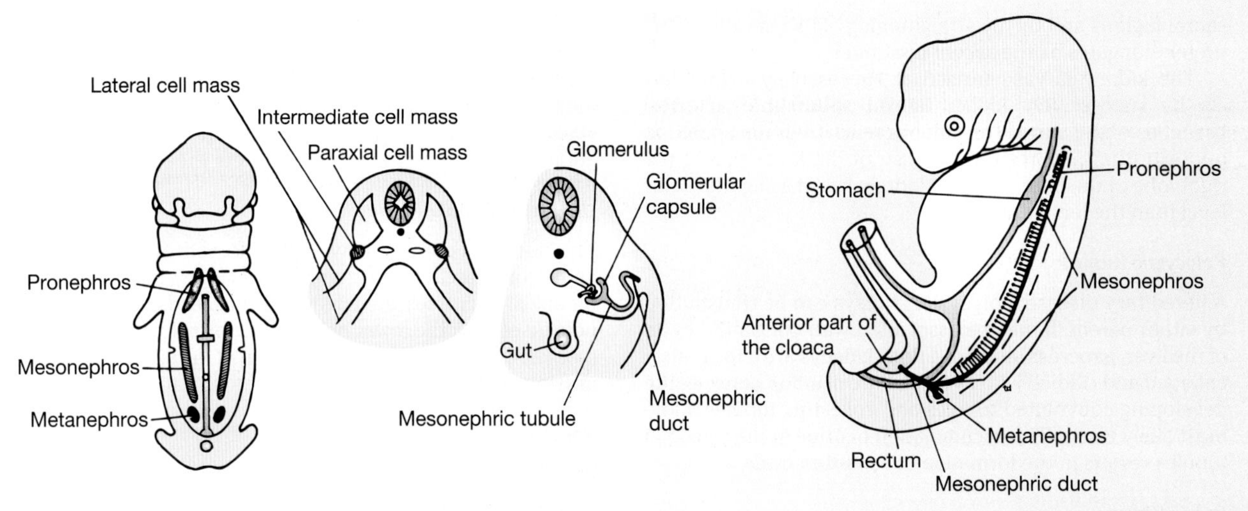

Figure 5.112 Origins and positions of the pronephros, mesonephros, and metanephros.

Metanephric Cap

The metanephric cap condenses around the ureteric bud (see Fig. 5.113) and forms the **glomerular capsules**, **proximal** and **distal convoluted tubules**, and the **loops of Henle**. The glomerular capsule becomes invaginated by a cluster of capillaries that form the **glomerulus**. Each distal convoluted tubule formed from the metanephric cap tissue becomes joined to a collecting tubule derived from the ureteric bud. The surface of the kidney is lobulated at first, but this lobulation usually disappears by the end of postnatal year 1.

The developing kidney is initially a pelvic organ and receives its blood supply from the pelvic continuation of the aorta, the middle sacral artery. Later, the kidneys "ascend" up the posterior abdominal wall. This so-called ascent is caused mainly by the growth of the body in the lumbar and

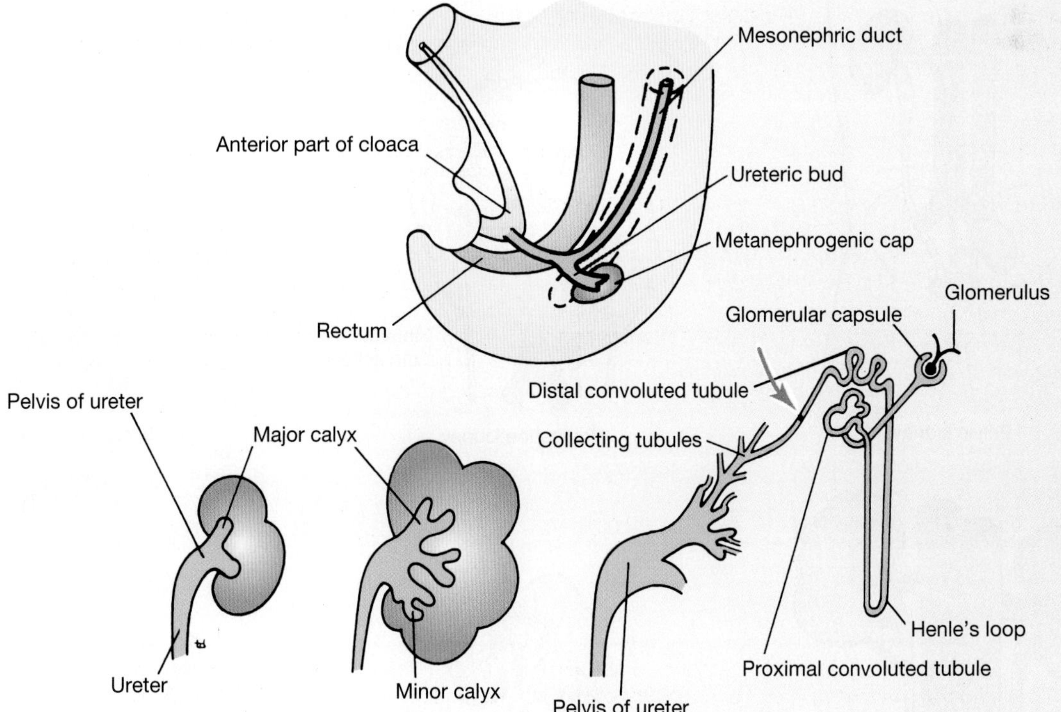

Figure 5.113 Origin of the ureteric bud from the mesonephric duct and the formation of the major and minor calyces and the collecting tubules. *Arrow* indicates the point of union between the collecting tubules and the convoluted tubules.

(continued)

sacral regions and by the straightening of its curvature. The ureter elongates as the ascent continues.

The kidney is vascularized at successively higher levels by successively higher **lateral splanchnic arteries**, branches of the aorta. The kidneys reach their final position opposite the L2 vertebra. Because of the large size of the right lobe of the liver, the right kidney lies at a slightly lower level than the left kidney.

Polycystic Kidney

A hereditary disease, polycystic kidneys can be transmitted by either parent. It may be associated with congenital cysts of the liver, pancreas, and lung. Both kidneys are enormously enlarged and riddled with cysts. Failure of union between the developing convoluted tubules and collecting tubules is the most likely cause. The accumulation of urine in the proximal tubules results in the formation of **retention cysts**.

Pelvic Kidney

In pelvic kidney, the kidney is arrested in some part of its normal ascent; it usually is found at the brim of the pelvis (Fig. 5.114). Such a kidney may present with no signs or symptoms and may function normally. However, if an ectopic kidney becomes inflamed, it may—because of its unusual position—give rise to a mistaken diagnosis.

Horseshoe Kidney

When the caudal ends of both kidneys fuse as they develop, the result is horseshoe kidney (see Fig. 5.114). Both kidneys commence to ascend from the pelvis, but the interconnecting bridge becomes trapped behind the **inferior mesenteric artery** so that the kidneys come to rest in the low lumbar region. Both ureters are kinked as they pass inferiorly over the bridge of renal tissue, producing **urinary stasis**, which may result in infection and stone formation. Surgical division of the bridge corrects the condition.

Unilateral Double Kidney

The kidney on one side may be double, with separate ureters and blood vessels. In unilateral double kidney, the ureteric bud on one side crosses the midline as it ascends, and its upper pole fuses with the lower pole of the normally placed kidney (see Fig. 5.114). Here again, angulation of the ureter may result in stasis of the urine and may require surgical treatment.

Rosette Kidney

Both kidneys may fuse together at their hila, and they usually remain in the pelvis. The two kidneys together form a rosette (see Fig. 5.114). This is the result of the early fusion of the two ureteric buds in the pelvis.

Supernumerary Renal Arteries

Supernumerary renal arteries are relatively common. They represent persistent fetal renal arteries, which grow in sequence from the aorta to supply the kidney as it ascends from the pelvis. Their occurrence is clinically important because a supernumerary artery may cross the pelviureteral junction and obstruct the outflow of urine, producing dilatation of the calyces and pelvis, a condition known as **hydronephrosis** (see Fig. 5.114).

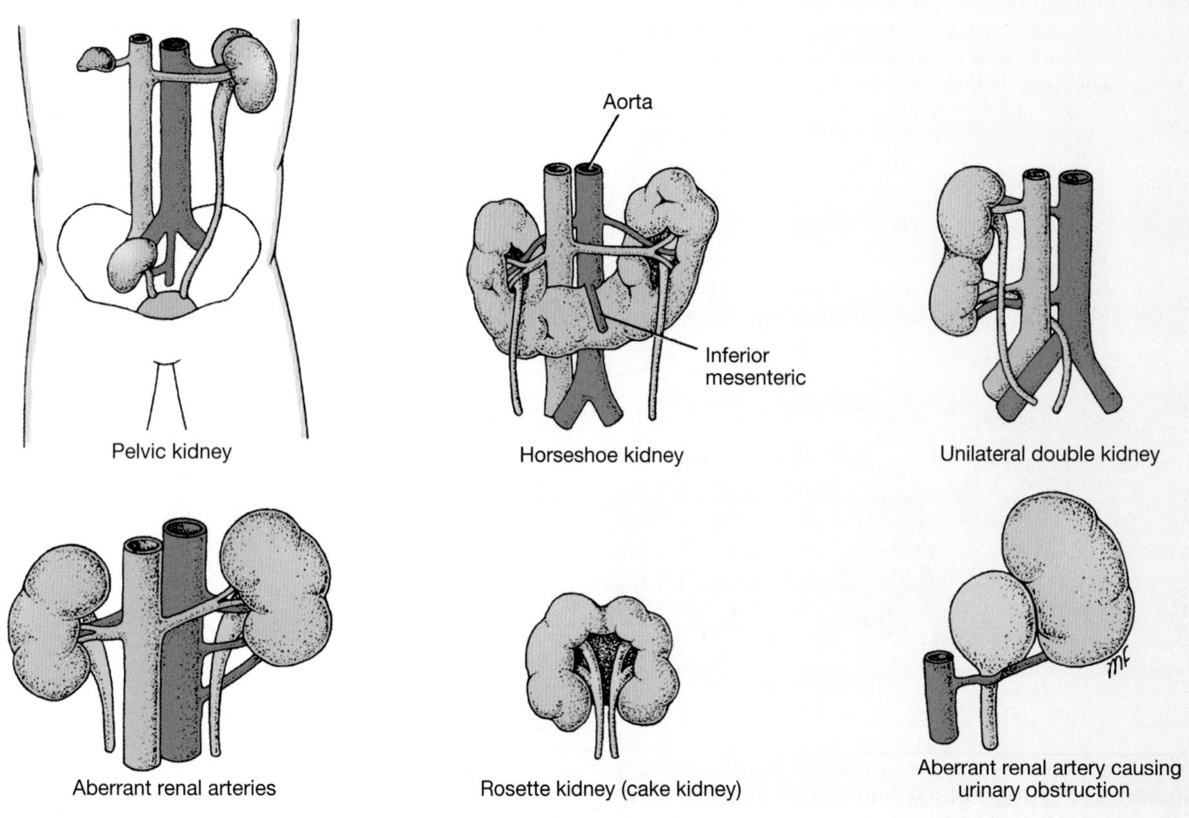

Figure 5.114 Some common congenital anomalies of the kidney.

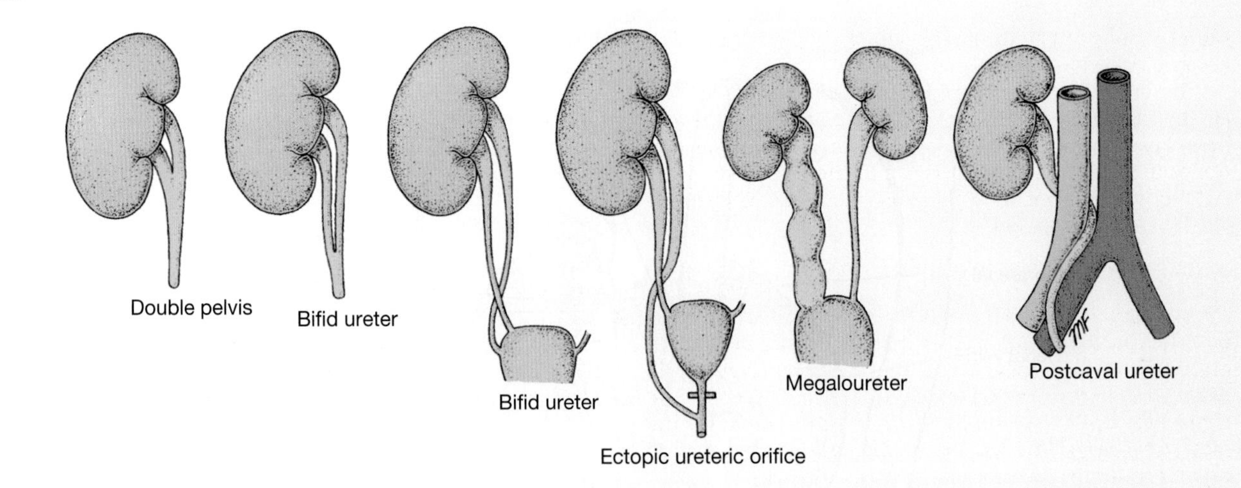

Figure 5.115 Some common congenital anomalies of the ureter.

Double Pelvis

Double pelvis of the ureter is usually unilateral (Fig. 5.115). The upper pelvis is small and drains the upper group of calyces; the larger lower pelvis drains the middle and lower groups of calyces. The cause is a premature division of the ureteric bud near its termination.

Bifid Ureter

In bifid ureter, the ureters may join in the lower third of their course, may open through a common orifice into the bladder, or may open independently into the bladder (see Fig. 5.115). In the latter case, one ureter crosses its fellow and may produce urinary obstruction. The cause of bifid ureter is a premature division of the ureteric bud.

Cases of double pelvis and double ureters may be found by chance on radiologic investigation of the urinary tract. They are more liable to become infected or to be the seat of calculus formation than a normal ureter.

Megaloureter

Megaloureter may be unilateral or bilateral and shows complete absence of motility (see Fig. 5.115). The cause is unknown. Because of urinary stasis, the ureter is prone to infection. Plastic surgery is required to improve the rate of drainage.

Postcaval Ureter

The right ureter may ascend posterior to the inferior vena cava and may be obstructed by it (see Fig. 5.115). Surgical rerouting of the ureter with reimplantation of the distal end into the bladder is the treatment of choice.

SUPRARENAL GLANDS

The two suprarenal glands are yellowish retroperitoneal organs that lie on the upper poles of the kidneys (Fig. 5.116). They are surrounded by renal fascia but are separated from the kidneys by the perirenal fat. Each gland has a yellow **cortex** and a dark brown **medulla**.

The cortex of the suprarenal glands secretes hormones that include **mineral corticoids** (concerned with the control of fluid and electrolyte balance), **glucocorticoids** (concerned with the control of the metabolism of carbohydrates), fats, proteins, and small amounts of sex hormones (which probably play a role in the prepubertal development of the sex organs). The medulla of the suprarenal glands secretes the **catecholamines epinephrine** and **norepinephrine**.

Location and Description

The **right suprarenal gland** is pyramid shaped and caps the upper pole of the right kidney (see Figs. 5.49, 5.71, 5.79. 5.107, and 5.116). It lies behind the right lobe of the liver and extends medially behind the inferior vena cava. It rests posteriorly on the diaphragm.

The **left suprarenal gland** is crescentic in shape and extends along the medial border of the left kidney from the upper pole to the hilus. It lies behind the pancreas, lesser sac, and stomach and rests posteriorly on the diaphragm.

Blood Supply

Multiple arteries supply each gland. The three typical vessels are a superior suprarenal artery (branch of the inferior phrenic artery), a middle suprarenal artery (branch of the aorta), and an inferior suprarenal artery (branch of the renal artery).

A single vein emerges from the hilum of each gland and drains into the **inferior vena cava** on the right and into the **renal vein** on the left.

Lymph Drainage

The lymph drains into the **lateral aortic nodes**.

Nerve Supply

Preganglionic sympathetic fibers derived from the **splanchnic nerves** supply the glands. Most of the nerves end in the medulla of the gland.

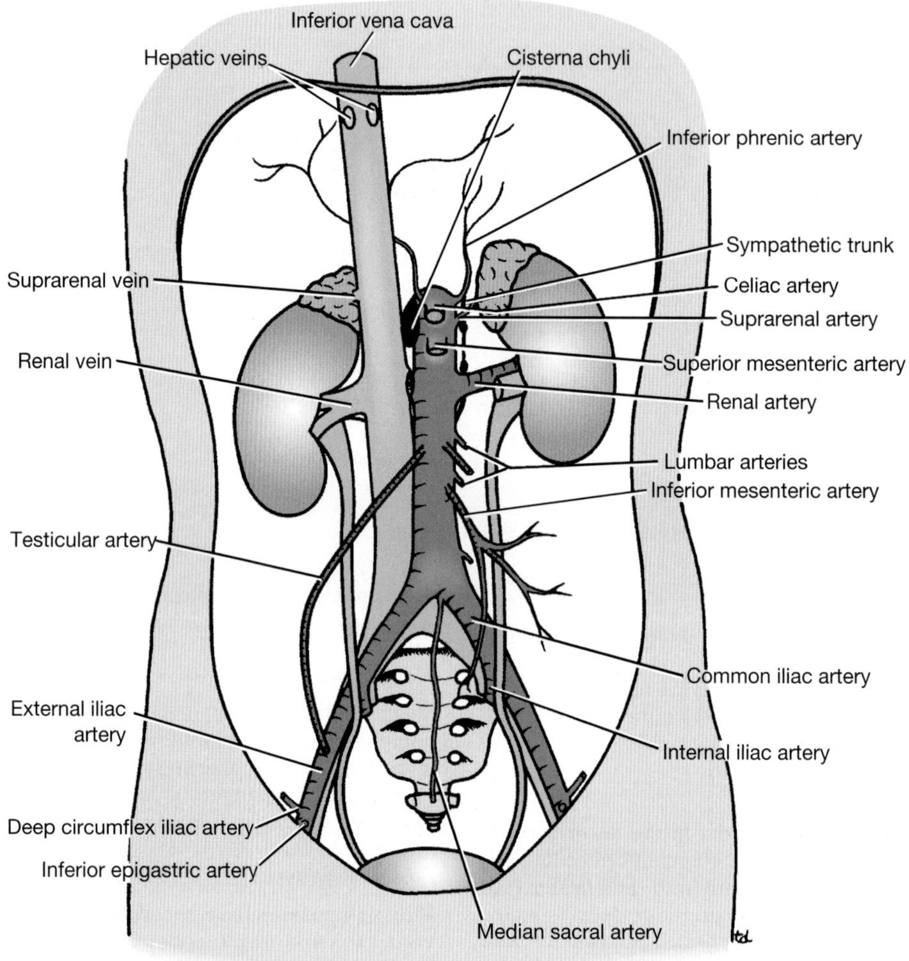

Figure 5.116 Aorta and inferior vena cava.

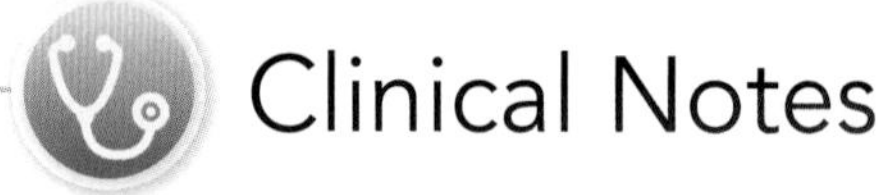

Clinical Notes

Cushing Syndrome

Suprarenal cortical hyperplasia is the most common cause of Cushing syndrome, the clinical manifestations of which include moon-shaped face, truncal obesity, abnormal hairiness (hirsutism), and hypertension. If the syndrome occurs later in life, it may result from an adenoma or carcinoma of the cortex.

Addison Disease

Adrenocortical insufficiency (Addison disease), which is characterized clinically by increased pigmentation, muscular weakness, weight loss, and hypotension, may be caused by tuberculous destruction or bilateral atrophy of both cortices.

Pheochromocytoma

Pheochromocytoma, a tumor of the medulla, produces a paroxysmal or sustained hypertension. The symptoms and signs result from the production of a large amount of catecholamines, which are then poured into the bloodstream.

Because of their position on the posterior abdominal wall, few tumors of the suprarenal glands can be palpated. CT scans can be used to visualize the glandular enlargement. However, when interpreting CT scans, remember the close relationship of the suprarenal glands to the crura of the diaphragm.

Surgical Significance of Renal Fascia

The suprarenal glands, together with the kidneys, are enclosed within the renal fascia. However, the suprarenal glands lie in a separate compartment, which allows the two organs to be separated easily at operation.

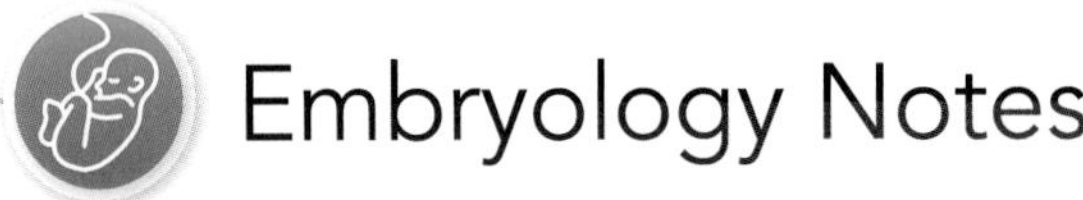

Suprarenal Gland Development

The **cortex** develops from the coelomic mesothelium covering the posterior abdominal wall. At first, a fetal cortex is formed; later, it becomes covered by a second final cortex. After birth, the fetal cortex retrogresses, and its involution is largely completed in the first few weeks of life.

The **medulla** is formed from the **sympathochromaffin cells** of the neural crest. These invade the cortex on its medial side. By this means, the medulla comes to occupy a central position and is arranged in cords and clusters. Preganglionic sympathetic nerve fibers grow into the medulla and influence the activity of the medullary cells.

Susceptibility to Trauma at Birth

The suprarenal glands are relatively large at birth because of the presence of the fetal cortex. Later, when this part of the cortex involutes, the gland becomes reduced in size. During the process of involution, the cortex is friable and susceptible to damage and severe hemorrhage.

POSTERIOR ABDOMINAL WALL

The posterior abdominal wall contains skeletal elements (lower ribs, lumbar vertebrae, and part of the pelvis), large muscles (psoas, iliacus, quadratus lumborum, and transversus abdominis), part of the urinary tract (kidneys and ureters), part of the GI tract (duodenum, ascending colon, and descending colon), and extensive neurovascular networks. It is formed in the midline by the L1 to L5 vertebrae and their intervertebral discs and laterally by rib 12 (left and right), the upper part of the bony pelvis, psoas muscles, quadratus lumborum muscles, and the aponeuroses of origin of the transversus abdominis muscles. The iliacus muscles lie in the upper part of the bony pelvis (Fig. 5.117; see also Fig. 5.1).

Posterior Abdominal Wall Muscles

The muscles of the posterior abdominal wall are summarized in Table 5.2.

Psoas Major

The fibers of the psoas major muscle run downward and laterally and leave the abdomen to enter the thigh by passing behind the inguinal ligament (see Fig. 5.117). The psoas is enclosed in a fibrous sheath that is derived from the lumbar fascia. The sheath is thickened above to form the **medial arcuate ligament**. The psoas major has a major action in the lower limb and will be discussed in more detail in Chapter 8. The **psoas minor** is a small, inconstant muscle of little

Figure 5.117 Muscles and bones forming the posterior abdominal wall.

Table 5.2 Posterior Abdominal Wall Muscles

NAME OF MUSCLE	ORIGIN	INSERTION	NERVE SUPPLY	ACTION
Psoas	Transverse processes, bodies, and intervertebral discs of T12 and L1 to L5 vertebrae	With iliacus into lesser trochanter of femur	Lumbar plexus	Flexes thigh on trunk; if thigh is fixed, it flexes trunk on thigh, as in sitting up from lying position
Quadratus lumborum	Iliolumbar ligament, iliac crest, tips of transverse processes of lower lumbar vertebrae	Rib 12	Lumbar plexus	Fixes rib 12 during inspiration; depresses rib 12 during forced expiration; abducts vertebral column of the same side
Iliacus	Iliac fossa	With psoas into lesser trochanter of femur	Femoral nerve	Flexes thigh on trunk; if thigh is fixed, it flexes the trunk on the thigh, as in sitting up from lying position

importance. When present (about 60% of individuals), it is located on the anterior surface of the psoas major and consists mainly of a long tendon. It may be present only unilaterally.

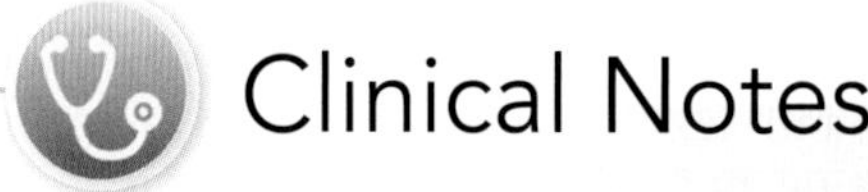

Clinical Notes

Psoas Fascia and Tuberculosis

The psoas fascia covers the anterior surface of the psoas muscle and can influence the direction taken by a tubercular abscess. Tubercular disease of the thoracolumbar region of the vertebral column results in the destruction of the vertebral bodies, with possible extension of pus laterally under the psoas fascia (Fig. 5.118). From there, the pus tracks downward, following the course of the psoas muscle, and appears as a swelling in the upper part of the thigh below the inguinal ligament. It may be mistaken for a femoral hernia.

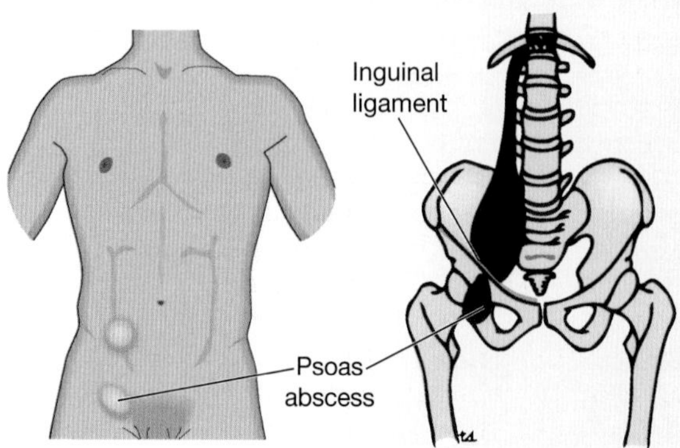

Figure 5.118 Case of advanced tubercular disease of the thoracolumbar region of the vertebral column. A psoas abscess is present, and swellings occur in the right groin above and below the right inguinal ligament.

Quadratus Lumborum

The quadratus lumborum is a flat, quadrilateral muscle that lies alongside the vertebral column (see Fig. 5.117). The fibers run upward and medially and are inserted into the lower border of rib 12 and the transverse processes of the L1 to L4 vertebrae. The anterior surface of the muscle is covered by lumbar fascia, which is thickened above to form the **lateral arcuate ligament** and below to form the **iliolumbar ligament**.

Transversus Abdominis

The transversus abdominis muscle was fully described earlier with the muscles of the anterolateral abdominal wall.

Iliacus

The iliacus muscle is fan shaped and arises from the upper part of the iliac fossa (see Fig. 5.117). Its fibers join the lateral side of the psoas major tendon, and the combined muscles are referred to as the **iliopsoas**. The iliopsoas is the major flexor of the thigh, or the major flexor of the trunk against the thigh.

The **posterior part of the diaphragm** also forms part of the posterior abdominal wall. The diaphragm was described earlier in this chapter.

Posterior Abdominal Wall Arteries

The major arteries on the posterior abdominal wall are the aorta, common iliac arteries, and external iliac arteries. The internal iliac arteries are in the pelvic cavity.

Aorta

The aorta enters the abdomen through the aortic opening (hiatus) of the diaphragm in front of the T12 vertebra (see Figs. 5.107 and 5.116). It descends behind the peritoneum on the anterior surface of the bodies of the lumbar vertebrae. At the level of the L4 vertebra, it divides into the two **common iliac arteries**. On its right side lie the inferior vena cava, the cisterna chyli, and the

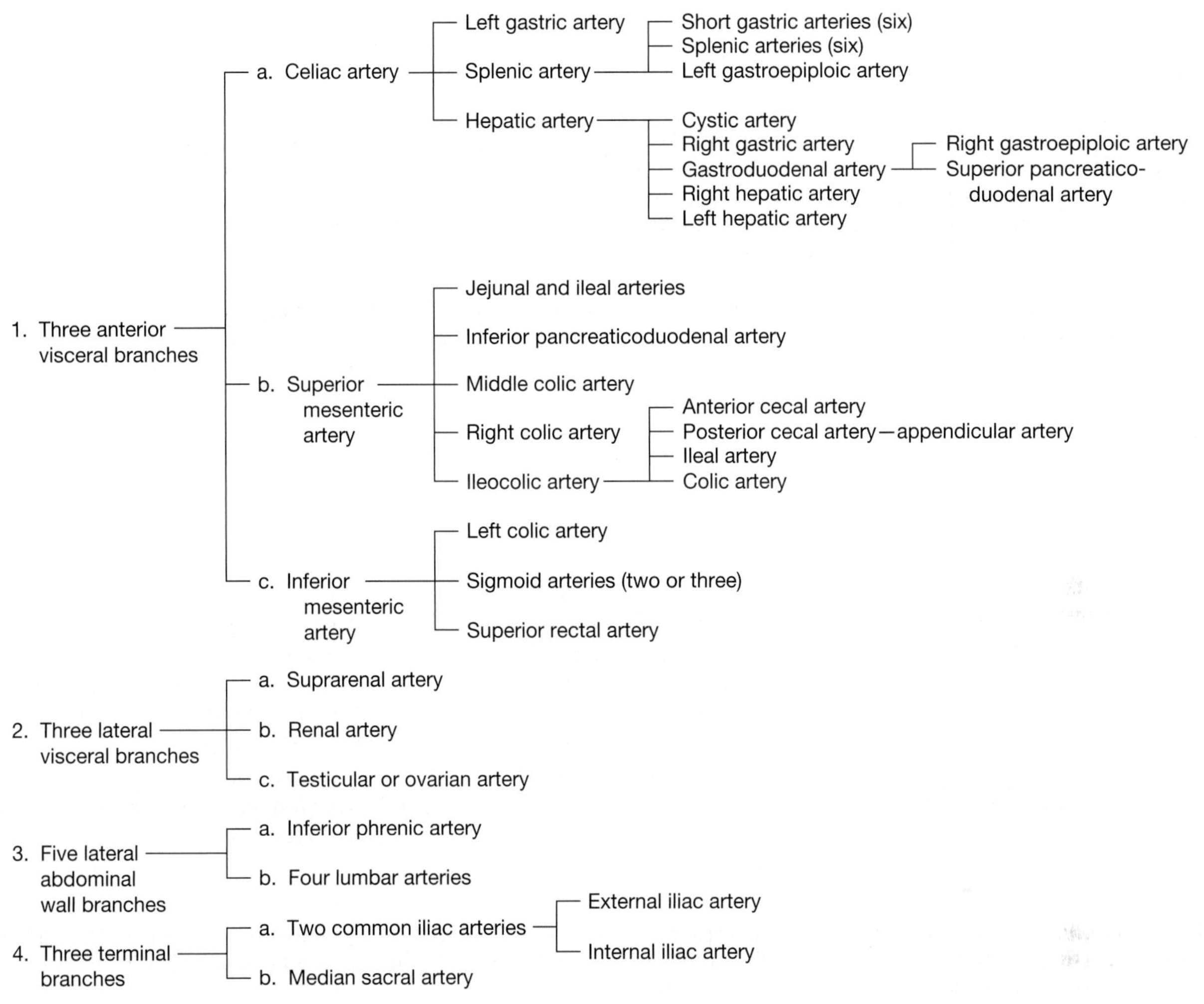

Diagram 5.1 Abdominal aorta branches.

beginning of the azygos vein. On its left side lies the left sympathetic trunk.

Branches (Summarized in Fig. 5.116 and Diagram 5.1)

- Three **anterior visceral branches:** celiac, superior mesenteric, and inferior mesenteric arteries
- Three **lateral visceral branches:** suprarenal, renal, and testicular or ovarian arteries
- Five **lateral abdominal wall branches:** inferior phrenic and four lumbar arteries
- Three **terminal branches:** two common iliac arteries and the median sacral artery

Common Iliac Arteries

Two of the terminal branches of the aorta are the right and left common iliac arteries. They arise at the level of the L4 vertebra and run downward and laterally along the medial border of the psoas muscle (see Figs. 5.107 and 5.116). Each artery ends in front of the sacroiliac joint by dividing into the **external** and **internal iliac arteries**. Each ureter crosses the anterior side of the common iliac artery at its bifurcation (see Fig. 5.116).

External Iliac Artery

The external iliac artery runs along the medial border of the psoas, following the pelvic brim (see Fig. 5.107). It gives off the **inferior epigastric** and **deep circumflex iliac branches** (see Fig. 5.116). The artery enters the thigh by passing under the inguinal ligament to become the **femoral artery**.

The inferior epigastric artery arises just above the inguinal ligament. It passes upward and medially along the medial margin of the deep inguinal ring (see Fig. 5.11) and enters the rectus sheath behind the rectus abdominis muscle. The deep circumflex iliac artery arises close to the inferior epigastric artery (see Fig. 5.116). It ascends laterally to the anterior superior iliac spine and the iliac crest, supplying the muscles of the anterior abdominal wall.

Internal Iliac Artery

The internal iliac artery passes down into the pelvis in front of the sacroiliac joint (see Fig. 5.116). Its further course is described in Chapter 6.

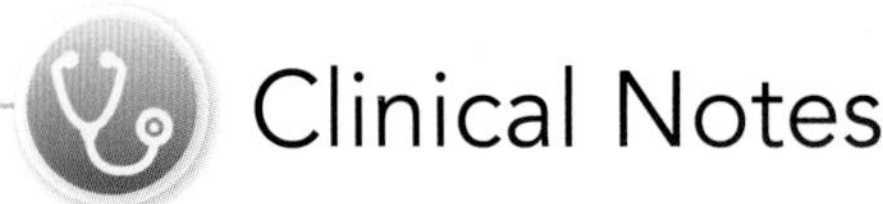

Clinical Notes

Aortic Aneurysms

Localized or diffuse dilatations of the abdominal part of the aorta (aneurysms) usually occur below the origin of the renal arteries. Most result from atherosclerosis, which causes weakening of the arterial wall, and occur most commonly in elderly males. Large aneurysms should be treated by open surgical repair. Endovascular repair can also be used by introducing a stent graft through a femoral artery in the groin and up through the external and common iliac arteries into the aorta.

Embolic Blockage of Abdominal Aorta

The bifurcation of the abdominal aorta where the lumen suddenly narrows may be a lodging site for an embolus discharged from the heart. The result is severe ischemia of the lower limbs.

Posterior Abdominal Wall Veins

The inferior vena cava is the major vein on the posterior abdominal wall. However, several of its tributaries have close relations to the posterior wall as well.

Inferior Vena Cava

The inferior vena cava conveys most of the blood from the body below the diaphragm to the right atrium of the heart. It is formed by the union of the **common iliac veins** behind the right common iliac artery at the level of the L5 vertebra (see Fig. 5.116). It ascends on the right side of the aorta, pierces the central tendon of the diaphragm at the level of the T8 vertebra, and drains into the right atrium.

The right sympathetic trunk lies behind its right margin and the right ureter lies close to its right border. The entrance into the lesser sac separates the inferior vena cava from the portal vein (see Fig. 5.55).

Tributaries

Tributaries are summarized in Figure 5.116 and Diagram 5.2. Remember that the venous blood from the abdominal portion of the GI tract drains to the liver by means of the tributaries of the portal vein, and that the left suprarenal and testicular or ovarian veins drain first into the left renal vein; thus, the tributaries of the inferior vena cava correspond closely to the branches of the abdominal portion of the aorta.

- Two **anterior visceral tributaries:** hepatic veins
- Three **lateral visceral tributaries:** right suprarenal vein (left vein drains into the left renal vein), renal veins, and right testicular or ovarian vein (left vein drains into the left renal vein)
- Five **lateral abdominal wall tributaries:** inferior phrenic and four lumbar veins
- Three **veins of origin:** two common iliac veins and the median sacral vein

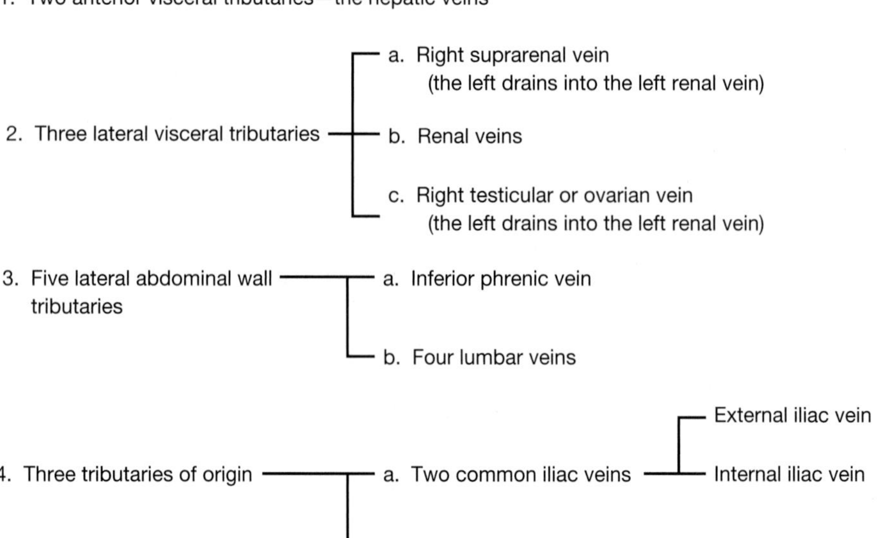

Diagram 5.2 Inferior vena cava tributaries.

Inferior Mesenteric Vein

The inferior mesenteric vein is a tributary of the portal circulation. It begins halfway down the anal canal as the **superior rectal vein** (see Figs. 5.65, 5.70, and 5.92). It passes up the posterior abdominal wall on the left side of the inferior mesenteric artery and the duodenojejunal flexure and joins the splenic vein behind the pancreas. It receives tributaries that correspond to the branches of the artery.

Splenic Vein

The splenic vein is a tributary of the portal circulation. It begins at the hilum of the spleen by the union of several veins and is then joined by the **short gastric** and **left gastro-omental veins** (see Figs. 5.65 and 5.92). It passes to the right within the splenorenal ligament and runs behind the pancreas. It joins the superior mesenteric vein behind the neck of the pancreas to form the **portal vein**. Veins from the pancreas and the inferior mesenteric vein join it.

Superior Mesenteric Vein

The superior mesenteric vein is a tributary of the portal circulation (see Figs. 5.65, 5.70, and 5.92). It begins at the ileocecal junction and runs upward on the posterior abdominal wall within the root of the mesentery of the small intestine and on the right side of the superior mesenteric artery. It passes in front of the third part of the duodenum and behind the neck of the pancreas, where it joins the **splenic vein** to form the **portal vein.** It receives tributaries that correspond to the branches of the superior mesenteric artery and also receives the inferior pancreaticoduodenal vein and the right gastroepiploic vein (see Fig. 5.65).

Portal Vein

The portal vein was described earlier in this chapter.

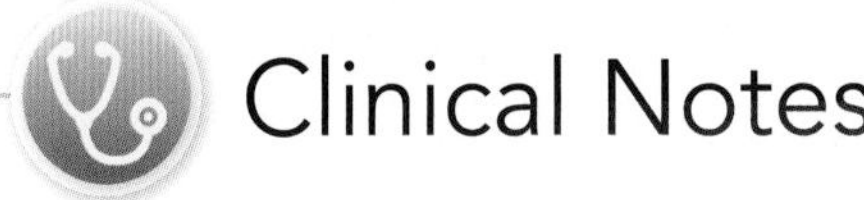

Clinical Notes

Abdominal Aorta Trauma

Blunt trauma to the aorta is most caused by head-on motor vehicle crashes. Rupture of the tunica intima and media occurs and is quickly followed by rupture of the tunica adventitia. The initial rupture of the intima and media is probably mainly caused by the sudden compression of the aorta against the vertebral column, whereas the delayed rupture of the adventitia is caused by the aortic blood pressure. Death follows unless quickly diagnosed by magnetic resonance imaging (MRI), and surgical treatment is instituted.

Obliteration of Abdominal Aorta and Iliac Arteries

Gradual occlusion of the bifurcation of the abdominal aorta, produced by atherosclerosis, results in the characteristic clinical symptoms of pain in the legs on walking (**claudication**) and erectile dysfunction, the latter caused by lack of blood in the internal iliac arteries. In otherwise healthy individuals, surgical treatment by thromboendarterectomy or a bypass graft should be considered. Because the progress of the disease is slow, some collateral circulation is established, but it is physiologically inadequate. However, the collateral blood flow does prevent tissue death in both lower limbs, although skin ulcers may occur.

The collateral circulation of the abdominal aorta is shown in Figure 5.119.

Inferior Vena Cava Trauma

Injuries to the inferior vena cava are commonly lethal, even though the contained blood is under low pressure. The anatomic inaccessibility of the vessel behind the liver, duodenum, and mesentery of the small intestine and the blocking presence of the right costal margin make a surgical approach difficult. Moreover, the thin wall of the vena cava makes it prone to extensive tears.

Because of the multiple anastomoses of the tributaries of the inferior vena cava (Fig. 5.120), it is impossible in an emergency to ligate the vessel. Most patients have venous congestion of the lower limbs.

Inferior Vena Cava Compression

The enlarged uterus commonly compresses the inferior vena cava during the later stages of pregnancy. This produces edema of the ankles and feet and temporary varicose veins.

Malignant retroperitoneal tumors can cause severe compression and eventual blockage of the inferior vena cava. This results in the dilatation of the extensive anastomoses of the tributaries (see Fig. 5.120). This alternative pathway for the blood to return to the right atrium of the heart is commonly referred to as the **caval–caval shunt**. The same pathway comes into effect in patients with a superior mediastinal tumor compressing the superior vena cava. Clinically, the enlarged subcutaneous anastomosis between the lateral thoracic vein, a tributary of the axillary vein, and the superficial epigastric vein, a tributary of the femoral vein, may be seen on the thoracoabdominal wall.

(continued)

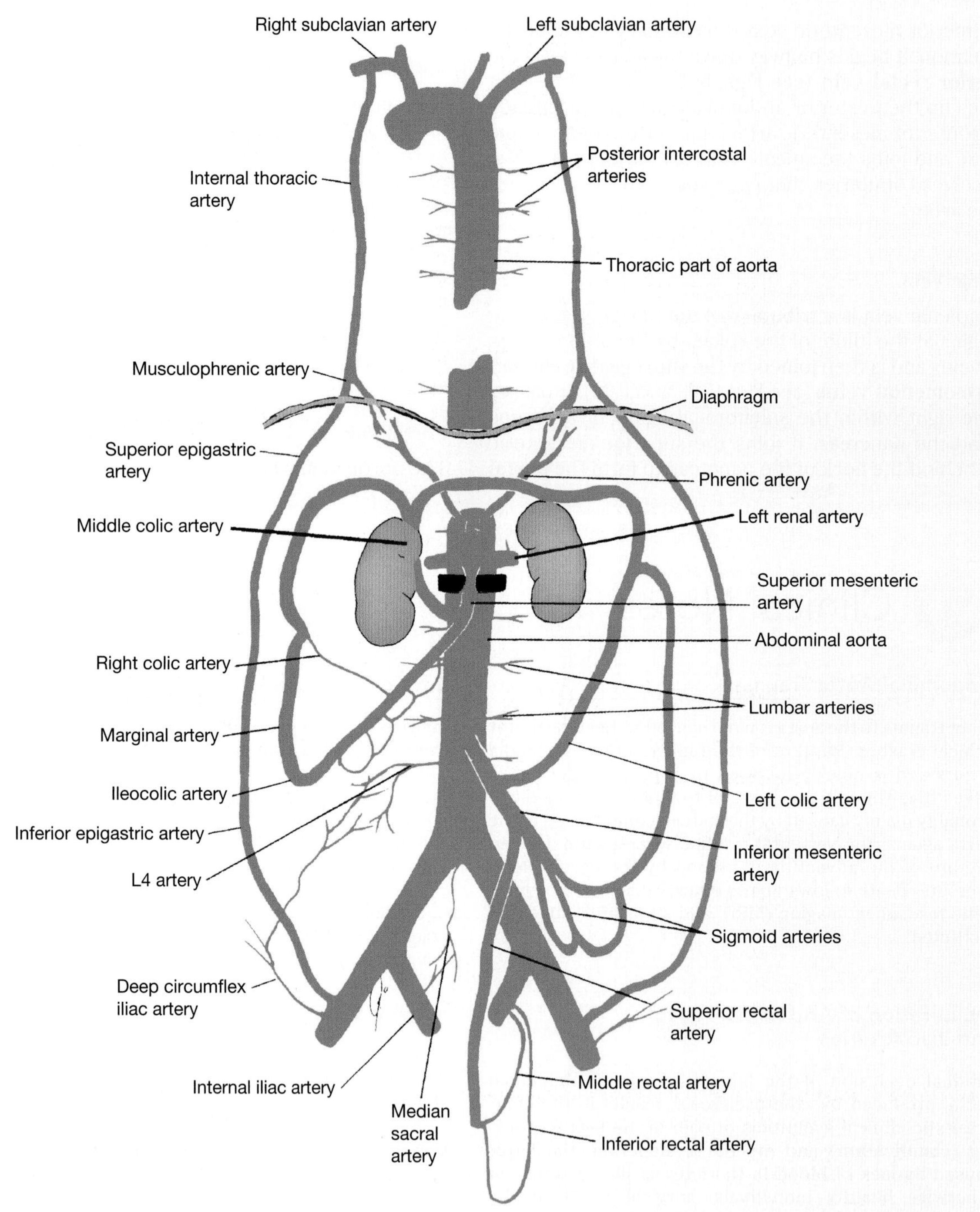

Figure 5.119 Possible collateral circulations of the abdominal aorta. Note the great dilatation of the mesenteric arteries and their branches, which occurs if the aorta is slowly blocked just below the level of the renal arteries (*black bar*).

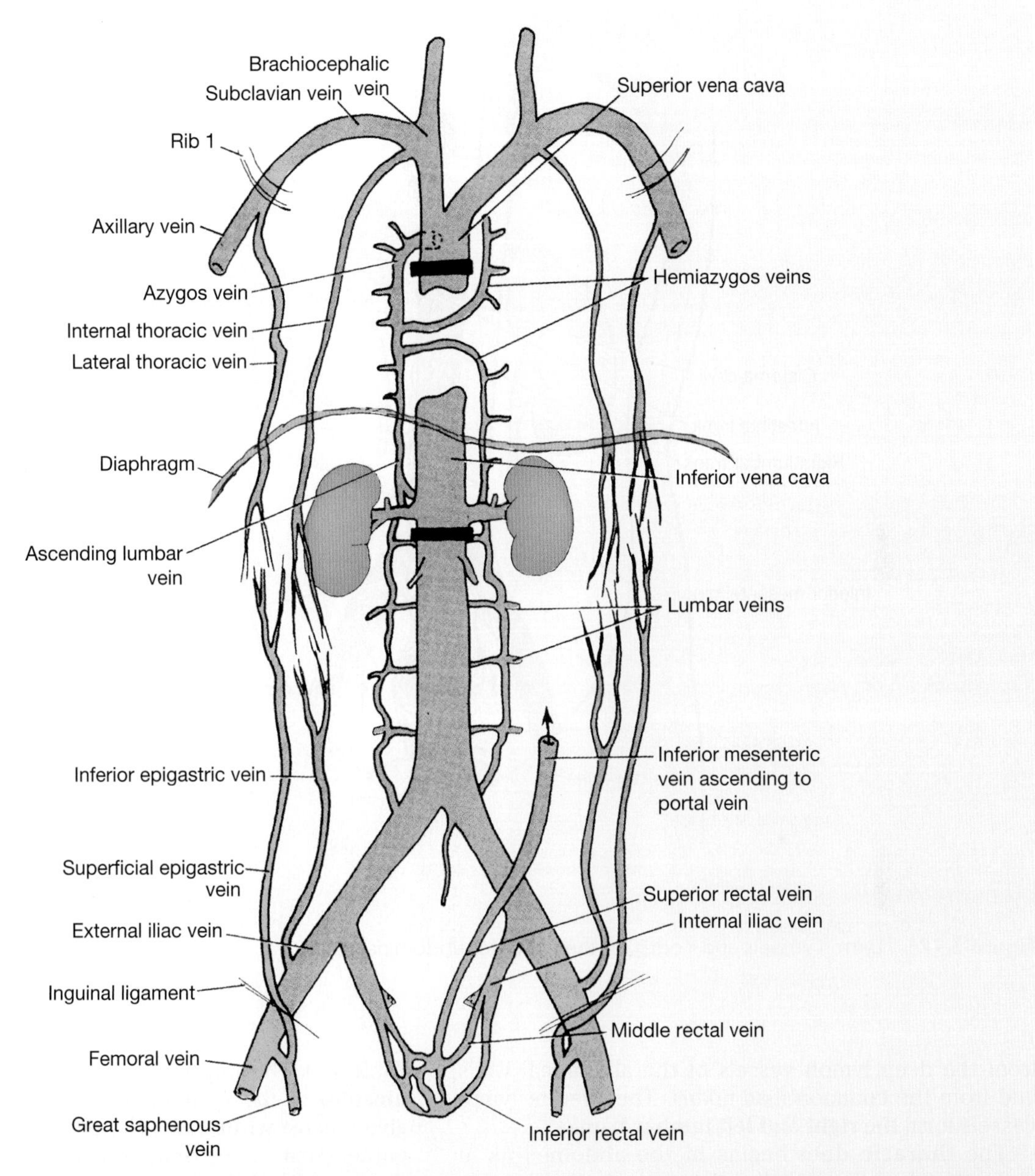

Figure 5.120 Possible collateral circulations of the superior and inferior venae cava. Note the alternative pathways that exist for blood to return to the right atrium of the heart if the superior vena cava becomes blocked below the entrance of the azygos vein (*upper black bar*). Similar pathways exist if the inferior vena cava becomes blocked below the renal veins (*lower black bar*). Also note the connections that exist between the portal circulation and systemic veins in the anal canal.

Posterior Abdominal Wall Lymphatics

The lymph nodes are closely related to the aorta and form a **preaortic** and a **right** and **left lateral aortic (para-aortic or lumbar) chain** (Fig. 5.121).

The **preaortic lymph nodes** lie around the origins of the celiac, superior mesenteric, and inferior mesenteric arteries and are referred to as the **celiac**, **superior mesenteric**, and **inferior mesenteric lymph nodes**, respectively. They drain the lymph from the GI tract, extending from the lower third of the esophagus to halfway down the anal canal, and from the spleen, pancreas, gallbladder, and greater part of the liver. The efferent lymph vessels form the large intestinal trunk (see Fig. 1.30A and below).

The **lateral aortic (para-aortic or lumbar) lymph nodes** drain lymph from the kidneys and suprarenal glands; from the testes in the male and from the ovaries, uterine tubes, and fundus of the uterus in the female;

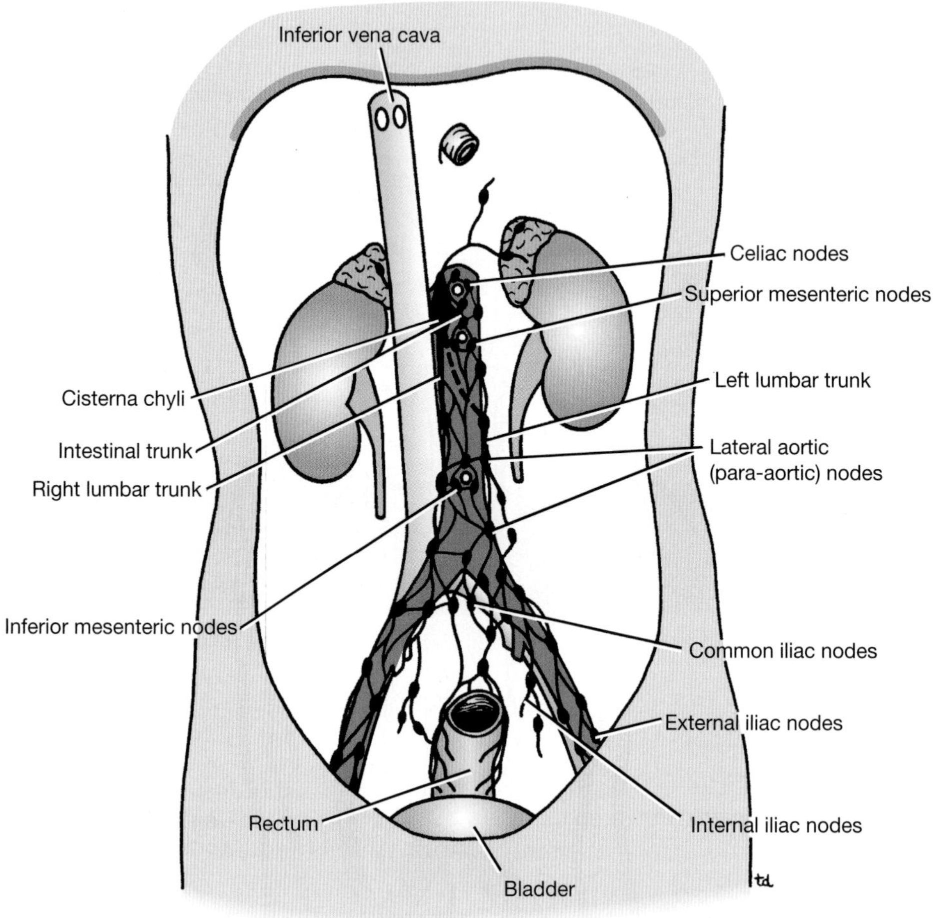

Figure 5.121 Lymph vessels and nodes on the posterior abdominal wall.

from the deep lymph vessels of the abdominal walls; and from the common iliac nodes. The efferent lymph vessels form the **right** and **left lumbar trunks**.

The **thoracic duct** begins in the abdomen as an elongated lymph sac, the **cisterna chyli**. This lies just below the diaphragm in front of the L1 and L2 vertebrae and on the right side of the aorta (see Fig. 5.121). The cisterna chyli receives the intestinal trunk, the right and left lumbar trunks, and some small lymph vessels that descend from the lower part of the thorax.

Posterior Abdominal Wall Nerves

The lumbar plexus and its branches, the sympathetic chain and its branches, and the aortic plexuses collectively form extensive nerve networks on the posterior wall.

Lumbar Plexus

The anterior rami of the L1 to L4 nerves form the lumbar plexus (one of the main nervous pathways supplying the lower limb) in the psoas muscle (Fig. 5.122 and Table 5.3). The anterior rami give off **gray rami communicantes** to the sympathetic trunk, and the upper two give receive **white rami communicantes** from the sympathetic trunk. The branches of the plexus emerge from the lateral and medial borders of the muscle and from its anterior surface.

The **iliohypogastric nerve**, **ilioinguinal nerve**, **lateral cutaneous nerve of the thigh**, and **femoral nerve** emerge from the lateral border of the psoas, in that order from above downward (see Fig. 5.78). The iliohypogastric and ilioinguinal nerves (L1) cross the quadratus lumborum muscle and enter the lateral and anterior abdominal walls (see "Nerves of the Anterior Abdominal Wall" earlier in this chapter). The lateral cutaneous nerve of the thigh crosses the iliac fossa in front of the iliacus muscle and enters the thigh behind the lateral end of the inguinal ligament. The femoral nerve (L2 to L4) is the largest branch of the lumbar plexus. It runs downward and laterally between the psoas and the iliacus muscles and enters the thigh behind the inguinal ligament and lateral to the femoral vessels and the femoral sheath. In the abdomen, it supplies the iliacus muscle.

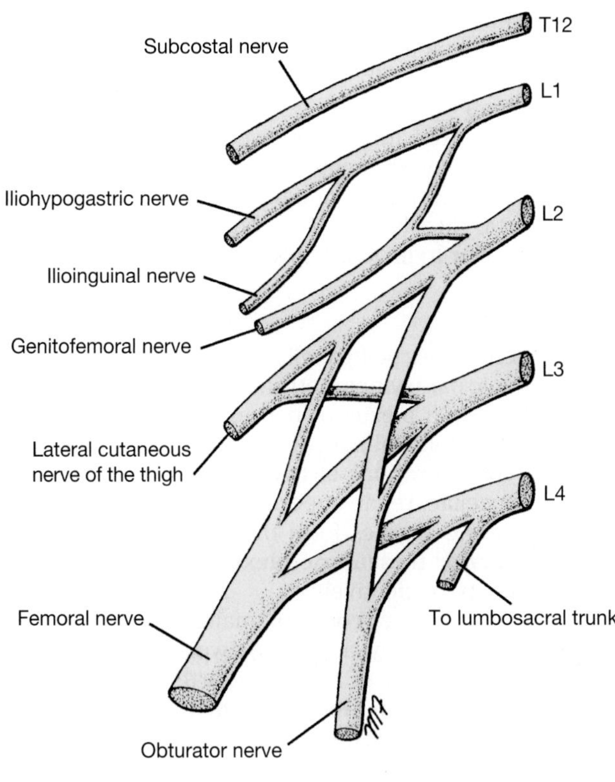

Figure 5.122 Lumbar plexus of nerves.

The **obturator nerve** and the L4 root of the **lumbosacral trunk** emerge from the medial border of the psoas at the brim of the pelvis. The obturator nerve (L2 to L4) crosses the pelvic brim in front of the sacroiliac joint and behind the common iliac vessels. It leaves the pelvis by passing through the obturator foramen into the thigh. The L4 root of the lumbosacral trunk takes part in the formation of the sacral plexus (see Chapter 6). It descends anterior to the ala of the sacrum and joins the S1 nerve.

The **genitofemoral nerve** (L1 and L2) emerges on the anterior surface of the psoas. It runs downward in front of the muscle and divides into a **genital branch**, which enters the spermatic cord and supplies the cremaster muscle, and a **femoral branch**, which supplies a small area of the skin of the thigh. It is the nervous pathway involved in the **cremasteric reflex**, in which stimulation of the skin of the thigh in the male results in reflex contraction of the cremaster muscle and the drawing upward of the testis within the scrotum.

Sympathetic Trunk (Abdominal Part)

The abdominal part of the sympathetic trunk is continuous above with the thoracic and below with the pelvic parts of the sympathetic trunk. It runs downward along the medial border of the psoas muscle on the bodies of the lumbar vertebrae (Fig. 5.123). It enters the abdomen from behind the medial arcuate ligament and gains entrance to the pelvis below by passing behind the common iliac vessels. The **right sympathetic trunk** lies behind the right border of the inferior vena cava; the **left sympathetic trunk** lies close to the left border of the aorta. The sympathetic trunk possesses four or five segmentally arranged ganglia, the first and second often being fused together.

Branches

- **White rami communicantes** join the first two ganglia to the L1 and L2 spinal nerves. A white ramus contains **preganglionic nerve fibers** and afferent sensory nerve fibers.

Table 5.3 Lumbar Plexus Branches and Distribution

BRANCHES	DISTRIBUTION
Iliohypogastric nerve	External oblique, internal oblique, transversus abdominis muscles of anterior abdominal wall; skin over the lower anterior abdominal wall and buttock
Ilioinguinal nerve	External oblique, internal oblique, transversus abdominis muscles of anterior abdominal wall; skin of upper medial aspect of the thigh; root of the penis and scrotum in the male; mons pubis and labia majora in the female
Lateral cutaneous nerve of the thigh	Skin of anterior and lateral surfaces of the thigh
Genitofemoral nerve (L1 and L2)	Cremaster muscle in the scrotum in male; skin over anterior surface of the thigh; nervous pathway for cremasteric reflex
Femoral nerve (L2 to L4)	Iliacus, pectineus, sartorius, quadriceps femoris muscles, and intermediate cutaneous branches to the skin of the anterior surface of the thigh and by saphenous branch to the skin of the medial side of the leg and foot; articular branches to hip and knee joints
Obturator nerve (L2 to L4)	Gracilis, adductor brevis, adductor longus, obturator externus, pectineus, adductor magnus (adductor portion), and skin on medial surface of thigh; articular branches to hip and knee joints
Segmental branches	Quadratus lumborum and psoas muscles

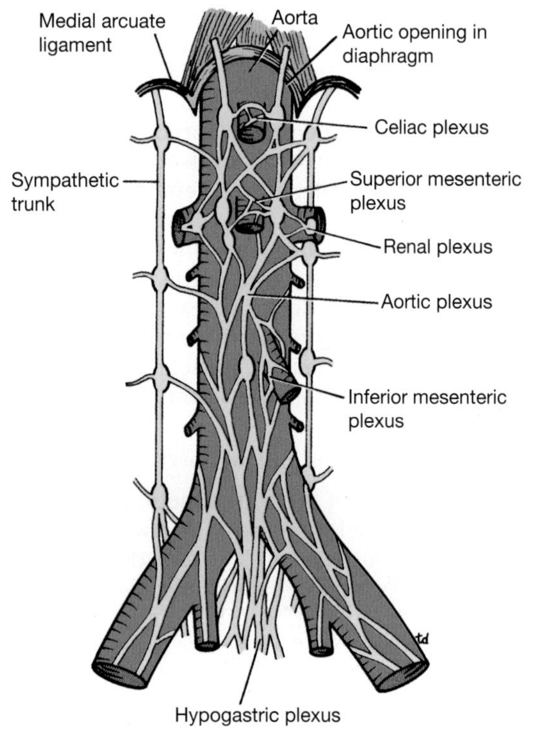

Figure 5.123 Aorta and related sympathetic plexuses.

- **Gray rami communicantes** join each ganglion to a corresponding lumbar spinal nerve. A gray ramus contains **postganglionic nerve fibers**. The postganglionic fibers are distributed through the branches of the spinal nerves to the blood vessels, sweat glands, and arrector pili muscles of the skin (see Chapter 1).
- Fibers pass medially to the sympathetic plexuses on the abdominal aorta and its branches. (These plexuses also receive fibers from splanchnic nerves and the vagus.)
- Fibers pass downward and medially in front of the common iliac vessels into the pelvis, where, together with branches from sympathetic nerves in front of the aorta, they form a large bundle of fibers called the **superior hypogastric plexus** (see Fig. 5.123).

Aortic Plexuses

Preganglionic and postganglionic sympathetic fibers, preganglionic parasympathetic fibers, and visceral afferent fibers form a plexus of nerves, the **aortic plexus**, around the abdominal part of the aorta (see Fig. 5.123). Regional concentrations of this plexus around the origins of the celiac, renal, superior mesenteric, and inferior mesenteric arteries form the **celiac plexus**, **renal plexus**, **superior mesenteric plexus**, and **inferior mesenteric plexus**, respectively.

The celiac plexus consists mainly of two **celiac ganglia** connected by a large network of fibers that surrounds the origin of the celiac artery. The ganglia receive the **greater** and **lesser splanchnic nerves** (preganglionic sympathetic fibers). Postganglionic branches accompany the branches of the celiac artery and follow them to their distribution. Parasympathetic **vagal fibers** also accompany the branches of the artery.

The renal and superior mesenteric plexuses are smaller than the celiac plexus. They are distributed along the branches of the corresponding arteries. The inferior mesenteric plexus is similar but receives parasympathetic fibers from the sacral parasympathetic nerves.

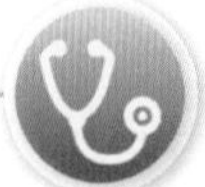

Clinical Notes

Lumbar Sympathectomy

Lumbar sympathectomy is performed mainly to produce a vasodilatation of the arteries of the lower limb in patients with vasospastic disorders. The preganglionic sympathetic fibers that supply the vessels of the lower limb leave the spinal cord from segments T11 to L2. They synapse in the lumbar and sacral ganglia of the sympathetic trunks. The postganglionic fibers join the lumbar and sacral nerves and distribute to the vessels of the limb as branches of these nerves. Additional postganglionic fibers pass directly from the lumbar ganglia to the common and external iliac arteries, but they follow the latter artery only down as far as the inguinal ligament. In the male, a bilateral lumbar sympathectomy may be followed by loss of ejaculatory power, but erection is not impaired.

Abdominal Pain

This section provides an anatomic basis for the different forms of abdominal pain found in clinical practice. Three distinct forms of pain exist: **somatic**, **visceral**, and **referred pain**.

Somatic Abdominal Pain

Somatic abdominal pain in the abdominal wall can arise from the skin, fascia, muscles, and parietal peritoneum. It can be severe and precisely localized. When the origin is on one side of the midline, the pain is also lateralized. The somatic pain impulses from the abdomen reach the central nervous system (CNS) in the following segmental spinal nerves:

- **Central part of the diaphragm:** Phrenic nerve (C3 to C5)
- **Peripheral part of the diaphragm:** Intercostal nerves (T7 to T11)
- **Anterior abdominal wall:** Thoracic nerves (T7 to T12) and the L1 nerve
- **Pelvic wall:** Obturator nerve (L2 to L4).

The inflamed parietal peritoneum is extremely sensitive, and because the same nerves innervate the full thickness of the abdominal wall, it is not surprising to find cutaneous hypersensitivity (hyperesthesia) and tenderness. Local reflexes involving the same nerves bring about a protective phenomenon in which the abdominal muscles increase in tone. This increased tone or rigidity, sometimes called **guarding**, is an attempt to rest and localize the inflammatory process.

Rebound tenderness occurs when the parietal peritoneum is inflamed. Any movement of that inflamed peritoneum, even when that movement is elicited by removing the examining hand from a site distant from the inflamed peritoneum, brings about tenderness.

Examples of acute, severe, localized pain originating in the parietal peritoneum are seen in the later stages of **appendicitis**. Cutaneous hyperesthesia, tenderness, and muscular spasm or rigidity occur in the lower right quadrant of the anterior abdominal wall. A **perforated peptic ulcer**, in which the parietal peritoneum is chemically irritated, produces the same symptoms and signs but involves the right upper and lower quadrants.

Visceral Abdominal Pain

Visceral abdominal pain arises in abdominal organs, visceral peritoneum, and the mesenteries. The causes of visceral pain include stretching of a viscus or mesentery, distention of a hollow viscus, impaired blood supply (**ischemia**) to a viscus, and chemical damage (eg, acid gastric juice) to a viscus or its covering peritoneum. Pain arising from an abdominal viscus is dull and poorly localized. Visceral pain is referred to the midline, probably because the viscera develop embryologically as midline structures and receive a bilateral nerve supply; many viscera later move laterally as development proceeds, taking their nerve supply with them.

Colic is a form of visceral pain produced by the violent contraction of smooth muscle. It is commonly caused by luminal obstruction as in intestinal obstruction, in the passage of a gallstone in the biliary ducts, or in the passage of a stone in the ureters.

Many visceral afferent fibers that enter the spinal cord participate in reflex activity. Reflex sweating, salivation, nausea, vomiting, and increased heart rate may accompany visceral pain.

The sensations that arise in viscera reach the CNS in afferent nerves that accompany the sympathetic nerves and enter the spinal cord through the posterior roots. The significance of this pathway is better understood in the following discussion on referred visceral pain.

Referred Abdominal Pain

Referred abdominal pain is the feeling of pain at a location other than the site of origin of the stimulus but in an area supplied by the same or adjacent segments of the spinal cord. Both somatic and visceral structures can produce referred pain.

In the case of **referred somatic pain**, the possible explanation is that the nerve fibers from the diseased structure and the area where the pain is felt ascend in the CNS along a common pathway, and the cerebral cortex is incapable of distinguishing between the sites. Examples of referred somatic pain follow. Pleurisy involving the lower part of the costal parietal pleura can give rise to referred pain in the abdomen because the lower parietal pleura receives its sensory innervation from the lower five intercostal nerves, which also innervate the skin and muscles of the anterior abdominal wall.

Visceral pain from the stomach is commonly referred to the epigastrium (Fig. 5.124). The afferent pain fibers

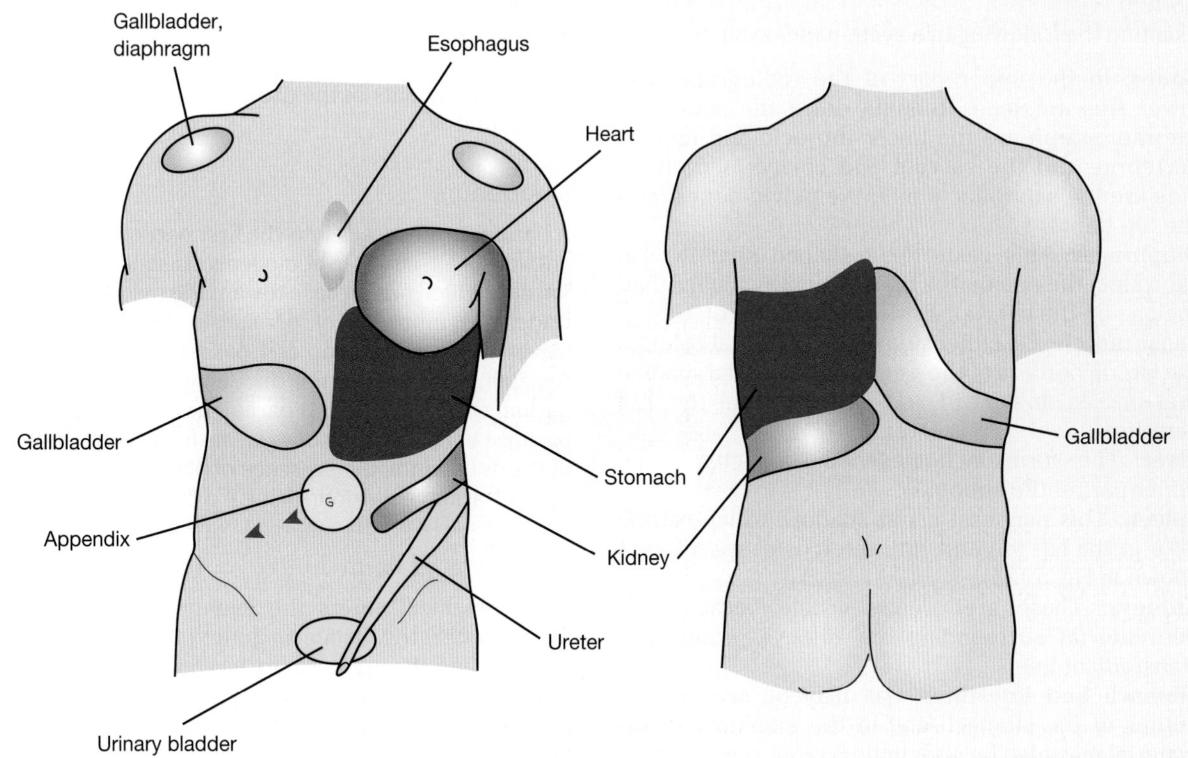

Figure 5.124 Some important skin areas involved in referred visceral pain.

(continued)

from the stomach ascend in company with the sympathetic nerves and pass through the celiac plexus and the **greater splanchnic nerves**. The sensory fibers enter the spinal cord at segments T5 to T9 and give rise to referred pain in dermatomes T5 to T9 on the lower chest and abdominal walls.

Visceral pain from the appendix, which is produced by distension of its lumen or spasm of its smooth muscle coat, travels in nerve fibers that accompany sympathetic nerves through the superior mesenteric plexus and the **lesser splanchnic nerve** to the spinal cord (T10 segment). The vague referred pain is felt in the region of the umbilicus (T10 dermatome). Later, if the inflammatory process involves the parietal peritoneum, the severe somatic pain dominates the clinical picture and is localized precisely in the right lower quadrant.

Visceral pain from the gallbladder, as occurs in patients with **cholecystitis** or **gallstone colic**, travels in nerve fibers that accompany sympathetic nerves. They pass through the celiac plexus and **greater splanchnic nerves** to the spinal cord (segments T5 to T9). The vague referred pain is felt in the dermatomes (T5 to T9) on the lower chest and upper abdominal walls. If the inflammatory process spreads to involve the parietal peritoneum of the anterior abdominal wall or peripheral diaphragm, the severe somatic pain is felt in the right upper quadrant and through to the back below the inferior angle of the scapula. Involvement of the central diaphragmatic parietal peritoneum, which is innervated by the phrenic nerve (C3 to C5), can give rise to referred pain over the shoulder because the supraclavicular nerves (C3 and C4) innervate the skin in this area.

RADIOGRAPHIC ANATOMY

The diverse nature of the abdominal contents (from hard to various degrees of soft structures) and the complexity of the topography in the abdomen make medical imaging a critical tool in evaluating the condition of this area. Plain film x-rays, CT, MRI, and ultrasound all provide unique insights.

Abdomen

Only the more important features seen in a standard anteroposterior radiograph of the abdomen, with the patient in the supine position, are described (Figs. 5.125 and 5.126).

Examine the following in a systematic order.

1. **Bones:** In the upper part of the radiograph, the lower ribs are seen. Running down the middle of the radiograph are the lower thoracic and lumbar vertebrae and the sacrum and coccyx. On either side are the sacroiliac joints, the pelvic bones, and the hip joints.
2. **Diaphragm:** This casts dome-shaped shadows on each side; the one on the right is slightly higher than the one on the left (not shown in Fig. 5.125).
3. **Psoas muscle:** On either side of the vertebral column, the lateral borders of the psoas muscle cast a shadow that passes downward and laterally from the T12 vertebra.
4. **Liver:** This forms a homogeneous opacity in the upper part of the abdomen.
5. **Spleen:** This may cast a soft shadow, which can be seen in the left 9th and 10th intercostal spaces (not shown in Fig. 5.125).
6. **Kidneys:** These are usually visible because the perirenal fat surrounding the kidneys produces a transradiant line.
7. **Stomach and intestines:** Gas may be seen in the fundus of the stomach and in the intestines. Fecal material may also be seen in the colon.
8. **Urinary bladder:** If this contains sufficient urine, it will cast a shadow in the pelvis.

Stomach

The stomach can be demonstrated radiologically (Figs. 5.127 and 5.128) by the administration of a watery suspension of barium sulfate (barium meal). With the patient in the erect position, the first few mouthfuls pass into the stomach and form a triangular shadow with the apex downward. The gas bubble in the fundus shows above the fluid level at the top of the barium shadow. As the stomach is filled, the greater and lesser curvatures are outlined, and the body and pyloric portions are recognized. The pylorus is seen to move downward and come to lie at the level of the L3 vertebra.

Fluoroscopic examination of the stomach as it is filled with the barium emulsion reveals peristaltic waves of contraction of the stomach wall, which commence near the middle of the body and pass to the pylorus. The respiratory movements of the diaphragm cause displacement of the fundus.

Duodenum

A barium meal passes into the first part of the duodenum and forms a triangular homogeneous shadow, the **duodenal cap**, which has its base toward the pylorus (Fig. 5.129). Under the influence of peristalsis, the barium quickly leaves the duodenal cap and passes rapidly through the remaining portions of the duodenum. The outline of the barium shadow in the first part of the duodenum is smooth because of the absence of mucosal folds. In the remainder of the duodenum, the presence of plicae circulares breaks up the barium emulsion, giving it a floccular appearance.

Jejunum and Ileum

A barium meal enters the jejunum in a few minutes and reaches the ileocecal junction in 30 minutes to 2 hours, and the greater part has left the small intestine in 6 hours. In the jejunum and upper part of the ileum, the mucosal folds and the peristaltic activity scatter the barium shadow (Fig. 5.130; see also Fig. 5.127). In the last part of the ileum, the barium meal tends to form a continuous mass of barium.

(text continue on page 406)

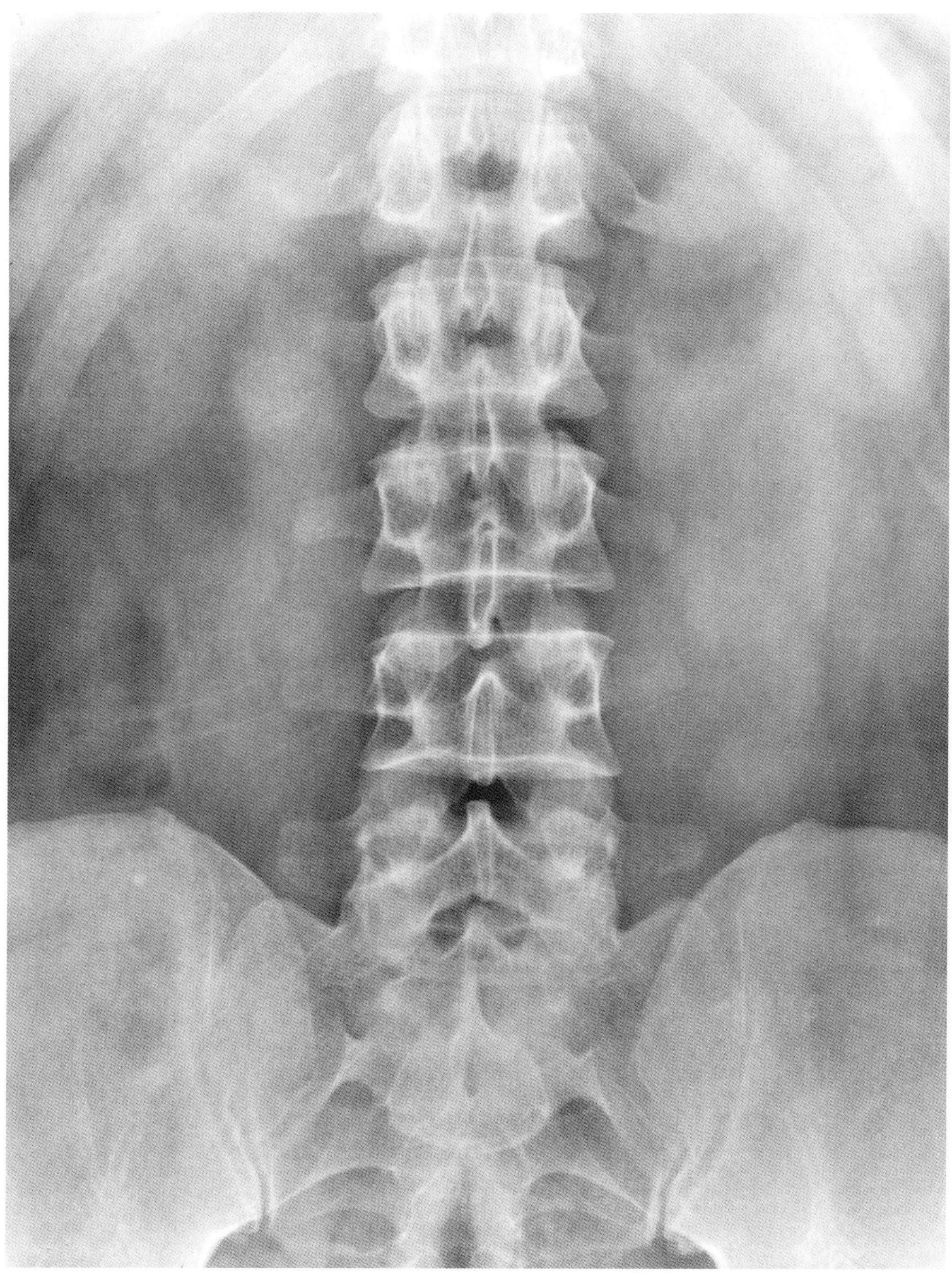

Figure 5.125 Anteroposterior radiograph of the abdomen.

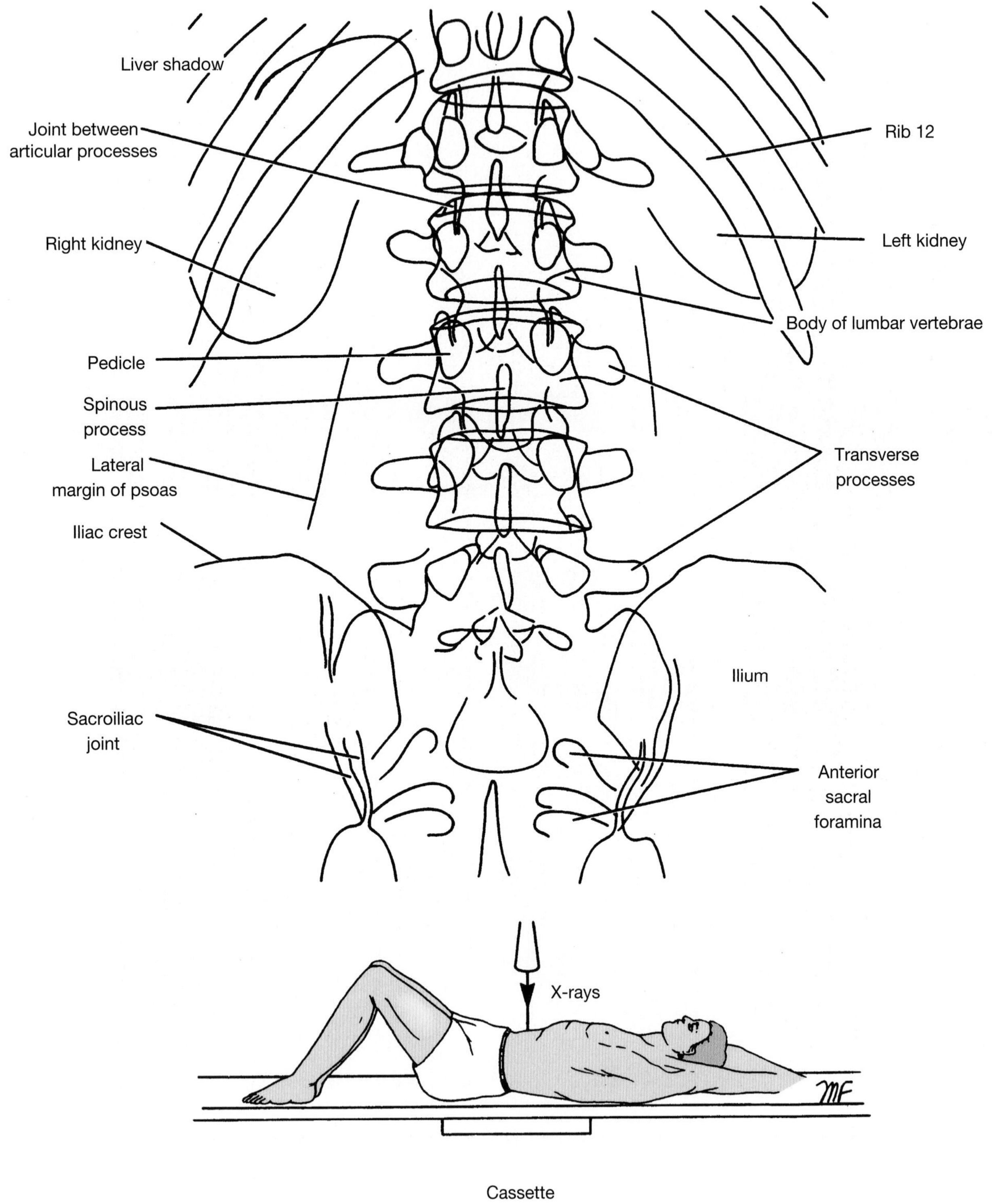

Figure 5.126 Representation of the main features seen in the anteroposterior radiograph in Figure 5.125.

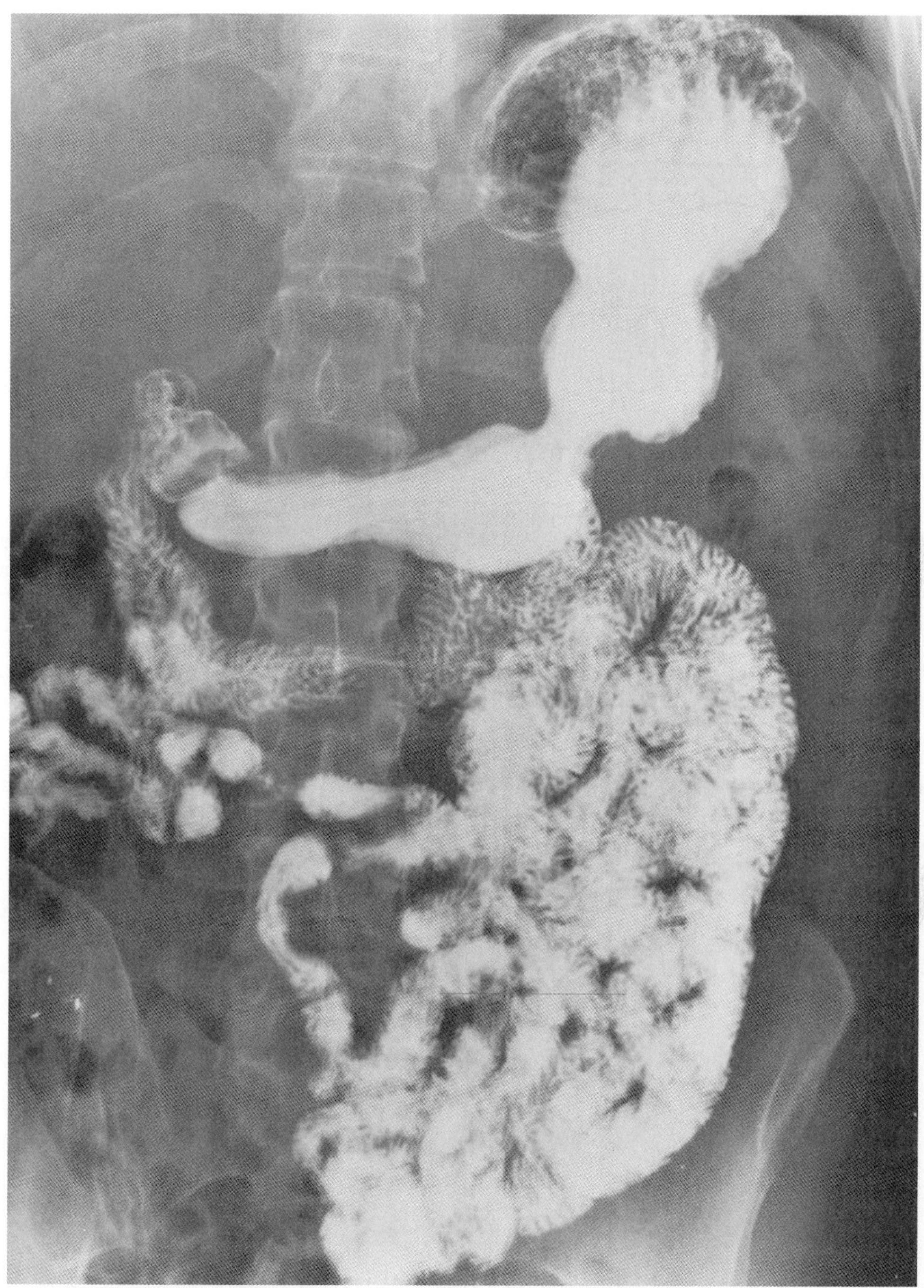

Figure 5.127 Anteroposterior radiograph of the stomach and the small intestine after ingestion of barium meal.

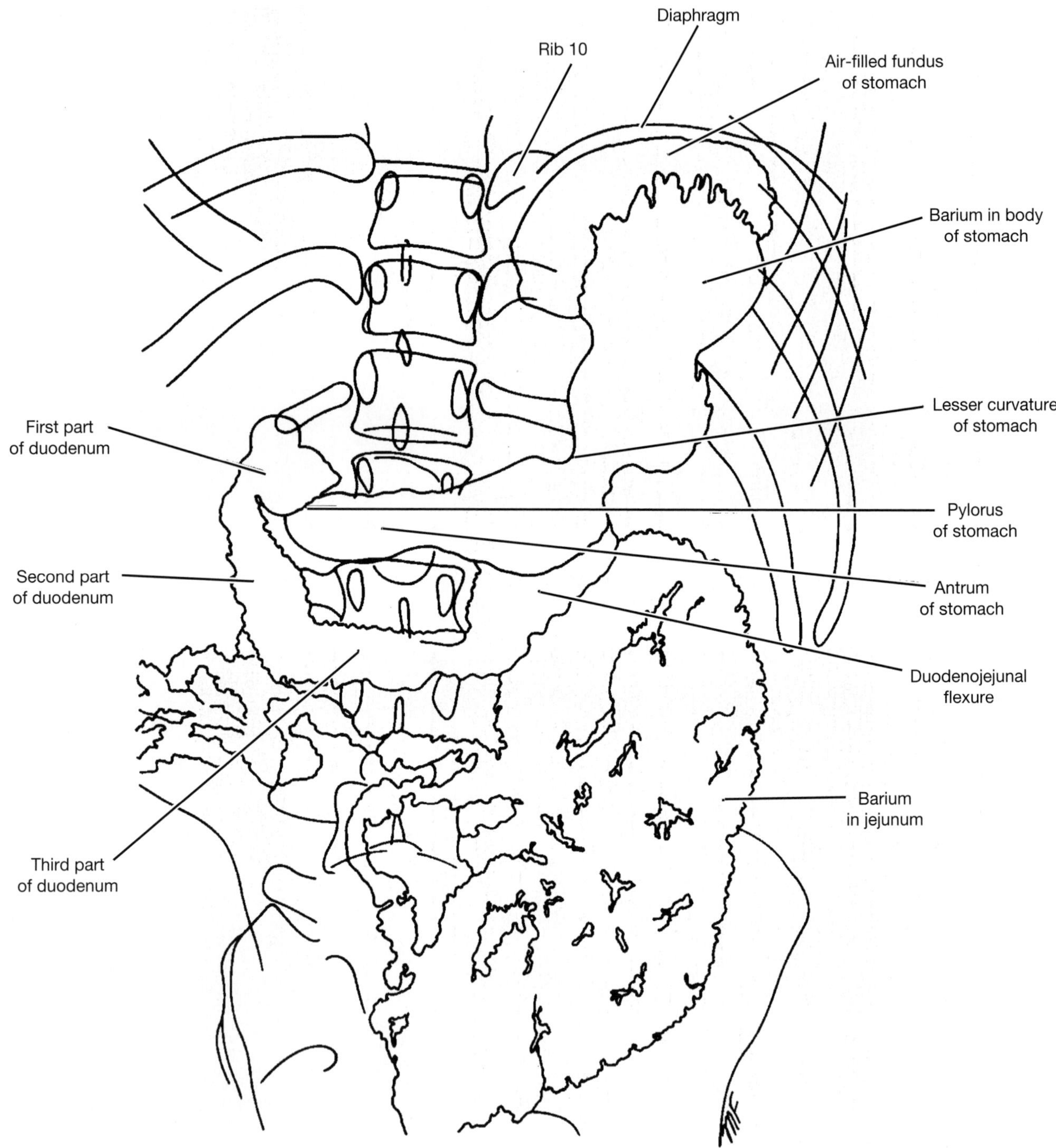

Figure 5.128 Representation of the main features seen in the radiograph in Figure 5.127.

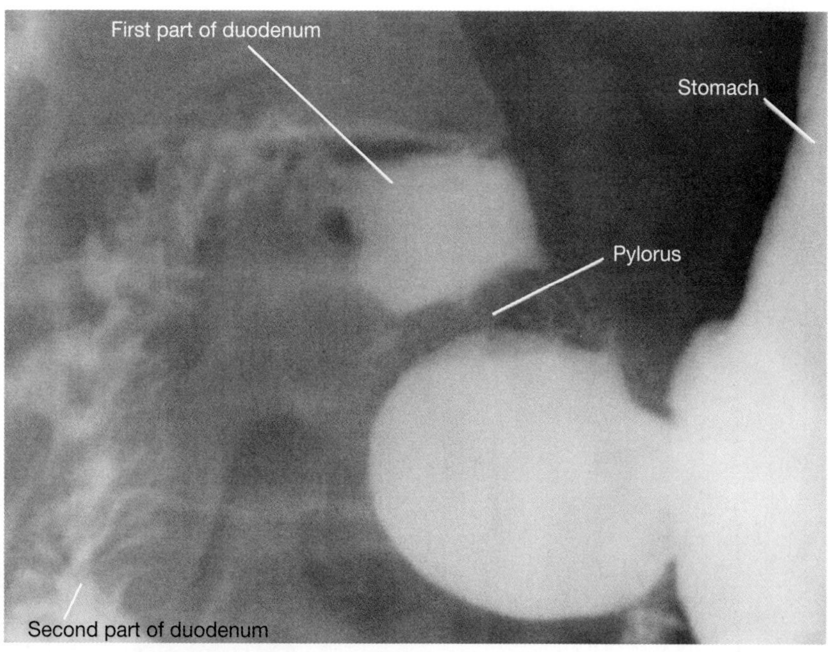

Figure 5.129 Anteroposterior radiograph of the duodenum after ingestion of barium meal.

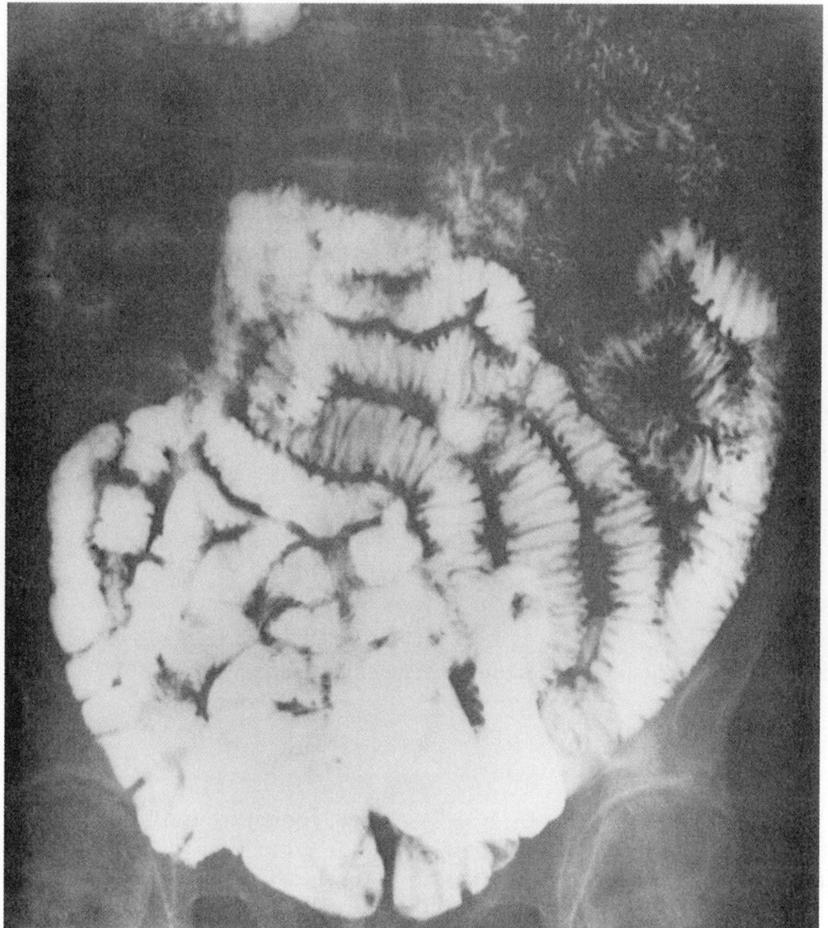

Figure 5.130 Anteroposterior radiograph of the small intestine after ingestion of barium meal.

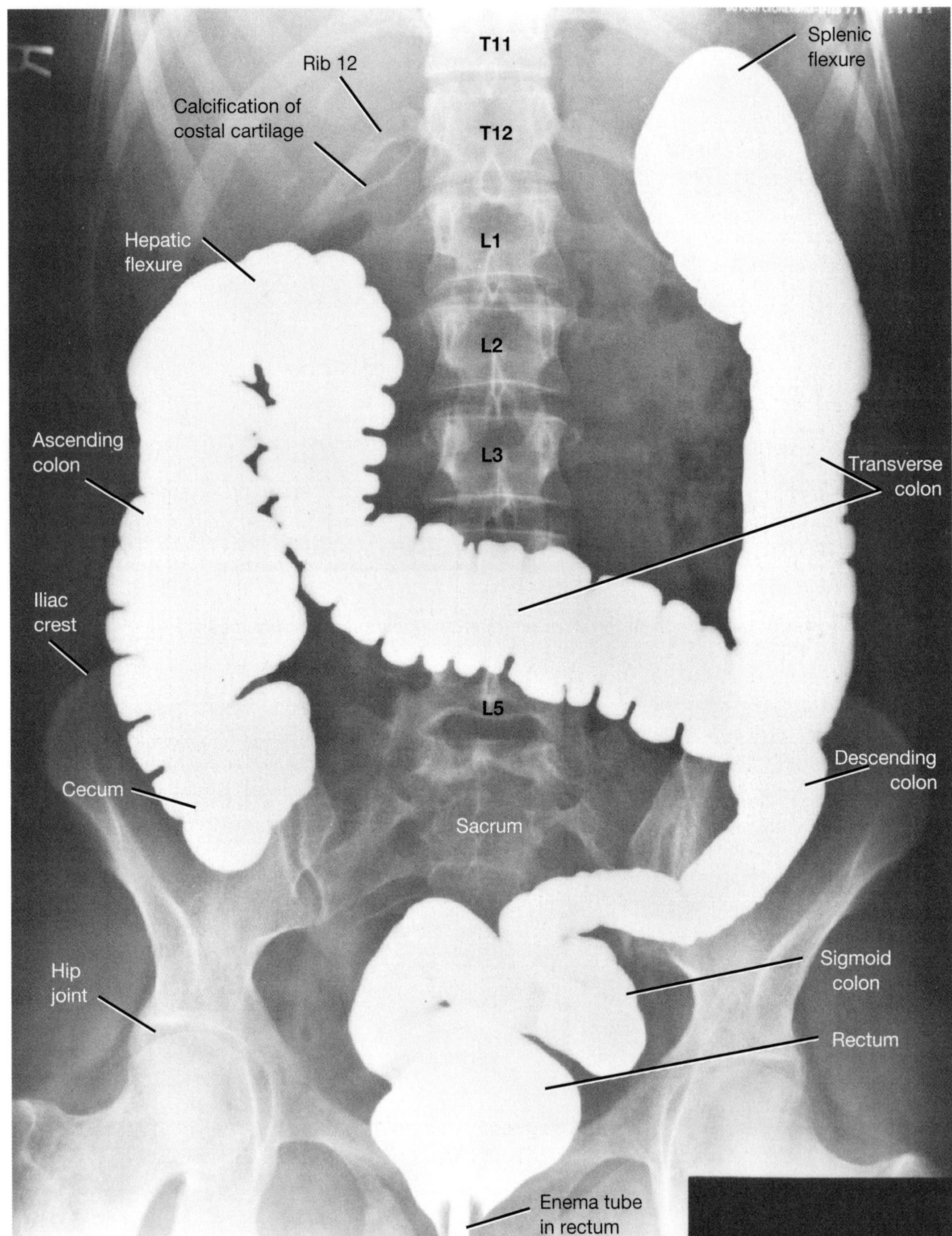

Figure 5.131 Anteroposterior radiograph of the large intestine after a barium enema.

Large Intestine

The large intestine can be demonstrated by the administration of a barium enema or a barium meal. The former is more satisfactory.

The bowel may be outlined by the administration of two to three pints (1 L) of barium sulfate emulsion through the anal canal. When the large intestine is filled, the entire outline can be seen in an anteroposterior projection (Figs. 5.131 and 5.132). Oblique and lateral views of the colic flexures may be necessary. The characteristic sacculations (haustra) are well seen when the bowel is filled, and after the enema has been evacuated, the mucosal pattern is clearly demonstrated.

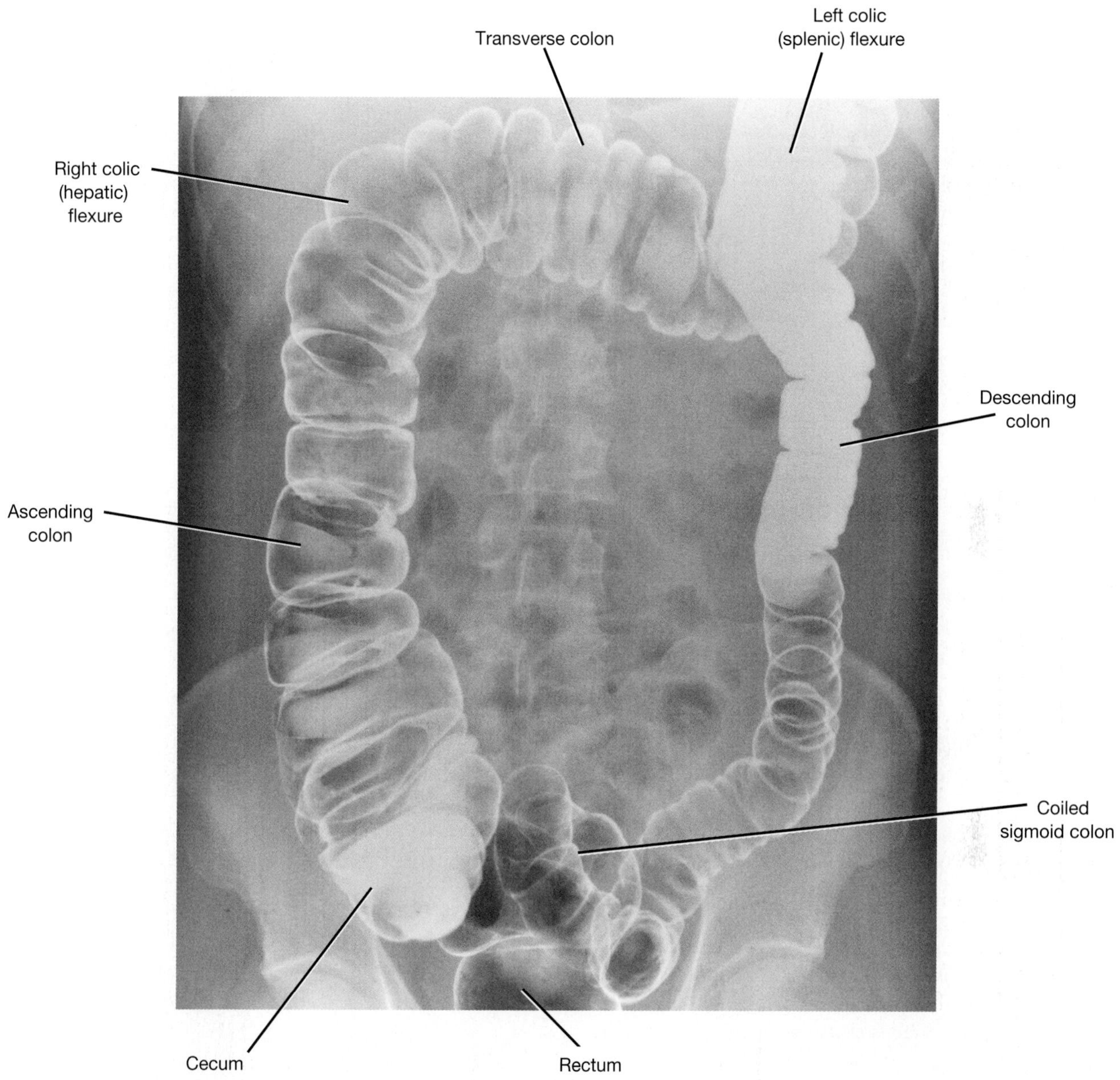

Figure 5.132 Anteroposterior radiograph of the large intestine after a barium enema. Air has been introduced into the intestine through the enema tube after evacuation of most of the barium. This procedure is referred to as a contrast enema.

The appendix frequently fills with barium after an enema. The radiographic appearances of the sigmoid colon and rectum are described in Chapter 6.

The arterial supply to the GI tract can be demonstrated by **arteriography**. A catheter is inserted into the femoral artery and threaded upward under direct vision on a screen into the abdominal aorta. The end of the catheter is then manipulated into the opening of the appropriate artery. Radiopaque material is injected through the catheter, and an arteriogram is obtained (Fig. 5.133).

Biliary Tree

The bile passages normally are not visible on a radiograph. Their lumina can be outlined by the administration of various iodine-containing compounds orally or by injection. When taken orally, the compound is absorbed from the small intestine, carried to the liver, and excreted with the bile. On reaching the gallbladder, it is concentrated with the bile. The concentrated iodine compound, mixed with the bile, is now radiopaque and reveals the gallbladder as a pear-shaped opacity in the angle between the right rib 12 and the vertebral column

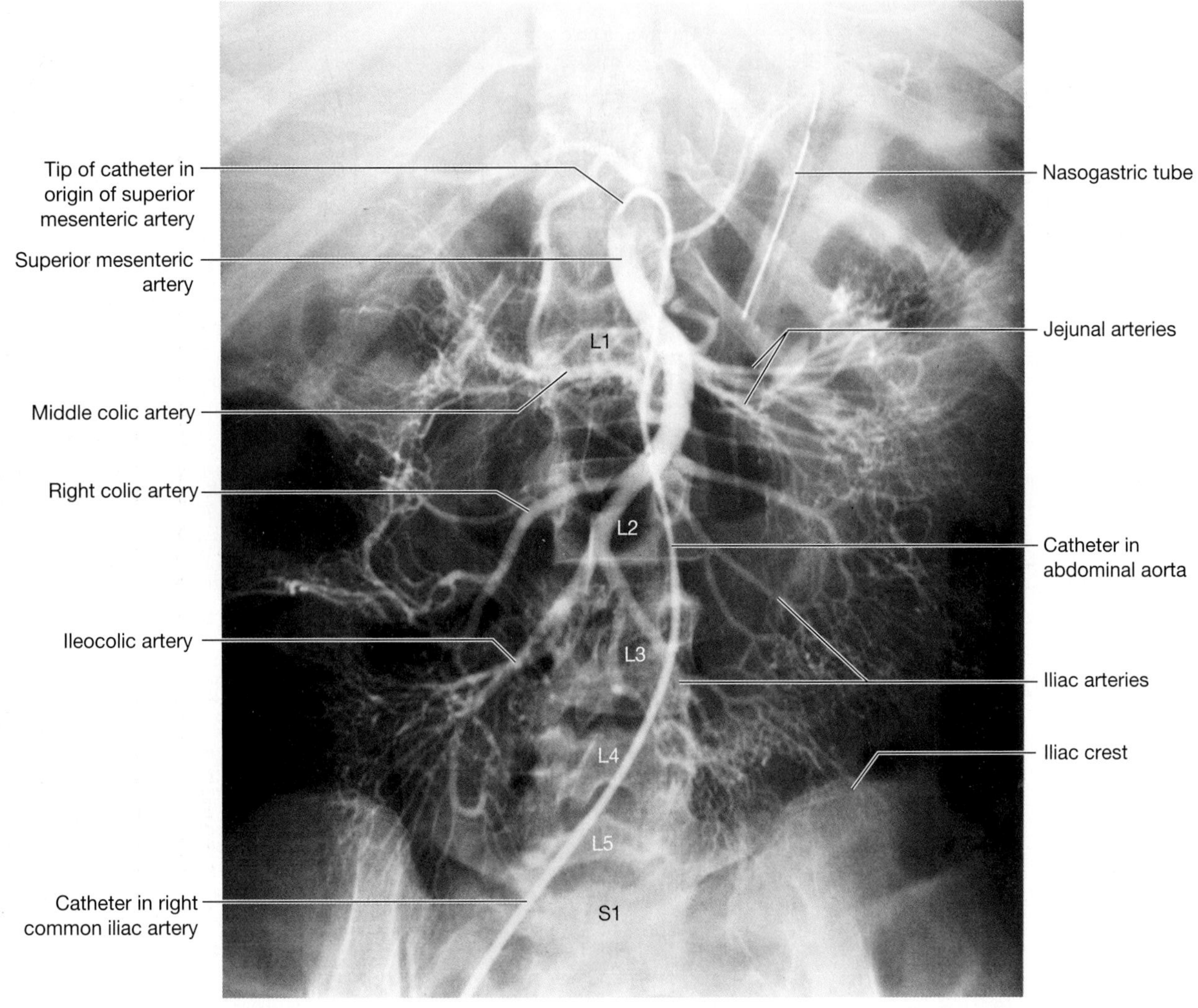

Figure 5.133 Arteriogram of the superior mesenteric artery. The catheter has been inserted into the right femoral artery and has passed up the external and common iliac arteries to ascend the aorta to the origin of the superior mesenteric artery. A nasogastric tube is also in position.

(Figs. 5.134 and 5.135). If the patient is given a fatty meal, the gallbladder contracts, and the cystic and bile ducts become visible as the opaque medium passes down to the second part of the duodenum. A sonogram of the upper part of the abdomen can be used to show the lumen of the gallbladder (see Fig. 5.97).

Urinary Tract

The **kidneys** are usually visible on a standard anteroposterior radiograph of the abdomen because the perirenal fat surrounding the kidneys produces a transradiant line.

Calyces, the **renal pelvis**, and the **ureter** are not normally visible on a standard radiograph. The lumen can be demonstrated by radiopaque compounds in intravenous pyelography or retrograde pyelography.

With **intravenous pyelography**, an iodine-containing compound is injected into a subcutaneous arm vein. It is excreted and concentrated by the kidneys, thus rendering the calyces and ureter opaque to x-rays (Figs. 5.136 to 5.138). When enough of the opaque medium has been excreted, the bladder is also revealed. The ureters are seen superimposed on the transverse processes of the lumbar vertebrae. They cross the sacroiliac joints and enter the pelvis. Near the ischial spines, they turn medially to enter the bladder. The three normal constrictions of the ureters (at the junction of the renal pelvis with the ureter, at the pelvic brim, and where the ureter enters the bladder) can be recognized.

With **retrograde pyelography**, a cystoscope is passed through the urethra into the bladder, and a ureteric catheter is inserted into the ureter. A solution of sodium iodide is then injected along the catheter

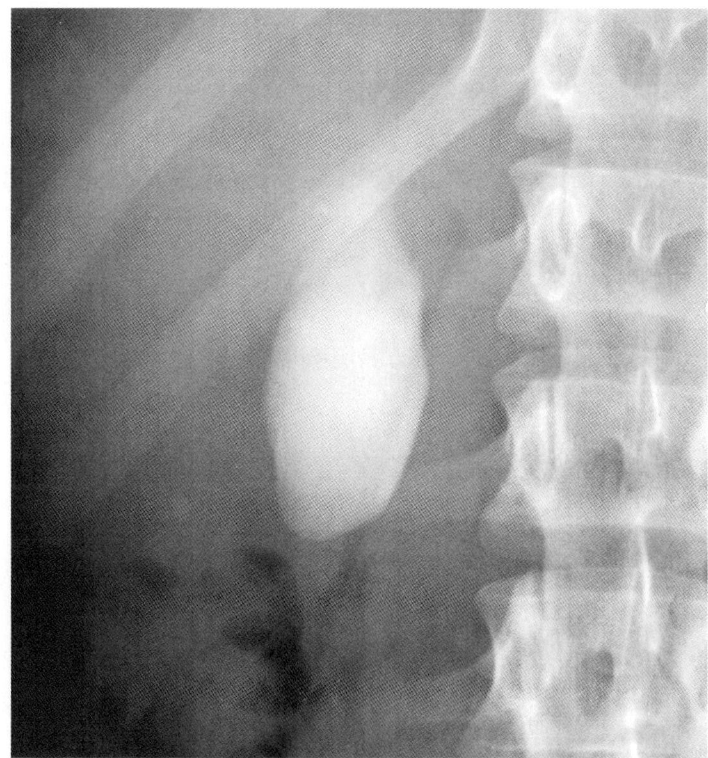

Figure 5.134 Anteroposterior radiograph of the gallbladder after administration of an iodine-containing compound.

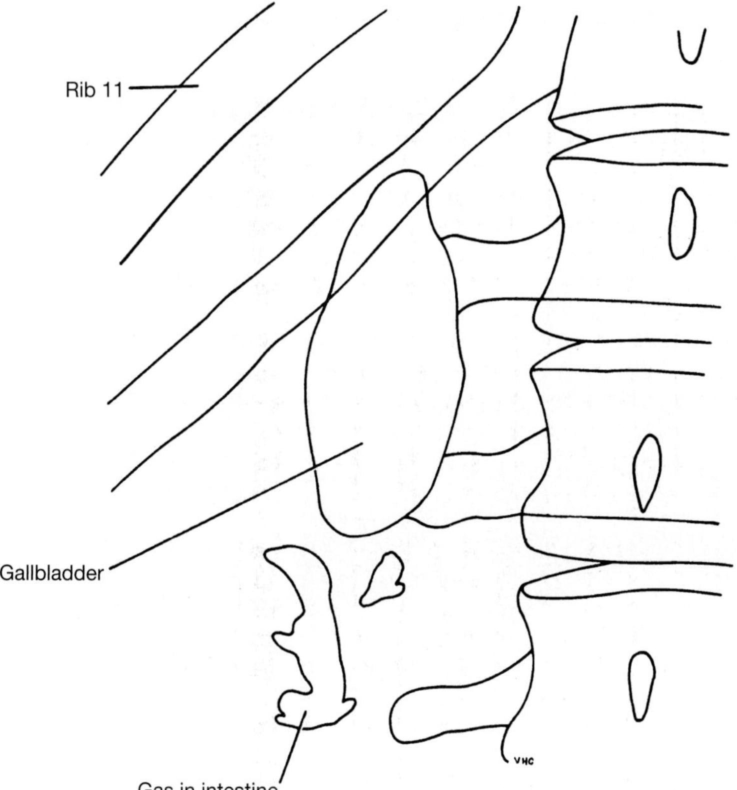

Figure 5.135 Representation of the main features seen in the radiograph in Figure 5.134.

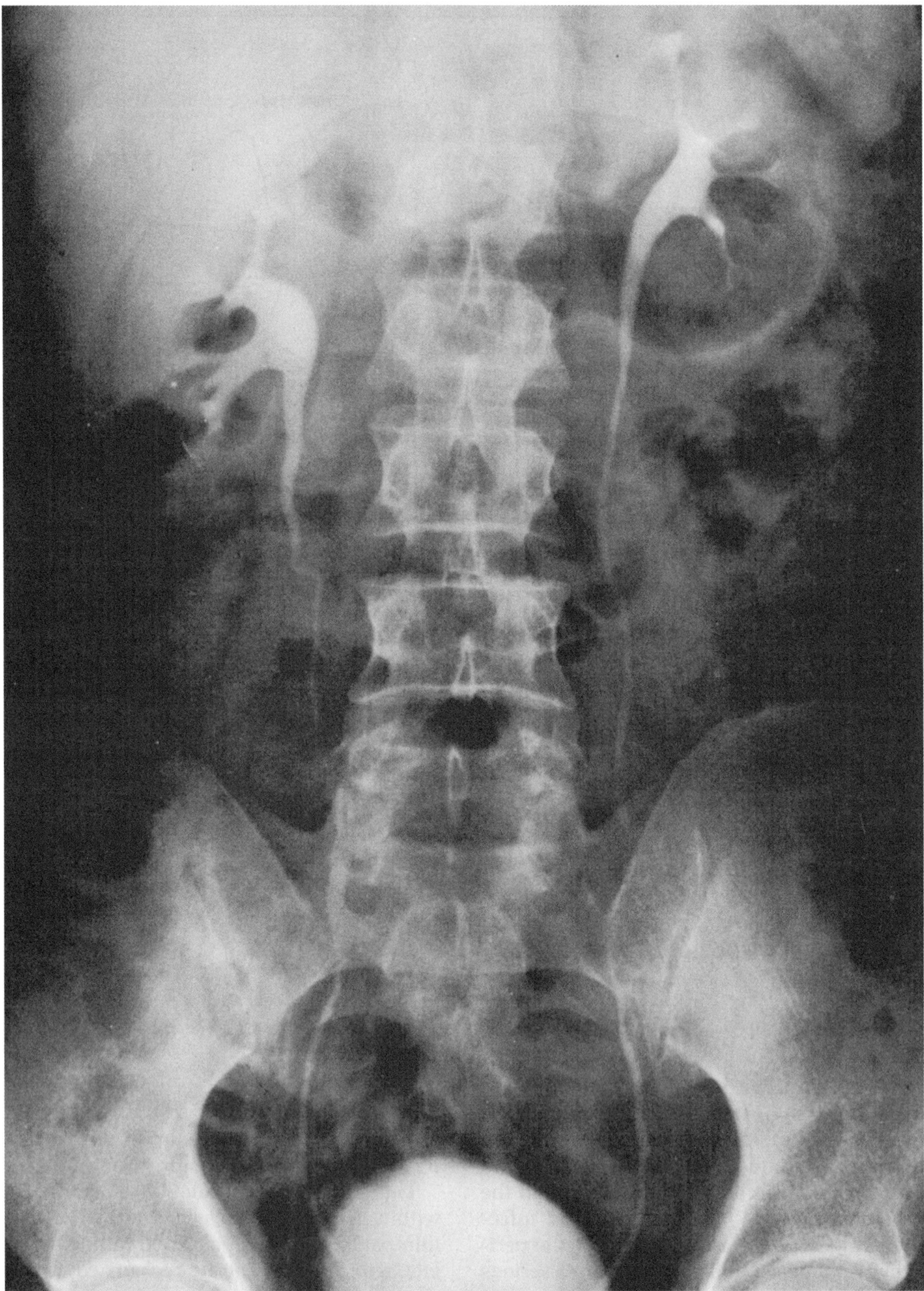

Figure 5.136 Anteroposterior radiograph of the ureter and renal pelvis after intravenous injection of an iodine-containing compound, which is excreted by the kidney. Major and minor calyces are also shown.

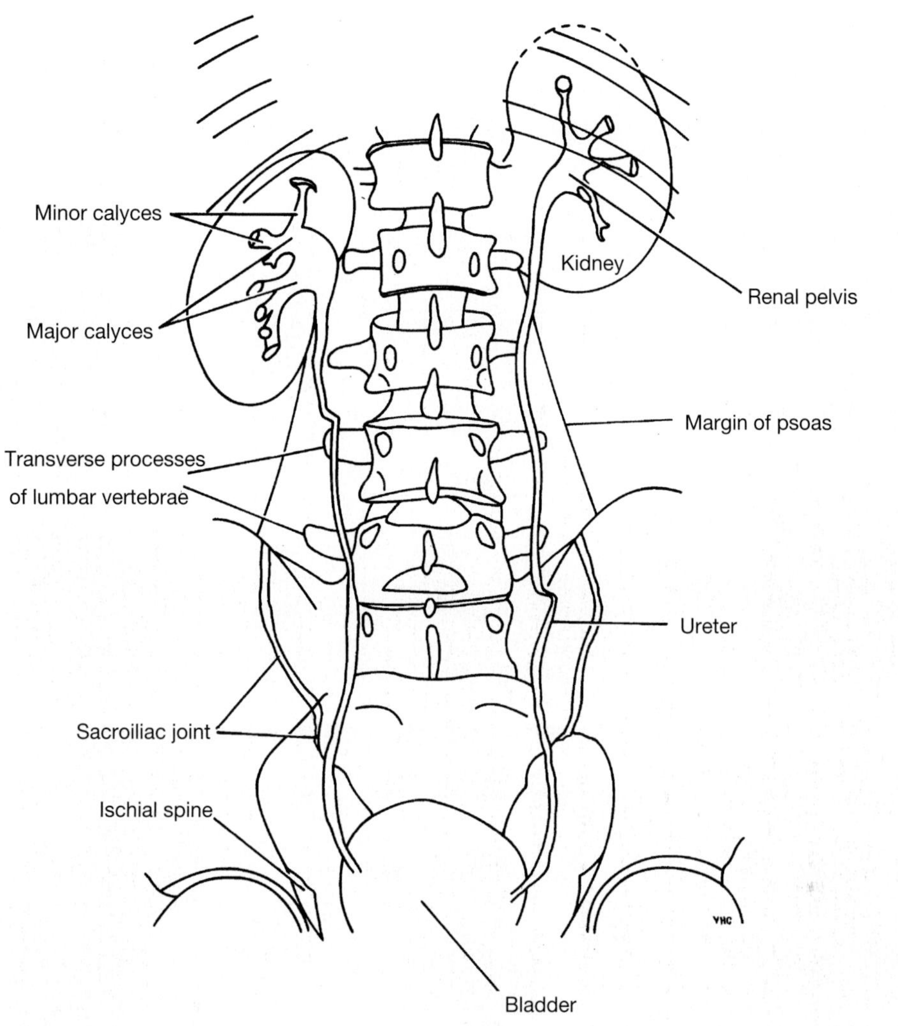

Figure 5.137 Representation of the main features seen in the radiograph in Figure 5.136.

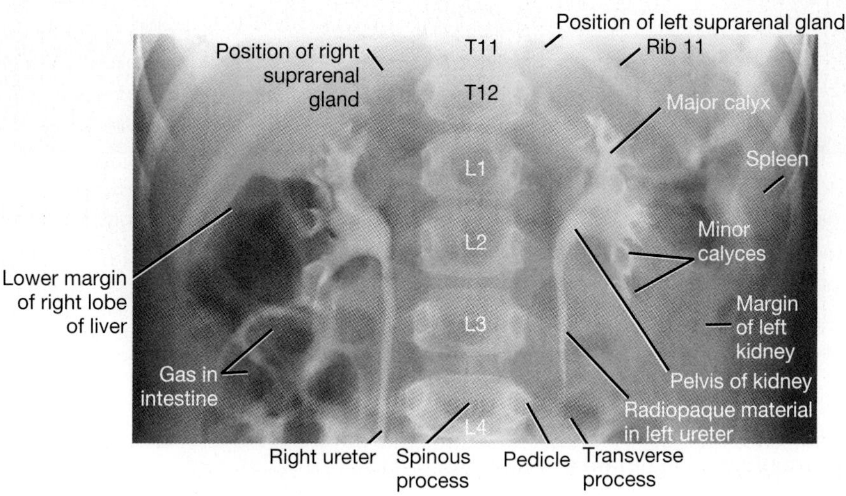

Figure 5.138 Anteroposterior radiograph of both kidneys 15 minutes after intravenous injection of an iodine-containing compound. The calyces, the renal pelvis, and the upper parts of the ureters are clearly seen (5-year-old female).

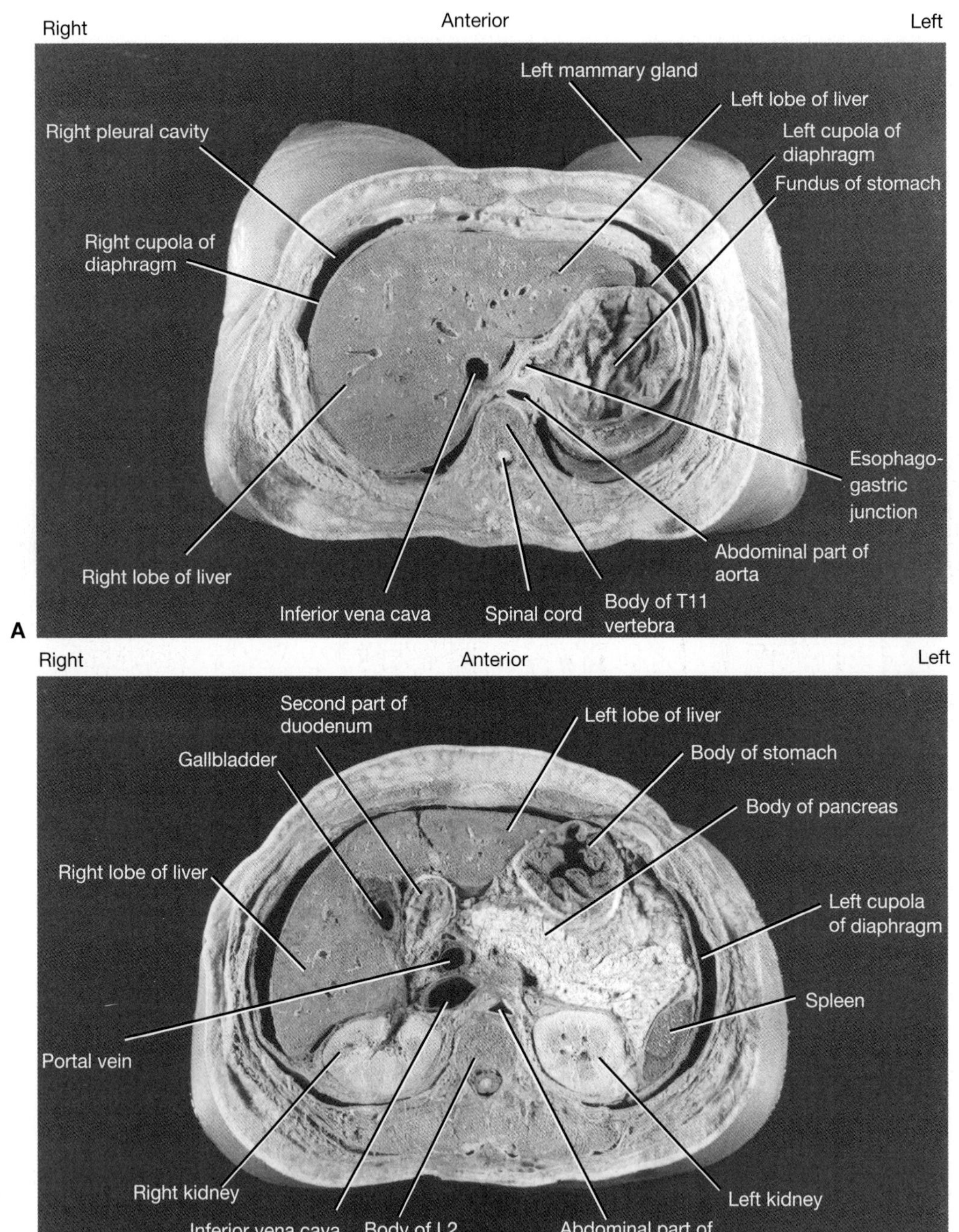

Figure 5.139 **A.** Cross section of the abdomen at the level of the body of the T11 vertebra, viewed from below. Note that the large size of the pleural cavity is an artifact caused by the embalming process. **B.** Cross section of the abdomen at the level of the body of the L2 vertebra, viewed from below.

into the ureter. When the minor calyces become filled with the radiopaque medium, the detailed anatomic features of the minor and major calyces and the pelvis of the ureter can be clearly seen. Each minor calyx has a cup-shaped appearance caused by the renal papilla projecting into it.

Cross-Sectional Abdominal Anatomy

Study the labeled cross sections of the abdomen shown in Figures 5.139 and 5.140 to assist in interpretation of CT scans of the abdomen (Fig. 5.141). The sections have been photographed on their inferior surfaces.

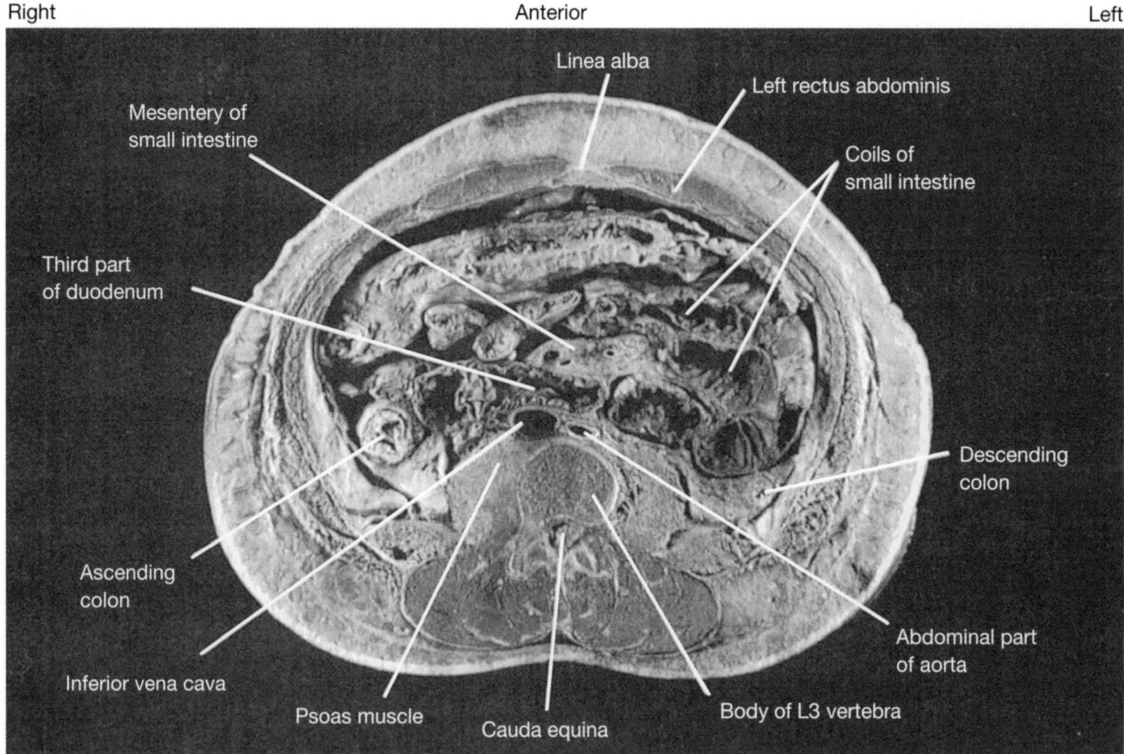

Figure 5.140 Cross section of the abdomen at the level of the body of the L3 vertebra, viewed from below.

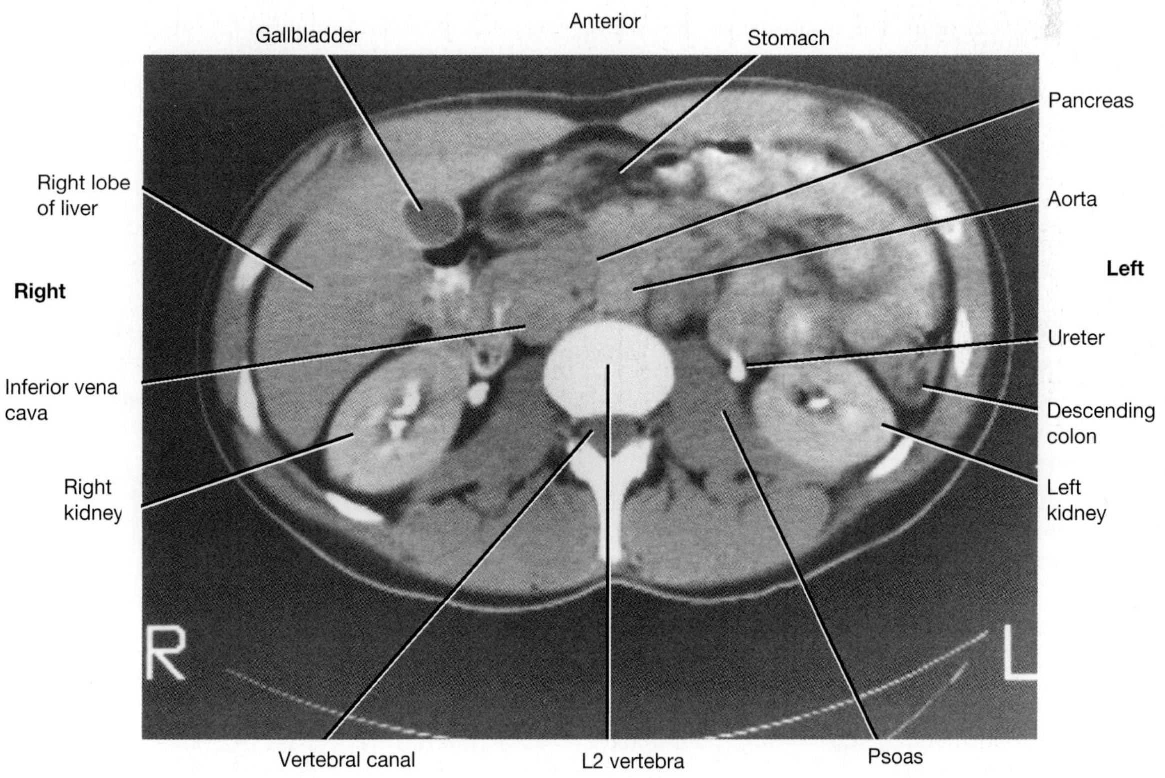

Figure 5.141 CT scan of the abdomen at the level of the L2 vertebra after intravenous pyelography. The radiopaque material can be seen in the renal pelvis and the ureters. The section is viewed from below.

SURFACE ANATOMY

Surface Landmarks of the Abdominal Wall

Several structures are readily palpable on the abdominal wall of a person with average body build. These are notable items in orientation for a basic physical examination.

Xiphoid Process

The xiphoid process is the thin cartilaginous lower part of the sternum. It is easily palpated in the depression where the costal margins meet in the upper part of the anterior abdominal wall (Fig. 5.142; see also Fig. 5.16). Feeling the lower edge of the body of the sternum identifies the **xiphisternal junction**, which lies opposite the body of the T9 vertebra.

Costal Margin

The costal margin is the curved lower margin of the thoracic wall and is formed in front by the cartilages of ribs 7 to 10 (see Figs. 5.16 and 5.142) and behind by the cartilages of ribs 11 and 12. The costal margin reaches its lowest level at the 10th costal cartilage, which lies opposite the body of the L3 vertebra. Rib 12 may be short and difficult to palpate.

Iliac Crest

The iliac crest is palpable along its entire length. It ends in front at the **anterior superior iliac spine** (see Figs. 5.16 and 5.142) and behind at the **posterior superior iliac spine**. Its highest point lies opposite the body of the L4 vertebra.

About 2 in. (5 cm) posterior to the anterior superior iliac spine, the outer margin projects to form the tubercle of the crest (see Fig. 5.142). The tubercle lies at the level of the body of the L5 vertebra.

Pubic Tubercle

The pubic tubercle is an important surface landmark. It may be identified as a small protuberance along the superior surface of the pubis (see Figs. 5.4, 5.10, and 5.142).

Symphysis Pubis

The symphysis pubis is the cartilaginous joint that lies in the midline between the bodies of the pubic bones (see Fig. 5.16). It is felt as a solid structure beneath the skin in the midline at the lower extremity of the anterior abdominal wall. The **pubic crest** is the ridge on the superior surface of the pubic bones medial to the pubic tubercle (see Fig. 5.4).

Inguinal Ligament

The inguinal ligament lies beneath a skin crease in the groin. It is the rolled-under inferior margin of the aponeurosis of the external oblique muscle (see Figs. 5.9, 5.13, and 5.16). It attaches laterally to the anterior superior iliac spine and curves downward and medially, to attach to the pubic tubercle.

Superficial Inguinal Ring

The superficial inguinal ring is a triangular aperture in the aponeurosis of the external oblique muscle and is situated above and medial to the pubic tubercle (see Figs. 5.9, 5.10, 5.15, and 5.142). In the adult male, the margins of the ring can be felt by invaginating the skin of the upper part of the scrotum with the tip of the little finger. The soft tubular **spermatic cord** can be felt

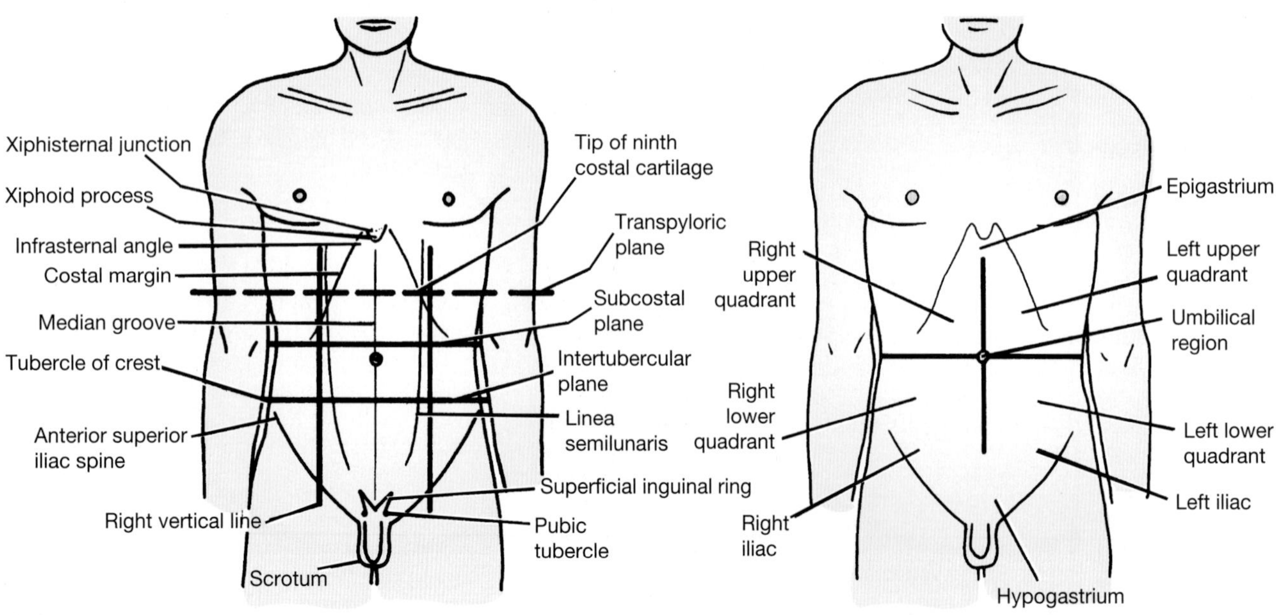

Figure 5.142 Surface landmarks and regions of the anterior abdominal wall.

emerging from the ring and descending over or medial to the pubic tubercle into the scrotum (see Fig. 5.15). Palpate the spermatic cord in the upper part of the scrotum between the finger and thumb and note the presence of the firm cordlike **vas deferens** in its posterior part (see Figs. 5.12 and 5.26).

In the female, the superficial inguinal ring is smaller and difficult to palpate; it transmits the round ligament of the uterus.

Scrotum

The scrotum is a pouch of skin and fascia containing the testes, the epididymides, and the lower ends of the spermatic cords. The skin of the scrotum is wrinkled and is covered with sparse hairs. The bilateral origin of the scrotum is indicated by the presence of a dark line in the midline, called the **scrotal raphe**, along the line of fusion. The **testis** on each side is a firm ovoid body surrounded on its lateral, anterior, and medial surfaces by the two layers of the **tunica vaginalis** (see Fig. 5.26). The testis should therefore lie free and not tethered to the skin or subcutaneous tissue. Posterior to the testis is an elongated structure, the **epididymis**. It has an enlarged upper end called the **head**, a **body**, and a narrow lower end, the **tail**. The vas deferens emerges from the tail and ascends medial to the epididymis to enter the spermatic cord at the upper end of the scrotum.

Linea Alba

The linea alba is a vertically running fibrous band that extends from the symphysis pubis to the xiphoid process and lies in the midline (see Fig. 5.10). It is formed by the fusion of the aponeuroses of the muscles of the anterior abdominal wall and is represented on the surface by a slight median groove (see Figs. 5.16 and 5.142).

Umbilicus

The umbilicus lies in the linea alba and is inconstant in position. It is a puckered scar and is the site of attachment of the umbilical cord in the fetus.

Rectus Abdominis

The rectus abdominis muscles lie on either side of the linea alba (see Fig. 5.16) and run vertically in the abdominal wall. They can be made prominent by asking the patient to raise their shoulders while in the supine position without using their arms.

Three tendinous intersections run across each rectus abdominis muscle. In muscular individuals, they can be palpated as transverse depressions at the level of the tip of the xiphoid process, at the umbilicus, and halfway between the two.

Linea Semilunaris

The linea semilunaris is the lateral edge of the rectus abdominis muscle and crosses the costal margin at the tip of the ninth costal cartilage (see Figs. 5.16 and 5.142). To accentuate the semilunar lines, the patient is asked to lie on their back and raise their shoulders off the couch without using their arms. To accomplish this, the patient contracts the rectus abdominis muscles so that their lateral edges stand out.

Abdominal Lines and Planes

A gridwork of vertical lines and horizontal planes (see Fig. 5.142) is commonly used to facilitate the description of the location of diseased structures or the performing of abdominal procedures.

Vertical Lines

Each vertical line (right and left) passes through the midpoint between the anterior superior iliac spine and the symphysis pubis (see Fig. 5.142, Left).

Transpyloric Plane

The horizontal transpyloric plane passes through the tips of the ninth costal cartilages on the two sides—that is, the point where the lateral margin of the rectus abdominis (linea semilunaris) crosses the costal margin (see Fig. 5.142, Left). It lies at the level of the body of the L1 vertebra. This plane passes through the pylorus of the stomach, duodenojejunal junction, neck of the pancreas, and hila of the kidneys.

Subcostal Plane

The horizontal subcostal plane joins the lowest point of the costal margin on each side—that is, the 10th costal cartilage (see Fig. 5.142, Left). This plane lies at the level of the L3 vertebra.

Intercristal Plane

The intercristal plane passes across the highest points on the iliac crests and lies on the level of the body of the L4 vertebra. This is commonly used as a surface landmark when performing a lumbar spinal tap (see Chapter 2).

Intertubercular Plane

The horizontal intertubercular plane joins the tubercles on the iliac crests (see Fig. 5.142, Left) and lies at the level of the L5 vertebra.

Abdominal Quadrants

It is common practice to divide the abdomen into quadrants by using a vertical and a horizontal line that intersect at the umbilicus (see Fig. 5.142, Right). The quadrants are the upper right, upper left, lower right, and lower left. The terms **epigastrium** and **periumbilical** are loosely used to indicate the area below the xiphoid process and above the umbilicus and the area around the umbilicus, respectively.

Surface Landmarks of the Abdominal Viscera

Importantly, the positions of most of the abdominal viscera show individual variations as well as variations in the same person at different times. Posture and respiration have a profound influence on the position of

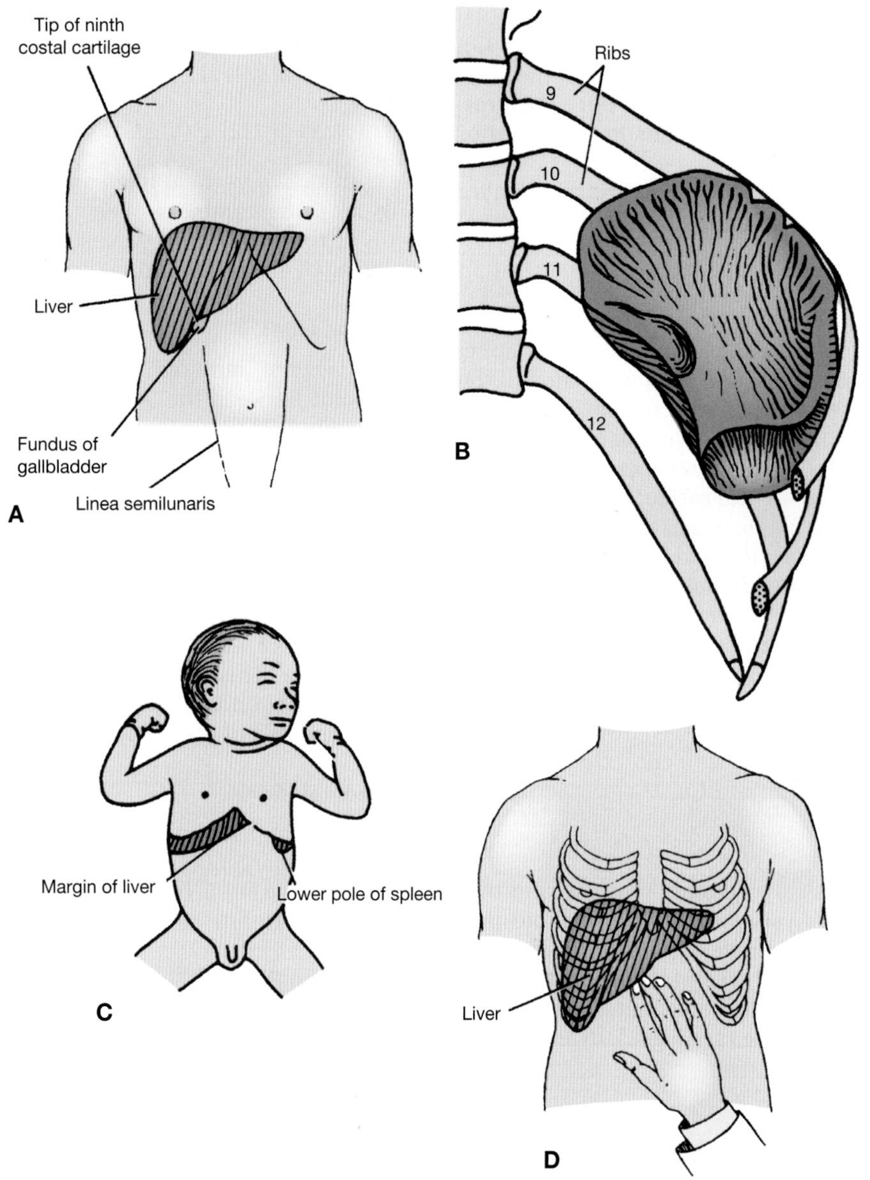

Figure 5.143 **A.** Surface markings of the liver and fundus of the gallbladder. **B.** Relation of the spleen to the ribs. **C.** In a young child, the lower margin of the normal liver and the lower pole of the normal spleen can be palpated. **D.** In a thin adult, the lower margin of the normal liver may just be felt at the end of deep inspiration.

viscera. The following organs are relatively fixed, and their surface markings are clinically valuable.

Liver

The liver lies under cover of the lower ribs, and most of its bulk lies on the right side (Fig. 5.143). In infants, until about the end of the 3rd year, the lower margin of the liver extends one or two fingerbreadths below the costal margin. In the adult who is obese or has a well-developed right rectus abdominis muscle, the liver is not palpable. In a thin adult, the lower edge of the liver may be felt a fingerbreadth below the costal margin. It is most easily felt when the patient inspires deeply and the diaphragm contracts and pushes down the liver.

Gallbladder

The fundus of the gallbladder lies opposite the tip of the right ninth costal cartilage—that is, where the lateral edge of the right rectus abdominis muscle crosses the costal margin (see Fig. 5.143).

Spleen

The spleen is situated in the left upper quadrant and lies under cover of ribs 9 to 12 (see Fig. 5.143). Its long axis corresponds to that of rib 10, and, in the adult, it does not normally project forward in front of the midaxillary line. In infants, the lower pole of the spleen may just be felt.

Pancreas

The pancreas lies across the transpyloric plane. The head lies below and to the right, the neck lies on the plane, and the body and tail lie above and to the left.

Kidneys

The right kidney lies at a slightly lower level than the left kidney because of the bulk of the right lobe of the liver (Fig. 5.144). The lower pole can be palpated in the right lumbar region at the end of deep inspiration in a person with poorly developed abdominal muscles. Each kidney moves about 1 in. (2.5 cm) in a vertical direction during full respiratory movement of the diaphragm. The normal left kidney, which is higher than the right kidney, is not palpable.

On the anterior abdominal wall, the hilum of each kidney lies on the transpyloric plane, about three fingerbreadths from the midline. On the back, the kidneys extend from the T12 spine to the L3 spine, and the hila are opposite the L1 vertebra.

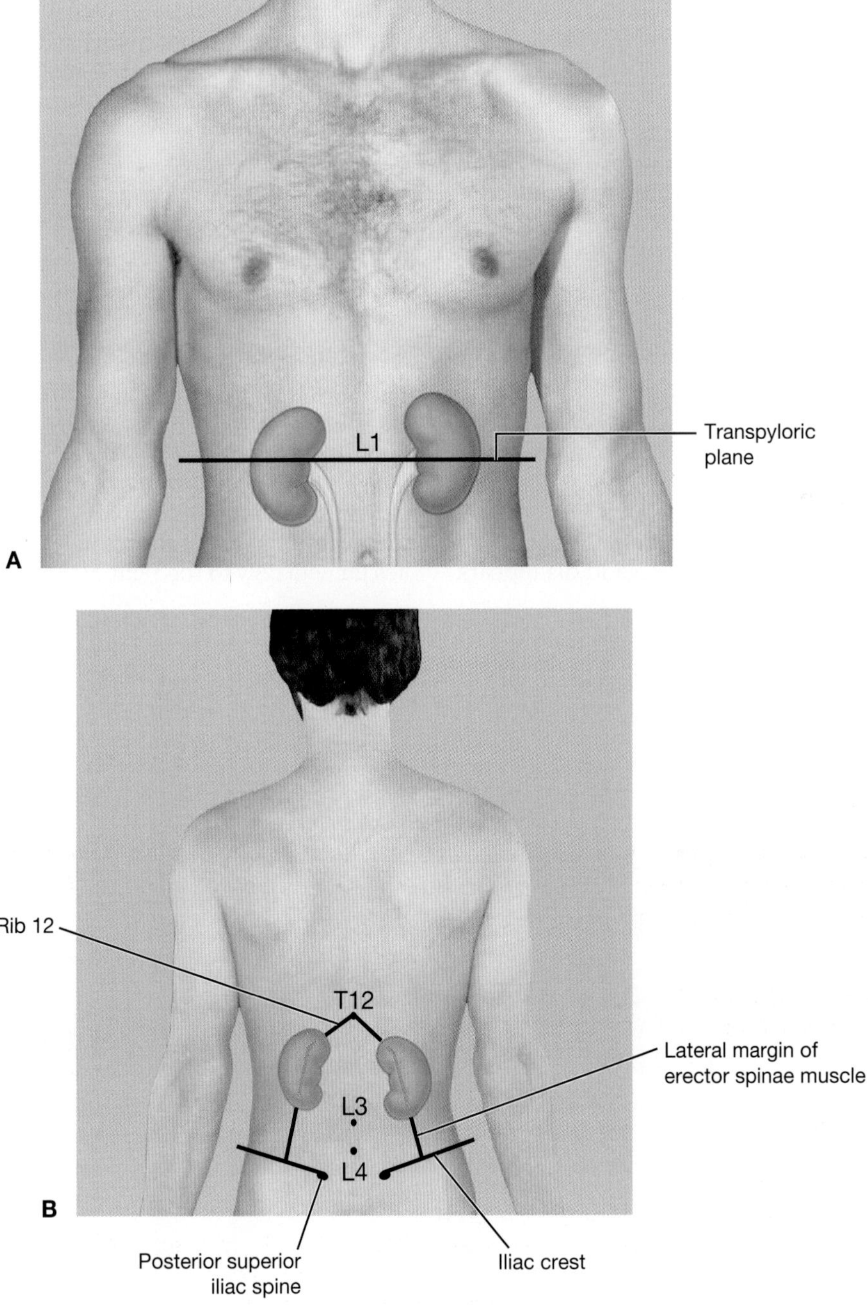

Figure 5.144 **A.** Surface anatomy of the kidneys and ureters on the anterior abdominal wall. Note the relationship of the hilum of each kidney to the transpyloric plane. **B.** Surface anatomy of the kidneys on the posterior abdominal wall.

Stomach

The **cardioesophageal junction** lies about three fingerbreadths below and to the left of the xiphisternal junction (the esophagus pierces the diaphragm at the level of the T10 vertebra).

The **pylorus** lies on the transpyloric plane just to the right of the midline. The **lesser curvature** lies on a curved line joining the cardioesophageal junction and the pylorus. The **greater curvature** has an extremely variable position in the umbilical region or below.

Duodenum (First Part)

The duodenum lies on the transpyloric plane about four fingerbreadths to the right of the midline.

Cecum

The cecum is situated in the right lower quadrant. It is often distended with gas and gives a resonant sound when percussed. It can be palpated through the anterior abdominal wall.

Appendix

The appendix lies in the right lower quadrant. The base of the appendix is situated one third of the way up the line joining the anterior superior iliac spine to the umbilicus (**McBurney's point**). The position of the free end of the appendix is variable.

Ascending Colon

The ascending colon extends upward from the cecum on the lateral side of the right vertical line and disappears under the right costal margin. It can be palpated through the anterior abdominal wall.

Transverse Colon

The transverse colon extends across the abdomen, occupying the umbilical region. It arches downward with its concavity directed upward. Because it has a mesentery, its position is variable.

Descending Colon

The descending colon extends downward from the left costal margin on the lateral side of the left vertical line. In the left lower quadrant, it curves medially and downward to become continuous with the sigmoid colon. The descending colon has a smaller diameter than the ascending colon and can be palpated through the anterior abdominal wall.

Urinary Bladder and Pregnant Uterus

The full bladder and pregnant uterus can be palpated through the lower part of the anterior abdominal wall above the symphysis pubis (see Chapter 6).

Aorta and Inferior Vena Cava

The aorta lies in the midline of the abdomen and bifurcates below into the right and left **common iliac arteries** opposite the L4 vertebra—that is, on the intercristal plane (Fig. 5.145). The pulsations of the aorta can be easily palpated through the upper part of the anterior abdominal wall just to the left of the midline. The inferior vena cava lies immediately to the right of the aorta.

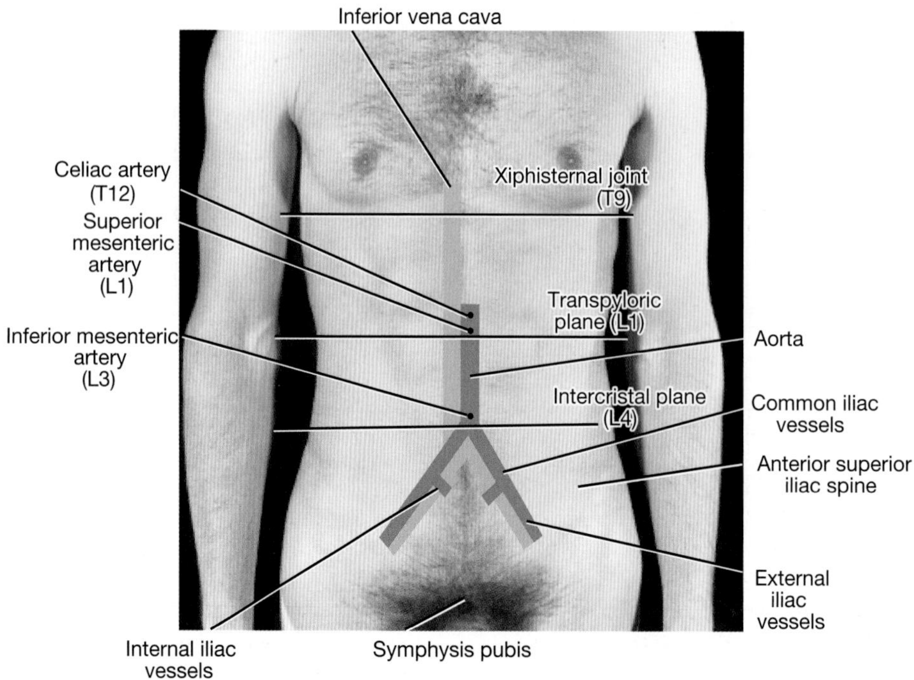

Figure 5.145 Surface projections of the aorta and its branches and the inferior vena cava on the anterior abdominal wall.

External Iliac Artery

The pulsations of this artery can be felt as it passes under the inguinal ligament to become continuous with the femoral artery. It can be located at a point halfway between the anterior superior iliac spine and the symphysis pubis.

Clinical Case 1 Discussion

An indirect inguinal hernia is caused by a congenital persistence of a sac formed from the lining of the abdomen. This sac has a narrow neck, and its cavity remains in free communication with the abdominal cavity. Hernias of the abdominal wall are common. It is necessary to know the anatomy of the abdomen in the region of the groin before the clinician can make a diagnosis or understand the different hernial types that can exist. Moreover, without this knowledge, it is impossible to appreciate the complications that can occur or to plan treatment. A hernia may start as a simple swelling, but it can end as a life-threatening problem.

Clinical Case 2 Discussion

Inflammation of the appendix initially is a localized disease giving rise to pain that is often referred to the umbilicus. Later, the inflammatory process spreads to involve the peritoneum covering the appendix, producing localized peritonitis. If the appendix ruptures, further spread occurs that produces a more generalized peritonitis. Inflammation of the parietal peritoneum lining the anterior abdominal wall causes pain and reflex spasm of the anterior abdominal muscles. This can be explained by the fact that the same segmental nerves supply the parietal peritoneum, the abdominal muscles, and the overlying skin. This is a protective mechanism to keep that area of the abdomen at rest so that the inflammatory process remains localized.

Understanding the symptoms and signs of appendicitis depends on having a working knowledge of the anatomy of the appendix, including its nerve supply, blood supply, and relationships with other abdominal structures.

Key Concepts

Osteology

- The thoracic cage covers all or parts of the upper abdominal organs (eg, liver stomach, spleen, and kidneys).
- The abdominal skeleton consists primarily of the lumbar vertebrae, costal margin of the thoracic cage, and iliac and pubic bone elements of the pelvis.

Anterolateral Abdominal Wall

- The anterolateral abdominal wall is made up of seven layers: skin, superficial fascia, deep fascia, muscles, transversalis fascia, extraperitoneal fascia, and parietal peritoneum.
- The superficial fascia is divided into two layers: a more superficial fatty layer and a deeper membranous layer.
- The abdominal wall houses three broad sheets of muscle: external oblique, internal oblique, and transversus abdominis. Additionally, the paired rectus abdominis muscles form vertical straps on either side of the anterior midline.
- The aponeuroses of the three sheets enclose the rectus abdominis to form the rectus sheath. The composition of the anterior and posterior walls of the sheath varies above and below the arcuate line.
- The external oblique aponeurosis contains a triangular defect, the superficial inguinal ring. The spermatic cord (males) or round ligament of the uterus (females) passes through this opening. The lower border of the external oblique aponeurosis forms the inguinal ligament.
- The tendinous fibers of the internal oblique and the transversus abdominis join to form the conjoint tendon.
- The anterior rami of the T7 to T12 and the L1 (iliohypogastric and ilioinguinal) nerves supply the anterolateral abdominal wall.
- Useful landmark dermatome references are that T7 is in the epigastrium over the xiphoid process, that of T10 includes the umbilicus, and that of L1 lies just above the symphysis pubis.
- The superior epigastric, inferior epigastric, deep circumflex iliac, lower two posterior intercostal, and lumbar arteries are the main arteries to the anterolateral abdominal wall.
- The superficial veins form a network that radiates out from the umbilicus. A few small paraumbilical veins connect the network through the umbilicus and along the ligamentum teres to the portal vein. This forms an important portal–systemic venous anastomosis. The deep veins follow the arteries of the same name.
- The lymph drainage of the skin of the anterior abdominal wall above the level of the umbilicus is upward to the anterior axillary (pectoral) group of nodes. Below the level of the umbilicus, the lymph drains downward and laterally to the superficial

inguinal nodes. The lymph of the skin of the back above the level of the iliac crests drains upward to the posterior axillary group of nodes. Below the level of the iliac crests, lymph drains downward to the superficial inguinal nodes. The deep lymph vessels follow the arteries.

- The inguinal canal is an oblique passage through the lower part of the anterior abdominal wall. The spermatic cord passes through the canal in males. The round ligament of the uterus runs through in females. The canal extends from the deep inguinal ring, a hole in the transversalis fascia, downward and medially to the superficial inguinal ring, a hole in the aponeurosis of the external oblique muscle. The inguinal canal has four walls: anterior, posterior, superior (roof), and inferior (floor).
- The spermatic cord is a bundle of structures that pass through the inguinal canal to and from the testis. The components are: vas deferens, testicular artery, testicular veins (pampiniform plexus), testicular lymph vessels, autonomic nerves, remains of the processus vaginalis, and genital branch of the genitofemoral nerve. Three concentric layers of fascia derived from the layers of the anterior abdominal wall enclose the cord.
- The scrotum houses the testes, epididymis, and spermatic cord. The parietal peritoneum and fasciae of the abdominal wall contribute to the layers of the scrotal wall. The labia majora are the female homologues of the scrotum.
- Lymph from the scrotal skin and fascia, including the tunica vaginalis, drains into the superficial inguinal lymph nodes. However, lymph from the testes drains upward to the lumbar nodes.
- The testis is the male gonad and lies within the scrotum. A tough fibrous capsule, the tunica albuginea, surrounds each testis. The epididymis has a head, body, and tail.
- There are several types of abdominal hernias, including inguinal (indirect and direct), femoral, umbilical, epigastric, rectus abdominis separation, incisional, linea semilunaris, lumbar, and internal.

General Arrangement of Organs

- The liver occupies the upper part of the abdominal cavity. The gallbladder adheres to the undersurface of the right lobe of the liver.
- The esophagus connects the pharynx with the stomach. It enters the right side of the stomach.
- The stomach occupies the left upper quadrant, epigastric, and umbilical regions.
- The duodenum of the small intestine is situated in the epigastric and umbilical regions. It extends from the stomach around the head of the pancreas. The jejunum occupies the upper left part of the abdominal cavity, whereas the ileum occupies the lower right part of the abdominal cavity and the pelvic cavity.
- The large intestine arches around and encloses the coils of the small intestine.
- The pancreas stretches obliquely across the posterior abdominal wall in the epigastric region, behind the stomach, and extends from the duodenum to the spleen.
- The spleen occupies the left upper part of the abdomen between the stomach and the diaphragm.
- The kidneys lie high up on the posterior abdominal wall. The left kidney lies slightly higher than the right. Each kidney gives rise to a ureter that runs downward to the urinary bladder. The suprarenal glands lie on the upper poles of the kidneys.

Peritoneum

- The peritoneum is a thin serous membrane that lines the walls of the abdominal and pelvic cavities and clothes the viscera. The parietal peritoneum lines the walls of the abdominopelvic cavity. The visceral peritoneum covers the organs. The potential space between the parietal and visceral layers is the peritoneal cavity.
- The peritoneal cavity is divided into two parts: greater sac and lesser sac. The greater sac is the main compartment. The lesser sac is smaller and lies behind the stomach. The greater and lesser sacs communicate with one another through the **epiploic foramen**.
- Retroperitoneal organs lie behind the peritoneum and are only partially covered with visceral peritoneum. Intraperitoneal organs are covered with visceral peritoneum and are attached to other organs or the abdominal wall by peritoneal bridges (eg, omenta, mesenteries, and ligaments).
- Subphrenic spaces and paracolic gutters may be sites for collection and movement of infected peritoneal fluid.
- The parietal peritoneum is sensitive to pain, temperature, touch, and pressure. Somatic nerves innervate it. The visceral peritoneum is sensitive to stretch and tearing and is not sensitive to touch, pressure, or temperature. Visceral afferent nerves supply it.

Gastrointestinal Tract

- The esophagus enters the abdomen through the diaphragm and connects to the stomach. The vagus nerves run along its sides. A physiologic sphincter, but not an anatomic sphincter, lies at the lower end of the esophagus. An important portal–systemic venous anastomosis occurs at the lower third of the esophagus.
- The stomach has two openings, the cardiac and pyloric orifices; two curvatures, the greater and lesser curvatures; and two surfaces, an anterior and a posterior surface. It is divided into the fundus,

body, pyloric antrum, and pylorus. Branches of the celiac artery supply it; it drains into the portal circulation. Lymph drainage is to the celiac nodes. Autonomic nerves supply the stomach.

- The small intestine is divided into duodenum, jejunum, and ileum. The duodenum is mostly retroperitoneal, has four parts, and receives the openings of the bile and pancreatic ducts. The jejunum and ileum are mobile and supported by the mesentery of the small intestine. Branches of the superior mesenteric artery supply most of the small intestine; it drains into the portal circulation. Lymph drainage is mostly to the superior mesenteric nodes. Autonomic nerves supply the small bowel.
- The abdominal part of the large intestine includes the cecum, appendix, ascending colon, transverse colon, descending colon, and sigmoid colon. The ascending and descending colon are retroperitoneal. The superior mesenteric artery supplies the cecum, appendix, ascending colon, and most of the transverse colon. The inferior mesenteric artery supplies the remainder. The entire abdominal large intestine drains to the portal circulation. Lymph drainage follows the arterial supply to either superior or inferior mesenteric nodes. Autonomic nerves supply the large bowel.

Accessory Organs of the Gastrointestinal Tract

- The liver is divided into right, left, quadrate, and caudate lobes. The porta hepatis (hilum) transmits all structures that enter or leave the liver except for the hepatic veins. The falciform, coronary, and triangular ligaments connect the liver to the body wall and diaphragm. The lesser omentum connects the liver to the stomach and duodenum. The hepatic artery (a branch of the celiac artery) and the portal vein supply blood to the liver. The hepatic veins drain the liver to the inferior vena cava. Lymph drainage is to the celiac nodes. Autonomic nerves supply the liver.
- The biliary tree consists of the right and left hepatic ducts, the common hepatic duct, the bile duct, the gallbladder, and the cystic duct. Ultimately, biliary drainage is into the duodenum at the major duodenal papilla.
- The pancreas is divided into a head, neck, body, and tail. It extends across the posterior abdominal wall from the concavity of the duodenum (head) to the hilum of the spleen (tail). The exocrine part primarily drains via the main pancreatic duct, which joins the bile duct and empties into the duodenum. An accessory pancreatic duct often occurs and drains separately. Branches of the celiac artery and some from the superior mesenteric artery supply the pancreas. Venous drainage is into the portal system. Lymph drainage is into celiac and superior mesenteric nodes. Autonomic nerves supply the pancreas.
- The spleen is a lymphoid organ, not a component of the gastrointestinal (GI) tract. It is connected to the stomach and left kidney by peritoneal ligaments. The splenic artery (branch of the celiac artery) supplies the spleen. The splenic vein drains the spleen and contributes to formation of the portal vein. Lymph drainage is to the celiac nodes. Autonomic nerves supply the spleen.

Urinary Tract

- The urinary tract consists of the kidneys, ureters, urinary bladder, and urethra.
- The kidneys are retroperitoneal and surrounded by layers of fat and fascia but are somewhat mobile. Each kidney has an outer cortex and inner medulla. The medulla is composed of renal pyramids. The gross level urinary drainage tract includes the renal pelvis, major calyces, and minor calyces. The renal artery (branch of the aorta) supplies the kidney. The renal vein drains the kidney into the inferior vena cava. Lymph drainage is to the para-aortic nodes.
- The ureters are retroperitoneal, lie largely on the psoas muscles, and extend from the kidneys to the posterior surface of the urinary bladder. Each has three constrictions where stones may lodge.

Suprarenal Glands

- The suprarenal glands lie on the upper poles of the kidneys. Each gland has an outer cortex and inner medulla.
- Three arteries supply the gland: superior suprarenal artery (branch of the inferior phrenic artery), middle suprarenal artery (branch of the aorta), and inferior suprarenal artery (branch of the renal artery).
- A single vein drains into the inferior vena cava on the right and into the renal vein on the left.
- The lymph drains into the para-aortic nodes.

Posterior Abdominal Wall

- L1 to L5 vertebrae and their intervertebral discs, rib 12 (right and left), and the upper part of the bony pelvis form the skeleton of the posterior abdominal wall.
- The muscles of the posterior wall include the psoas major, quadratus lumborum, aponeuroses of origin of the transversus abdominis, and the iliacus.
- The abdominal aorta runs from the aortic hiatus of the diaphragm to its termination as the common iliac arteries at the L4 level. It gives off multiple branches to the abdominal walls and viscera.
- The common iliac arteries terminate by dividing into external and internal iliac arteries.

- The inferior vena cava conveys most of the blood from the body below the diaphragm to the heart. It is formed by the union of the common iliac veins at the L5 level and ascends on the right side of the aorta.
- The lymph nodes are closely related to the aorta and form preaortic and right and left lateral aortic (para-aortic or lumbar) chains.
- The preaortic lymph nodes lie around the origins of the celiac, superior mesenteric, and inferior mesenteric arteries. They collect lymph from the viscera supplied by those arteries.
- The lateral aortic lymph nodes drain the lymph from the kidneys and suprarenal glands; from the testes in the male and from the ovaries, uterine tubes, and fundus of the uterus in the female; from the deep lymph vessels of the abdominal walls; and from the common iliac nodes.
- The pre- and lateral aortic nodes drain to the cisterna chyli.
- The anterior rami of the L1 to L4 nerves form the lumbar plexus. The branches of the plexus emerge from the lateral and medial borders and anterior surface of the psoas major muscle. The major branches of the plexus are the iliohypogastric nerve, ilioinguinal nerve, lateral cutaneous nerve of the thigh, femoral nerve, lumbosacral trunk, obturator nerve, and genitofemoral nerve.
- The abdominal part of the sympathetic trunk runs downward along the medial border of the psoas muscle on the bodies of the lumbar vertebrae. The right sympathetic trunk lies behind the right border of the inferior vena cava; the left sympathetic trunk lies close to the left border of the aorta. Branches include white and gray rami communicantes, branches to the aortic plexus, and branches to the superior hypogastric plexus.

Radiology

- Numerous skeletal and visceral structures can be demonstrated in plain film and CT scans of the abdomen. Contrast studies that utilize ingested barium sulfate suspensions are particularly useful in clarifying the GI tract. Iodine-containing compounds injected intravenously are helpful in visualizing the urinary tract.

Surface Anatomy

- Notable surface landmarks of the abdominal wall include the xiphoid process, costal margin, iliac crest, pubic tubercle, symphysis pubis, inguinal ligament, superficial inguinal ring, scrotum/labia majora, linea alba, umbilicus, and rectus abdominis.
- A grid of vertical and horizontal lines divides the abdominal wall into reference areas for purposes of describing the wall and the locations of abdominal contents.
- Structures that reliably project to landmark areas on the abdominal wall include the liver, gallbladder, spleen, pancreas, kidneys, stomach, colon, appendix, and aorta.

6 Pelvis

CLINICAL CASE 1

A 51-year-old male was involved in a light-plane accident. He was flying home from a business trip when, because of fog, he had to make a forced landing in a plowed field. On landing, the plane came abruptly to rest on its nose. His companion was killed on impact, and he was thrown from the cockpit. On admission to the emergency department, he was unconscious and showed signs of severe hypovolemic (loss of circulating blood) shock. He had extensive bruising of the lower part of the anterior abdominal wall, and the front of his pelvis was prominent on the right side. During examination of the penis, a drop of blood-stained fluid was expressed from the external orifice. No evidence of external hemorrhage was present.

CLINICAL CASE 2

A 62-year-old male visited his physician for an annual physical examination. He appeared to be in good health and had no issues to report. A general examination revealed nothing abnormal. The physician then told the patient that he was about to perform a rectal examination. At first, the patient objected, saying he did not feel it was necessary because nothing abnormal was found a year ago. The physician persisted, and, finally, the patient agreed to the examination.

The physician found a small, hard nodule projecting from the posterior surface of the prostate gland but no other abnormalities. He informed the patient of the findings and explained the possibility that the nodule could be malignant. The patient was upset, especially because he had no abnormal urinary symptoms.

See the Clinical Case Discussions at the end of this chapter for further insight.

CHAPTER OUTLINE

LEARNING OBJECTIVES

The purpose of this chapter is to review the basic anatomy of the pelvis and how that relates to common clinical conditions involving the pelvic organs.

1. Identify the bones of the pelvis and their major features in the context of the composition of the pelvic walls. Describe the functional aspects of these structures.
2. Identify the bony components, major supporting ligaments, key accessory structures (eg, intra-articular discs), and movements permitted at the joints of the pelvis. Relate these to the general mechanics of the pelvis.
3. Identify the specialized pelvic differences between males and females. Relate these to the mechanics of the pelvis, including the construction of the birth canal.
4. Identify the pelvic diaphragm, its components, and their innervation and basic functions. Indicate differences between males and females with respect to relationships to the urogenital tracts.
5. Identify the pelvic fasciae and peritoneum. Describe their relations with the abdominal fasciae and peritoneum.
6. Identify the lumbosacral plexuses, their segmental origins, and their major peripheral branches. Identify the sources of autonomic innervation to the pelvis. Describe the functional consequences of lesions of the main peripheral nerves.
7. Trace the flow of blood into and out of the pelvis by describing the courses, branching patterns, and distributions of the common iliac, external iliac, and internal iliac vessels. Note the relations of these vessels to neighboring organs, mesenteries, and neurovascular structures.
8. Trace the primary lymph drainage routes through the pelvis.
9. Identify the sigmoid colon and rectum. Describe the relationships of these structures with reference to their basic functions and to clinical examination.
10. Identify the ureters and the urinary bladder. Describe their gross features and relationships with the peritoneal cavity. Describe the position of the bladder in the pelvis in both full and empty states, the nature and source of its innervation, and its means of filling and drainage in both males and females.
11. Trace the courses of the male and female reproductive tracts. Identify accessory glands or organs in the pathway. Note the relationships of the individual components. Describe the nerves, muscles, and vasculature that are responsible for normal functioning in males and females.
12. Identify the major structures of the pelvis in standard radiographic and cross-sectional images.
13. Locate the surface projections and palpation points of major pelvic structures in a basic surface anatomy examination.

OVERVIEW

The pelvis is the region of the trunk that lies inferior to the abdomen. Although the abdominal and pelvic cavities are continuous, the two regions usually are described separately.

The term *pelvis* is loosely used to describe the region where the trunk and lower limbs meet. The word *pelvis* means "basin" and is more correctly applied to the skeleton of the region, that is, the pelvic girdle or bony pelvis. Thus, the pelvis is a bowl-shaped bony structure.

The main function of the bony pelvis is to transmit the weight of the body from the vertebral column to the femurs. In addition, it contains, supports, and protects the lower parts of the gastrointestinal (GI) and urinary tracts and the male and female internal organs of reproduction. It also contains important nerves, blood vessels, and lymphatic tissues and provides attachment for trunk and lower limb muscles.

Four bones make up the bony pelvis: the two **hip bones** (**os coxae**), which form the lateral and anterior walls, and the **sacrum** and **coccyx**, which are part of the vertebral column and form the posterior wall (Fig. 6.1). The two hip bones articulate with each other anteriorly at the **symphysis pubis** and posteriorly with the sacrum at the **sacroiliac joints**. The bony pelvis thus forms a strong basin-shaped structure.

The **pelvic cavity** (cavity of the true pelvis) is the area between the pelvic inlet and the pelvic outlet. The **pelvic diaphragm** subdivides this into the **main pelvic cavity** above and the **perineum** below (Fig. 6.2). This

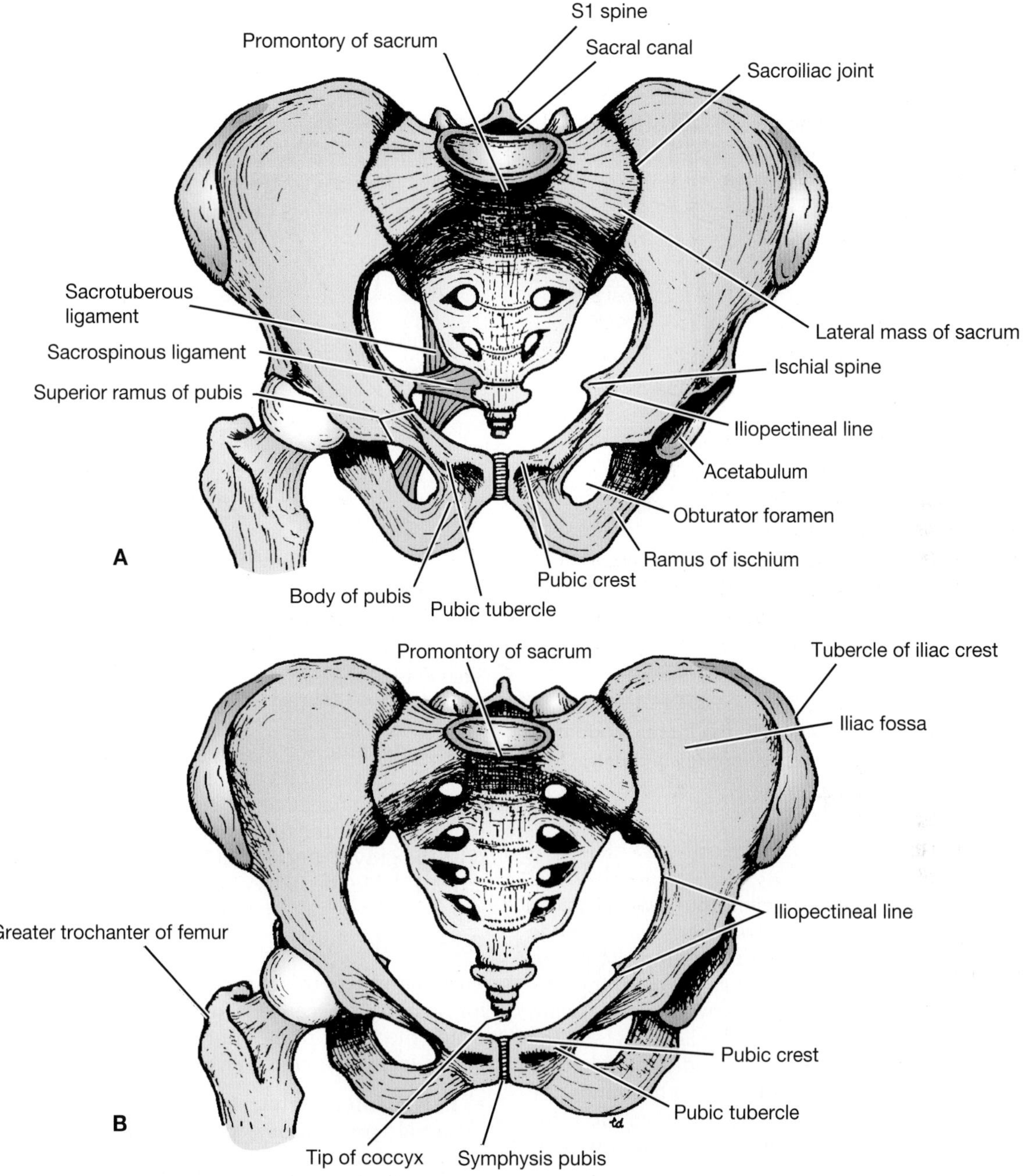

Figure 6.1 Anterior view of the male pelvis **(A)** and female pelvis **(B)**.

chapter examines the contents of the main pelvic cavity. The perineum is described in Chapter 7.

The pelvic cavity contains the lower ends of the GI and urinary tracts and the internal organs of reproduction as well as their nerve supply, blood supply, and lymphatic drainage. The sigmoid colon, rectum, and terminal coils of ileum occupy the posterior part of the pelvic cavity in both sexes. The urogenital organs fill the more anterior area. The organs project up into the peritoneal cavity, causing the peritoneum to drape over them in folds, producing important fossae that are the sites for the accumulation of blood and pus in different types of pelvic disease.

A physician is often confronted with problems involving infections, injuries, and prolapses of the rectum, uterus, and vagina. Emergency situations involving the bladder, the pregnant uterus, ectopic pregnancy, spontaneous abortion, and acute pelvic inflammatory disease are examples of problems found in the female. The urinary bladder and the prostate in the male are frequent sites of disease.

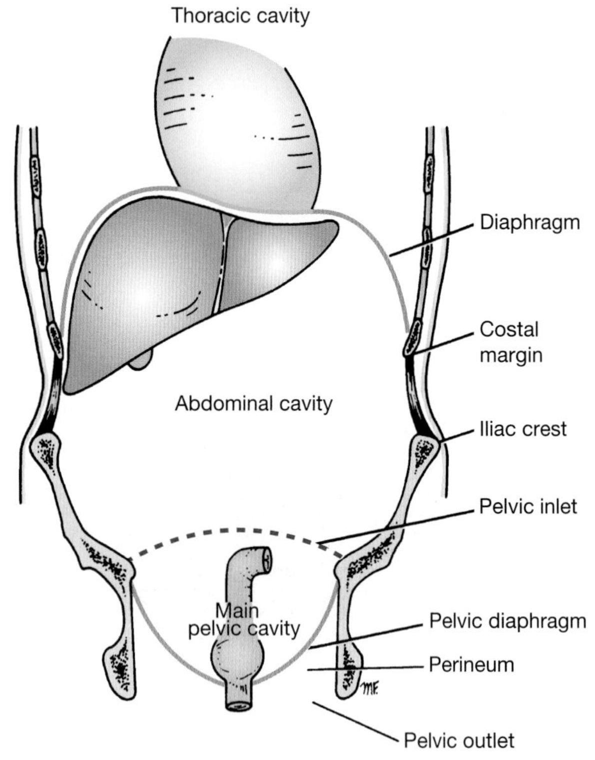

Figure 6.2 Coronal section through the thorax, abdomen, and pelvis showing the thoracic, abdominal, and pelvic cavities and the perineum.

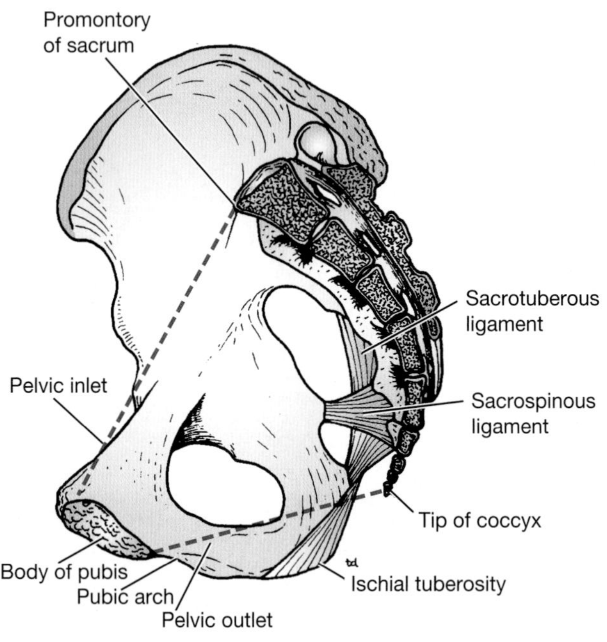

Figure 6.3 Right half of the pelvis showing the pelvic inlet, pelvic outlet, and sacrotuberous and sacrospinous ligaments.

PELVIC WALLS

The pelvic brim divides the pelvis into two parts: an upper false pelvis and a lower true pelvis. The **pelvic brim** is formed by the **sacral promontory** (anterior and upper margin of the S1 vertebra) behind, the **iliopectineal lines** (ridges that run downward and forward around the inner surface of the ileum) laterally, and the **symphysis pubis** (joint between the bodies of the pubic bones) anteriorly. The **false pelvis**, which bounds the lower part of the abdominal cavity, is above the brim. The **true pelvis**, which contains the pelvic cavity, is below the brim.

Pelvic Orientation

The correct orientation of the bony pelvis relative to the trunk is with the individual standing in the anatomic position. The front of the symphysis pubis and the **anterior superior iliac spines** lie in the same vertical plane (Fig. 6.3). This means the pelvic surface of the symphysis pubis faces upward and backward, and the anterior surface of the sacrum is directed forward and downward.

False Pelvis

The false pelvis is of little clinical importance. The boundaries are the lumbar vertebrae behind, the iliac fossae and the iliacus muscles laterally, and the lower part of the anterior abdominal wall in front. The false pelvis flares out at its upper end and is considered part of the abdominal cavity. It supports the abdominal contents and, after the third month of pregnancy, helps support the gravid uterus. During the early stages of labor, it helps guide the fetus into the true pelvis.

True Pelvis

The anatomy of the true pelvis in females is important for obstetrics because it forms the bony canal through which the infant passes during birth. The true pelvis in both sexes has an inlet, an outlet, and a cavity:

- **Pelvic inlet (pelvic brim):** its boundaries are the sacral promontory posteriorly, the iliopectineal lines laterally, and the symphysis pubis anteriorly (Figs. 6.4 and 6.5; see also Figs. 6.1 and 6.3).
- **Pelvic outlet:** its boundaries are the coccyx posteriorly, the **ischial tuberosities** laterally, and the **pubic arch** anteriorly (see Figs. 6.1 to 6.5). The pelvic outlet has three wide notches. The pubic arch lies anteriorly, between the **ischiopubic rami**. The sciatic notches lie laterally and are divided into the **greater** and **lesser sciatic foramina** by the **sacrotuberous** and **sacrospinous ligaments** (see Figs. 6.1A and 6.3). From an obstetric standpoint, because the sacrotuberous ligaments are strong and relatively inflexible, they are considered to form part of the perimeter of the pelvic outlet. Thus, the outlet is diamond shaped, with the ischiopubic rami and the symphysis pubis forming the boundaries in front and the sacrotuberous ligaments and the coccyx forming the boundaries behind.

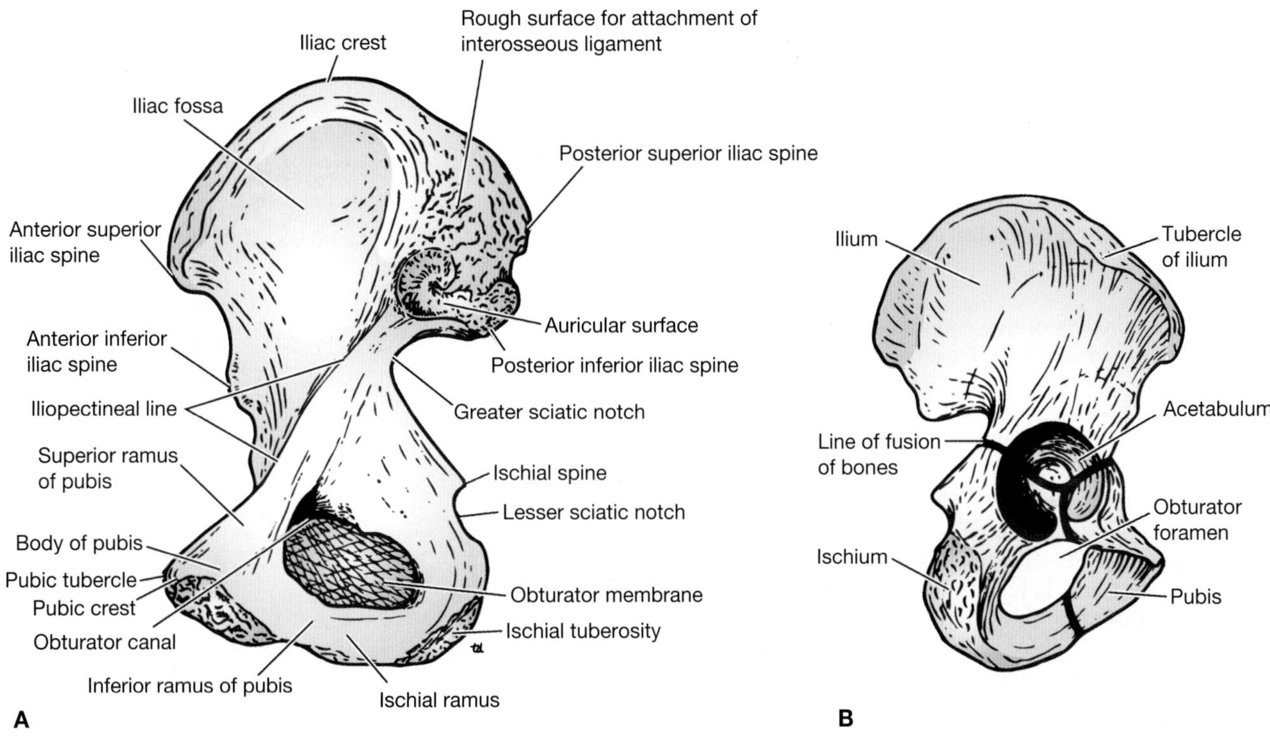

Figure 6.4 Right hip bone. **A.** Medial surface. **B.** Lateral surface. Note the lines of fusion between the three bones—ilium, ischium, and pubis.

- **Pelvic cavity:** this short, curved canal, with a shallow anterior wall and a much deeper posterior wall, lies between the inlet and the outlet (see Figs. 6.2, 6.3, and 6.5).

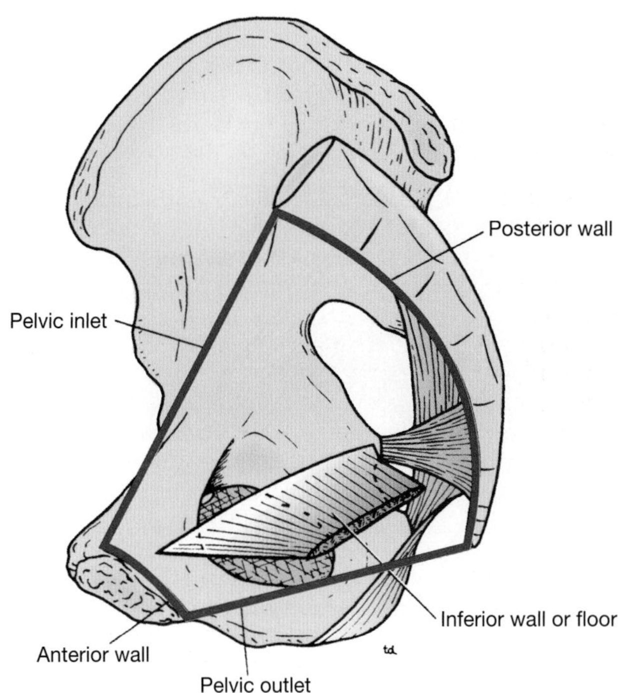

Figure 6.5 Right half of the pelvis showing the pelvic walls.

Pelvic Walls

Bones and ligaments that are partly lined with muscles covered with fascia and parietal peritoneum form the walls of the pelvic cavity. Because of its orientation, the pelvis has antero-inferior, posterior, and lateral walls and an inferior wall or floor (see Fig. 6.5).

Antero-Inferior Pelvic Wall

The antero-inferior pelvic wall is the smallest wall. It is formed by the bodies of the pubic bones, the pubic rami, and the symphysis pubis (Fig. 6.6). In the anatomic position, this wall assists in carrying the weight of the urinary bladder.

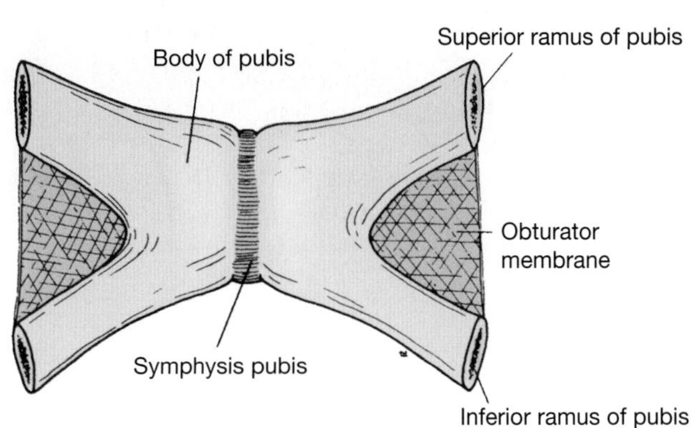

Figure 6.6 Anterior wall of the pelvis (posterior view).

Posterior Pelvic Wall

The posterior pelvic wall is extensive. It is formed by the sacrum and coccyx; piriformis muscles and their covering of parietal pelvic fascia; and the anterior sacroiliac, sacrospinous, and sacrotuberous ligaments (Figs. 6.7 and 6.8). Because of its size and orientation, this wall forms a roof-like cover over the posterior aspect of the pelvis and is sometimes referred to as the **pelvic roof**.

Sacrum

The sacrum consists of five rudimentary vertebrae fused together to form a single wedge-shaped bone with an anterior concavity (see Figs. 6.3 and 6.6). The upper border or **base** of the bone articulates with the L5 vertebra. The narrow inferior border articulates with the coccyx. Laterally, the sacrum articulates with the two iliac bones to form the **sacroiliac joints** (see Fig. 6.1). The anterior and upper margins of the S1 vertebra bulge forward to form the **sacral promontory** (see Fig. 6.3). This is the posterior margin of the pelvic inlet and is an important obstetric landmark used when measuring the size of the pelvis.

The sacral vertebral foramina together form the **sacral canal**. The laminae of the S5 vertebra, and sometimes those of S4, fail to meet in the midline, forming the **sacral hiatus** (see Fig. 6.7B). The sacral canal contains the anterior and posterior roots of the lumbar, sacral, and coccygeal spinal nerves; the filum terminale; and fibrofatty material. It also contains the lower part of the subarachnoid space down as far as the lower border of the S2 vertebra (Fig. 6.9).

The anterior and posterior surfaces of the sacrum possess four pairs of **anterior** and **posterior sacral foramina**, respectively, for the passage of the anterior and posterior rami of the S1 to S4 nerves (see Fig. 6.7).

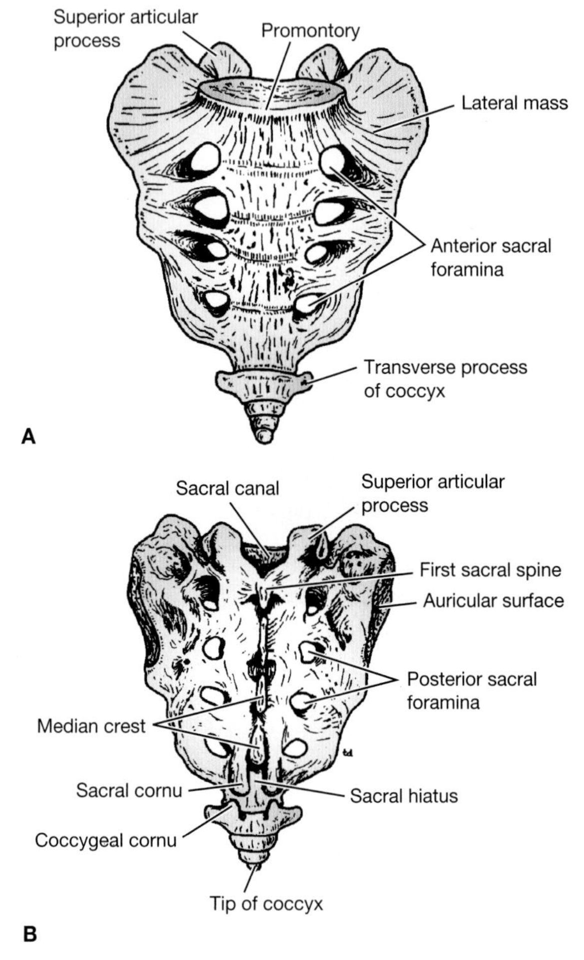

Figure 6.7 Sacrum. **A.** Anterior view. **B.** Posterior view.

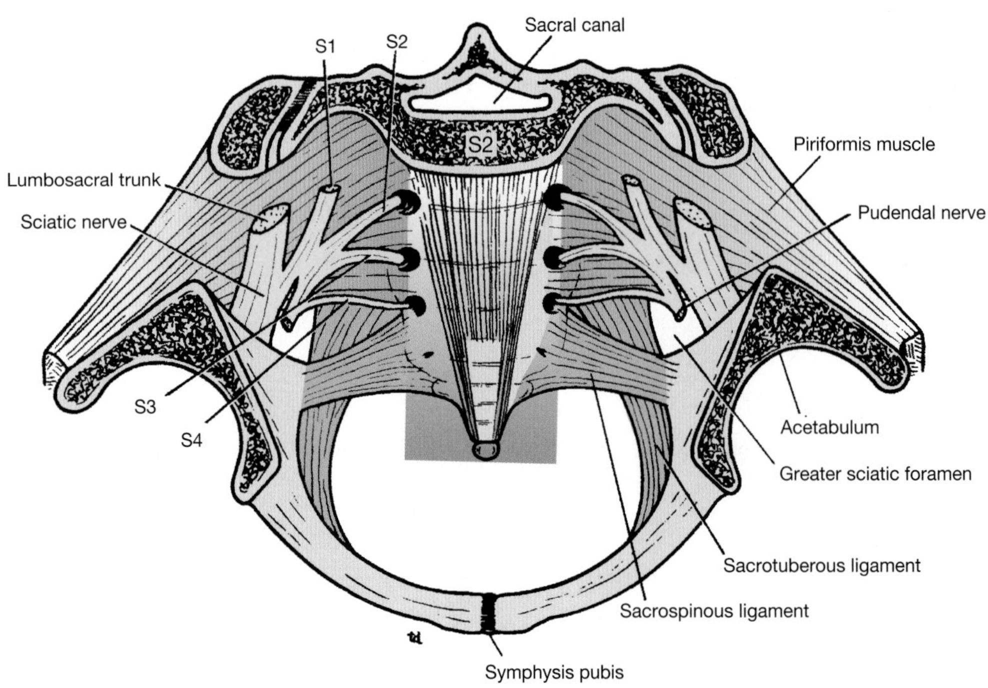

Figure 6.8 Horizontal section through the pelvis showing the posterior wall of the pelvis.

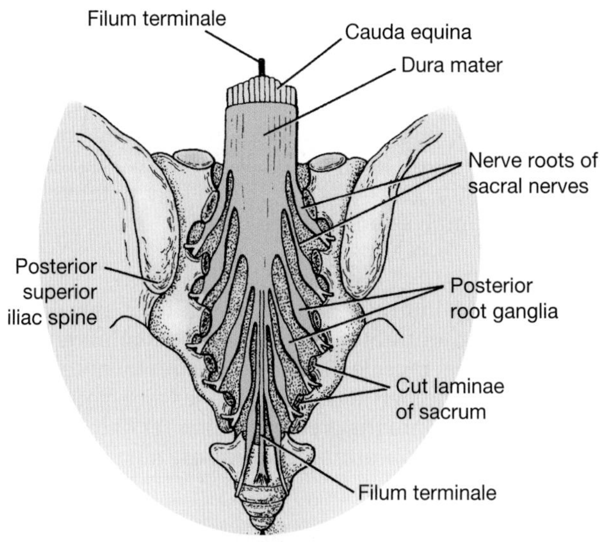

Figure 6.9 Sacrum from behind. Laminae have been removed to show the sacral nerve roots lying within the sacral canal. Note that in the adult the spinal cord ends below, at the level of the lower border of the L1 vertebra.

The sacrum is usually wider in proportion to its length in the female than in the male. The sacrum is tilted forward so that it forms an angle with the L5 vertebra, called the **lumbosacral angle**.

Coccyx

The coccyx consists of four vertebrae fused together to form a small triangular bone, which articulates at its base with the lower end of the sacrum (see Fig. 6.7).

The coccygeal vertebrae consist of bodies only, but the first vertebra possesses rudimentary **transverse processes** and **cornua**. The cornua are the remains of the pedicles and superior articular processes and project upward to articulate with the **sacral cornua**.

Piriformis Muscle

The piriformis muscle arises from the front of the sacrum and leaves the pelvis to enter the gluteal region by passing laterally through the greater sciatic foramen (see Fig. 6.8). Full details of the piriformis are summarized in Table 6.1.

Lateral Pelvic Wall

The lateral pelvic wall is formed by the part of the hip bone below the pelvic inlet, the obturator membrane, the sacrotuberous and sacrospinous ligaments, and the obturator internus muscle and its covering fascia.

Hip Bone

In children, each hip bone (os coxae) consists of the **ilium**, which lies superiorly; the **ischium**, which lies posteriorly and inferiorly; and the **pubis**, which lies anteriorly and inferiorly (see Fig. 6.4B). A **triradiate cartilage** joins the three separate bones at the **acetabulum**. At puberty, these three bones fuse together to form one large, irregular bone. The hip bones articulate with the sacrum at the sacroiliac joints and form the lateral walls of the pelvis. They also articulate with one another anteriorly at the symphysis pubis.

The **acetabulum** is a deep depression on the outer surface of the hip bone (*acetabulum* means "vinegar cup"), which articulates with the hemispherical head of the femur (see Figs. 6.1 and 6.4). The **greater sciatic notch** is a large, deep notch behind the acetabulum and is separated from the **lesser sciatic notch** by the **spine of the ischium**. The **sacrotuberous** and **sacrospinous ligaments** (see Fig. 6.3) convert the sciatic notches into the **greater** and **lesser sciatic foramina.**

The **ilium**, which is the upper flattened part of the hip bone, possesses the **iliac crest** (see Fig. 6.4). The iliac crest runs between the **anterior** and **posterior superior iliac spines**. Below these spines are the corresponding **anterior** and **posterior inferior iliac spines**. On the inner surface of the ilium is the large **auricular surface** for articulation with the sacrum. The **iliopectineal line** runs

Table 6.1 Pelvic Walls and Floor Muscles

NAME OF THE MUSCLE	ORIGIN	INSERTION	NERVE SUPPLY	ACTION
Piriformis	Front of lateral mass of the sacrum	Greater trochanter of the femur	Sacral plexus	Lateral rotator of the femur at the hip joint
Obturator internus	Obturator membrane and adjoining part of the hip bone	Greater trochanter of the femur	Nerve to obturator internus from sacral plexus	Lateral rotator of the femur at the hip joint
Levator ani	Body of the pubis, fascia of obturator internus, and spine of ischium	Perineal body; anococcygeal body; walls of the prostate, vagina, rectum, and anal canal	S4 nerve, pudendal nerve	Supports pelvic viscera; sphincter to the anorectal junction and vagina
Coccygeus	Spine of the ischium	Lower end of the sacrum; coccyx	S4 and S5 nerves	Assists levator ani to support the pelvic viscera; flexes coccyx

downward and forward around the inner surface of the ilium and serves to divide the false from the true pelvis.

The **ischium** is the inferior and posterior part of the hip bone and possesses an **ischial spine** and an **ischial tuberosity**.

The **pubis** is the anterior part of the hip bone and has a **body** and **superior** and **inferior pubic rami**. The body of the pubis bears the **pubic crest** and the **pubic tubercle** and articulates with the pubic bone of the opposite side at the **symphysis pubis** (see Fig. 6.1). The **obturator foramen**, which is bounded by the rami of the ischium and pubis, is a large opening in the lower part of the hip bone. The **obturator membrane** fills in most of the obturator foramen (see Fig. 6.4).

Obturator Membrane

The obturator membrane is a fibrous sheet that almost completely closes the obturator foramen, leaving a small gap, the **obturator canal**, for the passage of the obturator nerve and vessels as they leave the pelvis to enter the thigh (see Fig. 6.4).

Sacrotuberous Ligament

The sacrotuberous ligament is strong and extends from the lateral part of the sacrum and coccyx and the posterior inferior iliac spine to the ischial tuberosity (Figs. 6.10 and 6.11; see also Figs. 6.3 and 6.8).

Sacrospinous Ligament

The sacrospinous ligament is strong and triangle shaped. It is attached by its base to the lateral part of the sacrum and coccyx and by its apex to the spine of the ischium (see Figs. 6.1, 6.3, 6.8, 6.10, and 6.11).

The sacrotuberous and sacrospinous ligaments prevent the lower end of the sacrum and the coccyx from being rotated upward at the sacroiliac joint by the weight of the body (see Fig. 6.10B). The two ligaments also convert the greater and lesser sciatic notches into the **greater** and **lesser sciatic foramina**.

Obturator Internus Muscle

The obturator internus muscle arises from the pelvic surface of the obturator foramen and membrane (see Fig. 6.11). The muscle fibers converge to a tendon, which leaves the pelvis through the lesser sciatic foramen and inserts into the greater trochanter of the femur. Full details of the obturator internus are summarized in Table 6.1.

Inferior Pelvic Wall or Pelvic Floor

The floor of the pelvis supports the pelvic viscera and is formed by the funnel-like pelvic diaphragm and associated fascia.

The pelvic floor stretches across the pelvis and divides it into the main pelvic cavity above, which contains the pelvic viscera, and the perineum below. The perineum is considered in detail in Chapter 7.

Pelvic Diaphragm

The paired levator ani and coccygeus muscles and their covering fasciae form the pelvic diaphragm (Fig. 6.12). It

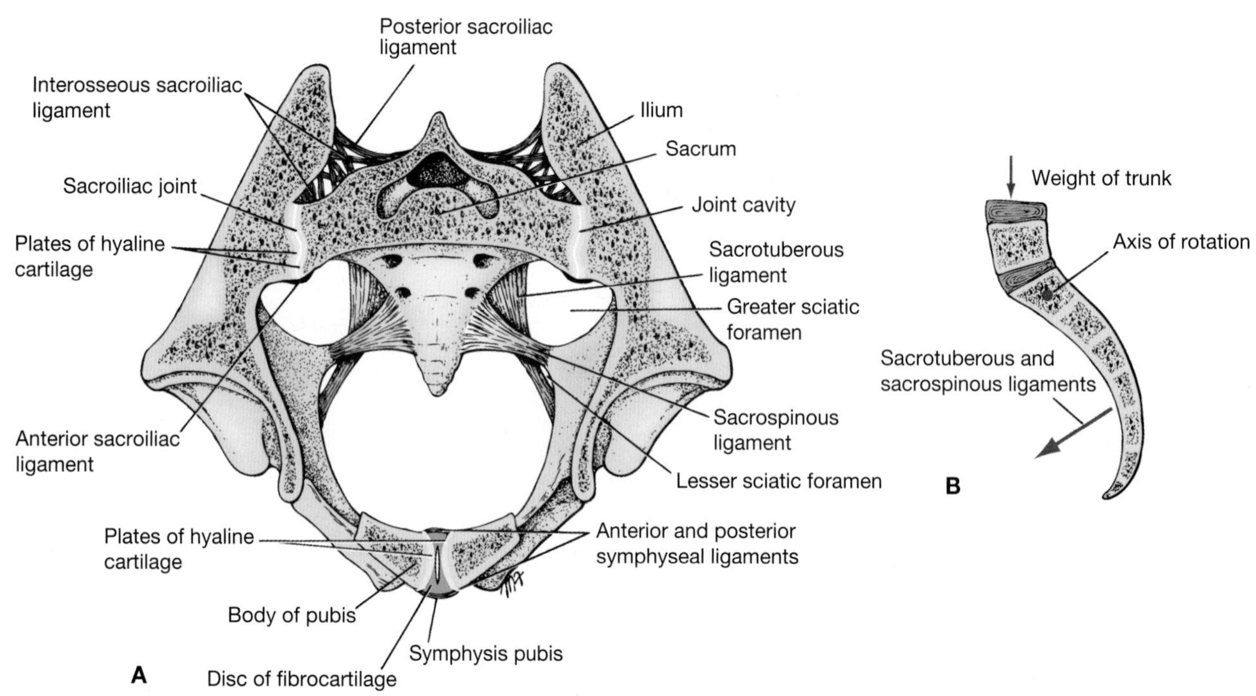

Figure 6.10 **A.** Horizontal section through the pelvis showing the sacroiliac joints and the symphysis pubis. **B.** Sagittal section through the L5 vertebra and the sacrum showing the function of the sacrotuberous and sacrospinous ligaments in resisting the rotation force exerted on the sacrum by the weight of the trunk.

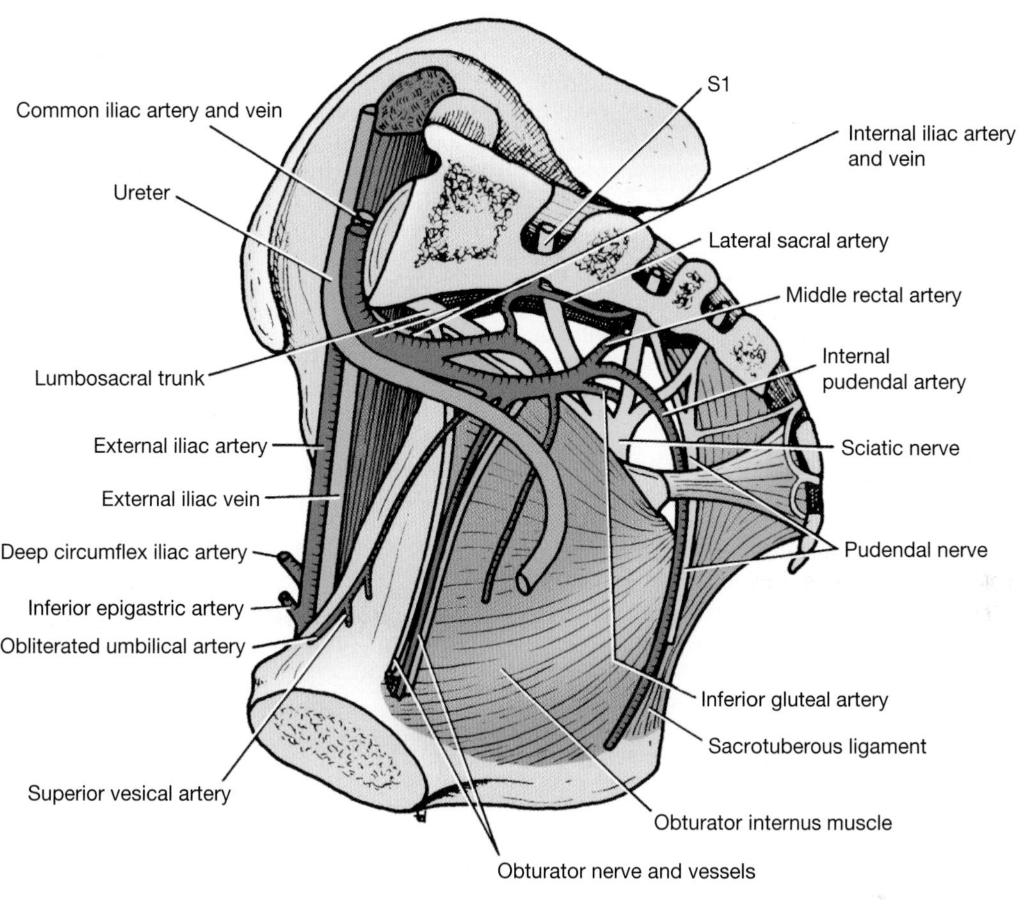

Figure 6.11 Lateral wall of the pelvis.

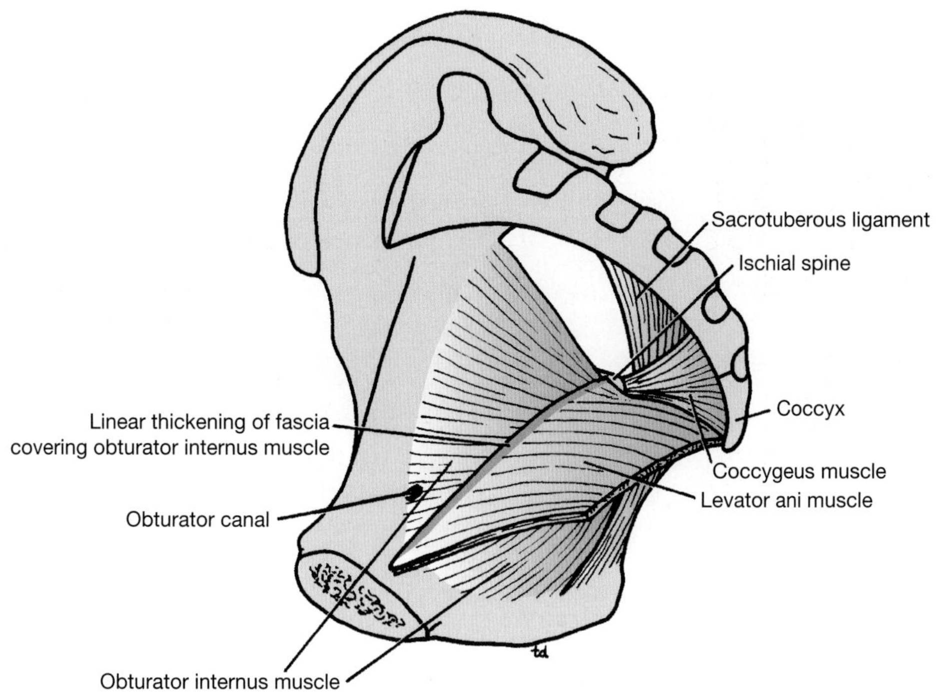

Figure 6.12 Inferior wall (floor) of the pelvis.

is incomplete anteriorly to allow passage of the urethra in males and the urethra and vagina in females. General details of both muscle components are summarized in Table 6.1.

Levator Ani Muscle

The levator ani muscle is a wide, thin sheet forming the larger, more anterior part of the pelvic diaphragm. It has a linear origin from the back of the body of the pubis, a **tendinous arch** formed by a thickening of the fascia covering the obturator internus, and the spine of the ischium (see Fig. 6.12). From this extensive origin, groups of fibers sweep downward and medially to their insertion (Fig. 6.13) as follows:

1. **Anterior fibers:** the **levator prostatae** (males) or **sphincter vaginae** (females) form a sling around the prostate gland or vagina and insert into a mass of fibrous tissue, called the **perineal body** (**central tendon of the perineum**), in front of the anal canal. The levator prostatae support the prostate and stabilize the perineal body. The sphincter vaginae constrict the vagina and stabilize the perineal body.
2. **Intermediate fibers:** the **puborectalis** forms a sling around the junction of the rectum and anal canal. The **pubococcygeus** passes posteriorly to insert into a small fibrous mass, called the **anococcygeal body**, between the tip of the coccyx and the anal canal.
3. **Posterior fibers:** the **iliococcygeus** inserts into the anococcygeal body and the coccyx.

Action

The levator ani muscles of the two sides form an efficient muscular sling that supports and maintains the pelvic viscera in position. They resist the rise in intrapelvic pressure during the straining and expulsive efforts of the abdominal muscles (as occurs in coughing). They also have an important sphincter action on the anorectal junction, and, in the female, they serve also as a sphincter of the vagina.

Coccygeus Muscle

This triangular muscle forms the smaller, more posterior portion of the pelvic diaphragm (see Figs. 6.12 and 6.13).

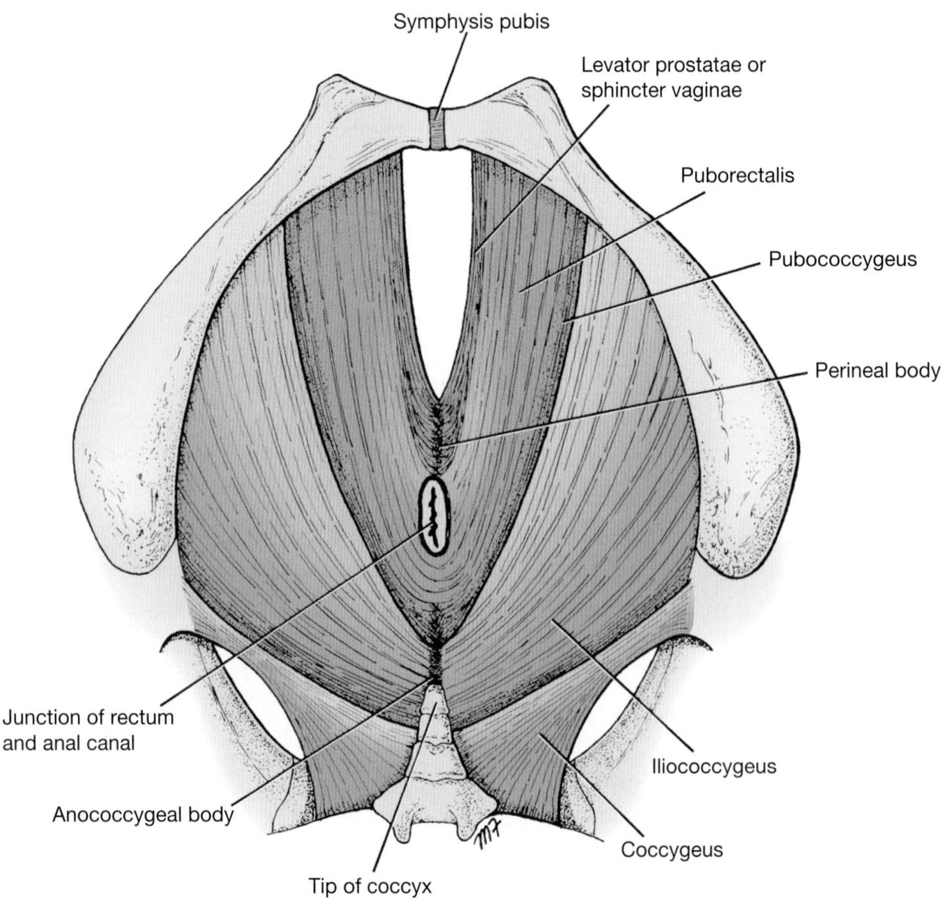

Figure 6.13 Levator ani and coccygeus muscles seen on their inferior aspects. Note the levator ani is made up of several different muscle groups. The levator ani and coccygeus muscles with their fascial coverings form a continuous muscular floor to the pelvis, known as the pelvic diaphragm.

Pelvic Joints

The four major joints in the adult pelvis include paired sacroiliac joints, the symphysis pubis, and the sacrococcygeal joint. Additional joints occur in the immature pelvis (eg, between the ilium, ischium, and pubis elements of the os coxae; between the sacral vertebrae in the sacrum). The vertebral joints are discussed in Chapter 2, and the joints within the hip bone are reviewed in Chapter 8.

Sacroiliac Joints

The sacroiliac joints are strong synovial joints and are formed between the **auricular surfaces** of the sacrum and the **iliac bones** (see Fig. 6.10). The sacrum carries the weight of the trunk, and, apart from the interlocking of the irregular articular surfaces, the shape of the bones contributes little to the stability of the joints. The strong **posterior** and **interosseous sacroiliac ligaments** suspend the sacrum between the two iliac bones. The **anterior sacroiliac ligament** is thin and lies in front of the joint.

The weight of the trunk tends to thrust the upper end of the sacrum downward and rotate the lower end of the bone upward (see Fig. 6.10B). The strong sacrotuberous and sacrospinous ligaments prevent this rotatory movement. The **iliolumbar ligament** connects the tip of the L5 transverse process to the iliac crest.

Movements

A small but limited amount of movement is possible at the sacroiliac joints. In older people, the synovial cavity disappears, and the joint becomes fibrosed. Their primary function is to transmit the weight of the body from the vertebral column to the bony pelvis.

Nerve Supply

The nerve supply is from branches of the sacral spinal nerves.

Symphysis Pubis

The symphysis pubis is a cartilaginous joint between the two pubic bones (see Fig. 6.10). The articular surfaces are covered by a layer of hyaline cartilage and connected by a fibrocartilaginous disc. Ligaments that extend from one pubic bone to the other surround the joint.

Movements

Almost no movement is possible at this joint.

Sacrococcygeal Joint

The sacrococcygeal joint is a cartilaginous joint between the bodies of the last sacral vertebra (S5) and the first coccygeal vertebra. Ligaments join the cornua of the sacrum and coccyx.

Movements

Extensive flexion and extension are possible at this joint.

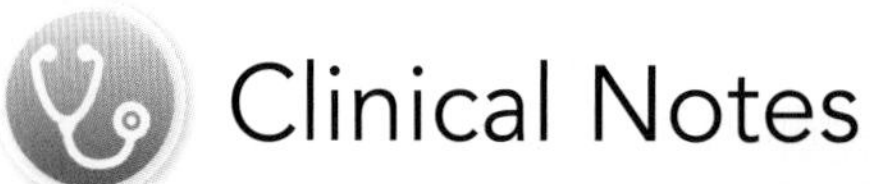

Joint Changes with Pregnancy

During pregnancy, the symphysis pubis and the ligaments of the sacroiliac and sacrococcygeal joints undergo softening in response to hormones, thus increasing their mobility and increasing the potential size of the pelvis during childbirth. The hormones responsible are estrogen and progesterone produced by the ovary and the placenta. An additional hormone, called relaxin, produced by these organs can also have a relaxing effect on the pelvic ligaments.

Joint Changes with Age

Obliteration of the cavity in the sacroiliac joint occurs in both sexes after middle age.

Sacroiliac Joint Disease

The sacroiliac joint is innervated by the lower lumbar and sacral nerves so that disease in the joint can produce low back pain and pain referred along the sciatic nerve (sciatica).

The sacroiliac joint is inaccessible to clinical examination. However, the joint comes closest to the surface at a small area located just medial to and below the posterior superior iliac spine. In disease of the lumbosacral region, movements of the vertebral column in any direction cause pain in the lumbosacral part of the column. In sacroiliac disease, pain is extreme on rotation of the vertebral column and is worst at the end of flexion. The latter movement causes pain because the hamstring muscles hold the hip bones in position, while the sacrum is rotating forward as the vertebral column is flexed.

Biologic Sex Differences

The bony pelvis exhibits several easily recognized anatomic differences related to biologic sex. The more obvious differences result from the adaptation of the female pelvis for childbearing. The stronger muscles in the male are responsible for the thicker bones and more prominent bony markings (Fig. 6.14; see also Fig. 6.1):

- The false pelvis is shallow in the female and deep in the male.
- The pelvic inlet is transversely oval in the female, but heart shaped in the male because of the indentation produced by the promontory of the sacrum in the male.
- The pelvic cavity is larger in the female, and the distance between the inlet and the outlet is much shorter.
- The pelvic outlet is larger in the female. The ischial spines are everted in the female but inverted in the male.
- The sacrum is shorter, wider, and flatter in the female.
- The subpubic angle, or pubic arch, is more rounded and wider in the female.

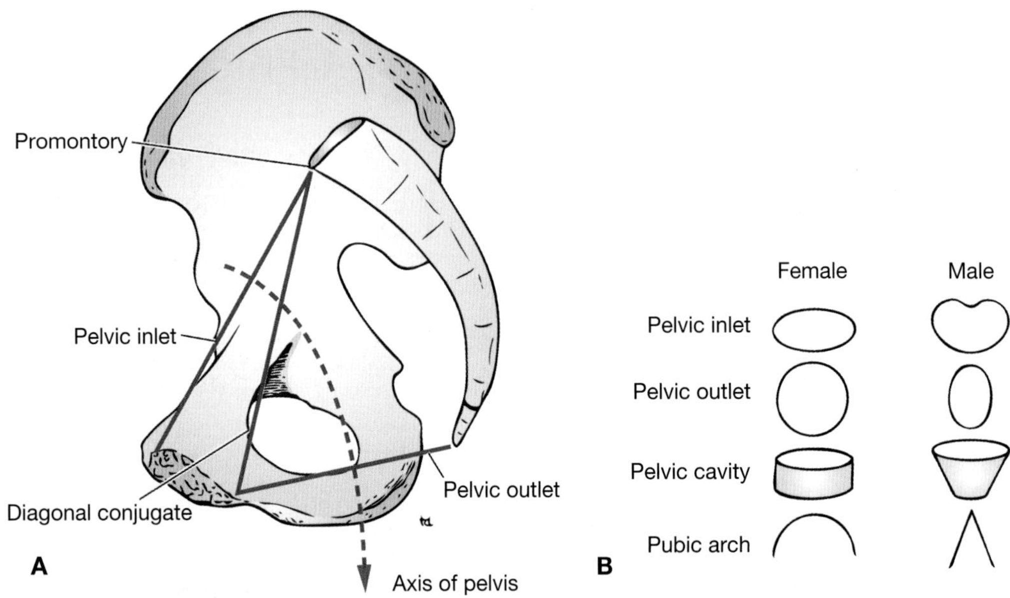

Figure 6.14 **A.** Pelvic inlet, pelvic outlet, diagonal conjugate, and axis of the pelvis. **B.** Some of the main differences between the female and the male pelvis.

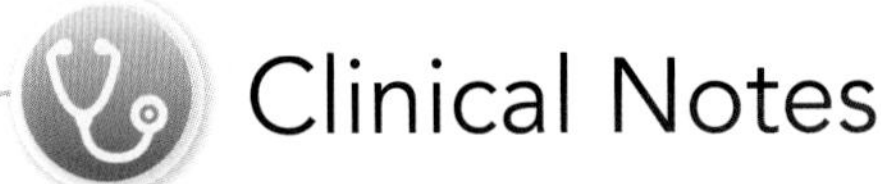

Clinical Notes

Clinical Concept: Pelvis Is a Basin with Holes in Its Walls

Bones and ligaments form much of the walls of the pelvis; these are partly lined with muscles (obturator internus and piriformis) covered with fascia and parietal peritoneum. The attachments of the gluteal muscles and the obturator externus muscle are on the outside of the pelvis. Thus, the greater part of the bony pelvis is sandwiched between inner and outer muscles.

The basin has anterior, posterior, and lateral walls and an inferior wall (floor) formed by the levator ani and coccygeus muscles and their covering fascia.

The basin has several holes. The posterior wall has holes on the anterior surface of the sacrum, the **anterior sacral foramina**, for the passage of the anterior rami of the sacral spinal nerves. The sacrotuberous and sacrospinous ligaments convert the greater and lesser sciatic notches into the **greater** and **lesser sciatic foramina**. The greater sciatic foramen provides an exit from the true pelvis into the gluteal region for the piriformis muscle, sciatic nerve, pudendal nerve, and gluteal nerves and vessels. The lesser sciatic foramen provides an entrance into the perineum from the gluteal region for the pudendal nerve and internal pudendal vessels.

The lateral pelvic wall has a large hole, the **obturator foramen**, which is closed by the obturator membrane, except for a small opening that permits the obturator nerve and vessels to leave the pelvis and enter the thigh.

Pelvic Measurements in Obstetrics

The capacity and shape of the female pelvis are of fundamental importance in obstetrics. The female pelvis is well adapted for the process of childbirth. The pelvis is shallower, and the bones are smoother than in the male. The size of the pelvic inlet is similar in the two sexes, but in the female, the cavity is larger and cylindrical, and the pelvic outlet is wider in both the anteroposterior and the transverse diameters.

Four terms relating to areas of the pelvis are commonly used in clinical practice:

- The **pelvic inlet (pelvic brim)** (see Fig. 6.14) is bounded anteriorly by the symphysis pubis, laterally by the iliopectineal lines, and posteriorly by the sacral promontory.
- The **pelvic outlet** of the true pelvis (see Fig. 6.14) is bounded in front by the pubic arch, laterally by the ischial tuberosities, and posteriorly by the coccyx. The sacrotuberous ligaments also form part of the margin of the outlet.
- The **pelvic cavity** is the space between the inlet and the outlet (see Fig. 6.14).
- The **axis of the pelvis** is an imaginary line joining the central points of the anteroposterior diameters from the inlet to the outlet and is the curved course taken by the infant's head as it descends through the pelvis during childbirth (Fig. 6.15; see also Fig. 6.14).

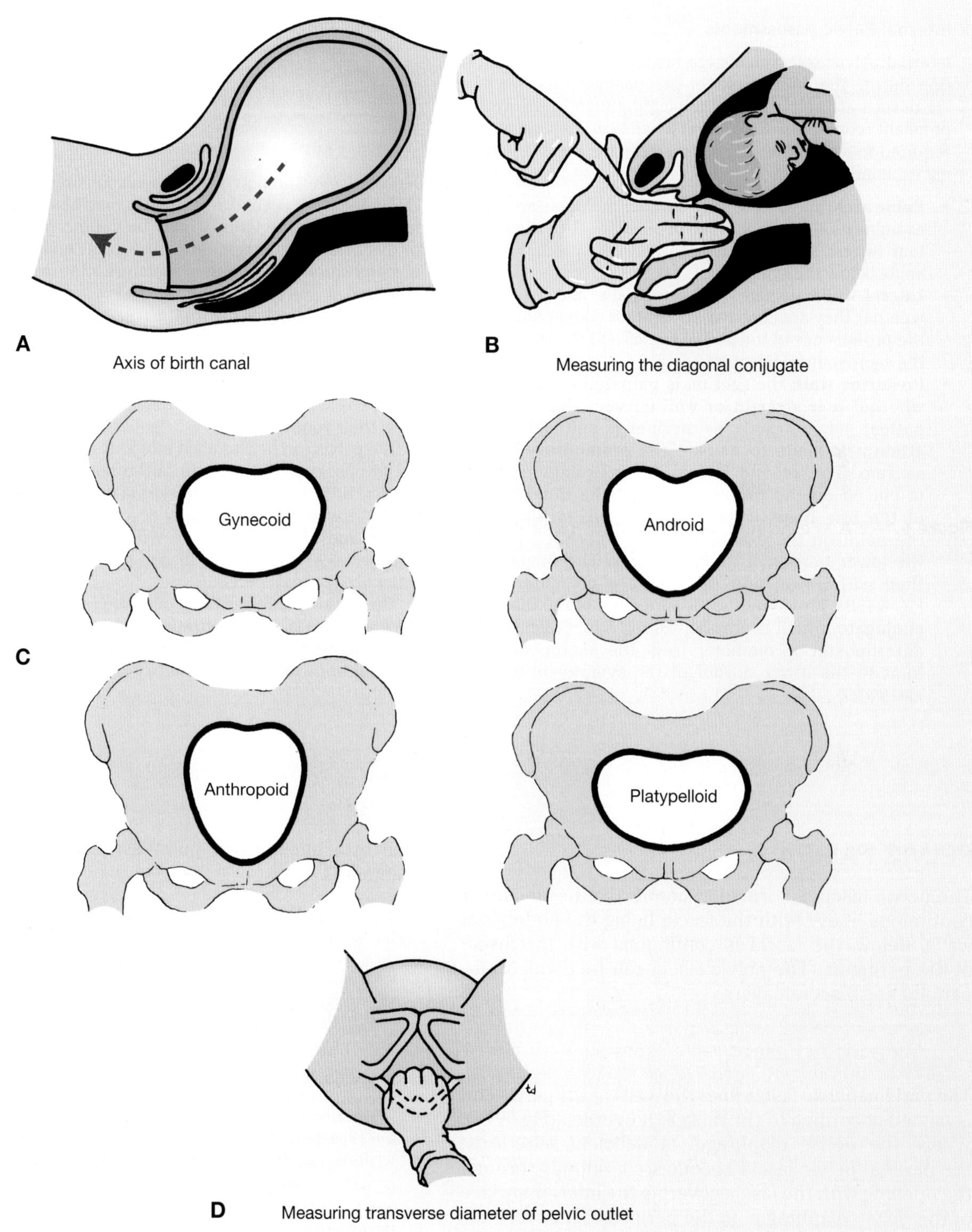

Figure 6.15 **A.** Birth canal. The *interrupted line* indicates the axis of the canal. **B.** Procedure used in measuring the diagonal conjugate. **C.** Different types of pelvic inlets, according to Caldwell and Moloy. **D.** Estimation of the width of the pelvic outlet by a closed fist.

(continued)

Internal Pelvic Assessments

Internal pelvic assessments are made by vaginal examination during the later weeks of pregnancy, when the pelvic tissues are softer and more yielding than in the newly pregnant condition. Considerable clinical experience is required to assess the shape and size of the pelvis by vaginal examination:

- **Pubic arch:** spread the fingers under the pubic arch and examine its shape. Is it broad or angular? The examiner's four fingers should be able to rest comfortably in the angle below the symphysis.
- **Lateral walls:** palpate the lateral walls, and determine whether they are concave, straight, or converging. Note the prominence of the ischial spines and the position of the sacrospinous ligaments.
- **Posterior wall:** the sacrum is palpated to determine whether it is straight or well curved. Finally, if the patient has relaxed the perineum sufficiently, an attempt is made to palpate the promontory of the sacrum. The second finger of the examining hand is placed on the promontory, and the index finger of the free hand, outside the vagina, is placed at the point on the examining hand where it contacts the lower border of the symphysis. The fingers are then withdrawn, and the distance measured (see Fig. 6.15B), providing the measurement of the **diagonal conjugate**, which is normally about 5 in. (13 cm). The anteroposterior diameter from the sacrococcygeal joint to the lower border of the symphysis is then estimated.
- **Ischial tuberosities:** the distance between the ischial tuberosities may be estimated by using the closed fist (see Fig. 6.15D). It measures about 4 in. (10 cm), but it is difficult to measure exactly.

Female Pelvis

Deformities of the pelvis may be responsible for **dystocia** (difficult labor). A contracted pelvis may obstruct the normal passage of the fetus. It may be indirectly responsible for dystocia by causing conditions such as malpresentation or malposition of the fetus, premature rupture of the fetal membranes, and uterine inertia.

The cause of pelvic deformities may be congenital (rare) or acquired from disease, poor posture, or fractures caused by injury. Pelvic deformities are more common in those who have grown up in a poor environment and are undernourished. These patients may have had minor degrees of rickets in their youth.

The pelvis can be classified into four general morphological groups: gynecoid, android, anthropoid, and platypelloid (see Fig. 6.15C). The **gynecoid** type is the typical female pelvis (41%), which was previously described.

The **android** type (33% of White females and 16% of Black females) is the funnel-shaped pelvis with a contracted outlet like the male pelvis.

The **anthropoid** type (24% of White females and 41% of Black females) is long, narrow, and oval shaped.

The **platypelloid** type (~2%) is a wide pelvis flattened at the brim, with the promontory of the sacrum pushed forward.

PELVIC FASCIA

The pelvic fascia is formed of connective tissue and is continuous above with the fascia lining the abdominal walls. Below, the fascia is continuous with the fascia of the perineum. The pelvic fascia can be divided into parietal and visceral layers.

Parietal Pelvic Fascia

The parietal pelvic fascia lines the walls of the pelvis and is named according to the muscle it overlies (Fig. 6.16). Where the pelvic diaphragm is deficient anteriorly, the parietal pelvic fascia becomes continuous through the opening with the fascia covering the inferior surface of the pelvic diaphragm. In the perineum, it covers the perineal membrane and forms the fascia deep to that structure.

Visceral Pelvic Fascia

The visceral layer of pelvic fascia covers and supports all the pelvic viscera. In certain locations, the fascia thickens and extends from the viscus to the pelvic walls and provides added support. These fascial condensations are termed *ligaments* and are named according to their attachments (eg, pubovesical and sacrocervical ligaments).

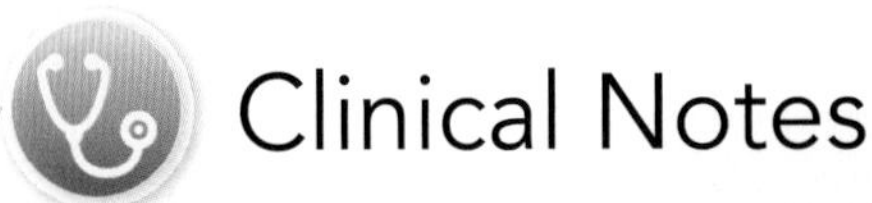

Cervical Fascial Ligaments

In the female, the fascial ligaments attached to the uterine cervix are of clinical importance because they assist with support of the uterus and thus prevent uterine prolapse. The visceral pelvic fascia around the uterine cervix and vagina is commonly referred to as the **parametrium**.

PELVIC PERITONEUM

The parietal peritoneum lines the pelvic walls and is reflected onto the pelvic viscera; it becomes continuous with the visceral peritoneum (see Fig. 6.16). Further details are provided later in this chapter.

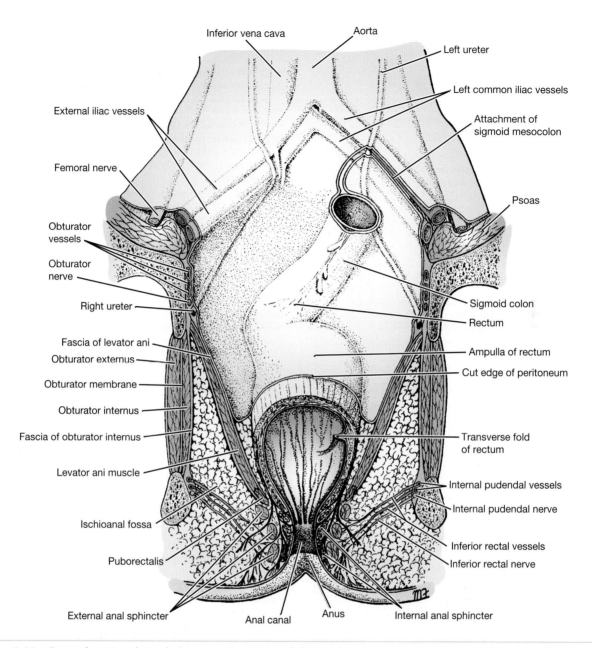

Figure 6.16 Coronal section through the posterior aspect of the pelvis.

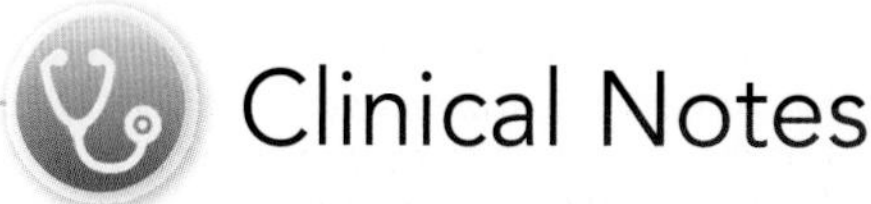

Clinical Notes

False Pelvis Fracture

Fractures of the false pelvis caused by direct trauma occasionally occur. The upper part of the ilium is seldom displaced because of the attachment of the iliacus muscle on the inside and the gluteal muscles on the outside.

True Pelvis Fracture

The mechanism of fractures of the true pelvis can be better understood if the pelvis is regarded not only as a basin but also as a rigid ring (Fig. 6.17). The ring is made up of the pubic rami, ischium, acetabulum, ilium, and sacrum, and it is joined by strong ligaments at the sacroiliac and symphyseal joints. If the ring breaks at any one point, the fracture will be stable, and no displacement will occur. However, if two breaks occur in the ring, the fracture will be unstable, and displacement will occur because the postvertebral and abdominal muscles will shorten and elevate the lateral part of the pelvis. The break in the ring may occur not as the result of a fracture but as the result of disruption of the sacroiliac or symphyseal joints. Fracture of the bone on

(continued)

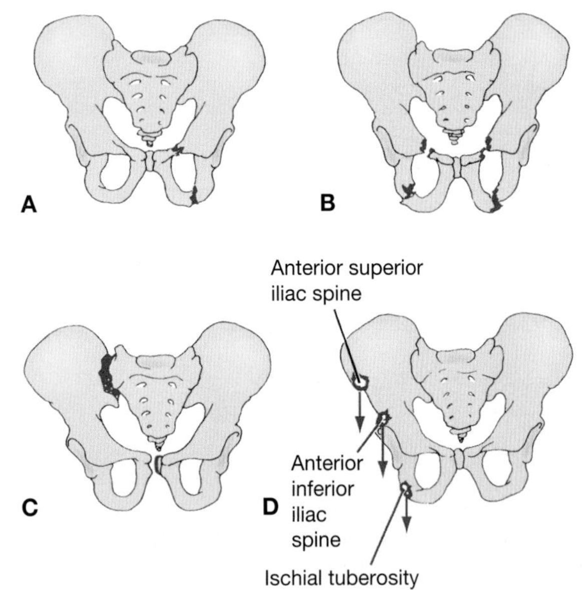

Figure 6.17 **A to C.** Different types of fractures of the pelvic basin. **D.** Avulsion fractures of the pelvis. The sartorius muscle is responsible for the avulsion of the anterior superior iliac spine; the straight head of the rectus femoris muscle, for the avulsion of the anterior inferior iliac spine; and the hamstring muscles, for the avulsion of the ischial tuberosity.

either side of the joint is more common than disruption of the joint.

The forces responsible for the disruption of the bony ring may be anteroposterior compression, lateral compression, or shearing.

Trauma to the true pelvis can result in fracture of the lateral mass of the sacrum. A heavy fall on the greater trochanter of the femur may drive the head of the femur through the floor of the acetabulum into the pelvic cavity.

Sacrococcygeal Fractures

Fractures of the lateral mass of the sacrum may occur as part of a pelvic fracture. Fractures of the coccyx are rare. However, **coccydynia** (coccygeal pain) is common and is usually caused by direct trauma to the coccyx, as in falling down a flight of stairs. The anterior surface of the coccyx can be palpated in a rectal examination.

Minor Pelvic Fractures

The anterior superior iliac spine may be pulled off by the forcible contraction of the sartorius muscle in athletes (see Fig. 6.17D). In a similar manner, the anterior inferior iliac spine may be avulsed by the contraction of the rectus femoris muscle. The ischial tuberosity can be avulsed by the contraction of the hamstring muscles. Healing may occur by fibrous union, possibly resulting in elongation of the muscle unit and some reduction in muscular efficiency.

Anatomy of Complications

Fractures of the true pelvis are commonly associated with injuries to the soft pelvic tissues.

If damaged, the thin pelvic veins—namely, the internal iliac veins and their tributaries—that lie in the parietal pelvic fascia beneath the parietal peritoneum can be the source of a massive hemorrhage, which may be life threatening.

The male urethra is often damaged, especially in vertical shear fractures that may disrupt the urogenital diaphragm (see Chapter 7).

The urinary bladder, which lies immediately behind the pubis in both sexes, is occasionally damaged by bone spicules. A full bladder is more likely to be injured than an empty bladder.

The rectum lies within the concavity of the sacrum and is protected and rarely damaged. However, fractures of the sacrum or ischial spine may be thrust into the pelvic cavity, tearing the rectum.

Nerve injuries can follow sacral fractures. The laying down of fibrous tissue around the anterior or posterior nerve roots or the branches of the sacral spinal nerves can result in persistent pain.

Damage to the sciatic nerve may occur in fractures involving the boundaries of the greater sciatic notch. The fibular (peroneal) part of the sciatic nerve is most often involved, resulting in the inability of a conscious patient to dorsiflex the ankle joint or failure of an unconscious patient to reflexively plantarflex (ankle jerk) the foot (see Chapter 8).

Pelvic Floor

The pelvic diaphragm is a gutter-shaped sheet of muscle formed by the levator ani and coccygeus muscles and their covering fasciae. The muscle fibers on the two sides slope downward and backward from their origins to the midline, producing a gutter that slopes downward and forward.

A rise in the intra-abdominal pressure, caused by the contraction of the diaphragm and the muscles of the anterior and lateral abdominal walls, is counteracted by the contraction of the muscles forming the pelvic floor. By this means, the pelvic viscera are supported and do not "drop out" through the pelvic outlet. Contraction of the puborectalis fibers greatly assists the anal sphincters in maintaining continence under these conditions by pulling the anorectal junction upward and forward. However, during the act of defecation, the levator ani continues to support the pelvic viscera, but the puborectalis fibers relax with the anal sphincters.

Female Pelvic Floor Functional Significance

The female pelvic floor serves an important function during the second stage of labor (Fig. 6.18). At the pelvic inlet, the widest diameter is transverse so that the longest axis of the infant's head (anteroposterior) takes up the transverse position. When the head reaches the pelvic floor, the gutter shape of the floor tends to cause the infant's head to rotate so that its long axis comes to lie in the anteroposterior position. The occipital part of the head now moves downward and forward along the gutter until it lies under the pubic arch. As the infant's head passes through the lower part of the birth canal, the small gap that exists in the anterior

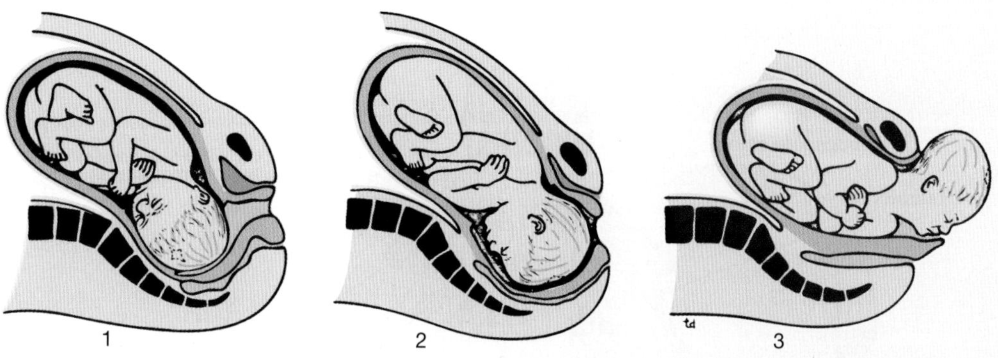

Figure 6.18 Stages in rotation of the infant's head during the second stage of labor. The shape of the pelvic floor plays an important part in this process.

part of the pelvic diaphragm becomes enormously enlarged so that the head may slip through into the perineum. Once the infant has passed through the perineum, the levator ani muscles recoil and take up their previous position.

Pelvic Floor Injury

Injury to the pelvic floor during a difficult delivery can result in loss of support for the pelvic viscera leading to **uterine** and **vaginal prolapse**, herniation of the bladder (**cystocele**), and alteration in the position of the bladder neck and urethra, leading to **stress incontinence**. In the latter condition, the patient dribbles urine whenever the intra-abdominal pressure is raised, as in coughing. **Prolapse of the rectum** may also occur.

Partial Fusion of Sacral Vertebrae

The S1 vertebra can be partly or completely separated from the S2 vertebra. Occasionally, on radiographs of the vertebral column, examples are seen in which the L5 vertebra has fused with the S1 vertebra (see Chapter 2, Sacralization of the L5 Vertebra).

PELVIC NERVES

Nerves derived from the lumbar and sacral plexuses and the sympathetic chain form extensive networks across the pelvic walls. These branches supply the pelvis and perineum, lower abdomen, and lower limb.

Lumbar Plexus

The lumbar plexus lies in the posterior abdominal wall (see Chapter 5). Two branches, the lumbosacral trunk and the obturator nerve, have notable relations to the pelvic walls.

Lumbosacral Trunk

Part of the anterior ramus of the L4 spinal nerve emerges from the medial border of the psoas muscle and joins the anterior ramus of the L5 nerve to form the **lumbosacral trunk** (Figs. 6.19 and 6.20). This trunk enters the pelvis by passing down in front of the sacroiliac joint and joins the sacral plexus.

Obturator Nerve

The obturator nerve is a branch of the lumbar plexus (L2 to L4). It emerges from the medial border of the psoas muscle in the abdomen and accompanies the lumbosacral trunk down into the pelvis (see Fig. 6.19). It crosses the front of the sacroiliac joint and runs forward on the lateral pelvic wall in the angle between the internal and external iliac vessels (see Fig. 6.11). On reaching the **obturator canal** (ie, the upper part of the obturator foramen, which is devoid of the obturator membrane), it splits into **anterior** and **posterior divisions** that pass through the canal to enter the adductor region of the thigh. The distribution of the obturator nerve in the thigh is considered in Chapter 8.

Pelvic Branches

Sensory branches supply the parietal peritoneum on the lateral wall of the pelvis.

Sacral Plexus

The sacral plexus lies on the posterior pelvic wall in front of the piriformis muscle (see Fig. 6.19). It is formed from the lumbosacral trunk (see above) and the anterior rami of the S1 to S4 nerves (see Fig. 6.20). The lumbosacral trunk passes down into the pelvis and joins the sacral nerves as they emerge from the anterior sacral foramina.

Relations

- **Anteriorly:** the internal iliac vessels and their branches and the rectum (see Fig. 6.11)
- **Posteriorly:** the piriformis muscle (see Fig. 6.19)

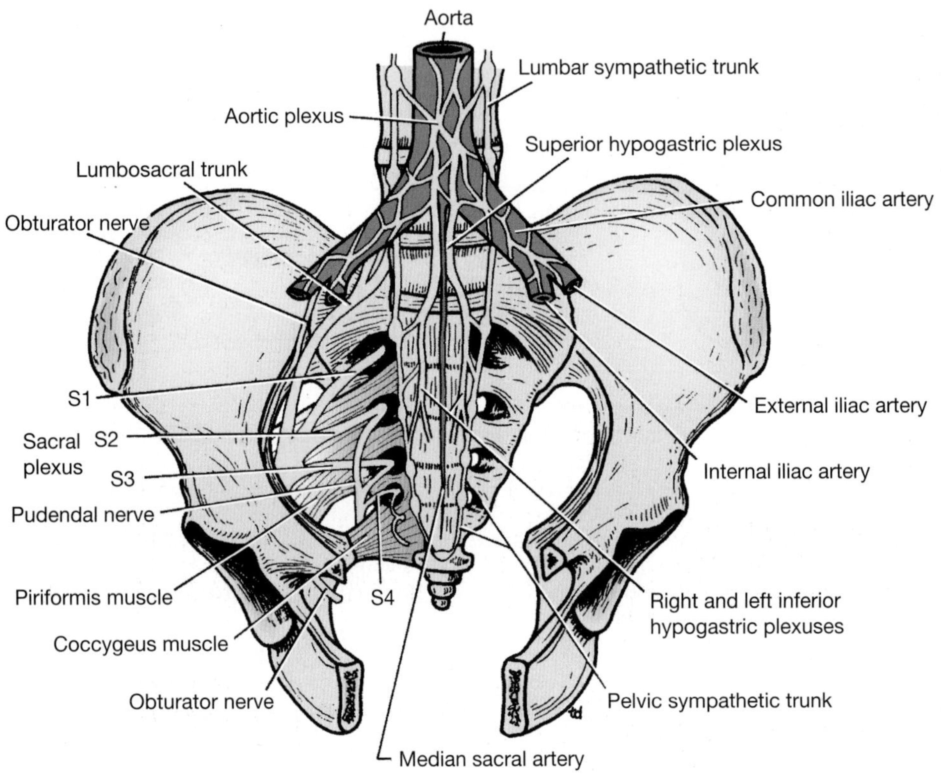

Figure 6.19 Posterior pelvic wall showing the sacral plexus, superior hypogastric plexus, and right and left inferior hypogastric plexuses. Pelvic parts of the sympathetic trunks are also shown.

Branches

The branches of the sacral plexus and their distribution are summarized in Table 6.2.

- Branches to the lower limb that leave the pelvis through the greater sciatic foramen (see Fig. 6.11):

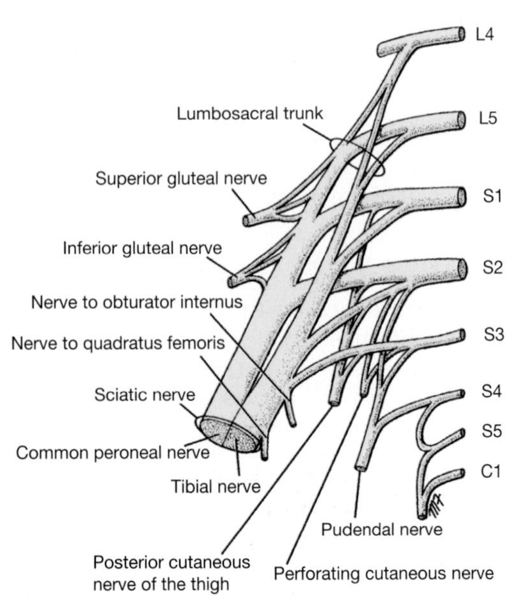

Figure 6.20 Sacral plexus.

1. **Sciatic nerve** (L4 and L5; S1 to S3) is the largest branch of the plexus and the largest nerve in the body (see Figs. 6.8 and 6.20).
2. **Superior gluteal nerve** supplies the gluteus medius and minimus and the tensor fasciae latae muscles.
3. **Inferior gluteal nerve** supplies the gluteus maximus muscle.
4. **Nerve to the quadratus femoris muscle** also supplies the inferior gemellus muscle.
5. **Nerve to the obturator internus muscle** also supplies the superior gemellus muscle.
6. **Posterior cutaneous nerve of the thigh** supplies the skin of the buttock and the back of the thigh.

- Branches to the pelvic muscles, pelvic viscera, and perineum (see Figs. 6.19 and 6.20):
  1. **Pudendal nerve** (S2 to S4) leaves the pelvis through the greater sciatic foramen and enters the perineum through the lesser sciatic foramen (see Fig. 6.11).
  2. **Nerve to the piriformis muscle** is a small branch to only this muscle.
  3. **Pelvic splanchnic nerves** constitute the sacral part of the parasympathetic system and arise from the S2 to S4 nerves. They are distributed mainly to the pelvic viscera.
- **Perforating cutaneous nerve** supplies the skin of the lower medial part of the buttock.

Table 6.2 Sacral Plexus Branches and Distribution

BRANCHES	DISTRIBUTION
Superior gluteal nerve	Gluteus medius, gluteus minimus, and tensor fasciae latae muscles
Inferior gluteal nerve	Gluteus maximus muscle
Nerve to piriformis	Piriformis muscle
Nerve to obturator internus	Obturator internus and superior gemellus muscles
Nerve to quadratus femoris	Quadratus femoris and inferior gemellus muscles
Perforating cutaneous nerve	Skin over medial aspect of the buttock
Posterior cutaneous nerve of the thigh	Skin over posterior surface of the thigh and popliteal fossa and also over the lower part of the buttock, scrotum, or labium majus
Sciatic nerve (L4 and L5; S1 to S3), tibial portion	Hamstring muscles (semitendinosus, biceps femoris [long head], adductor magnus [hamstring part]), gastrocnemius, soleus, plantaris, popliteus, tibialis posterior, flexor digitorum longus, flexor hallucis longus, and via medial and lateral plantar branches to muscles of sole of foot; sural branch supplies the skin on the lateral side of the leg and foot
Common fibular (peroneal) portion	Biceps femoris muscle (short head) and via deep fibular branch: tibialis anterior, extensor hallucis longus, extensor digitorum longus, fibularis tertius, and extensor digitorum brevis muscles; the skin over the cleft between the first and second toes. The superficial fibular branch supplies the fibularis longus and brevis muscles and the skin over the lower third of anterior surface of the leg and the dorsum of the foot
Pudendal nerve	Muscles of the perineum including the external anal sphincter, mucous membrane of the lower half of the anal canal, perianal skin, skin of the penis, scrotum, clitoris, and labia majora and minora

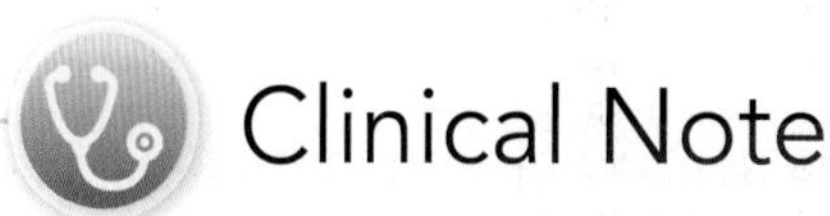

Nerve Pressure from Fetal Head

During the later stages of pregnancy, when the fetal head has descended into the pelvis, the patient often experiences discomfort or aching pain extending down one of the lower limbs. The discomfort, caused by pressure from the fetal head, is often relieved by changing position, such as lying on the side.

Nerve Invasion by Malignant Tumors

Malignant tumors extending from neighboring viscera can invade the sacral plexus or its branches. A carcinoma of the rectum, for example, can cause severe intractable pain down the lower limbs.

Referred Pain from Obturator Nerve

The obturator nerve lies on the lateral wall of the pelvis and supplies the parietal peritoneum. An inflamed appendix hanging down into the pelvic cavity could cause irritation of the obturator nerve endings, leading to referred pain down the inner side of the right thigh. Inflammation of the ovaries can produce similar symptoms.

Caudal Anesthesia (Analgesia)

Anesthetic solutions can be injected into the **sacral canal** through the **sacral hiatus**. The solutions then act on the spinal roots of the S2 to S5 and coccygeal segments of the cord as they emerge from the dura mater. The roots of higher spinal segments can also be blocked by this method. The needle must be confined to the lower part of the sacral canal because the meninges extend down as far as the lower border of the S2 vertebra. Caudal anesthesia is used in obstetrics to block pain fibers from the cervix and to anesthetize the perineum.

Autonomic Nerves

Sympathetic fibers derived from the sympathetic chain and parasympathetic fibers from the sacral nerves intertwine and form expansive plexuses on the pelvic walls and viscera. These autonomic fibers supply the pelvis, perineum, and hindgut.

Pelvic Part of Sympathetic Trunk

The pelvic part of the sympathetic trunk is continuous above, behind the common iliac vessels, with the abdominal part (see Fig. 6.19). It runs down behind the rectum on the front of the sacrum, medial to the anterior sacral foramina. The sympathetic trunk has four or five segmentally arranged ganglia. Below, the two trunks converge and finally unite in front of the coccyx.

Branches

- **Gray rami communicantes** to the sacral and coccygeal nerves
- **Fibers that join the hypogastric plexuses**

Pelvic Splanchnic Nerves

The pelvic splanchnic nerves form the parasympathetic part of the autonomic nervous system in the pelvis. The preganglionic fibers arise from the **S2 to S4 nerves** and synapse in ganglia in the inferior hypogastric plexus or in the walls of the viscera.

Some of the parasympathetic fibers ascend through the hypogastric plexuses and thence via the aortic plexus to the inferior mesenteric plexus. The fibers are then distributed along branches of the inferior mesenteric artery to supply the large bowel from the left colic flexure to the upper half of the anal canal.

Superior Hypogastric Plexus

The superior hypogastric plexus is situated in front of the promontory of the sacrum (see Fig. 6.19). It forms as a continuation of the aortic plexus and from branches of the L3 and L4 sympathetic ganglia. It contains sympathetic and sacral parasympathetic nerve fibers and visceral afferent nerve fibers. The superior hypogastric plexus divides inferiorly to form the **right** and **left hypogastric nerves**.

Inferior Hypogastric Plexuses

The inferior hypogastric plexuses lie on each side of the rectum, the base of the bladder, and the vagina (see Fig. 6.19). Each plexus is formed from a hypogastric nerve (from the superior hypogastric plexus) and from the pelvic splanchnic nerves. It contains postganglionic sympathetic fibers, preganglionic and postganglionic parasympathetic fibers, and visceral afferent fibers. Branches pass to the pelvic viscera via small subsidiary plexuses.

PELVIC ARTERIES

Several arteries stream across the pelvic walls. The common and external iliac arteries are related to the pelvic brim. The internal iliac, superior rectal, ovarian, and median sacral arteries run into the pelvic cavity. The arteries related to the pelvic walls are densely packed in the pelvic cavity and subject to significant variation in their branching patterns of origin. However, these vessels always terminate where they are supposed. Thus, identifying the individual arteries by their destinations is more reliable than by their origins.

Common Iliac Artery

Each common iliac artery ends at the pelvic inlet in front of the sacroiliac joint by dividing into the external and internal iliac arteries (see Figs. 6.11 and 6.19).

External Iliac Artery

The external iliac artery runs along the medial border of the psoas muscle, following the pelvic brim (see Fig. 6.11), and gives off the **inferior epigastric** and **deep circumflex iliac branches**. It leaves the false pelvis by passing under the inguinal ligament to become the **femoral artery**.

True Pelvis Arteries

The following arteries enter the pelvic cavity:

- **Internal iliac artery**
- **Superior rectal artery**
- **Ovarian artery**
- **Median sacral artery**

Internal Iliac Artery

The internal iliac artery passes down into the pelvis to the upper margin of the greater sciatic foramen, where it divides into anterior and posterior divisions (see Fig. 6.11). The branches of these divisions supply the pelvic viscera, perineum, pelvic walls, and the buttocks. The origin of the terminal branches is subject to variation, but the usual arrangement is shown in Diagram 6.1.

Anterior Division Branches

- **Umbilical artery:** the **superior vesical artery** arises from the proximal patent part of the umbilical artery. It supplies the upper portion of the bladder (see Fig. 6.11). It also gives off the **artery to the vas deferens**.
- **Obturator artery:** this artery runs forward along the lateral wall of the pelvis with the obturator nerve and leaves the pelvis through the obturator canal.

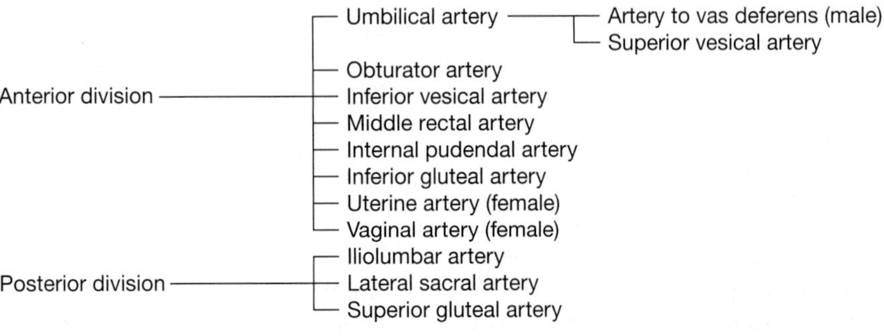

Diagram 6.1 Branches of the Internal Iliac Artery.

- **Inferior vesical artery:** this artery supplies the base of the bladder and the prostate and seminal vesicles in the male.
- **Middle rectal artery:** commonly, this artery arises with the inferior vesical artery (see Fig. 6.11). It supplies the muscle of the lower rectum and anastomoses with the **superior rectal** and **inferior rectal arteries**.
- **Internal pudendal artery:** this artery leaves the pelvis through the greater sciatic foramen and enters the gluteal region below the piriformis muscle (see Fig. 6.11). It then curls around the ischial spine (with the pudendal nerve) and enters the perineum by passing through the lesser sciatic foramen. It passes forward in the **pudendal canal** with the pudendal nerve. Its branches supply the musculature of the anal canal and the skin and muscles of the perineum.
- **Inferior gluteal artery:** this artery leaves the pelvis through the greater sciatic foramen below the piriformis muscle (see Fig. 6.11). It passes between the S1 and S2 or S2 and S3 nerves.
- **Uterine artery:** this artery runs medially on the floor of the pelvis and **crosses the ureter superiorly**. It passes above the **lateral fornix of the vagina** to reach the uterus. Here, it ascends between the layers of the broad ligament along the lateral margin of the uterus. It ends by following the uterine tube laterally, where it anastomoses with the ovarian artery. The uterine artery gives off a vaginal branch.
- **Vaginal artery:** this artery usually takes the place of the inferior vesical artery present in the male. It supplies the vagina and the base of the bladder.

Posterior Division Branches

- **Iliolumbar artery:** this artery ascends across the pelvic inlet posterior to the external iliac vessels, psoas, and iliacus muscles.
- **Lateral sacral arteries:** these arteries descend in front of the sacral plexus, giving off branches to neighboring structures and entering the anterior sacral foramina (see Fig. 6.11).
- **Superior gluteal artery:** this artery leaves the pelvis through the greater sciatic foramen above the piriformis muscle. It supplies the gluteal region.

Superior Rectal Artery

The superior rectal artery is a direct continuation of the **inferior mesenteric artery**. The name changes as the latter artery crosses the common iliac artery. It supplies the mucous membrane of the rectum and the upper half of the anal canal.

Ovarian Artery

The ovarian artery arises from the abdominal part of the aorta at the level of the L1 vertebra. The artery is long and slender and passes downward and laterally behind the peritoneum. It crosses the external iliac artery at the pelvic inlet and enters the **suspensory ligament of the ovary**. It then passes into the **broad ligament** and enters the ovary by way of the **mesovarium**. The **testicular artery** enters the inguinal canal and does not enter the pelvis.

Median Sacral Artery

The median sacral artery is a small artery that arises at the bifurcation of the aorta (see Fig. 6.19). It descends over the anterior surface of the sacrum and coccyx.

The distribution of the visceral branches of the pelvic arteries is discussed in detail with the individual viscera later in this chapter.

PELVIC VEINS

For the greater part, the pelvic veins correspond to the pelvic arteries. The **external iliac vein** begins behind the inguinal ligament as a continuation of the **femoral vein**. It runs along the medial side of the corresponding artery and joins the **internal iliac vein** to form the **common iliac vein** (see Fig. 6.11). It receives the **inferior epigastric** and **deep circumflex iliac veins**.

The **internal iliac vein** begins by the joining of tributaries that correspond to the branches of the internal iliac artery. It passes upward in front of the sacroiliac joint and joins the **external iliac vein** to form the **common iliac vein** (see Fig. 6.11).

The **median sacral veins** accompany the corresponding artery and end by joining the **left common iliac vein**.

PELVIC LYMPHATICS

The lymph nodes and vessels are arranged in a chain along the main blood vessels. The nodes are named after the blood vessels with which they are associated. Thus, there are external iliac nodes, internal iliac nodes, and common iliac nodes.

GASTROINTESTINAL TRACT

The sigmoid colon, rectum, and anal canal are the caudalmost parts of the GI tract. The sigmoid colon and rectum pass through the pelvic cavity, whereas the anal canal is largely contained in the perineum (and is reviewed in Chapter 7).

Sigmoid Colon

The sigmoid colon is 10 to 15 in. (25 to 38 cm) long and begins as a continuation of the **descending colon** in front of the pelvic brim (see Figs. 5.45, 5.131, and 5.132). It is continuous with the **rectum** below in front of the S3 vertebra. The sigmoid colon is mobile and hangs down into the pelvic cavity in the form of a roughly S-shaped loop. The fan-shaped **sigmoid mesocolon** attaches it to the posterior pelvic wall.

Relations

- **Anteriorly:** In the male, the urinary bladder. In the female, the posterior surface of the uterus and the upper part of the vagina.

- **Posteriorly:** The rectum and the sacrum. The sigmoid colon is also related to the lower coils of the terminal part of the ileum.

Blood Supply

Sigmoid branches of the inferior mesenteric artery supply the sigmoid colon (see Fig. 5.80). The accompanying veins drain into the **inferior mesenteric vein**, which joins the portal venous system (see Fig. 5.65).

Lymph Drainage

The lymph drains into nodes along the course of the sigmoid arteries. From these nodes, the lymph travels to the **inferior mesenteric nodes** (see Fig. 5.121).

Nerve Supply

The sympathetic and parasympathetic nerves from the **inferior hypogastric plexuses** (see Fig. 6.19).

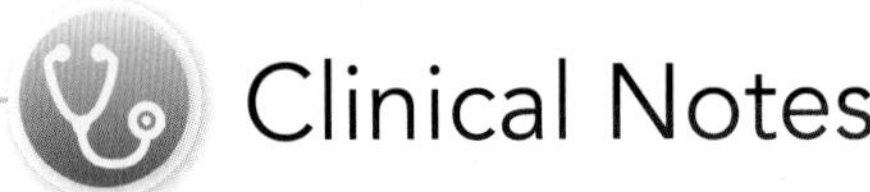

Clinical Notes

Sigmoid Colon Variation in Length and Location

The sigmoid colon shows great variation in length and may measure as much as 36 in. (91 cm). In the young child, because the pelvis is small, this segment of the colon may lie mainly in the abdomen.

Sigmoid Colon Cancer

The sigmoid colon is a common site for cancer of the large bowel. Because the lymphatic vessels of this segment of the colon drain ultimately into the inferior mesenteric nodes, an extensive resection of the gut and its associated lymphatic field is necessary to extirpate the growth and its local lymphatic metastases. The colon is removed from the left colic flexure to the distal end of the sigmoid colon, and the transverse colon is anastomosed to the rectum.

Volvulus

Because of its extreme mobility, the sigmoid colon sometimes rotates around its mesentery. This may correct itself spontaneously, or the rotation may continue until the blood supply of the gut is cut off completely. The rotation commonly occurs in a counterclockwise direction and is referred to as **volvulus**.

Diverticula

Diverticula of the mucous membrane along the course of the arteries supplying the sigmoid colon are a common clinical condition (see Chapter 5). In patients with diverticulitis or ulcerative colitis, the sigmoid colon may become adherent to the bladder, rectum, ileum, or ureter and produce an **internal fistula**.

Sigmoidoscopy

Examining the mucous membrane under direct vision for pathologic conditions is possible because the sigmoid colon lies only a short distance from the anus (6.5 in. [17 cm]). A flexible tube fitted with lenses and illuminated internally is introduced through the anus and carefully passed up through the anal canal, rectum, sigmoid colon, and descending colon. This examination, called **sigmoidoscopy**, can be carried out without an anesthetic in an outpatient clinic. Biopsy specimens of the mucous membrane can be obtained through this instrument.

Relevant Anatomic Facts

- The patient is placed in the left lateral position with their left knee flexed and their right knee extended (Fig. 6.21A). Alternatively, the patient is placed kneeling in the knee–chest position.
- The **sigmoidoscope** is gently inserted into the anus and anal canal in the direction of the umbilicus to ensure the instrument passes along the long axis of the canal (see Fig. 6.21B). Gentle but firm pressure is applied to overcome the resistance of the **anal sphincters** (Fig. 6.22).
- After about 1.5 in. (4 cm), the instrument enters the **ampulla of the rectum**. At this point, the tip of the sigmoidoscope

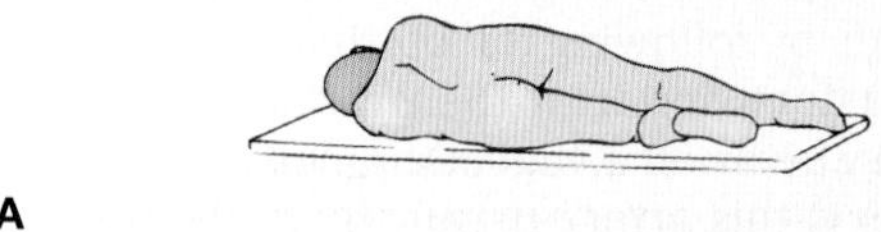

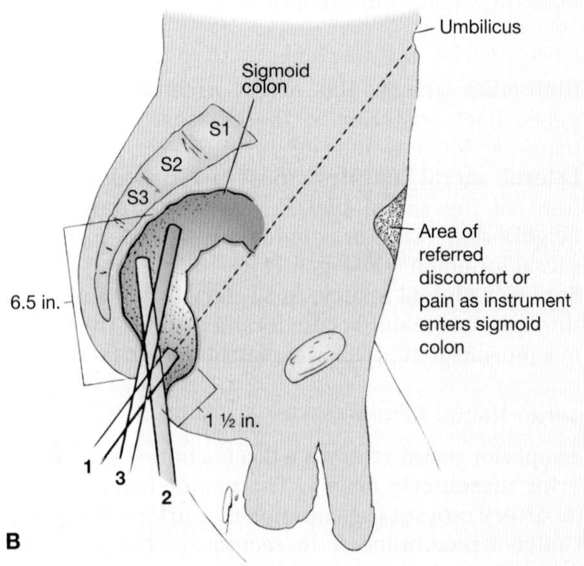

Figure 6.21 Sigmoidoscopy. **A.** Patient in the left lateral position with the left knee flexed and the right knee extended. **B.** Sagittal section of the male pelvis showing the positions (*1*, *2*, and *3*) of the tube of the sigmoidoscope relative to the patient as it ascends the anal canal and rectum. The area of discomfort or pain experienced by the patient as the tube is negotiated around the bend into the sigmoid colon is referred to the skin of the anterior abdominal wall below the umbilicus.

should be directed posteriorly in the midline to follow the **sacral curve of the rectum** (see Fig. 6.21B).
- Slow advancement is made under direct vision. Some slight side-to-side movement may be necessary to bypass the **transverse rectal folds** (see Fig. 6.22).
- At ~6.5 in. (16.25 cm) from the anal margin, the **rectosigmoid junction** will be reached. Here, the sigmoid colon bends forward and to the left, and the lumen appears to end in a blind cul-de-sac. To negotiate this angulation, the tip of the sigmoidoscope must be directed anteriorly and to the patient's left side. This maneuver can cause some discomfort in the anal canal from distortion of the anal sphincters by the shaft of the sigmoidoscope. Another possibility is that the point of the instrument may stretch the wall of the colon, giving rise to colicky pain in the lower abdomen.
- Once the instrument has entered the sigmoid colon, it should be possible to pass it smoothly along its full extent and, using the full length of the sigmoidoscope, enter the descending colon.
- The sigmoidoscope may now be slowly withdrawn, carefully inspecting the mucous membrane. The normal rectal and colonic mucous membrane is smooth and glistening and pale pink with an orange tinge, and blood vessels in the submucosa can be clearly seen. The mucous membrane is supple and moves easily over the end of the sigmoidoscope.

Anatomy of Complications

Perforation of the bowel at the rectosigmoid junction can occur. This is almost invariably caused by the operator failing to negotiate the curve between the rectum and the sigmoid colon. In some patients, the curve forms an acute angulation, which may frustrate the overzealous advancement of the sigmoidoscope. Perforation of the sigmoid colon results in the escape of colonic contents into the peritoneal cavity.

Colonoscopy

Direct visual inspection of the lining of the entire colon including the cecum (**colonoscopy**) has become an important weapon in the early diagnosis of mucosal polyps and large bowel cancer. Not only can the colon be observed and suspicious areas photographed for future reference, but also biopsy specimens can be removed for pathologic examination (see Fig. 5.82).

Following a regime in which the large bowel is thoroughly washed out, the patient is relaxed under a light anesthetic. The flexible endoscopic tube is introduced through the anus into the anal canal, rectum, and colon. Colonoscopy can also be used in the diagnosis and treatment of ulcerative colitis and Crohn disease.

Colostomy

The sigmoid colon is often selected as a site for performing a colostomy in patients with carcinoma of the rectum. Its mobility allows the surgeon to bring out a loop of colon, with its blood supply intact, through a small incision in the left iliac region of the anterior abdominal wall. Its mobility also makes it suitable for implantation of the ureters after surgical removal of the bladder.

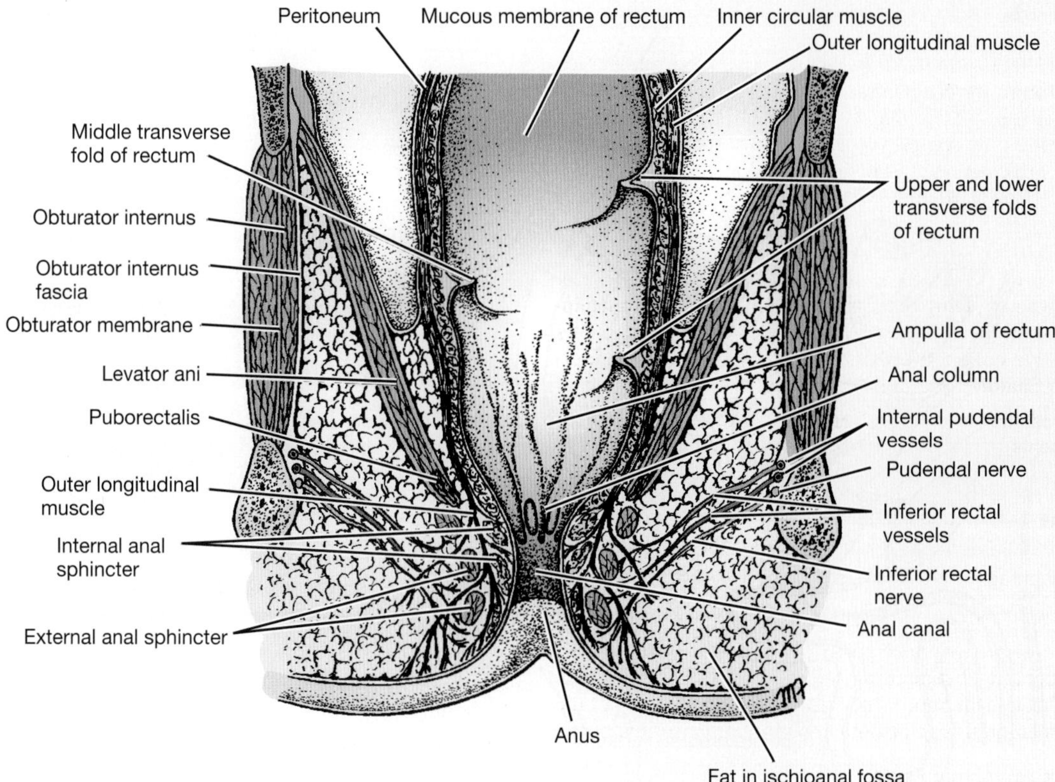

Figure 6.22 Coronal section through the pelvis showing the rectum and pelvic floor.

Rectum

The rectum is about 5 in. (13 cm) long and begins in front of the **S3 vertebra** as a continuation of the sigmoid colon (Figs. 6.23 and 6.24). It passes downward, following the curve of the sacrum and coccyx, and ends in front of the tip of the coccyx by piercing the pelvic diaphragm and becoming continuous with the **anal canal**. The lower part of the rectum is dilated to form the **rectal ampulla** (see Fig. 6.22).

The rectum deviates to the left but quickly returns to the median plane. On lateral view, the rectum follows the anterior concavity of the sacrum before bending downward and backward at its junction with the anal canal (see Figs. 6.23 and 6.24).

The puborectalis portion of the levator ani muscles forms a sling at the junction of the rectum with the anal canal and pulls this part of the bowel forward, producing the **anorectal angle** (also see Chapter 7).

The **peritoneum** covers the anterior and lateral surfaces of the first third of the rectum and only the anterior surface of the middle third, leaving the lower third devoid.

The **muscular coat** of the rectum is arranged in the usual outer longitudinal and inner circular layers of smooth muscle. However, the three **teniae coli** of the sigmoid colon come together so that the longitudinal fibers form a broad band on the anterior and posterior surfaces of the rectum.

The **mucous membrane** of the rectum, together with the circular muscle layer, forms two or three semicircular permanent folds called the **transverse folds of the rectum** (Fig. 6.25; see also Fig. 6.22). They vary in position.

Relations

- **Posteriorly:** The rectum is in contact with the sacrum and coccyx; piriformis, coccygeus, and levator ani muscles; sacral plexus; and sympathetic trunks (see Figs. 6.19, 6.23, and 6.24).
- **Anteriorly:** In the **male,** the upper two thirds of the rectum, which is covered by peritoneum, is related to the sigmoid colon and coils of ileum that occupy the **rectovesical pouch**. The lower third of the rectum, which is devoid of peritoneum, is related to the posterior surface of the bladder, to the termination of the vas deferens and the seminal vesicles on each side, and to the prostate (see Fig. 6.23). In the **female**, the upper two thirds of the rectum, which is covered by peritoneum, is related to the sigmoid colon and coils of ileum that occupy the **rectouterine pouch** (pouch of Douglas). The lower third of the rectum, which is devoid of peritoneum, is related to the posterior surface of the vagina (see Fig. 6.24).

Blood Supply

Multiple arteries from different sources and multiple veins with different terminations provide the rectal vasculature. Both the arteries and veins anastomose freely with their neighbors.

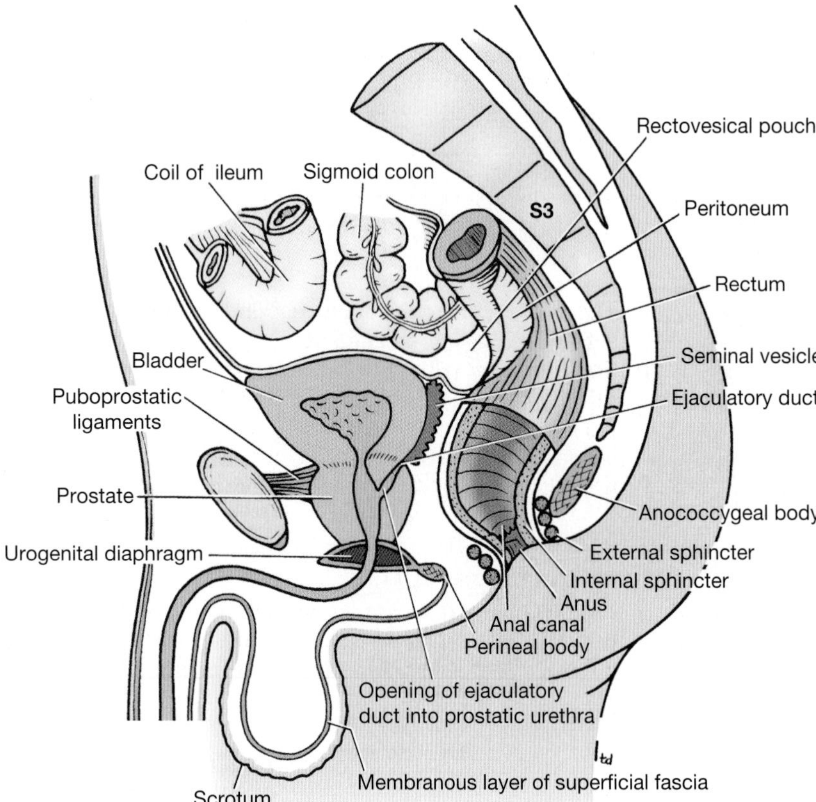

Figure 6.23 Sagittal section of the male pelvis.

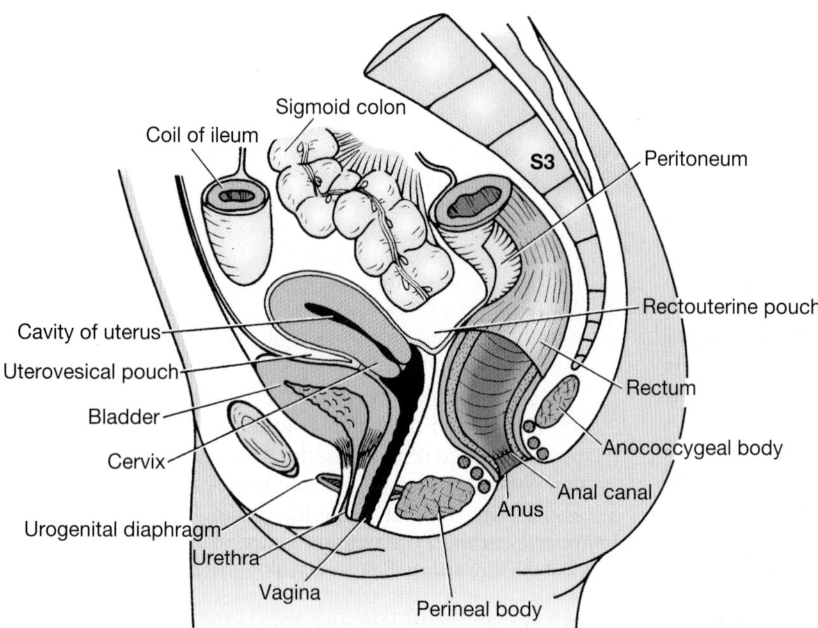

Figure 6.24 Sagittal section of the female pelvis.

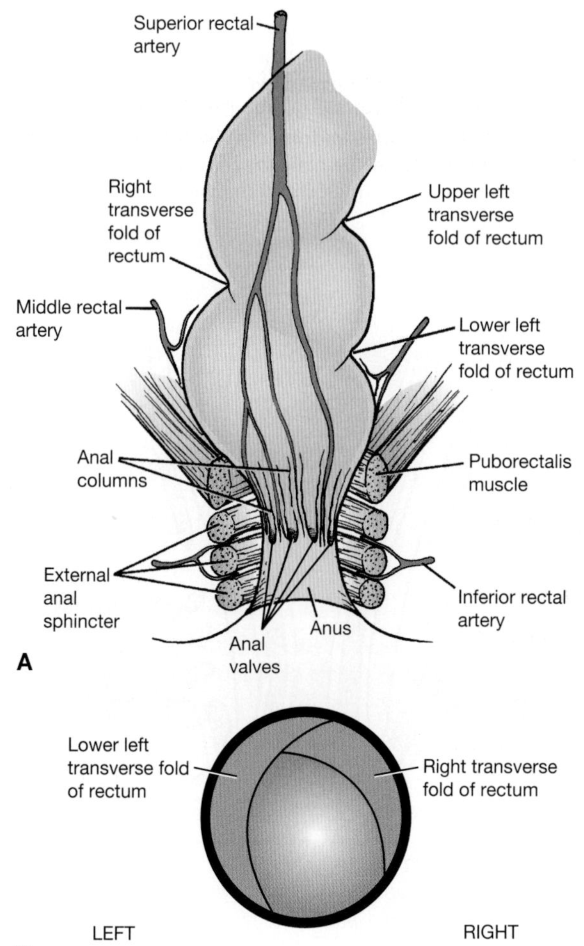

Figure 6.25 **A.** Blood supply to the rectum. **B.** Transverse folds of the rectum as seen through a sigmoidoscope.

Arteries

The superior, middle, and inferior rectal arteries (see Fig. 6.25) supply the rectum. The **superior rectal artery** is a direct continuation of the inferior mesenteric artery and is the chief artery supplying the mucous membrane. It enters the pelvis by descending in the root of the sigmoid mesocolon and divides into right and left branches, which pierce the muscular coat and supply the mucous membrane. They anastomose with one another and with the middle and inferior rectal arteries.

The **middle rectal artery** is a small branch of the internal iliac artery and is distributed mainly to the muscular coat.

The **inferior rectal artery** is a branch of the internal pudendal artery in the perineum. It anastomoses with the middle rectal artery at the anorectal junction.

Veins

The veins of the rectum correspond to the arteries. The **superior rectal vein** is a tributary of the portal circulation and drains into the inferior mesenteric vein. The **middle** and **inferior rectal veins** drain into the internal iliac and internal pudendal veins, respectively. The union between the rectal veins forms an important **anorectal portal–systemic anastomosis** (see Fig. 5.120).

Lymph Drainage

The lymph vessels of the upper rectum drain first into the pararectal nodes and then into **inferior mesenteric nodes**. Lymph vessels from the lower part of the rectum follow the middle rectal artery to the **internal iliac nodes**.

Nerve Supply

The nerve supply is from the sympathetic and parasympathetic nerves from the **inferior hypogastric plexuses** (see Fig. 6.19). The rectum is sensitive only to stretch.

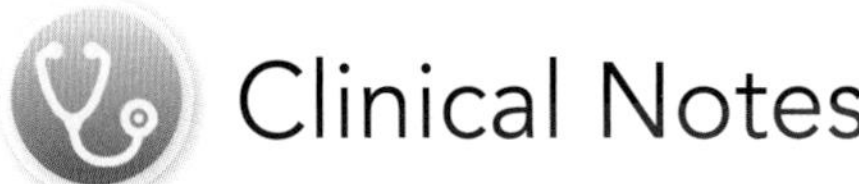

Clinical Notes

Rectal Curves and Mucosal Folds

To avoid causing the patient unnecessary discomfort when passing a sigmoidoscope, remember the anteroposterior flexure of the rectum, as it follows the curvature of the sacrum and coccyx, and the lateral flexures.

The crescentic **transverse mucosal folds of the rectum** must also be borne in mind when passing an instrument into the rectum. These folds likely serve to support the weight of the feces and to prevent excessive distention of the rectal ampulla.

Blood Supply and Internal Hemorrhoids

The chief arterial supply to the rectum is from the **superior rectal artery**, a continuation of the inferior mesenteric artery. In front of the S3 vertebra, the artery divides into right and left branches (see Fig. 6.25). Halfway down the rectum, the right branch divides into an anterior and a posterior branch. The tributaries of the **superior rectal vein** are arranged in a similar manner, so it is not surprising to find that **internal hemorrhoids** are arranged in three groups (see Chapter 7): two on the right side of the lower rectum and anal canal and one on the left.

Partial and Complete Rectal Prolapse

Partial and complete prolapses of the rectum through the anus are relatively common clinical conditions. In **partial prolapse**, the rectal mucous membrane and submucous coat protrude for a short distance outside the anus (Fig. 6.26A). In **complete prolapse**, the whole thickness of the rectal wall protrudes through the anus (Fig. 6.26B). In both conditions, many causative factors may be involved. However, damage to the levator ani muscles from childbirth and poor muscle tone in older adults are important contributing factors. A complete rectal prolapse may be regarded as a **sliding hernia** through the pelvic diaphragm.

Rectal Cancer

Cancer (carcinoma) of the rectum is a common clinical finding that remains localized to the rectal wall for a considerable time. At first, it tends to spread locally in the lymphatics around the circumference of the bowel. Later, it spreads upward and laterally along the lymph vessels, following the superior rectal and middle rectal arteries. Venous spread occurs late, and, because the superior rectal vein is a tributary of the portal vein, the liver is a common site for secondary deposits.

Once the malignant tumor has extended beyond the confines of the rectal wall, knowledge of the anatomic relations of the rectum enables a physician to assess the structures and organs likely to be involved. In both sexes, a **posterior penetration** involves the sacral plexus and can cause severe intractable pain down the leg in the distribution of the sciatic nerve. A **lateral penetration** may involve the ureter. An **anterior penetration** in the male may involve the prostate, seminal vesicles, or bladder; in the female, the vagina and uterus may be invaded.

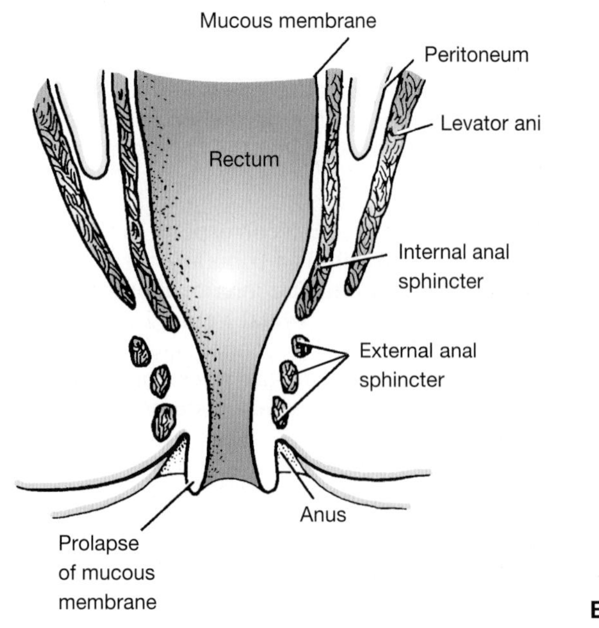

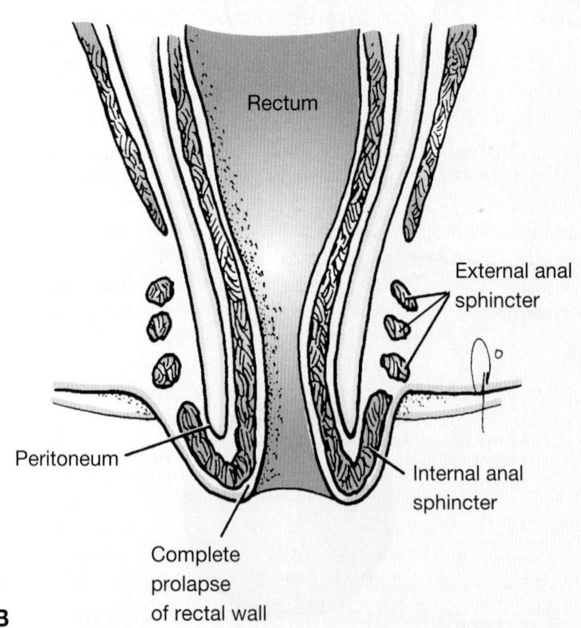

Figure 6.26 Coronal section of the rectum and anal canal. **A.** Incomplete rectal (mucosal) prolapse. **B.** Complete rectal prolapse.

It is clear from the anatomic features of the rectum and its lymph drainage that a wide resection of the rectum with its lymphatic field offers the best chance of cure. When the tumor has spread to contiguous organs and is of a low grade of malignancy, some form of pelvic evisceration may be justifiable.

It is most important for a medical student to remember that the interior of the lower part of the rectum can be examined by a gloved index finger introduced through the anal canal. The anal canal is about 1.5 in. (4 cm) long, so the pulp of the index finger can easily feel the mucous membrane lining the lower end of the rectum. Most cancers of the rectum can be diagnosed by this means. This examination can be extended in both sexes by placing the other hand on the lower part of the anterior abdominal wall. With the bladder empty, the anterior rectal wall can be examined bimanually. In the female, placing one finger in the vagina and another in the rectum may enable the physician to make a thorough examination of the lower part of the anterior rectal wall.

Rectal Injuries

The site of penetration relative to the peritoneal covering will determine the management of penetrating rectal injuries. The upper third of the rectum is covered by peritoneum on the anterior and lateral surfaces, the middle third is covered only on its anterior surface, and the lower third is devoid of a peritoneal covering (see Figs. 6.22 to 6.24). The treatment of penetration of the intraperitoneal portion of the rectum is identical to that of the colon because the peritoneal cavity has been violated. In the case of penetration of the extraperitoneal portion, the rectum is treated by diverting the feces through a temporary abdominal colostomy, administering antibiotics, and repairing and draining the tissue in front of the sacrum.

Pelvic Appendix

If an inflamed appendix is hanging down into the pelvis, abdominal tenderness in the right iliac region may not be felt, but deep tenderness may be experienced above the symphysis pubis. Rectal examination (males) or vaginal examination (females) may reveal tenderness of the peritoneum in the pelvis on the right side. If such an inflamed appendix perforates, a localized pelvic peritonitis may result.

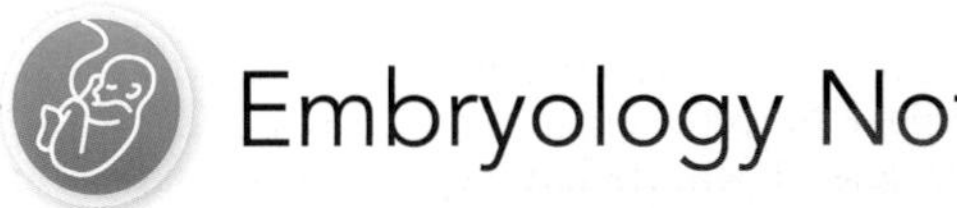

Embryology Notes

Distal Part of Large Bowel Development

The left colic flexure, descending colon, sigmoid colon, rectum, and upper half of the anal canal develop from the **hindgut**. Distally, this terminates as a blind sac of entoderm, which is in contact with a shallow ectodermal depression called the **proctodeum**. The apposed layers of ectoderm and entoderm form the **cloacal membrane**, which separates the cavity of the hindgut from the surface (Fig. 6.27). The hindgut sends off a diverticulum, the **allantois**, that passes into the umbilical cord. Distal to the allantois, the hindgut dilates to form the endodermal **cloaca**. A wedge of mesenchyme invaginates the entoderm in the interval between the allantois and the hindgut. With continued proliferation of the mesenchyme, a septum is formed that grows inferiorly and divides the cloaca into anterior and posterior parts. The septum is called the **urorectal septum**, the anterior part of the cloaca becomes the **primitive bladder** and the **urogenital sinus**, and the posterior part of the cloaca forms the **anorectal canal**. On reaching the cloacal membrane, the urorectal septum fuses with it and forms the future **perineal body**. Further development of the primitive bladder and the urogenital sinus in both sexes is considered in detail later in this chapter.

The anorectal canal forms the **rectum** and the **superior half of the anal canal**. The lining of the inferior half of the anal canal is formed from the ectoderm of the proctodeum (Fig. 6.28). The posterior part of the cloacal membrane breaks down so that the gut opens onto the surface of the embryo.

Hindgut Artery

The inferior mesenteric artery supplies the hindgut, which extends from the left colic flexure to halfway down the anal canal (see Fig. 5.91). Here, several ventral branches of the aorta fuse to form a single artery.

Meconium

At full term, the large intestine is filled with a mixture of intestinal gland secretions, bile, and amniotic fluid. This substance is dark green in color and is called **meconium**. It starts to accumulate at 4 months and reaches the rectum at 5 months.

Primary Megacolon (Hirschsprung Disease)

Hirschsprung disease shows a familial tendency and is more common in males. Symptoms usually appear during the first few days after birth. The newborn fails to pass meconium, and the abdomen becomes enormously distended. The sigmoid colon is greatly distended and hypertrophied, whereas the rectum and anal canal are constricted (Fig. 6.29). The constricted segment of the bowel causes the obstruction, usually because of a complete failure of development of the parasympathetic ganglion cells in this region. The treatment is operative excision of the aganglionic segment of the bowel.

(continued)

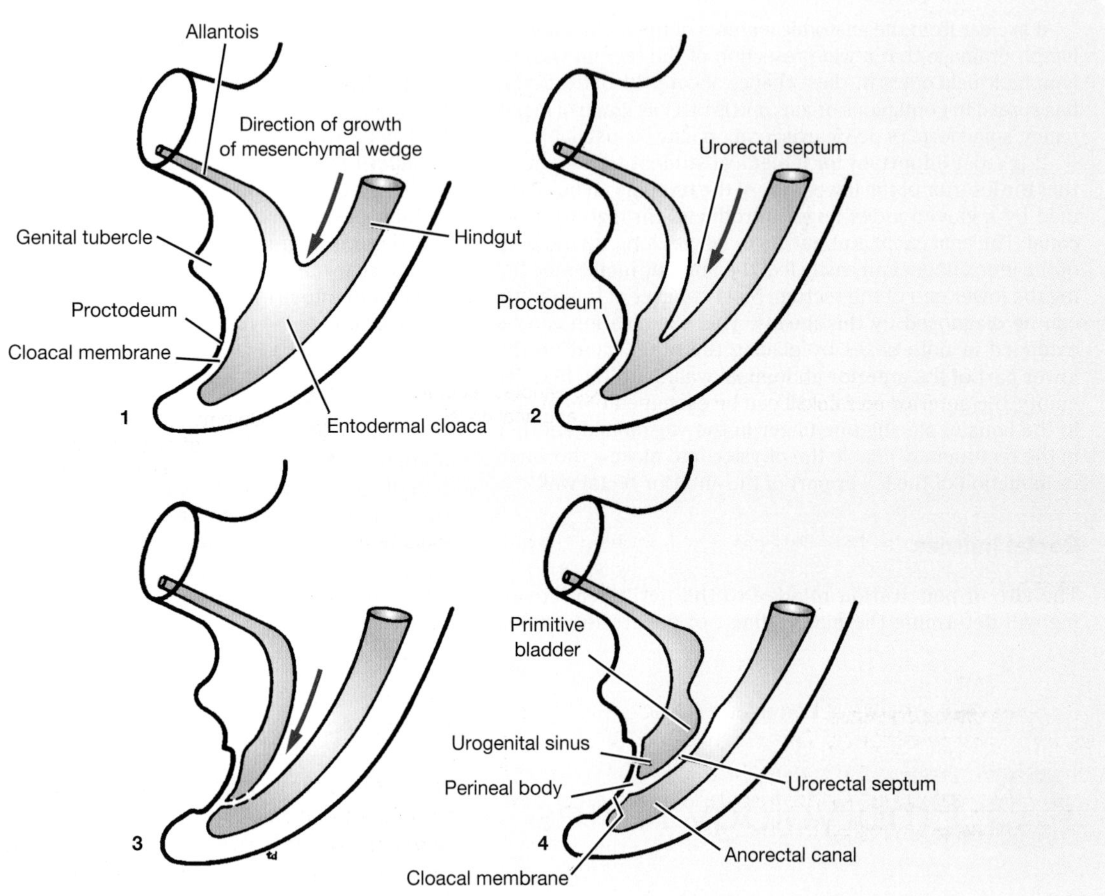

Figure 6.27 Progressive stages (1 to 4) in the formation of the urorectal septum, which divides the cloaca into an anterior part (primitive bladder and urogenital sinus) and a posterior part (anorectal canal).

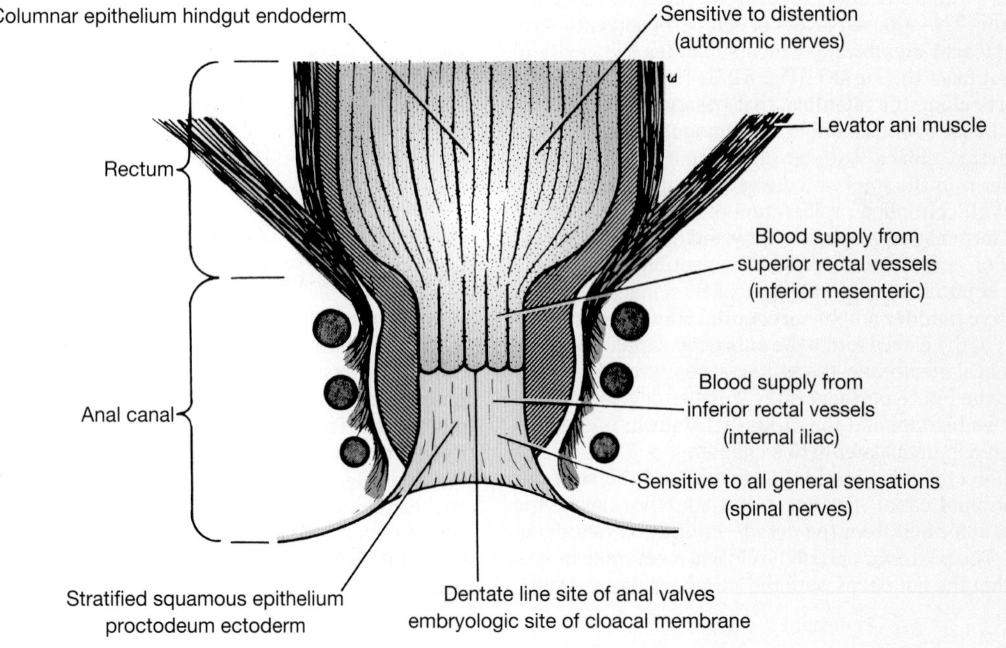

Figure 6.28 Structure of the anal canal and its embryologic origin.

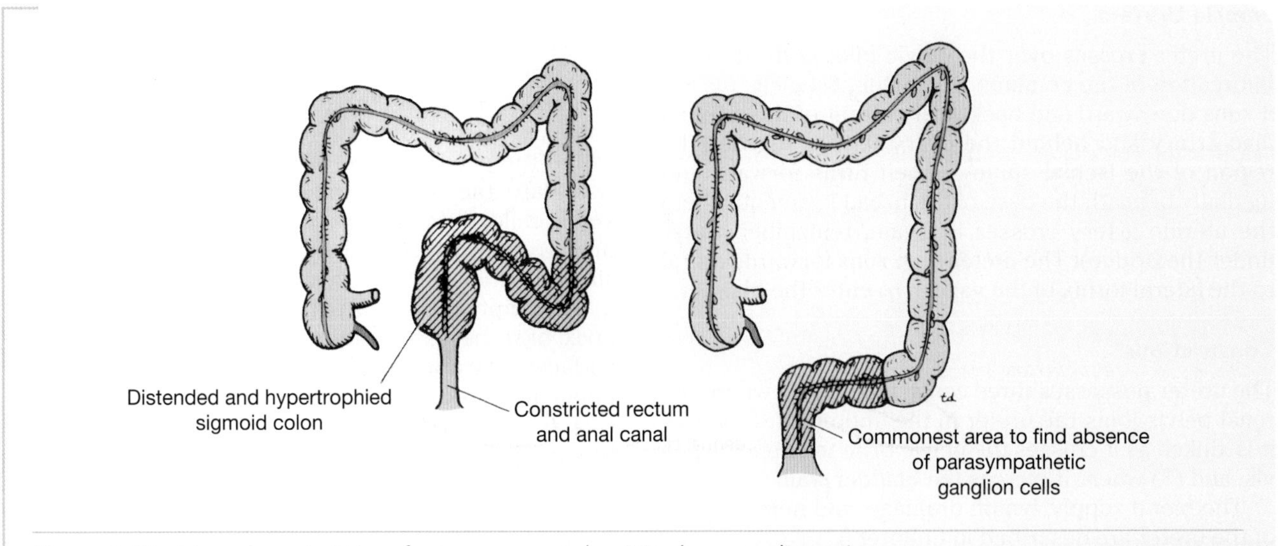

Figure 6.29 Main characteristics of primary megacolon (Hirschsprung disease).

URINARY TRACT

The pelvic components of the urinary tract are the ureters and urinary bladder. The urethra has both pelvic and perineal parts. Some aspects are covered in this chapter (eg, relations to the prostate), but most urethral anatomy is reviewed in Chapter 7.

Ureters

Each ureter is a muscular tube that extends from the kidney to the posterior surface of the bladder. Its abdominal course is described in Chapter 5.

Male Ureters

The ureter enters the pelvis by crossing the bifurcation of the common iliac artery in front of the sacroiliac joint (Fig. 6.30A). Each ureter then runs down the lateral wall of the pelvis in front of the internal iliac artery to the region of the ischial spine and turns forward to enter the lateral angle of the bladder. The vas deferens crosses over the ureter near the ureter's termination (remember, water under the bridge). The ureter passes obliquely through the wall of the bladder for about 0.75 in. (1.9 cm) before opening into the bladder.

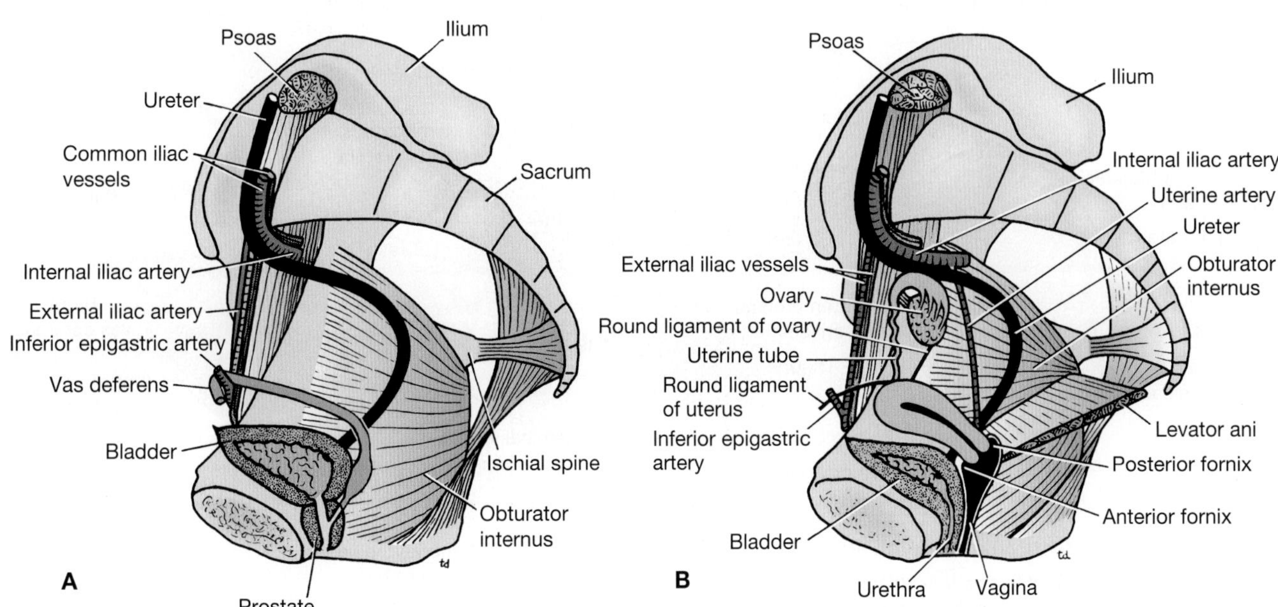

Figure 6.30 **A.** Right half of the male pelvis showing relations of the ureter and vas deferens. **B.** Right half of the female pelvis showing relations of the urinary and genital organs.

Female Ureters

The ureter crosses over the pelvic inlet in front of the bifurcation of the common iliac artery (see Fig. 6.30B). It runs downward and backward in front of the internal iliac artery and behind the ovary until it reaches the region of the ischial spine. It then turns forward and medially beneath the base of the broad ligament, where the uterine artery crosses it (again, remember, water under the bridge). The ureter then runs forward, lateral to the lateral fornix of the vagina, to enter the bladder.

Constrictions

The ureter possesses three constrictions: (1) where the renal pelvis joins the ureter in the abdomen, (2) where it is kinked as it crosses the pelvic brim to enter the pelvis, and (3) where it pierces the bladder wall.

The blood supply, lymph drainage, and nerve supply of the ureter are described in Chapter 5.

Urinary Bladder

The urinary bladder is situated immediately behind the pubic bones, within the pelvis, in both males and females (see Figs. 6.23, 6.24, and 6.30). It stores urine and, in the adult, has a maximum capacity of about 500 mL. The bladder has a strong muscular wall. Its shape and relations vary according to the amount of urine that it contains. In the adult, the empty bladder lies entirely within the pelvis. As the bladder fills, its superior wall rises into the hypogastric region (Fig. 6.31A). In the young child, the empty bladder projects above the pelvic inlet. Later, when the pelvic cavity enlarges, the bladder sinks into the pelvis to take up the adult position.

The empty bladder is pyramidal (Fig. 6.32), having an apex, base, neck, superior surface, and two inferolateral surfaces. The **apex** points anteriorly and lies behind the upper margin of the symphysis pubis (see Figs. 6.23, 6.24, 6.31, and 6.32A). It connects to the umbilicus by the **median umbilical ligament** (ie, the remains of the urachus).

The **base (posterior surface)** faces posteriorly and is triangular. The ureters join the **superolateral angles**, and the **inferior angle (neck)** gives rise to the **urethra** (see Fig. 6.32B).

Male Bladder

The two **vasa deferentia** lie side by side on the base of the bladder and separate the **seminal vesicles** from each other (see Fig. 6.32). The upper part of the base of the bladder is covered by peritoneum, which forms the anterior wall of the **rectovesical pouch**. The lower part

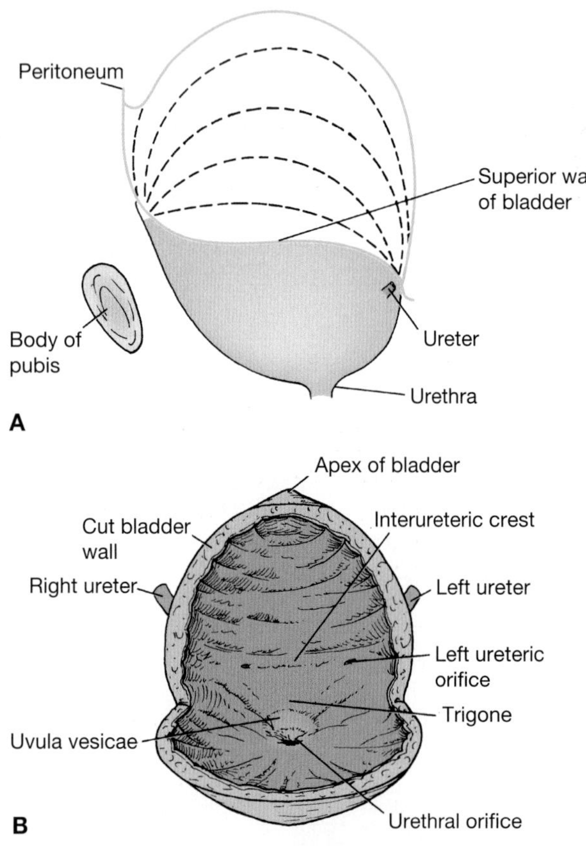

Figure 6.31 **A.** Lateral view of the bladder. Note that the superior wall rises as the viscus fills with urine. Note also that the peritoneum covering the superior surface of the bladder is peeled off from the anterior abdominal wall as the bladder fills. **B.** Interior of the bladder in the male as seen from in front.

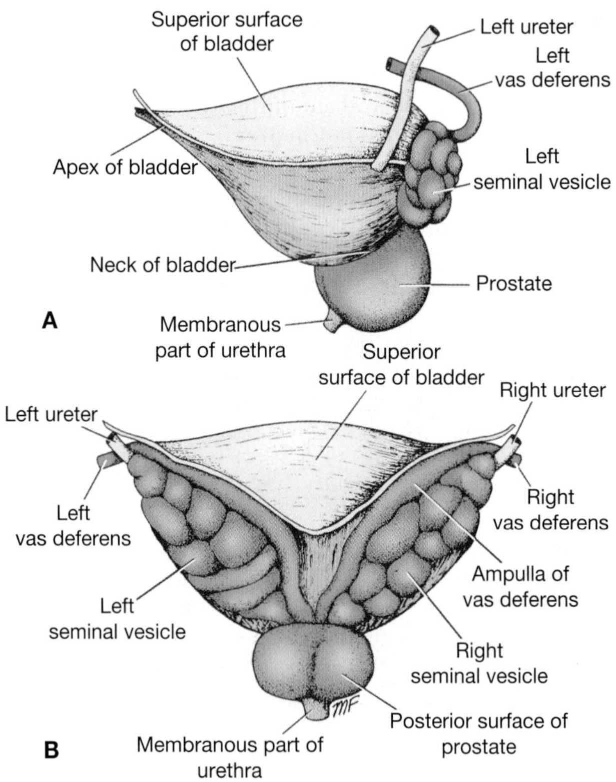

Figure 6.32 **A.** Lateral view of the bladder, prostate, and left seminal vesicle. **B.** Posterior view of the bladder, prostate, vasa deferentia, and seminal vesicles.

of the base is separated from the rectum by the vasa deferentia, seminal vesicles, and **rectovesical fascia** (see Fig. 6.23).

The **superior surface** of the bladder is covered with peritoneum and is related to coils of ileum or sigmoid solon. Along the lateral margins of this surface, the peritoneum passes to the lateral pelvic walls.

As the bladder fills, it becomes ovoid, and the superior surface bulges upward into the abdominal cavity (see Fig. 6.31A). The peritoneal covering is peeled off the lower part of the anterior abdominal wall so that the bladder comes into direct contact with the anterior abdominal wall.

The **inferolateral surfaces** are related in front to the **retropubic pad of fat** and the pubic bones. More posteriorly, they lie in contact with the obturator internus muscle above and the levator ani muscle below.

The **neck** of the bladder lies inferiorly and rests on the upper surface of the prostate gland (see Fig. 6.32). Here, the smooth muscle fibers of the bladder wall are continuous with those of the prostate. The neck of the bladder is held in position by the **puboprostatic ligaments** (males) or **pubovesical ligaments** (females). These ligaments are thickenings of the pelvic fascia.

When the bladder fills, the base and neck remain largely unchanged in position, but the superior surface rises into the abdomen, as described above.

The **mucous membrane** of the greater part of the empty bladder is thrown into folds that disappear when the bladder is full. The triangular area of mucous membrane covering the internal surface of the base of the bladder is called the **trigone**. Here, the mucous membrane is always smooth, even when the viscus is empty (see Fig. 6.31B), because the mucous membrane firmly adheres to the underlying muscular coat.

The **superior angles** of the trigone correspond to the openings of the ureters, and the **inferior angle** to the **internal urethral orifice**. The ureters pierce the bladder wall obliquely, and this provides a valvelike action, which prevents a reverse flow of urine toward the kidneys as the bladder fills.

The trigone is limited above by a muscular ridge, which runs from the opening of one ureter to that of the other and is known as the **interureteric crest** (**interureteric ridge**). The **uvula vesicae** are a small elevation situated immediately behind the urethral orifice, which is produced by the underlying median lobe of the prostate.

The muscular coat of the bladder is composed of smooth muscle and is arranged as three layers of interlacing bundles known as the **detrusor muscle**. The circular component of the muscle coat is thickened at the neck of the bladder to form the **sphincter vesicae** (**internal urethral sphincter**).

Female Bladder

The general shape and structure of the bladder, its blood supply, lymph drainage, nerve supply, and the process of micturition are identical to those in the male. Notable differences include the following.

Because of the absence of the prostate, the bladder lies at a lower level, and the neck rests directly on the upper surface of the urogenital diaphragm. The close relation of the bladder to the uterus and the vagina is of considerable clinical importance (see Fig. 6.24).

The apex of the bladder lies behind the symphysis pubis. The base is separated from the rectum by the vagina. The superior surface is related to the **uterovesical pouch** of peritoneum and to the body of the uterus.

Blood Supply

The **superior and inferior vesical arteries**, branches of the internal iliac arteries, supply the bladder (see Fig. 6.11).

The veins form the **vesical venous plexus** that drains into the internal iliac vein.

Lymph Drainage

The bladder drains to both the internal and external iliac nodes.

Nerve Supply

The sympathetic postganglionic fibers originate in the L1 and L2 chain ganglia and descend to the bladder via the **hypogastric plexuses** (see Fig. 6.19). The parasympathetic preganglionic fibers arise as the **pelvic splanchnic nerves** from the S2 to S4 nerves. They pass through the **inferior hypogastric plexuses** to reach the bladder wall, where they synapse with postganglionic neurons. Most **visceral afferent fibers** arising in the bladder reach the central nervous system (CNS) via the pelvic splanchnic nerves. Some afferent fibers travel with the sympathetic nerves via the hypogastric plexuses and enter the L1 and L2 segments of the spinal cord.

The parasympathetic nerves stimulate contraction of the detrusor muscle of the bladder wall and inhibit the action of the sphincter vesicae. The sympathetic nerves were once thought to inhibit contraction of the detrusor muscle and stimulate closure of the sphincter vesicae. However, current thought is that the sympathetic nerves to the detrusor muscle may have little or no action on the smooth muscle of the bladder wall and are distributed mainly to the blood vessels. In this case, the sympathetic nerves to the sphincter vesicae play only a minor role in causing contraction of the sphincter in maintaining urinary continence. However, in males, the sympathetic innervation of the sphincter causes active contraction of the bladder neck during ejaculation (brought about by sympathetic action), thus preventing seminal fluid from entering the bladder.

Micturition

Micturition is a reflex action controlled by higher centers in the brain in the toilet-trained individual. The reflex is initiated when the volume of urine reaches about 300 mL. This stimulates stretch receptors in the bladder wall, which transmit impulses to the CNS, resulting in

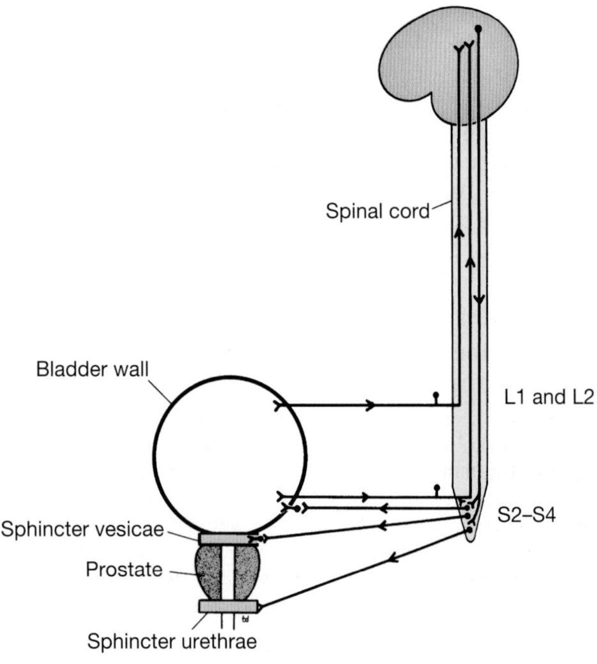

Figure 6.33 Nervous control of the bladder. Sympathetic fibers have been omitted for simplification.

a conscious desire to micturate. Most afferent impulses pass up the **pelvic splanchnic nerves** and enter the S2 to S4 segments of the spinal cord (Fig. 6.33). Some afferent impulses travel with the sympathetic nerves via the hypogastric plexuses and enter the L1 and L2 segments of the spinal cord.

Efferent parasympathetic impulses leave the spinal cord from the S2 to S4 segments and pass via the parasympathetic preganglionic nerve fibers through the **pelvic splanchnic nerves** and the **inferior hypogastric plexuses** to the bladder wall, where they synapse with postganglionic neurons. Postganglionic neurons then cause the smooth muscle of the bladder wall (the **detrusor muscle**) to contract, and the **sphincter vesicae** to relax. Somatic efferent impulses also pass to the external urethral sphincter via the pudendal nerve (S2 to S4), and this undergoes relaxation. Once urine enters the urethra, additional afferent impulses pass to the spinal cord from the urethra and reinforce the reflex action. Micturition can be assisted by contraction of the abdominal muscles to raise the intra-abdominal and pelvic pressures and exert external pressure on the bladder.

In young children, micturition is a simple reflex act and takes place whenever the bladder becomes distended. In the adult, this simple stretch reflex is inhibited by the activity of the cerebral cortex until the time and place for micturition are favorable. The inhibitory fibers pass downward with the corticospinal tracts to the S2 to S4 segments of the cord. Voluntary control of micturition is accomplished by contracting the sphincter urethrae, which closes the urethra. This is assisted by the sphincter vesicae, which compresses the bladder neck. Voluntary control of micturition normally develops around age 2 or 3 years.

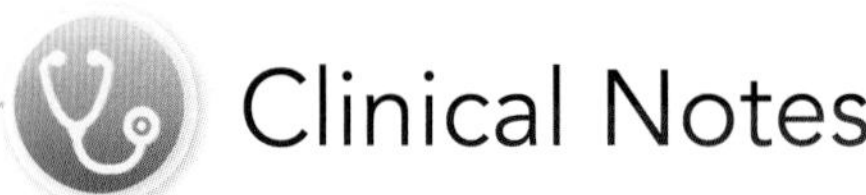

Clinical Notes

Ureteric Calculi

Ureteric calculi are discussed in Chapter 5. The ureter is narrowed anatomically at the junction of the renal pelvis and ureter, where the ureter bends down into the pelvis at the pelvic brim, and where it passes through the bladder wall. Urinary stones may be arrested at these sites.

When a calculus enters the lower pelvic part of the ureter, the pain is often referred to the testis and the tip of the penis in the male and the labium majus in the female.

Urinary Bladder Palpation

The full bladder in the adult projects up into the abdomen and may be palpated through the anterior abdominal wall above the symphysis pubis.

Bimanual palpation of the empty bladder with or without a general anesthetic is an important method of examining the bladder. In the male, one hand is placed on the anterior abdominal wall above the symphysis pubis, and the gloved index finger of the other hand is inserted into the rectum. The bladder wall can be palpated between the examining fingers. In the female, an abdominovaginal examination can be similarly made. In the child, the bladder is in a higher position than in the adult because of the relatively smaller size of the pelvis.

Bladder Distention

The normal adult bladder has a capacity of about 500 mL. In the presence of urinary obstruction in males, the bladder may become greatly distended without permanent damage to the bladder wall. In such cases, it is routinely possible to drain 1,000 to 1,200 mL of urine through a catheter.

Urinary Retention

In adult males, urinary retention is commonly caused by obstruction to the urethra by a benign or malignant enlargement of the prostate. Acute urethritis or prostatitis can also be responsible. Acute retention occurs much less frequently in females. The only anatomic cause of urinary retention in females is acute inflammation around the urethra (eg, from herpes).

Suprapubic Aspiration

As the bladder fills, the superior wall rises out of the pelvis and peels the peritoneum off the posterior surface of the anterior abdominal wall. In cases of acute retention of urine, when catheterization has failed, it is possible to pass a needle into the bladder through the anterior abdominal wall above the symphysis pubis, without entering the peritoneal cavity. This is a simple method of draining off the urine in an emergency.

Cystoscopy

The mucous membrane of the bladder, the two ureteric orifices, and the urethral meatus can easily be observed by means of a **cystoscope**. With the bladder distended with fluid, an illuminated tube fitted with lenses is introduced into the bladder through the urethra. The mucous membrane is pink and smooth over the trigone. If the bladder is partially emptied, the mucous membrane over the trigone remains smooth, but it is thrown into folds elsewhere. The ureteric orifices are slit like and eject a drop of urine at intervals of about 1 minute. The interureteric ridge and the uvula vesicae can easily be recognized.

Bladder Injuries

The bladder may rupture intraperitoneally or extraperitoneally. **Intraperitoneal rupture** usually involves the superior wall of the bladder and occurs most commonly when the bladder is full and has extended up into the abdomen. Urine and blood escape freely into the peritoneal cavity. **Extraperitoneal rupture** involves the anterior part of the bladder wall below the level of the peritoneal reflection. It most commonly occurs in fractures of the pelvis when bony fragments pierce the bladder wall. Lower abdominal pain and blood in the urine (hematuria) occur in most patients.

In young children, the bladder is an abdominal organ, so abdominal trauma can injure the empty bladder.

Stress Incontinence

The bladder is normally supported by the visceral pelvic fascia, which, in certain areas, is condensed to form ligaments. However, the most important support for the bladder is the tone of the levator ani muscles. In the female, a difficult labor, especially one in which forceps is used, excessively stretches the supports of the bladder neck, and the normal angle between the urethra and the posterior wall of the bladder is lost. This injury causes stress incontinence, a condition of partial urinary incontinence occurring when the patient coughs or strains or laughs excessively. Obese patients have twice the incidence of incontinence. The treatment of stress incontinence is directed to supporting the urethra so that the normal angle of the bladder and the urethra is restored. This may be accomplished with some success by the introduction of a vaginal appliance (**pessary**) that raises the upper end of the urethra. A more satisfactory permanent result may be achieved by raising the urethra and the bladder neck surgically by sutures or by a fascial sling or artificial tape.

Difficulty with Micturition after Spinal Cord Injury

Nervous control of micturition is disrupted after injuries to the spinal cord.

The normal bladder is innervated as follows:

- Sympathetic outflow is from the L1 and L2 segments of the spinal cord. The **sympathetic nerves** inhibit contraction of the detrusor muscle of the bladder wall and stimulate closure of the sphincter vesicae (however, note the earlier description of the nerve supply to the bladder).
- Parasympathetic outflow is from the S2 to S4 segments of the spinal cord. The **parasympathetic nerves** stimulate the contraction of the detrusor muscle of the bladder wall and inhibit the action of the sphincter vesicae.
- **Sensory nerve fibers** enter the spinal cord at the above segments.

Disruption of the process of micturition by spinal cord injuries may produce the following types of bladders.

The **atonic bladder** occurs during the phase of spinal shock, immediately after the injury, and may last for a few days to several weeks. The bladder wall muscle is relaxed, the sphincter vesicae tightly contracted, and the sphincter urethrae relaxed. The bladder becomes greatly distended and finally overflows. Depending on the level of the cord injury, the patient may or may not be aware that the bladder is full.

The **automatic reflex bladder** (Fig. 6.34A) occurs after the patient has recovered from spinal shock, provided that the

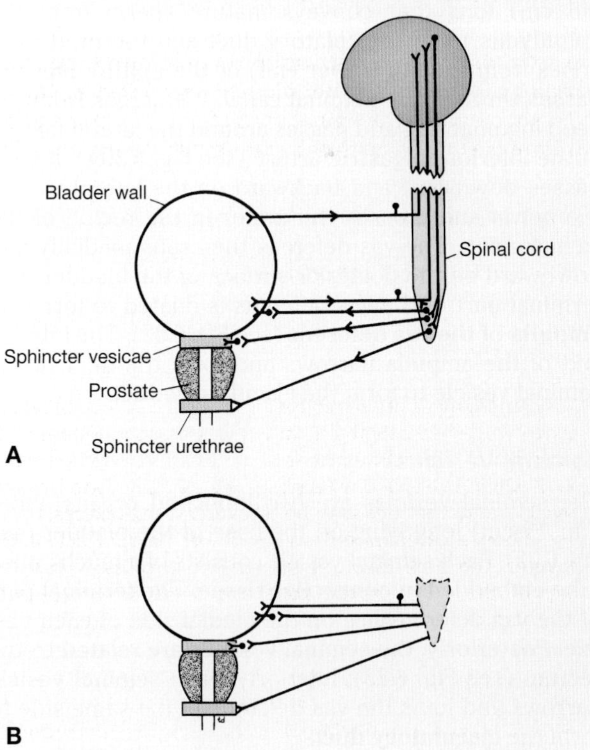

Figure 6.34 **A.** Nervous control of the bladder after section of the spinal cord in the upper thoracic region. **B.** Destruction of the sacral segments of the spinal cord. The afferent fibers from the bladder entering the central nervous system and the parasympathetic efferent fibers passing to the bladder are shown. The sympathetic fibers have been omitted for clarity.

(continued)

cord lesion lies above the level of the parasympathetic outflow (S2 to S4). It is the type of bladder normally found in infancy. The bladder fills and empties reflexively. Stretch receptors in the bladder wall are stimulated as the bladder fills, and the afferent impulses pass to the spinal cord (segments S2 to S4). Efferent impulses pass down to the bladder muscle, which contracts. The sphincter vesicae and the urethral sphincter both relax. This simple reflex occurs every 1 to 4 hours.

The **autonomous bladder** (see Fig. 6.34B) occurs if the sacral segments of the spinal cord are destroyed. The sacral segments of the spinal cord are situated in the upper part of the lumbar region of the vertebral column (see Chapter 2). The bladder is without any external reflex control. The bladder wall is flaccid, and the capacity of the bladder is greatly increased. It merely fills to capacity and overflows; continual dribbling is the result. The bladder may be partially emptied by manual compression of the lower part of the anterior abdominal wall, but infection of the urine and back pressure effects on the ureters and kidneys are inevitable.

MALE INTERNAL GENITAL ORGANS

The male internal genital organs are the vas deferens, seminal vesicles, ejaculatory ducts, prostate, prostatic urethra, and membranous urethra. The membranous urethra and the penis are described in Chapter 7. The testis and epididymis (both external genital organs) are described in Chapter 5.

Vas Deferens (Ductus Deferens)

The vas deferens is a thick-walled tube about 18 in. (45 cm) long that conveys mature sperm from the epididymis to the ejaculatory duct and the urethra. It arises from the **tail** (lower end) **of the epididymis** and passes through the inguinal canal. It emerges from the deep inguinal ring and passes around the lateral margin of the inferior epigastric artery (see Fig. 6.30A). It then passes downward and backward on the lateral wall of the pelvis and crosses the ureter in the region of the ischial spine. The vas deferens then runs medially and downward on the posterior surface of the bladder. The terminal part of the vas deferens is dilated to form the **ampulla of the vas deferens** (see Fig. 6.32). The inferior end of the ampulla narrows and joins the duct of the seminal vesicle to form the **ejaculatory duct**.

Seminal Vesicles

The seminal vesicles are two lobulated organs about 2 in. (5 cm) long lying on the base of the bladder (see Fig. 6.32). Each seminal vesicle consists of a much-coiled tube embedded in connective tissue. The terminal part of the vas deferens lies on the medial side of each vesicle. Posteriorly, the seminal vesicles are related to the rectum (see Fig. 6.23). Inferiorly, each seminal vesicle narrows and joins the vas deferens of the same side to form the **ejaculatory duct**.

Blood Supply

The **inferior vesicle** and **middle rectal arteries**, each of which is a branch of the internal iliac artery, supply the seminal vesicle.

The veins drain into the internal iliac veins.

Lymph Drainage

The seminal vesicles drain to the internal iliac nodes.

Function

The seminal vesicles produce a secretion that is added to the seminal fluid and accounts for about two thirds of the total ejaculate volume. The secretions nourish the spermatozoa and are important in sperm motility. During ejaculation, the seminal vesicles contract and expel their contents into the ejaculatory ducts, thus washing the spermatozoa out of the urethra.

Ejaculatory Duct

Each ejaculatory duct is <1 in. (2.5 cm) long and is formed by the union of the vas deferens and the duct of the seminal vesicle (Fig. 6.35). The ejaculatory duct pierces the posterior surface of the prostate and opens into the prostatic part of the urethra, close to the margin of the **prostatic utricle**. Its function is to drain the seminal fluid into the prostatic urethra.

Prostate Gland

The prostate is a walnut-size fibromuscular glandular organ that surrounds the prostatic urethra (see Figs. 6.23 and 6.35). It is about 1.25 in. (3 cm) long and lies between the neck of the bladder above and the urogenital diaphragm below (see Fig. 6.35).

A fibrous capsule surrounds the prostate. The somewhat conical prostate has a **base**, which lies against the bladder neck above, and an **apex**, which lies against the urogenital diaphragm below. The two ejaculatory ducts pierce the upper part of the posterior surface of the prostate to open into the prostatic urethra at the lateral margins of the **prostatic utricle**.

The numerous glands of the prostate are embedded in a mixture of smooth muscle and connective tissue, and their ducts open into the prostatic urethra (see Fig. 6.35C).

The prostate is incompletely divided into **five lobes** (see Fig. 6.35). The **anterior lobe** lies in front of the urethra and is devoid of glandular tissue. The **median (middle) lobe** is the wedge of gland situated between the urethra and the ejaculatory ducts. Its upper surface is related to the trigone of the bladder; it is rich in glands. The **posterior lobe** is situated behind the urethra and below the ejaculatory ducts and contains glandular tissue. The **right** and **left lateral lobes** lie on either side of the urethra and are separated by a shallow vertical groove on the posterior surface of the prostate. The lateral lobes contain many glands.

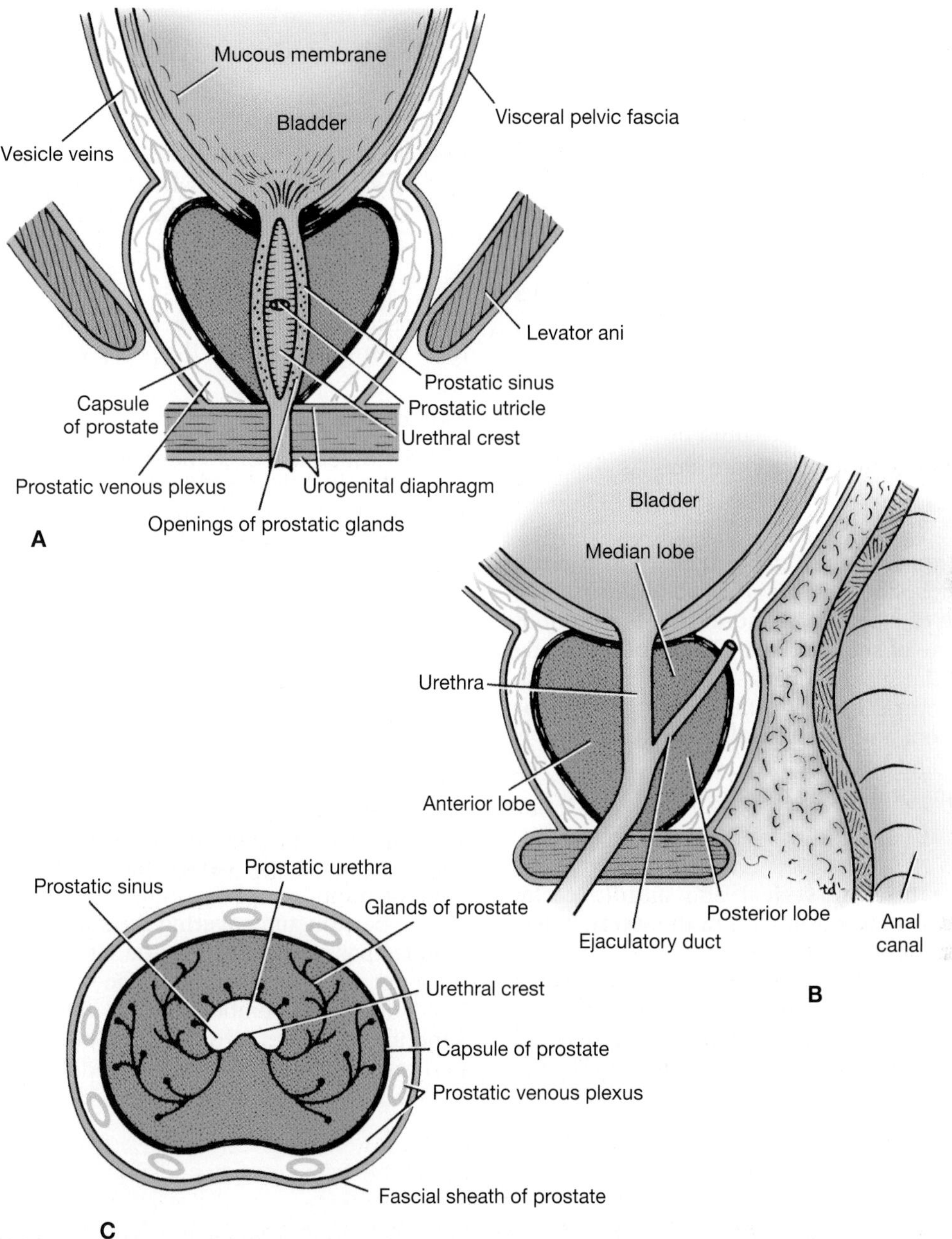

Figure 6.35 Prostate in coronal section **(A)**, sagittal section **(B)**, and horizontal section **(C)**. In the coronal section, note the openings of the ejaculatory ducts on the margin of the prostatic utricle.

Relations

- **Superiorly:** The base of the prostate is continuous with the neck of the bladder, the smooth muscle passing without interruption from one organ to the other. The urethra enters the center of the base of the prostate (see Figs. 6.23 and 6.35).
- **Inferiorly:** The apex of the prostate lies on the upper surface of the urogenital diaphragm. The urethra leaves the prostate just above the apex on the anterior surface (see Fig. 6.35B).
- **Anteriorly:** The prostate is related to the symphysis pubis, separated from it by the extraperitoneal fat in the **retropubic space** (**cave of Retzius**). The prostate is connected to the posterior aspect of the pubic bones by the fascial **puboprostatic ligaments** (see Fig. 6.23).
- **Posteriorly:** The prostate (see Figs. 6.23 and 6.35) is closely related to the anterior surface of the rectal ampulla and is separated from it by the **rectovesical septum** (**fascia of Denonvilliers**). This septum forms in fetal life by the fusion of the walls of the lower end of the rectovesical pouch of peritoneum, which originally extended down to the perineal body.
- **Laterally:** The prostate is embraced by the anterior fibers of the levator ani as they run posteriorly from the pubis (see Fig. 6.35A).

Prostatic Urethra

The prostatic urethra is about 1.25 in. (3 cm) long and begins at the neck of the bladder. It passes through the prostate from the base to the apex, where it becomes continuous with the membranous part of the urethra (see Fig. 6.35).

The prostatic urethra is the **widest and most dilatable portion of the entire urethra**. A longitudinal ridge called the **urethral crest** is located on the posterior wall. A groove called the **prostatic sinus** runs along each side of the crest; the prostatic glands open into these grooves. A small depression, the **prostatic utricle** (which is an analog of the uterus and vagina in females) lies on the summit of the urethral crest. The openings of the two ejaculatory ducts are located on each edge of the mouth of the utricle.

Prostate Function

The prostate produces thin, milky fluid rich in citric acid and acid phosphatase. This is added to the seminal fluid at the time of ejaculation and accounts for about 30% of the volume of seminal fluid. The smooth muscle that surrounds the gland squeezes the secretion into the prostatic urethra. Prostatic fluid is important for sperm nourishment and motility. Also, prostatic fluid is slightly alkaline and helps neutralize the acidity in the vaginal tract, thus prolonging the lifespan of sperm.

Blood Supply

Branches of the **inferior vesical** and **middle rectal arteries**, each of which is a branch of the internal iliac artery, supply the prostate.

The veins form the **prostatic venous plexus**, which lies outside the capsule of the prostate (see Fig. 6.35). The prostatic plexus receives the deep dorsal vein of the penis and numerous vesical veins and drains into the internal iliac veins.

Lymph Drainage

The prostate drains to the internal iliac nodes.

Nerve Supply

Branches of the inferior hypogastric plexuses innervate the prostate. The sympathetic nerves stimulate the smooth muscle of the prostate during ejaculation.

Visceral Pelvic Fascia

The visceral pelvic fascia is a layer of connective tissue that covers and supports the pelvic viscera (see Fig. 6.35).

Peritoneum

The peritoneum is best understood by tracing it around the pelvis in a sagittal plane (see Fig. 6.23).

The parietal peritoneum passes down from the anterior abdominal wall onto the upper surface of the urinary bladder. It then runs down on the posterior surface of the bladder for a short distance until it reaches the upper ends of the seminal vesicles. Here, it sweeps backward to reach the anterior aspect of the rectum, forming the shallow **rectovesical pouch**. The peritoneum then passes up on the front of the middle third of the rectum and the front and lateral surfaces of the upper third of the rectum. It then becomes continuous with the parietal peritoneum on the posterior abdominal wall. Thus, the rectovesical pouch is the lowest part of the abdominopelvic peritoneal cavity when the patient is in the erect position.

The peritoneum covering the superior surface of the bladder passes laterally to the lateral pelvic walls but does not cover the lateral surfaces of the bladder. It is important to remember that, as the bladder fills, the superior wall rises into the abdomen and peels off the peritoneum from the anterior abdominal wall so that the bladder directly contacts the abdominal wall.

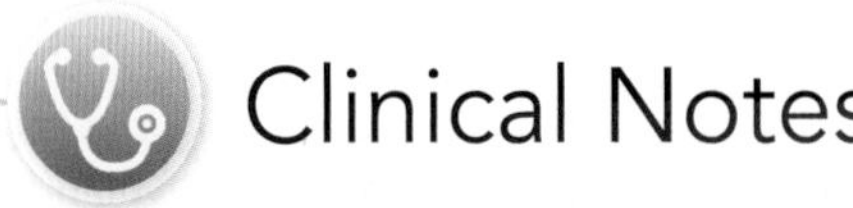

Prostate Examination

The prostate can be examined clinically by palpation by performing a rectal examination (see Chapter 7). The examiner's gloved finger can feel the posterior surface of the prostate through the anterior rectal wall.

Prostate Activity and Disease

Androgens and estrogens circulating in the bloodstream are thought to control the normal glandular activity of the prostate. The secretions of the prostate pour into the urethra during ejaculation and add to the seminal fluid. Acid phosphatase is an important enzyme present in the secretion in large amounts. When the glandular cells producing this enzyme cannot discharge their secretion into the ducts, as in carcinoma of the prostate, the serum acid phosphatase level of the blood rises.

Trace amounts of proteins produced specifically by prostatic epithelial cells are found in peripheral blood. In certain prostatic diseases, notably cancer of the prostate, this protein appears in the blood in increased amounts. The specific protein level can be measured by a simple laboratory test called the **prostate-specific antigen (PSA) test**.

Benign Prostatic Enlargement

Benign enlargement of the prostate is common in males older than age 50 years. The cause is possibly an imbalance in the hormonal control of the gland. The median lobe of the gland enlarges upward and encroaches within the sphincter vesicae, located at the neck of the bladder (Fig. 6.36). The leakage of urine into the prostatic urethra causes an intense reflex desire to micturate. The enlargement of the median and lateral lobes of the gland produces elongation and lateral compression and distortion of the urethra so that the patient has trouble passing urine, and the stream is weak. Back pressure effects on the ureters and both kidneys are common complications. The enlargement of the uvula vesicae (owing to the enlarged median lobe) results in the formation of a pouch of stagnant urine behind the urethral orifice within the bladder. The stagnant urine frequently becomes infected, and the inflamed bladder (**cystitis**) adds to the patient's symptoms.

The surgeon regards the prostatic venous plexus with respect in all operations on the prostate. The veins have thin walls, are valveless, and are drained by several large trunks directly into the internal iliac veins. Damage to these veins can result in severe hemorrhage.

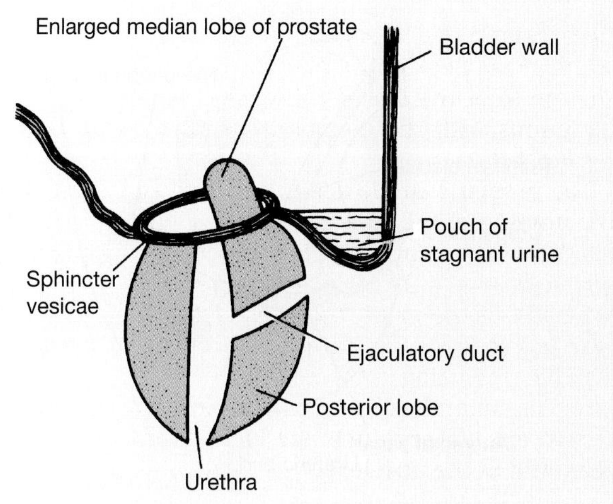

Figure 6.36 Sagittal section of a prostate that had undergone benign enlargement of the median lobe. Note the bladder pouch filled with stagnant urine behind the prostate.

Prostate Cancer and Prostatic Venous Plexus

Many connections exist between the prostatic venous plexus and the vertebral veins. During coughing, sneezing, or abdominal straining, it is possible for prostatic venous blood to flow in a reverse direction and enter the vertebral veins. This explains the frequent occurrence of skeletal metastases in the lower vertebral column and pelvic bones of patients with carcinoma of the prostate. Cancer cells enter the skull via this route by floating up the valveless prostatic and vertebral veins.

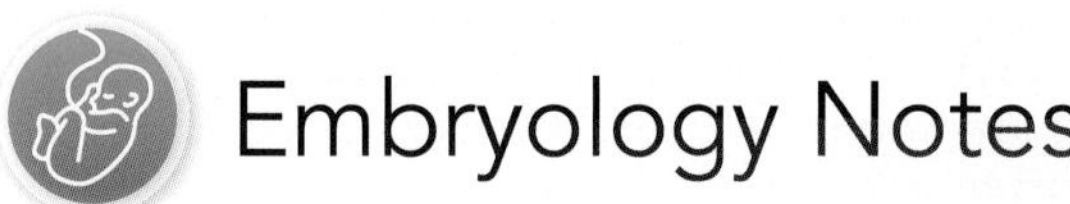

Embryology Notes

Bladder Development

The division of the cloaca into anterior and posterior parts by the development of the **urorectal septum** is described earlier in this chapter (see Fig. 6.27). The posterior portion forms the **anorectal canal** (Fig. 6.37). The entrance of the distal ends of the mesonephric ducts into the anterior part of the cloaca on each side permits, for purposes of description, the division of the anterior part of the cloaca into an area above the duct entrances called the **primitive bladder** and another area below called the **urogenital sinus**.

The caudal ends of the mesonephric ducts now become absorbed into the lower part of the bladder so that the ureters and ducts have individual openings in the dorsal wall. With differential growth of the dorsal bladder wall, the ureters come to open through the lateral angles of the bladder, and the mesonephric ducts open close together in what will be the urethra. That part of the dorsal bladder wall marked off by the openings of these four ducts forms the **trigone of the bladder** (Fig. 6.38). Thus, in the earliest stages, the lining of the bladder over the trigone is mesodermal in origin. Later, this mesodermal tissue is replaced by epithelium of endodermal origin. The smooth muscle of the bladder wall is derived from the splanchnopleuric mesoderm.

The primitive bladder is now divided into an upper dilated portion, the **bladder**, and a lower narrow portion, the **urethra** (see Fig. 6.37). The apex of the bladder is continuous with the **allantois**, which now becomes obliterated and forms a fibrous core, the **urachus**. The urachus persists throughout life as the **median umbilical ligament**, which runs from the apex of the bladder to the umbilicus.

Exstrophy of the bladder (**ectopia vesicae**) is a congenital anomaly that occurs three times more commonly in males. The posterior bladder wall protrudes through a defect in the anterior abdominal wall below the umbilicus (Fig. 6.39). The condition is caused by a failure of the embryonic mesenchyme to invade the embryonic disc caudal to the cloacal membrane. The absence of intervening mesenchyme between the ectoderm and entoderm produces an unstable state, which is followed by breakdown of this area.

Because of the urinary incontinence and almost certain occurrence of ascending urinary infection, surgical reconstruction of the bladder is attempted.

Mesonephric Duct Fate

In both biologic sexes, the mesonephric (Wolffian) duct gives origin on each side to the **ureteric bud**, which forms the **ureter**, the **pelvis** of the ureter, the **major** and **minor**

(continued)

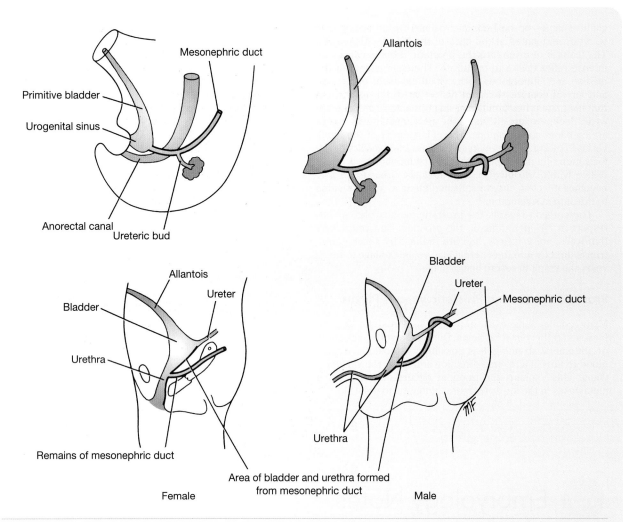

Figure 6.37 Formation of the urinary bladder from the anterior part of the cloaca and the terminal parts of the mesonephric ducts in both sexes. The mesonephric ducts and the ureteric buds are drawn into the developing bladder.

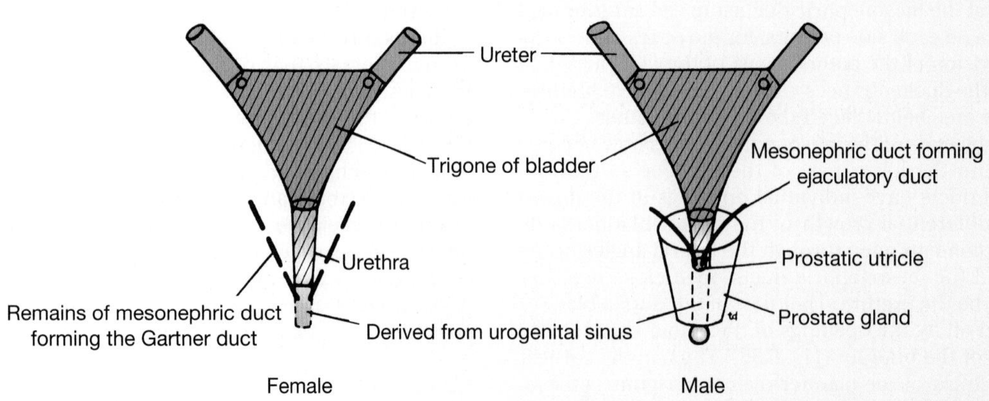

Figure 6.38 Parts of the bladder and urethra derived from the mesonephric ducts in both sexes (*hatch marks*). The lower end of the urethra in the female and the lower part of the prostatic urethra in the male form from the urogenital sinus.

calyces, and the **collecting tubules** of the kidney (see Chapter 5). Its inferior end is absorbed into the developing bladder and forms the **trigone** and part of the **urethra**.

In the male, its upper or cranial end is joined to the developing testis by the efferent ductules of the testis, and so it becomes the **duct of the epididymis**, the **vas deferens,** and the **ejaculatory duct**. A small diverticulum arises from the latter that forms the **seminal vesicle** (see Fig. 5.30).

In the female, the mesonephric duct largely disappears. Only small remnants persist—as the **duct of the epoophoron** and the **duct of the paroöphoron**. The caudal end may persist and extend from the epoophoron to the hymen as the **Gartner duct**.

Urethral Development

In the male, the **prostatic urethra** is formed from two sources. The proximal part, as far as the openings of the ejaculatory ducts, is derived from the mesonephric ducts. The distal part of the prostatic urethra is formed from the urogenital sinus (see Fig. 6.38). The **membranous urethra** and the greater part of the **penile urethra** also are formed from the urogenital sinus. The distal end of the penile urethra is derived from an ingrowth of ectodermal cells on the glans penis.

In the female, the upper two thirds of the urethra are derived from the mesonephric ducts. The lower end of the urethra is formed from the urogenital sinus.

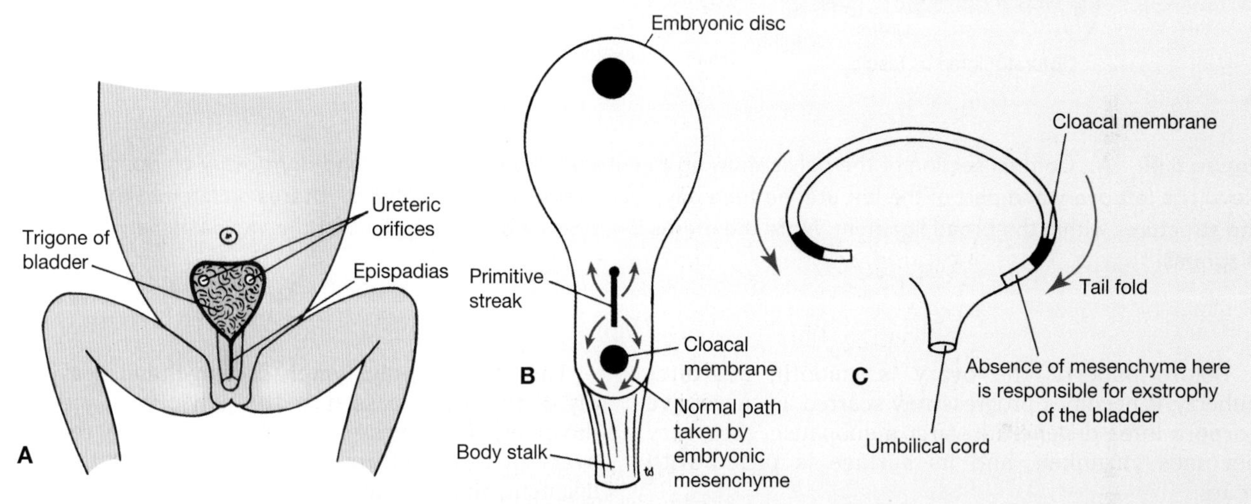

Figure 6.39 **A.** Exstrophy of the bladder. **B.** Dorsal view of the embryonic disc. The normal path taken by the growing embryonic mesenchyme in the region of the cloaca is shown. **C.** Fetus as seen from the side. The head and tail folds have developed, but the mesenchyme has failed to enter the ventral body wall between the cloaca and the umbilical cord.

FEMALE INTERNAL GENITAL ORGANS

The female internal genital organs are the ovaries, uterine tubes, uterus, and vagina. The external genitalia are described in Chapter 7.

Ovary

There is one ovary on each side of the pelvis. Each is oval shaped, measuring 1.5 × 0.75 in. (4 × 2 cm), and attaches to the back of the broad ligament by the **mesovarium** (Fig. 6.40).

That part of the broad ligament extending between the attachment of the mesovarium and the lateral wall of the pelvis is the **suspensory ligament of the ovary**.

The **round ligament of the ovary**, which represents the remains of the upper part of the gubernaculum, connects the lateral margin of the uterus to the ovary (see Figs. 6.30B and 6.40).

The ovary usually lies against the lateral wall of the pelvis in a depression called the **ovarian fossa**, bounded by the external iliac vessels above and by the internal iliac vessels behind (see Fig. 6.30B). However, the position of the ovary is extremely variable, and it often hangs down in the **rectouterine pouch (pouch of Douglas)**. During pregnancy, the enlarging uterus pulls the ovary up into the abdominal cavity. After childbirth, when the broad ligament is lax, the ovary takes up a variable position in the pelvis.

A thin fibrous capsule, the **tunica albuginea**, surrounds the ovaries. A modified area of peritoneum called the **germinal epithelium** covers this capsule externally. The term germinal epithelium is a misnomer because the layer does not give rise to ova. Oogonia develop before birth from primordial germ cells.

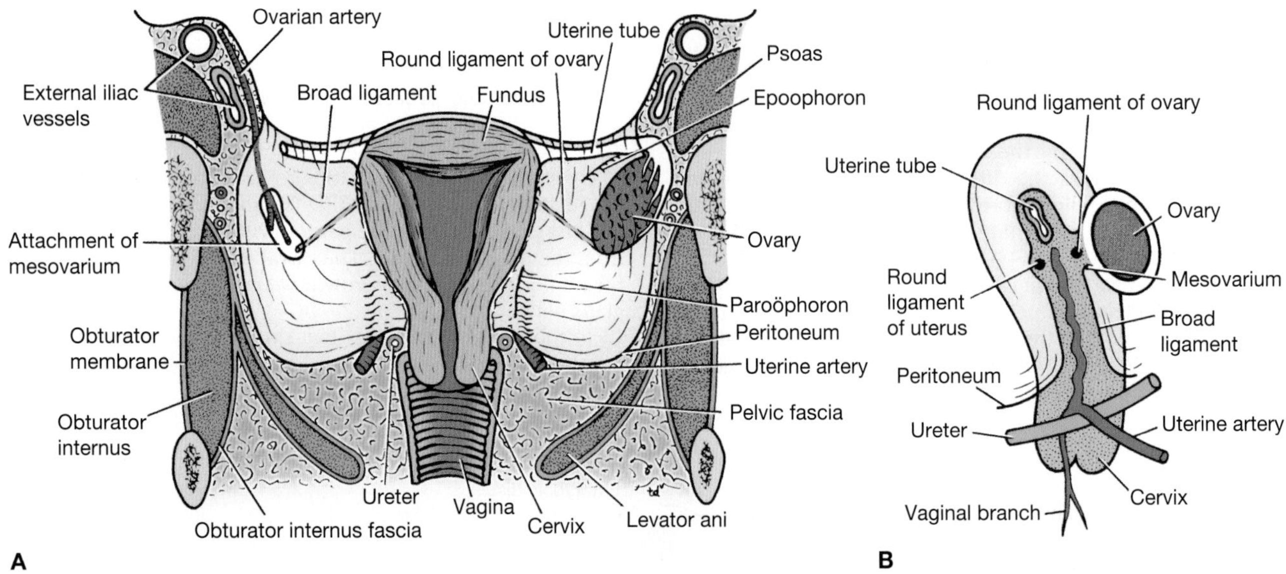

Figure 6.40 **A.** Coronal section of the pelvis showing the uterus, broad ligaments, and right ovary on posterior view. The left ovary and part of the left uterine tube have been removed for clarity. **B.** Uterus on lateral view. Note the structures within the broad ligament. Note the uterus is retroverted into the plane of the vaginal lumen in both diagrams.

Before puberty, the ovary is smooth, but after puberty, it becomes progressively scarred as successive corpora lutea degenerate. After menopause, the ovary becomes shrunken, and its surface is pitted with scars.

Function

The ovaries are the organs responsible for producing the female germ cells, the **ova**, and the female sex hormones, **estrogen** and **progesterone**, in the sexually mature female.

Blood Supply

The **ovarian arteries** arise from the abdominal aorta at the level of the L1 vertebra, in the same fashion as the testicular arteries (see Figs 5.78 and 5.116).

The ovarian vein drains into the **inferior vena cava** on the right side and into the **left renal vein** on the left side, in the same manner as the testicular veins.

Lymph Drainage

The lymph vessels of the ovary follow the ovarian artery and drain into the **paraaortic nodes** at the level of the L1 vertebra (see Fig. 5.121).

Nerve Supply

The nerve supply to the ovary is derived from the aortic plexus and accompanies the ovarian artery (see Fig. 5.123).

The blood supply, lymph drainage, and nerve supply of the ovary pass over the pelvic inlet and cross the external iliac vessels (see Fig. 6.40). They reach the ovary by passing through the lateral end of the broad ligament, the part known as the **suspensory ligament of the ovary**. The vessels and nerves finally enter the hilum of the ovary via the **mesovarium**.

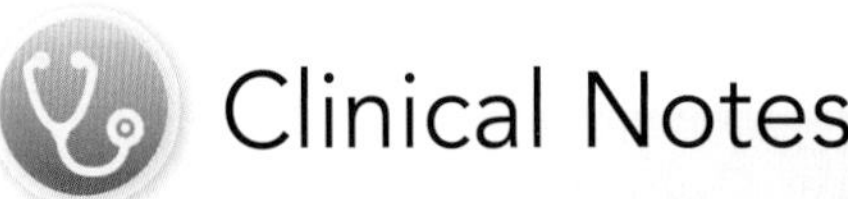

Clinical Notes

Ovary Position

The ovary is kept in position by the broad ligament and the mesovarium. After pregnancy, the broad ligament is lax, and the ovaries may prolapse into the rectouterine pouch. In these circumstances, the ovary may be tender and cause discomfort during sexual intercourse (**dyspareunia**). An ovary situated in the rectouterine pouch may be palpated through the posterior fornix of the vagina.

Ovarian Cysts

Follicular cysts are common and originate in unruptured graafian follicles; they rarely exceed 0.6 in. (1.5 cm) in diameter. **Luteal cysts** are formed in the corpus luteum. Fluid is retained, and the corpus luteum cannot become fibrosed. Luteal cysts rarely exceed 1.2 in. (3 cm) in diameter.

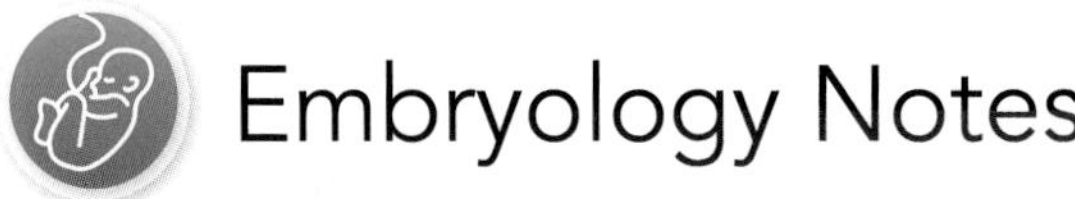

Embryology Notes

Ovarian Development

The female sex chromosome causes the **genital ridge** on the posterior abdominal wall to secrete estrogens. The presence of estrogen and the absence of testosterone induce the development of the ovary and the other female genital organs.

The **sex cords** contained within the genital ridges contain groups of **primordial germ cells**. These become broken up into irregular cell clusters by the proliferating mesenchyme (Fig. 6.41). The germ cells differentiate into **oogonia**, and, by the third month, they start to undergo mitotic divisions within the cortex of the ovary to form **primary oocytes**. A single layer of cells derived from the sex cords, called the **granulosa cells**, surrounds these primary oocytes. Thus, **primordial follicles** have been formed, but later, many degenerate. The mesenchyme that surrounds the follicles provides the **ovarian stroma**. The relationship of the ovary to the developing uterine tube is shown in Figure 6.42.

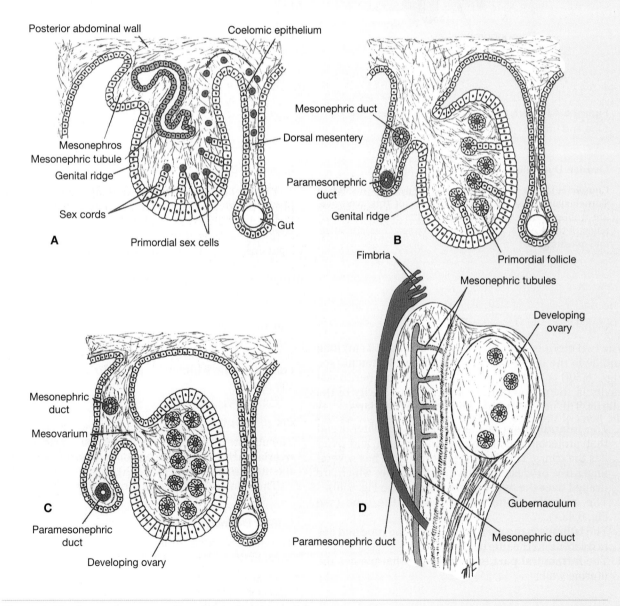

Figure 6.41 Successive stages **(A to D)** in formation of the ovary and its relationship to the mesonephric and paramesonephric ducts.

(continued)

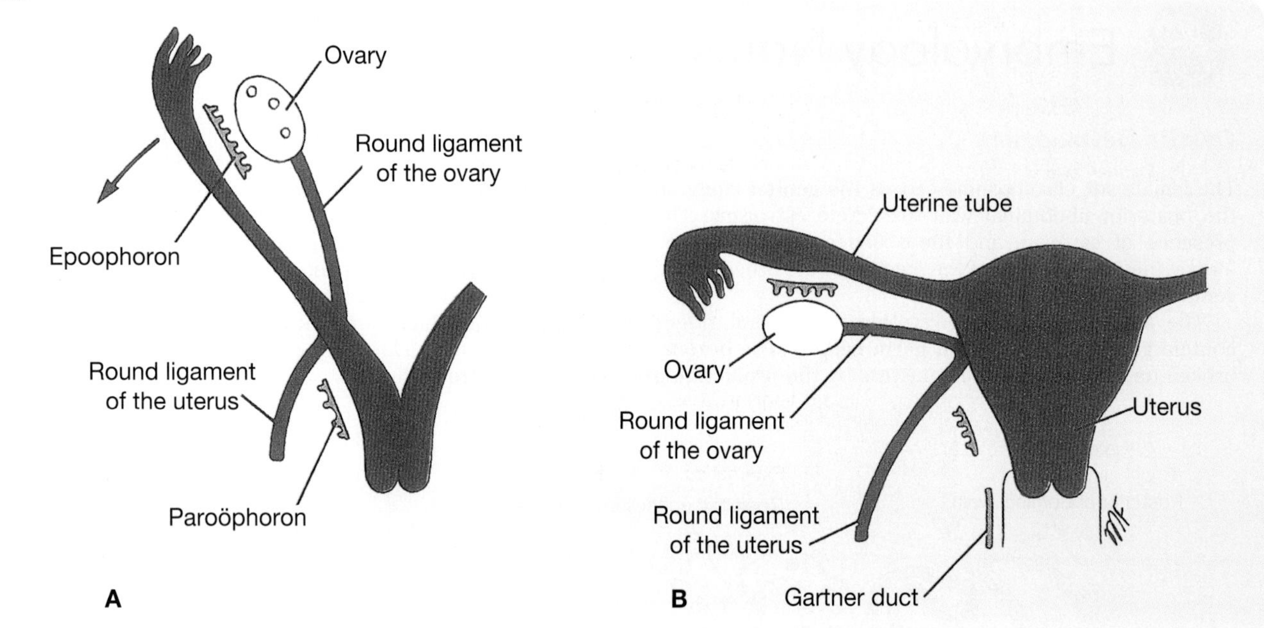

Figure 6.42 Early **(A)** and final **(B)** stages in the descent of the ovary and its relationship to the developing uterine tube and uterus.

Ovarian Dysgenesis

Complete failure of both ovaries to develop occurs in Turner syndrome. The classic features of this syndrome are webbed neck; short, stocky build; increased carrying angle of the elbows; lack of secondary sex characteristics; and amenorrhea.

Imperfect Descent of Ovary

The ovary may fail to descend into the pelvis or very rarely may be drawn downward with the round ligament of the uterus into the inguinal canal or even into the labium majus.

Uterine Tube

The two uterine tubes are each about 4 in. (10 cm) long and lie in the upper border of the **broad ligament** (see Figs. 6.30B and 6.40). Each connects the peritoneal cavity in the region of the ovary with the cavity of the uterus. The uterine tube is divided into four parts:

1. The **infundibulum** is the funnel-shaped lateral end that projects beyond the broad ligament and overlies the ovary. The free edge of the funnel has several finger-like processes, known as **fimbriae**, which are draped over the ovary (Fig. 6.43; see also Fig. 6.40).
2. The **ampulla** is the widest part of the tube (see Fig. 6.43A).
3. The **isthmus** is the narrowest part of the tube and lies just lateral to the uterus.
4. The **intramural part** is the segment that pierces the uterine wall.

Function

The uterine tube receives the ovum from the ovary and provides a site where fertilization of the ovum can take place (usually in the ampulla). It provides nourishment for the fertilized ovum and transports it to the cavity of the uterus. The tube serves as a conduit along which the spermatozoa travel to reach the ovum.

Blood Supply

The **uterine artery** from the internal iliac artery and the **ovarian artery** from the abdominal aorta both supply the uterine tube (see Fig. 6.43A).

The veins correspond to the arteries.

Lymph Drainage

The uterine tube drains to the **internal iliac** and **paraaortic nodes** (see Fig. 5.121).

Nerve Supply

Sympathetic and parasympathetic nerves from the **inferior hypogastric plexuses** innervate the uterine tube (see Fig. 6.19).

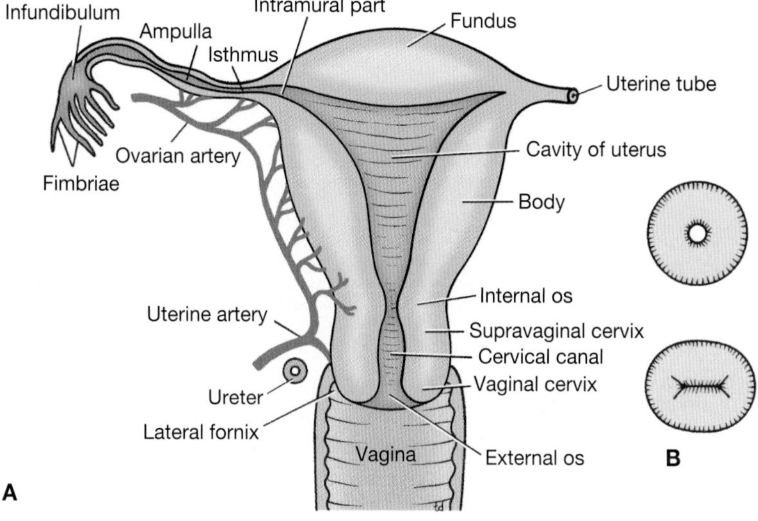

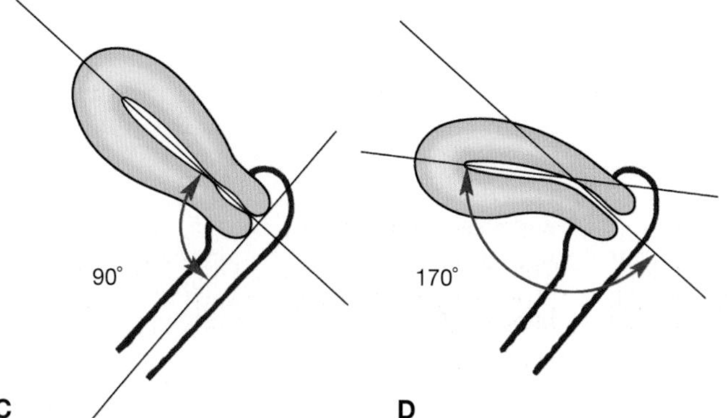

Figure 6.43 **A.** Different parts of the uterine tube and uterus. **B.** External os of the cervix: (*above*) nulliparous; (*below*) parous. **C.** Anteverted position of the uterus. **D.** Anteverted and anteflexed position of the uterus.

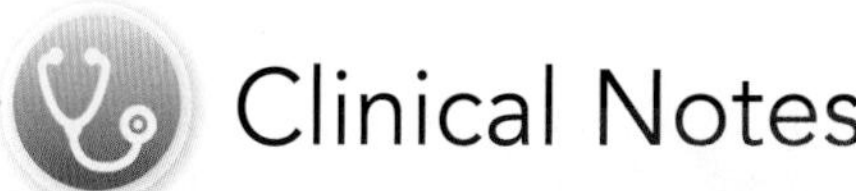

Clinical Notes

Clinical Concept: Uterine Tube as Conduit for Infection

The uterine tube lies in the upper free border of the broad ligament and is a direct route of communication from the vulva through the vagina and uterine cavity to the peritoneal cavity.

Pelvic Inflammatory Disease

Pathogenic organism(s) may enter the body through sexual contact and ascend through the uterus and enter the uterine tubes. **Salpingitis** may follow, with leakage of pus into the peritoneal cavity, causing pelvic peritonitis. A pelvic abscess usually follows, or the infection spreads farther, causing general peritonitis.

Ectopic Pregnancy

Implantation and growth of a fertilized ovum may occur outside the uterine cavity in the wall of the uterine tube (Fig. 6.44). This is a variety of ectopic pregnancy. Because there is no decidua formation in the tube, the eroding action of the trophoblast quickly destroys the wall of the tube. Tubal abortion or rupture of the tube, with the effusion of a large quantity of blood into the peritoneal cavity, is the common result.

The blood drains into the rectouterine pouch (pouch of Douglas) or into the uterovesical pouch. The blood may quickly ascend into the general peritoneal cavity, giving rise to severe abdominal pain, tenderness, and guarding. Irritation of the subdiaphragmatic peritoneum (supplied by phrenic nerves C3 to C5) may give rise to referred pain to the shoulder skin (via supraclavicular nerves C3 and C4).

Tubal Ligation

Ligation and division of the uterine tubes is a method of obtaining permanent birth control. The ova that are discharged from the ovarian follicles degenerate in the tube distal to the obstruction. If the patient later wishes to have children, restoration of the continuity of the uterine tubes can be attempted, and fertilization occurs in about 20% of patients.

(continued)

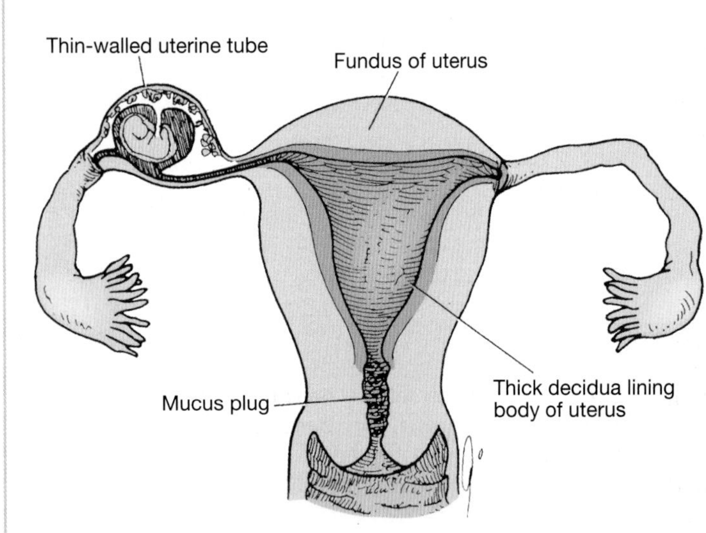

Figure 6.44 Ectopic pregnancy located where the ampulla of the uterine tube narrows to join the isthmus. Note the thin tubal wall compared to the thick decidua that lines the body of the uterus.

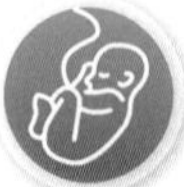

Embryology Notes

Uterine Tube Development

Early in development, the **paramesonephric ducts** appear on the posterior abdominal wall on the lateral side of the mesonephros. The uterine tube on each side is formed from the cranial vertical and middle horizontal parts of the paramesonephric duct (Fig. 6.45). The tube elongates and becomes coiled; differentiation of the muscle and mucous membrane takes place; the **fimbriae** develop; and the **infundibulum**, **ampulla**, and **isthmus** are identifiable.

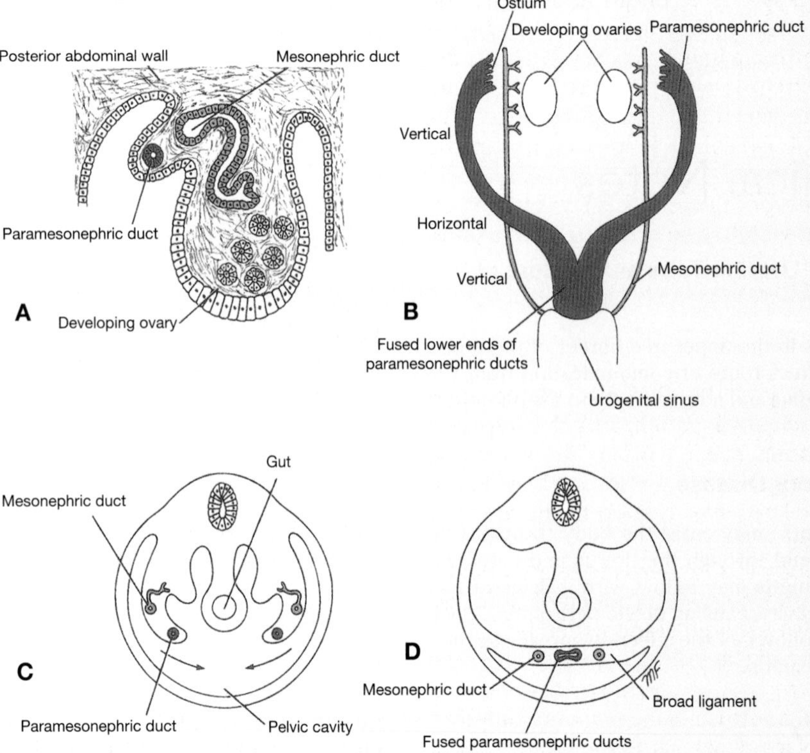

Figure 6.45 Relationship of the mesonephric and paramesonephric ducts to the developing ovary. **A.** Cross section of a developing ovary. **B.** Anterior view of ovaries and ducts. **C, D.** Mesonephric and paramesonephric ducts in a cross section of the pelvis. Note the developing broad ligament.

Uterus

The uterus is a hollow, pear-shaped organ with thick muscular walls. In the young nulliparous adult, it measures about 3 in. (8 cm) long, 2 in. (5 cm) wide, and 1 in. (2.5 cm) thick. It is divided into the fundus, body, and cervix (see Fig. 6.43A).

The **fundus** is the part of the uterus that lies above the entrance of the uterine tubes.

The **body** is the part of the uterus that lies below the entrance of the uterine tubes.

The **cervix** is the low, narrow part of the uterus. It pierces the anterior wall of the vagina and is divided into the **supravaginal** and **vaginal parts of the cervix**.

The **cavity of the uterine body** is triangular in coronal section, but it is merely a cleft in the sagittal plane. The **cavity of the cervix**, the **cervical canal**, communicates with the cavity of the body through the **internal os** and with that of the vagina through the **external os**. In a nulliparous patient, the external os is circular. In a parous patient, the vaginal part of the cervix is larger, and the external os becomes a transverse slit so that it possesses an anterior lip and a posterior lip (see Fig. 6.43B).

The uterus is covered with peritoneum except anteriorly, below the level of the internal os, where the peritoneum passes forward onto the bladder (see Fig. 6.24). Laterally, a space exists between the attachments of the layers of the broad ligament (see Fig. 6.40B).

The muscular wall, or **myometrium**, is thick and made up of smooth muscle supported by connective tissue.

The **endometrium** is the mucous membrane lining the body of the uterus. It is continuous above with the mucous membrane lining the uterine tubes and below with the mucous membrane lining the cervix. The endometrium is applied directly to the muscle; there is no submucosa. The endometrium undergoes extensive changes during the menstrual cycle in response to the ovarian hormones.

The supravaginal part of the cervix is surrounded by visceral pelvic fascia, which is referred to as the **parametrium**. The uterine artery crosses the ureter in this fascia on each side of the cervix (see Fig. 6.40B).

Relations

- **Anteriorly:** The body of the uterus is related anteriorly to the **uterovesical pouch** and the superior surface of the bladder (see Fig. 6.24). The supravaginal cervix is related to the superior surface of the bladder. The vaginal cervix is related to the anterior fornix of the vagina.
- **Posteriorly:** The body of the uterus is related posteriorly to the **rectouterine pouch** (pouch of Douglas) with coils of ileum or sigmoid colon within it.
- **Laterally:** The body of the uterus is related laterally to the broad ligament and the uterine artery and vein (see Fig. 6.40). The supravaginal cervix is related to the ureter as it passes forward to enter the bladder. The vaginal cervix is related to the lateral fornix of the vagina. The uterine tubes enter the superolateral angles of the uterus, and the round ligaments of the ovary and of the uterus are attached to the uterine wall just below this level.

Uterine Positions

In most females, the long axis of the uterus is bent forward at about a 90° angle to the long axis of the vagina. This position is referred to as **anteversion of the uterus** (see Fig. 6.43C). Furthermore, the long axis of the body of the uterus is bent forward at the level of the internal os with the long axis of the cervix. This position is termed **anteflexion of the uterus** (see Fig. 6.43D). Thus, in the erect position and with the bladder empty, the uterus lies in an almost horizontal plane.

In some females, the fundus and body of the uterus are bent backward on the vagina so that they lie in the rectouterine pouch (pouch of Douglas). In this situation, the uterus is said to be **retroverted**. If the body of the uterus is, in addition, bent backward on the cervix, it is said to be **retroflexed**.

Function

The uterus serves as a site for the reception, retention, and nutrition of the fertilized ovum.

Blood Supply

The arterial supply to the uterus is mainly from the **uterine artery**, a branch of the internal iliac artery. It reaches the uterus by running medially in the base of the broad ligament (see Fig. 6.40). It crosses above the ureter at right angles and reaches the cervix at the level of the internal os (see Fig. 6.43A). The artery then ascends along the lateral margin of the uterus within the broad ligament and ends by anastomosing with the **ovarian artery**, which also assists in supplying the uterus. The uterine artery gives off a small descending branch that supplies the cervix and the vagina.

The **uterine vein** follows the artery and drains into the internal iliac vein.

Lymph Drainage

The lymph vessels from the fundus of the uterus accompany the ovarian artery and drain into the **paraaortic nodes** at the level of the L1 vertebra (see Fig. 5.121). The vessels from the body and cervix drain into the **internal** and **external iliac lymph nodes**. A few lymph vessels follow the round ligament of the uterus through the inguinal canal and drain into the superficial inguinal lymph nodes.

Nerve Supply

Sympathetic and parasympathetic nerves from branches of the **inferior hypogastric plexuses** innervate the uterus (see Fig. 6.19).

Uterine Supports

The uterus is supported mainly by the tone of the levator ani muscles and by local condensations of pelvic fascia, which form three important ligaments.

Levator Ani Muscles and Perineal Body

The attachments of the levator ani muscles were described in Table 6.1. They form a broad muscular sheet stretching across the floor of the pelvic cavity,

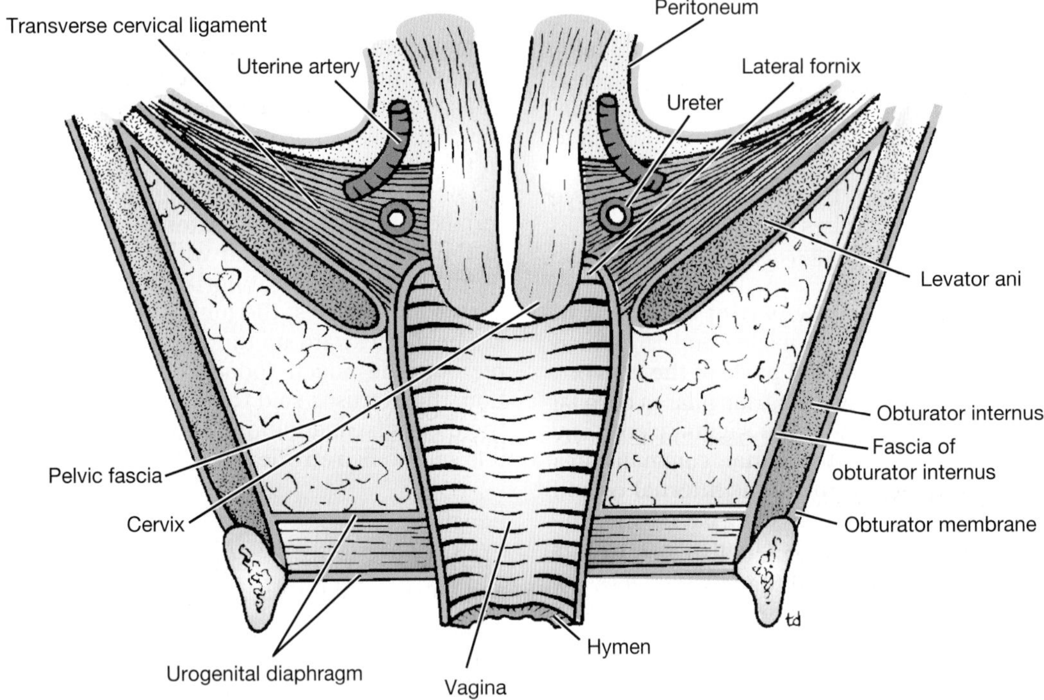

Figure 6.46 Coronal section of the pelvis showing relation of the levator ani muscles and the transverse cervical ligaments to the uterus and vagina. Note the transverse cervical ligaments are formed from a condensation of visceral pelvic fascia.

and, together with the pelvic fascia on their upper surface, they effectively support the pelvic viscera and resist the intra-abdominal pressure transmitted downward through the pelvis. The medial edges of the anterior parts of the levator ani muscles attach to the cervix of the uterus by the pelvic fascia (Fig. 6.46).

Some of the fibers of levator ani insert into a fibromuscular structure called the **perineal body** (see Fig. 6.24). This structure is important in maintaining the integrity of the pelvic floor. If the perineal body is damaged during childbirth, prolapse of the pelvic viscera may occur. The perineal body lies in the perineum between the vagina and the anal canal. It is slung up to the pelvic walls by the levatores ani and thus supports the vagina and, indirectly, the uterus.

Fascial Ligaments

Subperitoneal condensations of pelvic fascia on the upper surface of the levator ani muscles form three ligaments: transverse cervical, pubocervical, and sacrocervical. These attach to the cervix and the vault of the vagina and play an important role in supporting the uterus and keeping the cervix in its correct position (Fig. 6.47; see also Fig. 6.46).

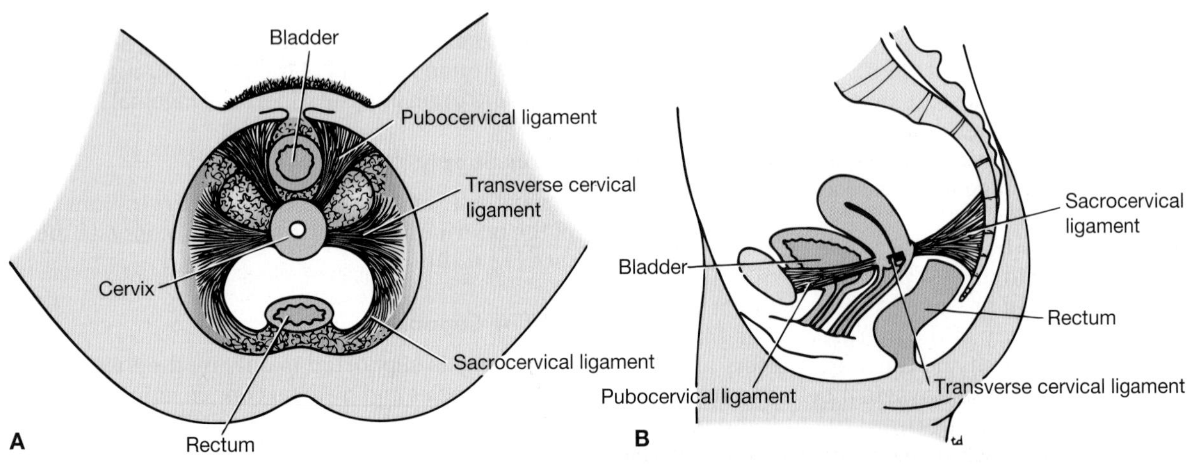

Figure 6.47 Ligamentous supports of uterus. **A.** As seen from below. **B.** Lateral view. These ligaments are formed from visceral pelvic fascia.

TRANSVERSE CERVICAL (CARDINAL) LIGAMENTS

The transverse cervical ligaments are fibromuscular condensations of pelvic fascia that pass to the cervix and the upper end of the vagina from the lateral walls of the pelvis.

PUBOCERVICAL LIGAMENTS

The pubocervical ligaments consist of two firm bands of connective tissue that pass to the cervix from the posterior surface of the pubis. They are positioned on either side of the neck of the bladder, to which they give some support (**pubovesical ligaments**).

SACROCERVICAL LIGAMENTS

The sacrocervical ligaments consist of two firm fibromuscular bands of pelvic fascia that pass to the cervix and the upper end of the vagina from the lower end of the sacrum. They form two ridges, one on either side of the rectouterine pouch.

The broad ligaments and the round ligaments of the uterus are lax structures, and the uterus can be pulled up or pushed down for a considerable distance before they become taut. Clinically, they are considered to play a minor role in supporting the uterus.

The round ligament of the uterus, which represents the remains of the lower half of the gubernaculum, extends between the superolateral angle of the uterus, through the deep inguinal ring and inguinal canal, to the subcutaneous tissue of the labium majus (see Fig. 6.30B). It may help keep the uterus anteverted (tilted forward) and anteflexed (bent forward) but is considerably stretched during pregnancy.

Prepuberty Uterus

The fundus and body of the uterus remain small until puberty, when they enlarge greatly in response to the estrogens secreted by the ovaries.

Postmenopausal Uterus

After menopause, the uterus atrophies and becomes smaller and less vascular. These changes occur because the ovaries no longer produce estrogens and progesterone.

Pregnant Uterus

During pregnancy, the uterus becomes greatly enlarged because of the increasing production of estrogens and progesterone, first by the corpus luteum of the ovary and later by the placenta. At first, it remains as a pelvic organ, but by the third month, the fundus rises out of the pelvis, and, by the ninth month, it has reached the xiphoid process (see Surface Anatomy below). The increase in size is largely a result of hypertrophy of the smooth muscle fibers of the myometrium, although some hyperplasia takes place.

Role of Uterus in Labor

Labor, or **parturition**, is the series of processes by which the infant, the fetal membranes, and the placenta are expelled from the genital tract of the mother. Normally, this process takes place after 39 gestational weeks, at which time, the pregnancy is said to be at **term**.

The cause of the onset of labor is not definitely known. By the end of pregnancy, the contractility of the uterus has been fully developed in response to estrogen, and it is particularly sensitive to the actions of oxytocin at this time. It is possible that the onset of labor is triggered by the sudden withdrawal of progesterone. Once the presenting part (usually the fetal head) starts to stretch the cervix, a nervous reflex mechanism is initiated and increases the force of the contractions of the uterine body.

The uterine muscular activity is largely independent of the extrinsic innervation. In women in labor, spinal anesthesia does not interfere with the normal uterine contractions. Severe emotional disturbance, however, can cause premature parturition.

Clinical Notes

Bimanual Uterine Pelvic Examination

A bimanual examination can provide a great deal of useful clinical information about the state of the uterus, uterine tubes, and ovaries. It may be performed under an anesthetic in patients in whom it causes distress. With the bladder empty, the vaginal portion of the cervix is first palpated with the index finger of the right hand. The external os is circular in the nulliparous woman but has anterior and posterior lips in the multiparous woman. The cervix normally has the consistency of the end of the nose, but in the pregnant uterus, it is soft and vascular and has the consistency of the lips. The left hand is then placed gently on the anterior abdominal wall above the symphysis pubis, and the fundus and body of the uterus may be palpated between the abdominal and vaginal fingers situated in the anterior fornix. The size, shape, and mobility of the uterus can then be ascertained.

In most patients, the uterus is anteverted and anteflexed. A retroverted, retroflexed uterus can be palpated through the posterior vaginal fornix.

Varicose Veins and Hemorrhoids in Pregnancy

Varicose veins and hemorrhoids are common conditions in pregnancy. The following factors probably contribute to their cause: pressure of the gravid uterus on the inferior vena cava and the inferior mesenteric vein, impairing venous return, and increased progesterone levels in the blood, leading to relaxation of the smooth muscle in the walls of the veins and venous dilatation.

Emergency Cesarean Section

An emergency cesarean section is rarely performed. However, a physician may need to perform this surgery in cases in

(continued)

which the mother may die after suffering a severe traumatic incident. Following maternal death, placental circulation ceases, and the child must be delivered within 10 minutes. Neonatal survival is rare after a delay of more than 20 minutes.

Anatomy of Technique

1. The bladder is emptied, and an indwelling catheter is left in position. This allows the empty bladder to sink down away from the operating field.
2. A midline skin incision is made that extends from just below the umbilicus to just above the symphysis pubis. The following structures are then incised: superficial fascia (fatty layer, then the membranous layer), deep fascia (thin layer), linear alba, transversalis fascia, extraperitoneal fatty layer, and parietal peritoneum. To avoid damaging loops of the small intestine or the greater omentum, which might be lying beneath the parietal peritoneum, a fold of peritoneum is raised between two hemostats; an incision is then made between the hemostats.
3. The bladder is identified, and a cut is made in the floor of the uterovesical pouch. The bladder is then separated from the lower part of the body of the uterus and depressed downward into the pelvis.
4. The uterus is palpated to identify the presenting part of the fetus.
5. A transverse incision about 1 in. (2.5 cm) long is made into the exposed lower segment of the body of the uterus. Care is taken that the uterine wall is not immediately penetrated, and the fetus injured.
6. When the uterine cavity is entered, the amniotic cavity is opened, and amniotic fluid spurts. The uterine incision is then enlarged sufficiently to deliver the head and trunk of the fetus. When possible, the large tributaries and branches of the uterine vessels in the myometrial wall are avoided. Great care must be taken to avoid the large uterine arteries that course along the lateral margin of the uterus.
7. Once the fetus is delivered, the umbilical cord is clamped and divided.
8. The contracting uterus will cause the placenta to bulge through the uterine incision. The placenta and fetal membranes are then delivered.
9. The uterine incision is closed with a full-thickness continuous suture. The peritoneum over the bladder and lower part of the uterine body is then repaired to restore the integrity of the uterovesical pouch. Finally, the abdominal wall incision is closed in layers.

Uterine Prolapse

The levator ani muscles and the subperitoneal fascial ligaments are critical in supporting the uterus and in positioning the cervix within the pelvic cavity. Damage to these structures during childbirth or general poor body muscular tone may result in downward displacement of the uterus called **uterine prolapse**. This condition occurs most commonly after menopause, when the visceral pelvic fascia tends to atrophy along with the pelvic organs. In advanced cases, the cervix descends the length of the vagina and may protrude through the orifice.

Because the cervix is attached to the vaginal vault, prolapse of the uterus is always accompanied by some degree of vaginal prolapse.

Hysterectomy and Damage to Ureters

During the surgical procedure of hysterectomy, great care must be exercised to not damage the ureters. When the surgeon is looking for the uterine artery on each side at the base of the broad ligament, it is essential that they first identify the ureter before clamping and tying off the artery. The uterine artery passes forward from the internal iliac artery and crosses the ureter at right angles to reach the cervix at the level of the internal os.

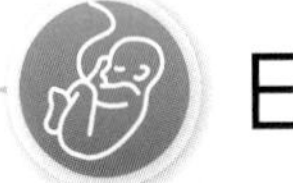

Embryology Notes

Uterine Development

The uterus is derived from the fused caudal vertical parts of the **paramesonephric ducts** (Fig. 6.48). The site of their angular junction becomes a convex dome and forms the **fundus** of the uterus. The fusion between the ducts is incomplete at first, and a septum persists between the lumina. Later, the septum disappears so that a single **cavity** remains. The upper part of the cavity forms the lumen of the **body** and **cervix** of the uterus. The **myometrium** is formed from the surrounding mesenchyme.

Uterine Agenesis

Rarely, the uterus will be absent as the result of a failure of the paramesonephric ducts to develop.

Infantile Uterus

Some adults may have an infantile uterus, a condition in which the uterus is much smaller than normal and resembles that present before puberty. Amenorrhea is present, but the vagina and ovaries may be normal.

Failure of Paramesonephric Duct Fusion

Failure of the paramesonephric ducts to fuse may cause a variety of uterine defects:

- The uterus may be **duplicated** with two bodies and two cervices.
- A complete septum may occur through the uterus, making two uterine cavities and two cervices.
- Two separate uterine bodies with one cervix may occur.
- One paramesonephric duct may fail to develop, leaving one uterine tube and half of the body of the uterus.

Clinically, the main problems with a double uterus may be seen when pregnancy occurs. Abortion is frequent, and the nonpregnant half of the uterus may cause obstruction at labor.

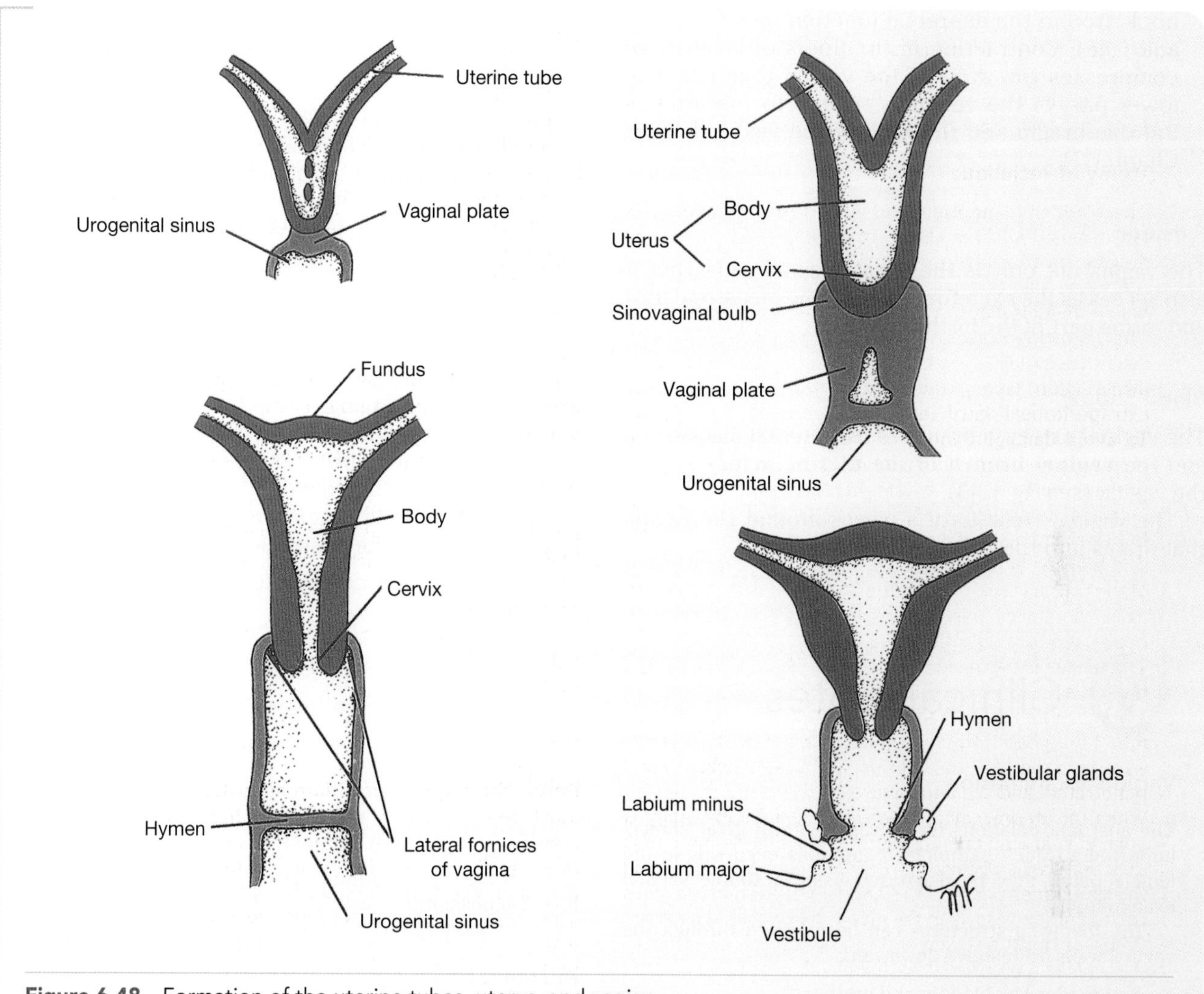

Figure 6.48 Formation of the uterine tubes, uterus, and vagina.

Vagina

The vagina is a muscular tube that extends upward and backward from the vulva to the uterus (see Fig. 6.24). It measures about 3 in. (8 cm) long and has **anterior** and **posterior walls**, which are normally in apposition. The cervix pierces the upper anterior wall of the vagina and projects downward and backward into the upper vagina. It is important to remember that the upper half of the vagina lies above the pelvic floor (ie, in the pelvic cavity), whereas the lower half lies within the perineum (see Figs. 6.24 and 6.46). The area of the vaginal lumen that surrounds the cervix is divided into four archlike regions, or **fornices**: anterior, posterior, right lateral, and left lateral. The vaginal orifice is covered or surrounded to a variable degree by a small, thin piece of mucosal tissue called the **hymen**, which forms during development and is present at birth. The hymen has no discernable function; it varies in size, shape, thickness, and degree of perforation and may change over time. However, it must be open enough for menstrual blood and normal secretions to exit the vagina. In time, it stretches or breaks because of various common activities (eg, inserting a tampon, vigorous exercise, and sexual activity). After childbirth, the hymen usually consists only of small, irregular remnants (tags).

Relations

- **Anteriorly:** The vagina is closely related to the bladder above and to the urethra below (see Fig. 6.24).
- **Posteriorly:** The upper third of the vagina is related to the rectouterine pouch (pouch of Douglas). The middle third is related to the ampulla of the rectum. The lower third is related to the perineal body, which separates it from the anal canal.
- **Laterally:** The upper part of the vagina is related to the ureter. The middle part is related to the anterior fibers (puborectalis) of the levator ani, as they run backward to reach the perineal body and

hook around the anorectal junction (see Figs. 6.40 and 6.46). Contraction of the fibers of levator ani compresses the walls of the vagina together. The lower part of the vagina is related to the urogenital diaphragm and the bulb of the vestibule (see Chapter 7).

Function

The vagina not only is the female genital canal, but it also serves as the excretory duct for the menstrual flow and forms part of the birth canal.

Blood Supply

The **vaginal artery**, a branch of the internal iliac artery, and the **vaginal branch of the uterine artery** supply the vagina (see Fig. 6.43).

The vaginal veins form a plexus around the vagina that drains into the internal iliac vein.

Lymph Drainage

The upper third of the vagina drains to the external and internal **iliac nodes**, the middle third drains to the **internal iliac nodes**, and the lower third drains to the **superficial inguinal nodes** (see Fig. 5.121).

Nerve Supply

Branches of the **inferior hypogastric plexuses** innervate the vagina (see Fig. 6.19).

Vaginal Supports

The levator ani muscles and the transverse cervical, pubocervical, and sacrocervical ligaments support the upper part of the vagina. These structures attach to the vaginal wall by pelvic fascia (see Figs. 6.46 and 6.47).

The urogenital diaphragm supports the middle part of the vagina (see Chapter 7).

The perineal body supports the lower part of the vagina, especially the posterior wall (see Fig. 6.24).

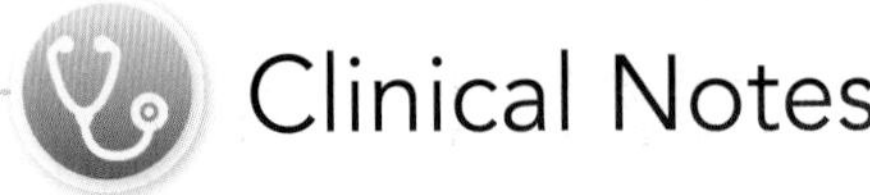

Clinical Notes

Vaginal Examination

The anatomic relations of the vagina are of great clinical importance. Many pathologic conditions occurring in the female pelvis may be diagnosed using a simple vaginal examination.

The following structures can be palpated through the vaginal walls from above downward:

- **Anteriorly:** The bladder and urethra
- **Posteriorly:** Loops of ileum and the sigmoid colon in the rectouterine peritoneal pouch (pouch of Douglas), the rectal ampulla, and the perineal body
- **Laterally:** The ureters, the pelvic fascia, the anterior fibers of the levator ani muscles, and the urogenital diaphragm

Vaginal Prolapse

The vaginal vault is supported by the same muscular and fascial structures that support the uterine cervix. Thus, prolapse of the uterus is necessarily associated with some degree of sagging of the vaginal walls. However, if the supports of the bladder, urethra, or anterior rectal wall are damaged in childbirth, prolapse of the vaginal walls occurs, with the uterus remaining in its correct position.

Bladder sagging results in the bulging of the anterior wall of the vagina, a condition known as a **cystocele**. When the ampulla of the rectum sags against the posterior vaginal wall, the bulge is called a **rectocele**.

Culdocentesis

The closeness of the peritoneal cavity to the posterior vaginal fornix enables the physician to drain a pelvic abscess through the vagina without performing a major operation. It is also possible to identify blood or pus in the peritoneal cavity by passing a needle through the posterior fornix.

Anatomic Structures through which Needle Passes

The needle passes through the mucous membrane of the vagina, muscular coat of the vagina, connective tissue coat of the vagina, visceral layer of pelvic fascia, and visceral layer of peritoneum.

Anatomic Features of Complications

The needle could impale the loops of ileum and the sigmoid colon, structures that are normally present within the rectouterine pouch. However, the presence of blood or pus within the pouch tends to deflect the viscera superiorly. Also, occasionally, when the uterus is somewhat retroflexed, the needle may enter the posterior wall of the body of the uterus.

Vaginal Trauma

Coital injury, picket fence type of impalement injury, and vaginal perforation caused by water under pressure, as occurs in water skiing, are common injuries. Lacerations of the vaginal wall involving the posterior fornix may violate the rectouterine pouch of the peritoneal cavity and cause prolapse of the small intestine into the vagina.

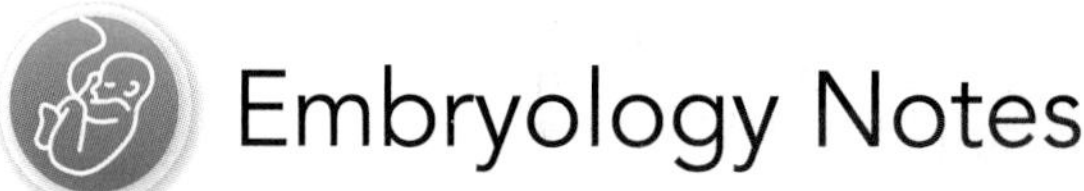

Embryology Notes

Vaginal Development

The vagina develops from the wall of the **urogenital sinus** (see Fig. 6.48). The fused lower ends of the paramesonephric ducts form the body and cervix of the uterus, and once the solid end of the fused ducts reaches the posterior wall of the urogenital sinus, two outgrowths occur from the sinus, the **sinovaginal bulbs**. The cells of the sinovaginal bulbs proliferate rapidly and form the **vaginal plate**. The vaginal plate thickens and elongates and extends around the solid end of the fused paramesonephric ducts. Later, the plate completely canalizes and forms the vaginal **fornices**.

Vaginal Agenesis

If the paramesonephric ducts fail to develop, the wall of the urogenital sinus will not form the vaginal plate. In these patients, the vagina, uterus, and uterine tubes are absent. Plastic surgical construction of a vagina may be attempted.

Double Vagina

A double vagina is caused by incomplete canalization of the vaginal plate.

Imperforate Vagina and Imperforate Hymen

Imperforate vagina is caused by a failure of the cells to degenerate in the center of the vaginal plates. Imperforate hymen is caused by a failure of the cells of the lower part of the vaginal plate and wall of the urogenital sinus to degenerate. These conditions lead to retention of the menstrual flow, a clinical condition called **hematocolpos**. Surgical incision of the obstruction, followed by dilatation, relieves the condition.

Visceral Pelvic Fascia

The visceral pelvic fascia is a layer of connective tissue, which, as in the male, covers and supports the pelvic viscera. It is condensed in specific areas to form the pubocervical, transverse cervical, and sacrocervical ligaments of the uterus (see Fig. 6.47).

Peritoneum

The peritoneum in the female, as in the male, is best understood by tracing it around the pelvis in a sagittal plane (see Fig. 6.24).

The parietal peritoneum passes down from the anterior abdominal wall onto the upper surface of the urinary bladder. It then turns back onto the anterior surface of the uterus, at the level of the internal os. This reflection creates the shallow **uterovesical pouch** between the superior wall of the bladder and the anterior wall of the uterus. The peritoneum now passes upward over the anterior surface of the body and fundus of the uterus and then downward over the posterior surface. It continues downward and covers the upper part of the posterior surface of the vagina and then passes onto the front of the rectum, as in the male. The contour of the peritoneal reflection from the vagina onto the rectum creates a deep recess, the **rectouterine pouch (pouch of Douglas)**. In the female, the rectouterine pouch is the lowest part of the abdominopelvic peritoneal cavity in the erect position.

Clinical Notes

Visceral Pelvic Fascia and Infection

Clinically, the pelvic fascia in the region of the uterine cervix is often referred to as the **parametrium**. It is a common site for the spread of acute infections from the uterus and vagina, and here the infection often becomes chronic (pelvic inflammatory disease).

Broad Ligaments

The broad ligaments are two-layered folds of peritoneum that extend across the pelvic cavity from the lateral margins of the uterus to the lateral pelvic walls, covering the body and fundus of the uterus, uterine tubes, and ovaries (see Fig. 6.40A). Superiorly, the two layers are continuous and form the upper **free edge**. Inferiorly, at the base of the ligament, the layers separate to cover the pelvic floor (see Fig. 6.40B). The connective tissue that fills the gap between the separated layers of the broad ligament is the **parametrium**. The part of the broad ligament that attaches to the lateral margins of the uterus is the **mesometrium**. The ovary attaches to the posterior layer of the broad ligament by the **mesovarium**. The part of the broad ligament that lies lateral to the attachment of the mesovarium forms the **suspensory ligament of the ovary**. The part of the broad ligament that attaches to the uterine tube and runs between the uterine tube and the mesovarium is the **mesosalpinx**.

The **uterine artery** crosses the **ureter** at the base of the broad ligament (see Figs. 6.40 and 6.46). This is a significant relationship in surgery in this area. Remember this by recalling that water (ureter) runs under the bridge (artery).

Each broad ligament contains the following:

- The **uterine tube** in its upper free border.
- The **round ligament of the ovary** and the **round ligament of the uterus**. These represent the remains of the **gubernaculum**.

- The uterine and ovarian blood vessels, lymph vessels, and nerves.
- The **epoophoron**, a vestigial structure that lies in the broad ligament above the attachment of the mesovarium. It represents the remains of the mesonephros (see Fig. 6.40A).
- The **paroöphoron**, also a vestigial structure that lies in the broad ligament just lateral to the uterus. It is also a mesonephric remnant.

RADIOGRAPHIC ANATOMY

The diverse nature of the pelvic contents (ranging from hard to various degrees of soft structures) and the dense packing of structures into the small space of the pelvic cavity make medical imaging a critical tool in evaluating the condition of this area. Plain film x-rays, CT, MRI, and ultrasound all provide unique insights.

Bony Pelvis

A routine anteroposterior (AP) view of the pelvis is taken with the patient in the supine position and with the cassette underneath the tabletop. A somewhat distorted view of the lower part of the sacrum and coccyx is obtained, and these bones may be partially obscured by the symphysis pubis. A better view of the sacrum and coccyx can be obtained by slightly tilting the x-ray tube.

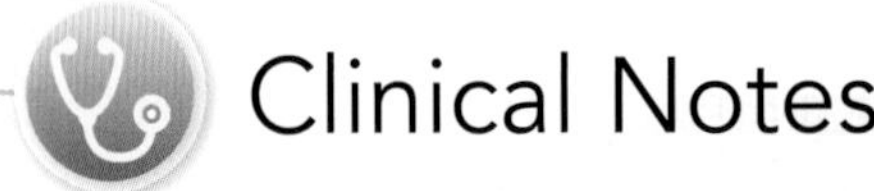

Clinical Notes

Rectouterine Pouch and Disease

Because the rectouterine pouch is the most inferior part of the entire peritoneal cavity (when the patient is in the standing position), it frequently becomes the site for the accumulation of blood (eg, from a ruptured ectopic pregnancy) or pus (eg, from a ruptured pelvic appendicitis or in gonococcal peritonitis).

Because the pouch lies directly behind the posterior fornix of the vagina, it is easily violated by misguided instruments that pierce the wall of the posterior fornix. Pelvic peritonitis is a danger that may ensue.

A needle may be passed into the pouch through the posterior fornix in a **culdocentesis.** Surgically, the pouch may be entered in a **posterior colpotomy** (vaginal incision).

The interior of the female pelvic peritoneal cavity may be viewed for evidence of disease through an endoscope. The instrument is introduced through a small colpotomy.

An AP radiograph should be systematically examined (Figs. 6.49 to 6.52). The lower lumbar vertebrae, sacrum, and coccyx may be looked at first, followed by the sacroiliac joints, the different parts of the hip bones, and finally the hip joints and upper ends of the femurs.

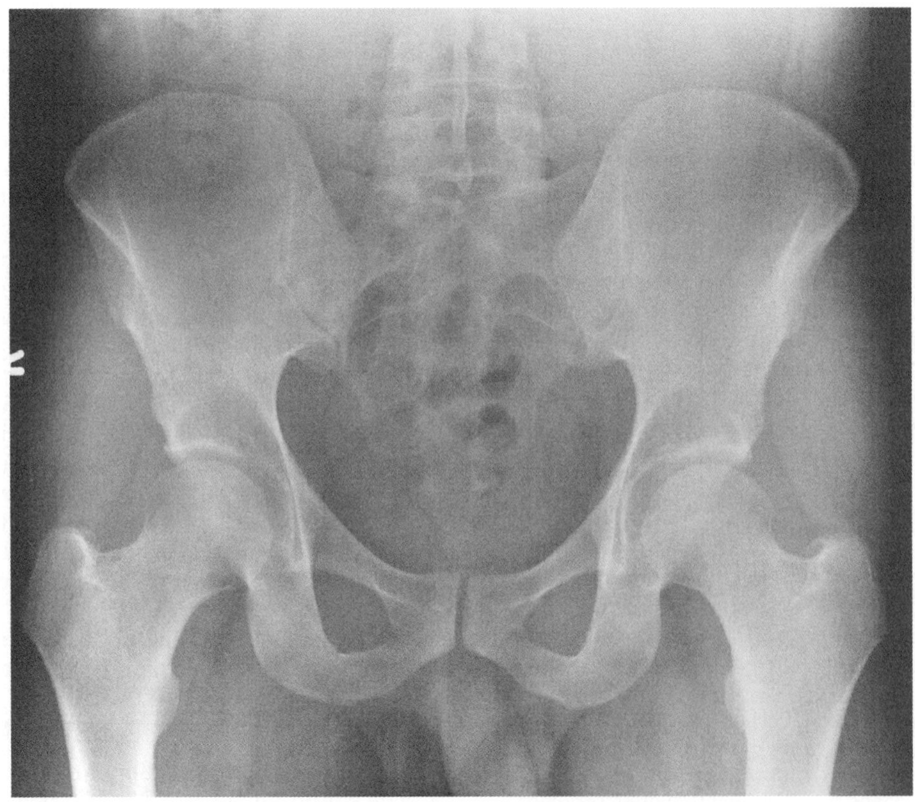

Figure 6.49 Anteroposterior radiograph of the male pelvis.

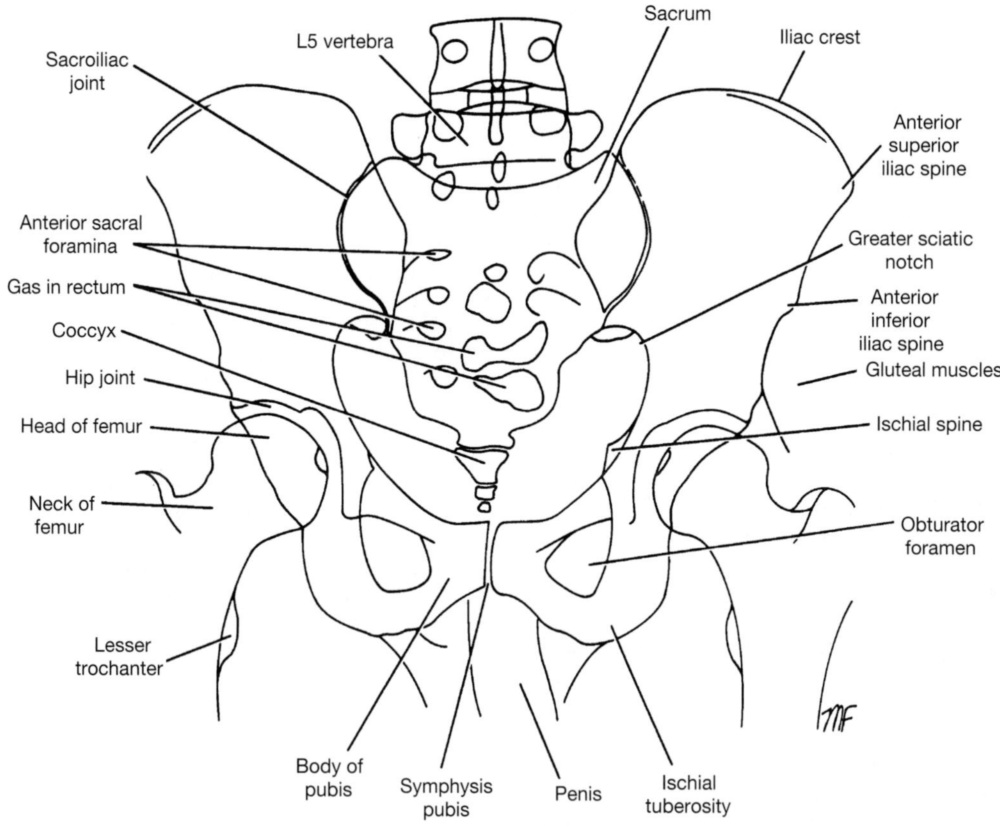

Figure 6.50 Representation of the radiograph of the pelvis seen in Figure 6.49.

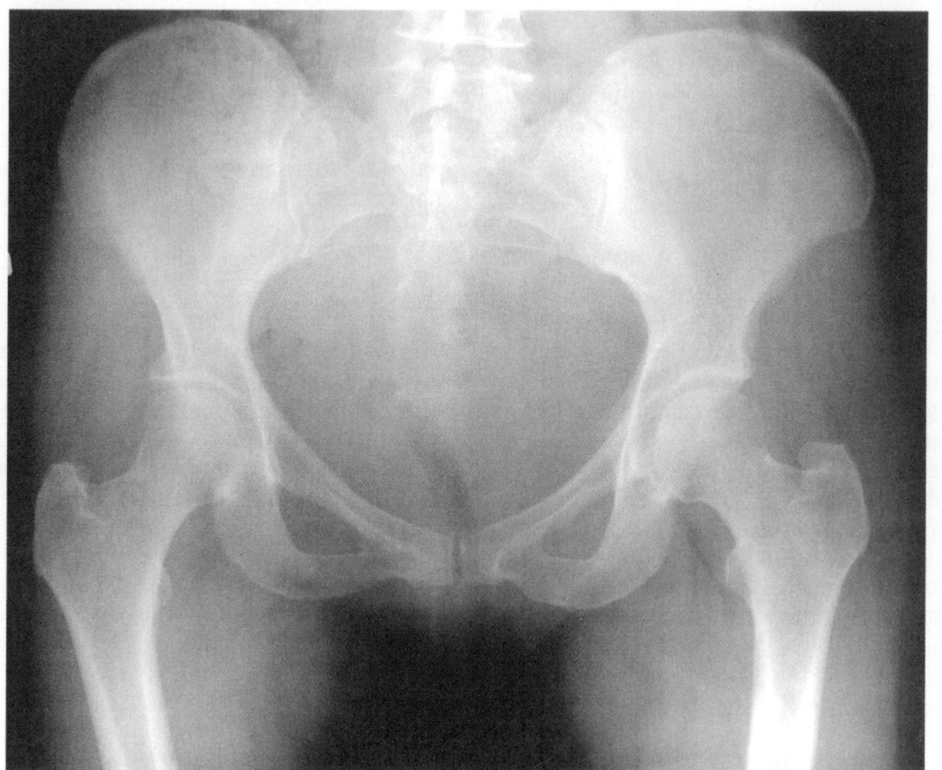

Figure 6.51 Anteroposterior radiograph of the adult female pelvis.

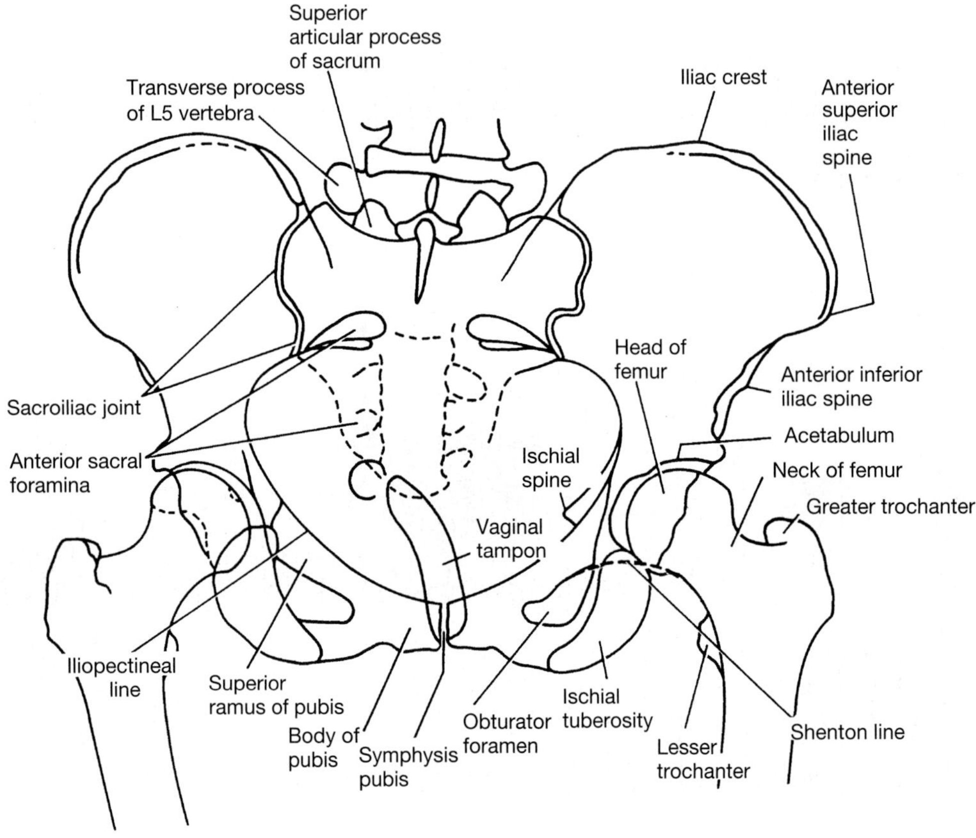

Figure 6.52 Representation of the radiograph of the pelvis seen in Figure 6.51.

Gas and fecal material may be seen in the large bowel, and soft tissue shadows of the skin and subcutaneous tissues may also be visualized. To demonstrate the sacrum and sacroiliac joints more clearly, lateral and oblique views of the pelvis are often taken.

Gastrointestinal Tract

The pelvic colon and rectum can be demonstrated effectively following a barium enema (ie, by the slow administration of 2 to 3 pints (1 L) of barium sulfate emulsion through the anus). The appearances of the pelvic colon are like those seen in the more proximal parts of the colon, but a distended sigmoid colon usually shows no haustra-like sacculations. The rectum has a wider caliber than the colon.

A contrast enema is sometimes useful for examining the mucous membrane of the sigmoid colon. The barium enema is partly evacuated, and air is injected into the colon. By this means, the walls of the colon are outlined (see Fig. 5.132).

Cross-Sectional Anatomy

Study the labeled cross sections of the pelvis shown in Figures 6.53 and 6.54 to assist in interpretation of computed tomography (CT) scans of the pelvis (Fig. 6.55). The sections have been photographed on their inferior surfaces.

Female Genital Tract

The instillation of viscous iodine preparations through the external os of the uterus allows visualization of the lumen of the cervical canal, the uterine cavity, and the different parts of the uterine tubes (Fig. 6.56). This procedure is known as **hysterosalpingography**. The patency of these structures is demonstrated by some of the opaque medium entering the peritoneal cavity.

A sonogram of the female pelvis can be used to visualize the pelvic organs and the developing fetus (Figs. 6.57 to 6.59).

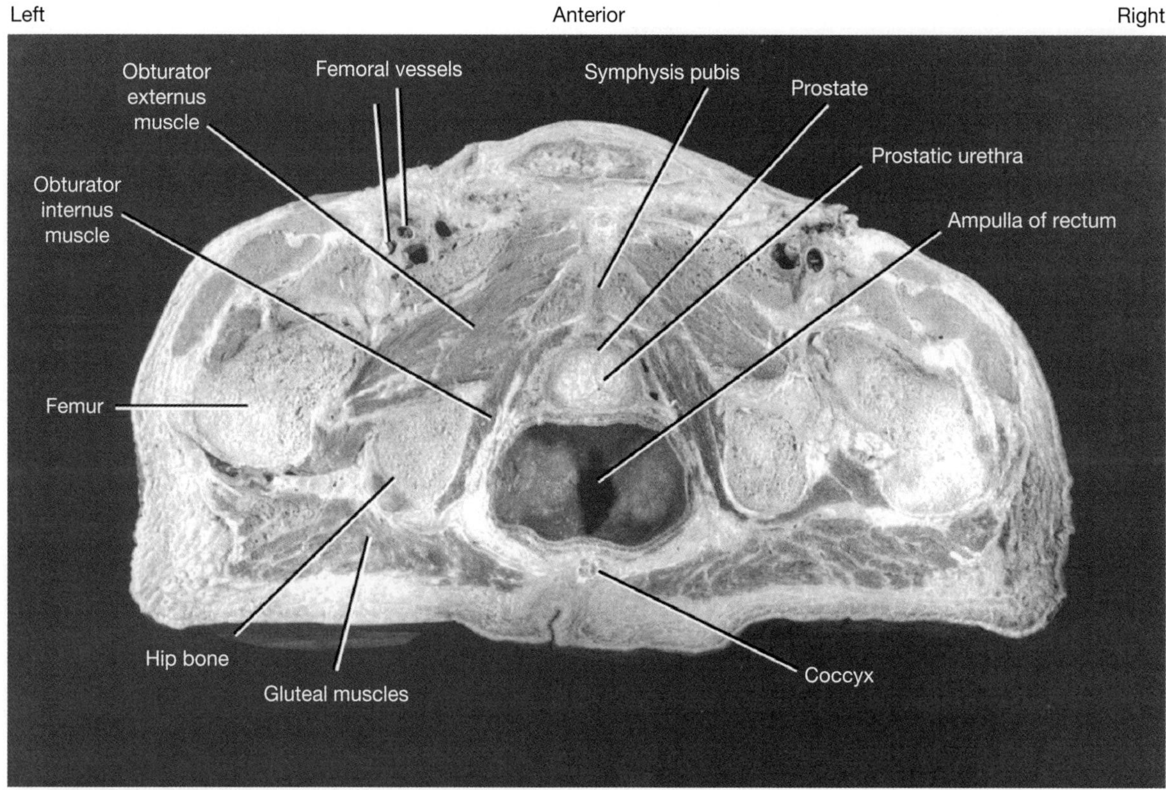

Figure 6.53 Cross section of the male pelvis as seen from above.

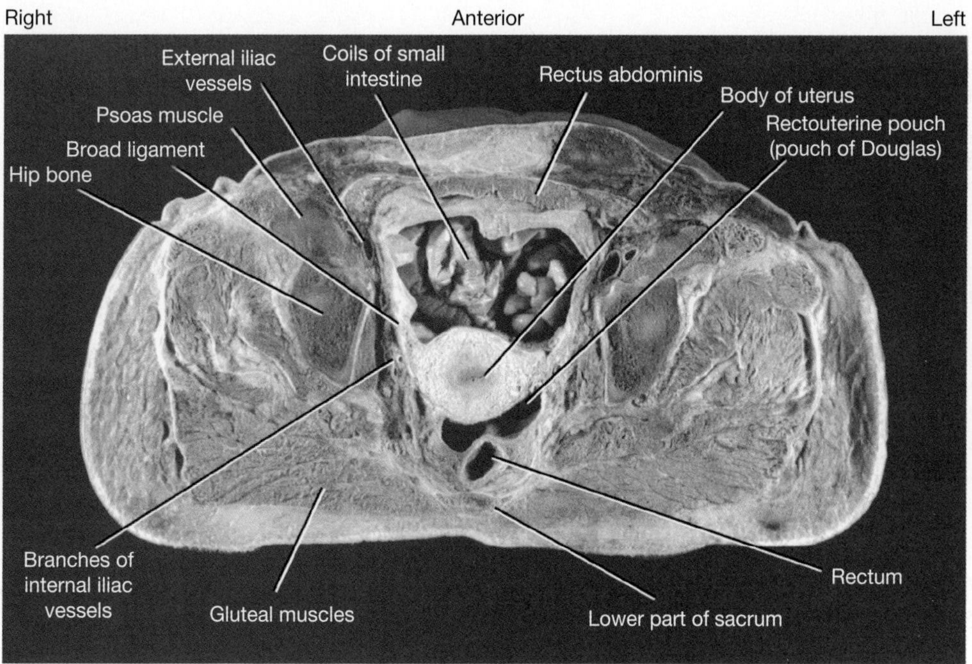

Figure 6.54 Cross section of the female pelvis as seen from below.

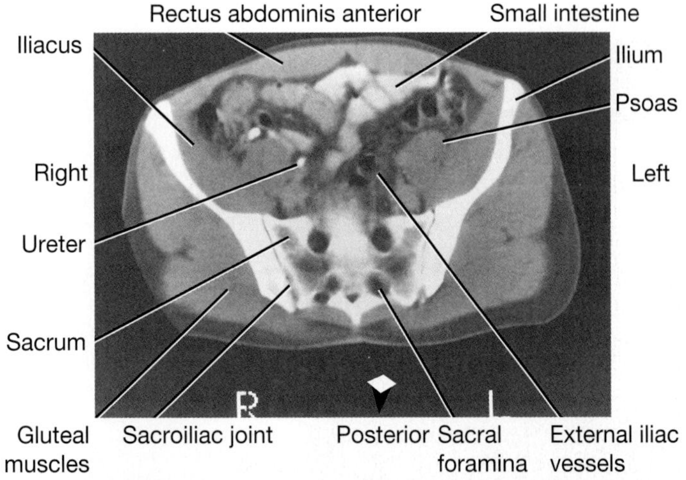

Figure 6.55 CT scan of the pelvis after a barium meal and intravenous pyelography. Note the presence of the radiopaque material in the small intestine and the right ureter. The section is viewed from below.

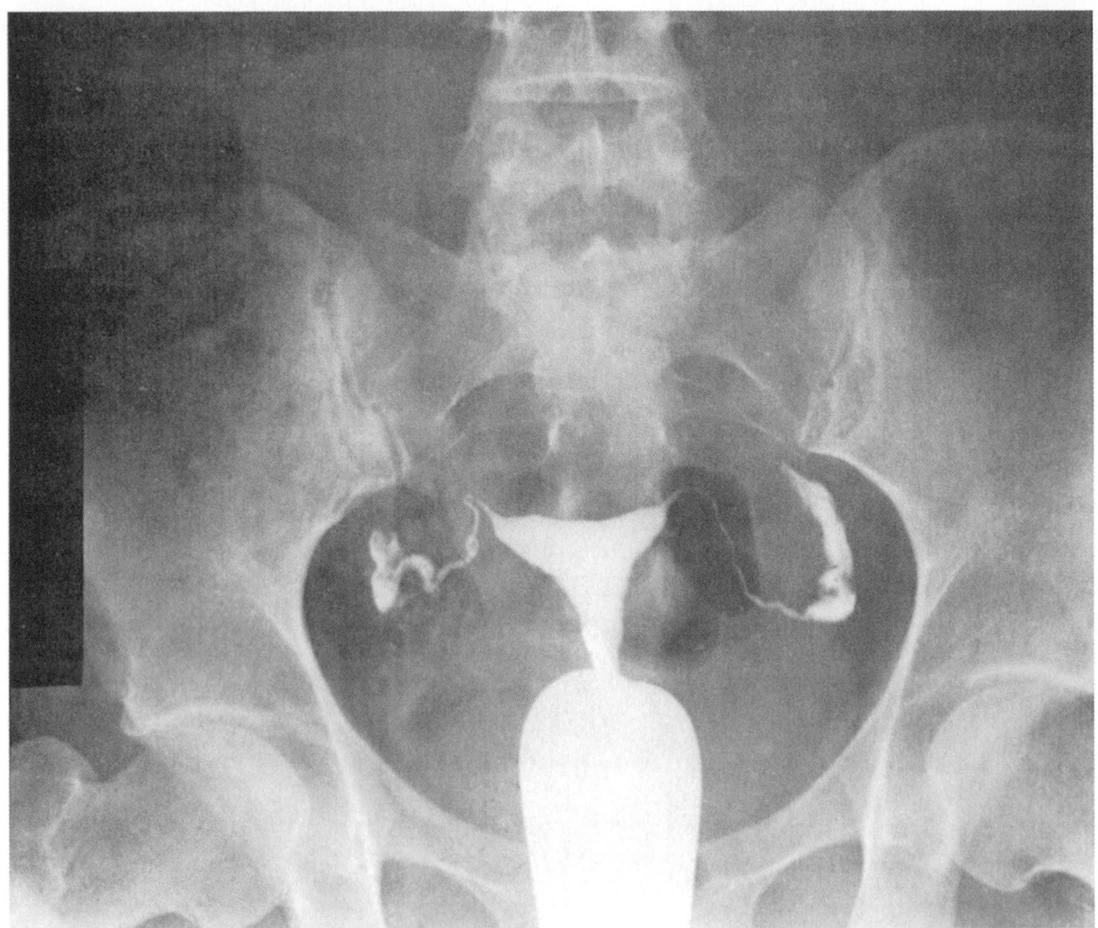

Figure 6.56 Anteroposterior radiograph of the female pelvis after injection of radiopaque compound into the uterine cavity (hysterosalpingogram).

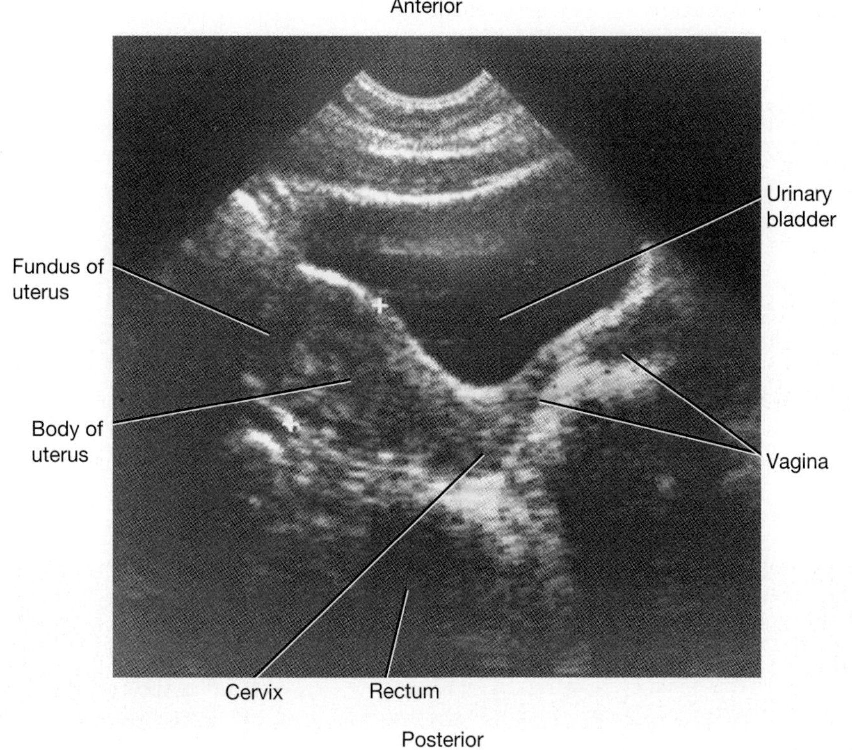

Figure 6.57 Longitudinal sonogram of the female pelvis showing the uterus, vagina, and bladder. (Courtesy of Dr. M. C. Hill.)

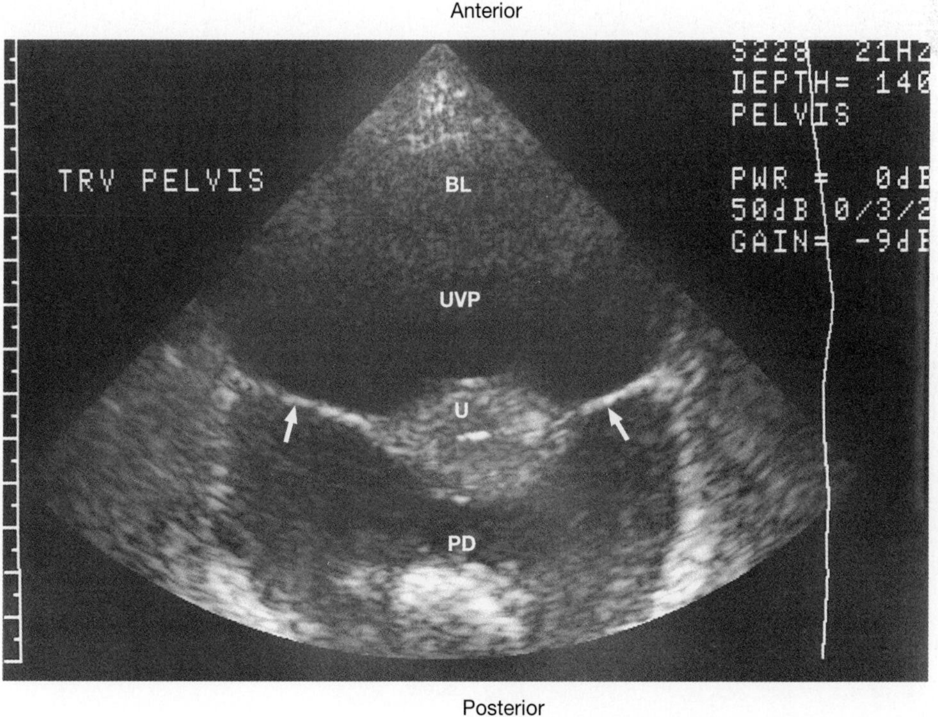

Figure 6.58 Transverse sonogram of the pelvis in a woman after an automobile accident, in which the liver was lacerated, and blood escaped into the peritoneal cavity. The bladder (*BL*), the body of the uterus (*U*), and the broad ligaments (*white arrows*) are identified. Note the presence of blood (*dark areas*) in the uterovesical pouch (*UVP*) and the pouch of Douglas (rectouterine pouch; *PD*). (Courtesy of L. Scoutt.)

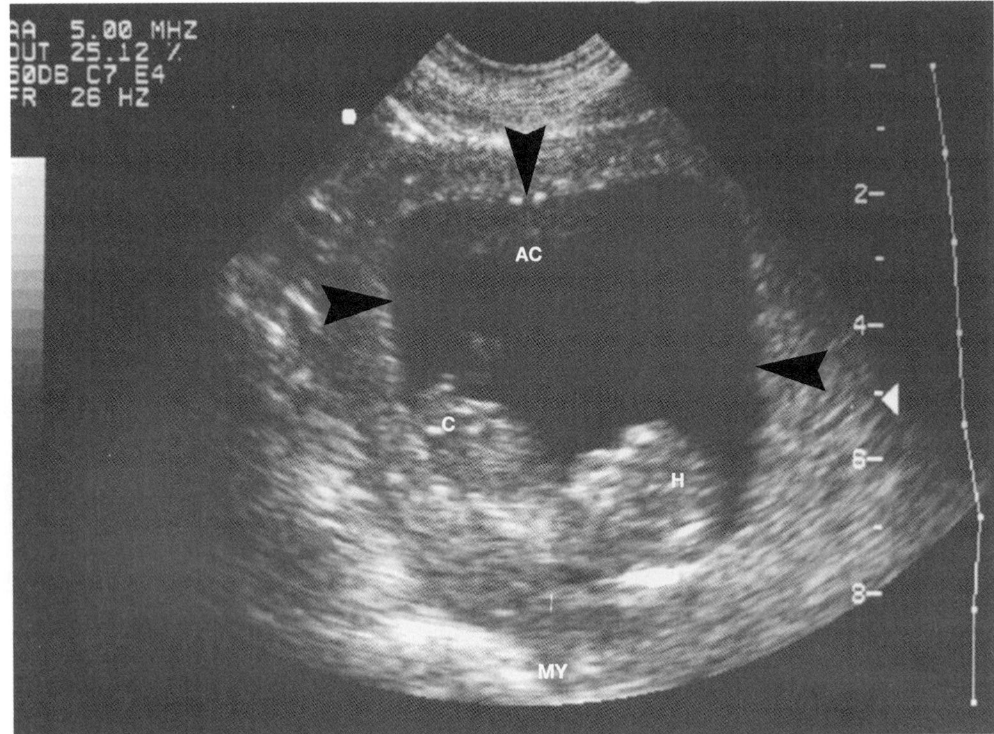

Figure 6.59 Longitudinal sonogram of a pregnant uterus at 11 weeks showing the intrauterine gestational sac (*black arrowheads*) and the amniotic cavity (*AC*) filled with amniotic fluid. The fetus is seen in longitudinal section with the head (*H*) and coccyx (*C*) well displayed. The myometrium (*MY*) of the uterus can be identified. (Courtesy of L. Scoutt.)

SURFACE ANATOMY

Several bony features of the pelvic walls are palpable in an adult of average body build. Additionally, significant parts of the underlying urogenital tracts are palpable with proper manipulation. Collectively, these form notable surface landmarks that help orient the clinician conducting a physical examination or procedure.

Iliac Crest

The iliac crest can be felt through the skin along its entire length (Figs. 6.60 to 6.62).

The **anterior superior iliac spine** is situated at the anterior end of the iliac crest and lies at the upper lateral end of the fold of the groin.

The **posterior superior iliac spine** is situated at the posterior end of the iliac crest (see Fig. 6.62). It lies at

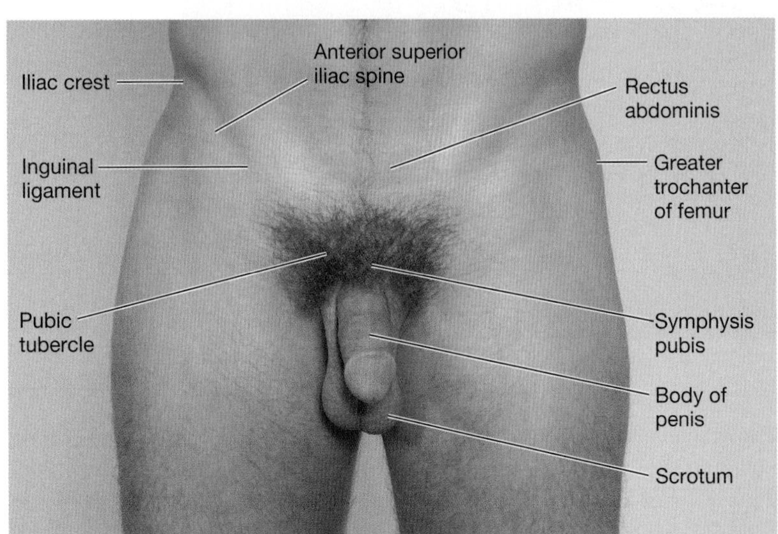

Figure 6.60 Anterior view of a young adult male showing the surface anatomy of the pelvic and inguinal regions and the groin. (Modified from *Moore's Essential Clinical Anatomy*, 7th ed; Fig. 6.58.)

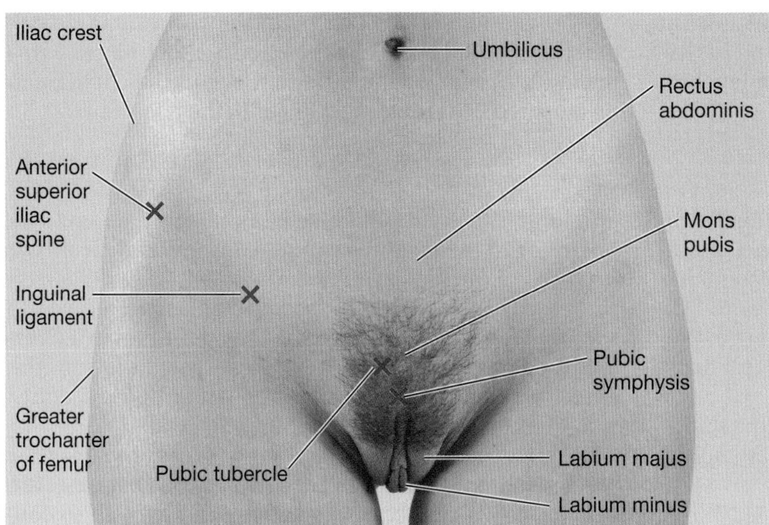

Figure 6.61 Anterior view of a young adult female showing the surface anatomy of the pelvic and inguinal regions and the groin. (Modified from *Moore's Essential Clinical Anatomy*, 7th ed; Fig. 6.52.)

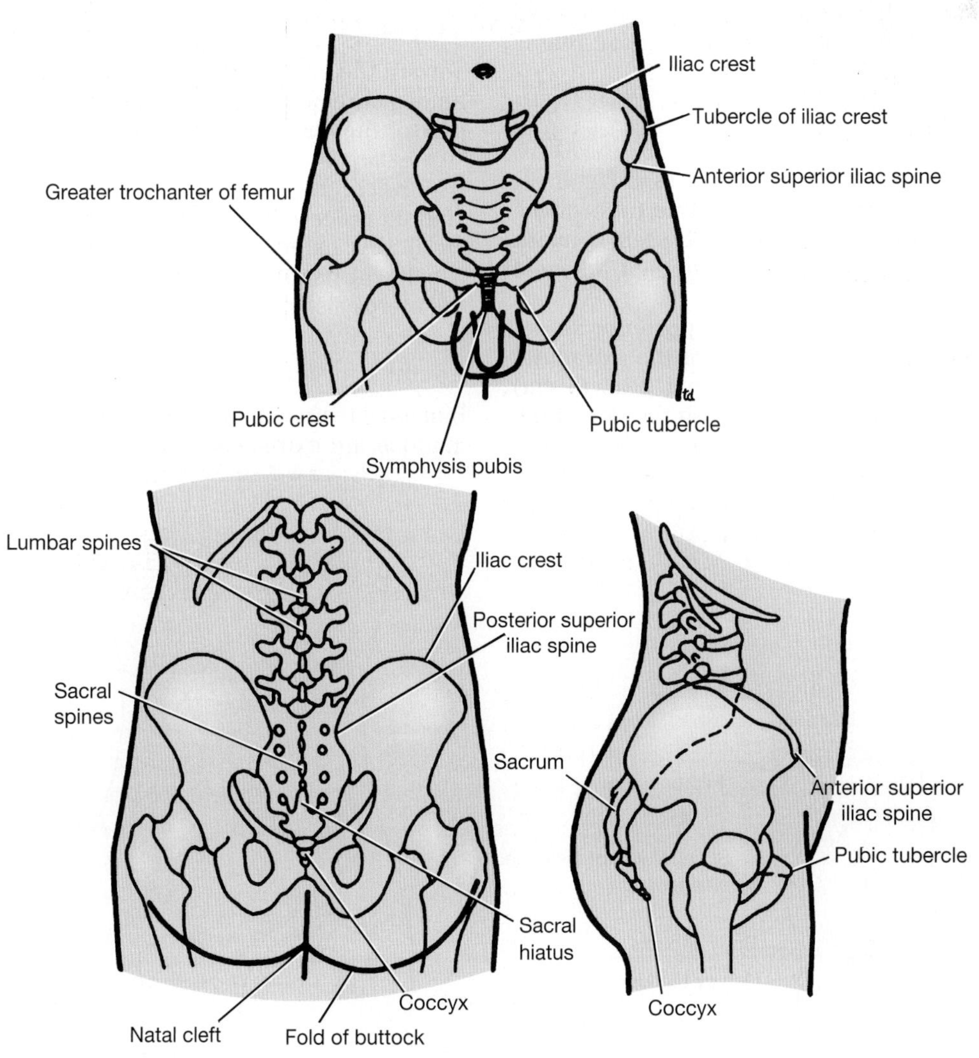

Figure 6.62 Relationship between different parts of the pelvis and the body surface.

the bottom of a small skin dimple and on a level with the S2 spine, which coincides with the lower limit of the subarachnoid space. It also coincides with the level of the middle of the sacroiliac joint.

Pubic Tubercle and Crest

The **pubic tubercle** can be felt on the upper border of the pubis (see Figs. 6.60 to 6.62). The medial end of the inguinal ligament is attached to it. The tubercle can be palpated easily in the male by invaginating the scrotum from below with the examining finger. In the female, the pubic tubercle can be palpated through the lateral margin of the labium majus.

The **pubic crest** is the ridge of the bone on the superior surface of the pubic bone, medial to the pubic tubercle (see Figs. 6.1 and 6.62).

Symphysis Pubis

The symphysis pubis (see Figs. 6.1 and 6.62) lies in the midline between the bodies of the pubic bones and can be palpated as a solid structure through the fat that is present in this region.

Sacrum and Coccyx

The **spinous processes** of the sacrum (see Fig. 6.62) are fused with each other in the midline to form the **median sacral crest**. The crest can be felt beneath the skin in the uppermost part of the cleft between the buttocks.

The **sacral hiatus** is situated on the posterior aspect of the lower end of the sacrum, where the extradural space terminates. The hiatus lies about 2 in. (5 cm) above the tip of the coccyx and beneath the skin of the cleft between the buttocks.

The inferior surface and tip of the **coccyx** can be palpated in the cleft between the buttocks about 1 in. (2.5 cm) behind the anus. The anterior surface of the coccyx can be palpated with the gloved finger in the anal canal.

Urinary Bladder

In adults, the empty bladder is a pelvic organ and lies posterior to the symphysis pubis. As the bladder fills, it rises out of the pelvis into the abdomen, where it can be palpated through the anterior abdominal wall above the symphysis pubis (Fig. 6.63A). The peritoneum covering the distended bladder becomes peeled off from the anterior abdominal wall so that the front of the bladder is in direct contact with the abdominal wall.

In children younger than age 6 years, the bladder is an abdominal organ even when empty because the capacity of the pelvic cavity is not great enough to contain it. The neck of the bladder lies just below the level of the upper border of the symphysis pubis.

Uterus

Toward the end of the second month of pregnancy, the fundus of the uterus can be palpated through the lower part of the anterior abdominal wall. With the progressive enlargement of the uterus, the fundus rises above the level of the umbilicus and reaches the region of the xiphoid process by the ninth month of pregnancy (see Fig. 6.63B). Later, when the presenting part of the fetus, usually the head, descends into the pelvis, the fundus of the uterus also descends.

Rectal and Vaginal Examinations

Bimanual rectoabdominal and vaginal–abdominal examinations are extremely valuable methods of palpating

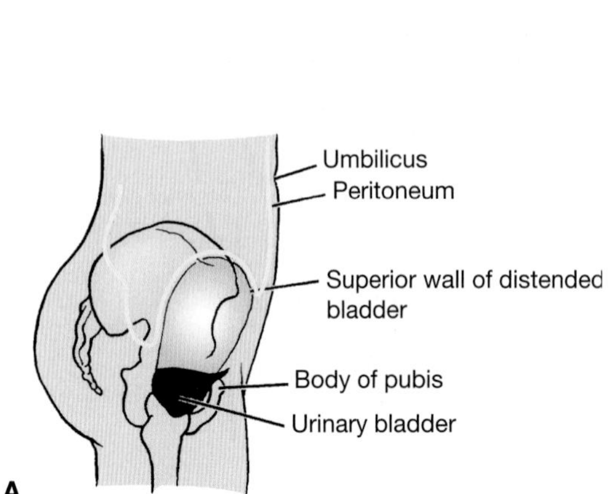

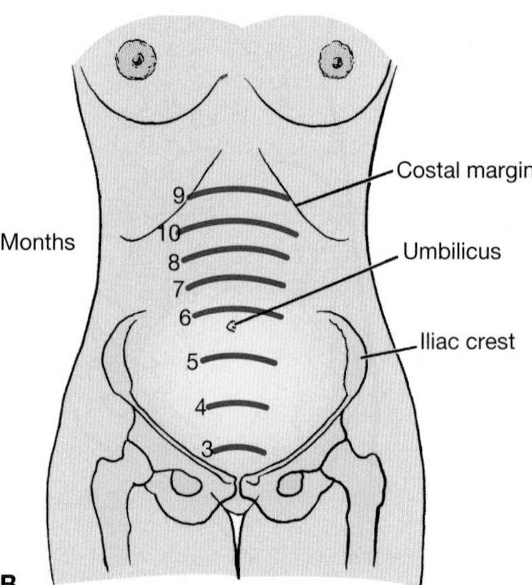

Figure 6.63 **A.** Surface anatomy of the empty and full bladder. **B.** Height of the fundus of the uterus at various months of pregnancy. Note that the peritoneum covering the distended bladder peels off from the anterior abdominal wall so that the front of the bladder comes to lie in direct contact with the abdominal wall.

the pelvic viscera. These procedures are described in detail in Chapter 7.

Clinical Case 1 Discussion

Radiographic examination of the pelvis showed a dislocation of the symphysis pubis and a linear fracture through the lateral part of the sacrum on the right side. The urethra was damaged by the shearing forces applied to the pelvic area, which explained the blood-stained fluid from the external orifice of the penis. The pelvic radiograph (later confirmed on CT scan) also revealed the presence of a large collection of blood in the loose connective tissue outside the peritoneum, which was caused by the tearing of the large, thin-walled pelvic veins by the fractured bone and accounted for the hypovolemic shock.

This patient illustrates the fact that in-depth knowledge of the anatomy of the pelvic region is necessary before a physician can even contemplate making an initial examination and start treatment in cases of pelvic injury.

Clinical Case 2 Discussion

The physician requested additional laboratory and radiologic tests. These indicated that the prostate-specific antigen (PSA) level in the blood was well above the normal range. Pelvic CT scans showed no evidence of pelvic lymphatic enlargement, and bone scans indicated no evidence of bone metastases. The diagnosis was early cancer of the prostate, which was later confirmed by a needle biopsy of prostatic tissue through the anterior wall of the rectum.

This case illustrates how a physician in general practice who has good knowledge of the relevant anatomic features of the pelvis can recognize an abnormal prostate when it is palpated through the anterior rectal wall. This patient later had the prostate removed, and the prognosis was excellent.

Key Concepts

Pelvis

- The bony pelvis consists of the paired hip bones (os coxae), sacrum, and coccyx. The pelvic brim divides the pelvis into an upper false pelvis containing the lower part of the abdominal cavity and a lower true pelvis containing the pelvic cavity.
- The true pelvis has an inlet (pelvic brim) above and an outlet below. The sacrotuberous and sacrospinous ligaments help form the greater and lesser sciatic foramina, which are parts of the pelvic outlet.
- The true pelvis has anterior, posterior, lateral, and inferior walls. The sacral promontory is the upper posterior margin of the pelvic inlet and is an important obstetric landmark used when measuring the size of the pelvis.
- The sacral canal contains the roots of the sacral and coccygeal spinal nerves and the lower part of the subarachnoid space. Caudal anesthesia can be administered via the sacral hiatus.
- The immature hip bone consists of the separate ilium, ischium, and pubis. These join by way of the triradiate cartilage in the acetabulum. Fusion of the hip bone occurs in puberty.
- The piriformis muscle contributes to the posterior pelvic wall. The obturator internus muscle forms part of the lateral pelvic wall. Both muscles act on the hip joint.
- The pelvic diaphragm forms a large part of the inferior pelvic wall (pelvic floor). The diaphragm consists of the levator ani and coccygeus muscles. The levator ani consists of several individual muscles.
- The pelvic joints are the sacroiliac joints, pubic symphysis, and the sacrococcygeal joint. These normally strong joints may loosen somewhat to accommodate childbirth.
- Several features of the pelvis reflect sexual dimorphism.

Fascia and Peritoneum

- The pelvic fascia consists of parietal and visceral layers that assist in supporting the pelvic viscera.

Nerves

- The lumbar and sacral plexuses and the sympathetic trunks provide the nerves of the pelvis.
- The lumbar plexus gives rise to the lumbosacral trunk and the obturator nerve.
- The sacral plexus gives rise to the sciatic nerve, gluteal nerves, pudendal nerve, and pelvic splanchnic nerves.
- The sympathetic trunks supply sympathetic innervation, and the pelvic splanchnic nerves provide parasympathetic fibers. The hypogastric plexuses convey both sympathetic and parasympathetic fibers.

Vasculature

- The common iliac artery supplies blood to the pelvis and lower limb. The common iliac divides into external and internal iliac arteries. The external iliac artery supplies the abdominal wall and lower limb.

- The internal iliac artery typically splits into anterior and posterior divisions, which give off the numerous branches supplying the pelvic viscera and the perineum.
- The superior rectal, ovarian, and median sacral arteries also enter the pelvis and supplement blood flow to the pelvic viscera and wall.
- Venous drainage of the pelvis parallels the arterial supply.
- Lymphatics of the pelvis parallel the main arteries.

Pelvic Cavity

- The pelvic cavity is the area between the pelvic inlet and the pelvic outlet. The pelvic diaphragm subdivides this into the main pelvic cavity above and the perineum below.
- The sigmoid colon, rectum, and terminal coils of ileum occupy the posterior part of the pelvic cavity in both sexes. The urogenital organs fill the more anterior area.

Gastrointestinal Tract

- The sigmoid colon is an S-shaped loop of large bowel supported by the sigmoid mesocolon.
- The rectum lies in front of the sacrum and coccyx. It has an expanded ampulla. The anorectal junction forms a sharp angle produced by the puborectalis muscle.

Urinary Tract

- The ureter possesses three constrictions where stones may lodge. The ureter enters the lateral angle of the urinary bladder.
- The bladder lies immediately behind the pubic bones, within the pelvis, in both males and females. The trigone is the internal triangular area demarcated by the openings of the ureters and the urethra. The general smooth muscle wall of the bladder is the detrusor muscle.
- In males, the vas deferentia and seminal vesicles lie on the base of the bladder. The neck of the bladder rests on the upper surface of the prostate gland. In females, the neck lies on the urogenital diaphragm.
- In males, the base of the bladder is related to the rectum. In females, the base is separated from the rectum by the vagina.
- In micturition, the neck and base of the bladder remain relatively fixed but the superior surface rises into the abdomen. Parasympathetic nerves stimulate contraction of the detrusor muscle and inhibit the action of the sphincter vesicae, thus allowing urination.
- Spinal cord injuries may disrupt the process of micturition and produce an atonic bladder, an automatic reflex bladder, or an autonomous bladder.

Male Internal Genital Organs

- The male internal genital organs are the vas deferens, seminal vesicles, ejaculatory ducts, prostate, prostatic urethra, and membranous urethra.
- The vas deferens arises from the tail of the epididymis, passes through the inguinal canal, crosses the pelvic wall and the base of the bladder, and joins the duct of the seminal vesicle to form the ejaculatory duct.
- The seminal vesicle lies on the base of the bladder. Its duct joins the vas deferens of the same side to form the ejaculatory duct.
- The ejaculatory duct forms by the union of the vas deferens and the duct of the seminal vesicle. It pierces the prostate and opens into the prostatic urethra.
- The prostate is an encapsulated gland situated below the neck of the bladder. It has five lobes and can be examined in a digital rectal exam. Enlargement or disease may obstruct urination and ejaculation.
- The prostatic urethra runs through the prostate from the bladder to the urogenital diaphragm. It is the widest and most dilatable portion of the entire urethra.
- The parietal peritoneum passes onto the upper surface of the bladder and sweeps backward to the anterior aspect of the rectum, forming the rectovesical pouch. The rectovesical pouch is the lowest part of the abdominopelvic peritoneal cavity when the male patient is in the erect position.

Female Internal Genital Organs

- The female internal genital organs are the ovaries, uterine tubes, uterus, and vagina.
- The ovary usually lies against the lateral wall of the pelvis. It has a thin fibrous capsule, the tunica albuginea.
- The uterine tube extends from the upper side of the uterus to the region of the ovary. It has four parts: infundibulum, ampulla, isthmus, and intramural part. Fertilization usually occurs in the ampulla. Ectopic tubal pregnancy may occur in the wall of the tube.
- The uterus is a hollow, pear-shaped organ divided into a fundus, body, and cervix. The cervix pierces and enters the upper end of the vagina. The long axis of the uterus is typically bent forward at about a 90° angle to the long axis of the vagina, in anteversion of the uterus. The uterus is supported by pelvic floor muscles (levator ani muscles) and pelvic fascia ligaments (transverse cervical, pubocervical, and sacrocervical ligaments).
- The vagina extends upward and backward from the vulva to the uterus. The upper half of the vagina lies above the pelvic floor, in the pelvic cavity, whereas the lower half lies within the perineum. The upper vaginal wall surrounds the cervix and forms the vaginal fornices. Significant aspects of the pelvic cavity are palpable in a digital vaginal exam.

- The parietal peritoneum continues down from the anterior abdominal wall onto the upper surface of the urinary bladder and then turns back onto the anterior surface of the uterus, creating the shallow uterovesical pouch. The peritoneum also runs over the uterus onto the upper part of the posterior surface of the vagina, and then onto the front of the rectum. This reflection creates the rectouterine pouch. In the female, the rectouterine pouch is the lowest part of the abdominopelvic peritoneal cavity in the erect position. The broad ligaments are folds of peritoneum that extend across the pelvic cavity from the lateral margins of the uterus to the lateral pelvic walls, covering the body and fundus of the uterus, uterine tubes, and ovaries. The broad ligament is composed of four parts: mesometrium, mesosalpinx, mesovarium, and suspensory ligament of the ovary.

Radiographic Anatomy

- Much of the bony pelvis can be visualized in routine plain radiographs.
- The pelvic organs are readily observed in contrast films and sonograms.

Surface Anatomy

- Several features of the bony pelvis are palpable through the skin.
- The distended urinary bladder is palpable through the anterior abdominal wall above the symphysis pubis. In young children, the bladder is an abdominal organ even when empty.
- The uterus is increasingly palpable through the anterior abdominal wall as pregnancy progresses.

7 Perineum

A 51-year-old female presented to her physician with breathlessness, which she noticed was worse on climbing stairs. On questioning, she said the problem started about 3 years ago and was getting worse. On examination, it was found that the patient had a healthy appearance, although her conjunctivae and lips were paler than normal, suggesting anemia. The cardiovascular and respiratory systems were normal. On further questioning, the patient said that she frequently passed bloodstained stools and was often constipated.

Digital examination of the anal canal revealed nothing abnormal apart from the presence of some bloodstained mucus on the glove. Proctoscopic examination of the patient in the lithotomy position revealed that the mucous membrane of the anal canal had three congested swellings that bulged into the lumen at the 3-, 7-, and 11-o'clock positions. Laboratory examination of the blood showed the red blood cells (RBCs) to be smaller than normal, and the RBC count was very low; the hemoglobin level was also low. The diagnosis was microcytic hypochromic anemia, secondary to prolonged bleeding from internal hemorrhoids.

See the Clinical Case Discussion at the end of this chapter for a further insight.

CHAPTER OUTLINE

LEARNING OBJECTIVES

The purpose of this chapter is to review the anatomy relative to significant clinical problems in the perineum. Because the descent of the testes and the structure of the scrotum are intimately related to the development of the inguinal canal, they are dealt with in detail in Chapter 5.

1. Define and delineate the boundaries and subdivisions of the perineum. Identify the contents of each.
2. Identify the anal canal and its components. Describe the relationships of these structures, with particular reference to the basis of a digital

anorectal exam in both males and females. Describe the anatomical basis for control of defecation and cause of hemorrhoids.

3. Delineate the ischioanal (ischiorectal) fossae. Identify the major contents of the fossae and describe the functional/clinical significance of the area.
4. Identify the urogenital diaphragm, its components, and their basic functions. Indicate sex differences with respect to relationships to the urogenital tracts.
5. Trace the courses of the male and female reproductive tracts. Identify accessory glands or organs and the relationships of components. Describe the roles of structures responsible for normal sexual functioning in males and females.
6. Identify the major nerves that supply the perineum. Identify the sources of autonomic innervation to the perineum. Trace the pathways of the main somatic and visceral nerves to the perineum and describe the clinical relevance of these routes. Describe the functional consequences of lesions of the main nerves supplying the perineum.
7. Trace the flow of blood into and out of the perineum by describing the courses, branching patterns, distributions, and major anastomoses of the main vessels. Note the relations of these vessels to neighboring organs.
8. Trace the primary drainage of lymph from the organs and walls of the perineum to their primary lymph nodes and points of venous connection.
9. Identify the major structures of the perineum in radiographic images.
10. Locate the surface projections and palpation points of major perineal structures in a basic surface anatomy examination.

OVERVIEW

The levatore ani and coccygeus muscles and their covering fasciae form the pelvic diaphragm (Figs. 7.1 and 7.2; see also Chapter 6). It is incomplete anteriorly (via the **urogenital hiatus**) to allow the passage of the urethra in males and the urethra and the vagina in females (see Fig. 7.2). The pelvic diaphragm divides the pelvic cavity into two parts: (1) the **main pelvic cavity** located above the diaphragm and (2) the **perineum** located below the diaphragm (see Fig. 6.2).

This chapter examines the perineum. The main pelvic cavity is described in Chapter 6. Be aware of anatomical directions. In the perineum, superficial equates

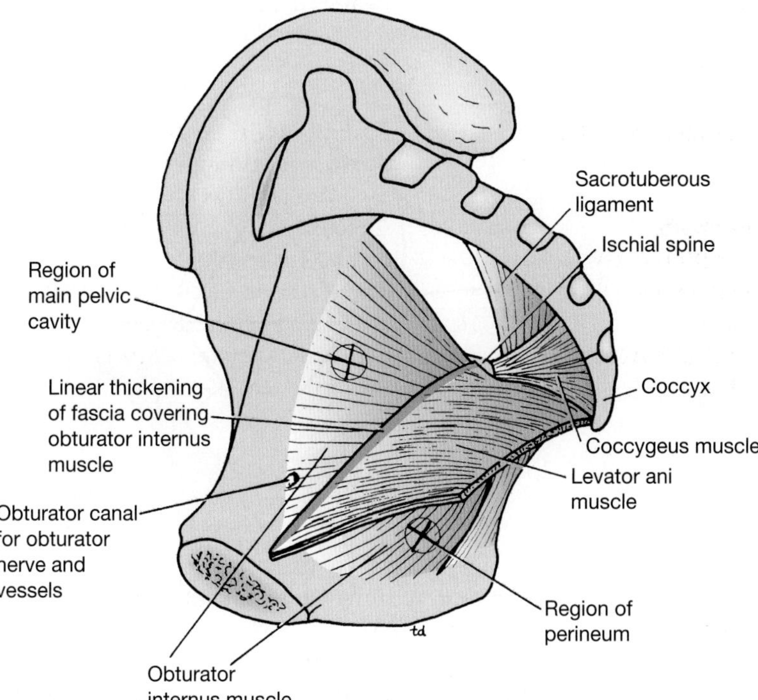

Figure 7.1 Right half of the pelvis showing the muscles forming the pelvic floor. Note that the levator ani and the coccygeus muscles and their covering fascia form the pelvic diaphragm. Note also that the region of the main pelvic cavity lies above the pelvic diaphragm, and the region of the perineum lies below the diaphragm.

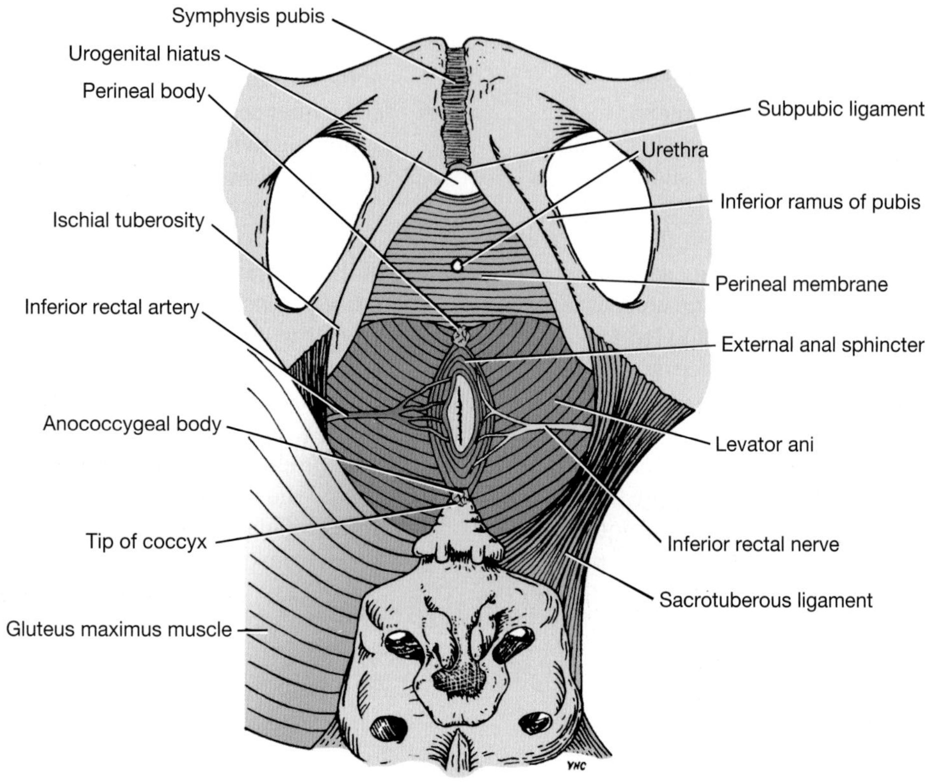

Figure 7.2 Anal triangle and urogenital triangle in the male as seen from below.

with inferior, and deep equates with superior. Thus, the perineum is inferior (superficial) to the pelvic diaphragm.

The perineum is diamond shaped when observed from below with the thighs abducted (Fig. 7.3). Its boundaries (from anterior to posterior) are the symphysis pubis, ischiopubic rami, ischial tuberosities, sacrotuberous ligaments, and the tip of the coccyx (see Figs. 7.2 and 7.3). An imaginary line connecting the ischial tuberosities divides the perineum into two triangles. The anterior triangle is the **urogenital triangle** that contains the urogenital orifices. The posterior triangle is the **anal triangle** that contains the anus.

In this view from below, the patient is in the **lithotomy position**, that is, the patient is supine with both hip joints flexed and abducted. The feet are in stirrups to hold them in a stable position. The lithotomy position is commonly used in females for examination of the perineum and pelvis.

The **perineal body (central tendon of the perineum)** is a fibromuscular mass located in the center of the perineum (see Fig. 7.2). This represents the embryonic site of attachment of the urorectal septum to the cloacal membrane. In males, it is located between the bulb of the penis and the anus. In females, it is located between the vagina and the anus. Functionally, the perineal body is a site of attachment for various muscles and fascial layers. Therefore, it is an important point of stability for perineal integrity and functions.

Common problems related to the perineum include infections, injuries, and prolapses involving the anal canal, urethra, and female external genitalia. Urethral obstruction, traumatic rupture of the penile urethra, and infections of the epididymis and testis frequently occur in the male.

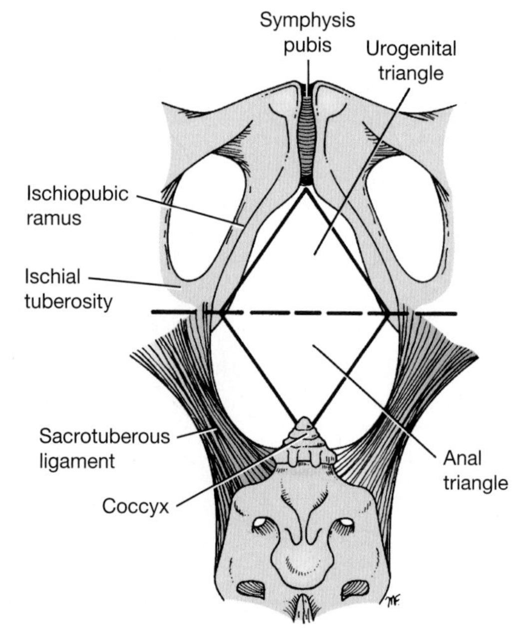

Figure 7.3 Diamond-shaped perineum divided by a *broken line* into the urogenital triangle and the anal triangle.

ANAL TRIANGLE

The anal triangle is the posterior half of the perineum (see Fig. 7.3). Its boundaries are the ischial tuberosities, sacrotuberous ligaments (overlapped by the borders of the gluteus maximus muscles), and the tip of the coccyx. The **anus**, or lower opening of the anal canal, lies in the midline, and an **ischioanal fossa** lies on each side. The anatomy of this region is virtually identical in males and females.

Anal Canal

The anal canal is about 1.5 in. (4 cm) long and passes downward and backward from the rectal ampulla to the anus (see Fig. 7.4). The levatore ani muscles and the

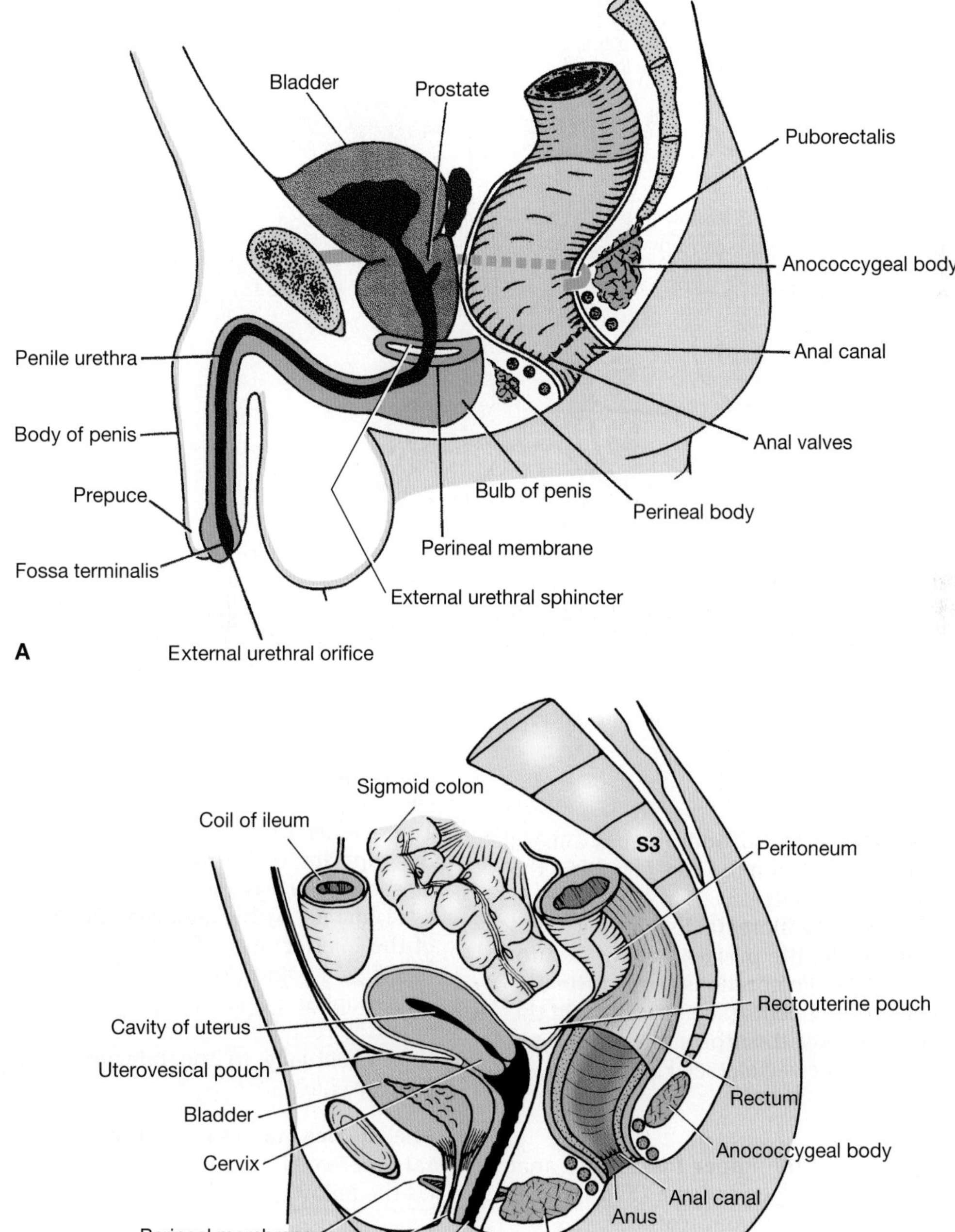

Figure 7.4 Sagittal sections of the male **(A)** and female **(B)** pelvis.

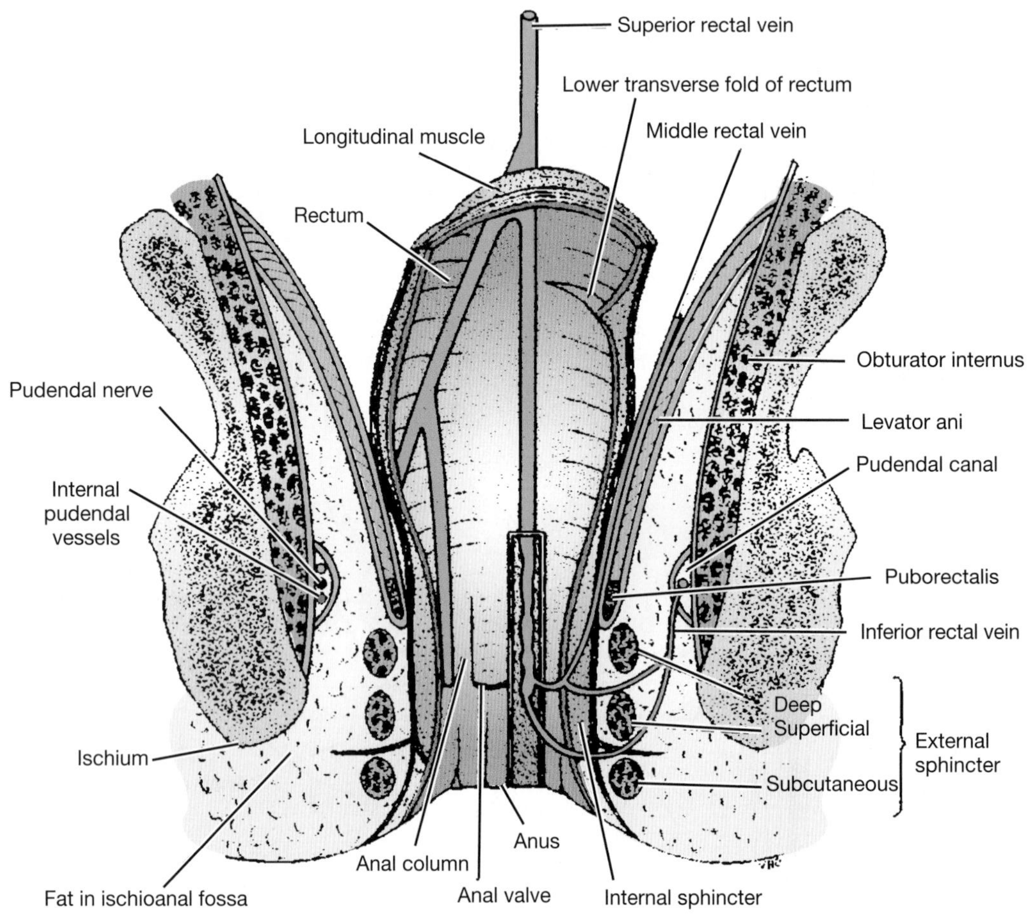

Figure 7.5 Coronal section of the pelvis and the perineum showing venous drainage of the anal canal.

anal sphincters keep their lateral walls in apposition, except during defecation.

Relations

- **Posteriorly:** The **anococcygeal body** that is a mass of fibrous tissue lying between the anal canal and the coccyx (see Figs. 7.2 and 7.4).
- **Laterally:** The fat-filled ischiorectal fossae (Fig. 7.5).
- **Anteriorly:** In the male, the perineal body, the urogenital diaphragm, the membranous part of the urethra, and the bulb of the penis (see Fig. 7.4A). In the female, the perineal body, the urogenital diaphragm, and the lower part of the vagina (see Fig. 7.4B).

Structure

The **mucous membrane of the upper half of the anal canal** is derived from **hindgut endoderm** (Fig. 7.6A). It has the following important anatomic features:

- It is lined by **columnar epithelium**.
- It is thrown into vertical folds called the **anal columns**, which are joined together at their lower ends by small semilunar folds called the **anal valves** (remains of proctodeal membrane) (Fig. 7.7; see also Fig. 7.5).
- The nerve supply is the same as that for the rectal mucosa and is derived from the autonomic **hypogastric plexuses**. It is sensitive only to stretch (see Fig. 7.6A).
- The arterial supply is that of the hindgut—namely, the **superior rectal artery**, a branch of the inferior mesenteric artery (see Fig. 7.6B). The venous drainage is mainly by the **superior rectal vein**, a tributary of the inferior mesenteric vein, and the portal vein (see Figs. 7.5 and 7.6C).
- The lymphatic drainage is mainly upward along the superior rectal artery to the pararectal nodes and then eventually to the **inferior mesenteric nodes** (see Fig. 7.6D).

The **mucous membrane of the lower half of the anal canal** is derived from the **ectoderm of the proctodeum**. It has the following important features:

- It is lined by the **stratified squamous epithelium**, which gradually merges at the anus with the perianal epidermis (see Fig. 7.6A).
- There are **no anal columns** (see Fig. 7.7).
- The nerve supply is from the somatic **inferior rectal nerve**. Thus, it is sensitive to pain, temperature, touch, and pressure (see Figs. 7.2 and 7.6A).

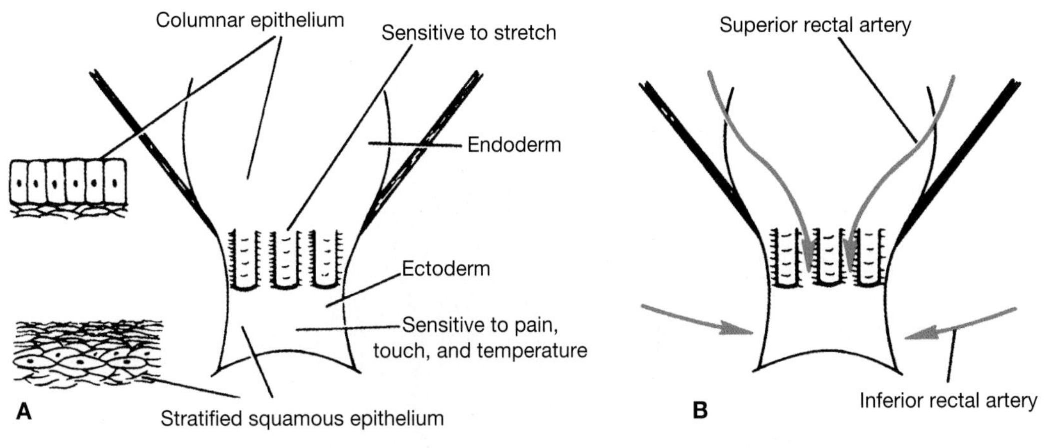

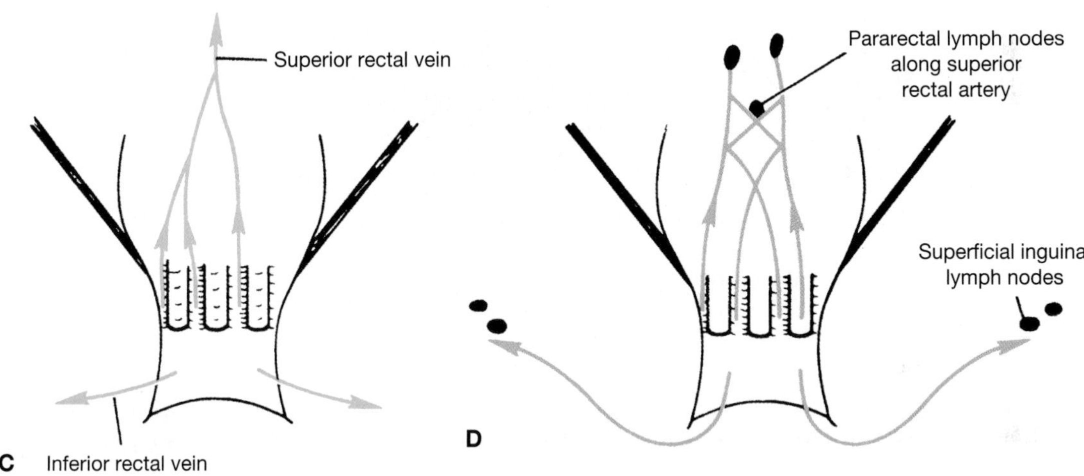

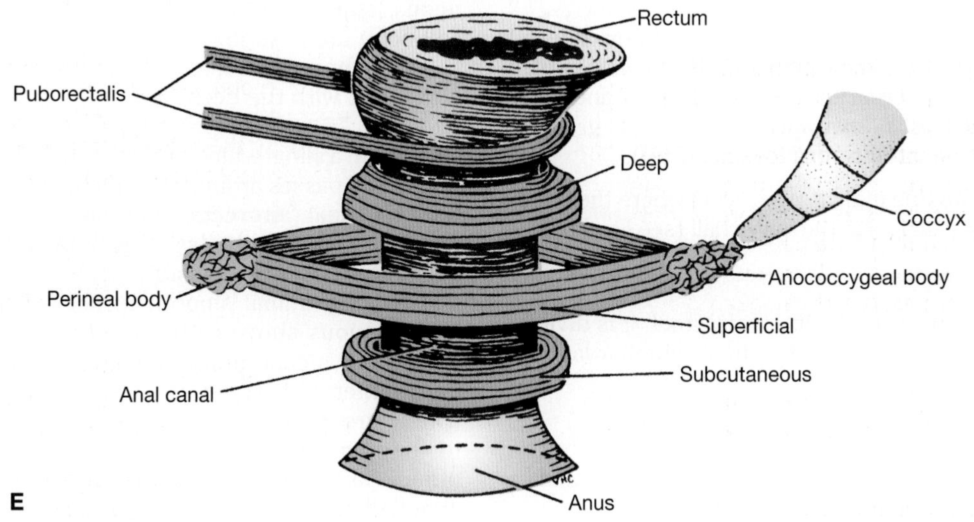

Figure 7.6 Upper and lower halves of the anal canal showing their embryologic origin and lining epithelium **(A)**, arterial supply **(B)**, venous drainage **(C)**, and lymph drainage **(D)**. Arrangement of the muscle fibers of the puborectalis muscle and different parts of the external anal sphincter **(E)**.

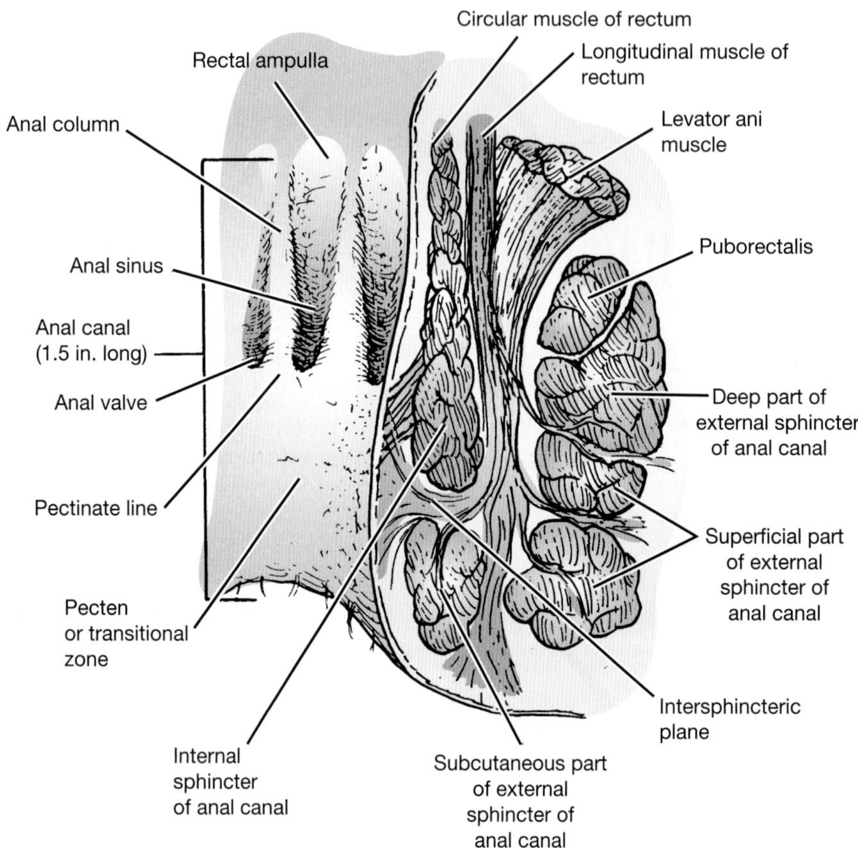

Figure 7.7 Coronal section of the anal canal showing the detailed anatomy of the mucous membrane and the arrangement of the internal and external anal sphincters. Note that the terms "pectinate line" (line at the level of the anal valves) and "pecten" (transitional zone between the skin and the mucous membrane) are sometimes used by clinicians.

- The arterial supply is from the **inferior rectal artery**, a branch of the internal pudendal artery (see Figs. 7.2 and 7.6B). The venous drainage is by the **inferior rectal vein**, a tributary of the internal pudendal vein, which drains into the internal iliac vein (see Figs. 7.5 and 7.6C).
- Lymph drainage is downward to the medial group of **superficial inguinal nodes** (see Fig. 7.6D).

The **pectinate line** indicates the level where the upper half of the anal canal joins the lower half (see Fig. 7.7).

Muscle Coat

As in the upper parts of the intestinal tract, it is divided into an outer longitudinal and an inner circular layer of smooth muscle (see Fig. 7.5).

Anal Sphincters

The anal canal has an involuntary internal sphincter and a voluntary external sphincter.

The **internal sphincter** is formed from a thickening of the smooth muscle of the circular coat at the upper end of the anal canal. A sheath of skeletal muscle that forms the voluntary external sphincter encloses the internal sphincter (see Figs. 7.5, 7.6E, and 7.7).

The **external sphincter** has three parts: **subcutaneous**, **superficial**, and **deep**. Details of the external sphincter are described in Table 7.1.

The **puborectalis** fibers of the two levatore ani muscles blend with the deep part of the external sphincter (see Figs. 7.5 to 7.7). The puborectalis fibers of the two sides form a sling, which in front is attached to the pubic bones and passes around the junction of the rectum and the anal canal (**anorectal junction**), pulling the two forward at an acute angle (see Figs. 7.4A and 7.6E). Further details are described in Table 7.1.

The longitudinal smooth muscle of the anal canal is continuous above with that of the rectum. It forms a continuous coat around the anal canal and descends in the interval between the internal and external anal sphincters. Some of the longitudinal fibers are attached to the mucous membrane of the anal canal, whereas others pass laterally into the ischioanal fossa or are attached to the perianal skin (see Fig. 7.5).

The internal sphincter, deep part of the external sphincter, and the puborectalis muscles form a distinct ring, called the **anorectal ring**, at the anorectal junction (see Fig. 7.6E). This can be felt on rectal examination.

Table 7.1 Perineal Muscles

MUSCLE	ORIGIN	INSERTION	NERVE SUPPLY	ACTION
External Anal Sphincter Muscles				
Subcutaneous part	Encircles anal canal, no bony attachments		Inferior rectal nerve and perineal branch of fourth sacral nerve	Together with puborectalis muscle forms voluntary sphincter of anal canal
Superficial part	Perineal body	Coccyx	Same as subcutaneous part	Same as subcutaneous part
Deep part	Encircles anal canal, no bony attachments		Same as subcutaneous part	Same as subcutaneous part
Puborectalis (part of levator ani)	Pubic bones	Sling around junction of rectum and anal canal	Perineal branch of fourth sacral nerve and from perineal branch of pudendal nerve	Together with external anal sphincter forms voluntary sphincter for anal canal
Male Urogenital Muscles				
Bulbospongiosus	Perineal body	Fascia of bulb of penis and corpus spongiosum and cavernosum	Perineal branch of pudendal nerve	Compresses urethra and assists in erection of penis
Ischiocavernosus	Ischial tuberosity	Fascia covering corpus cavernosum	Perineal branch of pudendal nerve	Assists in erection of penis
Sphincter urethrae	Pubic arch	Surrounds urethra	Perineal branch of pudendal nerve	Voluntary sphincter of urethra
Superficial transverse perineal muscle	Ischial tuberosity	Perineal body	Perineal branch of pudendal nerve	Fixes perineal body
Deep transverse perineal muscle	Ischial ramus	Perineal body	Perineal branch of pudendal nerve	Fixes perineal body
Female Urogenital Muscles				
Bulbospongiosus	Perineal body	Fascia of vestibular bulb	Perineal branch of pudendal nerve	Sphincter of vagina and assists in erection of clitoris
Ischiocavernosus	Ischial tuberosity	Fascia covering corpus cavernosum	Perineal branch of pudendal nerve	Assists in erection of clitoris
Sphincter urethrae	Same as in male			
Superficial transverse perineal muscle	Same as in male			
Deep transverse perineal muscle	Does not occur in females			

Blood Supply

The **superior rectal artery** supplies the upper half, and the **inferior rectal artery** supplies the lower half (see Fig. 7.6B).

The **superior rectal vein** drains the upper half into the inferior mesenteric vein. The **inferior rectal vein** drains the lower half into the internal pudendal vein (see Fig. 7.6C).

Lymph Drainage

The upper half of the anal canal drains into the pararectal nodes and then the **inferior mesenteric nodes**. The lower half drains into the **medial group of superficial inguinal nodes** (see Fig. 7.6D).

Nerve Supply

Visceral afferent fibers that ascend through the **hypogastric plexuses** innervate the mucous membrane of the upper half, which is sensitive to stretch. Somatic afferent fibers in the **inferior rectal nerves** supply the lower half, which is sensitive to pain, temperature, touch, and pressure. **Sympathetic fibers from the inferior hypogastric plexuses** innervate the involuntary internal sphincter. The **inferior rectal nerve**, a branch of the pudendal nerve (Fig. 7.8; see also Fig. 7.2), and the perineal branch of the S4 nerve supply the voluntary external sphincter. The inferior rectal nerve supplies the skin around the anus.

Defecation

The time, place, and frequency of defecation are a matter of habit. Some adults defecate once a day, some defecate several times a day, and some once in several days.

The desire to defecate is initiated by stimulation of the stretch receptors in the wall of the rectum by the presence of feces in the lumen. The act of defecation involves a coordinated reflex that results in the emptying of the descending colon, sigmoid colon, rectum, and anal canal. It is assisted by a rise in intra-abdominal pressure brought about by contraction of the muscles of the anterior abdominal wall. The tonic contraction of the internal and external anal sphincters, including the puborectalis muscles, is now voluntarily inhibited, and the feces are evacuated through the anal canal. Depending on the laxity of the submucous coat, the mucous membrane of the lower part of the anal canal is extruded through the anus ahead of the fecal mass. At the end of the act, the mucosa is returned to the anal canal by the tone of the longitudinal fibers of the anal walls and the contraction and upward pull of the puborectalis muscle. The empty lumen of the anal canal is now closed by the tonic contraction of the anal sphincters.

Ischioanal Fossa

The ischioanal fossa (ischiorectal fossa) is a wedge-shaped space located on each side of the anal canal (see Fig. 7.5). The skin is superficial and forms the base of the wedge. The junction of the medial and lateral walls forms the upper edge of the wedge. The sloping levator ani muscle and the anal canal form the medial wall. The lower part of the obturator internus muscle, covered with pelvic fascia, forms the lateral wall.

The paired ischioanal fossae communicate with one another posterior to the anal canal. Each fossa has a **posterior recess** that extends deep to the gluteus maximus muscle as well as an **anterior recess** that extends forward between the perineal membrane and pelvic diaphragm.

Fossa Contents

The ischioanal fossa is filled with dense fat, which supports the anal canal and allows it to distend during defecation. The pudendal nerve and internal pudendal vessels are embedded in a fascial canal, the **pudendal canal**, on the lateral wall of the ischioanal fossa, on the medial side of the ischial tuberosity (see Fig. 7.5). The inferior rectal vessels and nerve cross the fossa to reach the anal canal.

Pudendal Nerve

The pudendal nerve is a branch of the sacral plexus (S2 to S4 anterior rami). It leaves the main pelvic cavity through the **greater sciatic foramen**, enters the gluteal region of the lower limb, and curls around the attachment of the **sacrospinous ligament** at the **ischial spine** (see Fig. 7.8).

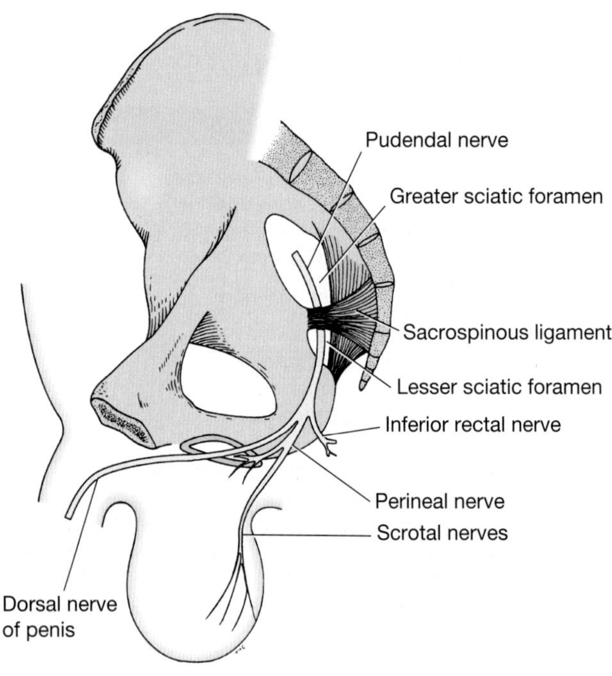

Figure 7.8 Course and branches of the pudendal nerve in the male.

After a brief course in the gluteal region, it passes through the **lesser sciatic foramen** and enters the posterior aspect of the perineum. The nerve then runs forward in the pudendal canal. Its branches supply the external anal sphincter and the muscles and skin of the perineum.

Branches

- **Inferior rectal nerve:** This runs medially across the ischioanal fossa and supplies the external anal sphincter, the mucous membrane of the lower half of the anal canal, and the perianal skin (see Fig. 7.2).
- **Dorsal nerve of the penis** (males) or **clitoris** (females): This is distributed to the penis in males or clitoris in females (see Fig. 7.8).
- **Perineal nerve:** This supplies the muscles in the urogenital triangle and the skin on the posterior surface of the scrotum (or labia majora).

Internal Pudendal Artery

The internal pudendal artery is a branch of the internal iliac artery. It travels with the pudendal nerve and passes from the pelvis through the greater sciatic foramen and enters the perineum through the lesser sciatic foramen.

Branches

- **Inferior rectal artery:** This supplies the lower half of the anal canal (see Figs. 7.2 and 7.6B).
- Branches to the penis in the male and to the labia and clitoris in the female.

Internal Pudendal Vein

The internal pudendal vein receives tributaries that correspond to the branches of the internal pudendal artery.

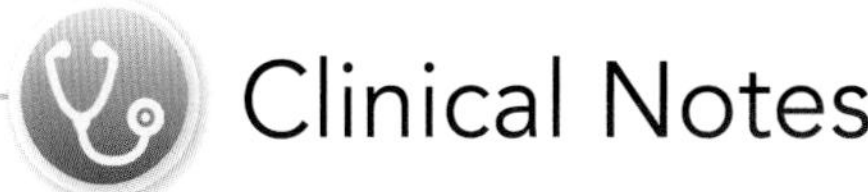

Clinical Notes

Portal–Systemic Anastomosis

The rectal veins form the important **anorectal portal–systemic anastomosis** (see Figs. 7.5 and 7.6C). The superior rectal vein is the portal component. It drains into the inferior mesenteric vein and ultimately into the portal vein. The inferior rectal vein is the systemic component, as it drains into the internal pudendal vein and ultimately into the internal iliac vein.

Internal Hemorrhoids (Piles)

Internal hemorrhoids are **varicosities of the tributaries of the superior rectal vein** and are covered by mucous membrane (see Fig. 7.9). The tributaries of the vein, which lie in the anal columns at the 3-, 7-, and 11-o'clock positions when the patient is viewed in the lithotomy position, are particularly liable to become varicose. Anatomically, a **hemorrhoid** is therefore a fold of mucous membrane and submucosa containing a varicose tributary of the superior rectal vein and a terminal branch of the superior rectal artery. **Internal hemorrhoids** are initially contained within the anal canal (**first degree**). As they enlarge, they extrude from the canal on defecation but return at the end of the act (**second degree**). With further elongation, they prolapse on defecation and remain outside the anus (**third degree**).

Because internal hemorrhoids occur in the upper half of the anal canal, where visceral afferent nerves innervate the mucous membrane, they are painless and are sensitive only to stretch. This may explain why large internal hemorrhoids give rise to an aching sensation rather than acute pain.

There are many causes of internal hemorrhoids. They frequently occur in members of the same family, which suggests a congenital weakness of the vein walls. Varicose veins of the legs and hemorrhoids often go together. The superior rectal vein is the most dependent part of the portal circulation and is valveless. The weight of the column of venous blood is thus greatest in the veins in the upper half of the anal canal. Here, the loose connective tissue of the submucosa gives little support to the walls of the veins. Moreover, the venous return is interrupted by the contraction of the muscular coat of the rectal wall during defecation. Chronic constipation, associated with prolonged straining at stool, is a common predisposing factor. Pregnancy hemorrhoids

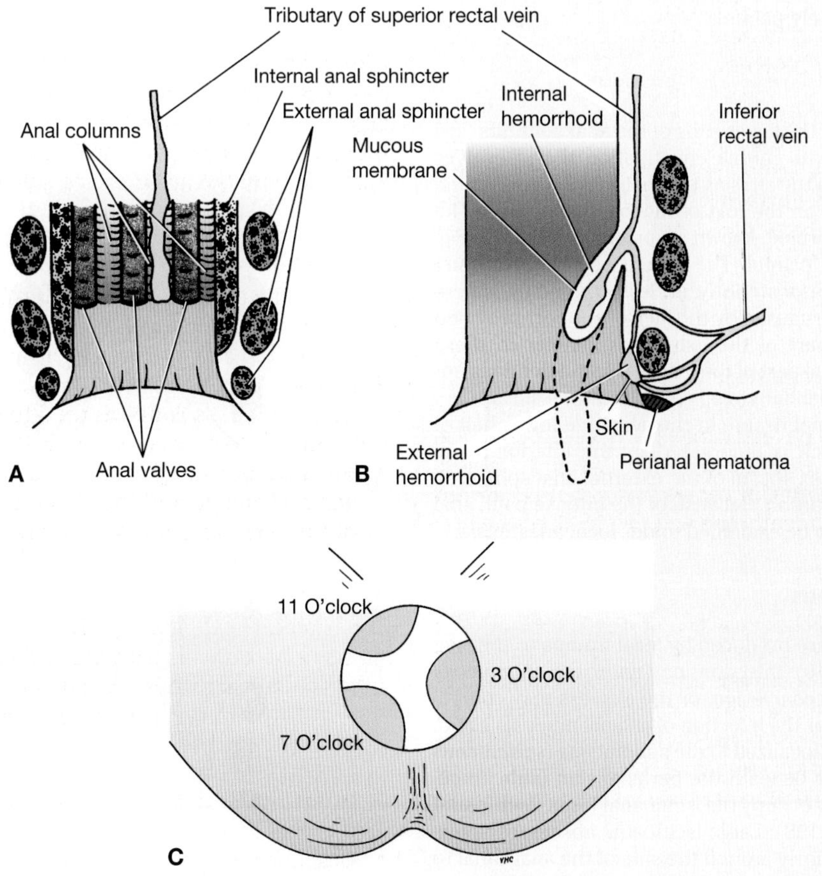

Figure 7.9 **A.** Normal tributary of the superior rectal vein within the anal column. **B.** Varicosed tributary of the superior rectal vein forming the internal hemorrhoid. *Dotted lines* indicate degrees of severity of condition. **C.** Positions of three internal hemorrhoids as seen through a proctoscope with the patient in the lithotomy position.

(continued)

are common owing to pressure on the superior rectal veins by the gravid uterus. Portal hypertension as a result of cirrhosis of the liver can also cause hemorrhoids. The possibility that cancerous tumors of the rectum are blocking the superior rectal vein must never be overlooked.

External Hemorrhoids

External hemorrhoids are varicosities of the tributaries of the inferior rectal vein as they run laterally from the anal margin. They are covered by skin (see Fig. 7.9B) and are commonly associated with well-established internal hemorrhoids.

The mucous membrane of the lower half of the anal canal or the skin covers external hemorrhoids. The inferior rectal nerves innervate them. They are sensitive to pain, temperature, touch, and pressure, which explains why external hemorrhoids tend to be painful. Thrombosis of an external hemorrhoid is common. Its cause is unknown, although coughing or straining may produce distention of the hemorrhoid followed by stasis. The patient immediately recognizes the presence of a small, acutely tender swelling at the anal margin.

Perianal Hematoma

A perianal hematoma is a small collection of blood beneath the perianal skin (see Fig. 7.9B). It is caused by a rupture of a small subcutaneous vein, possibly an external hemorrhoid, and is extremely painful.

Anal Fissure

Anal valves connect the lower ends of the **anal columns** (see Fig. 7.10). In people with chronic constipation, the anal valves may be torn down to the anus as the result of the edge of the fecal mass catching on the fold of mucous membrane. The elongated ulcer so formed, known as an **anal fissure** (see Fig. 7.10A), is extremely painful. The fissure occurs most commonly in the midline posteriorly or, less commonly, anteriorly, and this may be caused by the lack of support provided by the superficial part of the external sphincter in these areas. (The superficial part of the external sphincter does not encircle the anal canal but sweeps past its lateral sides.)

The site of the anal fissure in the sensitive lower half of the anal canal, which is innervated by the inferior rectal nerve, results in reflex spasm of the external anal sphincter, aggravating the condition. Because of the intense pain, anal fissures may have to be examined under local anesthesia.

Perianal Abscesses

Perianal abscesses are produced by fecal trauma to the anal mucosa (see Fig. 7.10). Infection may enter the submucosa through a small mucosal lesion, or the abscess may complicate an anal fissure or the infection of an anal mucosal gland. The abscess may be localized to the submucosa (**submucous abscess**), may occur beneath the perianal skin (**subcutaneous abscess**), or may occupy the ischioanal fossa (**ischioanal abscess**) (see Fig. 7.10B). Large ischioanal abscesses sometimes extend posteriorly around the side of the anal canal to invade the ischioanal fossa of the opposite side (**horseshoe abscess**). An abscess may be found in the space between the ampulla of the rectum and the upper surface of the levator ani (**pelvirectal abscess**). Anatomically, these abscesses are closely related to the different parts of the external sphincter and levator ani muscles, as seen in Figure 7.10B.

Anal fistulae develop as the result of spread or inadequate treatment of anal abscesses. The fistula opens at one end at the lumen of the anal canal or lower rectum and at the other end on the skin surface close to the anus (see Fig. 7.10C). If the abscess opens onto only one surface, it is known as a **sinus**, not a fistula. The high-level fistulae are rare and run from the rectum to the perianal skin. They are located above the anorectal ring; as a result, fecal material constantly soils the clothes. The low-level fistulae occur below the level of the anorectal ring (see Fig. 7.10C).

The most important part of the sphincteric mechanism of the anal canal is the **anorectal ring**. It consists of the deep

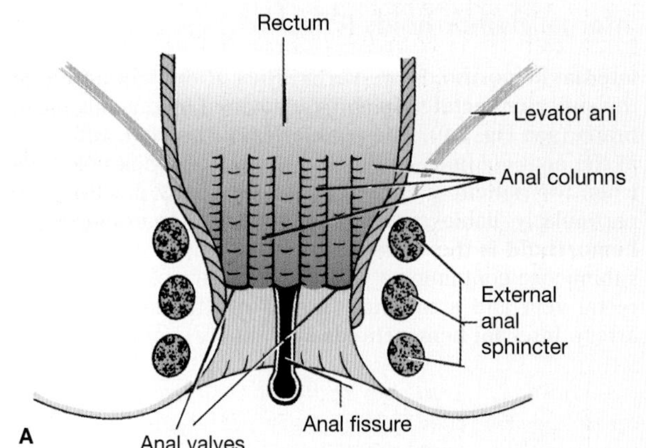

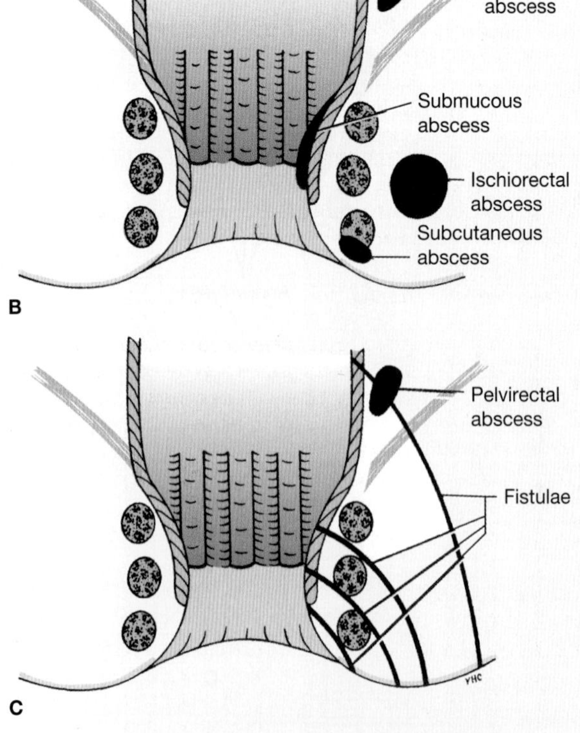

Figure 7.10 **A.** Tearing downward of the anal valve to form an anal fissure. **B.** Common locations of perianal abscesses. **C.** Common positions of perianal fistulae.

part of the external sphincter, the internal sphincter, and the puborectalis part of the levator ani. Surgical operations on the anal canal that result in damage to the anorectal ring produce fecal incontinence.

Removal of Anorectal Foreign Bodies

Normally, the anal canal is kept closed by the tone of the internal and external anal sphincters and the tone of the puborectalis part of the levator ani muscles. The levator ani muscles, possibly assisted by the transverse rectal mucosal folds, support the rectal contents. For these reasons, removing a large object that was inserted into the rectum may be a formidable problem.

The following procedure is usually successful:

1. The foreign body must first be fixed so that the sphincteric tone, together with external attempts to grab the object, does not displace the object farther up the rectum.
2. Large, irregular, or fragile foreign bodies may not be removed so easily, and it may be necessary to paralyze the anal sphincter by giving the patient a general anesthetic or by performing an anal sphincter nerve block.

Anal Sphincter Nerve Block and Anesthetizing Perianal Skin

By blocking the branches of the inferior rectal nerve and the perineal branch of the S4 nerve, the anal sphincters relax and the perianal skin is anesthetized.

The procedure is as follows:

1. An intradermal wheal is produced by injecting a small amount of anesthetic solution behind the anus in the midline.
2. A gloved index finger is inserted into the anal canal to serve as a guide.
3. A long needle attached to a syringe filled with anesthetic solution is inserted through the cutaneous wheal into the sphincter muscles along the posterior and lateral surfaces of the anal canal. The procedure is repeated on the opposite side. The purpose of the finger in the anal canal is to guide the needle and to prevent penetration of the anal mucous membrane.

Incontinence Associated with Rectal Prolapse

Fecal incontinence can accompany severe rectal prolapse of long duration. The prolonged and excessive stretching of the anal sphincters may be the cause of the condition. The condition can be treated by restoring the **anorectal angle** by tightening the puborectalis part of the levator ani muscles and the external anal sphincters behind the anorectal junction.

Incontinence after Trauma

Trauma, such as childbirth, or damage to the sphincters during surgery or perianal abscesses or fistulae can be responsible for incontinence after trauma.

Incontinence after Spinal Cord Injury

After severe spinal cord injuries, the patient is not aware of rectal distention. Moreover, the parasympathetic influence on the peristaltic activity of the descending colon, sigmoid colon, and rectum is lost. In addition, control over the abdominal musculature and sphincters of the anal canal may be severely impaired. The rectum, now an isolated structure, responds by contracting when the pressure within its lumen rises. This local reflex response is much more efficient if the sacral segments of the spinal cord are spared. At best, however, the force of the contractions of the rectal wall is small, and constipation and impaction of feces are the usual outcome.

Anorectal Examination

The following structures can be palpated by the gloved index finger inserted into the anal canal and rectum in the normal patient.

Anteriorly

In the male:

- Opposite the terminal phalanx: the contents of the rectovesical pouch, the posterior surface of the bladder, the seminal vesicles, and the vasa deferentia (see Fig. 7.11; see also Fig. 7.4)
- Opposite the middle phalanx: the rectoprostatic fascia and the prostate
- Opposite the proximal phalanx: the perineal body, the perineal membrane, and the bulb of the penis

In the female:

- Opposite the terminal phalanx: the rectouterine pouch, the vagina, and the cervix
- Opposite the middle phalanx: the perineal membrane and the vagina
- Opposite the proximal phalanx: the perineal body and the lower part of the vagina

Posteriorly

The sacrum, coccyx, and anococcygeal body can be felt in both sexes.

Laterally

The ischioanal fossae and ischial spines can be palpated in both sexes.

Cancer and Lymph Drainage of Anal Canal

The upper half of the mucous membrane of the anal canal is drained upward to lymph nodes along the course of the superior rectal artery. The lower half of the mucous membrane is drained downward to the medial group of superficial inguinal nodes. Many patients have thought they had an inguinal hernia, and the physician has found a cancer of the lower half of the anal canal, with secondary deposits in the inguinal lymph nodes.

Ischioanal Fossa and Infection

The ischioanal fossae are filled with poorly vascularized fat. The close proximity to the anal canal makes them particularly vulnerable to infection. Infection commonly tracks laterally from the anal mucosa through the external anal sphincter. Infection of the perianal hair follicles or sweat glands may also be the cause of infection in the fossae. Rarely, a perirectal abscess bursts downward through the levator ani muscle. An ischioanal abscess may involve the opposite fossa by the spread of infection across the midline behind the anal canal.

(continued)

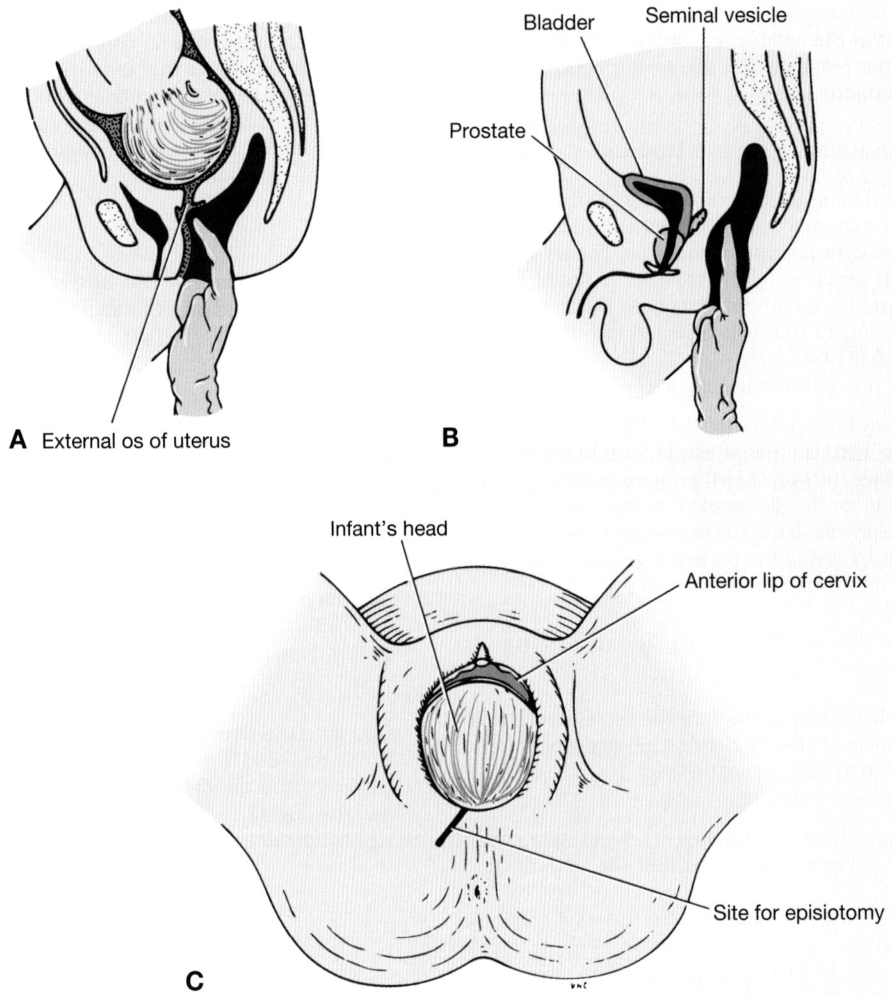

Figure 7.11 **A.** Rectal examination in a pregnant patient showing how it is possible to palpate the cervix through the anterior rectal wall. **B.** Rectal examination in the male showing how it is possible to palpate the prostate and the seminal vesicles through the anterior rectal wall. **C.** Position of the episiotomy incision in a woman during the second stage of labor. The infant's head is presenting at the vaginal orifice.

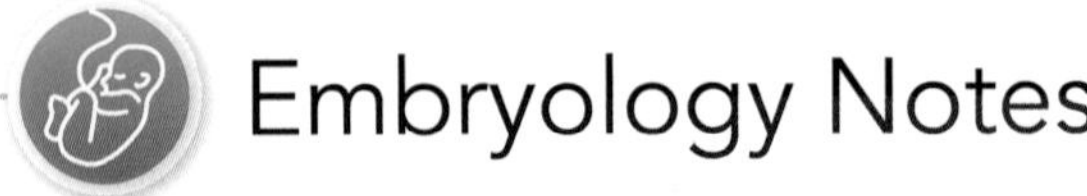

Embryology Notes

Anal Canal Development

The distal end of the hindgut terminates as a blind sac of endoderm called the **cloaca** (see Fig. 6.27). The cloaca lies in contact with a shallow ectodermal depression called the **proctodeum**. The apposed layers of ectoderm and entoderm form the **cloacal membrane**, which separates the cavity of the hindgut from the surface. The cloaca becomes divided into anterior and posterior parts by the **urorectal septum**; the posterior part of the cloaca is called the **anorectal canal**. The anorectal canal forms the rectum and the upper half of the anal canal. The lining of the superior half of the anal canal is formed from entoderm and that of the inferior half of the anal canal is formed from the ectoderm of the proctodeum. The sphincters of the anal canal are formed from the surrounding mesenchyme. The posterior part of the cloacal membrane breaks down so that the gut opens onto the surface of the embryo.

Imperforate Anus

About 1 child in 4,000 is born with imperforate anus caused by an imperfect fusion of the endodermal cloaca with the proctodeum.

UROGENITAL TRIANGLE

The urogenital triangle is the anterior half of the perineum (see Figs. 7.2 and 7.3). Its boundaries are the pubic arch anteriorly and the ischiopubic rami and ischial tuberosities laterally. The urogenital openings lie in the midline, in close relation to the external genitalia. The urogenital triangle is organized into several layers:

- Skin
- Superficial perineal fascia
- Deep perineal fascia
- Superficial (inferior) perineal space (pouch)
- Deep (superior) perineal space (pouch)

Superficial Fascia

The superficial fascia of the urogenital triangle is divided into a superficial fatty layer and a deep membranous layer. These are continuations of the superficial fascial layers of the anterior abdominal wall.

The **superficial fatty layer** (Camper fascia) is continuous with the fat of the ischioanal fossa (Fig. 7.12) and the superficial fascia of the thighs. In the scrotum, the fat is replaced by smooth muscle, the **dartos muscle**. The dartos muscle contracts in response to cold and reduces the surface area of the scrotal skin (see Chapter 5, Testis).

The **deep membranous layer** (Colles fascia) attaches posteriorly to the posterior border of the perineal membrane and the perineal body (see Fig. 7.12) and laterally to the margins of the pubic arch. It is continuous anteriorly with the membranous layer of superficial fascia of the anterior abdominal wall (Scarpa fascia). The fascia continues over the penis (males) or clitoris (females) as a tubular sheath continuous with the superficial fascia of the penis/clitoris (see Fig. 7.13A). It also forms a

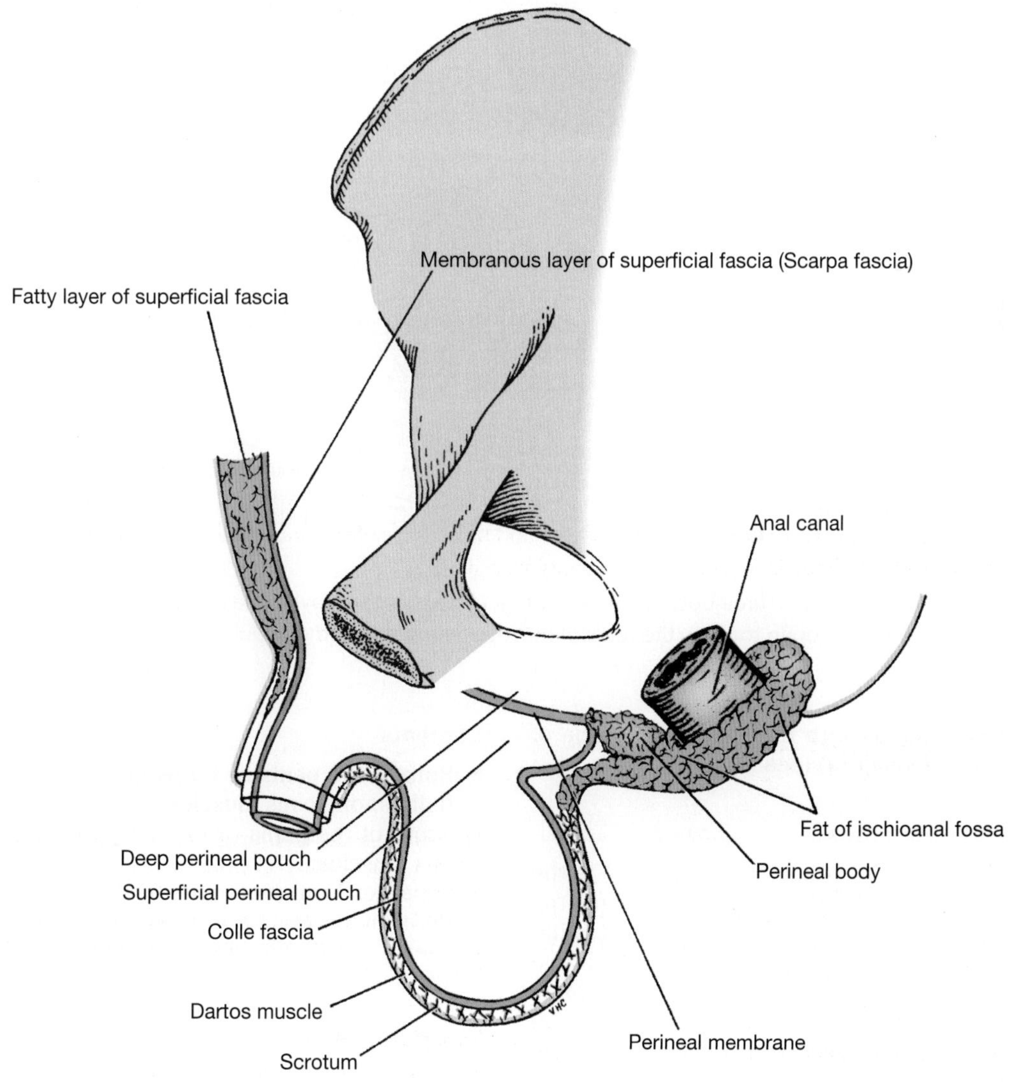

Figure 7.12 Arrangement of the superficial fascia in the urogenital triangle. Note the superficial and deep perineal spaces (pouches) relative to the perineal membrane.

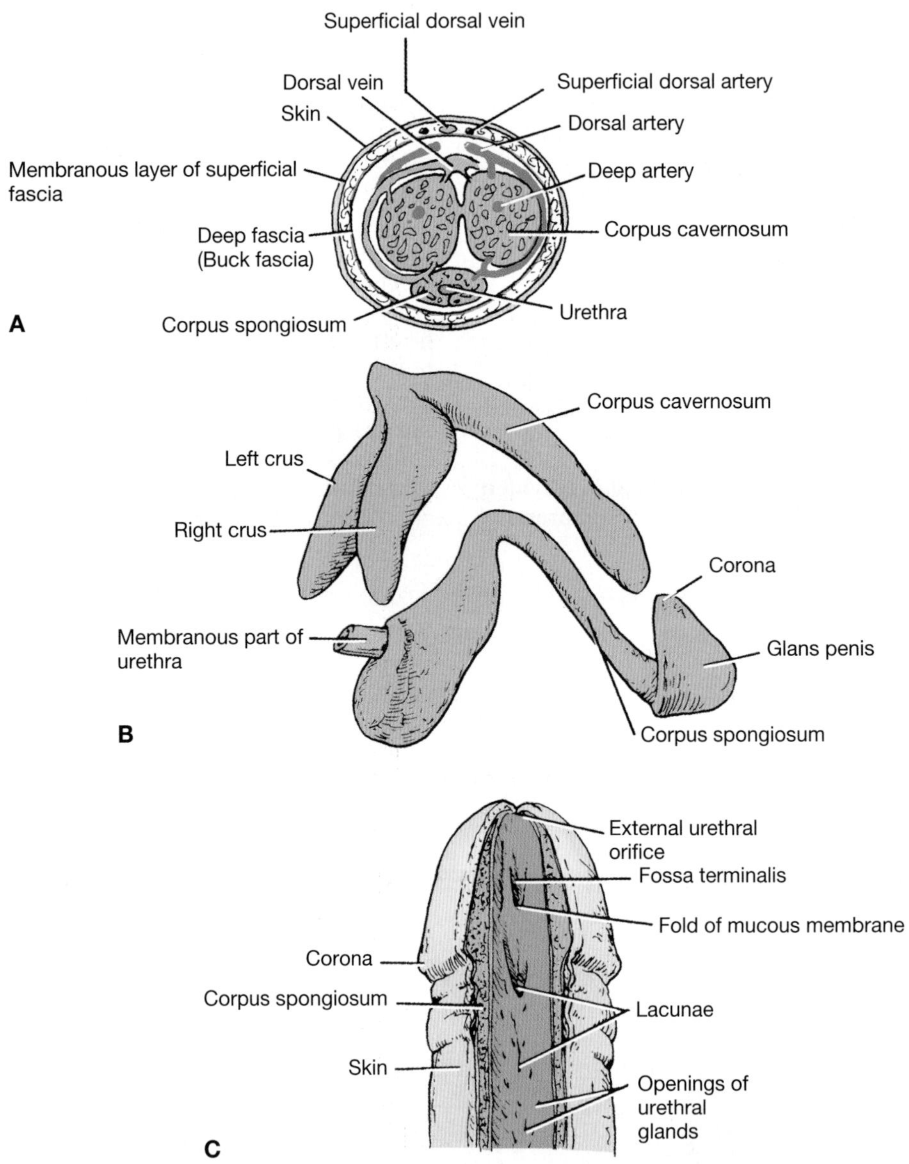

Figure 7.13 The penis. **A and B.** Three bodies of erectile tissue: two corpora cavernosa and the corpus spongiosum with the glans. **C.** Penile urethra slit open to show the folds of mucous membrane and glandular orifices in the roof of the urethra.

distinct layer continuous with the superficial fascia of the scrotum (or labia majora) (see Fig. 7.12).

Superficial Perineal Space

The superficial (inferior) perineal space (pouch) is the zone between the superficial perineal fascia and the perineal membrane (see Fig. 7.12). It is closed behind by the fusion of its walls with the perineal membrane and perineal body. Laterally, it is closed by the attachment of the membranous layer of superficial fascia and the perineal membrane to the margins of the pubic arch (see Figs. 7.14 and 7.15). Anteriorly, the space communicates freely with the potential space lying between the superficial fascia of the anterior abdominal wall and the anterior abdominal muscles.

Contents

- Bulb of the penis or bulbs of the vestibule plus the bulbospongiosus muscles
- Crura of the penis or clitoris plus the ischiocavernous muscles
- Superficial transverse perineal muscles
- Perineal nerves and vessels
- Greater vestibular glands (in females)

Deep Perineal Space and Urogenital Diaphragm

Traditional descriptions of the urogenital triangle identify a distinct **urogenital diaphragm** that lies deep (superior) to the superficial perineal space. This diaphragm is a three-layered, flat, triangular, musculofascial structure

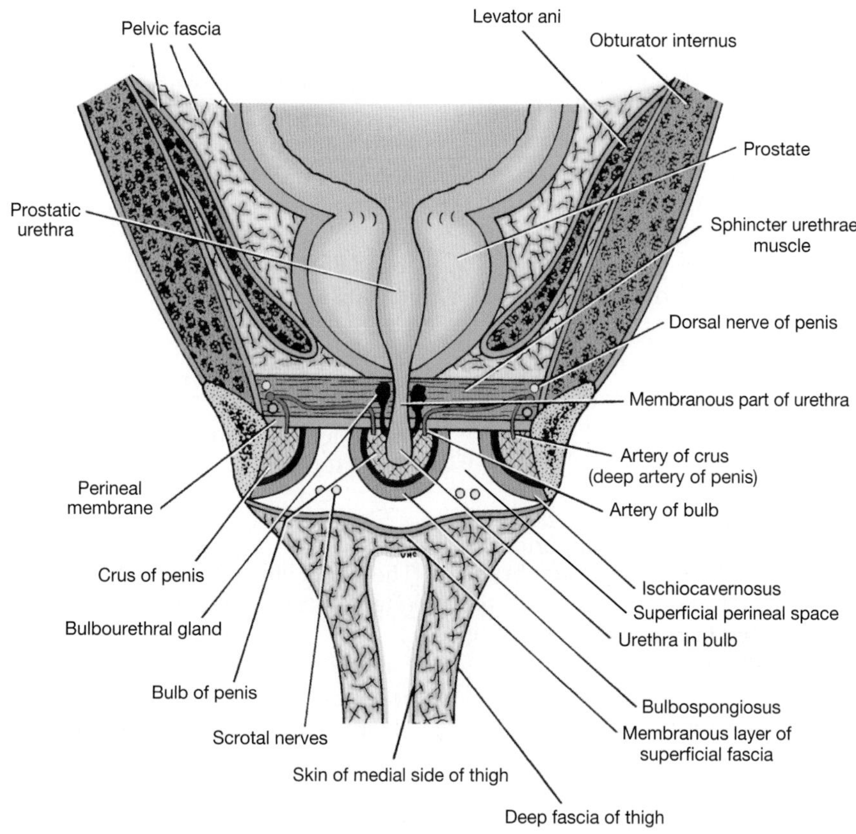

Figure 7.14 Coronal section of the male pelvis showing the prostate, perineal membrane, and the contents of the superficial perineal space (pouch).

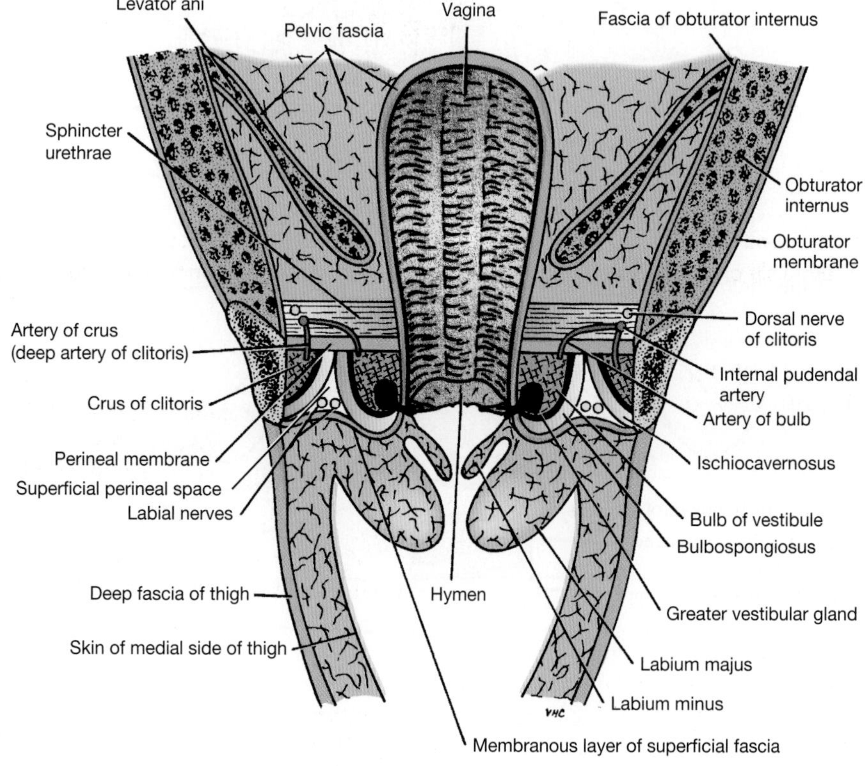

Figure 7.15 Coronal section of the female pelvis showing the vagina, perineal membrane, and the contents of the superficial perineal space (pouch).

situated in the anterior part of the perineum and fills in the **urogenital hiatus** (ie, the gap under the pubic arch where the levator ani is incomplete) (see Figs. 7.12, 7.14, and 7.15). The three layers are (from superficial to deep) as follows:

- **Inferior fascia of the urogenital diaphragm** (also termed the **perineal membrane**)
- **Deep perineal space** (pouch), formed by the sphincter urethrae and **deep transverse perineal muscles**
- **Superior fascia of the urogenital diaphragm**

However, current concepts describe a much more complex region, with the muscle and fascial components arranged in three-dimensional relations rather than the traditional flat, layered form. Some authors question if the urogenital diaphragm really exists as a distinct structure.

The contemporary view is that the **deep perineal space (pouch)** is the zone located deep (superior) to the superficial perineal space. The **perineal membrane** forms the inferior boundary of the deep space, and the inferior fascia of the **pelvic diaphragm** forms the superior boundary. The perineal membrane is a strong, thin, fibrous sheet that attaches along the ischiopubic rami. The deep space contains the following in both sexes:

- Part of the **urethra**
- Inferior part of the **external urethral sphincter**
- **Neurovascular branches** to the external genitalia
- **Anterior recesses of the ischioanal fossae**

The **external urethral sphincter** is a complex structure composed of multiple parts and is oriented more vertically than in the traditional description of a flat, disclike body. Only the inferior portion appears to form a true sphincter-like unit encircling the urethra. The **deep transverse perineal muscles** likely exist only in the male and are replaced by a smooth muscle mass in females.

MALE UROGENITAL TRIANGLE

In the male, the urogenital triangle contains the penis and scrotum.

Penis

The penis has a fixed **root** and a **body** that hangs free (Fig. 7.16; see also Fig. 7.4A).

Penile Root

The root of the penis is made up of three masses of erectile tissue: the **bulb of the penis** and the **right** and **left crura of the penis** (Fig. 7.17; see also Figs. 7.13 and 7.16). The bulb is situated in the midline and is attached

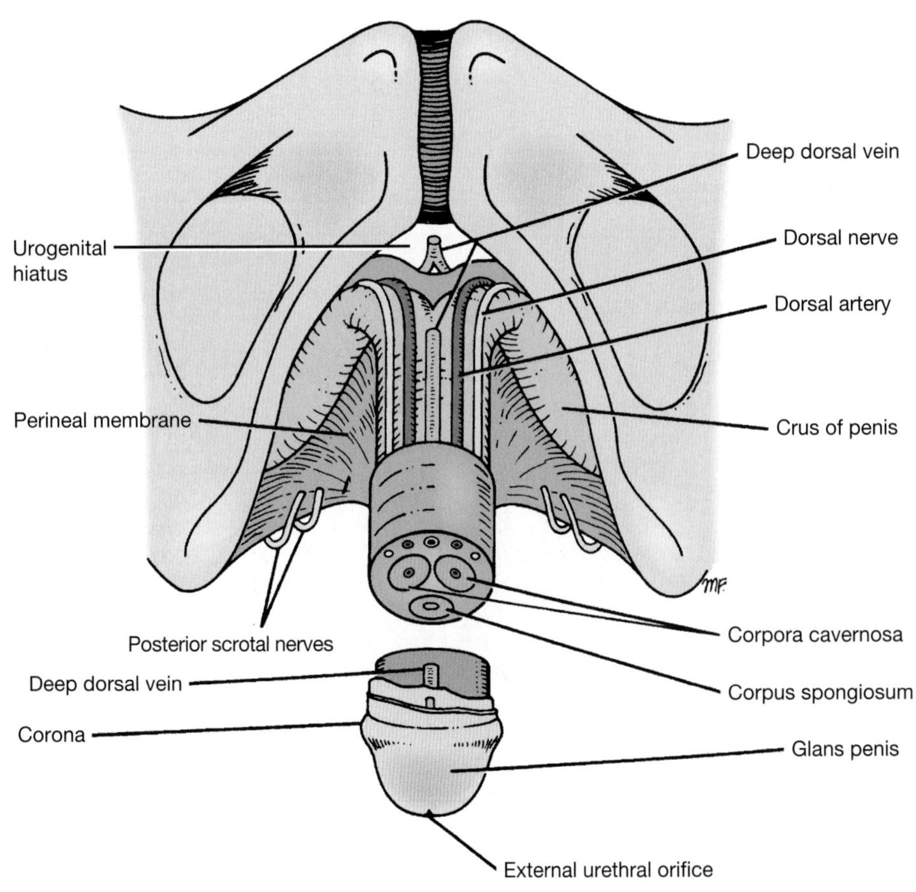

Figure 7.16 Root and body of the penis.

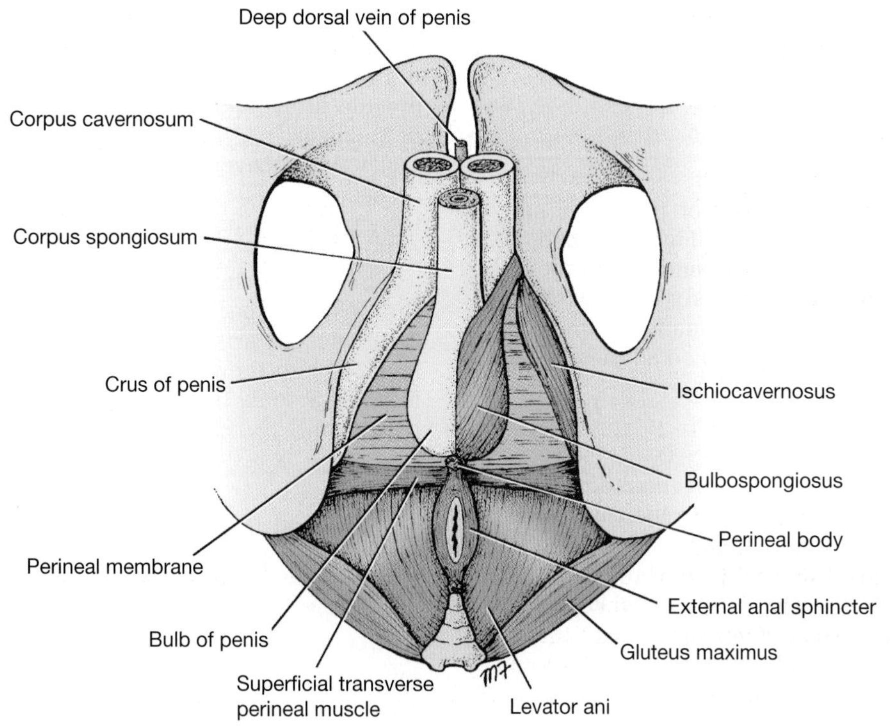

Figure 7.17 Root of penis and perineal muscles.

to the inferior (superficial) surface of the perineal membrane. The urethra traverses the bulb, and the **bulbospongiosus muscles** cover the exterior of the bulb. Each crus attaches to the side of the pubic arch, and the **ischiocavernosus muscle** covers its outer surface. The bulb continues forward into the body of the penis and forms the **corpus spongiosum** (see Fig. 7.17). The two crura converge anteriorly and come to lie side by side in the dorsal part of the body of the penis, forming the **corpora cavernosa** (see Figs. 7.13 and 7.16).

Penile Body

The essential components of the body of the penis are three cylinders of erectile tissue enclosed in a tubular sheath of deep fascia (**Buck fascia**). The erectile tissues are the two dorsally placed corpora cavernosa and the single corpus spongiosum that is applied to their ventral surface (see Figs. 7.13 and 7.16). The corpus spongiosum expands at its distal extremity to form the **glans penis**, which covers the distal ends of the corpora cavernosa. The pronounced posterior edge of the glans is the **corona**. The slit like orifice of the urethra, the **external urethral meatus**, is at the tip of the glans penis.

The **prepuce** (**foreskin**) is a hoodlike fold of skin that covers the glans. The **frenulum** is a tissue fold connecting the prepuce to the glans just below the urethral orifice.

Two condensations of deep fascia, the **suspensory ligament of the penis**, extend downward from the linea alba and symphysis pubis and attach to the fascia of the penis. This assists in supporting the body of the penis.

Blood Supply

The **external pudendal artery**, a branch of the **femoral artery**, supplies the skin and superficial fascia of the penis.

Branches of the **internal pudendal artery** supply the deeper parts of the penis. The **deep artery of the penis** supplies the crus and corpus cavernosum (see Fig. 7.13). This vessel gives off **helicine arteries** into the spongy erectile tissue of the corpus cavernosum. The **artery of the bulb** supplies the bulb, corpus spongiosum, and glans (see Fig. 7.14). Additionally, the **dorsal artery of the penis** runs along the posterior (dorsal) aspect of the penis, deep to the deep fascia, and supplies the skin and fasciae (see Figs. 7.13 and 7.16).

The veins largely correspond to the arteries. However, the erectile bodies drain into venous plexuses that empty into a single, large **deep dorsal vein** (see Figs. 7.13 and 7.16). This vein runs under the pubic symphysis, through the urogenital (genital) hiatus, and into the **prostatic venous plexus** in the deep aspect of the pelvic cavity.

Lymph Drainage

The skin of the penis drains mainly into the **medial group of superficial inguinal nodes**. The erectile bodies of the penis drain into the **internal iliac nodes**.

Nerve Supply

The **pudendal nerve** provides the somatic nerve supply to the skeletal muscles and skin of the penis (see Fig. 7.8). The **inferior hypogastric plexus** supplies autonomic fibers to the smooth muscle (including the vascular smooth muscle of the helicine arteries) of the penis.

Scrotum

The scrotum is an outpouching of the lower part of the anterior abdominal wall (see Figs. 7.4A and 7.12). It contains the testes, the epididymides, and the lower ends of the spermatic cords. The structure of the scrotum, descent of the testes, and formation of the inguinal canal are closely interrelated, and so all these are fully described in Chapter 5.

Blood Supply

Subcutaneous plexuses and arteriovenous anastomoses promote heat loss and thus assist in the environmental control of the temperature of the testes.

The **external pudendal branches** of the femoral and **scrotal branches** of the internal pudendal arteries supply the scrotum.

The veins accompany the corresponding arteries.

Lymph Drainage

The wall of the scrotum drains into the medial group of **superficial inguinal lymph nodes**. However, the contents of the scrotum (testis and epididymis) drain upward to the **lumbar (paraaortic) lymph nodes** at the level of the L1 vertebra. This arrangement makes sense in the context of the development of the region. Recall that the testis migrates from high up on the posterior abdominal wall, down through the inguinal canal, and into the scrotum, dragging its blood supply and lymph vessels after it.

Nerve Supply

The **ilioinguinal nerve** and the **genital branch of the genitofemoral nerve** supply the anterior scrotum. The **pudendal** and **posterior femoral cutaneous nerves** innervate the posterior scrotum. The pudendal nerve is the major nerve in terms of coverage.

Superficial Perineal Space Contents

The superficial perineal space (pouch) in the male contains the following (see Figs. 7.14, 7.16, and 7.17 and Table 7.1):

- Structures forming the root of the penis (bulb and crura)
- Muscles that cover the root structures (bulbospongiosus and ischiocavernosus)
- Superficial transverse perineal muscles
- Branches of the pudendal nerve and internal pudendal vessels

Muscles

The **bulbospongiosus muscles**, situated one on each side of the midline, cover the bulb of the penis and the posterior portion of the corpus spongiosum (see Fig. 7.17). Their function is to compress the penile part of the urethra and empty it of residual urine or semen. The anterior fibers also compress the deep dorsal vein of the penis, thus impeding the venous drainage of the erectile tissue and assisting in the process of erection of the penis.

The **ischiocavernosus muscles** cover the crus penis on each side. The action of each muscle is to compress the crus penis and assist in the process of erection of the penis.

The **superficial transverse perineal muscles** lie in the posterior part of the superficial perineal pouch. Each muscle arises from the ischial ramus and is inserted into the perineal body. The function of these muscles is to fix the perineal body in the center of the perineum.

Nerves

The **perineal branch of the pudendal nerve** on each side terminates in the superficial perineal pouch and supplies the muscles and skin (see Fig. 7.8).

Perineal Body

This small mass of fibrous tissue attaches to the center of the posterior margin of the perineal membrane (see Figs. 7.12 and 7.17). It serves as a point of attachment for the following muscles: external anal sphincter, bulbospongiosus muscle, and superficial transverse perineal muscles.

Deep Perineal Space Contents

As noted earlier, the contemporary view is that the deep perineal space (pouch) is the area located between the perineal membrane and the inferior fascia of the pelvic diaphragm. The deep perineal space (pouch) in the male contains the intermediate (membranous) part of the urethra, part of the external urethral sphincter (sphincter urethrae), bulbourethral glands, deep transverse perineal muscles, internal pudendal vessels and their branches, and the dorsal nerves of the penis.

Intermediate (Membranous) Part of Urethra

The intermediate (membranous) part of the urethra is about 0.5 in. (1.3 cm) long and lies within and is surrounded by the inferior part of the external urethral sphincter. It is continuous above with the **prostatic urethra** and below with the **penile urethra**. It is the shortest and least dilatable part of the urethra (see Fig. 7.14).

Sphincter Urethrae Muscle

The **external urethral sphincter** is a complex structure composed of multiple parts. Its upper, larger, more vertically oriented part extends up along the prostatic urethra as far as the neck of the bladder. The action of this section of muscle on the prostatic urethra is somewhat uncertain. Only the inferior portion of the external sphincter (ie, the part between the perineal membrane and the prostate) appears to form a true sphincter-like unit encircling the intermediate part of the urethra. This segment of the external sphincter may be referred to as the **sphincter urethrae muscle** (see Fig. 7.14). It compresses the intermediate part of the urethra and relaxes during micturition. This is the voluntary urethral sphincter. The **perineal branch of the pudendal nerve** supplies the sphincter urethrae.

Bulbourethral Glands

The bulbourethral glands are two small glands that lie in the deep perineal space, embedded in the sphincter urethrae muscle (see Fig. 7.14). Their ducts pierce the perineal membrane and enter the penile portion of the urethra. They pour their secretion into the urethra in response to erotic stimulation.

Deep Transverse Perineal Muscles

The deep transverse perineal muscles form a flat, sheetlike mass superior to the posterior part of the perineal membrane and posterior to the sphincter urethrae muscle. Each muscle arises from the ischial ramus and passes medially to insert into the perineal body. These muscles may help fix the perineal body but are clinically unimportant.

Internal Pudendal Artery

The internal pudendal artery (see Fig. 7.14) pierces the perineal membrane, enters the deep perineal space (pouch), and passes forward. It gives rise to the artery to the bulb of the penis; deep artery of the penis to the crus of the penis; and dorsal artery of the penis, which supplies the skin and fascia of the penis.

Dorsal Nerve of Penis

The dorsal nerve of the penis passes forward through the deep perineal space and supplies the skin of the penis (see Figs. 7.14 and 7.16).

Penile Erection

Erection in the male occurs from various sexual stimuli. Pleasurable sights, sounds, smells, and other psychic stimuli, fortified later by direct touch sensory stimuli from the general body skin and genital skin, result in a bombardment of the central nervous system (CNS) by afferent stimuli. Efferent nervous impulses pass down the spinal cord to the parasympathetic outflow in the **pelvic splanchnic nerves** (S2 to S4 segments). The parasympathetic preganglionic fibers enter the **inferior hypogastric plexuses** and synapse on the postganglionic neurons. The postganglionic fibers run through the **prostatic nerve plexus** (a subdivision of the inferior hypogastric plexus) join the **cavernous nerves** (branches of the prostatic plexus), pierce the pelvic floor, join the internal pudendal arteries, and distribute along their branches, which enter the erectile tissue at the root of the penis. Parasympathetic stimulation causes vasodilatation of the **helicine arteries**, producing a great increase in blood flow through the cavernous spaces of the erectile tissue. The corpora cavernosa and the corpus spongiosum become engorged with blood and expand, compressing their draining veins against the surrounding fascia. By this means, the outflow of blood from the erectile tissue is retarded so that the internal pressure is further accentuated and maintained. The penis thus increases in length and diameter and assumes the erect position.

Once the climax of sexual excitement is reached and ejaculation takes place, or the excitement passes off or is inhibited, the helicine arteries undergo vasoconstriction. The penis then returns to its flaccid state.

Ejaculation

With increasing sexual excitement, the external urethral meatus of the glans penis becomes moist because of the secretions of the bulbourethral glands.

Friction on the glans penis, reinforced by other afferent nervous impulses, results in a discharge along the sympathetic nerve fibers to the smooth muscle of the duct of the epididymis and the vas deferens on each side, seminal vesicles, and prostate. The smooth muscle contracts, and the spermatozoa, together with the secretions of the seminal vesicles and prostate, discharge into the prostatic urethra. The fluid now joins the secretions of the bulbourethral glands and penile urethral glands and is then ejected from the penile urethra because of the rhythmic contractions of the bulbospongiosus muscles, which compress the urethra. Meanwhile, the internal urethral sphincter of the bladder contracts and the detrusor muscle relaxes, preventing reflux of the spermatozoa into the bladder (**retrograde ejaculation**). The spermatozoa and the secretions of the several accessory glands constitute the **seminal fluid**, or **semen**.

At the climax of male sexual excitement, a mass discharge of nervous impulses takes place in the CNS. Impulses pass down the spinal cord to the sympathetic outflow (T1 to L2). The nervous impulses that pass to the genital organs are thought to leave the cord at the L1 and L2 segments in the preganglionic sympathetic fibers. Many of these fibers synapse with postganglionic neurons in the L1 to L2 ganglia. Other fibers may synapse in ganglia in the lower lumbar or pelvic parts of the sympathetic trunks. The postganglionic fibers distribute to the vas deferens, seminal vesicles, and the prostate via the inferior hypogastric plexuses.

Male Urethra

The male urethra is about 8 in. (20 cm) long and extends from the neck of the bladder to the external meatus on the glans penis (see Fig. 7.4). It is divided into three parts: prostatic, intermediate (membranous), and penile (spongy).

The **prostatic urethra** is described in Chapter 6. It is about 1.25 in. (3 cm) long and passes through the prostate from the base to the apex (see Figs. 7.4 and 7.14). This is the widest and most dilatable portion of the urethra.

The **intermediate (membranous)** urethra is about 0.5 in. (1.25 cm) long and passes through the sphincter urethrae muscle and the perineal membrane. This is the least dilatable portion of the urethra (see Figs. 7.4 and 7.14).

The **penile (spongy) urethra** is about 6 in. (15.75 cm) long and runs through the bulb and the corpus spongiosum of the penis (see Figs. 7.4, 7.14, and 7.16). The external meatus is the narrowest part of the entire urethra. The part of the urethra that lies within the glans penis is dilated to form the **fossa terminalis (navicular fossa)** (see Figs. 7.4 and 7.13). The bulbourethral glands open into the penile urethra below the perineal membrane.

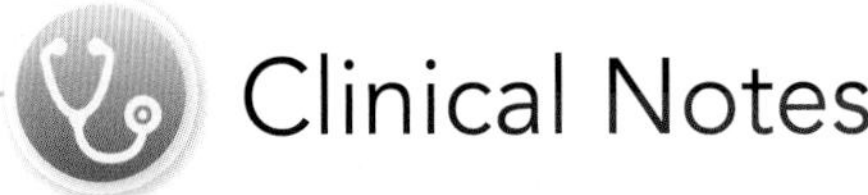

Clinical Notes

Circumcision

Circumcision is the operation of removing the greater part of the prepuce, or foreskin. In many newborn males, the prepuce cannot be retracted over the glans. This can result in infection of the secretions beneath the prepuce, leading to inflammation, swelling, and fibrosis of the prepuce. Repeated inflammation leads to constriction of the orifice of the prepuce (**phimosis**) with obstruction to urination. The current general belief is that chronic inflammation of the prepuce predisposes to carcinoma of the glans penis. For these reasons, prophylactic circumcision is commonly practiced. It is a rite in certain religions.

Catheterization

The following anatomic facts should be remembered before passing a catheter or other instrument along the male urethra:

- The external orifice at the glans penis is the narrowest part of the entire urethra.
- Within the glans, the urethra dilates to form the **fossa terminalis (navicular fossa)**.
- Near the posterior end of the fossa, a fold of mucous membrane projects into the lumen from the roof (see Fig. 7.13).
- The intermediate (membranous) part of the urethra is narrow and fixed.
- The prostatic part of the urethra is the widest and most dilatable part of the urethra.
- By holding the penis upward, the S-shaped curve to the urethra is converted into a J-shaped curve.

If the point of the catheter passes through the external orifice and is then directed toward the urethral floor until it has passed the mucosal fold, it should easily pass along a normal urethra into the bladder.

Anatomy of Procedure

The procedure is as follows:

1. The patient lies in a supine position.
2. With gentle traction, the penis is held erect at a right angle to the anterior abdominal wall. The lubricated catheter is passed through the narrow external urethral meatus. The catheter should pass easily along the penile urethra. On reaching the intermediate (membranous) part of the urethra, a slight resistance is felt because of the tone of the external urethral sphincter and the surrounding rigid perineal membrane.
3. The penis is then lowered toward the thighs, and the catheter is gently pushed through the sphincter.
4. Passage of the catheter through the prostatic urethra and bladder neck should not present any difficulty.

Urethral Infection

The most dependent part of the male urethra is that which lies within the bulb. Here, it is subject to chronic inflammation and stricture formation.

The many glands that open into the urethra—including those of the prostate, the bulbourethral glands, and many small penile urethral glands—are commonly the site of chronic gonococcal infection.

Injuries to the penis may occur as the result of blunt trauma, penetrating trauma, or strangulation. Amputation of the entire penis should be repaired by anastomosis using microsurgical techniques to restore continuity of the main blood vessels.

Urethral Rupture

Rupture of the urethra may complicate a severe blow on the perineum. The common site of rupture is within the bulb of the penis, just below the perineal membrane. The urine extravasates into the superficial perineal space and then passes forward over the scrotum beneath the membranous layer of the superficial fascia, as described in Chapter 5. If the intermediate (membranous) part of the urethra is ruptured, urine escapes into the deep perineal space and can extravasate upward around the prostate and bladder or downward into the superficial perineal space.

Erection and Ejaculation after Spinal Cord Injuries

The parasympathetic nerves that originate from the S2 to S4 segments of the spinal cord control erection of the penis. Bilateral damage to the reticulospinal nerve tracts in the spinal cord results in loss of erection. Later, when the effects of spinal shock have disappeared, spontaneous or reflex erection may occur if the sacral segments of the spinal cord are intact.

Sympathetic nerves that originate in the L1 and L2 segments of the spinal cord control ejaculation. As in the case of erection, severe bilateral damage to the spinal cord results in loss of ejaculation. Later, reflex ejaculation may be possible in patients with spinal cord transections in the thoracic or cervical regions.

FEMALE UROGENITAL TRIANGLE

In the female, the urogenital triangle contains the external genitalia and orifices of the urethra and the vagina.

Vulva

The term vulva is the collective name for the area of the female external genitalia (*vulv-* is Latin for a covering or wrapping; seed or womb covering). The external genitalia include the mons pubis, labia majora, labia minora, clitoris, vestibule, vestibular bulbs, greater vestibular glands, and the openings of the urethra and vagina. The **vestibule** is the specific space posterior to the glans clitoris and between the labia minora. It contains the openings of the urethra, vagina, and the ducts of the greater and lesser vestibular glands. The mons pubis, labia majora, and labia minora are described at the end of this chapter, under Surface Anatomy.

Blood Supply

Branches of the external and internal pudendal arteries on each side supply the vulva.

Lymph Drainage

The skin of the vulva drains into the medial group of superficial inguinal nodes.

Nerve Supply

The ilioinguinal nerves and the genital branch of the genitofemoral nerves supply the anterior parts of the vulva. The branches of the perineal nerves and the posterior femoral cutaneous nerves supply the posterior parts of the vulva.

Clitoris

The clitoris is the female phallic organ that corresponds to the penis in the male. It is situated anteriorly, at the apex of the vestibule. Its structure is similar to that of the penis.

Clitoral Root

The root of the clitoris is made up of two columns of erectile tissue, the **right** and **left corpora cavernosa**, plus the **ischiocavernosus muscle** that surrounds each (Fig. 7.18; see also Fig. 7.15). These paired units form the **crura** of the clitoris, which correspond to the crura of the penis.

Clitoral Body

The paired corpora cavernosa adjoin side by side below the pubic symphysis, enclosed in dense connective tissue, and form the body of the clitoris (see Fig. 7.18).

Glans of Clitoris

The glans of the clitoris is a small mass of erectile tissue that caps the body of the clitoris (see Fig. 7.18; see also Surface Anatomy later in this chapter). It connects to the vestibular bulbs by very small bands of erectile tissue. The **prepuce** is a small hoodlike fold of skin that partly covers the glans (Fig. 7.19A). The epithelium of the glans has numerous sensory endings and is the most sensitive part of the clitoris.

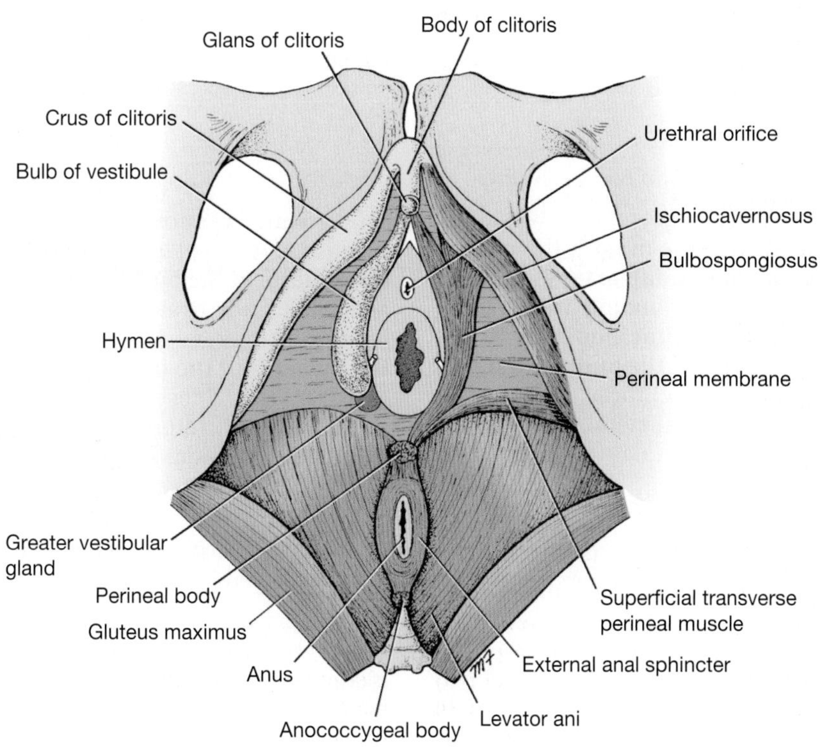

Figure 7.18 Root and body of the clitoris and the perineal muscles.

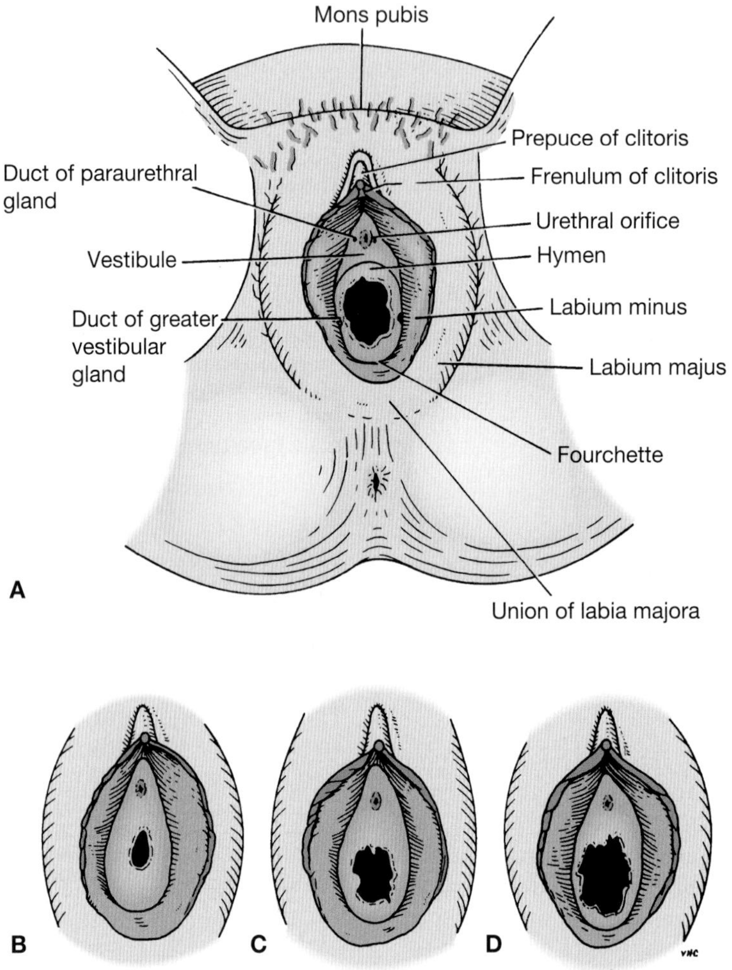

Figure 7.19 Vulva **(A)**. Note the different appearances of the hymen in a virgin **(B)**, a female who has had sexual intercourse **(C)**, and a multiparous female **(D)**.

Blood Supply, Lymph Drainage, and Nerve Supply

The blood supply, lymph drainage, and nerve supply follow virtually identical patterns in both the clitoris and penis. The **internal pudendal artery** supplies the clitoris and most of the surrounding area. Lymph drains directly to the **internal iliac nodes** or to the deep inguinal nodes. Branches of the **pudendal nerve** carry sensory fibers from the clitoris and provide motor supply to the associated skeletal muscles (eg, ischiocavernosus).

Vestibular Bulbs

The vestibular bulbs are paired erectile bodies located on each side of the vestibule, deep to the labia minora (see Fig. 7.18). A **bulbospongiosus muscle** covers each bulb. The bulbs attach to the inferior surface of the perineal membrane. Anteriorly, the bulbs connect to each other and to the glans of the clitoris via very small bands of erectile tissue. The two vestibular bulbs correspond to the single bulb of the penis separated by the vagina (see Embryology Notes below).

Greater Vestibular Glands

The greater vestibular glands are a pair of small mucus-secreting glands that lie under cover of the posterior parts of the bulbs of the vestibule (see Figs. 7.15 and 7.18). Each drains its secretion into the vestibule by a small duct, which opens into the groove between the hymen and the posterior part of the labium minus (see Fig. 7.19). These glands secrete lubricating mucus during sexual intercourse. The greater vestibular glands are the homologues of the male bulbourethral glands.

Superficial Perineal Space Contents

As in males, the superficial perineal space (pouch) in females is the zone between the superficial perineal fascia and the perineal membrane (see Figs. 7.15 and 7.12). It contains mainly structures comparable to those in the male superficial space. A notable sex difference is the presence of the greater vestibular glands in the female superficial space, whereas the male counterpart bulbourethral glands are in the deep perineal space.

Contents

- Bulbs of the vestibule plus the bulbospongiosus muscles
- Crura of the clitoris plus the ischiocavernosus muscles
- Superficial transverse perineal muscles
- Perineal nerves and vessels
- Greater vestibular glands

Muscles

The **bulbospongiosus muscle** surrounds the orifice of the vagina and covers the vestibular bulbs (see Figs. 7.15 and 7.18; see also Table 7.1). Its fibers extend forward to attach to the corpora cavernosa of the clitoris. The bulbospongiosus muscle reduces the size of the vaginal orifice and compresses the deep dorsal vein of the clitoris, thereby assisting in the mechanism of erection in the clitoris.

The **ischiocavernosus muscle** on each side covers the crus of the clitoris. Contraction of this muscle also assists in causing the erection of the clitoris.

The **superficial transverse perineal muscles** are identical in structure and function to those of the male.

Nerve Supply

The perineal branch of the pudendal nerve on each side terminates in the superficial perineal pouch where it supplies the muscles and most of the skin (see Fig. 7.8).

Perineal Body

The perineal body is larger than that of the male and is clinically important. It is a wedge-shaped mass of fibrous tissue situated between the lower end of the vagina and the anal canal (see Figs. 7.4 and 7.18). It is the point of attachment of many perineal muscles (as in the male), including the levatore ani muscles (see Table 7.1). The latter assist the perineal body in supporting the posterior wall of the vagina.

Deep Perineal Space Contents

As noted earlier, the contemporary view is that the deep perineal space (pouch) is the area located between the perineal membrane and the inferior fascia of the pelvic diaphragm (see Fig. 7.15). In females, the deep perineal space contains part of the urethra, the external urethral sphincter, part of the vagina, and branches of the internal pudendal vessels and pudendal nerve.

Recall that the **external urethral sphincter** is a complex structure composed of multiple parts. In females, the superior, more vertically oriented part extends up along the urethra as far as the neck of the bladder. The inferior portion forms a true sphincter-like unit encircling the urethra and may be referred to as the **sphincter urethrae muscle**. Additional parts extend from the sphincter and relate to the urethra and/or the vagina. These slips may be referred to as the compressor urethrae and urethrovaginal muscles. An organized **internal urethral sphincter** does not exist in females.

Typically, **deep transverse perineal muscles** are absent in females. Instead, a smooth muscle mass runs along the posterior margin of the perineal membrane and attaches to the perineal body.

The organization of the neurovascular supply to the deep perineal space is the same as in males (see the earlier text describing the contents of the deep perineal space).

Clitoral Erection

Sexual excitement produces engorgement of the erectile tissue within the clitoris in the same manner as in the male (see the earlier description of penile erection).

Female Orgasm

As sexual excitement builds, the vaginal walls become moist because of transudation of fluid through the congested mucous membrane. In addition, the greater vestibular glands at the vaginal orifice secrete lubricating mucus.

The upper part of the vagina, which resides in the pelvic cavity, has a visceral afferent innervation via the hypogastric plexuses and is sensitive only to stretch. However, the region of the vaginal orifice, the labia minora, and the clitoris have a somatic afferent supply through the ilioinguinal nerves and the dorsal nerves of the clitoris and are extremely sensitive to touch.

Appropriate sexual stimulation of these sensitive areas, reinforced by afferent nervous impulses from the breasts and other regions, results in a climax of pleasurable sensory impulses reaching the CNS. Impulses then pass down the spinal cord to the sympathetic outflow (T1 to L2).

The nervous impulses that pass to the genital organs are thought to leave the spinal cord at the L1 and L2 segments in preganglionic sympathetic fibers. Many of these fibers synapse with postganglionic neurons in the L1 and L2 ganglia; other fibers may synapse in ganglia in the lower lumbar or pelvic parts of the sympathetic trunks. The postganglionic fibers then distribute to the smooth muscle of the vaginal wall, which rhythmically contracts. In addition, nervous impulses travel in the pudendal nerve (S2 to S4) to reach the bulbospongiosus and ischiocavernosus muscles, which also undergo rhythmic contraction.

Female Urethra

The female urethra is about 1.5 in. (3.8 cm) long. It extends from the neck of the bladder (**internal urethral orifice**) to the vestibule (**external urethral orifice**) where it opens about 1 in. (2.5 cm) behind the clitoris (see Figs. 7.4B, 7.18, and 7.19). It passes through the genital hiatus of the pelvic diaphragm, the sphincter urethrae, and the perineal membrane. It lies immediately in front of the vagina and forms a palpable bulge on the anterior vaginal wall. The small openings of the ducts of the lesser vestibular (paraurethral) glands are at the sides of the external urethral orifice. The urethra can be dilated relatively easily.

Lesser Vestibular (Paraurethral) Glands

The lesser vestibular (paraurethral) glands lie on each side of the vestibule. They open into the vestibule by small ducts on either side of the external urethral orifice (see Fig. 7.19A). These glands correspond to the prostate in the male.

Vagina

The vagina is the female genital canal, the excretory duct for the menstrual flow from the uterus, and part of the birth canal. This muscular tube extends upward and backward between the vulva and the uterus (see Fig. 7.4B; see also the text section on Vagina in Chapter 6). It measures about 3 in. (8 cm) long. The cervix of the uterus pierces its upper anterior wall. The vaginal orifice in a virgin possesses a thin mucosal fold, called the **hymen**, which is perforated at its center (see Fig. 7.19B). The upper half of the vagina lies above the pelvic floor within the true pelvis between the bladder anteriorly and the rectum posteriorly (see Fig. 7.4B). The lower half lies within the perineum between the urethra anteriorly and the anal canal posteriorly (see Figs. 7.4B and 7.18).

Vaginal Supports

- **Upper third:** Levatore ani muscles and transverse cervical, pubocervical, and sacrocervical ligaments
- **Middle third:** Perineal membrane
- **Lower third:** Perineal body

Blood Supply

The **vaginal artery**, a branch of the internal iliac artery, and the **vaginal branch of the uterine artery** supply the vagina.

Vaginal veins drain into the internal iliac veins.

Lymph Drainage

- **Upper third:** Internal and external iliac nodes
- **Middle third:** Internal iliac nodes
- **Lower third:** Superficial inguinal nodes

Nerve Supply

Nerves from the inferior hypogastric plexuses supply the vagina.

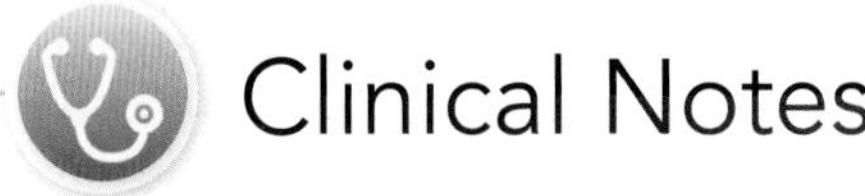

Clinical Notes

Vulval Infection

The presence of numerous glands and ducts opening onto the surface in the vulva makes this area prone to infection. The sebaceous glands of the labia majora, the ducts of the greater vestibular glands, the vagina (with its indirect communication with the peritoneal cavity), the urethra, and the lesser vestibular (paraurethral) glands can all become infected. The vagina itself has no glands and is lined with stratified squamous epithelium. Provided that the pH of its interior is kept low, it is capable of resisting infection to a remarkable degree.

Vulva and Pregnancy

An important sign in the diagnosis of pregnancy is the appearance of a bluish discoloration of the vulva and vagina because of venous congestion. This appears at the 8th to 12th week and increases as the pregnancy progresses.

Urethral Infection

The short length of the female urethra predisposes to ascending infection. Consequently, **cystitis** is more common in females than in males.

Urethral Injuries

Injuries are rare because of the short length of the urethra. In fractures of the pelvis, shearing forces may damage the urethra as it emerges from the fixed perineal membrane.

Catheterization

Because the female urethra is shorter, wider, and more dilatable, catheterization is much easier than in males. Moreover, the urethra is straight, and only minor resistance is felt as the catheter passes through the external urethral sphincter.

Vaginal Examination

Digital examination of the vagina may provide the physician with much valuable information concerning the health of the vaginal walls, uterus, and surrounding structures (see Fig. 7.4). Thus, the anatomic relations of the vagina must be known; they are considered in detail in Chapter 6.

Perineal Injury during Childbirth

The **perineal body** is a wedge of fibromuscular tissue that lies between the lower part of the vagina and the anal canal (see Figs. 7.4B and 7.18). It is held in position by the insertion of the perineal muscles and by the attachment of the levator ani muscles. It is a much larger structure in females than in males, and it serves to support the posterior wall of the vagina. Damage by laceration during childbirth can be followed by permanent weakness of the pelvic floor.

Few patients escape some injury to the birth canal during delivery. In most, this is little more than an abrasion of the posterior vaginal wall. Spontaneous delivery of the infant with the patient unattended can result in a severe tear of the lower third of the posterior wall of the vagina, perineal body, and overlying skin. In severe tears, the lacerations may extend backward into the anal canal and damage the external anal sphincter. In these cases, it is imperative that an accurate repair of the walls of the anal canal, vagina, and perineal body be undertaken as soon as possible.

In the management of childbirth, when it is obvious to the obstetrician that the perineum will tear before the infant's head emerges through the vaginal orifice, a planned surgical incision is made through the perineal skin in a posterolateral direction to avoid the anal sphincters. This procedure is known as an **episiotomy** (see Fig. 7.11C). Breech deliveries (buttocks or feet first) and forceps deliveries are usually preceded by an episiotomy.

Pudendal Nerve Block

The area anesthetized is the skin of the perineum. However, this nerve block does not completely abolish sensation from the anterior part of the perineum, which is also innervated by the ilioinguinal and genitofemoral nerves. It also does not abolish pain from uterine contractions that ascend to the spinal cord via the visceral afferent nerves that follow sympathetic nerves.

Indications

During the second stage of a difficult labor, when the presenting part of the fetus, usually the head, is descending through the vulva, forceps delivery and episiotomy may be necessary.

Transvaginal Procedure

The bony landmark used is the **ischial spine** (Fig. 7.20). The index finger is inserted through the vagina to palpate the ischial spine. The needle of the syringe is then passed through the vaginal mucous membrane toward the ischial spine. On passing through the **sacrospinous ligament**, the anesthetic solution is injected around the pudendal nerve.

Perineal Procedure

The bony landmark is the **ischial tuberosity** (see Fig. 7.20). The tuberosity is palpated subcutaneously through the buttock, and the needle is introduced into the **pudendal canal** along the medial side of the tuberosity. The canal lies about 1 in. (2.5 cm) deep to the free surface of the ischial tuberosity. The local anesthetic is then infiltrated around the pudendal nerve.

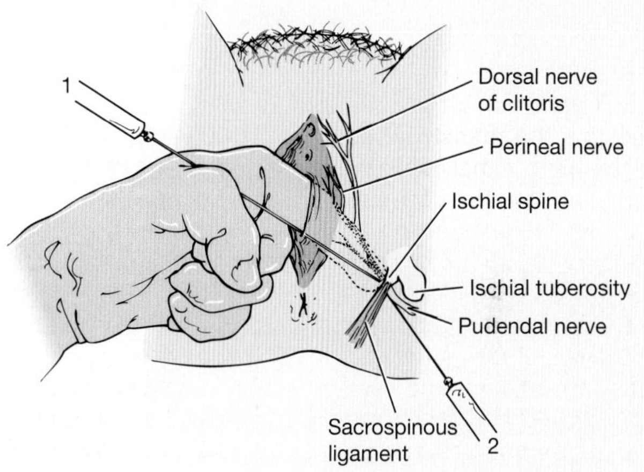

Figure 7.20 Pudendal nerve block. (1) Transvaginal method. The needle is passed through the vaginal mucous membrane toward the ischial spine. After the needle is passed through the sacrospinous ligament, the anesthetic solution is injected around the pudendal nerve. (2) Perineal method. The ischial tuberosity is palpated subcutaneously through the buttock. The needle is inserted on the medial side of the ischial tuberosity to a depth of about 1 in. (2.5 cm) from the free surface of the tuberosity. The anesthetic is injected around the pudendal nerve.

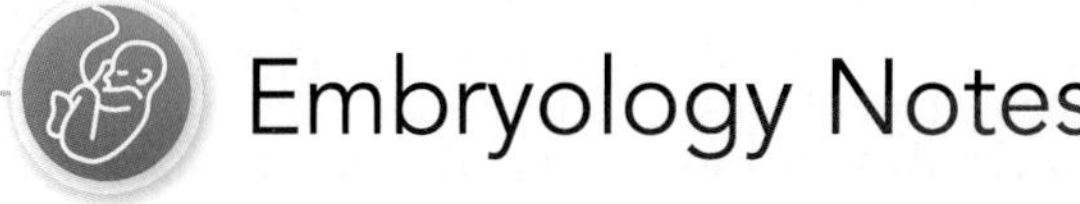

Embryology Notes

External Genitalia Development

The external genitalia develop from a common, sexually indifferent form. Early in development, the embryonic mesenchyme grows around the cloacal membrane and causes the overlying ectoderm to elevate and form three swellings. One swelling occurs between the cloacal membrane and the umbilical cord in the midline and is called the **genital tubercle** (Fig. 7.21). On each side of the membrane, another swelling, called the **genital fold**, appears. At week 7, the genital tubercle elongates to form the **glans**. The anterior part of the cloacal membrane, the **urogenital membrane**, now ruptures so that the urogenital sinus opens onto the surface. The endodermal cells of the urogenital sinus proliferate and grow into the root of the phallus, forming a **urethral plate**. Meanwhile, a second pair of lateral swellings, called the **genital swellings**, appears lateral to the genital folds. At this stage of development, the genitalia of the two sexes are identical.

Male Genitalia

In the male, the **phallus** rapidly elongates and pulls the genital folds anteriorly onto its ventral surface so that they form the lateral edges of a groove, the **urethral groove** (Fig. 7.22). The endodermal urethral plate forms the floor of the groove. The penile urethra develops as the result of the two genital folds fusing together progressively along the shaft of the phallus to the root of the glans penis. During month 4, the remainder of the urethra in the glans develops

(continued)

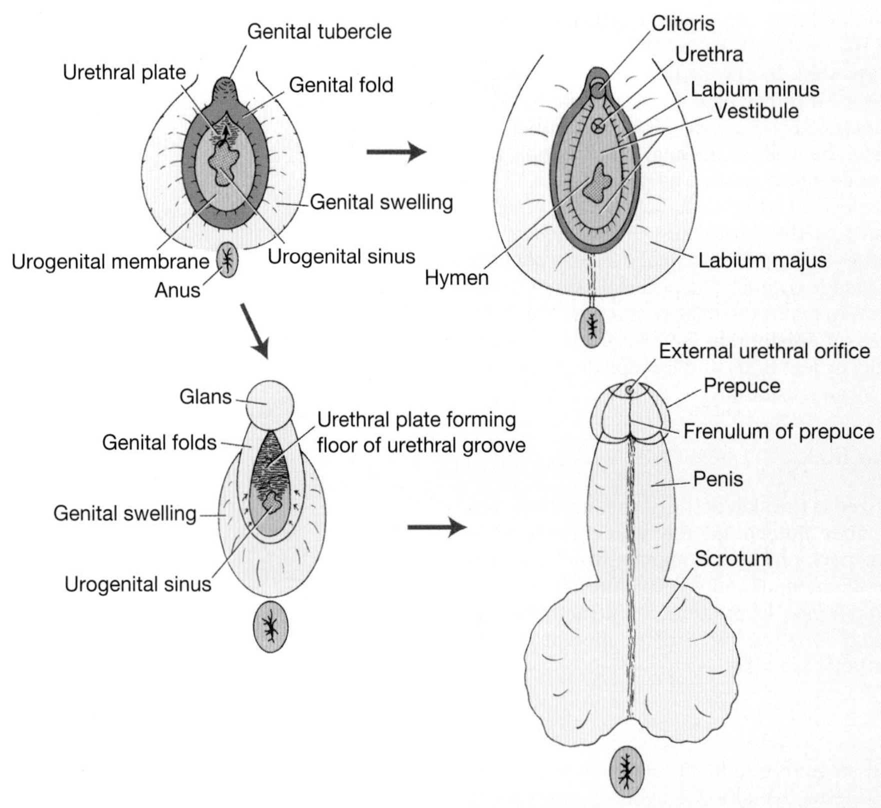

Figure 7.21 Development of the external genitalia in the female and male.

from a bud of ectodermal cells from the tip of the glans. This cord of cells later canalizes so that the penile urethra opens at the tip of the glans.

The **prepuce** (**foreskin**) forms from a fold of skin at the base of the glans (see Figs. 7.21 and 7.22). The fold of skin remains tethered to the ventral aspect of the root of the glans to form the **frenulum**. The erectile tissue—the corpus spongiosum and the corpora cavernosa—develops within the mesenchymal core of the penis.

Female Genitalia

The changes in the female are less extensive than those in the male. The phallus bends and forms the clitoris (see Fig. 7.21). The genital folds do not fuse to form the urethra, as in the male, but remain separate and develop into the **labia minora**. The genital swellings enlarge and form the **labia majora**.

Meatal Stenosis

The external urethral orifice (meatus) normally is the narrowest part of the male urethra, but occasionally the opening is excessively small and may cause a backpressure effect on the entire urinary system. In severe cases, dilatation of the orifice by incision is necessary.

Hypospadias

Hypospadias is the most common congenital anomaly affecting the male urethra. In this condition, the external urethral orifice is situated on the ventral or undersurface of the penis anywhere between the glans and the perineum. Five degrees of severity may occur, the first of which is the most common: (1) glandular, (2) coronal, (3) penile, (4) penoscrotal, and (5) perineal (Fig. 7.23). In all except the first type, the penis is curved in a downward or ventral direction, a condition referred to as **chordee**.

Types 1 and 2 are caused by a failure of the bud of ectodermal cells from the tip of the glans to grow into the substance of the glans and join the endodermal cells lining the penile urethra. Types 3, 4, and 5 are caused by a failure of the genital folds to unite on the undersurface of the developing penis and so convert the urethral groove into the penile urethra. In the penoscrotal variety, the genital swellings fail to fuse completely, so that the meatal orifice occurs in the midline of the scrotum.

Epispadias

Epispadias is a relatively rare condition and is more commonly found in the male. In this condition in the male, the external urethral orifice is situated on the dorsal or upper surface of the penis between the glans and the anterior abdominal wall (Fig. 7.24). The most severe type is associated with exstrophy of the bladder. In the female, the urethra is split dorsally and is associated with a double clitoris. It is thought that epispadias is caused by failure of the embryonic mesenchyme to develop in the lower part of the anterior abdominal wall, so that when the cloacal membrane breaks down, the urogenital sinus opens onto the surface of the cranial aspect of the penis.

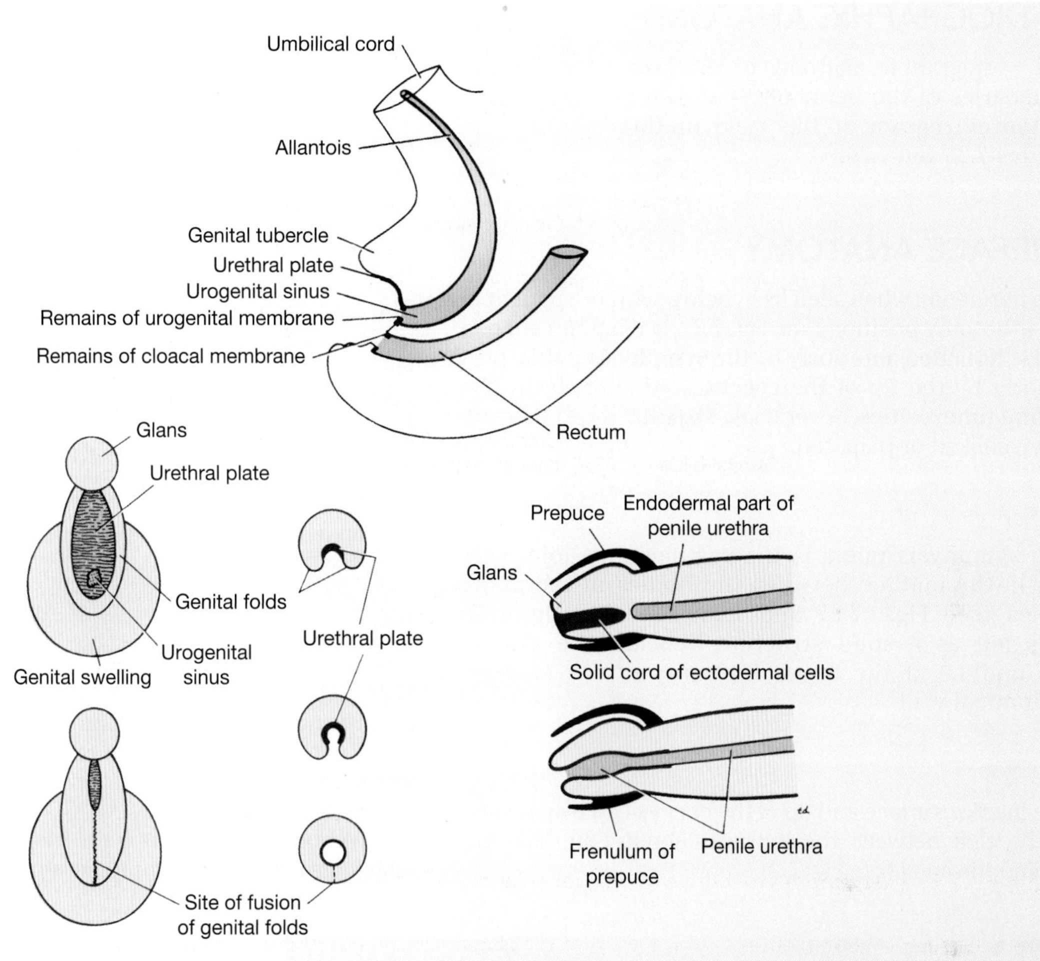

Figure 7.22 Development of the penile portion of the male urethra.

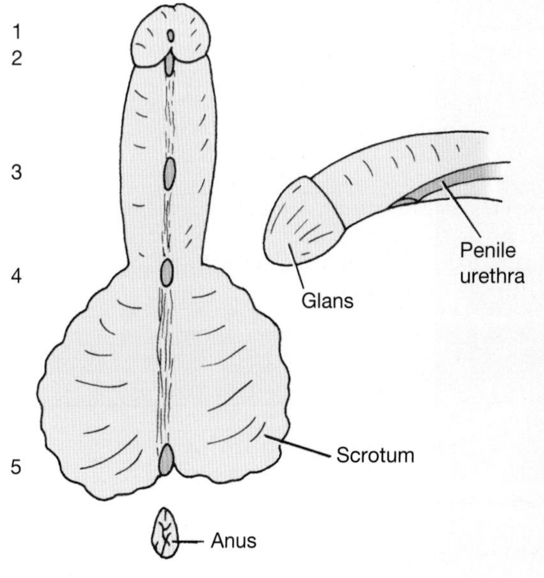

Figure 7.23 Types of hypospadias: (1) glandular, (2) coronal, (3) penile, (4) penoscrotal, and (5) perineal. Ventral flexion (chordee) of the penis is also present.

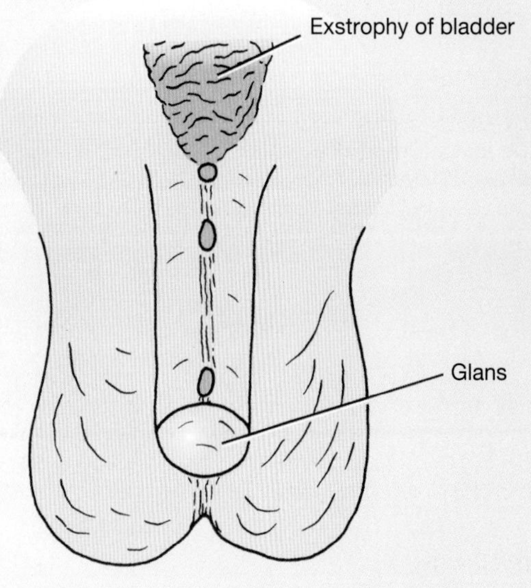

Figure 7.24 Types of epispadias.

RADIOGRAPHIC ANATOMY

The radiographic anatomy of the bones forming the boundaries of the perineum is shown in Chapter 6. A **cystourethrogram** of the male urethra is shown in Figures 7.25 and 7.26.

SURFACE ANATOMY

The perineum, when seen from below with the patient in the lithotomy position (see Fig. 7.3), is diamond shaped and is bounded anteriorly by the **symphysis pubis**, posteriorly by the tip of the **coccyx**, and laterally by the **ischial tuberosities**. Several key structures can be readily visualized or palpated.

Symphysis Pubis

The symphysis pubis is the cartilaginous joint that lies in the midline between the bodies of the pubic bones (see Figs. 7.27 and 7.28; see also Fig. 7.2). It is felt as a solid structure beneath the skin in the midline at the lower extremity of the anterior abdominal wall.

Coccyx

The inferior surface and tip of the coccyx can be palpated in the cleft between the buttocks about 1 in. (2.5 cm) behind the anus (see Fig. 7.2).

Ischial Tuberosity

The ischial tuberosity can be palpated in the lower part of the buttock (see Fig. 7.2). In the standing position, the tuberosity is covered by the gluteus maximus. In the sitting position, the ischial tuberosity emerges from beneath the lower border of the gluteus maximus and supports the weight of the body.

Anal Triangle

The anus is the lower opening of the anal canal and lies in the midline (see Fig. 7.28B). In the living, the anal margin is reddish brown and is puckered by the contraction of the **external anal sphincter**. Coarse hairs occur around the anal margin.

Male Urogenital Triangle

The male urogenital triangle contains the penis and the scrotum.

Penis

The penis consists of a root, a body, and a glans (see Figs. 7.13, 7.16, and 7.27). The **root of the penis** consists of three masses of erectile tissue, the **bulb** of the penis, and the right and left **crura** of the penis. The bulb can be felt on deep palpation in the midline of the perineum, posterior to the scrotum.

The **body of the penis** is the free portion of the penis, which is suspended from the symphysis pubis. Note

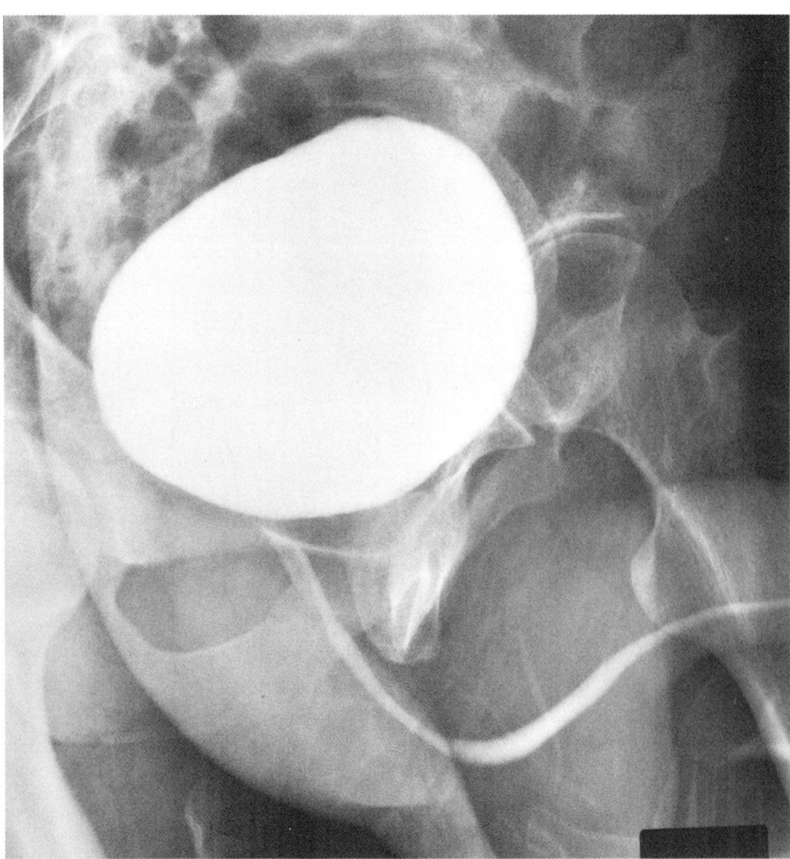

Figure 7.25 Cystourethrogram after intravenous injection of contrast medium (young adult male).

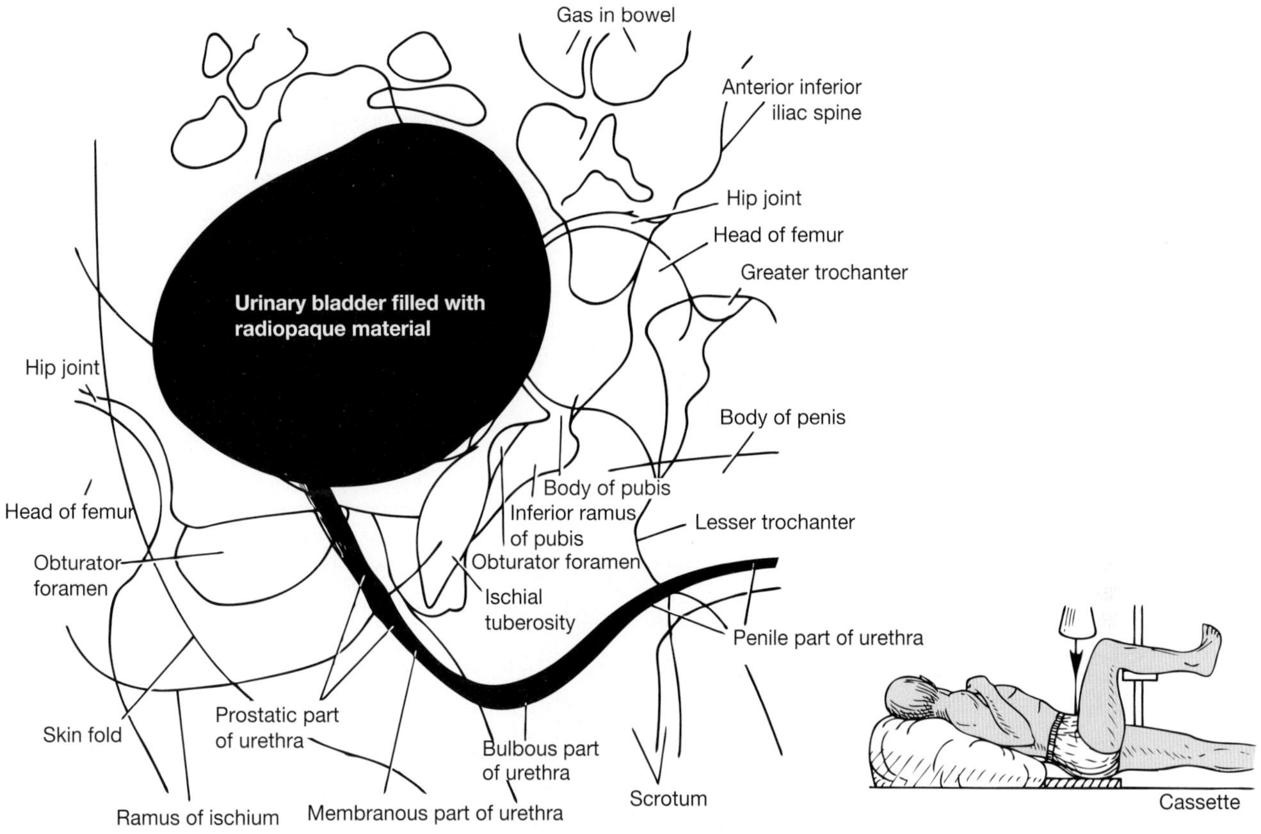

Figure 7.26 The main features seen in the cystourethrogram shown in Figure 7.25.

that the dorsal surface (anterior surface of the flaccid organ) usually possesses a **superficial dorsal vein** in the midline (see Fig. 7.13).

The **glans penis** forms the extremity of the body of the penis (see Figs. 7.13, 7.16, and 7.27). The **external urethral orifice (meatus)** is at the summit of the glans. A skin fold termed the **frenulum** extends from the lower margin of the external meatus and connects the glans to the **prepuce (foreskin)**. The edge of the base of the glans is called the **corona** (see Figs. 7.16 and 7.27). The prepuce is formed by a fold of skin attached to the neck of the penis. The prepuce covers the glans for a variable extent, and it should be possible to retract it over the glans.

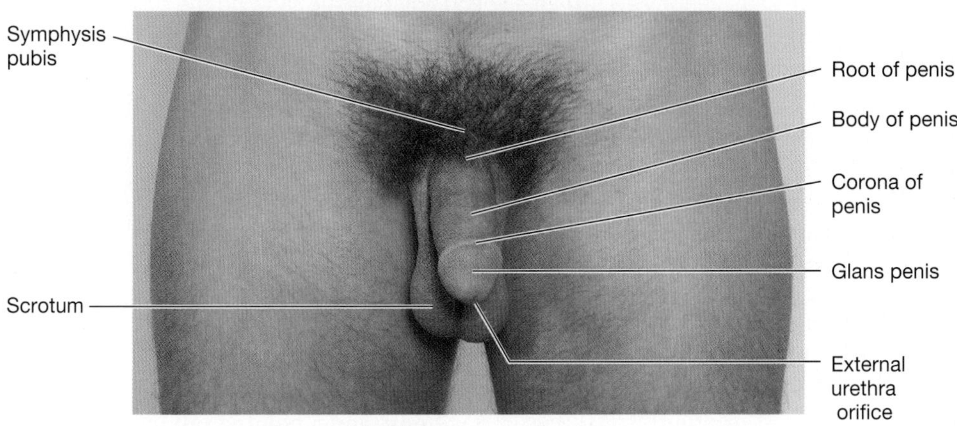

Figure 7.27 Anterior view of a young adult male showing the surface anatomy of the urogenital triangle, including the penis and scrotum. (Modified from *Moore's Essential Clinical Anatomy*, 7th ed; Fig. 6.58.)

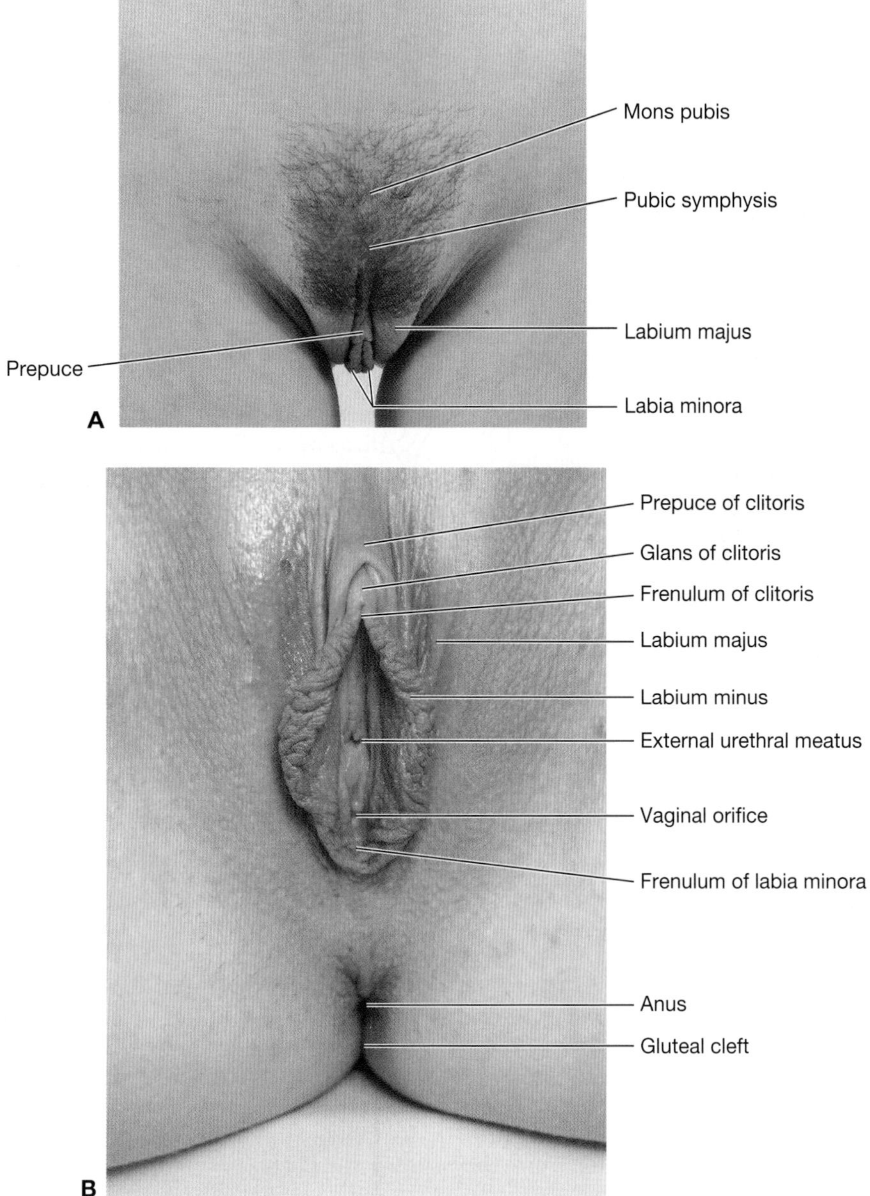

Figure 7.28 Anterior view **(A)** and inferior view **(B)** of a young adult female showing the surface anatomy of the perineum. **A.** The inferior abdominal wall and the urogenital triangle. **B.** The subject is in the lithotomy position with the labia minora separated. (Modified from *Moore's Essential Clinical Anatomy*, 7th ed; Fig. 6.52.)

Scrotum

The scrotum is a sac of skin and fascia (see Figs. 7.12 and 7.27) containing the testes and the epididymis. The skin of the scrotum is rugose and is covered with sparse hairs. The bilateral origin of the scrotum is indicated by the presence of a dark line in the midline, called the **scrotal raphe**, along the line of fusion.

Testes

The testes can be palpated easily. They are oval shaped and have a firm consistency. They lie free within the tunica vaginalis (see Fig. 5.26) and are not tethered to the subcutaneous tissue or skin.

Epididymis

Each epididymis can be palpated on the posterolateral surface of the testis. The epididymis is a long, narrow, firm structure having an expanded upper end or **head**, a **body**, and a pointed **tail** inferiorly (see Fig. 5.26). The cordlike **vas deferens** emerges from the tail and ascends medial to the epididymis to enter the spermatic cord at the upper end of the scrotum.

Female Urogenital Triangle

The female urogenital triangle contains the vulva and its component structures, including the labia majora, labia minora, and the clitoris.

Mons Pubis

The mons pubis is the rounded, hair-bearing elevation of skin found anterior to the pubis (see Figs. 7.19 and 7.28A). The mons is continuous posteriorly with the labia majora. The pubic hair in the female has an abrupt horizontal superior margin, whereas in the male it extends upward to the umbilicus.

Labia Majora

The labia majora are prominent, paired, fat-filled folds of skin extending posteriorly from the mons pubis (see Figs. 7.19 and 7.28). They unite in the anterior midline at the **anterior commissure** and in the posterior midline at the **posterior commissure**. The posterior commissure typically fades following the first vaginal birth. The lateral (external; outer) aspects of the labia majora have pigmented skin and coarse pubic hair, whereas the medial (internal) aspects are pink and hairless.

Labia Minora

The labia minora are two smaller, fat-free, hairless folds of soft skin that lie between the labia majora (see Figs. 7.19 and 7.28). The labia unite anteriorly to enclose the clitoris and form the more posterior **frenulum of the clitoris** and the more anterior **prepuce of the clitoris**. They also join posteriorly to form a small connecting fold, the **frenulum of the labia minora** (**fourchette**).

Vestibule

The vestibule is a smooth triangular area bounded laterally by the labia minora, with the clitoris at its apex and the fourchette at its base (see Figs. 7.19 and 7.28B).

Vaginal Orifice

The vaginal orifice lies in the vestibule, posterior to the external urethral meatus (see Figs. 7.19 and 7.28B). It is protected in virgins by a thin mucosal fold called the **hymen**, which is perforated at its center (see Fig. 7.19B). At the first coitus, the hymen tears, usually posteriorly or posterolaterally, and after childbirth only a few tags of the hymen remain (see Fig. 7.19C,D).

Orifices of the Ducts of the Greater Vestibular Glands

Small orifices, one on each side, are found in the groove between the hymen and the posterior part of the labium minus (see Fig. 7.19).

Clitoris

This is situated at the apex of the vestibule anteriorly (see Fig. 7.19). The glans of the clitoris is partly hidden by the prepuce (see Fig. 7.28).

Clinical Case Discussion

The severe anemia explained the patient's breathlessness. The constipation, anal canal swellings, and location of the anal bleeding suggested internal hemorrhoids. These hemorrhoids were dilatations of the tributaries of the superior rectal vein in the wall of the anal canal. Repeated abrasion of the hemorrhoids by hard stools caused the bleeding and loss of blood. Without knowledge of the anatomic position of the veins in the anal canal, the physician would not have been able to make a diagnosis.

Key Concepts

Perineum

- The perineum is the area inferior (superficial) to the pelvic diaphragm.
- The perineum is divided into two triangular regions: a more anterior urogenital triangle and a more posterior anal triangle. The urogenital triangle contains the urogenital orifices. The anal triangle contains the anus.
- The perineal body is a central fibromuscular mass that serves as the attachment for perineal muscles and fascia and aids in support of local viscera.

Anal Triangle

- The anal triangle contains the anal canal and the paired ischioanal fossae.
- The anal canal is the caudal end of the gastrointestinal tract. It runs from the rectal ampulla to the anal opening.
- The upper part of the anal canal is related to the embryonic hindgut in structure, vasculature, lymph drainage, and innervation. The lower part is related to the embryonic proctodeum. The pectinate line marks the interface of the two parts.
- The anal canal has an involuntary internal sphincter and a voluntary external sphincter. The smooth muscle of the anal canal forms the internal sphincter. The external sphincter is skeletal muscle and has three parts. Autonomic nerves supply the internal sphincter. The inferior rectal nerves supply the external sphincter.
- The ischioanal fossae are fat-filled spaces on each side of the anal canal. The fat supports the anal

canal and allows it to distend during defecation. The pudendal nerve and internal pudendal vessels are embedded in the pudendal canal, on the lateral wall of the ischioanal fossa.

- The pudendal nerve and internal pudendal vessels are the primary supply to the entire perineum. The significant anorectal portal–systemic anastomosis occurs between the superior and inferior rectal veins. Varicosities of branches of these veins cause hemorrhoids.
- Digital anorectal exams allow palpable inspection of the anal canal and neighboring structures in all directions.

Urogenital Triangle

- The urogenital triangle is organized in layers, two of which are the superficial perineal space and the deep perineal space.
- The superficial perineal space is the area between the superficial perineal fascia and the perineal membrane. It houses the external genitalia, part of the urethra, and the neurovascular supplies of those structures.
- The deep perineal space is located deep to the superficial perineal space and extends from the perineal membrane to the pelvic diaphragm. It contains part of the urethra, the inferior part of the external urethral sphincter, and neurovascular branches to those structures.
- The external urethral sphincter is the voluntary sphincter for urination. Only the inferior portion appears to form a true sphincter-like unit encircling the urethra.

Male Urogenital Triangle

- Contains the penis and scrotum.
- The penis consists of a root and body. The root is made up of three masses of erectile tissue: the bulb and the right and left crura. The bulb forms the corpus spongiosum and each crus forms a corpus cavernosum. The bulbospongiosus muscle surrounds the bulb, and the ischiocavernosus muscle surrounds each crus. The bulb and crura join to form the body of the penis. The expanded end of the corpus spongiosum forms the glans of the penis. Branches of the internal pudendal arteries supply the erectile tissues of the penis. The pudendal nerves provide the nerve supply.
- The scrotum is an outpouching of the lower part of the anterior abdominal wall. It houses the testes, epididymides, and spermatic cords.
- The superficial perineal space contains the bulb and crura of the penis and their covering muscles and the superficial transverse perineal muscles.
- The deep perineal space contains the intermediate part of the urethra, sphincter urethrae and deep transverse perineal muscles, and bulbourethral glands.
- The male urethra has three parts: prostatic (in the prostate), intermediate (running through the sphincter urethrae and perineal membrane), and penile (in the bulb and corpus spongiosum).

Female Urogenital Triangle

- The female urogenital triangle contains the external genitalia and urethral and vaginal orifices.
- The clitoris corresponds to the penis. It consists of a root, body, and glans. The root consists of the paired crura (corpora cavernosa plus ischiocavernosus muscles). The body is the adjoined corpora cavernosa. The glans is a cap of erectile tissue at the end of the body.
- The vestibular bulbs are paired erectile bodies that correspond to the bulb of the penis. A bulbospongiosus muscle covers each bulb.
- The greater vestibular glands are a pair of small mucus-secreting glands that lie at the posterior ends of the vestibular bulbs. They are the homologues of the male bulbourethral glands.
- The superficial perineal space contains the crura of the clitoris with their muscles, the vestibular bulbs with their muscles, the superficial transverse perineal muscles, the greater vestibular glands, and the lower end of the urethra.
- The deep perineal space contains part of the urethra, the external urethral sphincter, and part of the vagina.
- The female urethra pierces the sphincter urethrae and the perineal membrane and lies along the anterior vaginal wall.
- The lesser vestibular glands lie on each side of the vestibule. They correspond to the prostate.
- The vagina runs from the vulva to the uterus. Its lower half lies within the perineum between the urethra anteriorly and the anal canal posteriorly.

Surface Anatomy

- Several key structures in the perineum can be readily visualized or palpated. These include much of the bony boundaries of the perineum, the anal canal, and much of the external genitalia.

8 Lower Limb

An 18-year-old student was doing part-time work delivering pizzas on his motorcycle. His boss insisted on quick delivery, so the student tended to weave in and out of traffic whenever there was a holdup. On one occasion, he misjudged the gap between two vehicles, and forcefully struck the outer surface of his left knee against a car bumper. Examination in the emergency department showed he had extensive paralysis of the muscles in the anterior and lateral aspects of the left leg. As a result, he was unable to dorsiflex and evert the foot, which showed footdrop. In addition, he had diminished sensation down the anterior and lateral sides of the leg and tops of the foot and toes, including the medial side of the great toe. A series of radiographs of the knee region showed no evidence of bone fractures.

See the Clinical Case Discussion at the end of this chapter for further insights.

CHAPTER OUTLINE

LEARNING OBJECTIVES

The purpose of this chapter is to review the anatomy of the lower limb in relation to common clinical conditions.

1. Identify the primary regions of the lower limb and the defining boundaries of each.
2. Identify the bones of the lower limb and their major features in skeletal specimens and standard radiographic images. Describe the functional aspects of these structures.
3. Identify the bony components, major supporting ligaments, key accessory structures, and movements of the hip, knee, and ankle joints. Describe the features of major traumas to each joint.
4. Identify the medial and lateral longitudinal and transverse arches of the foot. Describe the roles of bones, ligaments, and muscles in maintaining these arches.
5. Identify the muscles of the gluteal region, indicating their attachments, innervation, and major actions. Note the roles of the gluteal muscles during locomotion.
6. Describe the topographic relationships of the neurovascular structures in the gluteal region and the consequences of intragluteal injections into specific quadrants of the region.
7. Describe the arrangement and mechanical significance of the deep fascia in the lower limb. Identify the fascia lata, iliotibial tract, and intermuscular septa in the hip and thigh.
8. Define the osseofascial compartments of the lower limb.
    a. Identify the muscles contained in each compartment.
    b. Describe the attachments, innervation, and major actions of each muscle.
    c. Describe the innervation and major actions of each compartment.
    d. Predict the functional consequences of loss of action of each muscle and each compartment.
9. Trace the course of cutaneous and motor innervation in the lower limb.
    a. Identify the lumbosacral plexus and its component parts, from spinal segmental sources to major terminal branches.
    b. Identify the spinal segmental level(s) of origin and relationship of each major peripheral nerve to the lumbosacral plexus.
    c. Predict the functional consequences of lesions to specific spinal levels and individual peripheral nerves.
10. Define the boundaries and contents of the femoral triangle. Describe the composition of the femoral sheath, canal, and ring. Describe the anatomical basis of a femoral hernia.
11. Define the boundaries of the popliteal fossa and describe its contents. Note the spatial relationships of the major neurovascular structures in the fossa. Identify the main components of the arterial anastomoses around the knee.
12. Trace the flow of blood from the common iliac artery through the lower limb. Note:
    a. The different sources of arterial supply, their pathways, and their major branches
    b. The significance of the obturator canal, femoral sheath, adductor canal, adductor hiatus, greater sciatic foramen, and lesser sciatic foramen
    c. The composition and significance of the cruciate anastomosis
    d. The territories supplied by and the pathways of the major peripheral vessels
13. Trace the venous drainage of the lower limb through the saphenous tract to the pelvic cavity. Describe the significance of the saphenous veins in terms of common clinical conditions.
14. Describe the pattern of lymphatic drainage of the lower limb, including the relationship of this drainage with those of the abdominal wall and groin regions.
15. Determine the movements that occur at the knee joint during normal locomotion. Describe the mechanics of "locking" and "unlocking" of the knee.
16. Identify the extrinsic and intrinsic muscles of the foot, indicating their attachments, innervation, and major actions. Compare and contrast the patterning and functions of muscles of the hand and foot.
17. Describe the arrangements of flexor, extensor, and peroneal retinacula, and major tendons around the ankle, including the functional significance of these arrangements.
18. Compare and contrast the pattern of development of the lower limb with that of the upper limb.
19. Locate the projections and palpation points of the major structures of the lower limb in a basic surface examination.

OVERVIEW

The primary functions of the lower limbs are to support body weight and produce locomotion. The lower limbs are very stable and can bear the weight of the body because the two hip bones articulate posteriorly with the trunk at the strong sacroiliac joints and anteriorly with each other at the symphysis pubis. This stability also provides the foundation for standing in the upright posture, walking, and running.

Each lower limb is organized into the **gluteal region**, **thigh**, **popliteal fossa**, **leg**, **ankle**, and **foot**. The thigh and leg are compartmentalized, and each compartment has its own muscles that perform group functions and its own distinct nerve and blood supply.

Lower limb problems are some of the most common problems dealt with by health professionals, whether working in general practice, surgery, or an emergency department. Some of the many conditions physicians encounter are arthritis, varicose veins, vascular deficiencies, fractures, dislocations, sprains, lacerations, knee effusions, leg pain, ankle injuries, and peripheral nerve injuries.

OSTEOLOGY

The bones of the lower limb are the os coxae (hip bone), femur, patella, tibia, fibula, metatarsal bones, tarsal bones, and phalanges. The general arrangement of the bones is similar to that in the upper limb.

Os Coxae

The os coxae (*os coxae* is Latin for "hip bone") is topographically and functionally the equivalent of the upper limb clavicle and scapula. It forms the lower limb girdle that attaches the limb to the vertebral column.

Three skeletal elements, the ilium, ischium, and pubis, form the os coxae (Figs. 8.1 to 8.3). These bones meet one another at the acetabulum via the Y-shaped **triradiate cartilage**. The os coxae articulate with the sacrum at the sacroiliac joints and form the anterolateral walls of the pelvis. They also articulate with one another anteriorly at the symphysis pubis. The detailed structure of the internal (pelvic) aspect of the bony pelvis is considered in Chapter 6. The important features found on the outer (gluteal) surface of the os coxae in the gluteal region are as follows.

The **ilium**, which is the upper flattened part of the bone, possesses the **iliac crest** (see Figs. 8.1 and 8.2). This can be felt through the skin along its entire length. It ends in front at the **anterosuperior iliac spine** and behind at the **posterosuperior iliac spine**. The **iliac tubercle** lies about 2 in. (5 cm) behind the anterosuperior spine. Below the anterosuperior iliac spine is the **anteroinferior iliac spine**. A similar prominence, the **posteroinferior iliac spine**, is located below the posterosuperior iliac spine. The ilium possesses a large notch, the **greater sciatic notch**, above and behind the acetabulum.

The **ischium** is L shaped, possessing an upper thicker part, the **body**, and a lower thinner part, the **ramus**. The **ischial spine** projects from the posterior border of the ischium and intervenes between the **greater** and **lesser sciatic notches**. The **ischial tuberosity** is the large, roughened area that forms the posterior aspect of the lower part of the body of the bone. The greater and lesser sciatic notches are converted into greater and lesser sciatic foramina by the presence of the sacrospinous and sacrotuberous ligaments (see below).

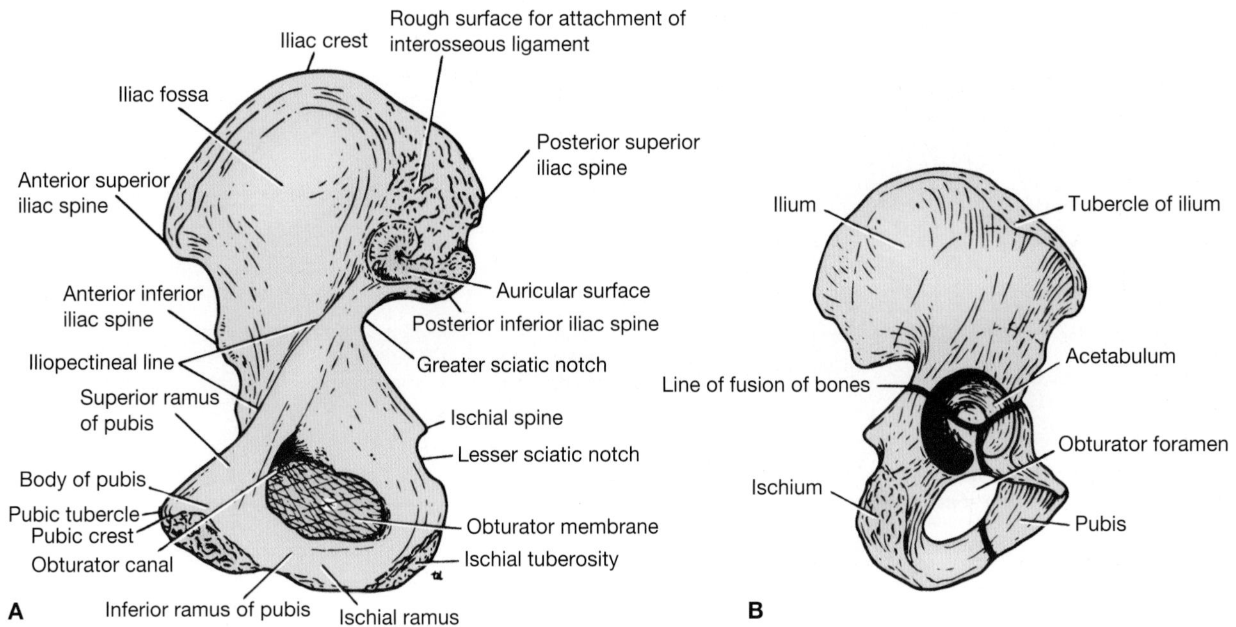

Figure 8.1 Medial surface **(A)** and lateral surface **(B)** of the right os coxae. Note the lines of fusion between the three bones (ilium, ischium, and pubis) along the triradiate cartilage.

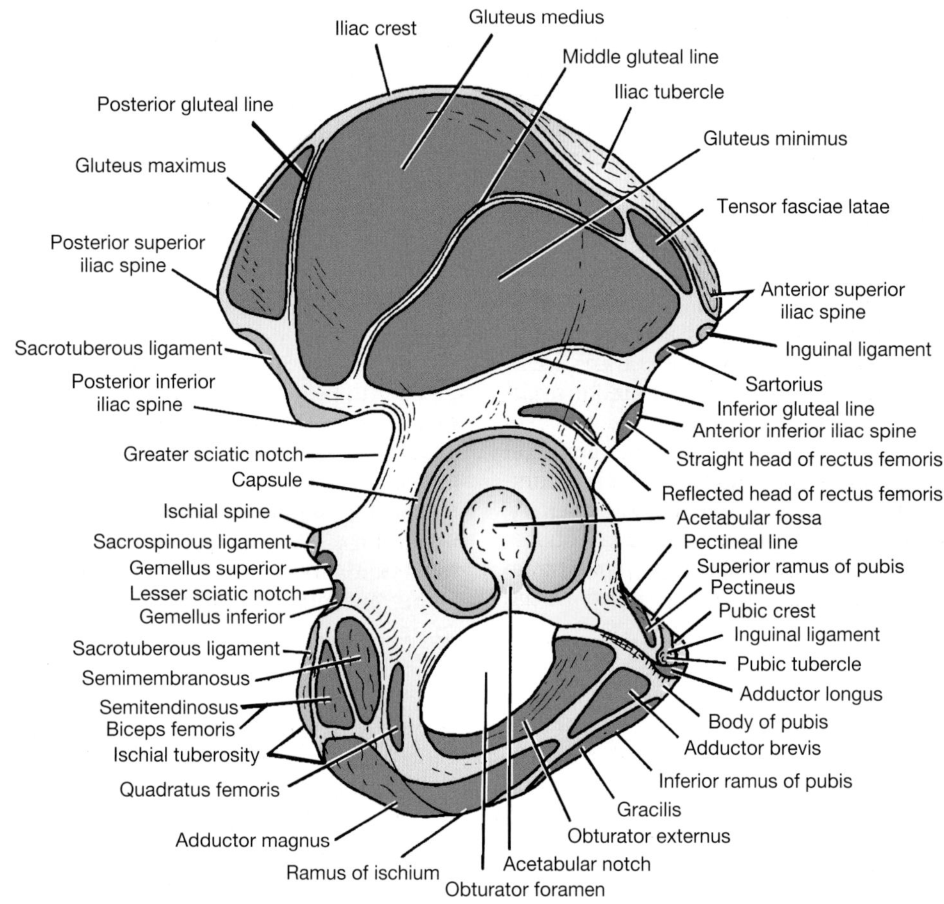

Figure 8.2 Muscles and ligaments attached to the external surface of the right os coxae.

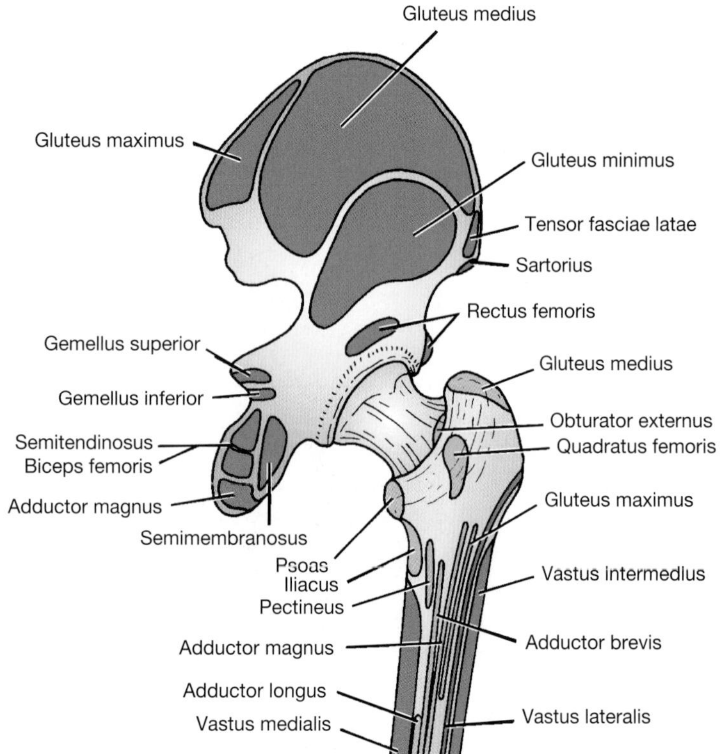

Figure 8.3 Muscles attached to the external surface of the right os coxae and the posterior surface of the femur.

The **pubis** is divided into a **body**, **superior ramus**, and **inferior ramus**. The bodies of the two pubic bones articulate with each other in the midline anteriorly at the **symphysis pubis**. The superior ramus joins the ilium and ischium at the acetabulum, and the inferior ramus joins the ischial ramus below the **obturator foramen**. The **obturator membrane** fills in the obturator foramen in life (see Chapter 6). The **pubic crest** forms the upper border of the body of the pubis, and it ends laterally as the **pubic tubercle**.

The outer surface of the hip bone has a deep depression termed the **acetabulum**. This articulates with the almost spherical head of the femur to form the hip joint. The inferior margin of the acetabulum is deficient and is marked by the **acetabular notch** (see Fig. 8.2). The **articular surface** of the acetabulum is limited to a horseshoe-shaped area and is covered with hyaline cartilage. The floor of the acetabulum is nonarticular and is called the **acetabular fossa**.

In the anatomic position, the front of the symphysis pubis and the anterosuperior iliac spines lie in the same vertical plane. This means that the pelvic surface of the symphysis pubis faces upward and backward, and the anterior surface of the sacrum is directed forward and downward.

The important muscle and ligament attachments to the outer surface of the hip bone are shown in Figures 8.2 and 8.3.

Femur

The femur (*femur* is Latin for "thigh") articulates above with the acetabulum to form the hip joint and below with the tibia and the patella to form the knee joint.

The upper end of the femur has a head, neck, and greater and lesser trochanters (Fig. 8.4). The **head** forms about two thirds of a sphere and articulates with the acetabulum of the os coxae to form the hip joint (see Fig. 8.3). In the center of the head is a small depression, called the **fovea capitis**, for the attachment of the **ligament of the head** (see Fig. 8.4). Part of the blood supply to the head of the femur from the obturator artery is conveyed along this ligament and enters the bone at the fovea.

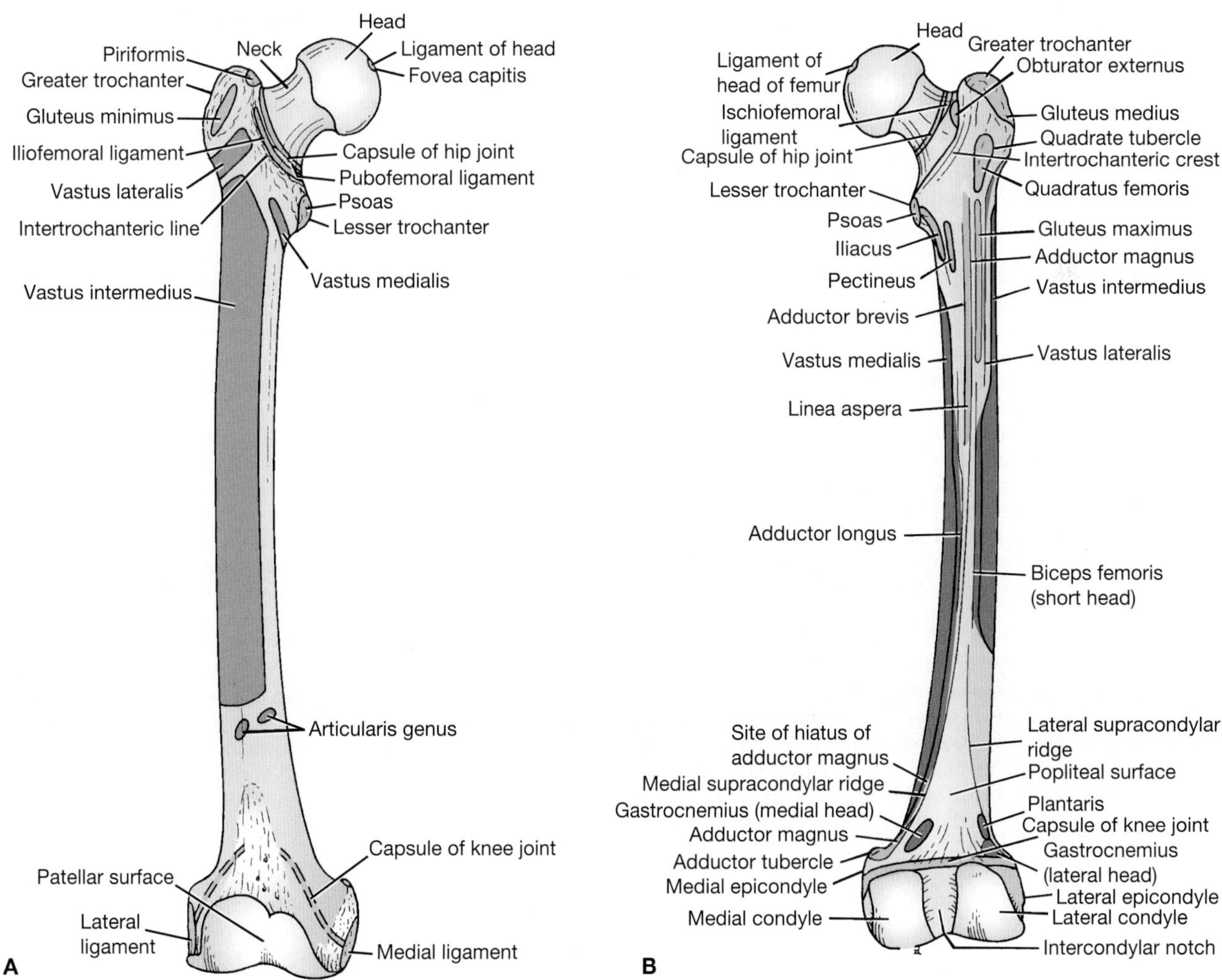

Figure 8.4 Bony features and muscle and ligament attachments on the anterior **(A)** and posterior **(B)** surfaces of the right femur.

The **neck**, which connects the head to the shaft, passes downward, backward, and laterally and makes an angle of about 125° (slightly less in the female) with the long axis of the shaft. Disease can alter the size of this angle.

The **greater** and **lesser trochanters** are large eminences situated at the junction of the neck and the shaft. The **intertrochanteric line** connects the trochanters anteriorly, where the iliofemoral ligament attaches. A prominent **intertrochanteric crest** connects the trochanters posteriorly.

The **shaft** of the femur is smooth and rounded on its anterior surface but posteriorly has a ridge, the **linea aspera**, where muscles and intermuscular septa attach. The margins of the linea aspera diverge above and below. The medial margin continues below as the **medial supracondylar ridge** to the **adductor tubercle** on the **medial condyle**. The lateral margin becomes continuous below with the **lateral supracondylar ridge**. The **gluteal tuberosity** is on the posterior surface of the shaft below the greater trochanter. The shaft becomes

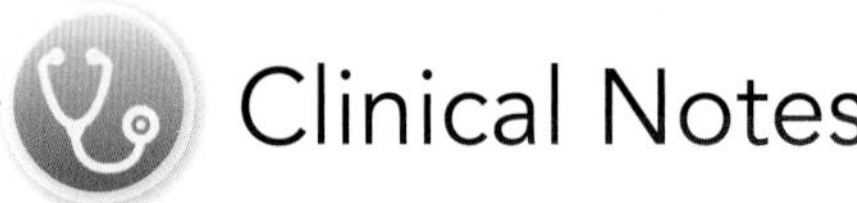

Clinical Notes

Head of Femur Tenderness and Hip Joint Arthritis

The part of the head of the femur that is not intra-acetabular can be palpated on the anterior aspect of the thigh just inferior to the inguinal ligament and just lateral to the pulsating femoral artery. Tenderness over the head of the femur usually indicates the presence of arthritis of the hip joint.

Blood Supply to Femoral Head and Neck Fractures

Avascular necrosis of the head of the femur can occur after fractures of the neck of the femur. Prior to adulthood, the epiphysis of the head is supplied by a small branch of the **obturator artery**, which passes to the head along the **ligament of the femoral head**. The upper part of the neck of the femur receives a profuse blood supply from the **medial femoral circumflex artery**. These branches pierce the joint capsule and ascend the neck deep to the synovial membrane. As long as the epiphyseal cartilage remains, no communication occurs between the two sources of blood. In the adult, after the epiphyseal cartilage disappears, an anastomosis between the two sources of blood supply is established. Fractures of the femoral neck interfere with or completely interrupt the blood supply from the root of the femoral neck to the femoral head. The scant blood flow along the small artery that accompanies the ligament of the head may be insufficient to sustain the viability of the femoral head, and ischemic necrosis gradually takes place.

Neck of the Femur and Coxa Valga and Vara

The neck of the femur is inclined at an angle with the shaft. This angle is about 160° in children and about 125° in adults. An increase in this angle is referred to as **coxa valga**, and it occurs, for example, in cases of congenital dislocation of the hip. In this condition, adduction of the hip joint is limited. A decrease in this angle is referred to as **coxa vara**, and it occurs in fractures of the neck of the femur and in slipping of the femoral epiphysis. In this condition, abduction of the hip joint is limited. The Shenton line is a useful means of assessing the angle of the femoral neck on a radiograph of the hip region (see Fig. 8.14 legend).

Femur Fractures

Fractures of the neck of the femur are common and are of two types, subcapital and trochanteric. The **subcapital fracture** occurs in the elderly and is usually produced by a minor trip or stumble. Subcapital femoral neck fractures are particularly common in postmenopausal females. This sex predisposition is because of a thinning of the cortical and trabecular bone caused by estrogen deficiency. Avascular necrosis of the head is a common complication. If the fragments are not impacted, considerable displacement occurs. The strong muscles of the thigh, including the rectus femoris, adductor muscles, and hamstring muscles, pull the distal fragment upward, shortening the leg (as measured from the anterosuperior iliac spine to the adductor tubercle or medial malleolus) (Fig. 8.5). The gluteus maximus, piriformis, obturator internus, gemelli, and quadratus femoris rotate the distal fragment laterally, as seen by the toes pointing laterally.

Trochanteric fractures occur in individuals of any age but are more common in elderly females with osteoporosis. The fracture line is extracapsular, and both fragments have a profuse blood supply. If the bone fragments are not impacted, the pull of the strong muscles will produce shortening and lateral rotation of the leg, as previously explained.

Fractures of the shaft of the femur usually occur in young and healthy persons. In fractures of the **upper third of the shaft of the femur**, the proximal fragment is flexed by the iliopsoas; abducted by the gluteus medius and minimus; and laterally rotated by the gluteus maximus, piriformis, obturator internus, gemelli, and quadratus femoris (Fig. 8.6). The lower fragment is adducted by the adductor muscles, pulled upward by the hamstrings and quadriceps, and laterally rotated by the adductors and the weight of the foot.

In fractures of the **middle third of the shaftof the femur**, the distal fragment is pulled upward by the hamstrings and the quadriceps, resulting in considerable shortening. The distal fragment is also rotated backward by the pull of the two heads of the gastrocnemius.

In fractures of the **distal third of the shaftof the femur**, the same displacement of the distal fragment occurs as seen in fractures of the middle third of the shaft. However, the distal fragment is smaller and is rotated backward by the gastrocnemius muscle to a greater degree and may exert pressure on the popliteal artery and interfere with the blood flow through the leg and foot.

Knowledge of the different actions of the muscles of the leg is necessary to understand the displacement of the fragments of a fractured femur. Considerable traction on the distal fragment is usually required to overcome the powerful muscles and restore the limb to its correct length before manipulation and operative therapy to bring the proximal and distal fragments into correct alignment.

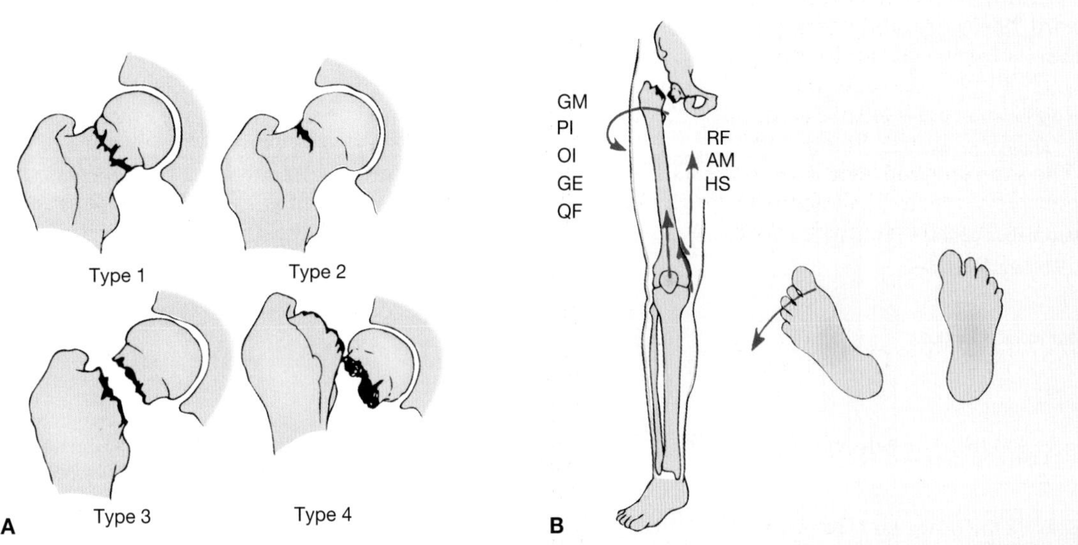

Figure 8.5 **A.** Fractures of the neck of the femur. **B.** Displacement of the lower bone fragment caused by the pull of the powerful muscles. Note the outward rotation of the leg so that the foot characteristically points laterally. AM, adductor muscles; GE, gemelli; GM, gluteus maximus; HS, hamstring muscles; OI, obturator internus; PI, piriformis; QF, quadratus femoris; RF, rectus femoris.

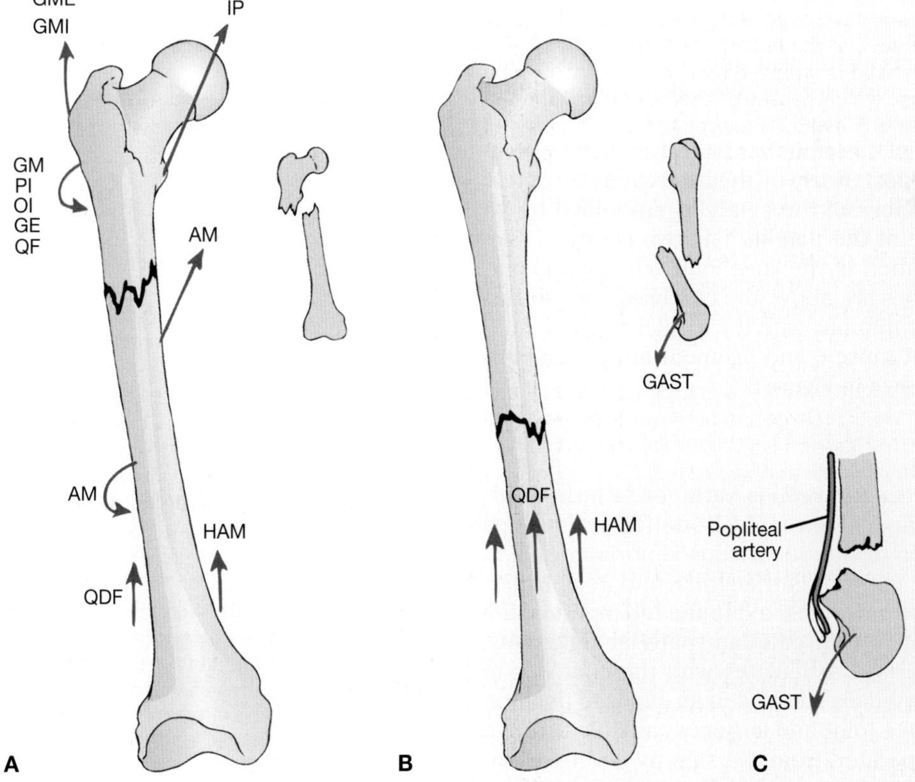

Figure 8.6 Fractures of the shaft of the femur. **A.** Upper third of the femoral shaft. Note the displacement caused by the pull of the powerful muscles. **B.** Middle third of the femoral shaft. Note the posterior displacement of the lower fragment caused by the gastrocnemius muscle. **C.** Lower third of the femoral shaft. Note the excessive displacement of the lower fragment caused by the pull of the gastrocnemius muscle, threatening the integrity of the popliteal artery. AM, adductor muscles; GAST, gastrocnemius; GE, gemelli; GM, gluteus maximus; GME, gluteus medius; GMI, gluteus minimus; HAM, hamstrings; IP, iliopsoas; OI, obturator internus; PI, piriformis; QDF, quadriceps femoris; QF, quadratus femoris.

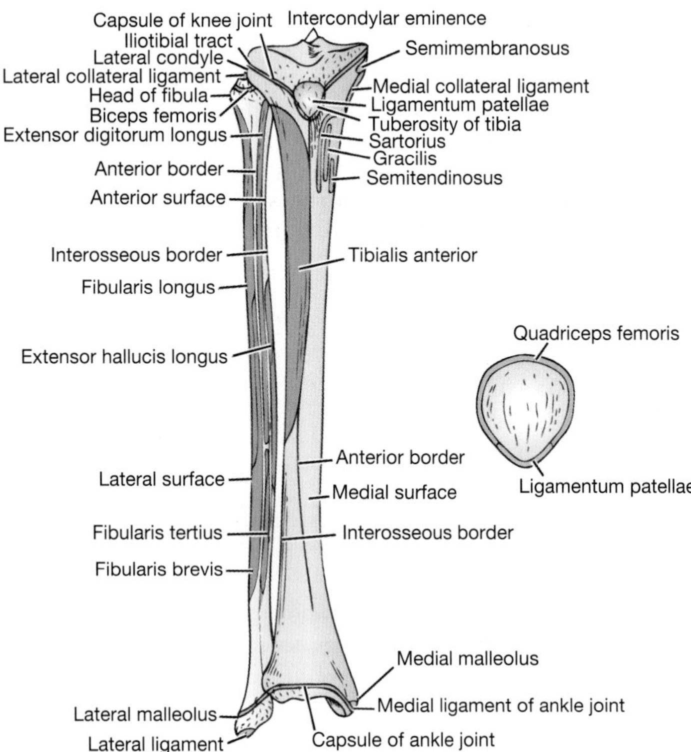

Figure 8.7 Muscles and ligaments attached to the anterior surfaces of the right tibia and fibula. Attachments to the patella are also shown.

broader toward its distal end and forms a flat, triangular area on its posterior surface called the **popliteal surface**.

The lower end of the femur has **lateral** and **medial condyles**, separated posteriorly by the **intercondylar notch**. The anterior surfaces of the condyles are joined by an **articular surface of the patella**. The two condyles take part in the formation of the knee joint. The **medial** and **lateral epicondyles** are above the condyles. The **adductor tubercle** is continuous with the medial epicondyle.

The important muscle and ligament attachments to the femur are shown in Figure 8.4.

Patella

The patella (kneecap; *patella* is Latin for "a little dish"; Fig. 8.7) is the largest **sesamoid bone** (ie, it develops within the tendon of the quadriceps femoris muscle in front of the knee joint). It is triangular, and its apex lies inferiorly. The **apex** is connected to the tuberosity of the tibia by the **ligamentum patellae (patellar ligament)**. The posterior surface articulates with the condyles of the femur. The patella is situated in an exposed position in front of the knee joint and is easily palpable through the skin. It is separated from the skin by an important subcutaneous bursa, the **prepatellar bursa** (see Knee Joint below). The upper, lateral, and medial margins give attachment to the different parts of the quadriceps femoris muscle.

Tibia

The tibia (*tibia* is Latin for "shin bone") is the large weight-bearing medial bone of the leg (Fig. 8.8; see also

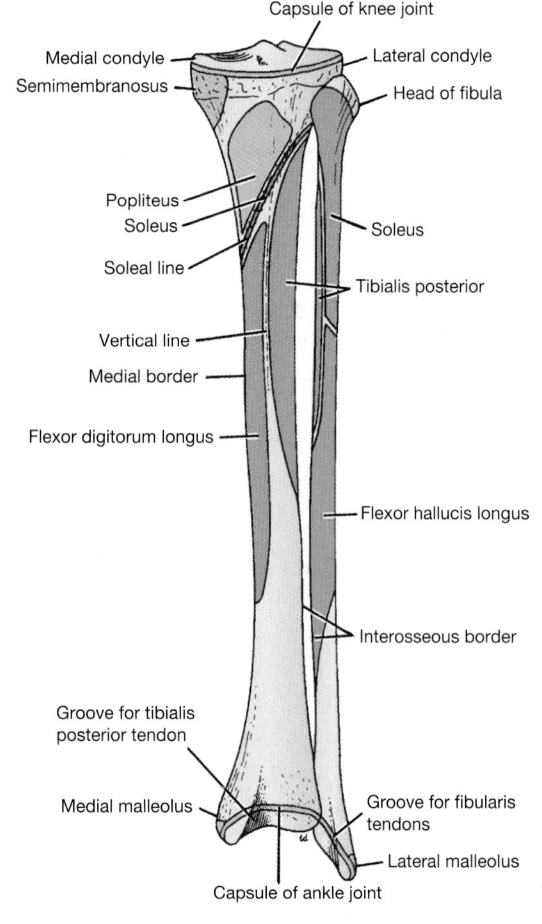

Figure 8.8 Muscles and ligaments attached to the posterior surfaces of the right tibia and the fibula.

Fig. 8.7). It articulates with the condyles of the femur and the head of the fibula above and with the talus and the distal end of the fibula below. It has an expanded upper end, a smaller lower end, and a shaft.

The **lateral** and **medial condyles** (sometimes called **lateral** and **medial tibial plateaus**) are at the upper end. These articulate with the lateral and medial condyles of the femur and the intervening **lateral** and **medial menisci**. **Anterior** and **posterior intercondylar areas** separate the upper articular surfaces of the tibial condyles. The **intercondylar eminence** lies between these areas (see Fig. 8.7). The lateral condyle possesses a small circular articular **facet for the head of the fibula** on its lateral aspect.

The **shaft** of the tibia is triangular in cross section, presenting three borders and three surfaces. Its **anterior** and **medial borders**, with the medial surface between them, are subcutaneous. The anterior border is prominent and forms the **shin**. The **tuberosity of the tibia** is at the junction of the anterior border with the upper end of the tibia and receives the attachment of the ligamentum patellae. The anterior border becomes rounded below, where it is continuous with the medial malleolus. The **lateral (interosseous) border** gives attachment to the interosseous membrane. The posterior surface of the shaft shows an oblique line, the **soleal line**, for the attachment of the soleus muscle.

The **lower end of the tibia** is slightly expanded and shows a saddle-shaped articular surface for the talus on its inferior aspect. The lower end is prolonged downward medially to form the large **medial malleolus**. The lateral surface of the medial malleolus articulates with the talus. The lower end of the tibia shows a wide, rough depression on its lateral surface for articulation with the fibula.

The important muscles and ligaments attached to the tibia are shown in Figures 8.7 and 8.8.

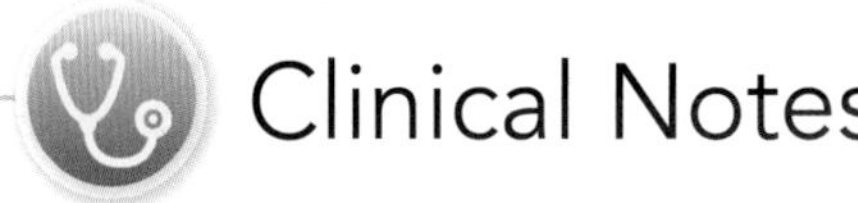

Patellar Dislocations

The patella is a sesamoid bone lying within the quadriceps tendon. The lower horizontal fibers of the vastus medialis muscle and the large size of the lateral condyle of the femur prevent the patella from being displaced laterally during the action of the quadriceps muscle. Congenital recurrent dislocations of the patella are caused by underdevelopment of the lateral femoral condyle. Traumatic dislocation of the patella results from direct trauma to the quadriceps attachments of the patella (especially the vastus medialis), with or without fracture of the patella.

Patellar Fractures

A patella fractured because of direct violence, as in a vehicular accident, breaks into several small fragments. Little separation of the fragments takes place because the bone lies within the quadriceps femoris tendon. The close relationship of the patella to the overlying skin may result in the fracture being open. Fracture of the patella as a result of indirect violence is caused by the sudden contraction of the quadriceps snapping the patella across the front of the femoral condyles. The knee is in the semiflexed position, and the fracture line is transverse. Separation of the fragments usually occurs in this case.

Tibia and Fibula Fractures

Fractures of the tibia and fibula are common. If only one bone is fractured, the other acts as a splint, and displacement is minimal. Fractures of the shaft of the tibia are often open because the entire length of the medial surface is covered only by skin and superficial fascia. Fractures of the distal third of the shaft of the tibia are prone to delayed union or nonunion. This can be because the nutrient artery is torn at the fracture line, with a consequent reduction in blood flow to the distal fragment. It is also possible that the splintlike action of the intact fibula prevents the proximal and distal fragments from coming into apposition.

Fractures of the proximal end of the tibia, at the tibial condyles (tibial plateau), are common. They usually result from direct violence to the lateral side of the knee joint, as when a person is hit by the bumper of a vehicle. The tibial condyle may show a split fracture or be broken up, or the fracture line may pass between both condyles in the region of the intercondylar eminence. Fractures of the distal end of the tibia are considered with the ankle joint (see below).

Intraosseous Tibia Infusion in Infants

This technique may be used for the infusion of fluids and blood when obtaining an intravenous line is not possible. The procedure is quick and easy to perform, as follows:

1. With the distal leg adequately supported, the anterior subcutaneous surface of the tibia is palpated.
2. The skin is anesthetized about 1 in. (2.5 cm) distal to the tibial tuberosity, thus blocking the infrapatellar branch of the saphenous nerve.
3. The bone marrow needle is directed at right angles through the skin, superficial fascia, deep fascia, tibial periosteum, and the cortex of the tibia. Once the needle tip reaches the medulla and bone marrow, the operator senses a feeling of "give." The position of the needle in the marrow can be confirmed by aspiration. The needle should be directed slightly caudad to avoid injury to the epiphyseal plate of the proximal end of the tibia. The transfusion may then commence.

Fibula

The fibula (*fibul* is Latin for "clasp" or "buckle") is the slender lateral bone of the leg (see Figs. 8.7 and 8.8). It takes no part in articulation at the knee joint, but it participates in the ankle joint below. It takes no part in the transmission of body weight, but it provides attachment for muscles. The fibula has an expanded upper end, a shaft, and a lower end.

The upper end, or **head**, possesses a **styloid process** and an **articular surface** for articulation with the lateral condyle of the tibia.

The **shaft** of the fibula is long and slender. Typically, it has four borders and four surfaces. The **medial (interosseous) border** gives attachment to the interosseous membrane.

The **lower end** of the fibula forms the triangular **lateral malleolus**, which is subcutaneous. A triangular **articular facet** for articulation with the lateral aspect of the talus is on the medial surface of the lateral malleolus. A depression called the **malleolar fossa** lies below and behind the articular facet.

The important muscles and ligaments attached to the fibula are shown in Figures 8.7 and 8.8.

Foot Bones

The bones of the foot are the **tarsal bones**, **metatarsals**, and **phalanges**. The general groupings are like that of the carpals, metacarpals, and phalanges in the wrist and hand.

Tarsal Bones

The tarsal bones (*tars* is Greek for "ankle") are the **calcaneum**, **talus**, **navicular**, **cuboid**, and the **three cuneiform bones**. Only the talus articulates with the tibia and the fibula at the ankle joint.

The tarsal bones, unlike those of the carpus, start to ossify before birth. Centers of ossification for the calcaneum and the talus, and often for the cuboid, are present at birth. Ossification takes place in all the tarsal bones by age 5 years.

Calcaneum

The calcaneum (*calcan* is Latin for "heel") is the largest bone of the foot and forms the prominence of the heel (Figs. 8.9 to 8.11). It articulates above with the talus and in front with the cuboid. It has six surfaces.

- The **anterior surface** is small and forms the articular facet that articulates with the cuboid bone.
- The **posterior surface** forms the prominence of the heel and gives attachment to the tendo calcaneus (Achilles tendon).
- Two articular facets for the talus, separated by a roughened groove, the **sulcus calcanei**, dominate the **superior surface**.
- The **inferior surface** has an **anterior tubercle** in the midline and a large **medial** and a smaller **lateral tubercle** at the junction of the inferior and posterior surfaces.
- The **medial surface** possesses a large, shelflike process, termed the **sustentaculum tali**, which assists in the support of the talus.
- The **lateral surface** is almost flat. Its anterior part has a small elevation called the **peroneal tubercle**, which separates the tendons of the fibularis longus and brevis muscles.

The important muscles and ligaments attached to the calcaneum are shown in Figures 8.10 and 8.11.

Talus

The talus (*talus* is Latin for "ankle") articulates above at the ankle joint with the tibia and fibula, below with the calcaneum, and in front with the navicular bone. It possesses a head, neck, and body (see Figs. 8.9 to 8.11). Numerous important ligaments attach to the talus, but no muscles attach to this bone.

The **head** of the talus is directed distally and has an oval convex articular surface for articulation with the navicular bone. This articular surface is continued on its inferior surface, where it rests on the sustentaculum tali behind and the calcaneonavicular ligament in front.

The **neck** of the talus lies posterior to the head and is slightly narrowed. Its upper surface is roughened and gives attachment to ligaments, and its lower surface shows a deep groove, the **sulcus tali**. The sulcus tali and the sulcus calcanei in the articulated foot form a tunnel, the **sinus tarsi**, which is occupied by the strong interosseous talocalcaneal ligament.

The **body** of the talus is cuboidal. Its superior surface articulates with the distal end of the tibia. Its lateral surface presents a triangular **articular facet** for articulation with the lateral malleolus of the fibula. Its medial surface has a small, comma-shaped **articular facet** for articulation with the medial malleolus of the tibia. The posterior surface is marked by two small **tubercles**, separated by a groove for the flexor hallucis longus tendon.

Navicular Bone

The **tuberosity** of the navicular bone (*navicul* is Latin for "little ship"; see Figs. 8.9 to 8.11) can be seen and felt on the medial border of the foot 1 in. (2.5 cm) in front of and below the medial malleolus. It gives attachment to the main part of the tibialis posterior tendon.

Cuboid Bone

A deep **groove** on the inferior aspect of the cuboid bone (*cubo* is Greek for "cube"; see Figs. 8.9 to 8.11) lodges the tendon of the fibularis longus muscle.

Cuneiform Bones

The three small, wedge-shaped cuneiform bones (*cune* is Latin for "wedge"; see Figs. 8.10 and 8.11) articulate proximally with the navicular bone and distally with the first three metatarsal bones. Their wedge shape contributes greatly to the formation and maintenance of the transverse arch of the foot.

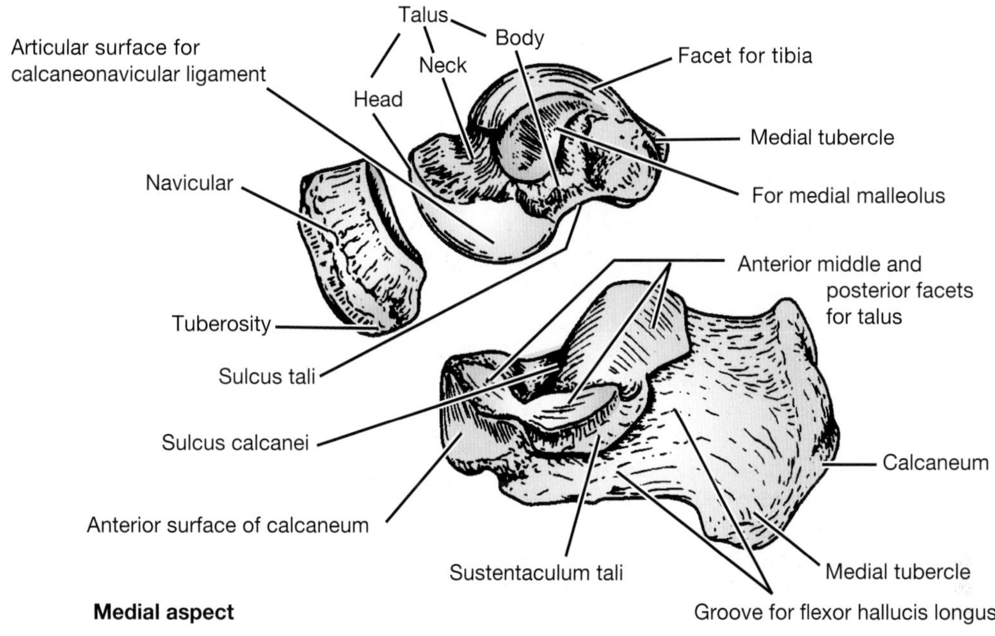

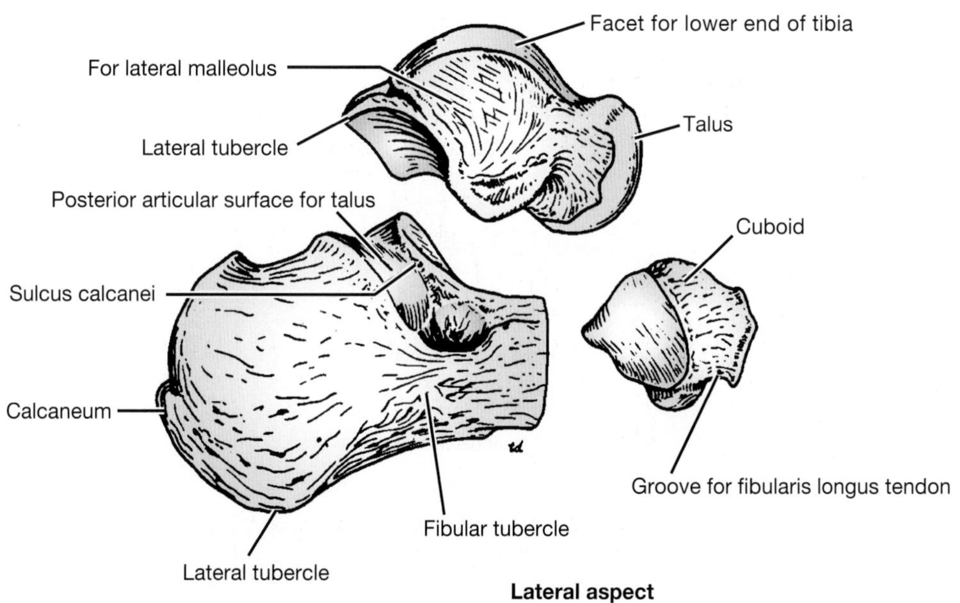

Figure 8.9 Calcaneum, talus, navicular, and cuboid bones.

Metatarsal Bones and Phalanges

The metatarsal bones (*meta* is Latin for "a boundary"; in this case, a boundary at the tarsus) and phalanges (*phalan* is Greek for "a battle line"; see Figs. 8.10 and 8.11) resemble the metacarpals and phalanges of the hand in that each possesses a **head** distally, a **shaft**, and a **base** proximally. The five metatarsals are numbered from the medial to the lateral side; that is, the first metatarsal aligns with the great toe (hallux) and so forth across the foot.

The **first metatarsal** bone is large and strong and plays an important role in supporting the weight of the body. The head is grooved on its inferior aspect by the **medial** and **lateral sesamoid bones** in the tendons of the flexor hallucis brevis.

The **fifth metatarsal** has a prominent **tubercle** on its base that can be easily palpated along the lateral border of the foot. The fibularis brevis tendon attaches to the tubercle.

As with the digits in the hand, each toe has three phalanges except the great toe, which possesses only two.

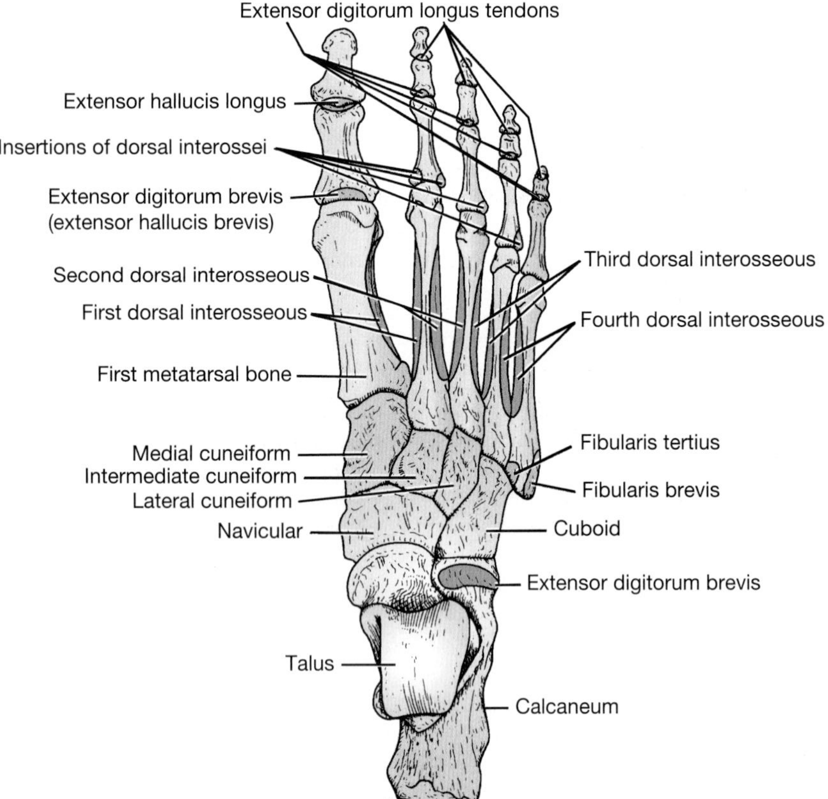

Figure 8.10 Muscle attachments on the dorsal aspect of the bones of the right foot.

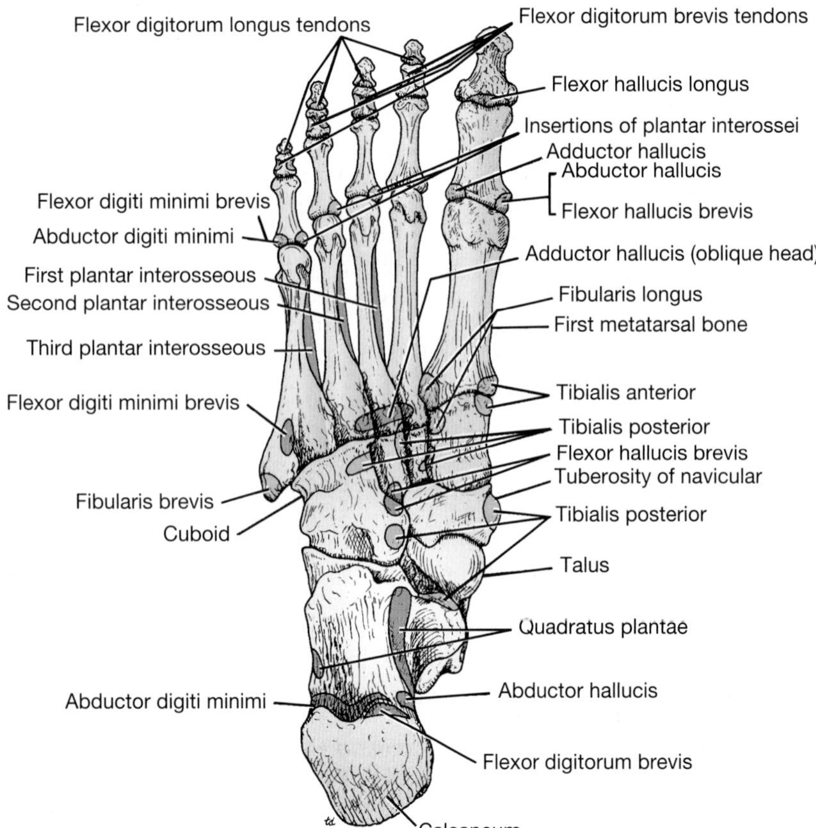

Figure 8.11 Muscle attachments on the plantar aspect of the bones of the right foot.

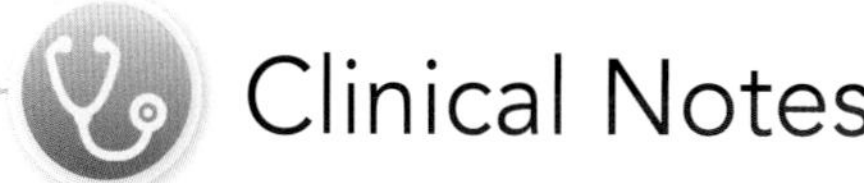

Clinical Notes

Talus Fractures

Fractures occur at the neck or body of the talus. Neck fractures occur during violent dorsiflexion of the ankle joint when the neck is driven against the anterior edge of the distal end of the tibia. Jumping from a height can fracture the body of the talus, although the two malleoli prevent the displacement of the fragments.

Calcaneum Fractures

Compression fractures of the calcaneum result from falls from a height. The weight of the body drives the talus downward into the calcaneum, crushing it in such a way that it loses vertical height and becomes wider laterally. The posterior portion of the calcaneum above the insertion of the tendo calcaneus can be fractured by posterior displacement of the talus. The sustentaculum tali can be fractured by forced inversion of the foot.

Metatarsal Fractures

The base of the fifth metatarsal can be fractured during forced inversion of the foot, at which time the tendon of insertion of the fibularis brevis muscle pulls off the base of the metatarsal.

Stress fracture of a metatarsal bone is common in runners and after long periods of walking. It occurs most frequently in the distal third of the second, third, or fourth metatarsal bone. Minimal displacement occurs because of the attachment of the interosseous muscles.

JOINTS

The major joints in the lower limb are the hip, knee, and ankle. Additionally, numerous joints occur in the foot. Tarsal joints couple the individual tarsal bones, tarsometatarsal joints bind tarsal elements with the metatarsal bones, intermetatarsal joints connect the metatarsal bones, metatarsophalangeal joints link the metatarsals with the proximal phalanges, and interphalangeal joints tie the phalanges. The sacroiliac joints and pubic symphysis are pelvic joints (see Chapter 6).

Because of opposite developmental rotations, certain movements in the lower limb are specialized or seemingly contradictory compared to the upper limb. In the upper limb, the joints **flex** anteriorly and **extend** posteriorly (except the thumb). In the lower limb, the hip flexes anteriorly and extends posteriorly; however, the knee does the opposite (Fig. 8.12). In the foot, **dorsiflexion** (the equivalent to extension) refers to lifting the top of the foot superiorly, toward the shin, whereas **plantar flexion** (the equivalent to flexion) refers to moving the sole inferiorly, as in standing on the toes. **Inversion** describes turning the foot so the sole faces in a medial direction, toward the midline, whereas **eversion** is the opposite movement in which the sole faces laterally, away from the midline. Abduction and adduction are movements away from or toward the midline of the body, respectively. In the fingers and toes, **abduction** is spreading apart the digits and **adduction** is drawing them together. In the fingers, this occurs relative to the long axis of the hand that runs through the third digit. However, in the toes, these movements are relative to the long axis of the foot that runs through the second digit.

Hip Joint

The hip joint is the articulation between the hemispherical **head of the femur** and the cup-shaped **acetabulum** of the os coxae (hip bone; Figs. 8.13 and 8.14). The articular surface of the acetabulum is horseshoe shaped and is deficient inferiorly at the **acetabular notch**. The cavity of the acetabulum is deepened by the presence of a fibrocartilaginous rim called the **acetabular labrum**. The labrum bridges across the acetabular notch and is here called the **transverse acetabular ligament**. The articular surfaces are covered with hyaline cartilage.

Type

The hip joint is a synovial ball-and-socket joint.

Capsule

The capsule encloses the joint and attaches to the acetabular labrum medially (see Fig. 8.13). Laterally, it attaches to the intertrochanteric line of the femur in front and halfway along the posterior aspect of the neck of the bone behind. At its attachment to the intertrochanteric line in front, some of its fibers, accompanied by blood vessels, reflect upward along the neck as bands called retinacula. These blood vessels supply the head and neck of the femur.

Ligaments

The **iliofemoral ligament** is a strong, inverted Y-shaped ligament (Fig. 8.15). Its base attaches to the anteroinferior iliac spine above. Below, the two limbs of the Y attach to the upper and lower parts of the intertrochanteric line of the femur. This strong ligament prevents overextension during standing.

The **pubofemoral ligament** is triangular (see Fig. 8.15A). The base of the ligament attaches to the superior ramus of the pubis, and the apex attaches below to the lower part of the intertrochanteric line. This ligament limits extension and abduction.

The **ischiofemoral ligament** is spiral shaped and is attached to the body of the ischium near the acetabular margin (see Fig. 8.15B). The fibers pass upward and

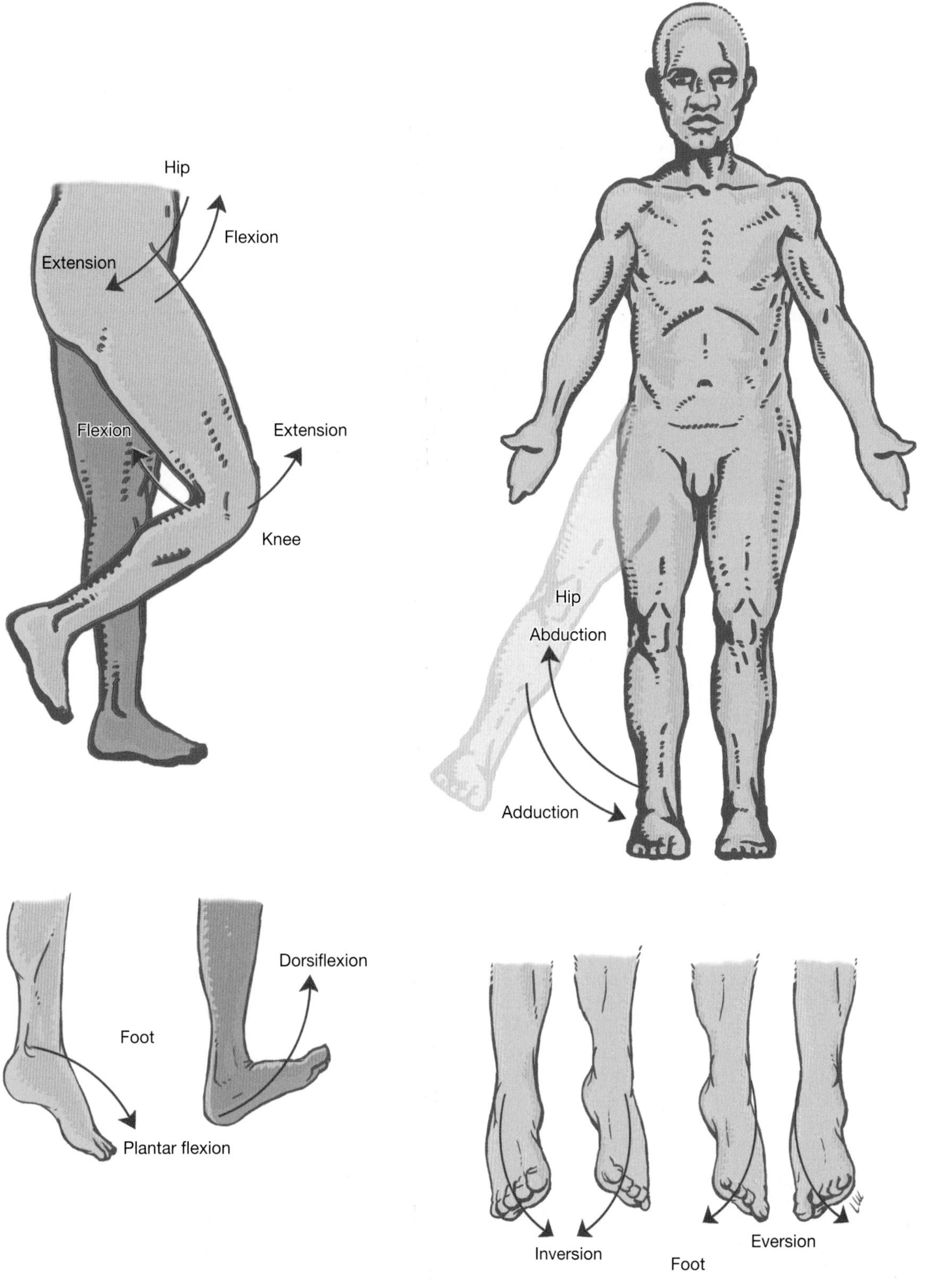

Figure 8.12 Anatomic terms used to describe movements of the lower limb.

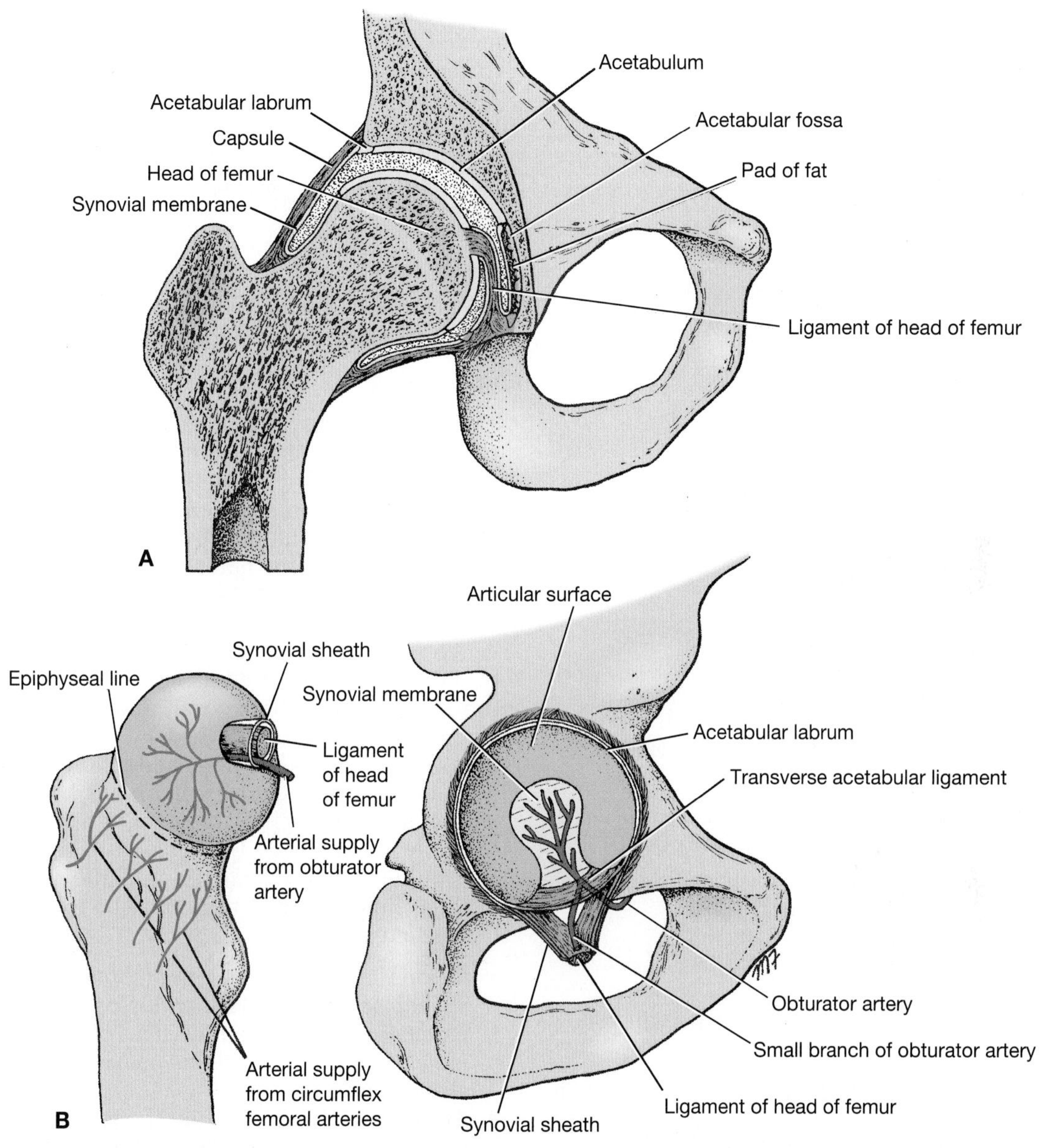

Figure 8.13 Coronal section of the right hip joint **(A)** and articular surfaces of the right hip joint and arterial supply of the head of the femur **(B)**.

laterally and attach to the greater trochanter. This ligament limits extension.

The **transverse acetabular ligament** is formed by the acetabular labrum as it bridges the acetabular notch (see Fig. 8.13B). The ligament converts the notch into a tunnel through which the blood vessels and nerves enter the joint.

The **ligament of the head of the femur** is flat and triangular (see Fig. 8.13). It attaches by its apex to the pit on the head of the femur (**fovea capitis**) and by its base to the transverse ligament and the margins of the acetabular notch. It lies within the joint and is ensheathed by synovial membrane.

Synovial Membrane

The synovial membrane lines the capsule and attaches to the margins of the articular surfaces (see Fig. 8.13). It covers the portion of the neck of the femur that lies within the joint capsule. It ensheathes the ligament of the head of the femur and covers the pad of fat contained in the acetabular fossa. A pouch of synovial membrane frequently protrudes through a gap in the anterior wall of the capsule, between the pubofemoral and iliofemoral ligaments, and forms the **psoas bursa** deep to the psoas tendon (Fig. 8.16; see also Fig. 8.15).

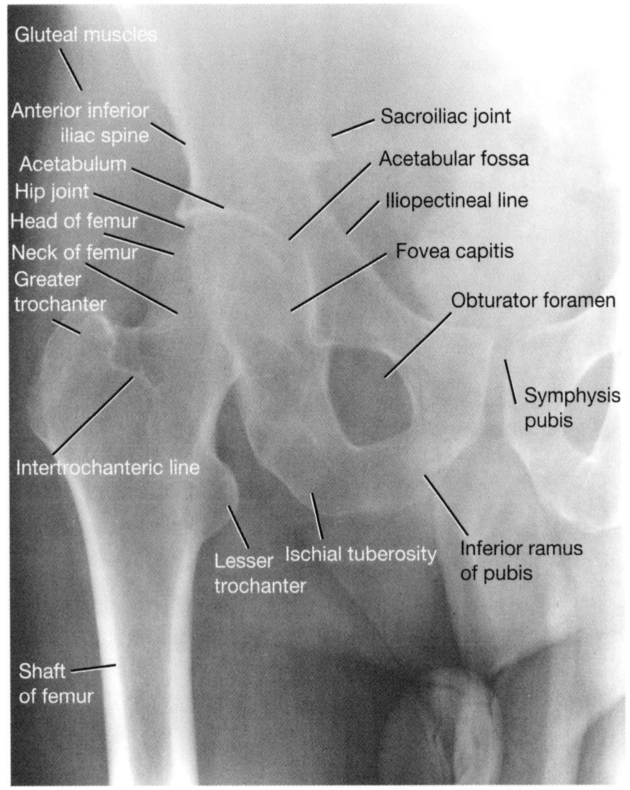

Figure 8.14 Anteroposterior radiograph of the hip joint. Note that the inferior margin of the neck of the femur should form a continuous curve with the upper margin of the obturator foramen (the **Shenton line**).

Blood Supply

The arteries supplying the hip joint include the following (see Fig. 8.13B):

- **Retinacular branches** of the medial and lateral circumflex femoral arteries
- **Artery to the head of the femur** (acetabular branch of the obturator artery)

The retinacular arteries, especially those from the medial circumflex femoral artery, are the major supply to the head and neck of the femur and the hip joint. The artery to the head of the femur is a variably sized branch of the obturator artery. It traverses the ligament of the head of the femur and supplies the head of the femur. It may form anastomoses with the retinacular arteries.

Nerve Supply

Femoral, obturator, and sciatic nerves and the nerve to the quadratus femoris supply the area.

Movements

The hip joint has a wide range of movements. The strength of the joint depends largely on the shape of the bones taking part in the articulation and on the strong ligaments. When the knee is flexed, flexion of the hip is limited by the anterior surface of the thigh meeting the anterior abdominal wall. When the knee is extended, flexion is limited by the tension of the hamstring group of muscles. Extension, which is the movement of the flexed thigh backward to the anatomic position, is limited by the tension of the iliofemoral, pubofemoral, and ischiofemoral ligaments. Abduction is limited by the tension of the pubofemoral ligament, and adduction is limited by contact with the opposite limb and by the tension in the ligament of the head of the femur. Lateral rotation is limited by the tension in the iliofemoral and pubofemoral ligaments, and the ischiofemoral ligament limits medial rotation. The following movements take place:

- **Flexion** is performed by the iliopsoas, rectus femoris, and sartorius and the adductor muscles.
- **Extension** (backward movement of the flexed thigh) is performed by the gluteus maximus and the hamstring muscles.
- **Abduction** is performed by the gluteus medius and minimus, assisted by the sartorius, tensor fasciae latae, and piriformis.

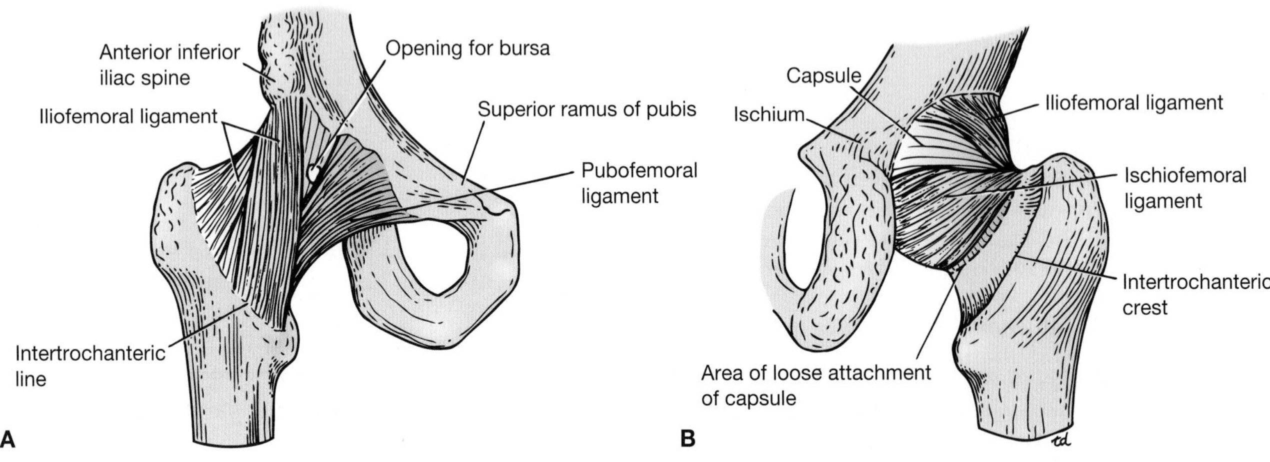

Figure 8.15 Anterior aspect **(A)** and posterior aspect **(B)** of the right hip joint.

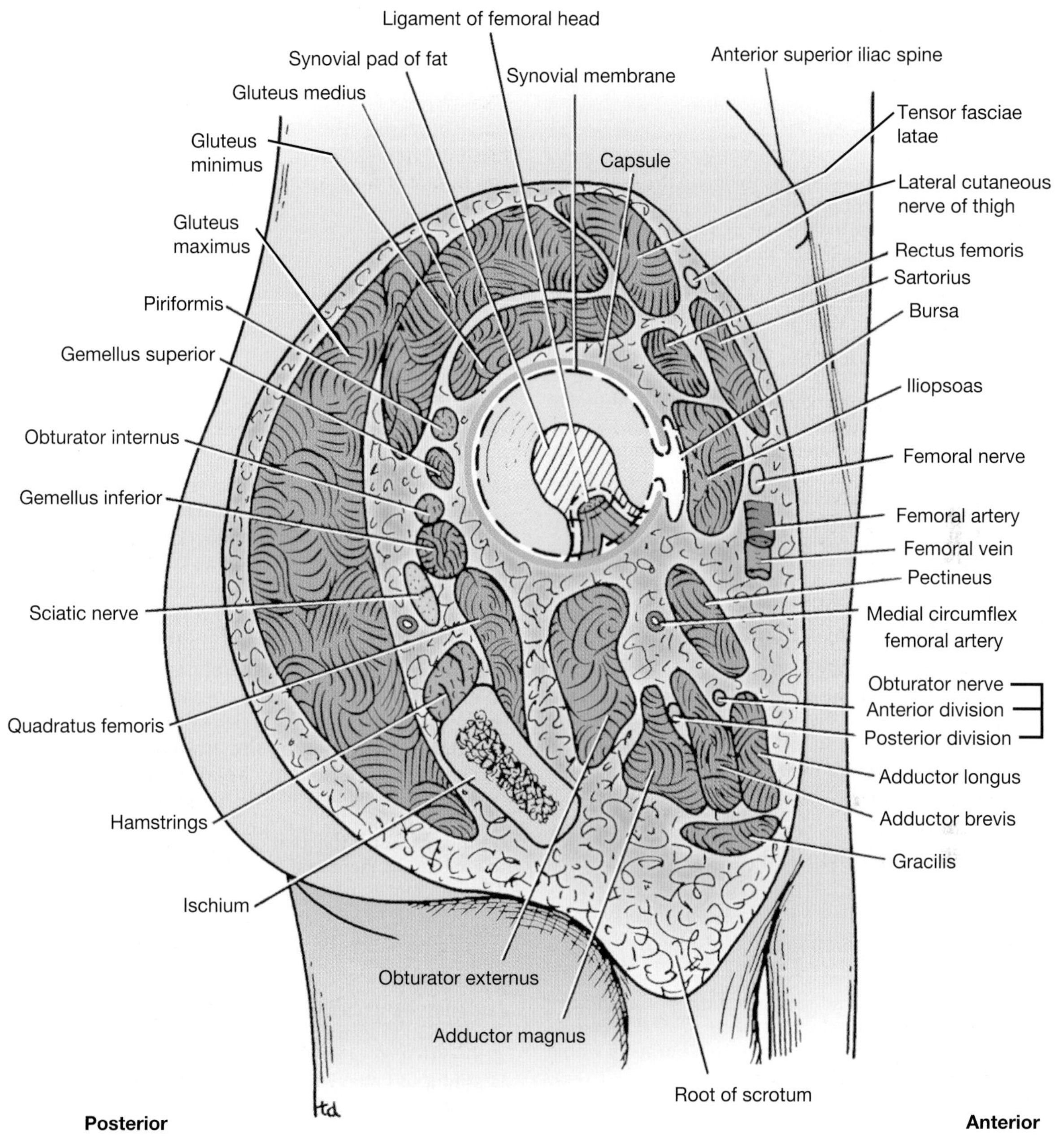

Figure 8.16 Structures surrounding the right hip joint.

- **Adduction** is performed by the adductor longus and brevis and the adductor fibers of the adductor magnus. These muscles are assisted by the pectineus and the gracilis.
- **Lateral rotation** is performed by the piriformis, obturator internus and externus, superior and inferior gemelli, and quadratus femoris, assisted by the gluteus maximus.
- **Medial rotation** is performed by the anterior fibers of the gluteus medius and gluteus minimus and the tensor fasciae latae.
- **Circumduction** is a combination of the previous movements (see Chapter 1).

The extensor group of muscles is more powerful than the flexor group, and the lateral rotators are more powerful than the medial rotators.

Important Relations

- **Anteriorly:** Iliopsoas, pectineus, and rectus femoris muscles. The iliopsoas and pectineus separate the femoral vessels and nerve from the joint (see Fig. 8.16).
- **Posteriorly:** The obturator internus, gemelli, and quadratus femoris muscles separate the joint from the sciatic nerve.
- **Superiorly:** Piriformis and gluteus minimus.
- **Inferiorly:** Obturator externus tendon.

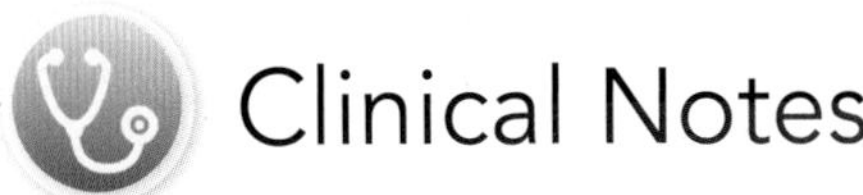

Clinical Notes

Referred Hip Joint Pain

The femoral nerve supplies the hip joint and the skin of the front and medial sides of the thigh. Thus, pain originating in the hip joint may refer to the front and medial side of the thigh. The posterior division of the obturator nerve supplies both the hip and knee joints. This explains why hip joint disease sometimes gives rise to pain in the knee joint.

Congenital Hip Dislocation

The stability of the hip joint depends on the ball-and-socket arrangement of the articular surfaces and the strong ligaments. In congenital dislocation of the hip (see Embryology Notes later in this chapter), the upper lip of the acetabulum fails to develop adequately, and the head of the femur, having no stable platform under which it can lodge, rides up out of the acetabulum onto the gluteal surface of the ilium.

Traumatic Hip Dislocation

Traumatic dislocation of the hip is rare because of the joint's strength; it is usually caused by vehicle accidents. It usually occurs when the joint is flexed and adducted. The head of the femur is displaced posteriorly out of the acetabulum, and it comes to rest on the gluteal surface of the ilium (**posterior dislocation**). The close relation of the sciatic nerve to the posterior surface of the joint makes it prone to injury in posterior dislocations.

Hip Joint Stability and Trendelenburg Sign

The stability of the hip joint when a person stands on one leg with the foot of the opposite leg raised above the ground depends on three factors:

- The gluteus medius and minimus must be functioning normally.
- The head of the femur must be located normally within the acetabulum.
- The neck of the femur must be intact and must have a normal angle with the shaft of the femur.

If any one of these factors is defective, the pelvis will sink downward on the opposite, unsupported side. The patient is then said to exhibit a **positive Trendelenburg sign** (Fig. 8.17).

When walking normally, a person alternately contracts the gluteus medius and minimus, first on one side, then the other. By this means, they can alternately raise the pelvis on one side, then the other, allowing the leg to be flexed at the hip joint and moved forward—that is, the leg is raised clear of the ground before it is thrust forward in taking the forward step. A patient with a left-sided congenital dislocation of the hip or paralysis of the left-side gluteus medius and/or minimus, when asked to stand on the left leg and raise the opposite leg off the ground, will exhibit a positive Trendelenburg sign, and the unsupported (right) side of the pelvis will sink below the horizontal. When walking, they show the characteristic "dipping" gait. In patients with bilateral congenital dislocation of the hip, the gait is typically "waddling" in nature.

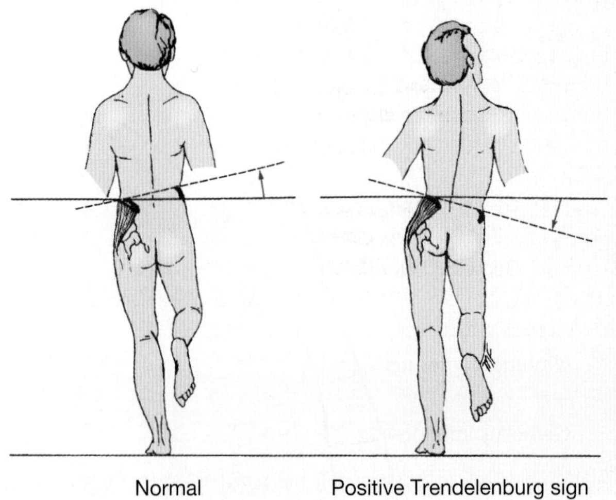

Figure 8.17 Trendelenburg test.

Hip Joint Arthritis

A patient with an inflamed hip joint will place the femur in the position that gives minimum discomfort—that is, the position in which the joint cavity has the greatest capacity to contain the increased amount of synovial fluid secreted. The hip joint is partially flexed, abducted, and externally rotated.

Osteoarthritis, the most common disease of the hip joint in the adult, causes pain, stiffness, and deformity. The pain may be in the hip joint itself or referred to the knee (the obturator nerve supplies both joints). The stiffness is caused by the pain and reflex spasm of the surrounding muscles. The deformity is flexion, adduction, and external rotation, and is produced initially by muscle spasm and later by muscle contracture.

Femoral Head Avascular Necrosis

Fractures of the neck of the femur occur commonly in older adults, especially females, because of osteoporosis-related degeneration in bone structure. Such fractures often include tearing of the retinacular branches of the medial circumflex femoral artery, resulting in compromised blood flow to the head of the femur. In some cases, the artery to the head of the femur may be the sole remaining source of blood to the femoral head. However, if the artery to the head is absent or inadequate for sufficient blood flow (common), the femoral head may undergo avascular necrosis.

In children, traumatic dislocations of the hip or fractures that disrupt the femoral epiphysis between the head and neck may result in damage to the artery of the head or the retinacular arteries. Again, the outcome may be avascular necrosis of the femoral head.

Knee Joint

The knee joint is the largest and most complicated joint in the body. It consists of two main parts: (1) paired condylar joints between the rounded medial and lateral condyles of the femur above and the corresponding condyles of the tibia and their cartilaginous menisci below and (2) a gliding joint between the patella and the patellar surface of the femur (Figs. 8.18 to 8.21). Note that the fibula is not directly involved in the joint.

The articular surfaces of the femur, tibia, and patella are covered with hyaline cartilage. Note that the articular surfaces of the medial and lateral condyles of the tibia are often referred to clinically as the **medial** and **lateral tibial plateaus**.

Type

The joint between the femur and tibia is a synovial joint of the hinge variety, but some degree of rotatory movement is possible. The joint between the patella and femur is a synovial joint of the plane gliding variety.

Capsule

The capsule is attached to the margins of the articular surfaces and surrounds the sides and posterior aspect of the joint. On the front of the joint, the capsule is absent, permitting the synovial membrane to pouch upward beneath the quadriceps tendon, forming the **suprapatellar bursa** (Fig. 8.22). On each side of the patella, the capsule is strengthened by expansions from the tendons of vastus lateralis and medialis. Behind the joint, the capsule is strengthened by an expansion of the semimembranosus muscle called the **oblique popliteal ligament**. An opening in the capsule behind the lateral tibial condyle permits the tendon of the popliteus to emerge.

Ligaments

The ligaments are divided into those that lie outside the joint capsule (extracapsular ligaments) and those that lie within (intracapsular ligaments).

Extracapsular Ligaments

The **ligamentum patellae** attaches above to the lower border of the patella and below to the tuberosity of the tibia (see Figs. 8.7 and 8.22A). It is a continuation of the central portion of the common tendon of the quadriceps femoris muscle.

The **lateral collateral ligament** is cordlike and attaches above to the lateral condyle of the femur and below to the head of the fibula (see Fig. 8.22). The tendon of the popliteus muscle intervenes between the ligament and the lateral meniscus (Figs. 8.23 and 8.24).

The **medial collateral ligament** is a flat band and attaches above to the medial condyle of the femur and below to the medial surface of the shaft of the tibia (see Fig. 8.22). It is firmly attached to the edge of the medial meniscus (see Figs. 8.22 and 8.23).

The **oblique popliteal ligament** is a tendinous expansion derived from the semimembranosus muscle. It strengthens the posterior aspect of the capsule.

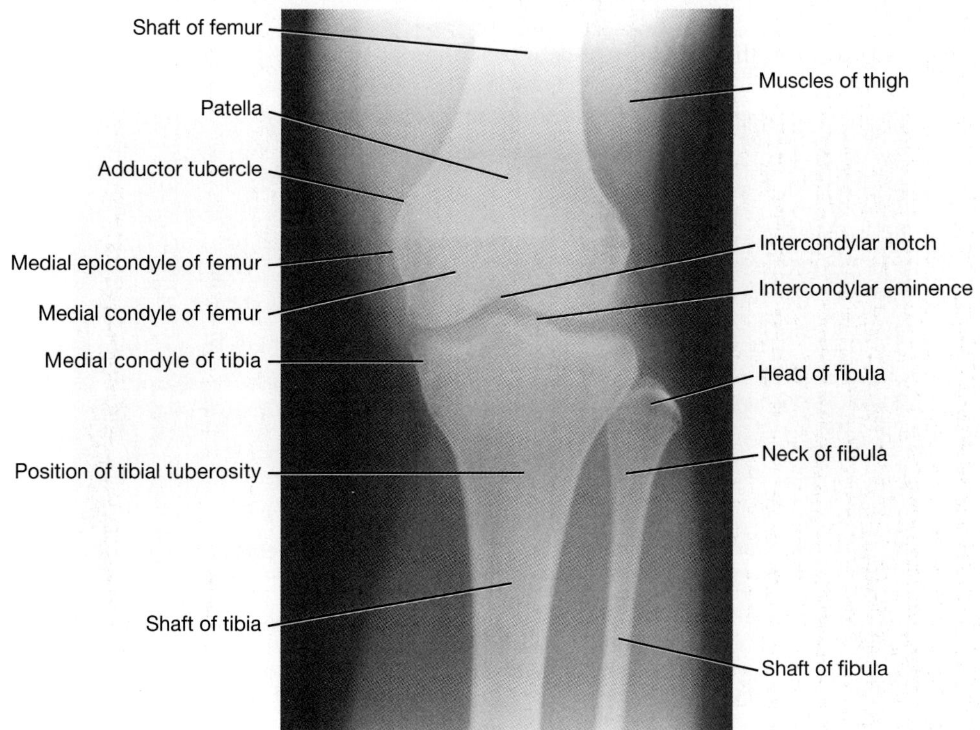

Figure 8.18 Anteroposterior radiograph of the adult knee.

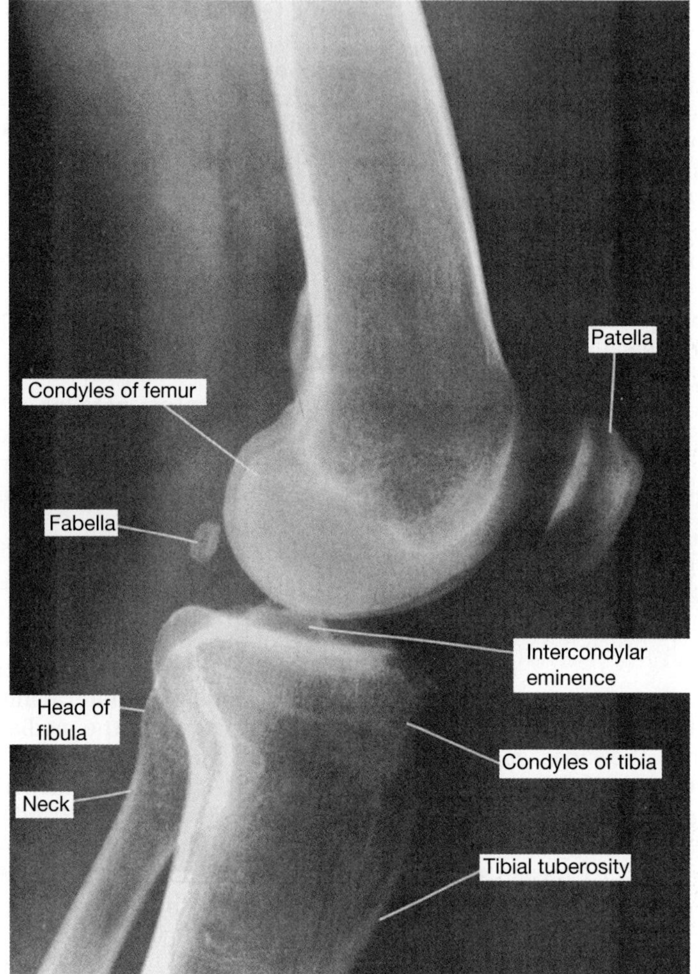

Figure 8.19 Lateral radiograph of the adult knee.

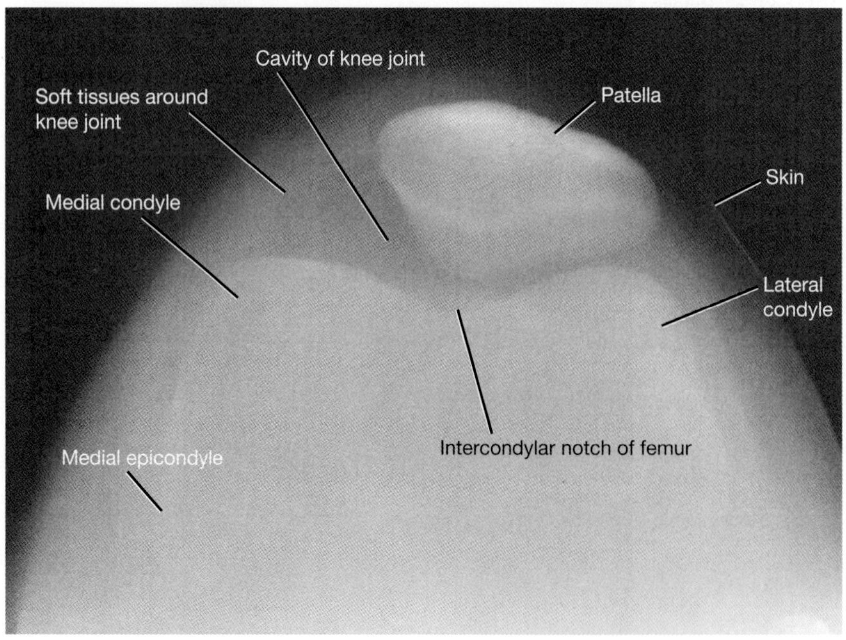

Figure 8.20 Tangential view of the patella.

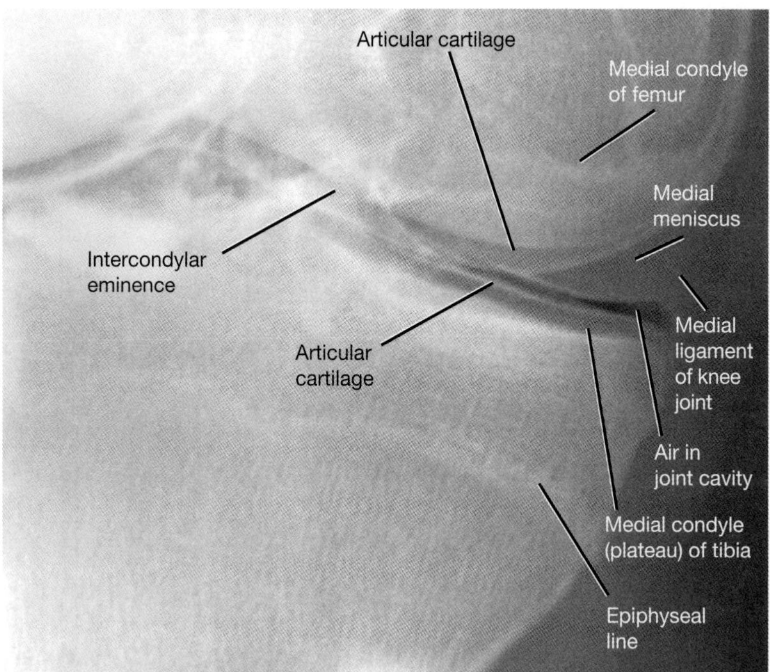

Figure 8.21 Pneumoarthrography of the knee.

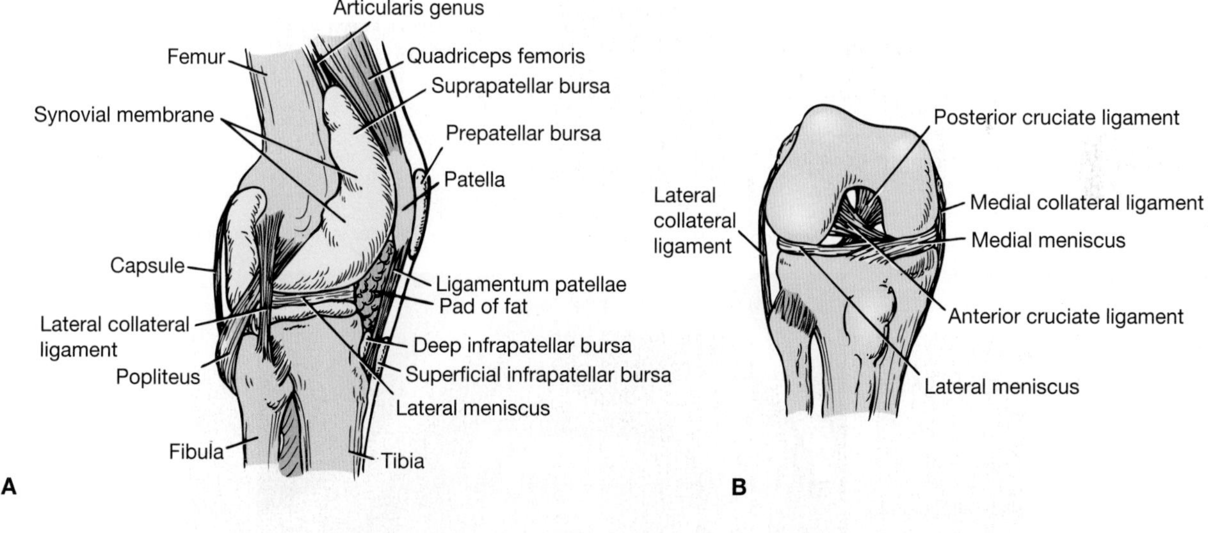

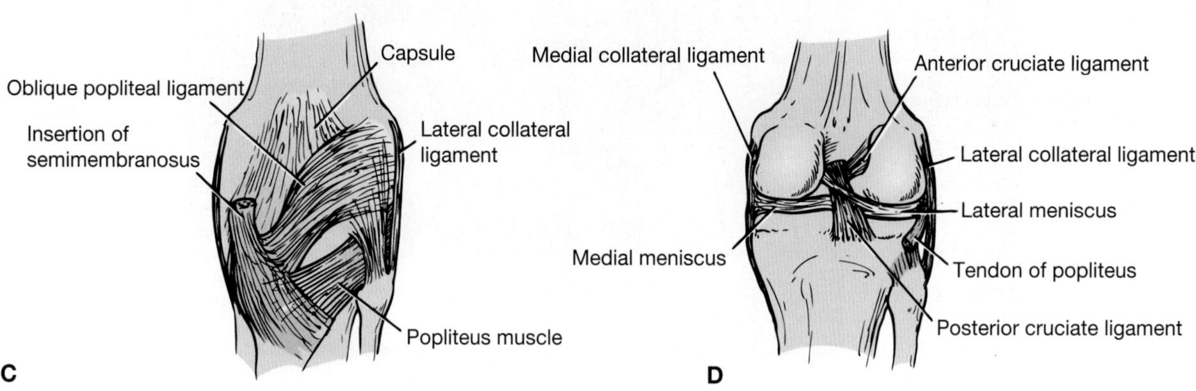

Figure 8.22 **A.** Right knee joint as seen from the lateral aspect. **B.** Anterior aspect, with the joint flexed. **C, D.** Posterior aspect.

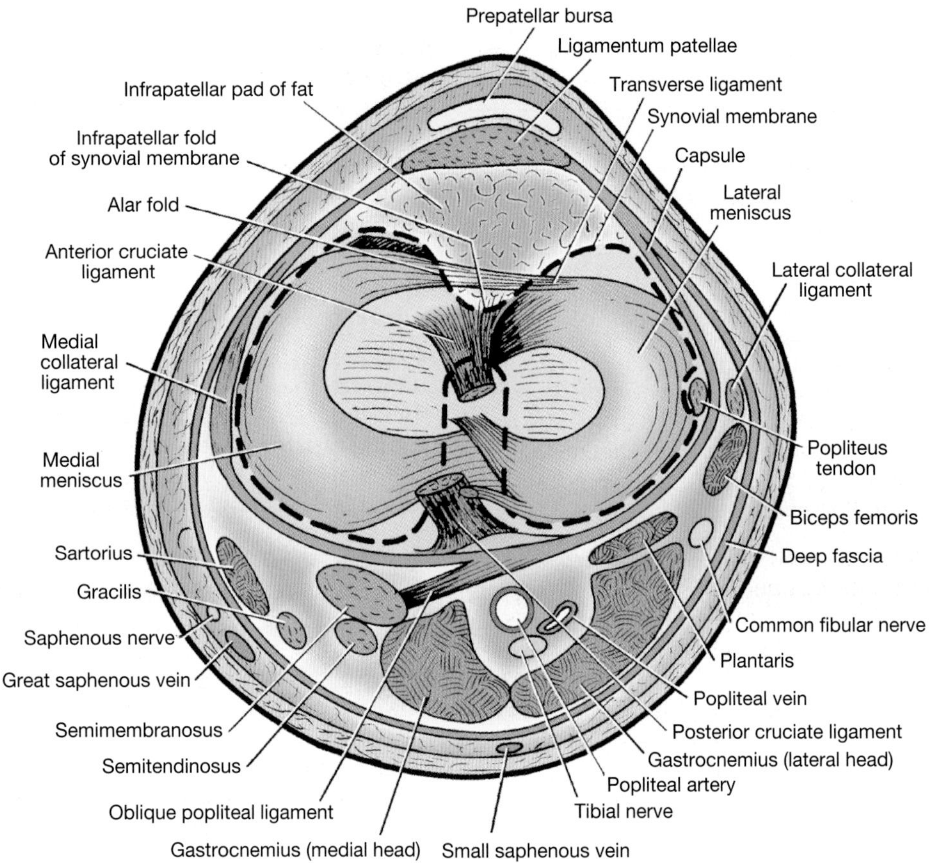

Figure 8.23 Relations of the right knee joint.

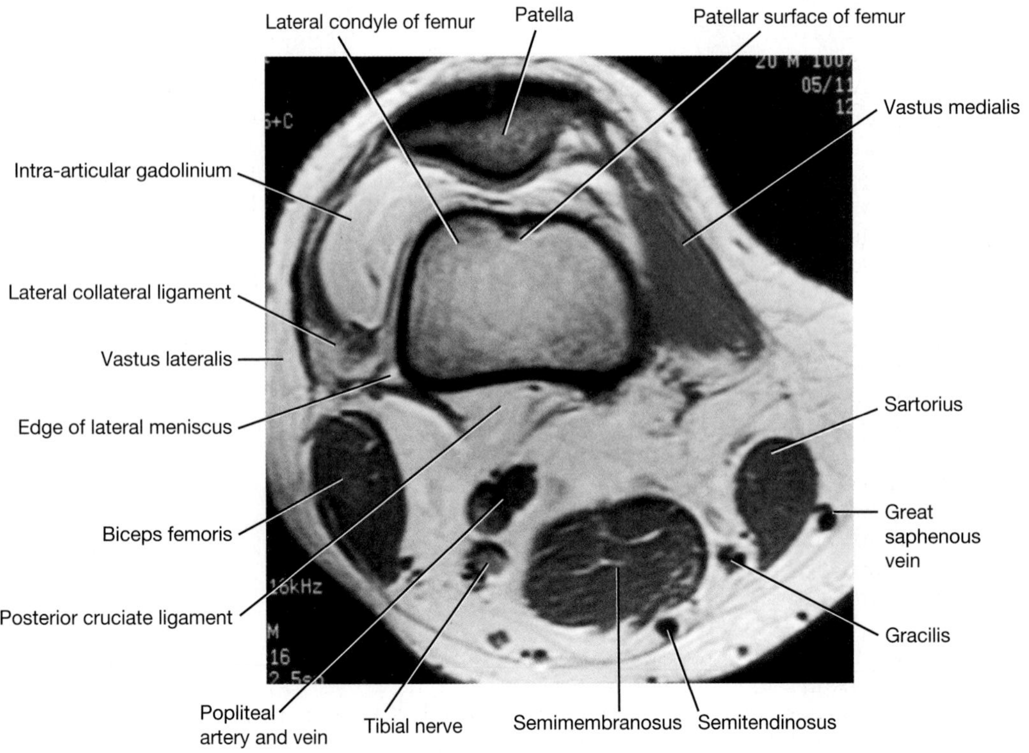

Figure 8.24 Transverse (axial) proton density magnetic resonance image of the right knee with intra-articular gadolinium to saline solution (as seen from below).

Intracapsular Ligaments

The cruciate ligaments (*cruci* is Latin for "a cross") are two strong intracapsular ligaments that cross each other within the joint cavity (see Figs. 8.22 to 8.24). They are named anterior and posterior according to their tibial attachments. These important ligaments are the main bond between the femur and the tibia throughout the joint's range of movement.

ANTERIOR CRUCIATE LIGAMENT

The **anterior cruciate ligament** (**ACL**) attaches to the anterior intercondylar area of the tibia and passes upward, backward, and laterally to attach to the posterior part of the medial surface of the lateral femoral condyle. The ACL prevents posterior displacement of the femur on the tibia. Conversely, with the knee joint flexed, the ACL prevents the tibia from being pulled anteriorly relative to the femur.

POSTERIOR CRUCIATE LIGAMENT

The **posterior cruciate ligament** (**PCL**) attaches to the posterior intercondylar area of the tibia and passes upward, forward, and medially to attach to the anterior part of the lateral surface of the medial femoral condyle. The PCL prevents anterior displacement of the femur on the tibia. With the knee joint flexed, the PCL prevents the tibia from being pulled posteriorly relative to the femur.

Menisci

The menisci are C-shaped sheets of fibrocartilage. The peripheral border is thick and attached to the capsule, and the inner border is thin and concave and forms a free edge (see Figs. 8.21 to 8.23). The upper surfaces are in contact with the femoral condyles. The lower surfaces are in contact with the tibial condyles. Their function is to deepen the articular surfaces of the tibial condyles to receive the convex femoral condyles; they also serve as cushions between the two bones and distribute forces transmitted through the joint.

Each meniscus is attached to the upper surface of the tibia by **anterior** and **posterior horns**. Because the medial meniscus also attaches to the medial collateral ligament, it is relatively immobile.

Synovial Membrane

The synovial membrane lines the capsule and attaches to the margins of the articular surfaces (see Figs. 8.22 and 8.23). On the front and above the joint, it forms a pouch, which extends up beneath the quadriceps femoris muscle for three fingerbreadths above the patella, forming the **suprapatellar bursa**. This is held in position by the attachment of a small portion of the vastus intermedius muscle, called the **articularis genus** muscle.

At the back of the joint, the synovial membrane is prolonged downward on the deep surface of the tendon of the popliteus, forming the **popliteal bursa**. A bursa is interposed between the medial head of the gastrocnemius and the medial femoral condyle and the semimembranosus tendon; this is termed the **semimembranosus bursa**, and it frequently communicates with the synovial cavity of the joint.

The synovial membrane is reflected forward from the posterior part of the capsule around the front of the cruciate ligaments. As a result, the cruciate ligaments lie behind the synovial cavity and are not bathed in synovial fluid.

In the anterior part of the joint, the synovial membrane is reflected backward from the posterior surface of the ligamentum patellae to form the **infrapatellar fold**; the free borders of the fold are termed the **alar folds**.

Bursae Related to Knee Joint

Numerous bursae are related to the knee joint. They are found wherever skin, muscle, or tendon rubs against bone. Four are situated in front of the joint, six behind. The suprapatellar bursa and the popliteal bursa always communicate with the joint, and the semimembranosus bursa may communicate with the joint.

Anterior Bursae

- The **suprapatellar bursa** lies beneath the quadriceps muscle and communicates with the joint cavity (see Fig. 8.22A). It is described above.
- The **prepatellar bursa** lies in the subcutaneous tissue between the skin and the front of the lower half of the patella and the upper part of the ligamentum patellae (see Figs. 8.22A and 8.23).
- The **superficial infrapatellar bursa** lies in the subcutaneous tissue between the skin and the front of the lower part of the ligamentum patellae (see Fig. 8.22A).
- The **deep infrapatellar bursa** lies between the ligamentum patellae and the tibia.

Posterior Bursae

- The **popliteal bursa** is found in association with the tendon of the popliteus and communicates with the joint cavity. It was described previously.
- The **semimembranosus bursa** is found related to the insertion of the semimembranosus muscle and may communicate with the joint cavity. It was described previously.

The remaining four posterior bursae are related to the tendon of insertion of the biceps femoris; related to the tendons of the sartorius, gracilis, and semitendinosus muscles as they pass to their insertion on the tibia; beneath the lateral head of origin of the gastrocnemius muscle; and beneath the medial head of origin of the gastrocnemius muscle.

Nerve Supply

The femoral, obturator, common fibular, and tibial nerves supply the knee joint.

Movements

The knee joint can flex, extend, and rotate. When the foot is planted on the ground with the knee joint in full extension, the femur medially rotates on the tibia resulting in a twisting and tightening of all the major ligaments of the joint, and the knee becomes a mechanically rigid structure. However, if the foot is off the ground, the tibia may laterally rotate on the femur. In both instances, the cartilaginous menisci are compressed like rubber cushions between the femoral and tibial condyles. The fully extended knee is said to be in the locked and stabilized position.

Before flexion of the knee joint can occur, it is essential that the major ligaments be untwisted and slackened to permit movements between the joint surfaces. This unlocking or untwisting process is accomplished by the **popliteus** muscle, which laterally rotates the femur on the tibia. Once again, the menisci must adapt their shape to the changing contour of the femoral condyles. The attachment of the popliteus to the lateral meniscus results in that structure being also pulled backward.

When the knee joint is flexed to a right angle, a considerable range of rotation is possible. In the flexed position, the tibia can also be moved passively forward and backward on the femur. This is possible because the major ligaments, especially the cruciate ligaments, are slack in this position.

The stability of the knee joint depends on the tone of the strong muscles acting on the joint and the strength of the ligaments. Of these factors, the tone of the muscles is the most important. After injury to a patient's knee joint, a physiotherapist must build up the strength of these muscles, especially the quadriceps femoris. The following muscles produce movements of the knee joint.

Flexion

The biceps femoris, semitendinosus, and semimembranosus muscles, assisted by the gracilis, sartorius, and popliteus muscles, produce flexion. Flexion is limited by the contact of the back of the leg with the thigh.

Extension

The quadriceps femoris produces extension. Extension is limited by the tension of all the major ligaments of the joint.

Medial Rotation

The sartorius, gracilis, and semitendinosus produce medial rotation.

Lateral Rotation

The biceps femoris produces lateral rotation.

Important Relations

- **Anteriorly:** Prepatellar bursa (see Fig. 8.23)
- **Posteriorly:** Popliteal vessels; tibial and common fibular nerves; lymph nodes; and the muscles that form the boundaries of the popliteal fossa, namely, the semimembranosus, semitendinosus, biceps femoris, the two heads of the gastrocnemius, and the plantaris (see Figs. 8.23 and 8.24)
- **Medially:** Sartorius, gracilis, and semitendinosus muscles
- **Laterally:** Biceps femoris and common fibular nerve

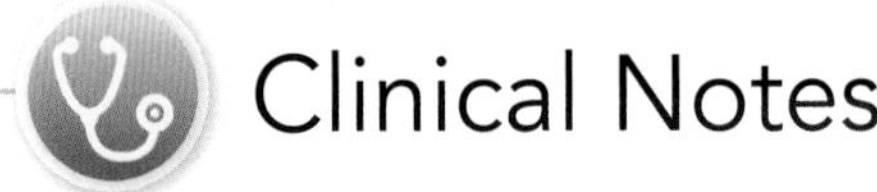

Knee Joint Strength

The strength of the knee joint depends on the strength of the ligaments that bind the femur to the tibia and on the tone of the muscles acting on the joint. The most important muscle group is the quadriceps femoris. If well developed, it can stabilize the knee in the presence of torn ligaments.

Knee Injury and Synovial Membrane

The synovial membrane of the knee joint is extensive, and, if the articular surfaces, menisci, or ligaments of the joint are damaged, the large synovial cavity becomes distended with fluid. The wide communication between the suprapatellar bursa and the joint cavity results in this structure also becoming distended. The swelling of the knee extends three or four fingerbreadths above the patella and laterally and medially beneath the aponeuroses of insertion of the vastus lateralis and medialis, respectively.

Ligamentous Injury of Knee Joint

Four ligaments—the medial collateral ligament, lateral collateral ligament, ACL, and PCL—are commonly injured in the knee. Sprains or tears occur depending on the degree of force applied.

Medial Collateral Ligament

Forced abduction of the tibia on the femur can result in partial tearing of the medial collateral ligament, which can occur at its femoral or tibial attachments. Remember that tears of the menisci result in localized tenderness on the joint line, whereas sprains of the medial collateral ligament result in tenderness over the femoral or tibial attachments of the ligament.

Lateral Collateral Ligament

Forced adduction of the tibia on the femur can result in injury to the lateral collateral ligament. This occurs less commonly than medial ligament injury.

Cruciate Ligaments

Injury to the cruciate ligaments can occur when excessive force is applied to the knee joint.

Tears of the ACL are common. It is the most frequently injured ligament in the body, for which surgery is performed. The condition is more common in females, and this may be explained by the different alignment of the thigh on the leg in females associated with the wider pelvis. There is also an increased risk in females during the preovulatory phase of the menstrual cycle, possibly because of the influence of the female sex hormones. **Tears of the PCL** are less common.

Injury to the cruciate ligaments is always accompanied by damage to other knee structures: the collateral ligaments are commonly torn, or the capsule may be damaged. The joint cavity quickly fills with blood (**hemarthrosis**), so the joint is swollen. Examination of patients with a ruptured ACL shows that the tibia can be pulled excessively forward on the femur; with rupture of the posterior cruciate ligament, the tibia can be made to move excessively backward on the femur (Fig. 8.25). Such excessive movement is referred to as a **positive drawer sign** because the tibial motion is like that of opening or closing a drawer. Because the stability of the knee joint depends largely on the tone of the quadriceps femoris muscle and the integrity of the collateral ligaments, operative repair of isolated torn cruciate ligaments is not always attempted. The knee is immobilized in slight flexion in a cast, and active physiotherapy on the quadriceps femoris muscle is begun at once. However, if the capsule of the joint and the collateral ligaments are also torn, early operative repair is essential.

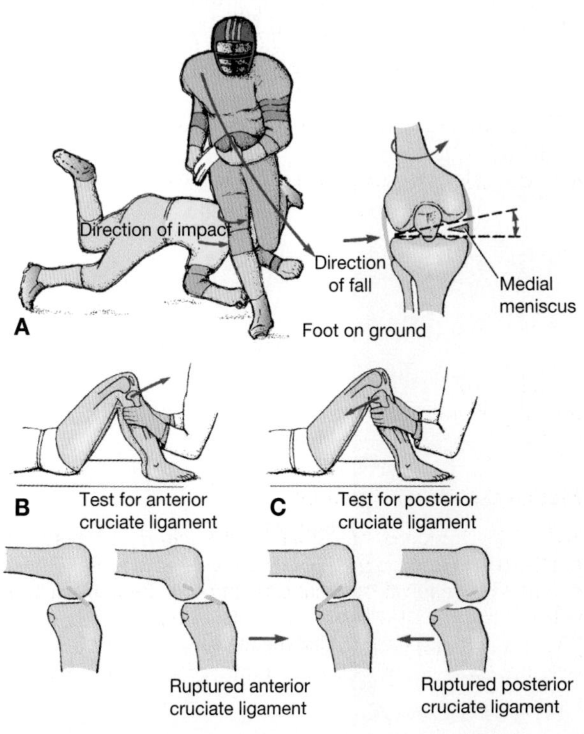

Figure 8.25 **A.** Mechanism involved in damage to the medial meniscus of the knee joint from playing football. Note that the right knee joint is semiflexed and that medial rotation of the femur on the tibia occurs. The impact causes forced abduction of the tibia on the femur, and the medial meniscus is pulled into an abnormal position. The cartilaginous meniscus is then ground between the femur and the tibia. **B.** Test for integrity of the anterior cruciate ligament (ACL). **C.** Test for integrity of the posterior cruciate ligament (PCL).

Meniscal Injury

Injuries of the menisci are common. The medial meniscus is damaged much more frequently than the lateral, which is probably because of its strong attachment to the medial collateral ligament of the knee joint, which restricts its mobility. The injury occurs when the femur is rotated on the tibia, or the tibia is rotated on the femur, with the knee joint partially flexed and taking the weight of the body. The tibia is usually abducted on the femur, and the medial meniscus is pulled into an abnormal position between the femoral and tibial condyles (see Fig. 8.25A). A sudden movement between the condyles results in the meniscus being subjected to a severe grinding force, and it splits along its length (Fig. 8.26). When the torn part of the meniscus becomes wedged between the articular surfaces, further movement is impossible, and the joint is said to "lock."

Injury to the lateral meniscus is less common, probably because it is not attached to the lateral collateral ligament of the knee joint and is consequently more mobile. The popliteus muscle sends a few of its fibers into the lateral meniscus, and these can pull the meniscus into a more favorable position during sudden movements of the knee joint.

Pneumoarthrography

Air can be injected into the synovial cavity of the knee joint so that soft tissues can be studied. This technique is based on the fact that air is less radiopaque than structures such as the medial and lateral menisci, so their outline can be visualized on a radiograph (see Fig. 8.21).

Arthroscopy

Arthroscopy involves the introduction of a lighted instrument into the synovial cavity of the knee joint through a small incision. This technique permits the direct visualization of structures, such as the cruciate ligaments and the menisci, for diagnostic purposes.

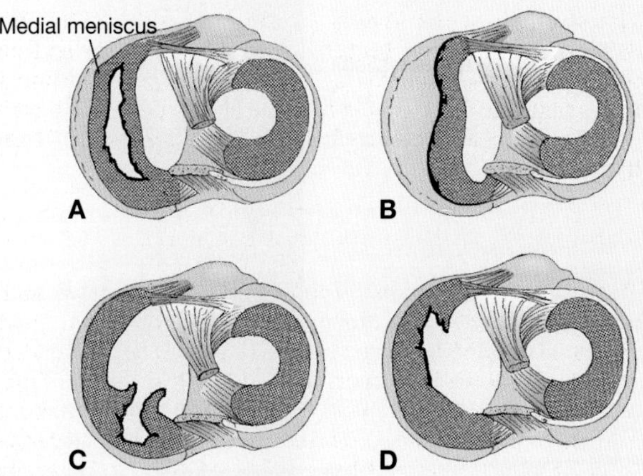

Figure 8.26 Tears of the medial meniscus of the knee joint. **A.** Complete bucket handle tear. **B.** The meniscus is torn from its peripheral attachment. **C.** Tear of the posterior portion of the meniscus. **D.** Tear of the anterior portion of the meniscus.

Proximal Tibiofibular Joint

Articulation is between the lateral condyle of the tibia and the head of the fibula (see Figs 8.7 and 8.18). The articular surfaces are flattened and covered by hyaline cartilage.

Type

This is a synovial, plane, gliding joint.

Capsule

The capsule surrounds the joint and is attached to the margins of the articular surfaces.

Ligaments

Anterior and **posterior ligaments** strengthen the capsule. The **interosseous membrane**, which connects the shafts of the tibia and fibula together, also greatly strengthens the joint.

Synovial Membrane

The synovial membrane lines the capsule and is attached to the margins of the articular surfaces.

Nerve Supply

The common fibular nerve supplies the joint.

Movements

A small amount of gliding movement takes place during movements at the ankle joint.

Distal Tibiofibular Joint

Articulation is between the fibular notch at the lower end of the tibia and the lower end of the fibula (Fig. 8.27). The opposed bony surfaces are roughened.

Type

The distal tibiofibular joint is a fibrous joint.

Capsule

There is no capsule.

Ligaments

The **interosseous ligament** is a strong, thick band of fibrous tissue that binds the two bones together. The **interosseous membrane**, which connects the shafts of the tibia and fibula together, also greatly strengthens the joint (Figs. 8.28 and 8.29).

The **anterior** and **posterior ligaments** are flat bands of fibrous tissue connecting the two bones together in front and behind the interosseous ligament.

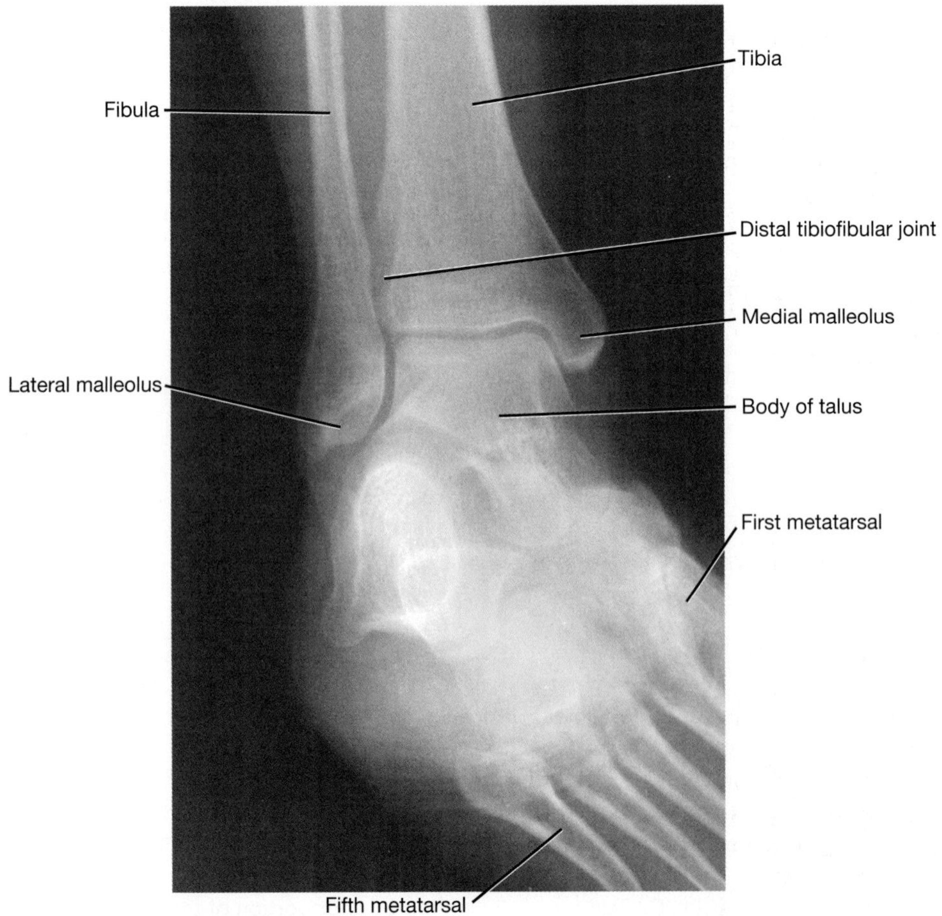

Figure 8.27 Anteroposterior radiograph of the adult ankle.

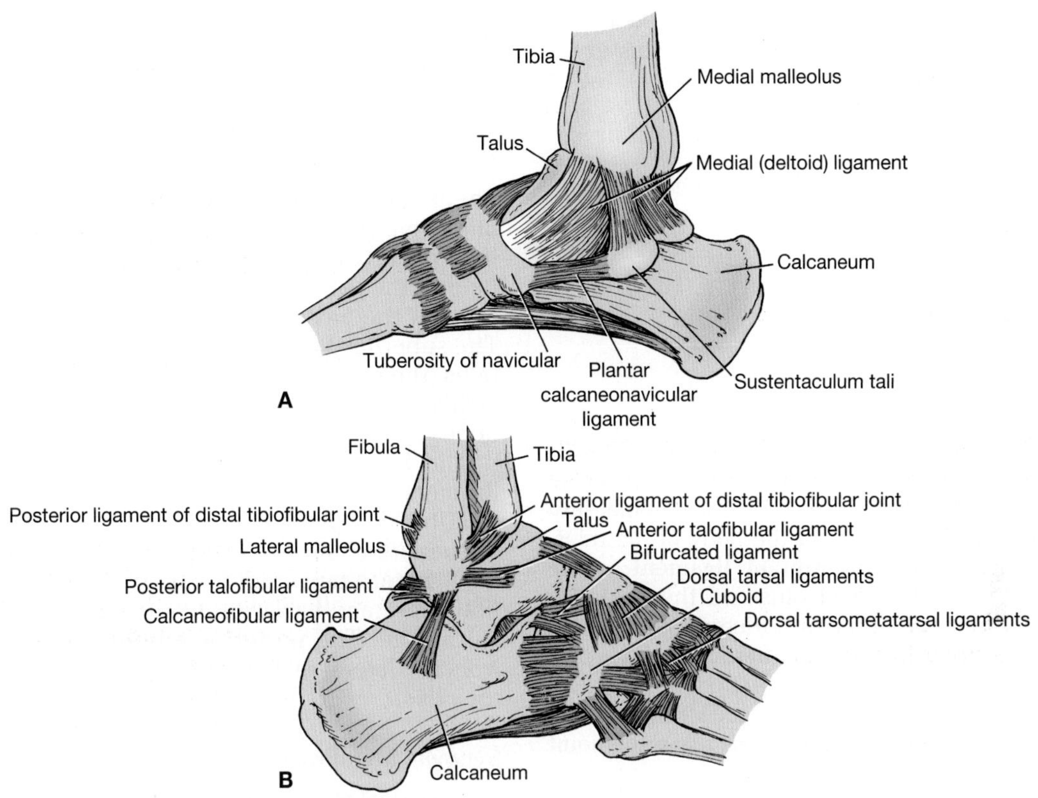

Figure 8.28 Right ankle joint as seen from the medial aspect **(A)** and the lateral aspect **(B)**.

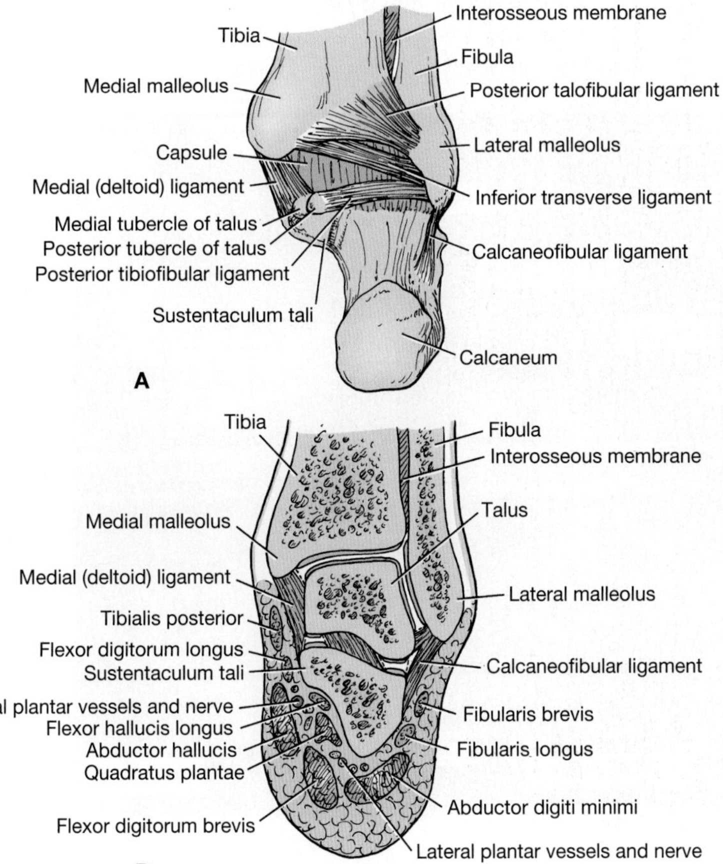

Figure 8.29 Right ankle joint as seen from the posterior aspect **(A)** and in coronal section **(B)**.

The **inferior transverse ligament** runs from the medial surface of the upper part of the lateral malleolus to the posterior border of the lower end of the tibia.

Nerve Supply

Deep fibular and tibial nerves supply the joint.

Movements

A small amount of movement takes place during movements at the ankle joint.

Ankle Joint

The ankle joint is between the lower end of the tibia, the two malleoli, and the body of the talus (Fig. 8.30; see also Figs. 8.27 to 8.29). It consists of a deep socket formed by the lower ends of the tibia and fibula, into which is fitted the upper part of the body of the talus. The **inferior transverse tibiofibular ligament**, which runs between the lateral malleolus and the posterior border of the lower end of the tibia, deepens the socket into which the body of the talus fits snugly (see Fig. 8.29). The articular surfaces are covered with hyaline cartilage. The shape of the bones and the strength of the ligaments and the surrounding tendons make this joint strong and stable.

Type

The ankle is a synovial joint. The talus moves on a transverse axis in a hinge-like manner.

Capsule

The capsule encloses the joint and attaches to the bones near their articular margins.

Ligaments

The **medial (deltoid) ligament** is a strong triangular unit composed of three parts (see Figs. 8.28 and 8.29). Its apex attaches to the tip of the medial malleolus. Below, the deep fibers attach to the nonarticular area on the medial surface of the body of the talus. The superficial fibers attach to the medial side of the talus, the sustentaculum tali, the plantar calcaneonavicular ligament, and the tuberosity of the navicular bone.

The **lateral ligament** is weaker than the medial ligament and consists of three bands. The **anterior talofibular ligament** runs from the lateral malleolus to the lateral surface of the talus. The **calcaneofibular ligament** runs from the tip of the lateral malleolus downward and backward to the lateral surface of the calcaneum. The **posterior talofibular ligament** runs from the lateral malleolus to the posterior tubercle of the talus.

Synovial Membrane

The synovial membrane lines the capsule.

Nerve Supply

Deep fibular and tibial nerves supply the ankle joint.

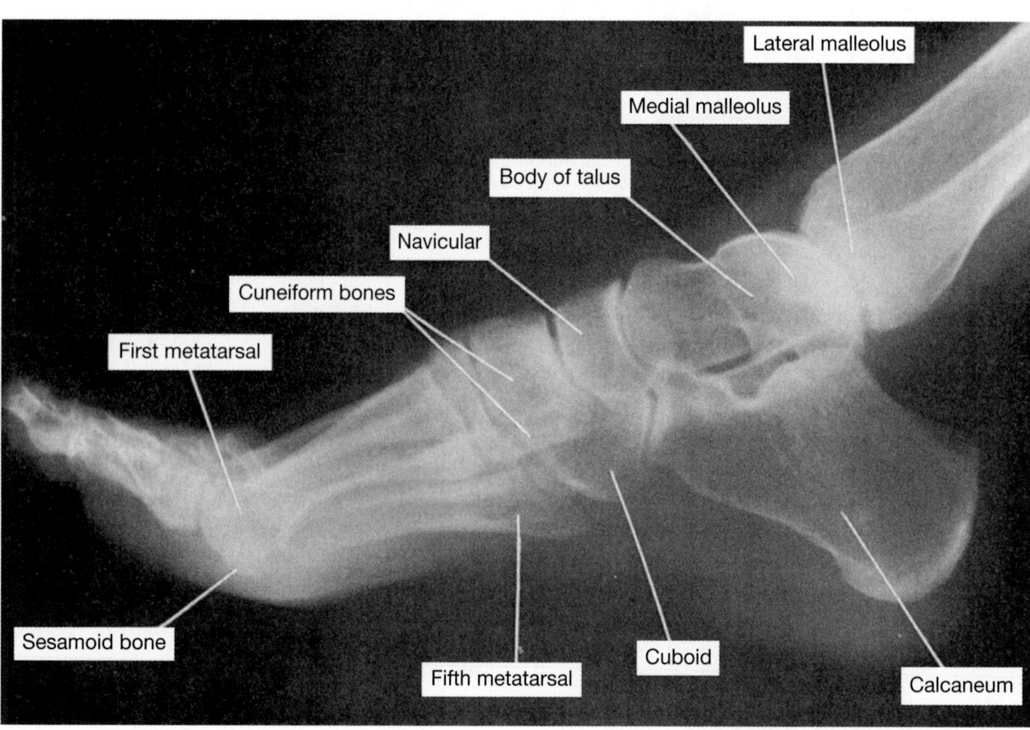

Figure 8.30 Lateral radiograph of the adult ankle.

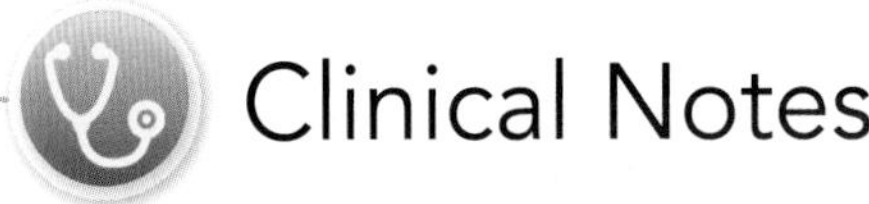

Ankle Joint Stability

The ankle joint is a hinge joint possessing great stability. The deep mortise formed by the lower end of the tibia and the medial and lateral malleoli securely holds the talus in position.

"Lateral Ankle" Acute Sprains

Acute sprains of the lateral ankle are usually caused by excessive inversion of the foot with plantar flexion of the ankle. The anterior talofibular ligament and the calcaneofibular ligament are partially torn, giving rise to great pain and local swelling.

"Medial Ankle" Acute Sprains

Acute sprains of the medial ankle are similar to but less common than those of the lateral ankle. They may occur to the medial (deltoid) ligament because of excessive eversion. The great strength of the medial ligament usually results in the ligament pulling off the tip of the medial malleolus.

Ankle Joint Fracture Dislocations

Fracture dislocations of the ankle are common and caused by forced external rotation and overeversion of the foot. The talus is externally rotated forcibly against the lateral malleolus of the fibula. The torsion effect on the lateral malleolus causes it to fracture spirally. If the force continues, the talus moves laterally, and the medial ligament of the ankle joint becomes taut and pulls off the tip of the medial malleolus. If the talus is forced to move still farther, its rotary movement results in its violent contact with the posteroinferior margin of the tibia, which shears off.

Other less common types of fracture dislocation are caused by forced overeversion (without rotation), in which the talus presses the lateral malleolus laterally and causes it to fracture transversely. Overinversion (without rotation), in which the talus presses against the medial malleolus, produces a vertical fracture through the base of the medial malleolus.

Movements

Dorsiflexion (toes pointing upward) and plantar flexion (toes pointing downward) are the primary movements. The movements of inversion and eversion take place at the tarsal joints and not at the ankle joint.

Dorsiflexion is performed by the tibialis anterior, extensor hallucis longus, extensor digitorum longus, and fibularis tertius. It is limited by the tension of the tendo calcaneus, posterior fibers of the medial ligament, and the calcaneofibular ligament.

Plantar flexion is performed by the gastrocnemius, soleus, plantaris, fibularis longus, fibularis brevis, tibialis posterior, flexor digitorum longus, and flexor hallucis longus. It is limited by the tension of the opposing muscles, anterior fibers of the medial ligament, and the anterior talofibular ligament.

Note that during dorsiflexion of the ankle joint, the wider anterior part of the articular surface of the talus is forced between the medial and lateral malleoli, causing them to separate slightly and tighten the ligaments of the distal tibiofibular joint. This arrangement greatly increases the stability of the ankle joint when the foot is in the initial position for major thrusting movements in walking, running, and jumping.

Note also that when the ankle joint is fully plantar flexed, the ligaments of the distal tibiofibular joint are less taut and small amounts of rotation, abduction, and adduction are possible.

Important Relations

- **Anteriorly:** Tibialis anterior, extensor hallucis longus, anterior tibial vessels, deep fibular nerve, extensor digitorum longus, and fibularis tertius
- **Posteriorly:** Tendo calcaneus and plantaris
- **Posterolaterally (behind the lateral malleolus):** Fibularis longus and brevis
- **Posteromedially (behind the medial malleolus):** Tibialis posterior, flexor digitorum longus, posterior tibial vessels, tibial nerve, and flexor hallucis longus

Tarsal Joints

The tarsal joints are between the tarsal bones. They are all synovial joints. Multiple joints and numerous ligaments occupy this area (Figs. 8.31 and 8.32; see also Figs. 8.28 to 8.30).

Subtalar Joint

The subtalar joint is the posterior joint between the talus and the calcaneum. Articulation is between the inferior surface of the body of the talus and the facet on the middle of the upper surface of the calcaneum (see Figs. 8.9 and 8.29). The articular surfaces are covered with hyaline cartilage.

Type

This is a plane joint.

Capsule

The capsule encloses the joint and is attached to the margins of the articular areas of the two bones.

Ligaments

Medial and **lateral** (**talocalcaneal**) **ligaments** strengthen the capsule. The **interosseous** (**talocalcaneal**) **ligament**

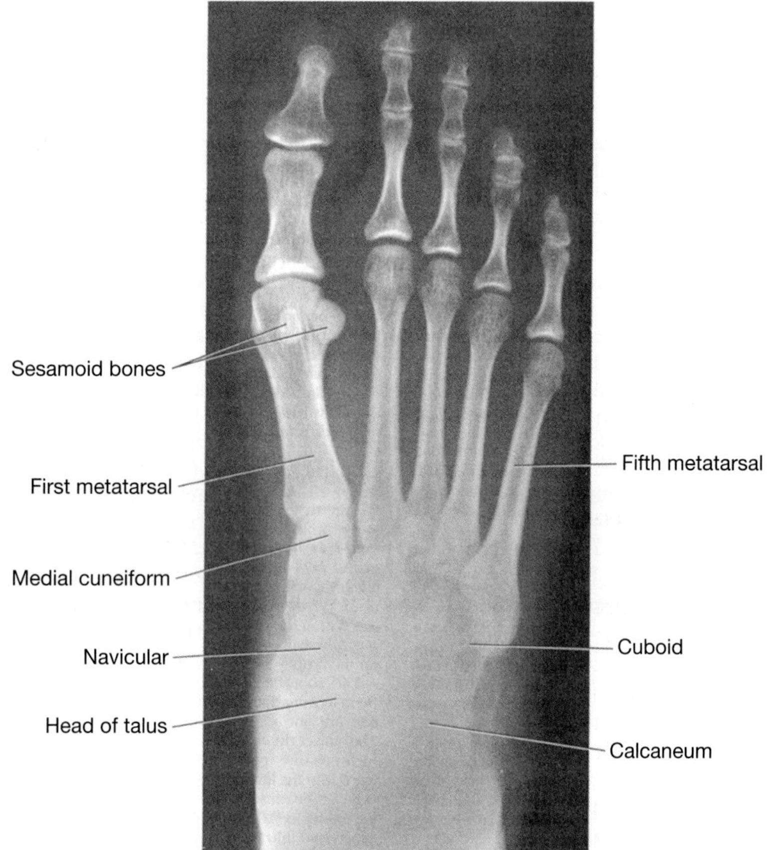

Figure 8.31 Anteroposterior radiograph of the adult foot.

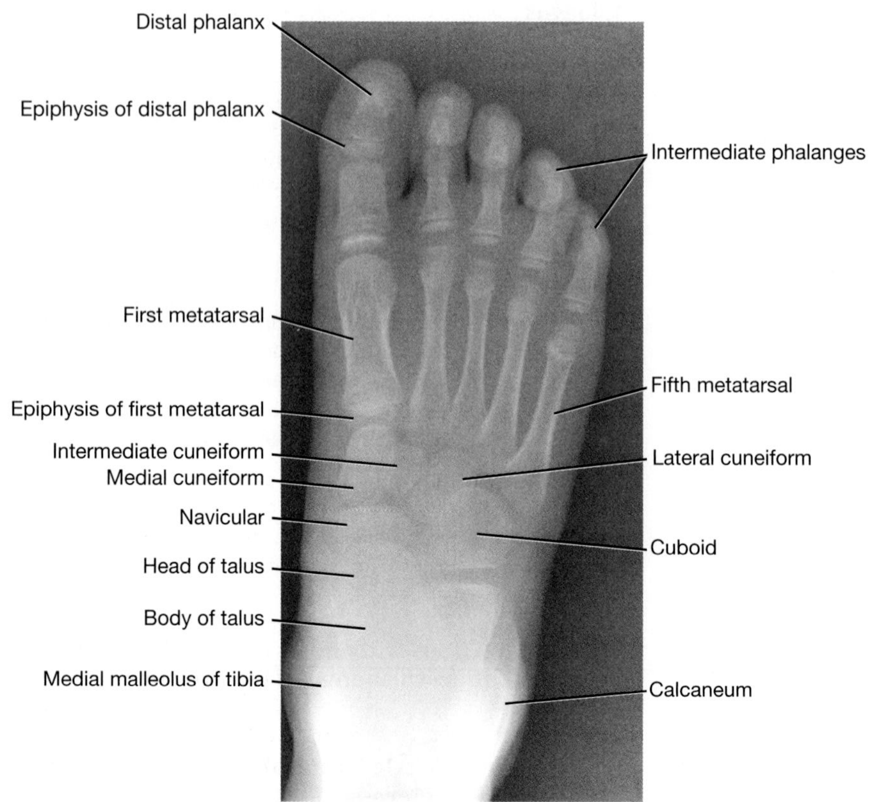

Figure 8.32 Anteroposterior radiograph of the foot showing the epiphyses of the phalanges and metatarsal bones (10-year-old male).

(see Fig. 8.29) is strong and is the main bond of union between the two bones. It attaches above to the sulcus tali and below to the sulcus calcanei.

Synovial Membrane

The synovial membrane lines the capsule.

Movements

Gliding and rotatory movements are possible.

Talocalcaneonavicular Joint

The talocalcaneonavicular joint is the anterior joint between the talus and the calcaneum and involves the navicular bone (see Fig. 8.9). Articulation is between the rounded head of the talus, the upper surface of the sustentaculum tali, and the posterior concave surface of the navicular bone. The articular surfaces are covered with hyaline cartilage.

Type

The joint is a plane type.

Capsule

The capsule incompletely encloses the joint.

Ligaments

The **plantar calcaneonavicular ligament** is strong and runs from the anterior margin of the sustentaculum tali to the inferior surface and tuberosity of the navicular bone (see Fig. 8.28A). The superior surface of the ligament is covered with fibrocartilage and supports the head of the talus.

Synovial Membrane

The synovial membrane lines the capsule.

Movements

Gliding and rotatory movements are possible.

Calcaneocuboid Joint

Articulation is between the anterior end of the calcaneum and the posterior surface of the cuboid (see Fig. 8.9). The articular surfaces are covered with hyaline cartilage.

Type

The calcaneocuboid joint is a plane type.

Capsule

The capsule encloses the joint.

Ligaments

The **bifurcated ligament** is a strong ligament on the upper surface of the joint (see Fig. 8.28B). It is Y shaped, and the stem attaches to the upper surface of the anterior part of the calcaneum. The lateral limb attaches to the upper surface of the cuboid and the medial limb to the upper surface of the navicular bone.

The **long plantar ligament** is a strong ligament on the lower surface of the joint (see Sole Muscles). It attaches to the undersurface of the calcaneum behind and to the undersurface of the cuboid and the bases of the third, fourth, and fifth metatarsal bones in front. It bridges over the groove for the fibularis longus tendon, converting it into a tunnel.

The **short plantar ligament** is a wide, strong ligament that attaches to the anterior tubercle on the undersurface of the calcaneum and to the adjoining part of the cuboid bone.

Synovial Membrane

The synovial membrane lines the capsule.

Movements in Subtalar, Talocalcaneonavicular, and Calcaneocuboid Joints

The talocalcaneonavicular and the calcaneocuboid joints are together referred to as the **midtarsal** or **transverse tarsal joints**.

The important movements of inversion and eversion of the foot take place at the subtalar and transverse tarsal joints. **Inversion** is the movement of the foot so that the sole faces medially. **Eversion** is the opposite movement of the foot so that the sole faces in the lateral direction. The movement of inversion is more extensive than eversion.

The tibialis anterior, extensor hallucis longus, and medial tendons of extensor digitorum longus perform inversion; the tibialis posterior also assists.

The fibularis longus, brevis, and tertius muscles perform eversion; the lateral tendons of the extensor digitorum longus also assist.

Cuneonavicular Joint

The cuneonavicular joint is the articulation between the navicular bone and the three cuneiform bones (see Fig. 8.10). It is a gliding joint. **Dorsal** and **plantar ligaments** strengthen the capsule. The joint cavity is continuous with those of the intercuneiform and cuneocuboid joints and with the cuneometatarsal and intermetatarsal joints, between the bases of the second and third and third and fourth metatarsal bones.

Cuboideonavicular Joint

The cuboideonavicular joint is usually a fibrous joint, with the two bones connected by dorsal, plantar, and interosseous ligaments.

Intercuneiform and Cuneocuboid Joints

The intercuneiform and cuneocuboid joints are plane types. Their joint cavities are continuous with that of the cuneonavicular joint. Dorsal, plantar, and interosseous ligaments connect the bones.

Tarsometatarsal and Intermetatarsal Joints

The tarsometatarsal and intermetatarsal joints are synovial joints of the plane variety. Dorsal, plantar, and interosseous ligaments connect the bones. The tarsometatarsal joint of the great toe has a separate joint cavity.

Metatarsophalangeal and Interphalangeal Joints

The metatarsophalangeal and interphalangeal joints closely resemble those of the hand. The deep transverse ligaments connect the joints of the five toes.

The movements of abduction and adduction of the toes, performed by the interossei muscles, are minimal and take place from the **midline of the second digit** and not the third, as in the hand.

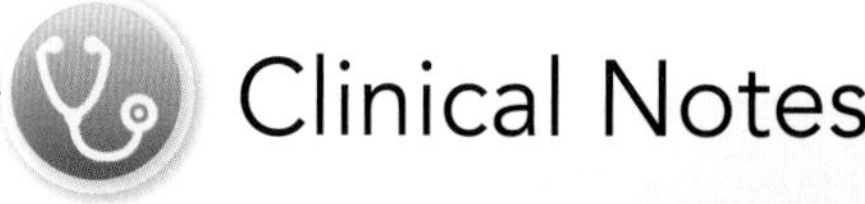

Clinical Notes

Metatarsophalangeal Joint of Great Toe

Hallux valgus, which is a lateral deviation of the great toe at the metatarsophalangeal joint, is a common condition. Its incidence is greater in females and is associated with badly fitting shoes. It is often accompanied by the presence of a short first metatarsal bone. Once the deformity is established, it is progressively worsened by the pull of the flexor hallucis longus and extensor hallucis longus muscles. Later, osteoarthritic changes occur in the metatarsophalangeal joint, which then becomes stiff and painful; the condition is then known as **hallux rigidus**.

FOOT AS FUNCTIONAL UNIT

The foot has two important functions: to support body weight and serve as a lever to propel the body forward in walking and running. If the foot possessed a single strong bone instead of a series of small bones, it could sustain the body weight and serve well as a rigid lever for forward propulsion (Fig. 8.33). However, with such an arrangement, the foot could not adapt itself to uneven surfaces, and the forward propulsive action would depend entirely on the activities of the gastrocnemius and soleus muscles. Because the lever is segmented with multiple joints, the foot is pliable and can adapt itself to uneven surfaces. Moreover, the long flexor muscles and the small muscles of the foot can exert their action on the bones of the forepart of the foot and toes (ie, the takeoff point of the foot) and greatly assist the forward propulsive action of the gastrocnemius and soleus muscles.

Arches

A segmented structure can hold up weight only if it is built in the form of an arch. The foot has three such arches, which are present at birth: the **medial longitudinal**, **lateral longitudinal**, and **transverse arches** (Fig. 8.34). In the young child, the foot appears to be flat because of the presence of a large amount of subcutaneous fat on the sole.

The imprint of a wet foot on the floor made with the person in the standing position, shows that the heel, lateral margin of the foot, pad under the metatarsal heads, and the pads of the distal phalanges are in contact with the ground (see Figs. 8.33 and 8.34). The medial margin of the foot, from the heel to the first metatarsal head, is arched above the ground because of the important medial longitudinal arch. The pressure exerted on the ground by the lateral margin of the foot is greatest at the heel and the fifth metatarsal head and least between these areas because of the presence of the low-lying lateral longitudinal arch. The transverse arch involves the bases of the five metatarsals and the cuboid and cuneiform bones. This is only half an arch, with its base on the lateral border of the foot and its summit on the foot's medial border. The foot has been likened to a half-dome, so that when the medial borders of the two feet are placed together, a complete dome is formed. Thus,

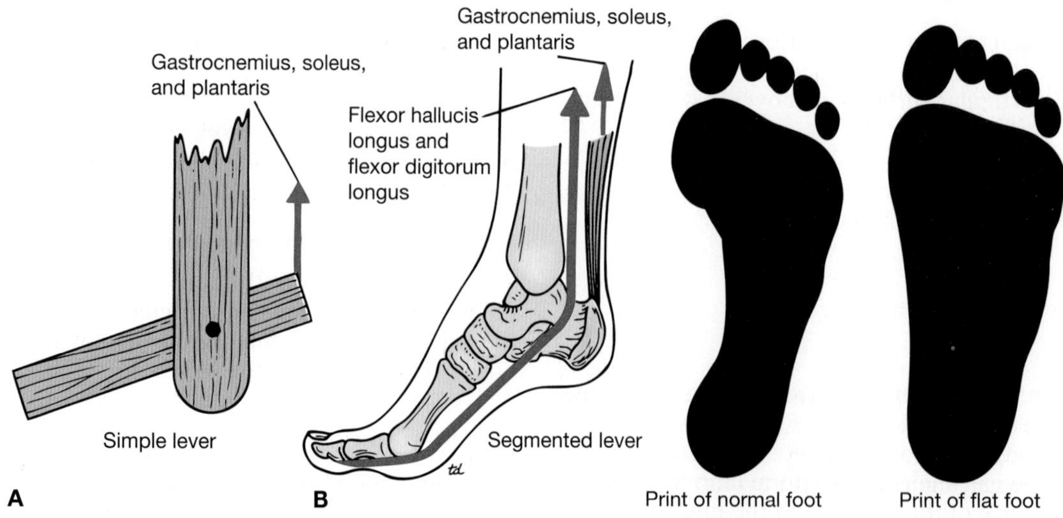

Figure 8.33 Foot as a simple lever **(A)** and as a segmented lever **(B)**. Floor prints of a normal foot and a flatfoot are also shown.

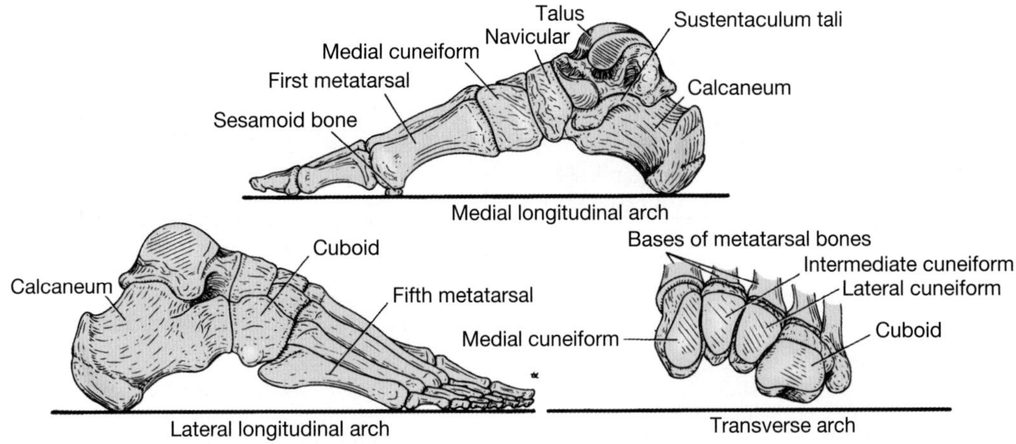

Figure 8.34 Bones forming the medial longitudinal, lateral longitudinal, and transverse arches of the right foot.

the body weight on standing is distributed through the foot via the heel behind and six points of contact with the ground in front: the two sesamoid bones under the head of the first metatarsal and the heads of the remaining four metatarsals.

Arch Bones

Examination of an articulated foot or a lateral radiograph of the foot shows the bones that form the arches (see Figs. 8.30 and 8.34).

- **Medial longitudinal arch:** This consists of the calcaneum, talus, navicular bone, the three cuneiform bones, and the first three metatarsal bones.
- **Lateral longitudinal arch:** This consists of the calcaneum, cuboid, and the fourth and fifth metatarsal bones.
- **Transverse arch:** This consists of the bases of the metatarsal bones and the cuboid and the three cuneiform bones.

Arch Support Mechanisms

The following engineering methods underlie the support of a stone bridge and help explain the methods used to support the arches of the feet (Fig. 8.35):

- **Shape of stones:** The most effective way of supporting the arch is to make the stones wedge shaped, with the thin edge of the wedge lying inferiorly. This applies particularly to the important stone that occupies the center of the arch and is referred to as the **keystone**.
- **Inferior edges of stones tied together:** Interlocking the stones or binding their lower edges together with metal staples accomplishes this. This method effectively counteracts the tendency of the lower edges of the stones to separate when the arch is weight bearing.
- **Use of tie beams:** When the span of the bridge is large and the foundations at either end are insecure, a tie beam connecting the ends effectively prevents separation of the pillars and consequent sagging of the arch.
- **Suspension bridge:** Here, the maintenance of the arch depends on multiple supports suspending the arch from a cable above the level of the bridge.

Medial Longitudinal Arch Maintenance

- **Shape of bones:** The sustentaculum tali holds up the talus, the concave proximal surface of the navicular bone receives the rounded head of the talus, and the slight concavity of the proximal surface of the medial cuneiform bone receives the navicular. The rounded head of the talus is the keystone in the center of the arch.
- **Inferior edges of bones tied together:** This is accomplished by the plantar ligaments, which are larger and stronger than the dorsal ligaments. The most important ligament is the plantar calcaneonavicular ligament. The tendinous extensions of the insertion of the tibialis posterior muscle play an important role in this respect.
- **Tying ends of arch together:** This is accomplished by the plantar aponeurosis, medial part of the flexor digitorum brevis, abductor hallucis, flexor hallucis longus, medial part of the flexor digitorum longus, and the flexor hallucis brevis.
- **Suspending arch from above:** The tibialis anterior and posterior and the medial ligament of the ankle joint accomplish this.

Lateral Longitudinal Arch Maintenance

- **Shape of bones:** Minimal shaping of the distal end of the calcaneum and the proximal end of the cuboid. The cuboid is the keystone.
- **Inferior edges of bones tied together** by the long and short plantar ligaments and the origins of the short muscles from the forepart of the foot.
- **Tying ends of arch together** are the plantar aponeurosis, the abductor digiti minimi, and the lateral part of the flexor digitorum longus and brevis.
- **Suspending arch from above** are the fibularis longus and brevis.

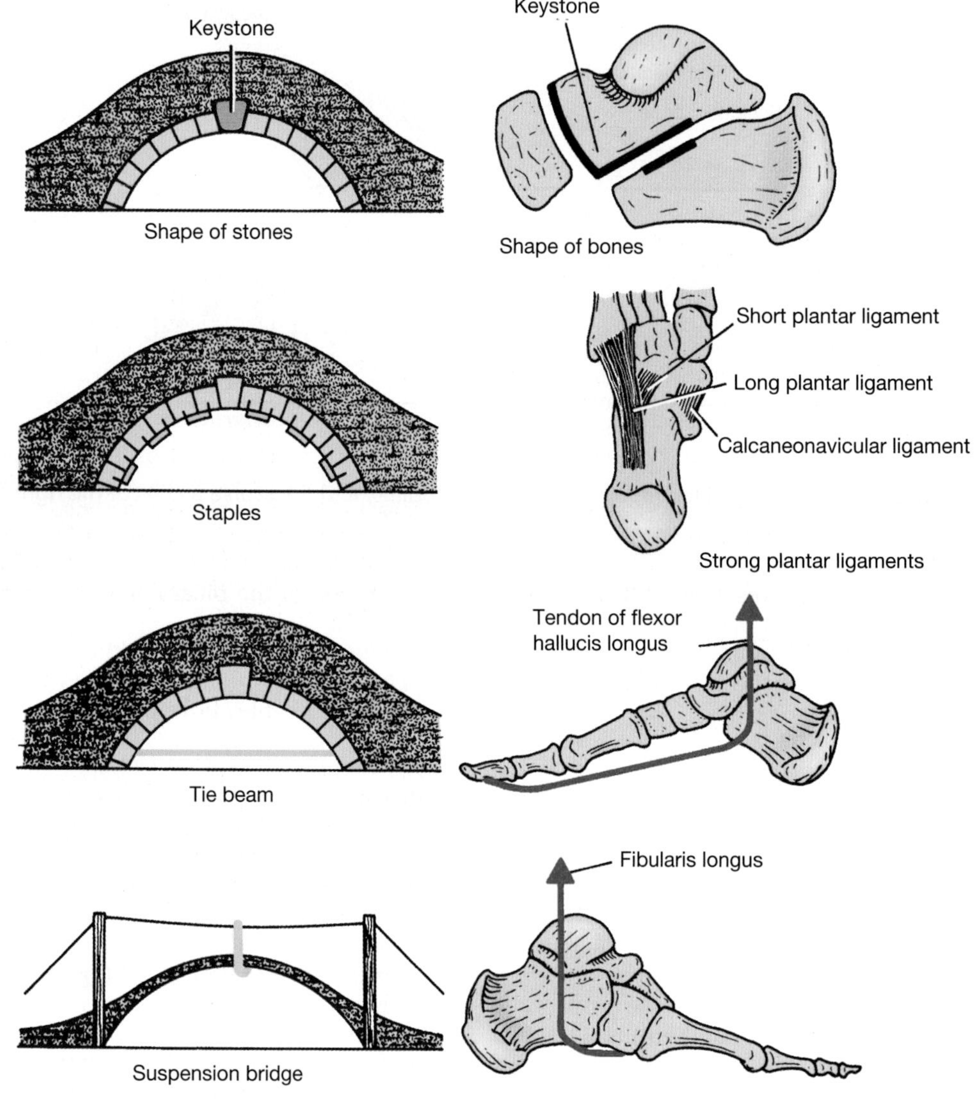

Figure 8.35 Different methods by which the arches of the foot may be supported.

Transverse Arch Maintenance

- **Shape of bones:** The marked wedge shaping of the cuneiform bones and the bases of the metatarsal bones (see Fig. 8.34).
- **Inferior edges of bones tied together** by the deep transverse ligaments, the strong plantar ligaments, and the origins of the plantar muscles from the forepart of the foot; the dorsal interossei and the transverse head of the adductor hallucis are particularly important in this respect.
- **Tying ends of arch together** is the fibularis longus tendon.
- **Suspending arch from above** are the fibularis longus tendon and the fibularis brevis.

The shape of the bones, strong ligaments, and muscle tone maintains the arches of the feet. Which of these factors is the most important? Active muscle testing demonstrated that the tibialis anterior, fibularis longus, and the small muscles of the foot play no important role in the normal static support of the arches. They are commonly totally inactive. However, during walking and running, all these muscles become active. Standing immobile for long periods, especially if the person is overweight, places excessive strain on the bones and ligaments of the feet and results in fallen arches or flatfeet. People that stand upright for long periods can sustain their arches provided they receive adequate training to develop their muscle tone.

Foot Propulsive Action

When standing immobile, body weight is distributed via the heel behind and the heads of the metatarsal bones in front (including the two sesamoid bones under the head of the first metatarsal).

Walking

As the body weight is thrown forward, the weight is borne successively on the lateral margin of the foot and the

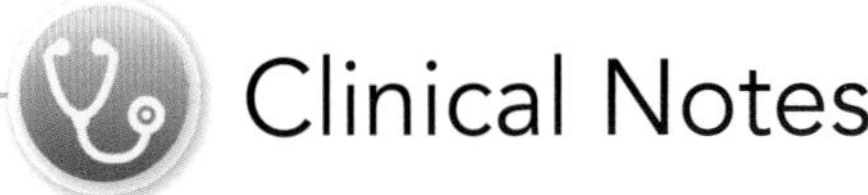

Clinical Notes

Clinical Problems Associated with Foot Arches

Of the three arches, the medial longitudinal is the largest and clinically the most important. The shape of the bones; the strong ligaments, especially those on the plantar surface of the foot; and the tone of muscles all play an important role in supporting the arches. The tone of muscles is an important factor in arch support in the active foot. When the muscles are fatigued by excessive exercise (eg, during long hikes), standing for long periods (eg, from occupations such as hospitality or health care), overweight, or illness, the muscular support gives way, the ligaments are stretched, and pain is produced.

Pes planus (**flatfoot**) is a condition in which the medial longitudinal arch is depressed or collapsed. As a result, the forefoot is displaced laterally and everted. The head of the talus is no longer supported, and the body weight forces it downward and medially between the calcaneum and the navicular bone. When the deformity has existed for some time, the plantar, calcaneonavicular, and medial ligaments of the ankle joint become permanently stretched, and the bones change shape. The muscles and tendons are also permanently stretched. The causes of flatfoot are both congenital and acquired.

Pes cavus (**claw foot**) is a condition in which the medial longitudinal arch is unduly high. Most cases are caused by muscle imbalance, in many instances resulting from poliomyelitis.

Lower Limb Bursae and Bursitis

A variety of bursae are found in the lower limb where skin, tendons, ligaments, or muscles repeatedly rub against bony points or ridges.

Bursitis, or inflammation of a bursa, can be caused by acute or chronic trauma, crystal disease, infection, or disease of a neighboring joint that communicates with the bursa. An inflamed bursa becomes distended with excessive amounts of fluid. The following bursae are prone to inflammation: the bursa over the ischial tuberosity; greater trochanter bursa; prepatellar and superficial infrapatellar bursae; the bursa between the tendons of insertion of the sartorius, gracilis, and semitendinosus muscles on the medial proximal aspect of the tibia; and the bursa between the tendo calcaneus and the upper part of the calcaneum (long-distance runner's ankle).

Two important bursae communicate with the knee joint, and they can become distended if excessive amounts of synovial fluid accumulate within the joint. The suprapatellar bursa extends proximally about three fingerbreadths above the patella beneath the quadriceps femoris muscle. The bursa, which is associated with the insertion of the semimembranosus muscle, may enlarge in patients with osteoarthritis of the knee joint.

The anatomic bursae described should not be confused with **adventitious bursae**, which develop in response to abnormal and excessive friction. For example, a subcutaneous bursa sometimes develops over the tendo calcaneus in response to badly fitting shoes. A **bunion** is an adventitial bursa located over the medial side of the head of the first metatarsal bone.

heads of the metatarsal bones. As the heel rises, the toes extend at the metatarsophalangeal joints, and the plantar aponeurosis is pulled on, thus shortening the tie beams, and heightening the longitudinal arches. The "slack" in the long flexor tendons is taken up, thereby increasing their efficiency. The body is then thrown forward by the actions of the gastrocnemius and soleus (and plantaris) on the ankle joint, using the foot as a lever, and by the toes being strongly flexed by the long and short flexors of the foot, providing the final thrust forward. The lumbricals and interossei contract and keep the toes extended so that they do not fold under because of the strong action of the flexor digitorum longus. In this action, the long flexor tendons also assist in plantar flexing the ankle joint.

Running

In running, weight is borne on the forepart of the foot, and the heel does not touch the ground. The forward thrust to the body is provided by the mechanisms described for walking (above).

GLUTEAL REGION

The gluteal region, or buttock, is bounded superiorly by the iliac crest and inferiorly by the fold of the buttock. The region is largely made up of the gluteal muscles and a thick layer of superficial fascia.

Skin

Both anterior and posterior rami of spinal nerves supply **cutaneous nerves** in the following pattern (Figs. 8.36 and 8.37):

- **Upper medial quadrant:** supplied by the posterior rami of the L1 to L3 and S1 to S3 nerves
- **Upper lateral quadrant:** supplied by the lateral branches of the anterior rami of the iliohypogastric (L1) and T12 nerves
- **Lower lateral quadrant:** supplied by branches from the lateral cutaneous nerve of the thigh (L2 and L3, anterior rami)
- **Lower medial quadrant:** supplied by branches from the posterior cutaneous nerve of the thigh (S1 to S3, anterior rami)

Small branches of the lower sacral and coccygeal nerves supply the skin over the coccyx in the floor of the cleft between the buttocks.

The **lymph vessels** drain into the **lateral group of the superficial inguinal nodes** (Figs. 8.38 and 8.39).

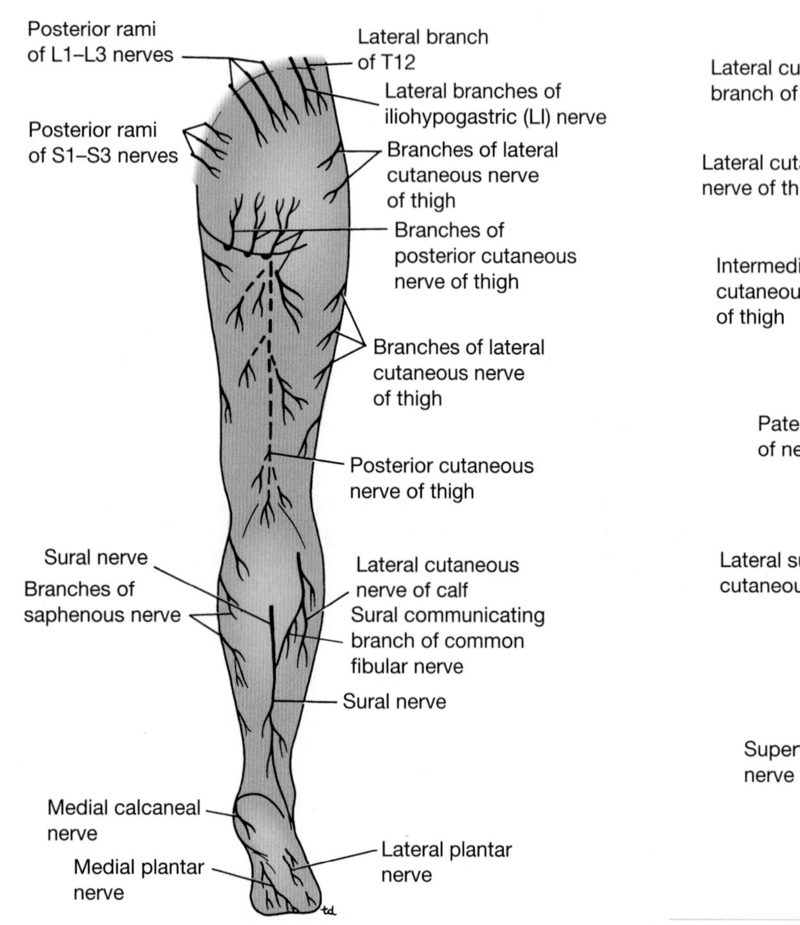

Figure 8.36 Cutaneous nerves of the posterior surface of the right lower limb.

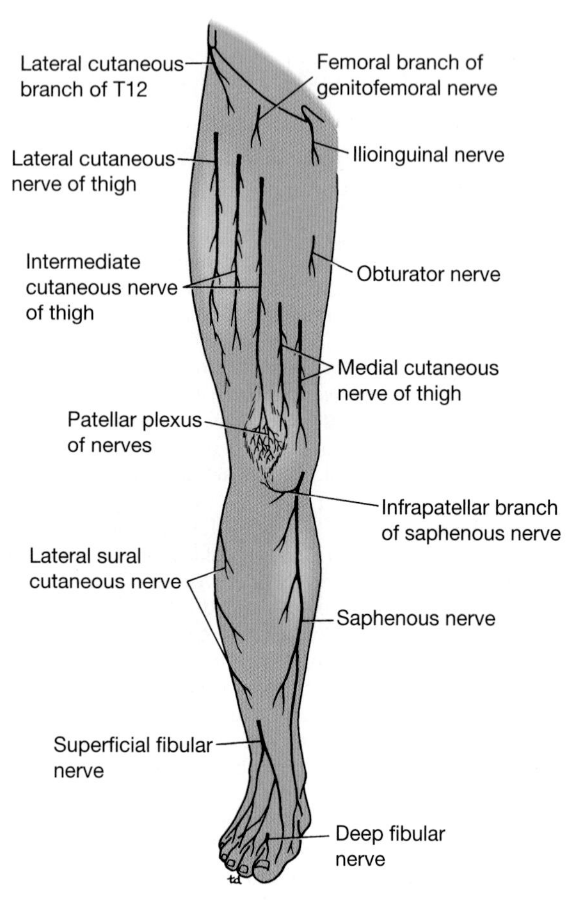

Figure 8.37 Cutaneous nerves of the anterior surface of the right lower limb.

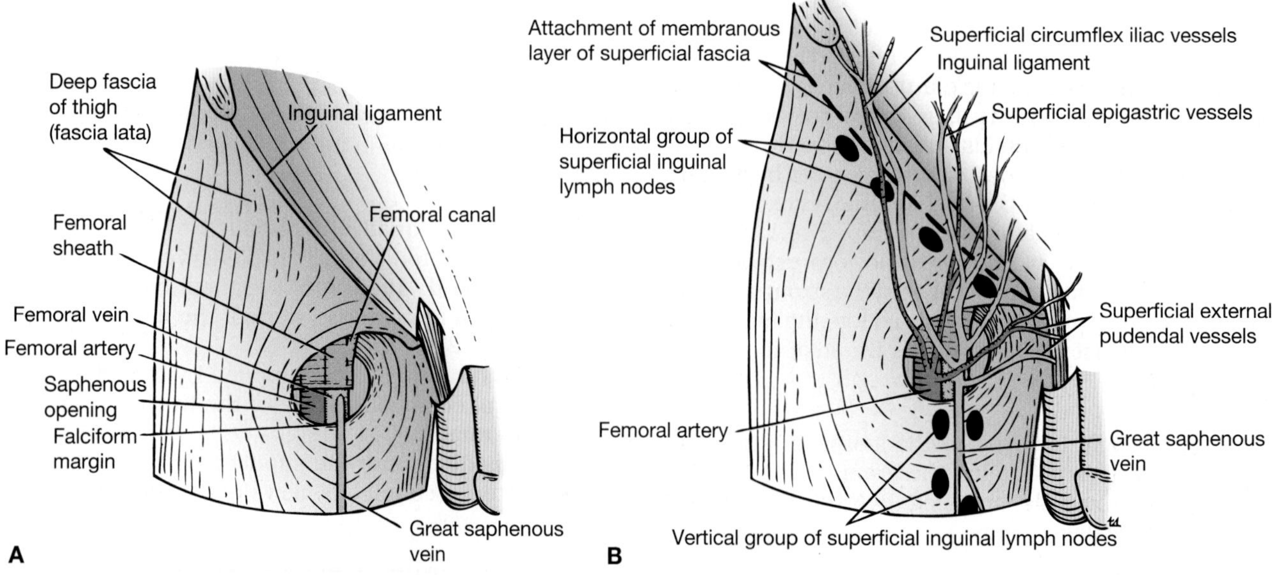

Figure 8.38 A and B. Superficial veins, arteries, and lymph nodes over the right femoral triangle. Note the saphenous opening in the deep fascia and its relationship to the femoral sheath. Also note the line of attachment of the membranous layer of superficial fascia to the deep fascia, about a fingerbreadth below the inguinal ligament.

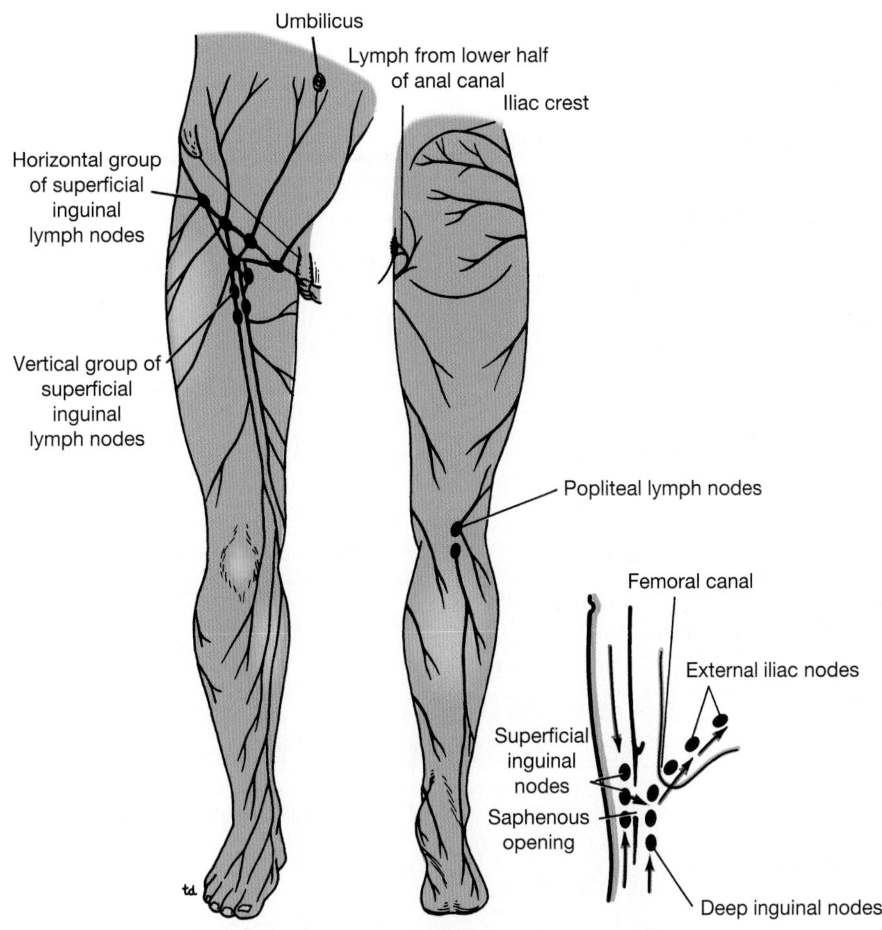

Figure 8.39 Lymph drainage for the superficial tissues of the right lower limb and the abdominal walls below the level of the umbilicus. Note the arrangement of the superficial and deep inguinal lymph nodes and their relationship to the saphenous opening in the deep fascia. Also note that all lymph from these nodes ultimately drains into the external iliac nodes via the femoral canal.

Fascia

The **superficial fascia** is thick, especially in females. It is impregnated with large quantities of fat that contribute to the prominence of the buttock.

The **deep fascia** is continuous below with the deep fascia, or **fascia lata**, of the thigh. In the gluteal region, it splits to enclose the gluteus maximus muscle (Fig. 8.40). Above the gluteus maximus, it continues as a single layer that covers the outer surface of the gluteus medius and attaches to the iliac crest. On the lateral surface of the thigh, the fascia lata is thickened to form a strong, wide band, the **iliotibial tract (iliotibial band)**. This is attached above to the tubercle of the iliac crest and below to the lateral condyle of the tibia. The iliotibial tract forms a sheath for the tensor fasciae latae muscle and receives the greater part of the insertion of the gluteus maximus.

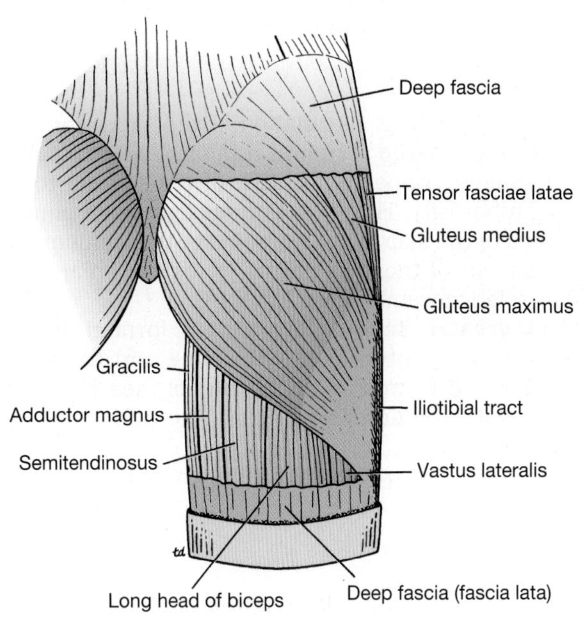

Figure 8.40 Right gluteus maximus muscle.

Ligaments and Foramina

The sacrotuberous and sacrospinous ligaments are two prominent structures in the gluteal region (Figs. 8.41 and 8.42; see also Fig. 6.1A). These function to stabilize the

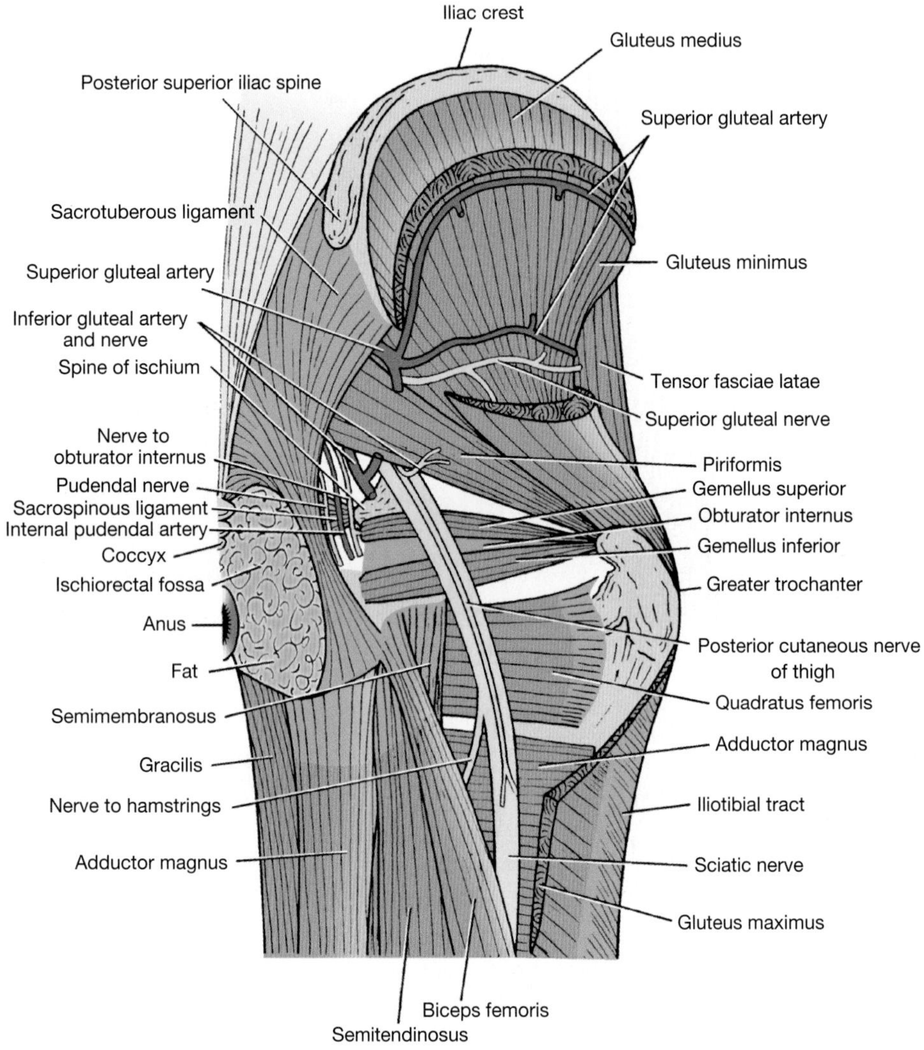

Figure 8.41 Structures in the right gluteal region. The greater part of the gluteus maximus and part of the gluteus medius have been removed.

sacrum and prevent its rotation at the sacroiliac joint by the weight of the vertebral column. The **sacrotuberous ligament** connects the back of the sacrum to the ischial tuberosity. The **sacrospinous ligament** connects the back of the sacrum to the spine of the ischium. The arrangement of these ligaments forms the greater and lesser sciatic foramina (see Fig. 6.10).

The **greater sciatic foramen** is formed by the greater sciatic notch of the hip bone and the sacrotuberous and sacrospinous ligaments (see Figs. 6.1A and 8.1). It provides an exit from the pelvis into the gluteal region.

The following structures exit the greater sciatic foramen (see Figs. 8.41 and 8.42):

- Piriformis muscle
- Sciatic nerve
- Posterior cutaneous nerve of the thigh
- Superior and inferior gluteal nerves
- Superior and inferior gluteal arteries and veins
- Nerves to the obturator internus and quadratus femoris
- Pudendal nerve
- Internal pudendal artery and vein

The **lesser sciatic foramen** (see Fig. 5.11) is formed by the lesser sciatic notch of the hip bone and the sacrotuberous and sacrospinous ligaments (see Figs. 6.1A and 8.1). It provides an entrance into the perineum from the gluteal region. Its presence enables nerves and blood vessels that have left the pelvis through the greater sciatic foramen above the pelvic floor to enter the perineum below the pelvic floor.

The following structures pass through the lesser sciatic foramen (see Figs. 8.41 and 8.42):

- Tendon of obturator internus muscle
- Nerve to obturator internus
- Pudendal nerve
- Internal pudendal artery and vein

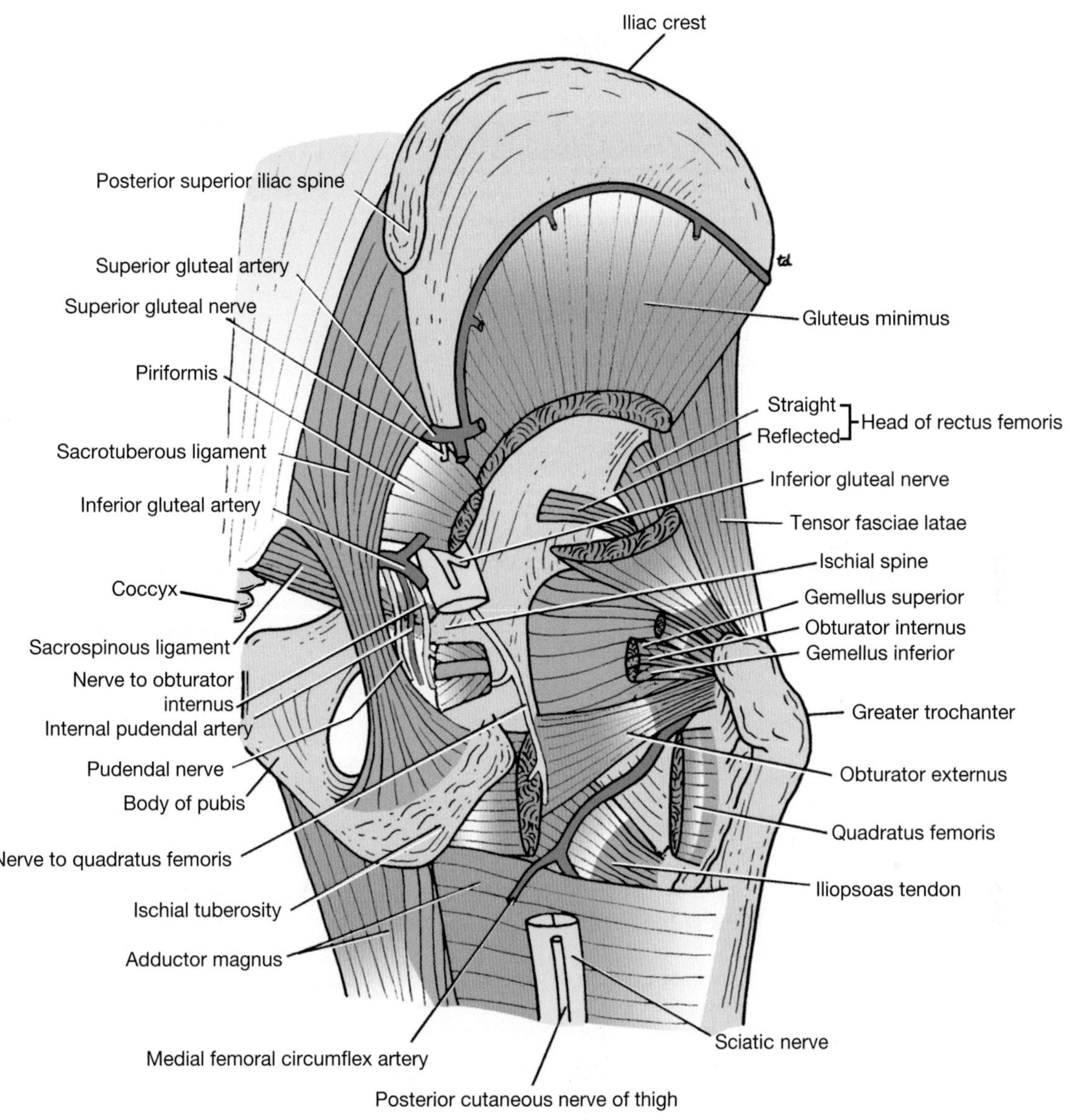

Figure 8.42 Deep structures in the right gluteal region; the gluteus maximus and the gluteus medius muscles have been completely removed.

Gluteal Region Muscles

The muscles of the gluteal region include the gluteus maximus, gluteus medius, gluteus minimus, tensor fasciae latae, piriformis, obturator internus, superior and inferior gemelli, and the quadratus femoris. The muscles are shown in Figures 8.40 through 8.42 and summarized in Table 8.1.

Note the following:

- The gluteus maximus (see Fig. 8.40) is the largest muscle in the body. It lies superficial in the gluteal region and is largely responsible for the prominence of the buttock.
- The tensor fasciae latae (see Figs. 8.40 to 8.42) runs downward and backward to its insertion in the iliotibial tract and thus assists the gluteus maximus muscle in maintaining the knee in the extended position.
- The piriformis (see Fig. 8.41) lies partly within the pelvis at its origin. It emerges through the greater sciatic foramen to enter the gluteal region. Its position serves to separate the superior gluteal vessels and nerves from the inferior gluteal vessels and nerves.
- The obturator internus is a fan-shaped muscle that originates within the pelvis. Its tendon emerges through the lesser sciatic foramen to enter the gluteal region (see Figs. 8.41 and 8.42). The tendon is joined by the superior and inferior gemelli and inserts into the greater trochanter of the femur.
- Three bursae are usually associated with the gluteus maximus: between the tendon of insertion and the greater trochanter, between the tendon of insertion and the vastus lateralis, and overlying the ischial tuberosity.

Table 8.1 Gluteal Region Muscles

MUSCLE	ORIGIN	INSERTION	NERVE SUPPLY	NERVE ROOT[a]	ACTION
Gluteus maximus	Outer surface of ilium, sacrum, coccyx, sacrotuberous ligament	Iliotibial tract and gluteal tuberosity of femur	Inferior gluteal nerve	L5; **S1**, **S2**	Extends and laterally rotates hip joint; through iliotibial tract, it extends knee joint
Gluteus medius	Outer surface of ilium	Lateral surface of greater trochanter of femur	Superior gluteal nerve	**L5**; S1	Abducts thigh at hip joint; tilts pelvis when walking to permit opposite leg to clear ground
Gluteus minimus	Outer surface of ilium	Anterior surface of greater trochanter of femur	Superior gluteal nerve	**L5**; S1	Abducts thigh at hip joint; tilts pelvis when walking to permit opposite leg to clear ground
Tensor fasciae latae	Iliac crest	Iliotibial tract	Superior gluteal nerve	**L5**; S1	Assists gluteus maximus in extending the knee joint
Piriformis	Anterior surface of sacrum	Upper border of greater trochanter of femur	First and second sacral nerves	**S1**, S2	Lateral rotator of thigh at hip joint
Obturator internus	Inner surface of obturator membrane	Upper border of greater trochanter of femur	Sacral plexus	L5; **S1**	Lateral rotator of thigh at hip joint
Gemellus superior	Spine of ischium	Upper border of greater trochanter of femur	Sacral plexus	L5; **S1**	Lateral rotator of thigh at hip joint
Gemellus inferior	Ischial tuberosity	Upper border of greater trochanter of femur	Sacral plexus	L5; S1	Lateral rotator of thigh at hip joint
Quadratus femoris	Lateral border of ischial tuberosity	Quadrate tubercle of femur	Sacral plexus	L5; S1	Lateral rotator of thigh at hip joint

[a]The predominant nerve root supply is in bold.

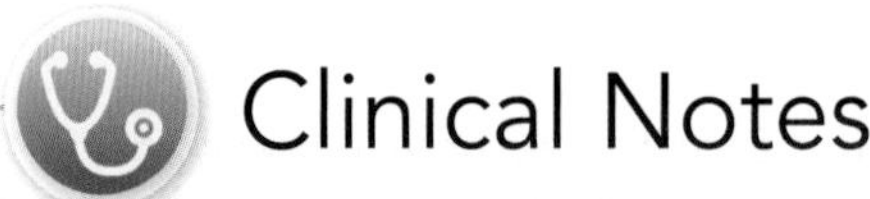

Clinical Notes

Gluteus Maximus and Intramuscular Injections

The gluteus maximus is a large, thick muscle with coarse fasciculi that can be easily separated without damage. The great thickness of this muscle makes it ideal for intramuscular injections. The injection should be given well forward on the upper outer quadrant of the buttock to avoid injury to the underlying sciatic nerve.

Gluteus Maximus and Bursitis

Bursitis, or inflammation of a bursa, can be caused by acute or chronic trauma. An inflamed bursa becomes distended with excessive amounts of fluid and can be extremely painful. The bursae associated with the gluteus maximus are prone to inflammation.

Gluteus Medius and Minimus and Poliomyelitis

The superior gluteal nerve (L4 to S1) supplies the gluteus medius and minimus muscles. They may be paralyzed when poliomyelitis involves the lower lumbar and sacral segments of the spinal cord. Paralysis of these muscles seriously interferes with the ability to tilt the pelvis when walking.

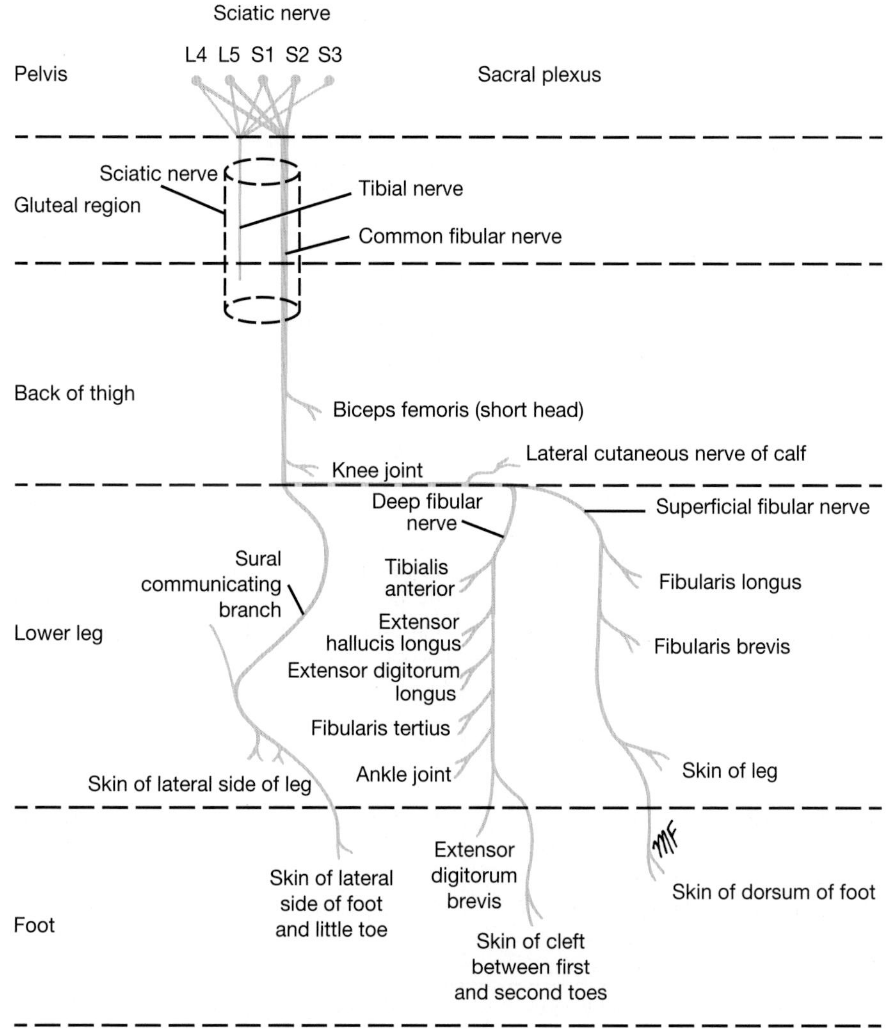

Figure 8.43 Summary of the origin of the sciatic nerve and the main branches of the common fibular (peroneal) nerve.

Gluteal Region Nerves

All the following nerves of the gluteal region originate from the sacral plexus.

Sciatic Nerve

The sciatic nerve (L4 to S3) emerges from the pelvis through the lower part of the greater sciatic foramen (see Figs. 8.41 and 8.42). It is the largest nerve in the body and consists of the **tibial** and **common fibular (peroneal) nerves** bound together with fascia (Figs. 8.43 and 8.44). The nerve appears below the piriformis muscle and curves downward and laterally, lying successively on the root of the ischial spine, superior gemellus, obturator internus, inferior gemellus, and quadratus femoris to reach the back of the adductor magnus muscle (see Fig. 8.41). It is related posteriorly to the posterior cutaneous nerve of the thigh and the gluteus maximus. It leaves the buttock region by passing deep to the long head of the biceps femoris to enter the back of the thigh.

Occasionally, the common fibular nerve leaves the sciatic nerve high in the pelvis and appears in the gluteal region by passing above or through the piriformis muscle.

The sciatic nerve usually gives no branches in the gluteal region.

Posterior Cutaneous Nerve of the Thigh

The posterior cutaneous nerve of the thigh enters the gluteal region through the lower part of the greater sciatic foramen below the piriformis muscle (see Fig. 8.41). It passes downward on the posterior surface of the sciatic nerve and runs down the back of the thigh beneath the deep fascia. It supplies the skin over the popliteal fossa.

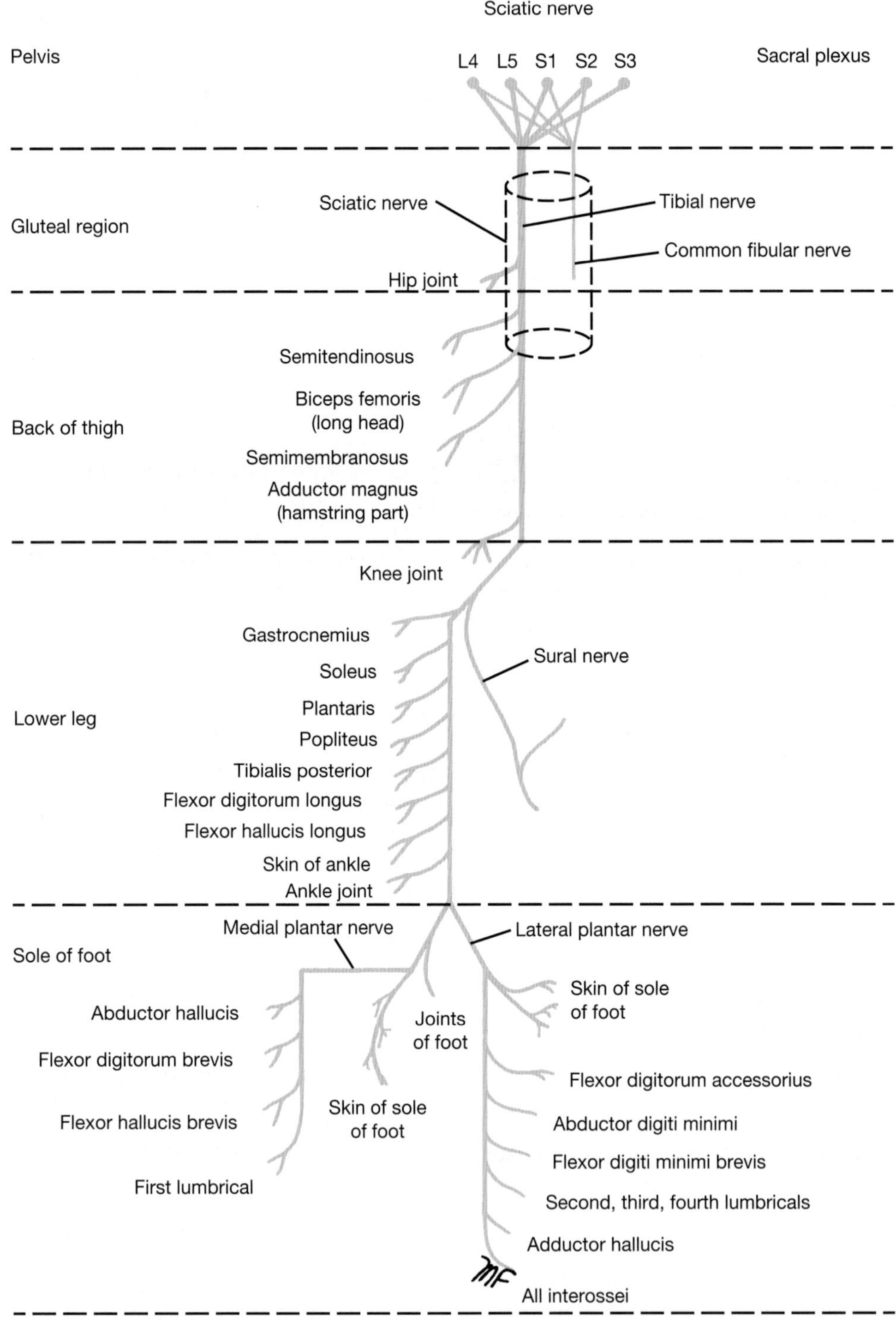

Figure 8.44 Summary of the origin of the sciatic nerve and the main branches of the tibial nerve.

Branches

- **Gluteal branches** to the skin over the lower medial quadrant of the buttock (see Fig. 8.36)
- **Perineal branch** to the skin of the back of the scrotum or labium majus
- **Cutaneous branches** to the back of the thigh and the upper part of the leg

Superior Gluteal Nerve

The superior gluteal nerve leaves the pelvis through the upper part of the greater sciatic foramen above the piriformis (see Fig. 8.41). It runs forward between the gluteus medius and minimus, supplies both, and ends by supplying the tensor fasciae latae.

Inferior Gluteal Nerve

The inferior gluteal nerve leaves the pelvis through the lower part of the greater sciatic foramen below the piriformis (see Figs. 8.41 and 8.42). It supplies the gluteus maximus muscle.

Nerve to Quadratus Femoris

The nerve to the quadratus femoris leaves the pelvis through the lower part of the greater sciatic foramen (see Fig. 8.42). It ends by supplying the quadratus femoris and the inferior gemellus.

Pudendal Nerve and Nerve to Obturator Internus

The pudendal nerve and nerve to the obturator internus leave the pelvis through the lower part of the greater sciatic foramen, below the piriformis (see Figs. 8.41 and 8.42). They cross the ischial spine with the internal pudendal artery and immediately reenter the pelvis through the lesser sciatic foramen. They then lie in the posterior aspect of the ischioanal fossa (see Chapter 7). The pudendal nerve supplies structures in the perineum. The nerve to the obturator internus supplies the obturator internus muscle on its pelvic surface.

Gluteal Region Arteries

The superior and inferior gluteal arteries are the primary vessels supplying the gluteal region. Both are branches of the internal iliac artery within the pelvic cavity. Both contribute to major collateral networks around the hip.

Superior Gluteal Artery

The superior gluteal artery enters the gluteal region through the upper part of the greater sciatic foramen above the piriformis (see Figs. 8.41 and 8.42). It divides into branches that distribute throughout the gluteal region, but has a primary flow through the fascial space between the gluteus medius and minimus muscles.

Inferior Gluteal Artery

The inferior gluteal artery enters the gluteal region through the lower part of the greater sciatic foramen, below the piriformis (see Figs. 8.41 and 8.42). It distributes branches that run throughout the gluteal region, including a major supply to the gluteus maximus muscle.

Trochanteric Anastomosis

The trochanteric anastomosis provides the main blood supply to the head of the femur. The nutrient arteries pass along the femoral neck beneath the capsule. The following arteries take part in the anastomosis: the superior gluteal artery, inferior gluteal artery, medial femoral circumflex artery, and lateral femoral circumflex artery.

Cruciate Anastomosis

The cruciate anastomosis is situated at the level of the lesser trochanter of the femur and, together with the trochanteric anastomosis, provides a collateral connection between the internal iliac and the femoral arteries. The following arteries take part in the anastomosis: the inferior gluteal artery, medial femoral circumflex artery, lateral femoral circumflex artery, and the first perforating artery, a branch of the profunda artery.

THIGH

The thigh is the proximal segment of the lower limb proper, from the hip to the knee. The femur is the bony core of the thigh.

Fascia

The **fatty layer of the superficial fascia** on the anterior abdominal wall extends into the thigh and continues down over the lower limb without interruption.

The **membranous layer of the superficial fascia** of the anterior abdominal wall extends into the thigh and attaches to the deep fascia (fascia lata) about a fingerbreadth below the inguinal ligament (see Fig. 8.38). This relationship is important in connection with extravasation of urine after a rupture of the urethra (see Chapter 5).

The **deep fascia** (**fascia lata**) encloses the thigh like a spandex legging (Fig. 8.45). Its upper end attaches to the pelvis and the inguinal ligament. It is thickened on its lateral aspect to form the **iliotibial tract** (see Figs. 8.40 and 8.45), which is attached above to the iliac tubercle and below to the lateral condyle of the tibia. The iliotibial tract receives the insertion of the tensor fasciae latae and the greater part of the gluteus maximus muscle. In the gluteal region, the deep fascia forms investing sheaths that enclose the tensor fasciae latae and gluteus maximus muscles.

The **saphenous opening** is a gap in the deep fascia in the front of the thigh just below the inguinal ligament. It is filled with loose connective tissue called the **cribriform fascia**. It transmits the great saphenous vein, some small branches of the femoral artery, and lymph vessels (see Fig. 8.38). The saphenous opening is situated about 1.5 in. (4 cm) below and lateral to the pubic tubercle. The **falciform margin** is the lower lateral border of the opening, which lies anterior to the femoral vessels (see Fig. 8.38A). The border of the opening then curves upward and medially, and then laterally behind the femoral vessels, to attach to the pectineal line of the superior ramus of the pubis.

Cutaneous Nerves

The **lateral cutaneous nerve of the thigh**, a branch of the lumbar plexus (L2 and L3), enters the thigh behind the lateral end of the inguinal ligament (see Fig. 8.37). Having divided into anterior and posterior branches, it supplies the skin of the lateral aspect of the thigh and

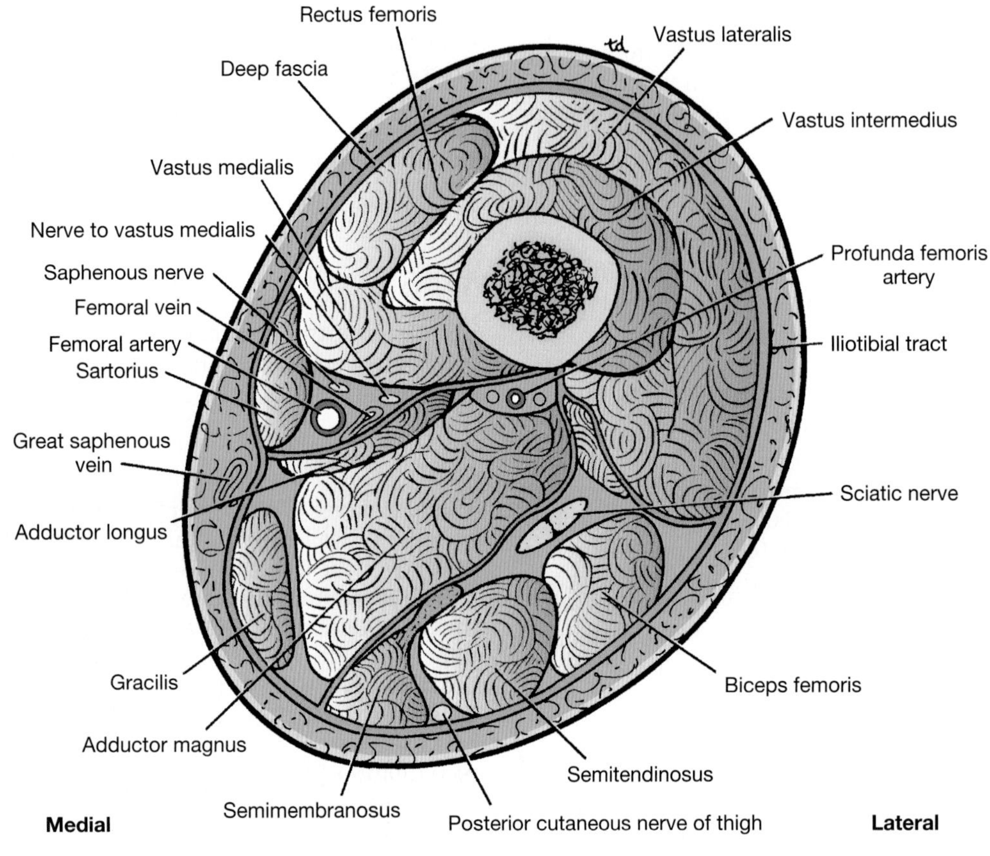

Figure 8.45 Transverse section through the middle of the right thigh as seen from above.

knee. It also supplies the skin of the lower lateral quadrant of the buttock (see Fig. 8.36).

The **femoral branch of the genitofemoral nerve**, a branch of the lumbar plexus (L1 and L2), enters the thigh behind the middle of the inguinal ligament and supplies a small area of skin (see Fig. 8.37). The **genital branch** supplies the cremaster muscle.

The **ilioinguinal nerve**, a branch of the lumbar plexus (L1), enters the thigh through the superficial inguinal ring. It distributes to the skin of the root of the penis and adjacent part of the scrotum (or root of the clitoris and adjacent part of the labium majus in the female) and to a small skin area below the medial part of the inguinal ligament.

The **medial cutaneous nerve of the thigh**, a branch of the femoral nerve, supplies the medial aspect of the thigh and joins the patellar plexus.

The **intermediate cutaneous nerve of the thigh**, a branch of the femoral nerve, divides into two branches that supply the anterior aspect of the thigh and joins the patellar plexus.

Branches from the **anterior division of the obturator nerve** supply a variable area of skin on the medial aspect of the thigh.

The **patellar plexus** lies in front of the knee and is formed from the terminal branches of the lateral, intermediate, and medial cutaneous nerves of the thigh and the infrapatellar branch of the saphenous nerve.

The **posterior cutaneous nerve of the thigh**, a branch of the sacral plexus, leaves the gluteal region by emerging from beneath the lower border of the gluteus maximus muscle (see Fig. 8.36). It descends on the back of the thigh, and in the popliteal fossa, it pierces the deep fascia and supplies the skin. It gives off numerous branches to the skin on the back of the thigh and the upper part of the leg.

Superficial Veins

The superficial veins of the leg are the great and small saphenous veins and their tributaries (Fig. 8.46). They are comparable to the basilic and cephalic veins in the upper limb and have significant clinical importance.

The **great saphenous vein** drains the medial end of the **dorsal venous arch** of the foot and passes upward directly in front of the medial malleolus. It then ascends in company with the saphenous nerve in the superficial fascia over the medial side of the leg. The vein passes behind the knee and curves forward around the medial side of the thigh. It passes through the lower part of the saphenous opening in the deep fascia and joins the femoral vein about 1.5 in. (4 cm)

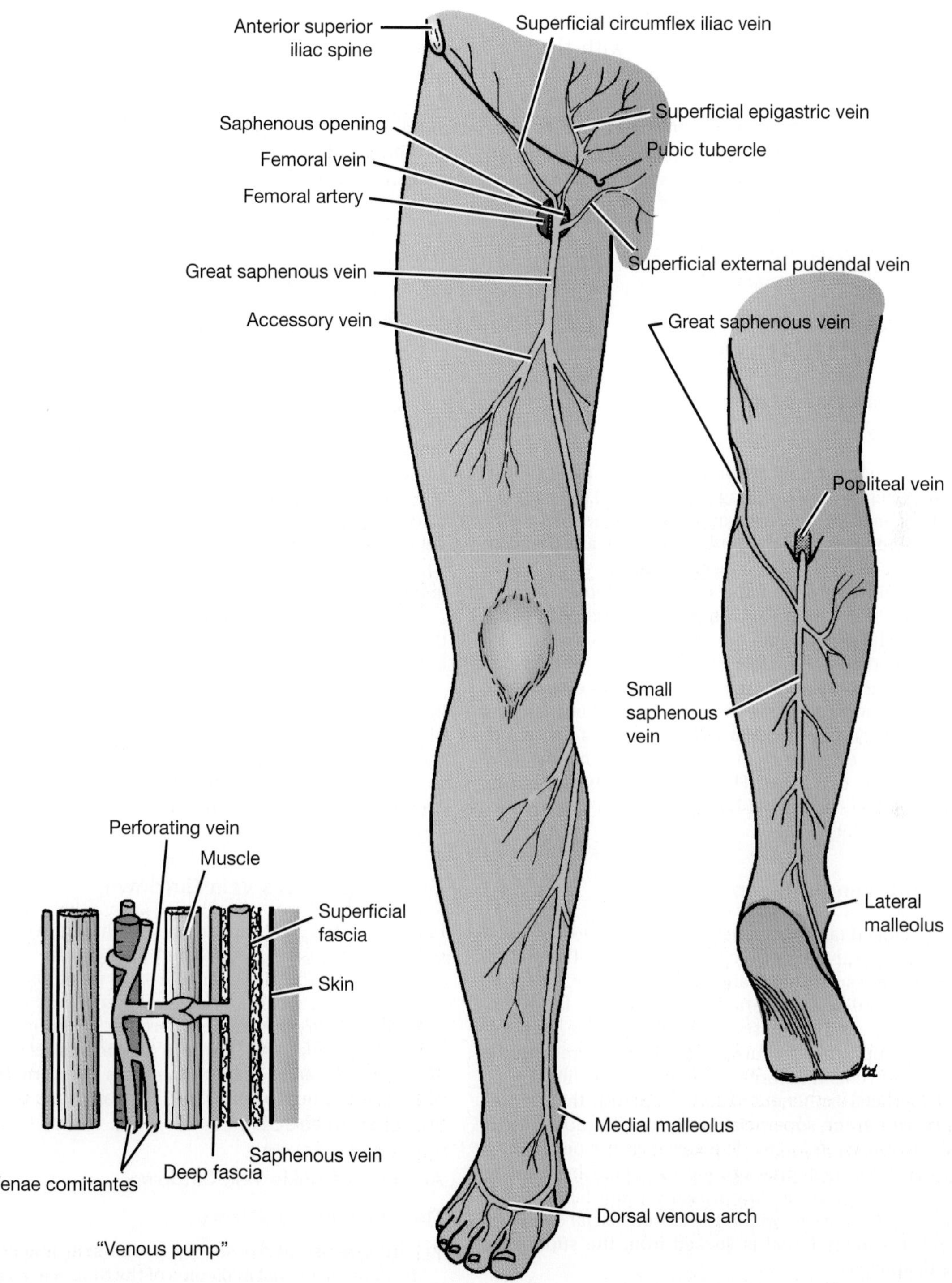

Figure 8.46 Superficial veins of the right lower limb. Note the importance of the valved perforating veins in the "venous pump."

below and lateral to the pubic tubercle (see Figs. 8.38 and 8.46).

The great saphenous vein possesses **numerous valves** and is connected to the small saphenous vein by one or two branches that pass behind the knee. Several **perforating veins** connect the great saphenous vein with the deep veins along the medial side of the calf (see Fig. 8.46).

The great saphenous vein usually receives three tributaries that are variable in size and arrangement at the saphenous opening in the deep fascia: the **superficial circumflex iliac vein**, **superficial epigastric vein**, and the **superficial external pudendal vein** (see Figs. 8.38 and 8.46). These veins correspond with the like-named three branches of the femoral artery found in this region.

An additional vein, known as the **accessory vein**, usually joins the main vein about the middle of the thigh or higher up at the saphenous opening (see Fig. 8.46).

Many small veins from the back of the thigh curve around the medial and lateral aspects of the thigh and ultimately drain into the great saphenous vein. Superficial veins from the lower part of the back of the thigh join the small saphenous vein in the popliteal fossa.

The **small saphenous vein** is described later in this chapter, with the back of the leg.

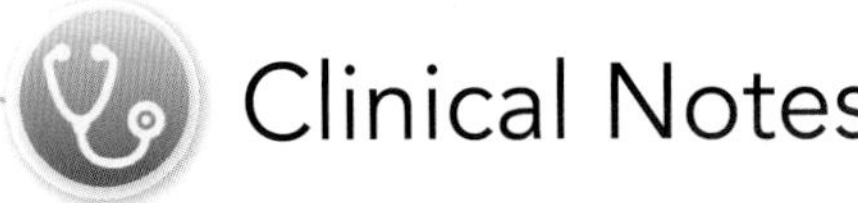

Clinical Notes

Lower Limb Veins

The veins of the lower limb are organized into three groups: superficial, deep, and perforating (see Fig. 8.46). The **superficial veins** consist of the great and small saphenous veins and their tributaries, which are situated beneath the skin in the superficial fascia. The constant position of the great saphenous vein in front of the medial malleolus should be remembered for patients requiring emergency blood transfusion. The **deep veins** are the venae comitantes to the anterior and posterior tibial arteries, the popliteal vein, and the femoral veins and their tributaries. The **perforating veins** are communicating vessels that run between the superficial and deep veins. Many of these veins are found particularly in the region of the ankle and the medial side of the lower part of the leg. They possess **valves** that are arranged to allow the flow of blood only from the superficial veins to the deep veins.

Lower Limb Venous Pump

Within the closed fascial compartments of the lower limb, the thin-walled, valved venae comitantes are subjected to intermittent pressure at rest and during exercise. The pulsations of the adjacent arteries help move the blood up the limb. However, the contractions of the large muscles within the compartments during exercise compress these deeply placed veins and force the blood up the limb.

The superficial saphenous veins, except near their termination, lie within the superficial fascia and are not subject to these compression forces. The valves in the perforating veins prevent the high-pressure venous blood from being forced outward into the low-pressure superficial veins. Moreover, as the muscles within the closed fascial compartments relax, venous blood is sucked from the superficial into the deep veins.

Varicose Veins

A varicosed vein has a larger diameter than normal and is elongated and tortuous. This condition commonly occurs in the superficial veins of the lower limb and, although not life threatening, may cause considerable discomfort.

Varicose veins have many causes, including hereditary weakness of the vein walls, incompetent valves, elevated intra-abdominal pressure as a result of multiple pregnancies or abdominal tumors, and thrombophlebitis of the deep veins, which results in the superficial veins becoming the main venous pathway for the lower limb. It is easy to understand how this condition can be produced by incompetence of a valve in a perforating vein. Every time the patient exercises, high-pressure venous blood escapes from the deep veins into the superficial veins and produces a varicosity, which might be localized to begin with but becomes more extensive later.

The successful operative treatment of varicose veins depends on the ligation and division of all the main tributaries of the great or small saphenous veins to prevent a collateral venous circulation from developing, and the ligation and division of all the perforating veins responsible for the leakage of high-pressure blood from the deep to the superficial veins. In addition, a common practice is now to remove or strip the superficial veins. It is imperative to ascertain that the deep veins are patent before taking operative measures.

Great Saphenous Vein Cutdown

Exposure of the great saphenous vein through a skin incision (**cutdown**) is usually performed at the ankle (Fig. 8.47A). This site has the disadvantage that phlebitis (inflammation of the vein wall) is a potential complication. The great saphenous vein also can be entered at the groin in the femoral triangle (Fig. 8.47C), where phlebitis is relatively rare. The larger diameter of the vein at this site permits the use of large-diameter catheters and the rapid infusion of large volumes of fluids.

Anatomy of Ankle Vein Cutdown

The procedure is as follows:

1. The sensory nerve supply to the skin immediately in front of the medial malleolus of the tibia is from branches of the **saphenous nerve**, a branch of the femoral nerve. The saphenous nerve branches are blocked with local anesthetic.
2. A transverse incision is made through the skin and subcutaneous tissue across the long axis of the vein just anterior and superior to the medial malleolus (see Fig. 8.47A,B). The vein is constantly found at this site, even though it may not be visible through the skin.
3. The vein is easily identified, and the saphenous nerve should be recognized. The nerve usually lies just anterior to the vein.

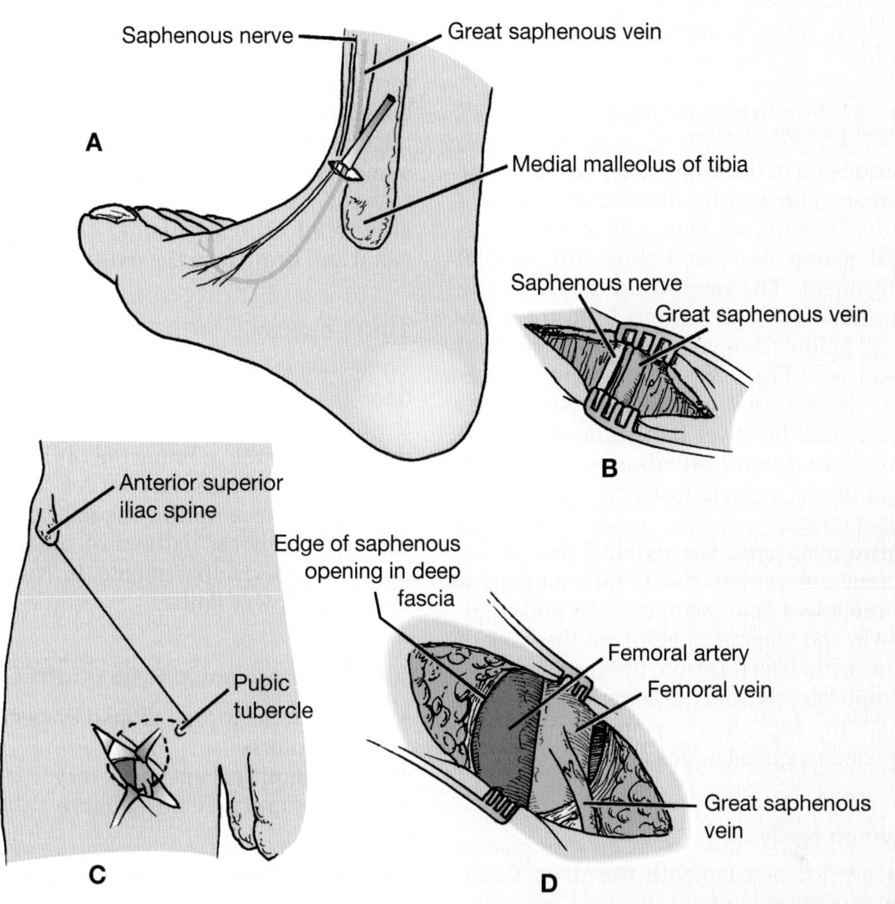

Figure 8.47 Great saphenous vein cutdown. **A and B.** At the ankle. The great saphenous vein is constantly found in front of the medial malleolus of the tibia. **C and D.** At the groin. The great saphenous vein drains into the femoral vein two fingerbreadths below and lateral to the pubic tubercle.

Anatomy of Groin Vein Cutdown

1. Branches of the **ilioinguinal nerve** and the **intermediate cutaneous nerve of the thigh** supply the area of thigh skin below and lateral to the scrotum or labium majus. The branches of these nerves are blocked with local anesthetic.
2. A transverse incision is made through the skin and subcutaneous tissue centered on a point about 1.5 in. (4 cm) below and lateral to the pubic tubercle (Fig. 8.47C,D). If the femoral pulse can be felt (it may be absent in patients with severe shock), the incision is carried medially just medial to the pulse.
3. The great saphenous vein lies in the subcutaneous fat and passes posteriorly through the saphenous opening in the deep fascia to join the femoral vein about 1.5 in. (4 cm), or two fingerbreadths below and lateral to the pubic tubercle. It is important to understand that the great saphenous vein passes through the saphenous opening to gain entrance to the femoral vein. However, the size and shape of the opening are subject to variation.

Great Saphenous Vein in Coronary Bypass Surgery

In patients with occlusive coronary disease caused by atherosclerosis, the diseased arterial segment can be bypassed by inserting a graft consisting of a portion of the great saphenous vein. The venous segment is reversed so that its valves do not obstruct the arterial flow. Following removal of the great saphenous vein at the donor site, the superficial venous blood ascends the lower limb by passing through the perforating veins and entering the deep veins.

The great saphenous vein can also be used to bypass obstructions of the brachial or femoral arteries.

Inguinal Lymph Nodes

The inguinal lymph nodes are divided into superficial and deep groups.

Superficial Inguinal Lymph Nodes

The superficial nodes lie in the superficial fascia below the inguinal ligament and can be divided into a horizontal and a vertical group (see Figs. 8.38 and 8.39).

The **horizontal group** lies just below and parallel to the inguinal ligament. The **medial members** of the group receive superficial lymph vessels from the anterior abdominal wall below the level of the umbilicus and from the perineum (see Fig. 8.39). The lymph vessels from the urethra, the external genitalia of both sexes (but not the testes), and the lower half of the anal canal drain by this route. The **lateral members** of the group receive superficial lymph vessels from the back below the level of the iliac crests.

The **vertical group** lies along the terminal part of the great saphenous vein and receives most of the superficial lymph vessels of the lower limb (see Figs. 8.38 and 8.39). Lymph from the skin and superficial fascia on the back of the thigh drains upward and forward into the vertical group.

The efferent lymph vessels from the superficial inguinal nodes pass through the saphenous opening in the deep fascia and join the deep inguinal nodes (see Fig. 8.39).

Deep Inguinal Lymph Nodes

The deep nodes are located beneath the deep fascia and lie along the medial side of the femoral vein (see Femoral Sheath below). The efferent vessels from these nodes enter the abdomen by passing through the femoral canal to lymph nodes along the external iliac artery (see Fig. 8.39).

The deep inguinal lymph nodes are variable in number, but there are commonly three. They lie along the medial side of the terminal part of the femoral vein, and the most superior is usually located in the femoral canal. They receive all the lymph from the superficial inguinal nodes via lymph vessels that pass through the cribriform fascia of the saphenous opening. They also receive lymph from the deep structures of the lower limb that have ascended in lymph vessels alongside the arteries, some having passed through the popliteal nodes. The efferent lymph vessels from the deep inguinal nodes ascend into the abdominal cavity through the femoral canal and drain into the external iliac nodes.

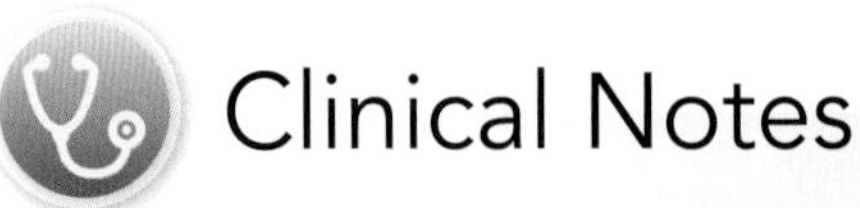

Lower Limb Lymphatics

The superficial and deep inguinal lymph nodes not only drain all the lymph from the lower limb but also drain lymph from the skin and superficial fascia of the anterior and posterior abdominal walls below the level of the umbilicus. Lymph from the external genitalia and the mucous membrane of the lower half of the anal canal also drains into these nodes. Remember the large distances the lymph has had to travel in some instances before it reaches the inguinal nodes. For example, a patient may present with an enlarged, painful inguinal lymph node caused by lymphatic spread of pathogenic organisms that entered the body through a small scratch on the undersurface of the great toe.

Thigh Fascial Compartments and Muscles

Three fascial septa pass from the inner aspect of the deep fascial sheath of the thigh to the linea aspera of the femur (see Fig. 8.45). This arrangement divides the thigh into three compartments, each having its own complement of muscles, nerves, and arteries. The compartments are anterior, medial, and posterior in position. This general pattern of organization of the limb into defined compartments is the same in both the upper and lower limbs.

Anterior Fascial Compartment Contents

- **Muscles:** Sartorius, iliopsoas, pectineus, and quadriceps femoris
- **Blood supply:** Femoral artery
- **Nerve supply:** Femoral nerve

Anterior Fascial Compartment Muscles

The muscles are illustrated in Figures 8.45 and 8.48 through 8.51 and summarized in Table 8.2. Recall that the iliacus and psoas major are separate muscles in the abdomen, but merge together in the thigh to form a single iliopsoas muscle.

Action of Quadriceps Femoris Muscle (Quadriceps Mechanism)

The quadriceps femoris muscle (consisting of the rectus femoris, vastus intermedius, vastus lateralis, and vastus medialis) inserts into the patella and, via the **ligamentum patellae (patellar ligament)**, attaches to the tibial tuberosity (Fig. 8.52). Together, they provide a powerful extensor of the knee joint. Some of the tendinous fibers of the vastus lateralis and vastus medialis form bands, or **retinacula**, which join the capsule of the knee joint and strengthen it. The lowest muscle fibers of the vastus medialis are almost horizontal and prevent the patella from being pulled laterally during contraction of the quadriceps muscle. The tone of the quadriceps muscle greatly strengthens the knee joint. The rectus femoris muscle is the only component of the quadriceps that crosses the hip joint, and it flexes the hip in addition to extending the knee. Some authors now describe a new, separate, fifth component of the quadriceps mass named the tensor vastus intermedius. This lies between the vastus intermedius and vastus lateralis and inserts into the patella via the quadriceps tendon. Its functional significance remains uncertain at present.

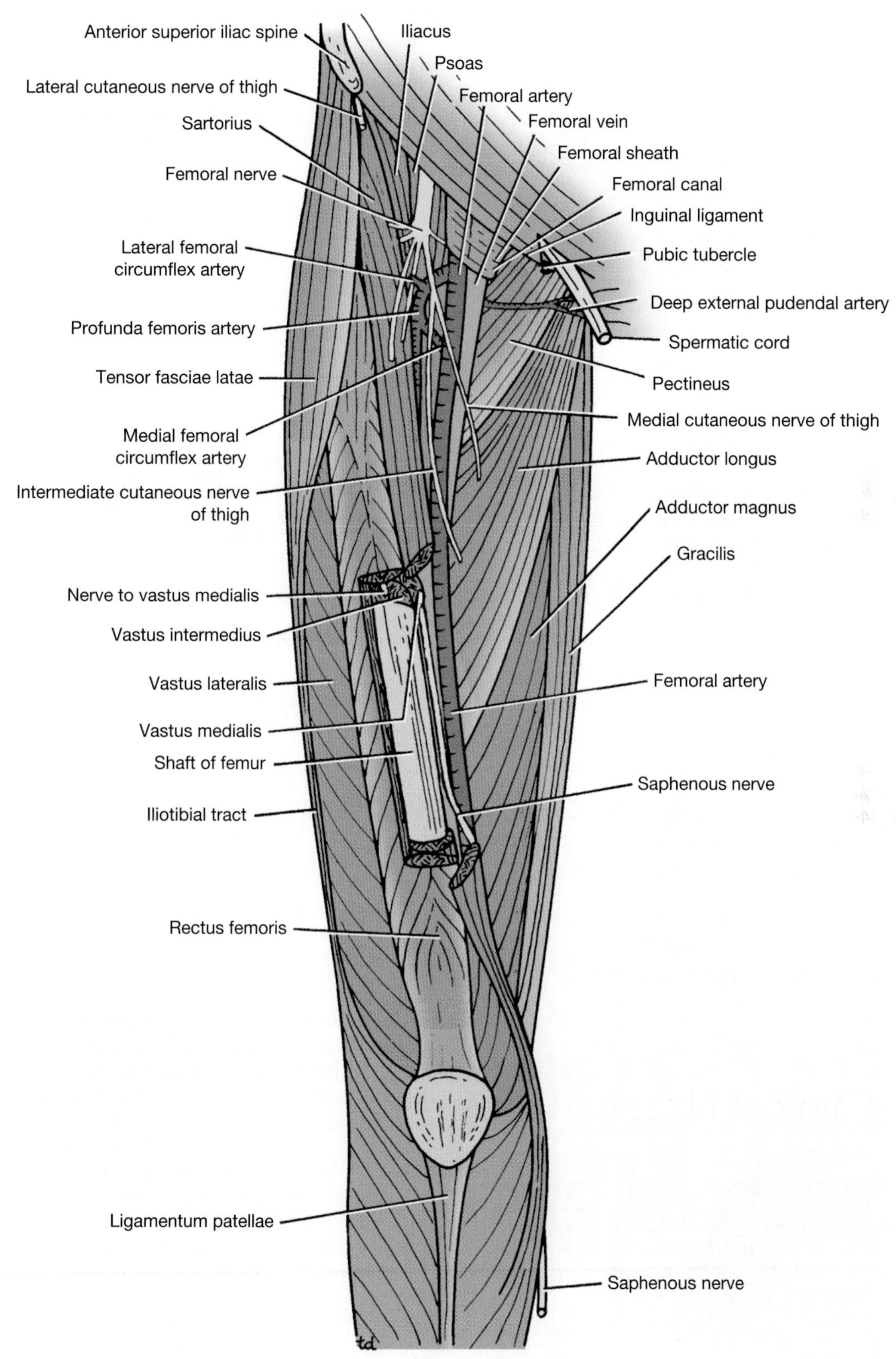

Figure 8.48 Femoral triangle and adductor (subsartorial) canal in the right lower limb.

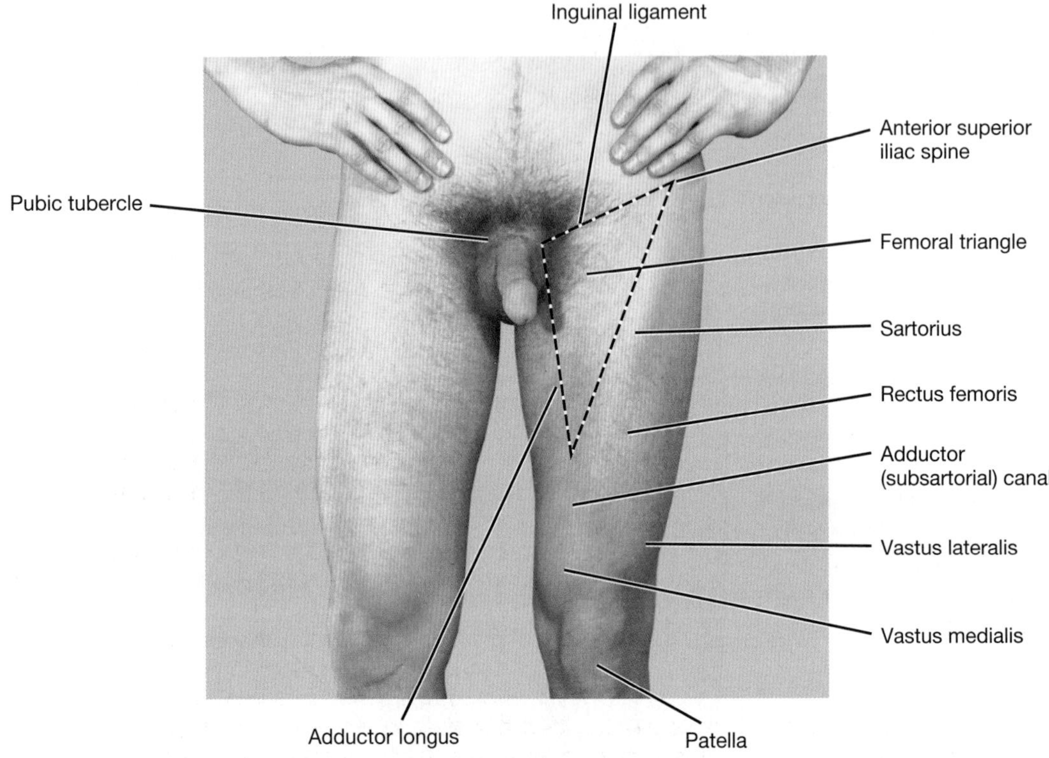

Figure 8.49 Femoral triangle and adductor canal in the left thigh of a young adult male. The broken lines indicate the boundaries of the femoral triangle.

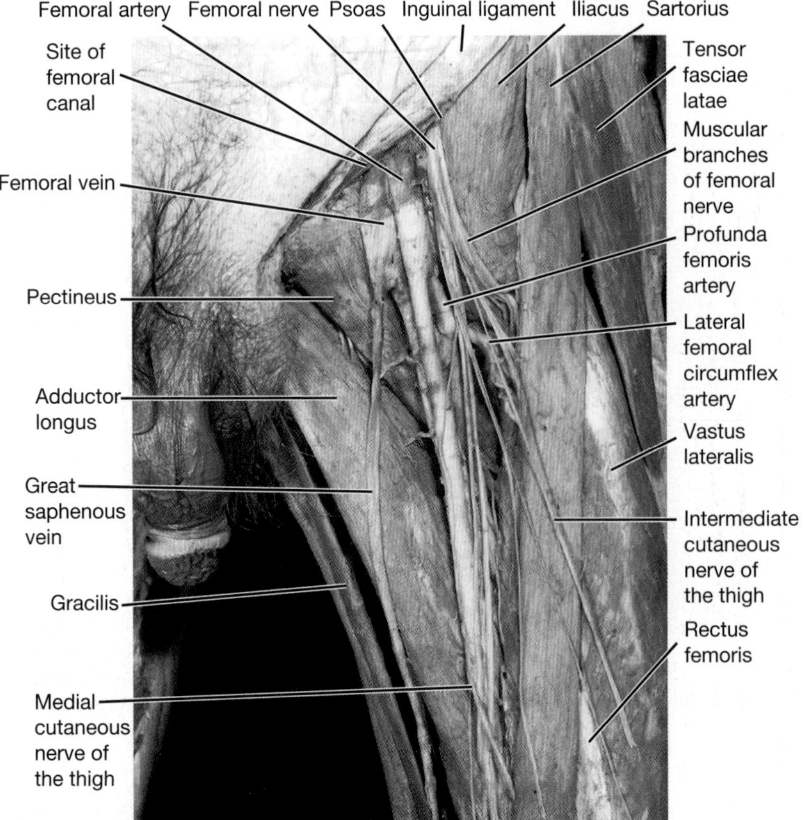

Figure 8.50 Dissection of the femoral triangle in the left lower limb.

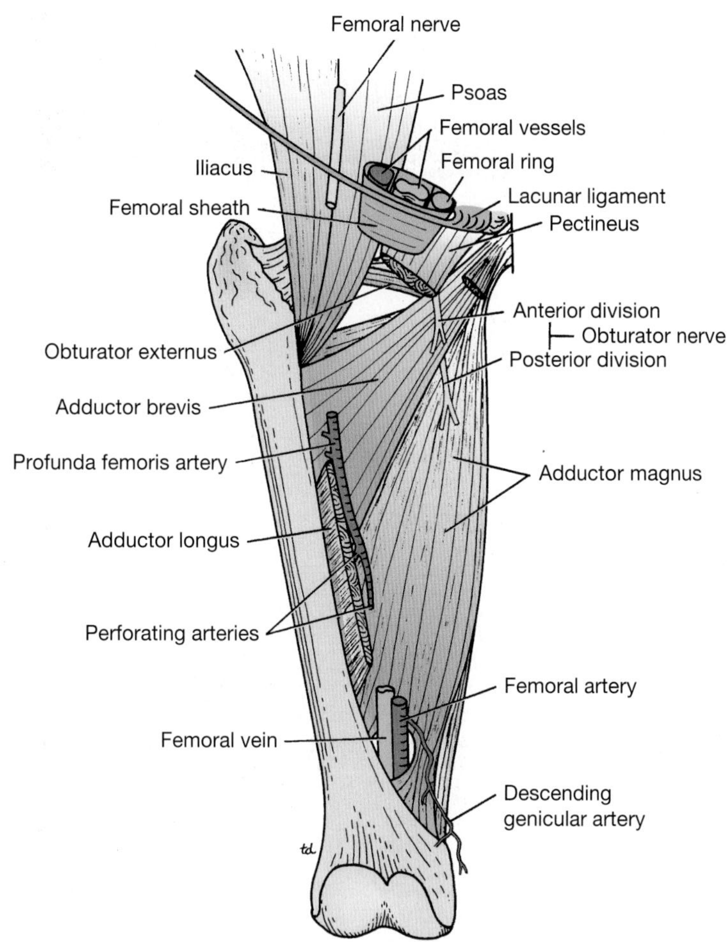

Figure 8.51 Relationship between the obturator nerve and the adductor muscles in the right lower limb.

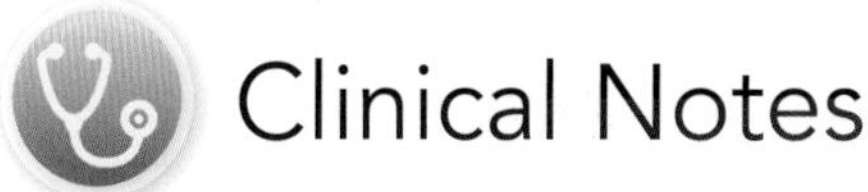

Clinical Notes

Quadriceps Femoris as Knee Joint Stabilizer

The quadriceps femoris is the most important extensor muscle for the knee joint. Its tone greatly strengthens the joint; therefore, this muscle mass must be carefully examined when the disease of the knee joint is suspected. Both thighs should be examined, and the size, consistency, and strength of the quadriceps muscles should be tested. Reduction in size caused by muscle atrophy can be evaluated by measuring the circumference of each thigh a fixed distance above the superior border of the patella.

The vastus medialis muscle extends farther distally than the vastus lateralis. The vastus medialis is the first part of the quadriceps muscle to atrophy in knee joint disease and the last to recover.

Rectus Femoris Rupture

The rectus femoris muscle can rupture in sudden violent extension movements of the knee joint. The muscle belly retracts proximally, leaving a gap that may be palpable on the anterior surface of the thigh. Surgical repair is indicated in complete rupture of the muscle.

Ligamentum Patellae Rupture

Very strong force is required to tear the patellar ligament. This can occur when the knee is flexed and the foot planted, such as during forceful running or jumping. Also, direct impact to the front of the knee, deep lacerations, and ligament weakness are common causes. In a complete tear, the patella is detached from the tibia and the patient cannot fully extend (straighten) their knee. Sometimes, the ligament does not tear, but rather avulses the tibial tuberosity with the attached ligament. In both cases, the patella may retract proximally owing to reactive muscle spasticity and locate above the knee.

Table 8.2 Muscles of Anterior Fascial Compartment of Thigh

MUSCLE	ORIGIN	INSERTION	NERVE SUPPLY	NERVE ROOT[a]	ACTION
Sartorius	Anterosuperior iliac spine	Upper medial surface of shaft of tibia	Femoral nerve	L2, L3	Flexes, abducts, laterally rotates thigh at hip joint; flexes and medially rotates leg at knee joint
Iliacus	Iliac fossa of hip bone	With psoas into lesser trochanter of femur	Femoral nerve	**L2**, L3	Flexes thigh on trunk; if thigh is fixed, it flexes the trunk on the thigh as in sitting up from lying down
Psoas	Transverse processes, bodies, and intervertebral discs of the 12th thoracic and five lumbar vertebrae	With iliacus into lesser trochanter of femur	Lumbar plexus	**L1**, **L2**, L3	Flexes thigh on trunk; if thigh is fixed, it flexes the trunk on thigh as in sitting up from lying down
Pectineus	Superior ramus of pubis	Upper end of linea aspera of shaft of femur	Femoral nerve (sometimes obturator nerve)	**L2**, L3	Flexes and adducts thigh at hip joint
Quadriceps Femoris					
Rectus femoris	Straight head: anteroinferior iliac spine Reflected head: ilium above acetabulum	Quadriceps tendon into patella, then via ligamentum patellae into tubercle of tibia	Femoral nerve	L2, **L3**, **L4**	Extension of leg at knee joint; flexes thigh at hip joint
Vastus lateralis	Upper end and shaft of femur	Quadriceps tendon into patella, then via ligamentum patellae into tubercle of tibia	Femoral nerve	L2, **L3**, **L4**	Extension of leg at knee joint
Vastus medialis	Upper end and shaft of femur	Quadriceps tendon into patella, then via ligamentum patellae into tubercle of tibia	Femoral nerve	L2, **L3**, **L4**	Extension of leg at knee joint; stabilizes patella
Vastus intermedius	Anterior and lateral surfaces of shaft of femur	Quadriceps tendon into patella, then via ligamentum patellae into tubercle of tibia	Femoral nerve	L2, **L3**, **L4**	Extension of leg at knee joint; articularis genus retracts synovial membrane

[a]The predominant nerve root supply is in bold.

Femoral Triangle

The femoral triangle is a triangular depression situated in the upper part of the medial aspect of the thigh just below the inguinal ligament (see Figs. 8.48 to 8.50). Its boundaries are as follows:

- **Superiorly:** Inguinal ligament
- **Laterally:** Sartorius muscle
- **Medially:** Adductor longus muscle
- **Floor:** Gutter shaped and formed from lateral to medial by the iliopsoas, pectineus, and adductor longus muscles
- **Roof:** Skin and fasciae of the thigh

The major contents of the femoral triangle are as follows:

- Femoral nerve and its terminal branches
- Femoral sheath
- Femoral artery and its branches
- Femoral vein and its tributaries
- Deep inguinal lymph nodes

Adductor (Subsartorial) Canal

The adductor canal is an intermuscular cleft situated on the medial aspect of the middle third of the thigh deep to the sartorius muscle (see Figs. 8.45, 8.48, and 8.49).

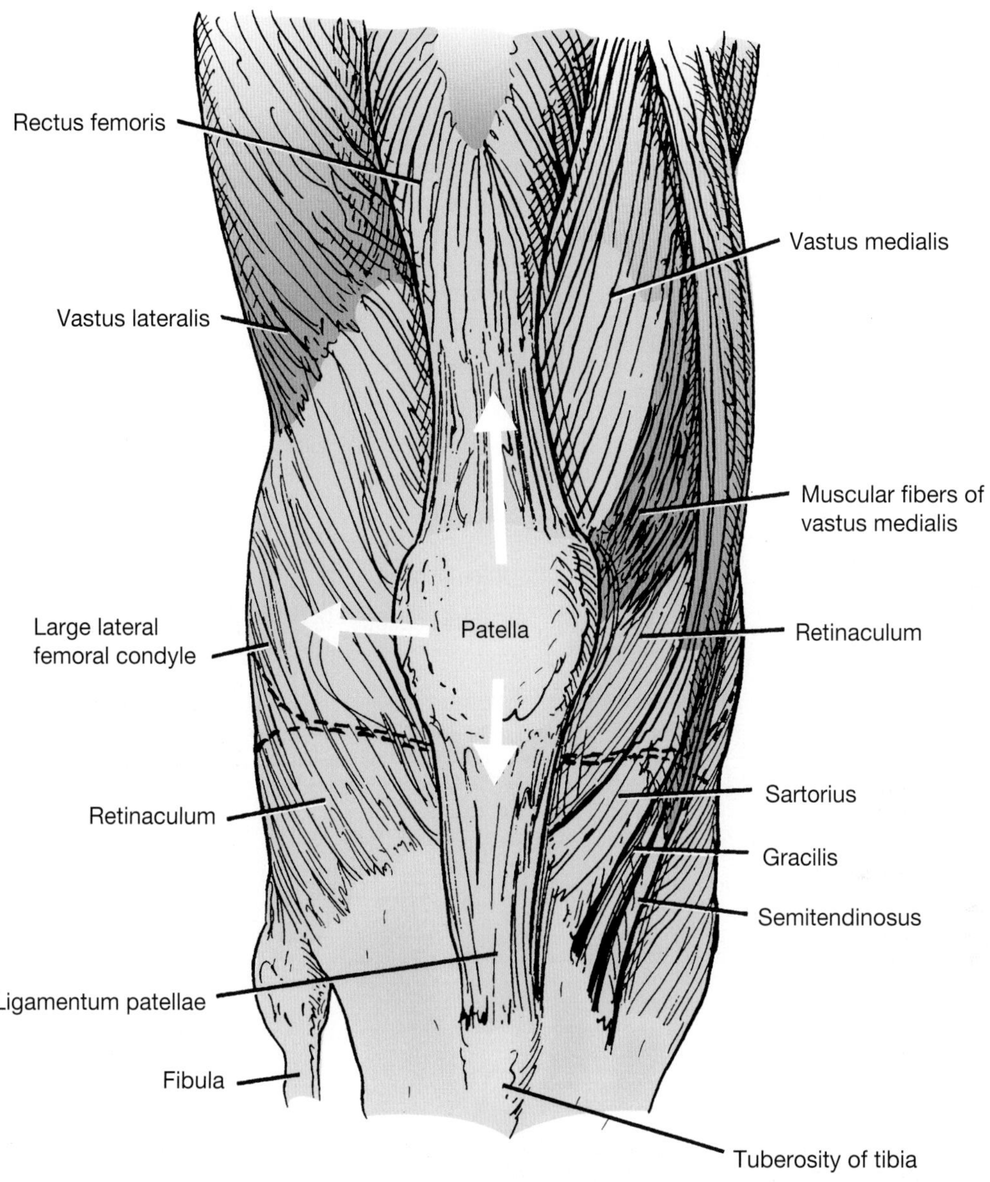

Figure 8.52 Quadriceps femoris mechanism. The lateral and upward pull of the powerful rectus femoris and the vastus lateralis muscles on the patella is counteracted by the lowest horizontal muscular fibers of the vastus medialis and the large lateral condyle of the femur, which projects forward.

It begins above at the apex of the femoral triangle and ends below at the adductor hiatus (the opening in the adductor magnus). In cross section, it is triangular and has three walls:

- The **anteromedial wall** is formed by the sartorius muscle and fascia.
- The **posterior wall** is formed by the adductor longus and magnus.
- The **lateral wall** is formed by the vastus medialis.

The adductor canal contains the following:

- Terminal part of the femoral artery
- Femoral vein
- Deep lymph vessels
- Saphenous nerve, the nerve to the vastus medialis, and the terminal part of the obturator nerve

Femoral Sheath

The femoral sheath (Fig. 8.53; see also Figs. 8.38, 8.48, and 8.51) is a downward protrusion of the fascial lining of the abdominal walls into the thigh. Its anterior wall is continuous above with the transversalis fascia and its posterior wall with the fascia iliaca. The sheath surrounds the femoral vessels and lymphatics for about 1 in. (2.5 cm) below the inguinal ligament. Thin fibrous

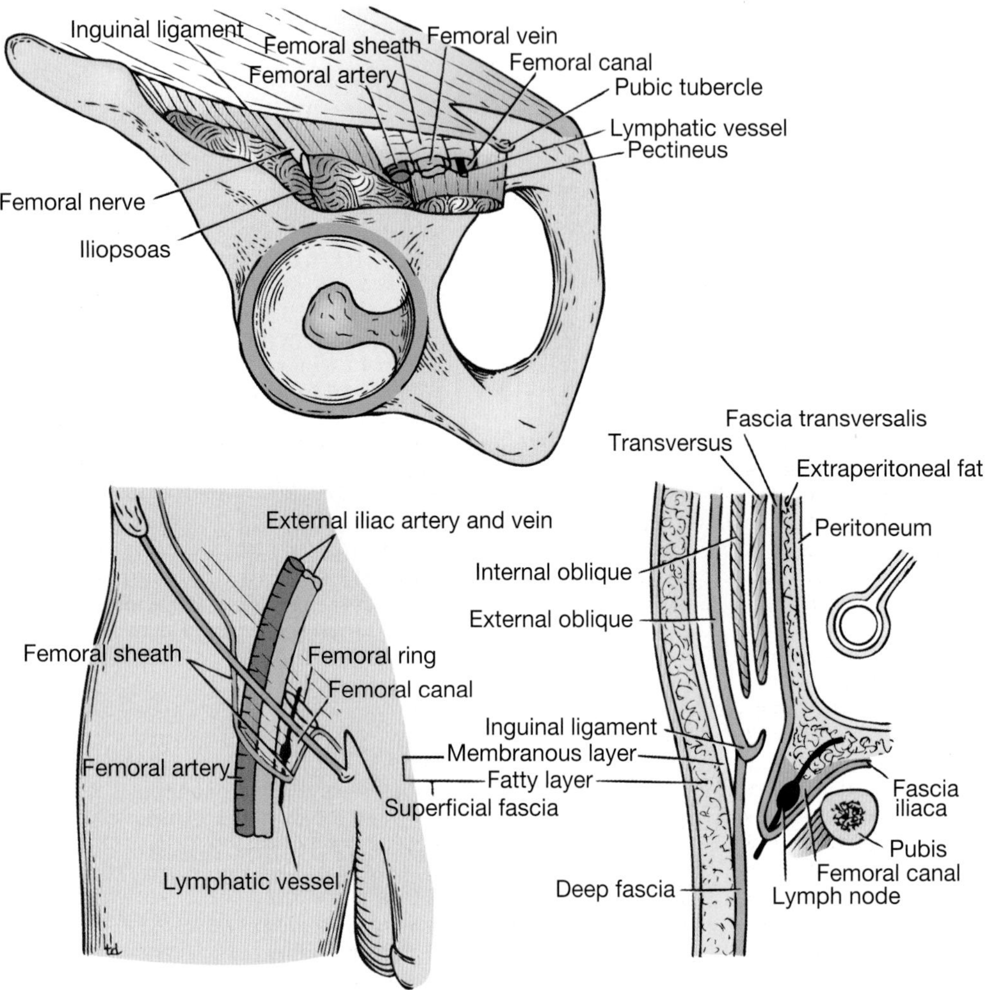

Figure 8.53 Right femoral sheath and its contents.

septa divide the sheath into three compartments: lateral, intermediate, and medial.

The **femoral artery**, as it enters the thigh beneath the inguinal ligament, occupies the **lateral compartment** of the sheath. The **femoral vein**, as it leaves the thigh, lies medial to the artery and occupies the **intermediate compartment**. Lymph vessels occupy the most **medial compartment** as they leave the thigh (see Fig. 8.53). Notice that the femoral nerve does not occupy the femoral sheath.

The small medial compartment for the lymph vessels is termed the **femoral canal**. It is about 0.5 in. (1.3 cm) long, and its upper opening is called the **femoral ring**. The **femoral septum**, which is a condensation of extraperitoneal tissue, plugs the opening of the femoral ring and closes the ring. The femoral canal contains fatty connective tissue, all the efferent lymph vessels from the deep inguinal lymph nodes, and one of the deep inguinal lymph nodes.

The femoral sheath adheres to the walls of the blood vessels and inferiorly blends with the tunica adventitia of these vessels. The part of the femoral sheath that forms the medially located femoral canal does not adhere to the walls of the small lymph vessels. Therefore, this site is a potentially weak area in the abdominal wall. A protrusion of peritoneum could be forced down the femoral canal, pushing the femoral septum before it. Such a condition is known as a **femoral hernia** and is described below.

The femoral ring has the following important relations: the inguinal ligament anteriorly, superior ramus of the pubis posteriorly, lacunar ligament medially and the femoral vein laterally.

The lower end of the femoral canal is normally closed by the adherence of its medial wall to the tunica adventitia of the femoral vein. It lies close to the saphenous opening in the deep fascia of the thigh (see Fig. 8.38).

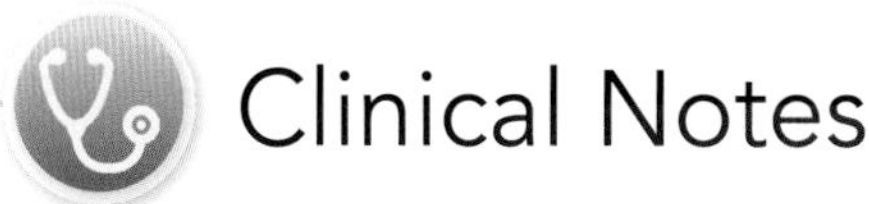

Femoral Sheath and Femoral Hernia

A femoral hernia is more common in females (possibly because of their wider pelvis and femoral canal). The **hernial sac** descends through the femoral canal within the femoral sheath, pushing the femoral septum before it. On escaping through the lower end of the femoral canal, it expands to form a swelling in the upper part of the thigh deep to the deep fascia. With further expansion, the hernial sac may turn upward to cross the anterior surface of the inguinal ligament (see Femoral Hernia in Chapter 5).

The **neck of the sac** always lies **below and lateral to the pubic tubercle** (see Figs. 5.39 and 5.40). This serves to distinguish it from an inguinal hernia, which lies above and medial to the pubic tubercle. The neck of the sac is narrow and lies at the **femoral ring**. The ring is related anteriorly to the inguinal ligament, posteriorly to the pectineal ligament and the superior ramus of the pubis, medially to the sharp free edge of the lacunar ligament, and laterally to the femoral vein. Because of these anatomic structures, the neck of the sac is unable to expand. Once an abdominal viscus has passed through the neck into the **body of the sac**, it may be difficult to push it up and return it to the abdominal cavity (**irreducible hernia**). Furthermore, after the patient strains or coughs, a piece of bowel may be forced through the neck, and its blood vessels may be compressed by the femoral ring, seriously impairing its blood supply (**strangulated hernia**). A femoral hernia is a dangerous condition and should always be treated surgically.

When considering the differential diagnosis of a femoral hernia, it is important to consider diseases that may involve other anatomic structures close to the inguinal ligament. For example:

- **Inguinal canal:** The swelling of an inguinal hernia lies above the medial end of the inguinal ligament. If the hernial sac emerges through the superficial inguinal ring to start its descent into the scrotum, the swelling will lie above and medial to the pubic tubercle. The sac of a femoral hernia lies below and lateral to the pubic tubercle.
- **Superficial inguinal lymph nodes:** Usually, more than one lymph node is enlarged. In patients with inflammation of the nodes (**lymphadenitis**), carefully examine the entire area of the body that drains its lymph into these nodes. A small, unnoticed skin abrasion may be found. Never forget the mucous membrane of the lower half of the anal canal—it may have an undiscovered carcinoma.
- **Great saphenous vein:** A localized dilation of the terminal part of the great saphenous vein, a **saphenous varix**, can cause confusion, especially because a hernia and a varix increase in size when the patient is asked to cough. (Elevated intra-abdominal pressure drives the blood downward.) The presence of varicose veins elsewhere in the leg should help in the diagnosis.
- **Psoas sheath:** Tuberculous infection of a lumbar vertebra can result in the extravasation of pus down the psoas sheath into the thigh. The presence of a swelling above and below the inguinal ligament, together with clinical signs and symptoms referred to the vertebral column, should enable a correct diagnosis.
- **Femoral artery:** An expansile swelling lying along the course of the femoral artery that fluctuates in time with the pulse rate should indicate a diagnosis of aneurysm of the femoral artery.

Anterior Fascial Compartment Blood Supply

The femoral artery and vein supply and drain the anterior compartment of the thigh. The artery is the continuation of the **external iliac artery** from the pelvis. The vein drains into the **external iliac vein**.

Femoral Artery

The femoral artery is the main arterial supply to the lower limb. It enters the thigh deep to the inguinal ligament (Fig. 8.54; see also Figs. 8.48 and 8.50). Here, it lies midway between the anterosuperior iliac spine and the symphysis pubis. It descends almost vertically toward the adductor tubercle of the femur and ends at the **adductor hiatus** (opening in the adductor magnus muscle) by entering the popliteal space as the **popliteal artery** (see Fig. 8.51).

RELATIONS

- **Anteriorly:** In the upper part of its course, it is superficial and is covered by the skin and fascia roofing the femoral triangle. In the lower part of its course, it passes deep to the sartorius muscle in the adductor canal (see Fig. 8.48).
- **Posteriorly:** The artery lies on the iliopsoas muscle, which separates it from the hip joint, the pectineus, and the adductor longus. The femoral vein intervenes between the artery and the adductor longus.
- **Medially:** It is related to the femoral vein in the upper part of its course (see Figs. 8.48 and 8.50).
- **Laterally:** The femoral nerve and its branches (see Fig. 8.48).

BRANCHES

- The **superficial circumflex iliac artery** is a small branch that runs up to the region of the anterosuperior iliac spine (see Fig. 8.38B).
- The **superficial epigastric artery** is a small branch that crosses the inguinal ligament and runs to the region of the umbilicus.
- The **superficial external pudendal artery** is a small branch that runs medially to supply the skin of the scrotum (males) or labium majus (females).

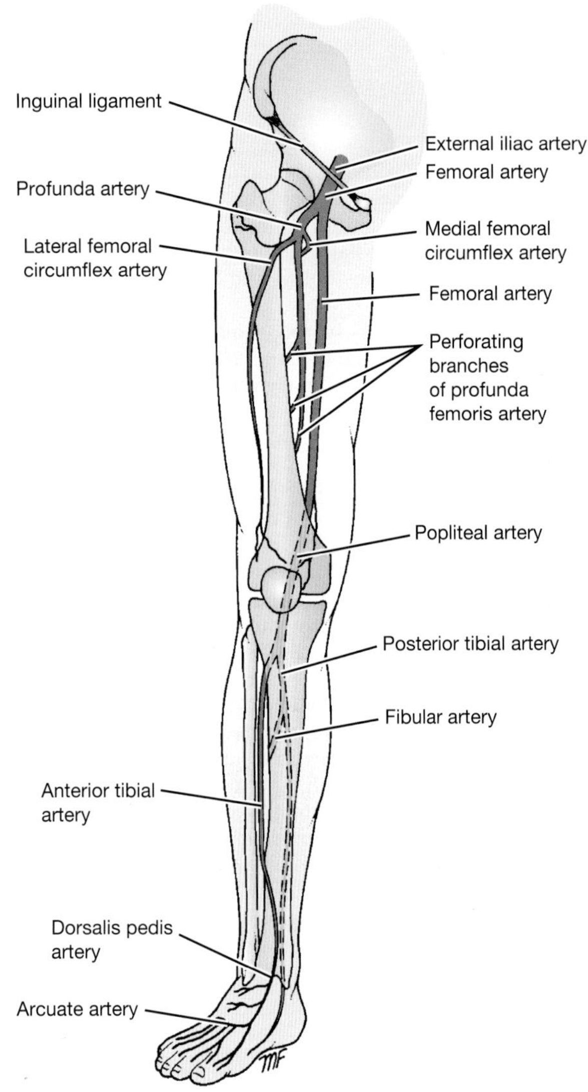

Figure 8.54 Major arteries of the lower limb.

- The **deep external pudendal artery** (see Fig. 8.48) runs medially and supplies the skin of the scrotum or labium majus.
- The **profunda femoris artery** is a large and important branch that arises from the lateral side of the femoral artery about 1.5 in. (4 cm) below the inguinal ligament (see Figs. 8.48, 8.50, and 8.54). It passes medially behind the femoral vessels and enters the medial fascial compartment of the thigh (Fig. 8.55; see also Figs. 8.50 and 8.51). At its origin, it gives off the **medial** and **lateral femoral circumflex arteries**; during its course, it gives off **three perforating arteries** (see Figs. 8.54 and 8.55). It ends by becoming the **fourth perforating artery** (see Fig. 8.55).
- The **descending genicular artery** is a small branch that arises from the femoral artery near its termination (see Fig. 8.51). It assists in supplying the knee joint.

Femoral Vein

The femoral vein enters the thigh by passing through the **adductor hiatus** (opening in the adductor magnus muscle) as a continuation of the **popliteal vein** (see Fig. 8.51). It ascends through the thigh, lying at first on the lateral side of the artery, then posterior to it, and finally on its medial side (see Fig. 8.48). It leaves the thigh in the intermediate compartment of the femoral sheath and passes behind the inguinal ligament to become the **external iliac vein** (see Fig. 8.53).

The tributaries of the femoral vein are the **great saphenous vein** and the veins that correspond to the branches of the femoral artery (see Fig. 8.38). The superficial circumflex iliac vein, superficial epigastric vein, and external pudendal veins drain into the great saphenous vein.

Anterior Fascial Compartment Nerve Supply

The **femoral nerve** is the largest branch of the lumbar plexus (L2 to L4). It emerges from the lateral border of

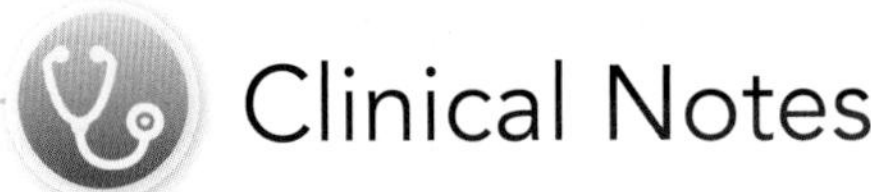

Clinical Notes

Femoral Artery Catheterization

A long, fine catheter can be inserted into the femoral artery as it descends through the femoral triangle. The catheter is guided under fluoroscopic view along the external and common iliac arteries into the aorta. The catheter can then be passed into the inferior mesenteric, superior mesenteric, celiac, or renal arteries. Contrast medium can then be injected into the artery under examination and a permanent record obtained by taking a radiograph. Pressure records can also be obtained by guiding the catheter through the aortic valve into the left ventricle.

Femoral Vein Catheterization

Femoral vein catheterization is used when rapid access to a large vein is needed. The femoral vein has a constant relationship to the medial side of the femoral artery just below the inguinal ligament and is easily cannulated. However, because of the high incidence of thrombosis with the possibility of fatal pulmonary embolism, the catheter should be removed once the patient is stabilized.

Anatomy of the Procedure

1. The genitofemoral nerve supplies the skin of the thigh below the inguinal ligament. This nerve is blocked with a local anesthetic.
2. The femoral pulse is palpated midway between the anterosuperior iliac spine and the symphysis pubis, and the femoral vein lies immediately medial to it.
3. At a site about two fingerbreadths below the inguinal ligament, the needle is inserted into the femoral vein.

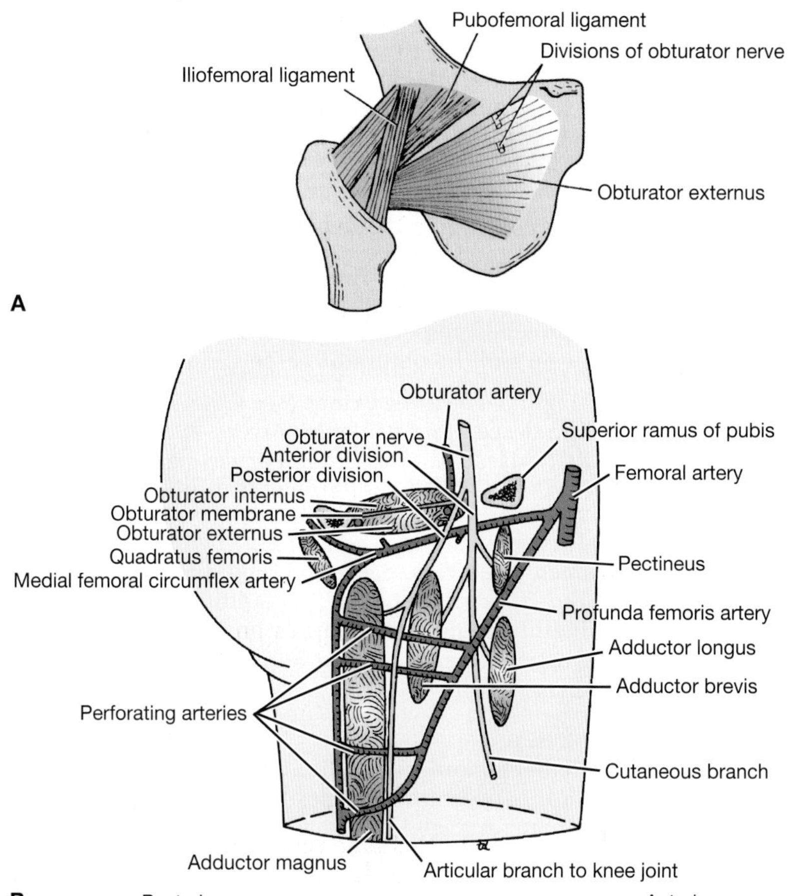

Figure 8.55 **A.** Obturator externus muscle in anterior view. **B.** Vertical section (lateral view) of the medial compartment of the thigh. Note the courses taken by the obturator nerve and its divisions and the profunda femoris artery and its branches. Also, note the anastomosis between the perforating arteries and the medial femoral circumflex artery.

the psoas major muscle within the abdomen and passes downward in the interval between the psoas major and iliacus. It lies behind the fascia iliaca and enters the thigh lateral to the femoral artery and the femoral sheath, behind the inguinal ligament (see Figs. 8.48, 8.50, and 8.53). About 1.5 in. (4 cm) below the inguinal ligament, it terminates by dividing into anterior and posterior divisions. The femoral nerve supplies all the muscles of the anterior compartment of the thigh and has a significant cutaneous territory along the length of the limb (Fig. 8.56; see also Figs. 8.36, 8.37, and 8.48). **Note that the femoral nerve does not enter the thigh within the femoral sheath.**

Branches

ANTERIOR DIVISION

The anterior division (see Fig. 8.56) gives off two cutaneous and two muscular branches. The cutaneous branches are the **medial cutaneous nerve of the thigh** and the **intermediate cutaneous nerve** that supply the skin of the medial and anterior surfaces of the thigh, respectively (see Figs. 8.37 and 8.48). The muscular branches supply the sartorius and the pectineus. However, sometimes the **obturator nerve** supplies the pectineus.

POSTERIOR DIVISION

The posterior division (see Fig. 8.56) gives off one cutaneous branch, the **saphenous nerve**, and muscular

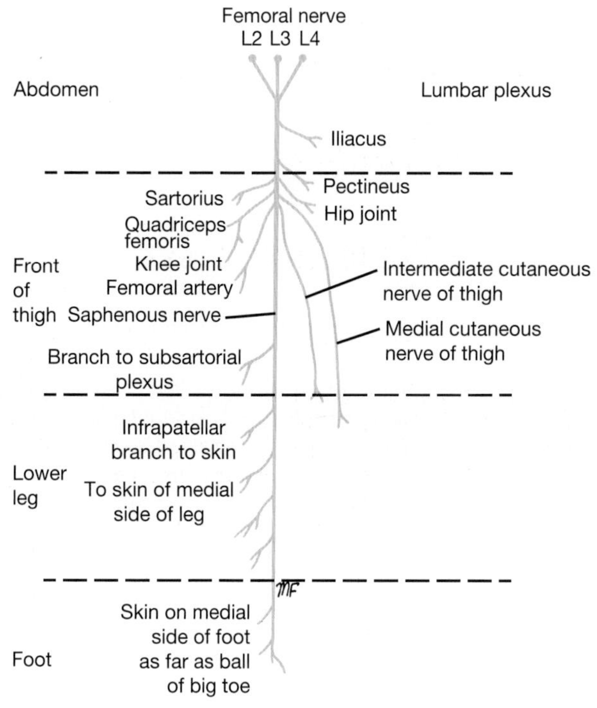

Figure 8.56 Summary of the main branches of the femoral nerve.

branches to the quadriceps muscle. The saphenous nerve runs downward and medially and crosses the femoral artery from its lateral to its medial side (see Fig. 8.48). It emerges on the medial side of the knee between the tendons of sartorius and gracilis. It then runs down the medial side of the leg in company with the great saphenous vein (see Fig. 8.37). It passes in front of the medial malleolus and along the medial border of the foot, where it terminates in the region of the ball of the great toe.

The muscular branch of the rectus femoris also supplies the hip joint. The branches to the three vasti muscles also supply the knee joint.

Medial Fascial Compartment Contents

- **Muscles:** Gracilis, adductor longus, adductor brevis, adductor magnus, and obturator externus
- **Blood supply:** Profunda femoris artery and obturator artery
- **Nerve supply:** Obturator nerve

Medial Fascial Compartment Muscles

The muscles of the medial fascial compartment are illustrated in Figures 8.45, 8.48 through 8.51, and 8.55 and summarized in Table 8.3.

Note that the **adductor magnus** is a large, triangular muscle consisting of upper adductor and lower hamstring portions (see Figs. 8.48 and 8.51). The obturator nerve innervates the adductor portion, whereas the tibial nerve supplies the hamstring portion. This duel neural organization reflects the separate developmental origins of the two parts. The **adductor hiatus** is a gap in the attachment of this muscle to the femur, which permits the femoral vessels to pass from the adductor canal downward into the popliteal space (see Fig. 8.51).

Medial Fascial Compartment Blood Supply

The profunda femoris and obturator vessels are the vascular channels for the medial compartment of the thigh. The profunda vessels are related to the femoral artery and vein and the obturator vessels to the internal iliac artery and vein.

Profunda Femoris Artery

The profunda femoris is a large artery that arises from the lateral side of the femoral artery in the femoral triangle, about 1.5 in. (4 cm) below the inguinal ligament (see Figs. 8.48, 8.54, and 8.55). It descends in the interval between the adductor longus and adductor brevis and then lies on the adductor magnus, where it ends as the fourth perforating artery (see Fig. 8.55).

BRANCHES

- **Medial femoral circumflex artery:** This passes backward between the muscles that form the floor of the femoral triangle and gives off muscular branches in the medial fascial compartment of the thigh (see Figs. 8.54 and 8.55). It takes part in the formation of the cruciate anastomosis.

Table 8.3 Muscles of the Medial Fascial Compartment of Thigh

MUSCLE	ORIGIN	INSERTION	NERVE SUPPLY	NERVE ROOT[a]	ACTION
Gracilis	Inferior ramus of pubis, ramus of ischium	Upper part of shaft of tibia on medial surface	Obturator nerve	**L2**, L3	Adducts thigh at hip joint; flexes leg at knee joint
Adductor longus	Body of pubis, medial to pubic tubercle	Posterior surface of shaft of femur (linea aspera)	Obturator nerve	L2, **L3**, **L4**	Adducts thigh at hip joint and assists in medial rotation
Adductor brevis	Inferior ramus of pubis	Posterior surface of shaft of femur (linea aspera)	Obturator nerve	L2, **L3**, **L4**	Adducts thigh at hip joint
Adductor magnus	Inferior ramus of pubis, ramus of ischium, ischial tuberosity	Posterior surface of shaft of femur, adductor tubercle of femur	Adductor portion: obturator nerve Hamstring portion: sciatic nerve	L2, **L3**, **L4**	Adducts thigh at hip joint and assists in medial rotation; hamstring portion extends thigh at hip joint
Obturator externus	Outer surface of obturator membrane and pubic and ischial rami	Medial surface of greater trochanter	Obturator nerve	L3, **L4**	Laterally rotates thigh at hip joint

[a]The predominant nerve root supply is in bold.

- **Lateral femoral circumflex artery:** This passes laterally between the terminal branches of the femoral nerve (see Figs. 8.48 and 8.54). It breaks up into branches that supply the muscles of the region and takes part in the formation of the cruciate anastomosis.
- **Four perforating arteries:** Three of these arise as branches of the profunda femoris artery. The **fourth perforating artery** is the terminal part of the profunda femoris artery (see Fig. 8.55). The perforating arteries run backward, piercing the various muscle layers. They supply the muscles and terminate by anastomosing with one another and with the inferior gluteal artery and the circumflex femoral arteries above and the muscular branches of the popliteal artery below.

Profunda Femoris Vein

The profunda femoris vein receives tributaries that correspond to the branches of the artery. It drains into the femoral vein in the femoral triangle.

Obturator Artery

The obturator artery is a branch of the internal iliac artery. It passes forward on the lateral wall of the pelvis and accompanies the obturator nerve through the **obturator canal** (ie, the upper part of the obturator foramen) (see Fig. 8.55). On entering the medial fascial compartment of the thigh, it divides into medial and lateral branches, which pass around the margin of the outer surface of the obturator membrane. It gives off muscular branches and an articular branch to the hip joint.

Obturator Vein

The obturator vein receives tributaries that correspond to the branches of the artery. It drains into the internal iliac vein.

Medial Fascial Compartment Nerve Supply

The **obturator nerve** supplies most of the medial compartment. It arises from the lumbar plexus (L2 to L4) and emerges on the medial border of the psoas major muscle within the abdomen. It runs forward on the lateral wall of the pelvis to reach the upper part of the obturator foramen, where it divides into anterior and posterior divisions (Fig. 8.57; see also Fig. 8.55). The **tibial nerve** component of the sciatic nerve supplies part of the adductor magnus muscle (see the muscle descriptions above).

Obturator Nerve Branches

- The **anterior division** passes downward in front of the obturator externus and the adductor brevis and behind the pectineus and adductor longus (see Fig. 8.55). It gives muscular branches to the gracilis, adductor brevis, and adductor longus, and occasionally to the pectineus. It gives articular branches to the hip joint and terminates as a small nerve that supplies the femoral artery. It contributes a variable branch to the subsartorial plexus and supplies the skin on the medial side of the thigh.
- The **posterior division** pierces the obturator externus and passes downward behind the adductor brevis and in front of the adductor magnus. It terminates by descending through the adductor hiatus to supply the knee joint. It gives muscular branches to the obturator externus, to the adductor part of the adductor magnus, and occasionally to the adductor brevis.

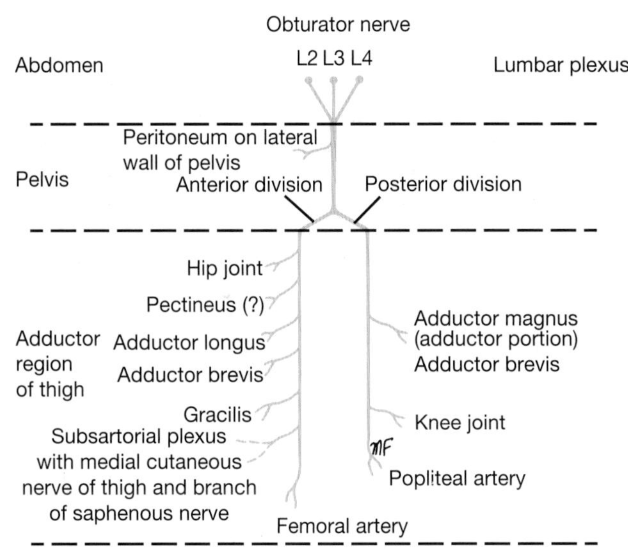

Figure 8.57 Summary of the main branches of the obturator nerve.

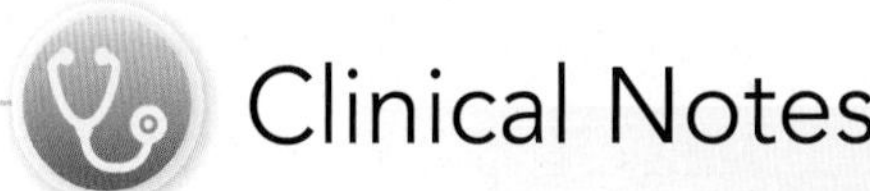

Adductor Muscles and Cerebral Palsy

In patients with cerebral palsy who have marked spasticity of the adductor group of muscles, it is common practice to perform a **tenotomy** of the adductor longus tendon and to divide the anterior division of the obturator nerve. In addition, in some severe cases, the posterior division of the obturator nerve is crushed. This operation overcomes the spasm of the adductor group of muscles and permits slow recovery of the muscles supplied by the posterior division of the obturator nerve.

Posterior Fascial Compartment Contents

- **Muscles:** Biceps femoris, semitendinosus, semimembranosus, and a small part of the adductor magnus (hamstring portion)
- **Blood supply:** Branches of the profunda femoris artery
- **Nerve supply:** Sciatic nerve (both tibial and common fibular components)

Posterior Fascial Compartment Muscles

The muscles of the posterior fascial compartment collectively are called the **hamstrings**. They are illustrated in Figures 8.58 and 8.59 and summarized in Table 8.4.

Note the following:

- The **biceps femoris** muscle has two heads: a **long head** (hamstring portion) and a **short head** (gluteal or adductor portion). It also receives a dual nerve supply from the sciatic nerve. The **tibial nerve** component innervates the long head, and the **common fibular (peroneal)** component supplies the short head.
- As noted earlier, the **adductor magnus** muscle also has two parts (upper adductor part and lower hamstring part) and a dual innervation. The **tibial nerve** component of the sciatic nerve supplies the hamstring portion, and the **obturator nerve** supplies the adductor part.
- The **semimembranosus** insertion sends a fibrous expansion upward and laterally, which reinforces the capsule on the back of the knee joint. This expansion is called the **oblique popliteal ligament** (see Figs. 8.22C and 8.23).

Posterior Compartment Blood Supply

The four **perforating branches of the profunda femoris artery** provide a rich blood supply to this compartment (see Figs. 8.54 and 8.55). The profunda femoris vein drains the greater part of the blood from the compartment.

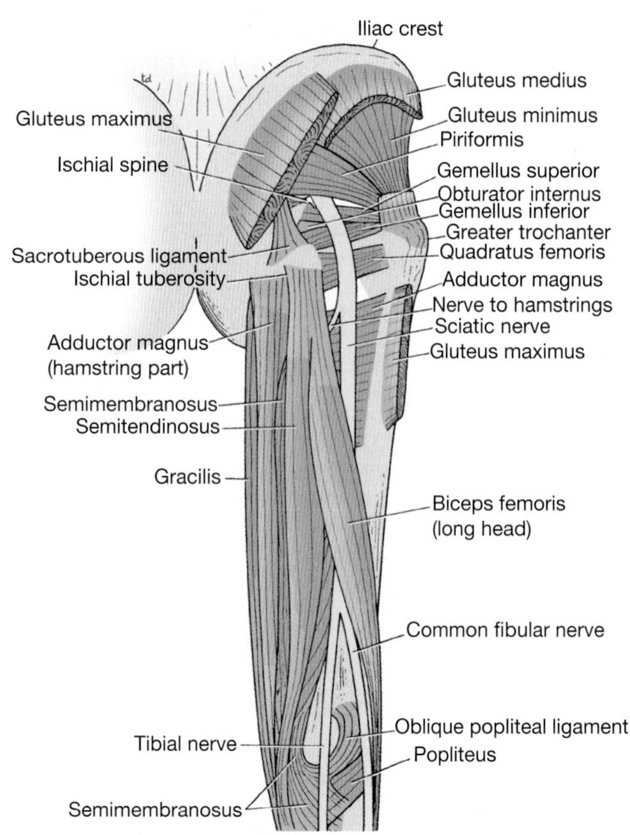

Figure 8.58 Structures in the posterior aspect of the right thigh.

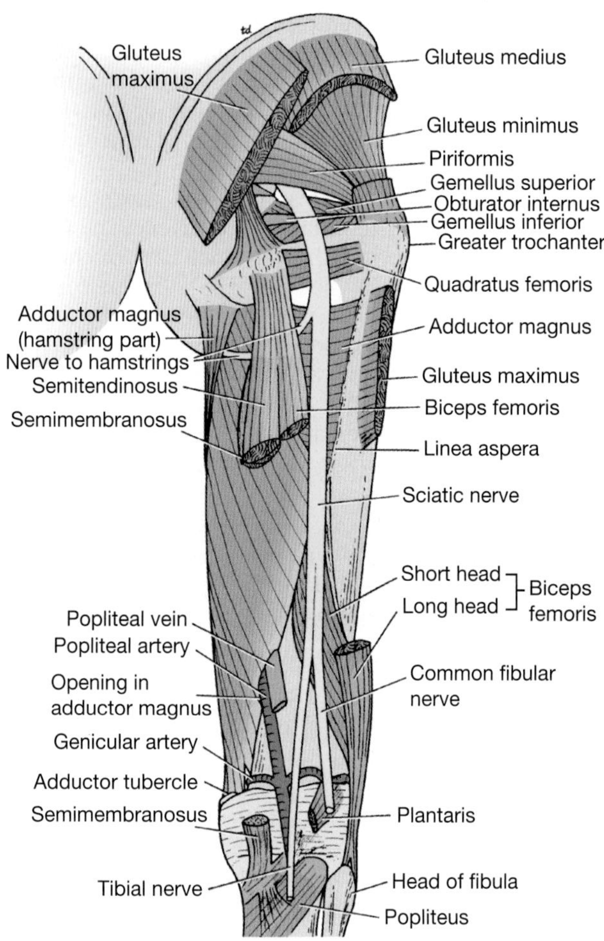

Figure 8.59 Deep structures in the posterior aspect of the right thigh.

Posterior Compartment Nerve Supply

The **sciatic nerve** leaves the gluteal region (see Gluteal Region Nerves) and descends in the midline of the posterior compartment of the thigh (see Figs. 8.58 and 8.59). It is overlapped posteriorly by the adjacent margins of the biceps femoris and semimembranosus muscles and lies on the posterior aspect of the adductor magnus muscle. It ends in the lower third of the thigh by dividing into the separate **tibial** and **common fibular (peroneal) nerves**. Occasionally, the sciatic nerve divides into its two terminal parts at a higher level—in the upper part of the thigh, gluteal region, or even inside the pelvis.

The tibial nerve supplies most of the posterior compartment of the thigh (see Fig. 8.44), whereas the common fibular nerve innervates only the short head of the biceps (see Fig. 8.43). Both the tibial and common fibular nerves enter the popliteal fossa and continue into the leg (see Figs. 8.43 and 8.44).

Table 8.4 Muscles of Posterior Fascial Compartment of Thigh

MUSCLE	ORIGIN	INSERTION	NERVE SUPPLY	NERVE ROOT[a]	ACTION
Biceps femoris	Long head: ischial tuberosity	Head of fibula	Long head: tibial portion of sciatic nerve	L5; **S1**, S2	Flexes and laterally rotates leg at knee joint; long head also extends thigh at hip joint
	Short head: linea aspera, lateral supracondylar ridge of shaft of femur		Short head: common fibular portion of sciatic nerve	L5; **S1**, S2	
Semitendinosus	Ischial tuberosity	Upper part of medial surface of shaft of tibia	Tibial portion of sciatic nerve	**L5**; **S1**, S2	Flexes and medially rotates leg at knee joint; extends thigh at hip joint
Semimembranosus	Ischial tuberosity	Medial condyle of tibia	Tibial portion of sciatic nerve	**L5**; **S1**, S2	Flexes and medially rotates leg at knee joint; extends thigh at hip joint
Adductor magnus (hamstring portion)	Ischial tuberosity	Adductor tubercle of femur	Tibial portion of sciatic nerve	L**4**, L5; S1	Extends thigh at hip joint

[a]The predominant nerve root supply is in bold.

POPLITEAL FOSSA

The popliteal fossa is a diamond-shaped intermuscular space situated at the back of the knee (Figs. 8.60 and 8.61). The fossa is most prominent when the knee joint is flexed. It contains the popliteal vessels, small saphenous vein, common fibular (peroneal) and tibial nerves, posterior cutaneous nerve of the thigh, genicular branch of the obturator nerve, connective tissue, and lymph nodes. The popliteal fossa is comparable to the cubital fossa in the upper limb, in that both connect the upper and lower segments of the limb. However, these fossae face opposite directions because of opposite developmental rotations of the limbs.

Boundaries

- **Laterally:** Biceps femoris above and the lateral head of the gastrocnemius and plantaris below
- **Medially:** Semimembranosus and semitendinosus above and the medial head of the gastrocnemius below
- **Anterior wall (floor):** Popliteal surface of the femur, capsule of the knee joint, and popliteus muscle (Fig. 8.62)
- **Roof:** Skin, the superficial fascia, and the deep fascia of the thigh

Muscles

The biceps femoris, semimembranosus, and semitendinosus muscles are described earlier in Posterior Fascial Compartment Muscles. The gastrocnemius and plantaris muscles are described later in Posterior Fascial Compartment Muscles: Superficial Group.

The **popliteus muscle** plays a key role in the movements of the knee joint. It is illustrated in Figures 8.62 and 8.63 and summarized in Table 8.7 (with the muscles of the posterior fascial compartment of the leg). The muscle arises within the capsule of the knee joint, and its tendon separates the lateral meniscus from the lateral ligament of the joint. It emerges through the lower part of the posterior surface of the capsule of the joint to pass to its insertion. The popliteus acts to flex the knee and to produce medial rotation of the tibia on the femur or, if the foot is on the ground, lateral rotation of the femur on the tibia. The latter action occurs at the commencement of flexion of the extended knee, and its rotatory action slackens the ligaments of the knee joint. This action is sometimes referred to as **unlocking the knee joint**. Because of its attachment to the lateral meniscus, it also pulls the cartilage backward at the commencement of flexion of the knee.

Popliteal Artery

The popliteal artery is the continuation of the femoral artery (see Fig. 8.54). It is deeply placed and enters the popliteal fossa through the **adductor hiatus** (see Figs. 8.51, 8.59, and 8.62). It ends at the level of the lower border of the popliteus muscle by dividing into anterior and posterior tibial arteries (see Fig. 8.62).

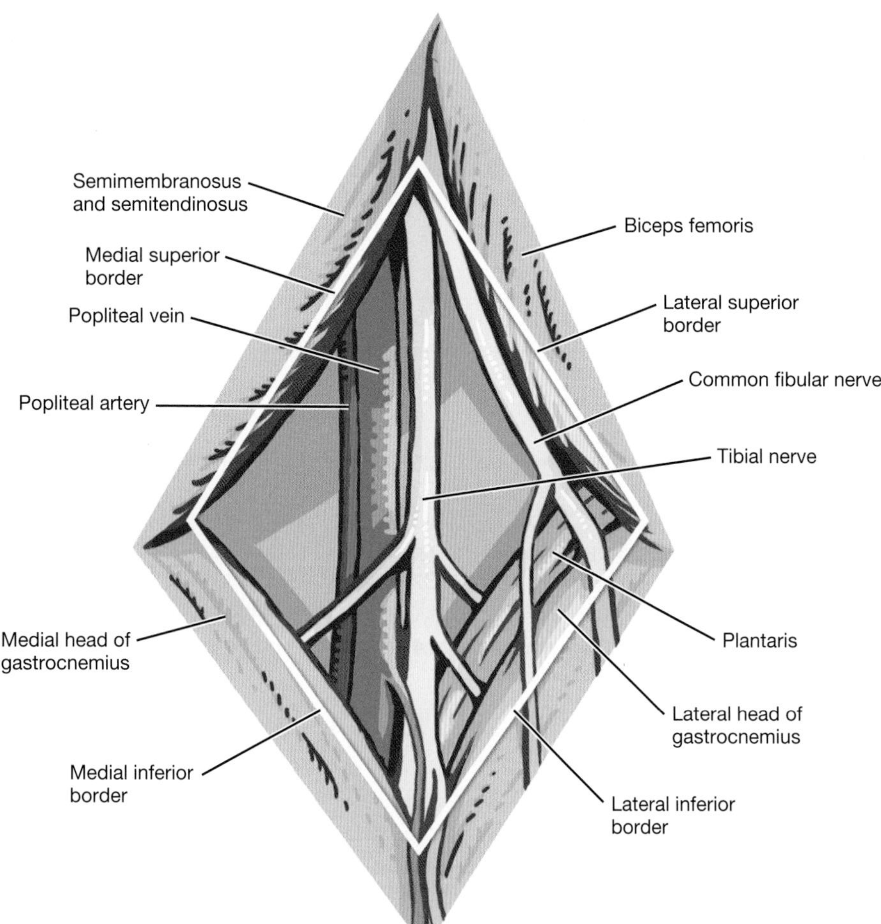

Figure 8.60 Schematic illustration of the boundaries and major contents of the right popliteal fossa. The white diamond indicates the borders of the fossa.

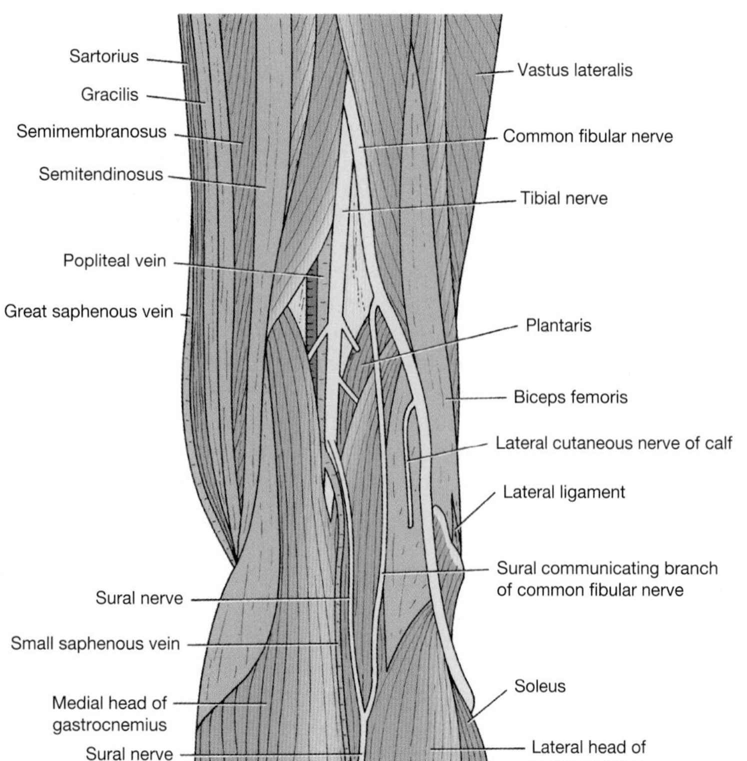

Figure 8.61 Boundaries and contents of the right popliteal fossa.

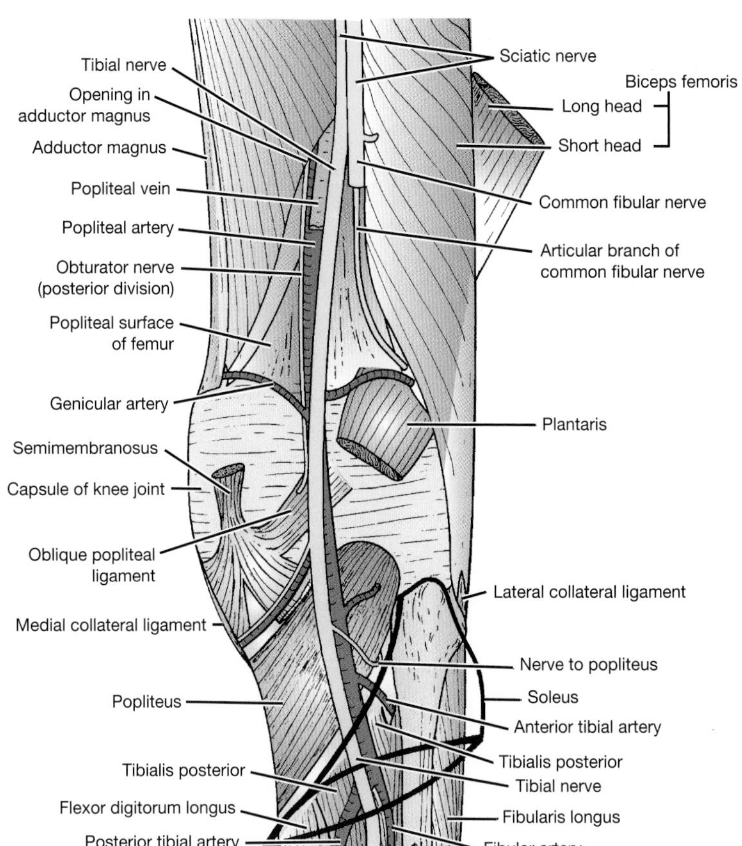

Figure 8.62 Deep structures in the right popliteal fossa. The proximal end of the soleus muscle is shown in outline only.

Relations

- **Anteriorly:** Popliteal surface of the femur, knee joint, and popliteus muscle (see Fig. 8.62)
- **Posteriorly:** Popliteal vein, tibial nerve, fascia, and skin (see Figs. 8.60 and 8.61)

Branches

The popliteal artery has muscular branches and multiple genicular branches to the knee joint (see Fig. 8.62).

Arterial Anastomosis around Knee Joint

There is a profuse anastomosis of small branches of the femoral artery with muscular and articular branches of the popliteal artery and with branches of the anterior and posterior tibial arteries. This network is necessary to compensate for the narrowing of the popliteal artery that occurs during extreme flexion of the knee.

Popliteal Vein

The popliteal vein is formed by the junction of the **venae comitantes** of the anterior and posterior tibial arteries at the lower border of the popliteus muscle on the medial side of the popliteal artery. As it ascends through the fossa, it crosses behind the popliteal artery so that it comes to lie on its lateral side (see Figs. 8.61 and 8.62). It passes through the adductor hiatus to become the femoral vein.

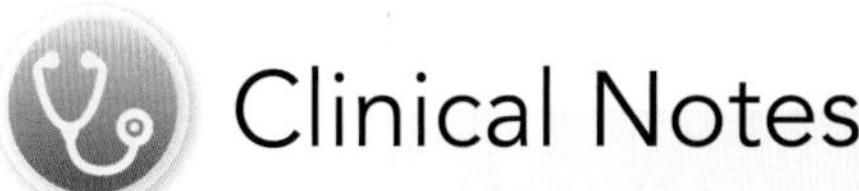

Clinical Notes

Popliteal Aneurysm

The pulsations of the wall of the femoral artery against the tendon of the adductor magnus at the opening of the adductor hiatus are thought to contribute to the cause of popliteal aneurysms.

Semimembranosus Bursa Swelling

Semimembranosus bursa swelling is the most common swelling found in the popliteal space. It is made tense by extending the knee joint and becomes flaccid when the joint is flexed. It should be distinguished from a Baker cyst, which is centrally located and arises as a pathologic (osteoarthritis) diverticulum of the synovial membrane through a hole in the back of the capsule of the knee joint.

Tributaries

The tributaries of the popliteal vein are as follows:

- Veins that correspond to branches given off by the popliteal artery
- **Small saphenous vein,** which perforates the deep fascia and passes between the two heads of the gastrocnemius muscle to end in the popliteal vein (see Fig. 8.61)

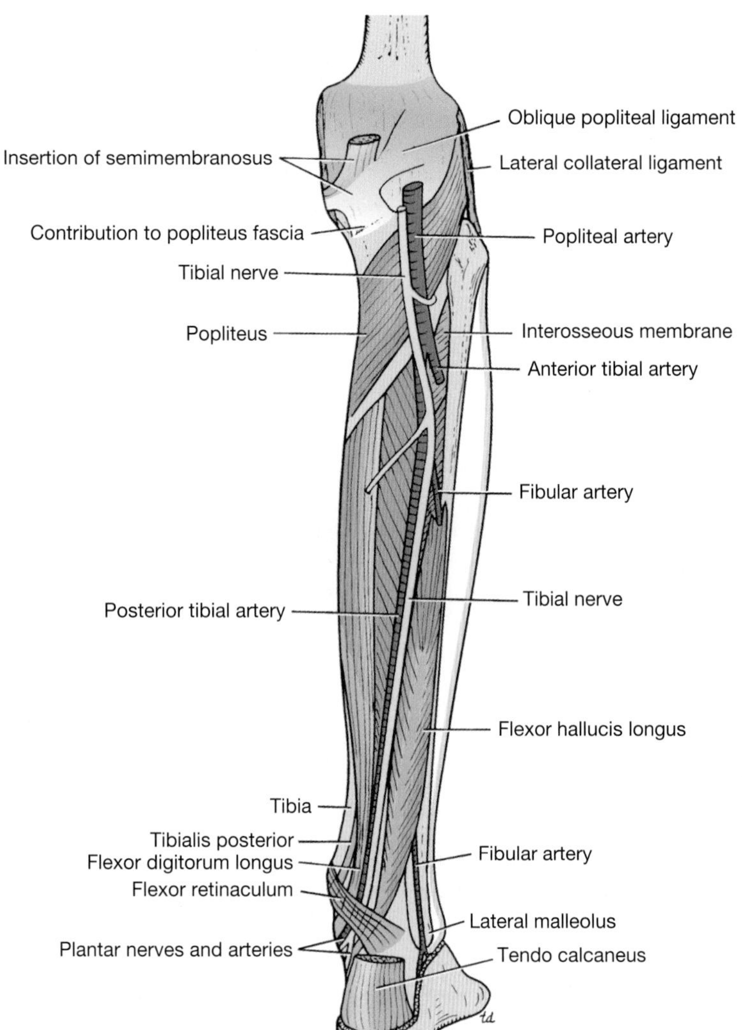

Figure 8.63 Deep structures in the posterior aspect of the right leg.

Popliteal Lymph Nodes

About six lymph nodes are embedded in the fatty connective tissue of the popliteal fossa (see Fig. 8.39). They receive superficial lymph vessels from the lateral side of the foot and leg. These accompany the small saphenous vein into the popliteal fossa. They also receive lymph from the knee joint and from deep lymph vessels accompanying the anterior and posterior tibial arteries.

Nerves

The sciatic nerve divides into its tibial and common fibular components above the popliteal fossa, and each nerve passes through the fossa as it descends into the leg.

Tibial Nerve

The larger terminal branch of the sciatic nerve, the tibial nerve, arises in the lower third of the thigh. It runs downward through the popliteal fossa, lying first on the lateral side of the popliteal artery, then posterior to it, and finally medial to it (see Figs. 8.61 and 8.62). The popliteal vein lies between the nerve and the artery throughout its course. The nerve enters the posterior compartment of the leg by passing beneath the soleus muscle.

Branches

- **Cutaneous:** The **sural nerve** descends between the two heads of the gastrocnemius muscle and is usually joined by the **sural communicating branch of the common fibular nerve** (see Figs. 8.44 and 8.61). Numerous small branches arise from the sural nerve to supply the skin of the calf and the back of the leg. The sural nerve accompanies the small saphenous vein behind the lateral malleolus and distributes to the skin along the lateral border of the foot and the lateral side of the little toe.
- **Muscular** branches supply both heads of the gastrocnemius and the plantaris, soleus, and popliteus (see Figs. 8.44, 8.61, and 8.62).
- **Articular** branches supply the knee joint.

Common Fibular (Peroneal) Nerve

The smaller terminal branch of the sciatic nerve, the common fibular (peroneal) nerve, arises in the lower third of the thigh. It runs downward through the popliteal fossa, closely following the medial border of the biceps femoris muscle (see Figs. 8.61 and 8.62). It leaves the fossa by crossing superficial to the lateral head of the gastrocnemius muscle. It then passes behind the head of the fibula, winds laterally around the neck of the bone, pierces the fibularis (peroneus) longus muscle, and divides into two terminal branches: the **superficial fibular (peroneal) nerve** and the **deep fibular (peroneal) nerve** (see Fig. 8.43). As the nerve lies on the lateral aspect of the neck of the fibula, it is subcutaneous and can easily be rolled against the bone.

Branches

- **Cutaneous:** The **sural communicating branch** (see Figs. 8.43 and 8.61) runs downward and joins the sural nerve. The **lateral cutaneous nerve of the calf** supplies the skin on the lateral side of the back of the leg (see Figs. 8.36 and 8.61).
- **Muscular** branch to the short head of the biceps femoris muscle, which arises high up in the popliteal fossa (see Fig. 8.62).
- **Articular** branches to the knee joint.

Posterior Cutaneous Nerve of the Thigh

The posterior cutaneous nerve of the thigh terminates by supplying the skin over the popliteal fossa (see Fig. 8.36).

Obturator Nerve

The posterior division of the obturator nerve leaves the adductor (subsartorial) canal with the femoral artery by passing through the adductor hiatus (see Fig. 8.62). The nerve terminates by supplying the knee joint.

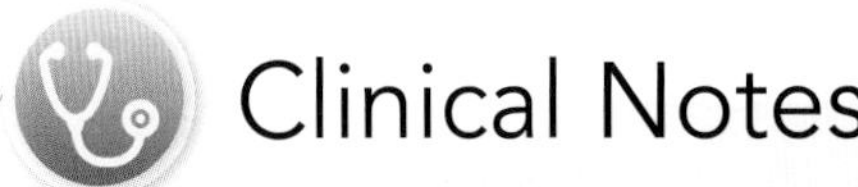

Common Fibular (Peroneal) Nerve Injury

The common fibular nerve is extremely vulnerable to injury as it winds around the neck of the fibula. At this site, it is exposed to direct trauma or is involved in fractures of the upper part of the fibula. Injury to the common fibular nerve causes **footdrop** (see Clinical Notes on Lower Limb Nerves below).

LEG

The leg is the middle part of the lower limb proper, that is the part between the knee and the ankle. Conversely, the arm is the proximal segment of the upper limb, that is the part between the shoulder and the elbow. Thus, "arm" and "leg" refer to very different locations within the limbs.

Fascia

The deep fascia of the leg forms the compartments of the leg (see below) and also forms a series of retinacula that aid the mechanical efficiency of the muscles of the leg.

Interosseous Membrane

The interosseous membrane binds the tibia and fibula together and provides attachment for neighboring muscles (Fig. 8.64; see also Fig. 8.63).

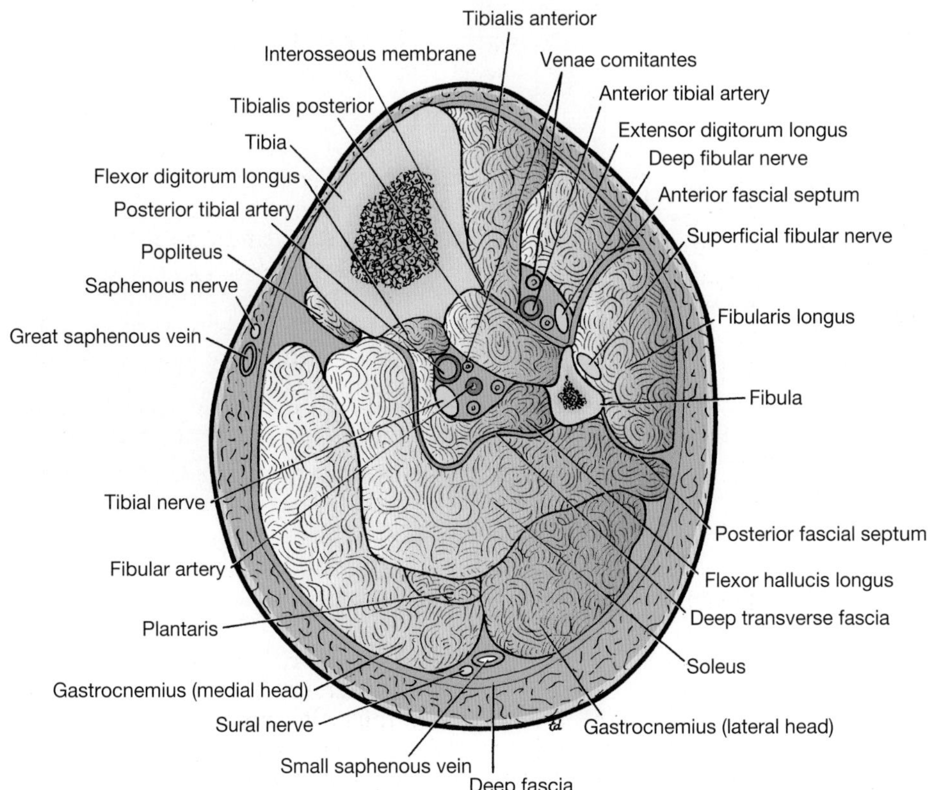

Figure 8.64 Transverse section through the middle of the right leg as seen from above.

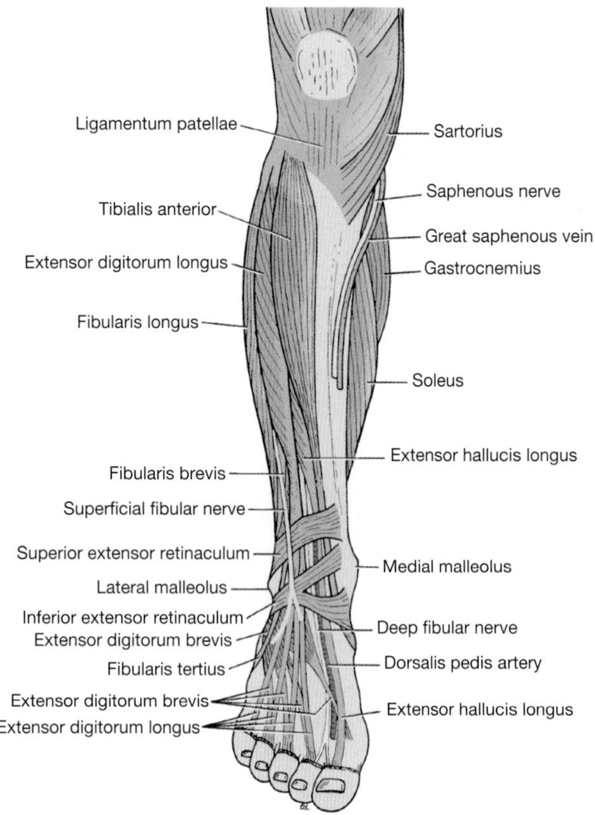

Figure 8.65 Structures in the anterior and lateral aspects of the right leg and the dorsum of the foot.

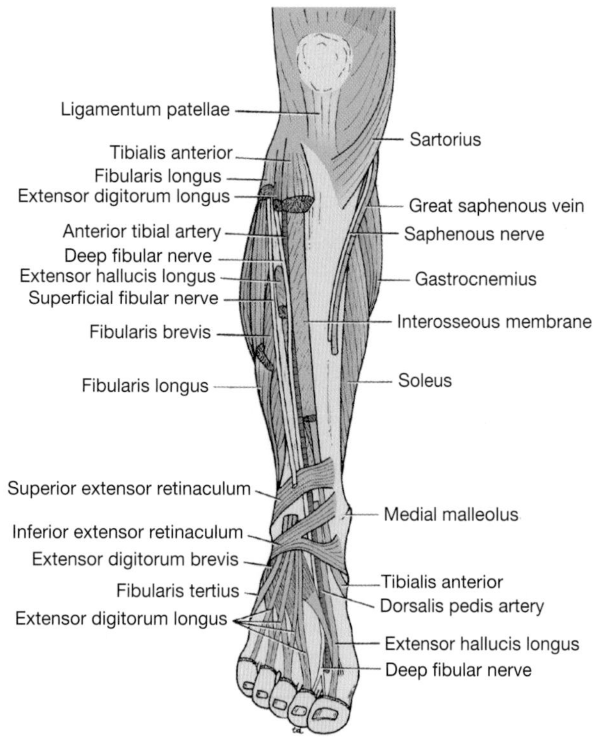

Figure 8.66 Deep structures in the anterior and lateral aspects of the right leg and the dorsum of the foot.

Ankle Retinacula

The retinacula are thickenings of the deep fascia that keep the long tendons around the ankle joint in position, prevent the long tendons from bowstringing, and act as pulleys. Details of the arrangement of the tendons beneath the different retinacula are described later, with the ankle.

Superior Extensor Retinaculum

The superior extensor retinaculum is attached to the distal ends of the anterior borders of the fibula and the tibia (Figs. 8.65 to 8.68).

Inferior Extensor Retinaculum

The inferior extensor retinaculum is a Y-shaped band located in front of the ankle joint (see Figs. 8.65 to 8.68). Fibrous bands separate the tendons into compartments (Fig. 8.69), each of which is lined by a synovial sheath.

Flexor Retinaculum

The flexor retinaculum extends downward and backward from the medial malleolus to attach to the medial surface of the calcaneum (Fig. 8.70B; see also Fig. 8.63). It binds the tendons of the deep muscles of the back of the leg to the back of the medial malleolus as they pass forward to enter the sole. The tendons lie in compartments (see Fig. 8.69), each of which is lined by a synovial sheath.

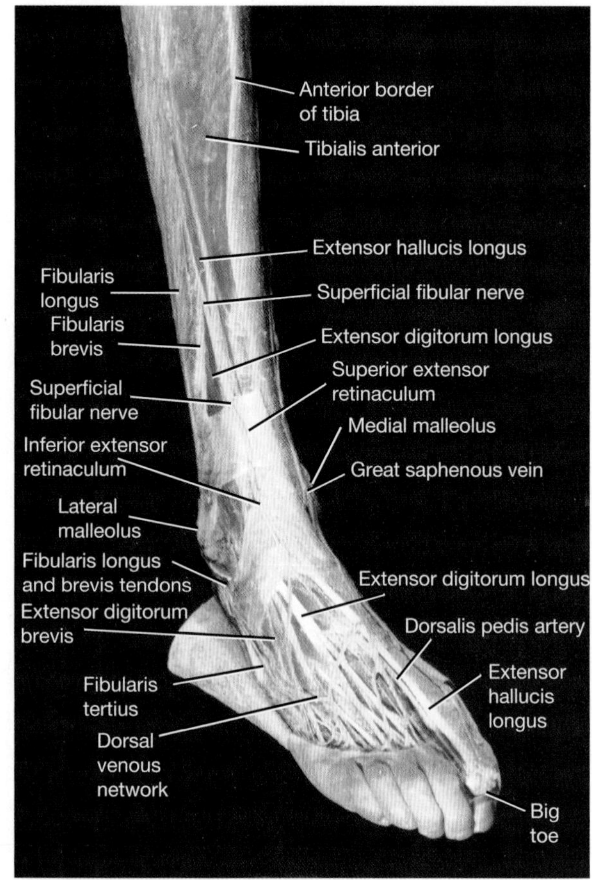

Figure 8.67 Dissection of the front of the right leg and dorsum of the foot.

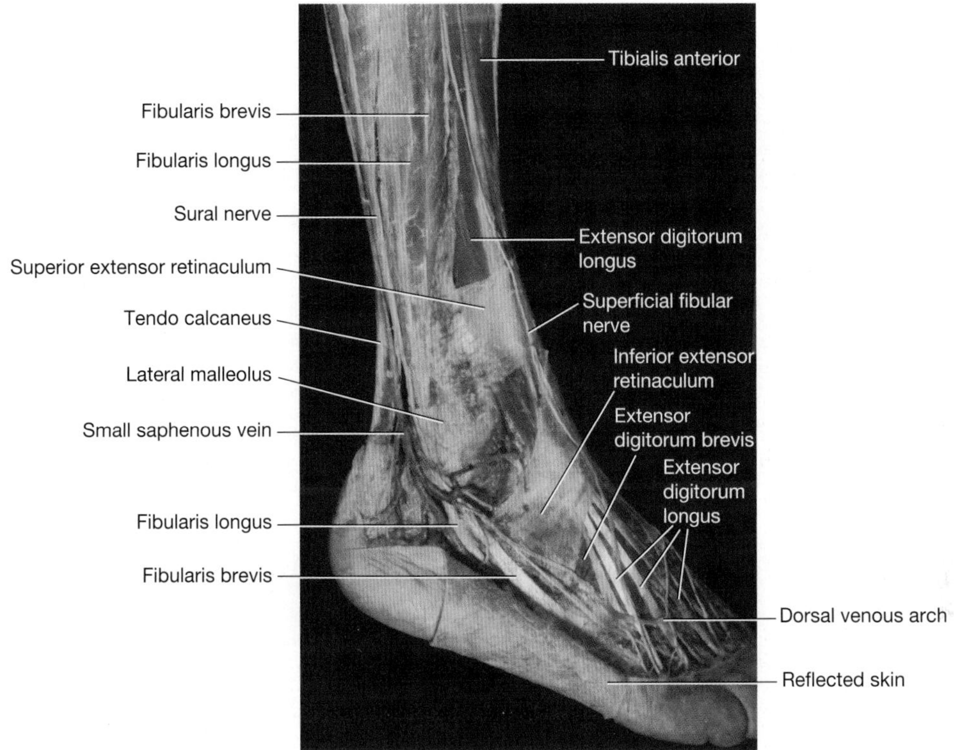

Figure 8.68 Dissection of the right ankle region showing the structures passing behind the lateral malleolus. Note the position of the retinacula.

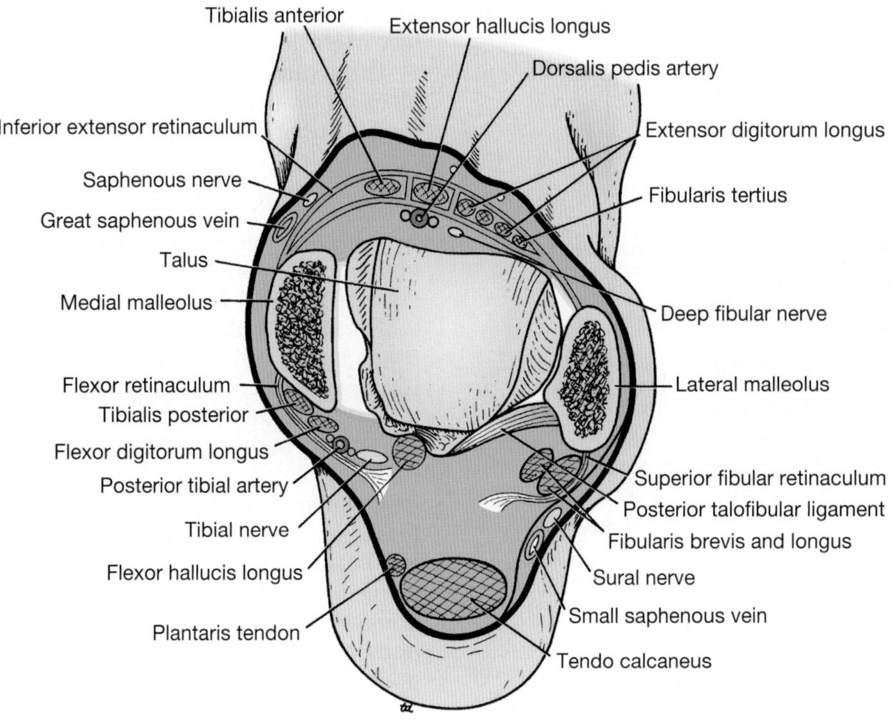

Figure 8.69 Relations of the right ankle joint.

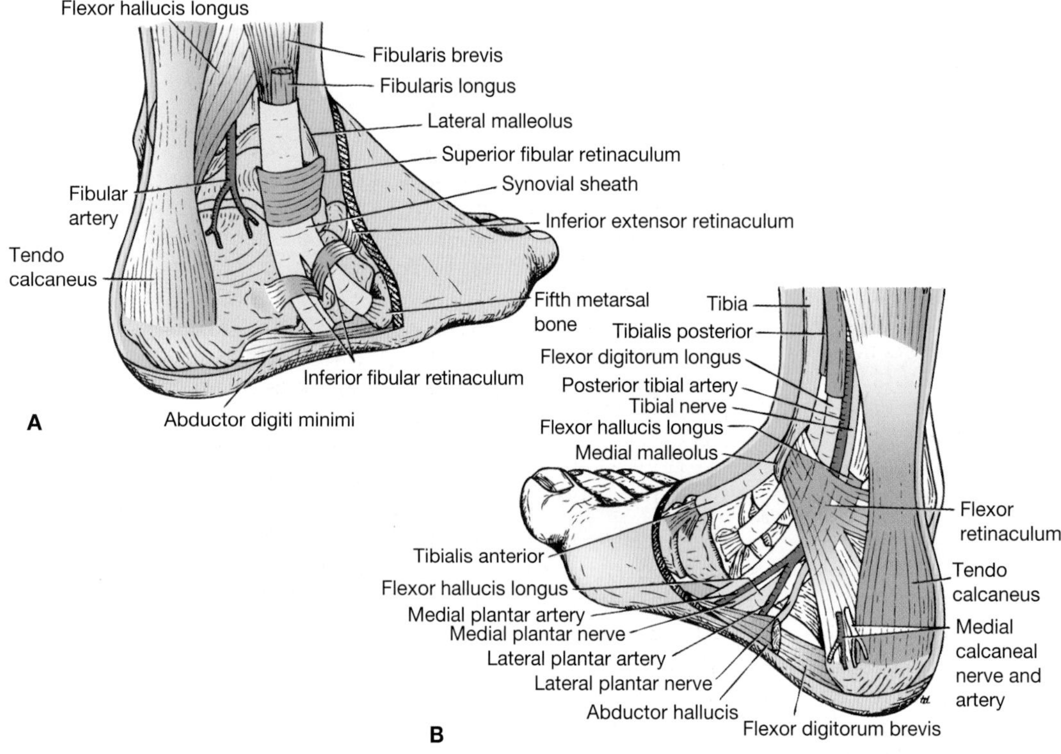

Figure 8.70 Structures passing behind the lateral malleolus **(A)** and the medial malleolus **(B)**. Synovial sheaths of the tendons are shown in *blue*. Note the positions of the retinacula.

Superior Fibular (Peroneal) Retinaculum

The superior fibular (peroneal) retinaculum connects the lateral malleolus to the lateral surface of the calcaneum (see Figs. 8.69 and 8.70A). It binds the tendons of the fibularis longus and brevis to the back of the lateral malleolus. The tendons have a common synovial sheath.

Inferior Fibular (Peroneal) Retinaculum

The inferior fibular (peroneal) retinaculum binds the tendons of the fibularis longus and brevis muscles to the lateral side of the calcaneum (see Fig. 8.70A). The tendons each possess a synovial sheath, which is continuous above with the common sheath.

Cutaneous Nerves

The **lateral cutaneous nerve of the calf**, a branch of the common fibular (peroneal) nerve, supplies the skin on the upper part of the lateral surface of the leg (see Fig. 8.36).

The **superficial fibular (peroneal) nerve**, a branch of the common fibular (peroneal) nerve, supplies the skin of the lower part of the anterolateral surface of the leg (see Fig. 8.37).

The **saphenous nerve**, a branch of the femoral nerve, supplies the skin on the anteromedial surface of the leg (see Fig. 8.37).

The **posterior cutaneous nerve of the thigh** descends on the back of the thigh. It supplies the skin over the popliteal fossa and the upper part of the back of the leg (see Fig. 8.36).

The **lateral cutaneous nerve of the calf**, a branch of the common fibular (peroneal) nerve, supplies the skin on the upper part of the posterolateral surface of the leg (see Fig. 8.36).

The **sural nerve**, a branch of the tibial nerve, supplies the skin on the lower part of the posterolateral surface of the leg (see Fig. 8.36).

The **saphenous nerve**, a branch of the femoral nerve, gives off branches that supply the skin on the posteromedial surface of the leg (see Fig. 8.37).

Superficial Veins

Numerous small veins curve around the medial aspect of the leg and ultimately drain into the great saphenous vein (see Fig. 8.46).

The **small saphenous vein** arises from the lateral part of the dorsal venous arch of the foot. It ascends behind the lateral malleolus in company with the sural nerve, follows the lateral border of the tendo calcaneus, and then runs up the middle of the back of the leg. The vein pierces the deep fascia, passes between the two heads of the gastrocnemius muscle in the lower part of the popliteal fossa, and ends in the popliteal vein (see Figs. 8.46 and 8.61). The small saphenous vein has numerous valves along its course. The termination of this vein is variable. It may join the popliteal vein. It may join the great saphenous vein. Or, it may split in two, one division joining the popliteal and the other joining the great saphenous vein.

Tributaries

- Numerous **small veins** from the back of the leg
- **Communicating veins** with the deep veins of the foot

- Important **anastomotic branches** that run upward and medially and join the great saphenous vein (see Fig. 8.46)

Lymph Vessels

The greater part of the lymph from the skin and superficial fascia on the **front of the leg** drains upward and medially in vessels that follow the great saphenous vein, to end in the **vertical group of superficial inguinal lymph nodes** (see Fig. 8.39). A small amount of lymph from the upper lateral part of the front of the leg may pass via vessels that accompany the small saphenous vein and drain into the popliteal nodes.

Lymph vessels from the skin and superficial fascia on the **back of the leg** drain upward and either pass forward around the medial side of the leg to end in the vertical group of superficial inguinal nodes or drain into the popliteal nodes.

Leg Fascial Compartments and Muscles

The deep fascia tightly surrounds the leg and is continuous above with the deep fascia of the thigh. Below the tibial condyles, it is attached to the periosteum on the anterior and medial borders of the tibia (see Fig. 8.64). **Two intermuscular septa** pass from its deep aspect to attach to the fibula. These, together with the **interosseous membrane**, divide the leg into **three compartments**: anterior, lateral, and posterior. As with the thigh, each compartment has its own muscles, blood supply, and nerve supply.

Anterior Fascial Compartment Contents

- **Muscles:** Tibialis anterior, extensor digitorum longus, fibularis tertius, and extensor hallucis longus
- **Blood supply:** Anterior tibial artery
- **Nerve supply:** Deep fibular (peroneal) nerve

Anterior Fascial Compartment Muscles

The muscles are illustrated in Figures 8.64 through 8.69 and summarized in Table 8.5.

Note the following:

- **Extension (dorsiflexion)** at the ankle is the movement of the foot away from the ground, as in lifting the foot up toward the shin (see Fig. 8.12). **Flexion (plantar flexion)** is movement of the foot toward the ground, as in standing on the toes.
- **Inversion** of the foot is the movement of turning the sole of the foot medially, toward the midline (Fig. 8.71; see also Fig. 8.12). **Eversion** of the foot is turning the sole laterally, away from the midline.
- The **fibularis tertius** muscle extends/dorsiflexes the foot at the ankle joint along with the other muscles in this compartment and is supplied by the deep fibular (peroneal) nerve. The muscle also everts the foot at the subtalar and transverse tarsal joints along with the fibularis longus and brevis muscles but receives no innervation from the superficial fibular (peroneal) nerve.
- The **extensor digitorum longus tendons** on the dorsal surface of each toe become incorporated into a fascial expansion called the **extensor expansion**. The central part of the expansion is inserted into the base of the middle phalanx, and the two lateral parts converge to be inserted into the base of the distal phalanx. This is similar to the insertion of the extensor digitorum in the hand.

Anterior Fascial Compartment Artery

The **anterior tibial artery** is the smaller of the terminal branches of the popliteal artery (see Fig. 8.54). It arises at the level of the lower border of the popliteus muscle and passes forward into the anterior compartment of the leg through an opening in the upper part of the interosseous membrane (see Fig. 8.62). It descends

Table 8.5 Muscles of Anterior Fascial Compartment of Leg

MUSCLE	ORIGIN	INSERTION	NERVE SUPPLY	NERVE ROOT[a]	ACTION
Tibialis anterior	Lateral surface of shaft of tibia and interosseous membrane	Medial cuneiform and base of first metatarsal bone	Deep fibular nerve	**L4**, L5	Extends[b] foot at ankle joint; inverts foot at subtalar and transverse tarsal joints; holds up medial longitudinal arch of foot
Extensor digitorum longus	Anterior surface of shaft of fibula	Extensor expansion of lateral four toes	Deep fibular nerve	L5; S1	Extends toes; extends foot at ankle joint
Fibularis tertius	Anterior surface of shaft of fibula	Base of fifth metatarsal bone	Deep fibular nerve	L5; S1	Extends foot at ankle joint; everts foot at subtalar and transverse tarsal joints
Extensor hallucis longus	Anterior surface of shaft of fibula	Base of distal phalanx of great toe	Deep fibular nerve	L5; S1	Extends great toe; extends foot at ankle joint; inverts foot at subtalar and transverse tarsal joints

[a]The predominant nerve root supply is in bold.

[b]Extension, or dorsiflexion, of the ankle is the movement of the foot away from the ground.

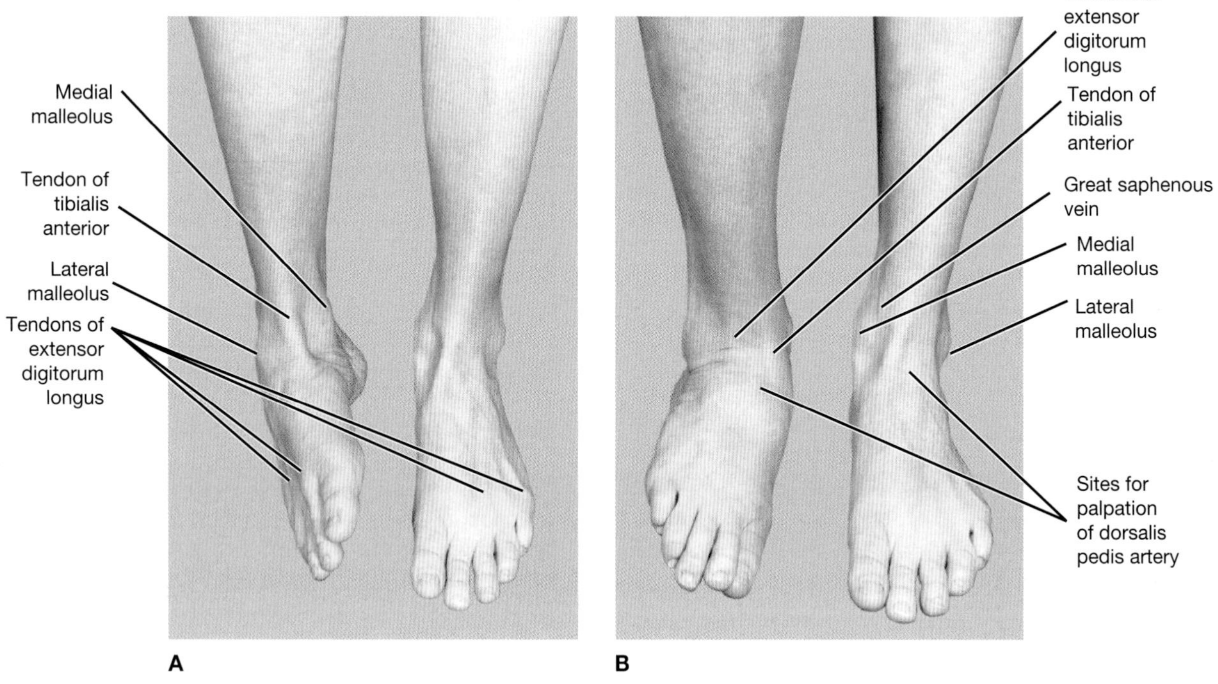

Figure 8.71 Anterior view of the ankles and feet showing inversion **(A)** and eversion **(B)** of the right foot.

on the anterior surface of the interosseous membrane, accompanied by the deep fibular (peroneal) nerve (see Figs. 8.64 and 8.66). In the upper part of its course, it lies deep beneath the muscles of the compartment. In the lower part of its course, it lies superficial, in front of the lower end of the tibia. After passing deep to the superior extensor retinaculum, it has the tendon of the extensor hallucis longus on its medial side and the deep fibular (peroneal) nerve and the tendons of extensor digitorum longus on its lateral side. Here, its pulsations can easily be felt in the living subject. The artery becomes the **dorsalis pedis artery** in front of the ankle joint, after passing the level of the malleoli (see Figs. 8.65 and 8.66).

Branches

- **Muscular branches** to neighboring muscles.
- **Anastomotic branches** that anastomose with branches of other arteries around the knee and ankle joints.
- **Venae comitantes** of the anterior tibial artery join those of the posterior tibial artery in the popliteal fossa to form the popliteal vein.

Anterior Fascial Compartment Nerve Supply

The **deep fibular (peroneal) nerve** is one of the terminal branches of the common fibular (peroneal) nerve (see Fig. 8.43). It arises in the substance of the fibularis longus muscle on the lateral side of the neck of the fibula (see Fig. 8.66). The nerve enters the anterior compartment by piercing the anterior fascial septum. It then descends deep to the extensor digitorum longus muscle, first lying lateral, then anterior, and finally lateral to the anterior tibial artery. The nerve passes deep to the extensor retinacula and continues into the foot.

Branches

- **Muscular branches** to the anterior compartment (tibialis anterior, extensor digitorum longus, fibularis tertius, and extensor hallucis longus)
- **Articular branch** to the ankle joint

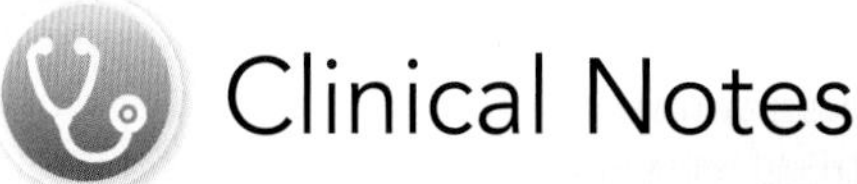

Anterior Compartment Syndrome

Anterior compartment syndrome of the leg is produced by an increase in the intracompartmental pressure that results from an increased production of tissue fluid. Soft tissue injury associated with bone fractures is a common cause, and early diagnosis is critical. The deep, aching pain in the anterior compartment of the leg that is characteristic of this syndrome can become severe. Dorsiflexion of the foot at the ankle joint increases the severity of the pain. Stretching of the muscles that pass through the compartment by passive plantar flexion of the ankle also increases the pain. As the pressure rises, the venous return is diminished, thus producing a further rise in pressure. In severe cases, the arterial supply is eventually cut off by compression, and the dorsalis pedis arterial pulse disappears. The tibialis anterior, extensor digitorum longus, and extensor hallucis longus muscles are paralyzed. Loss of sensation is limited to the area supplied by the deep fibular (peroneal) nerve, that is the skin cleft between the first and second toes. The surgeon can open the anterior compartment of the leg by making a longitudinal incision through the deep fascia and thus decompress the area and prevent anoxic necrosis of the muscles.

Table 8.6 Muscles of Lateral Fascial Compartment of Leg

MUSCLE	ORIGIN	INSERTION	NERVE SUPPLY	NERVE ROOT[a]	ACTION
Fibularis longus	Lateral surface of shaft of fibula	Base of first metatarsal and the medial cuneiform	Superficial fibular nerve	**L5**; **S1**, S2	Plantar flexes foot at ankle joint; everts foot at subtalar and transverse tarsal joints; supports lateral longitudinal and transverse arches of foot
Fibularis brevis	Lateral surface of shaft of fibula	Base of fifth metatarsal bone	Superficial fibular nerve	**L5**; **S1**, S2	Plantar flexes foot at ankle joint; everts foot at subtalar and transverse tarsal joint; supports lateral longitudinal arch of foot

[a]The predominant nerve root supply is in bold.

Lateral Fascial Compartment Contents

- **Muscles:** Fibularis longus and fibularis brevis
- **Blood supply:** Branches from the fibular artery
- **Nerve supply:** Superficial fibular (peroneal) nerve

Lateral Fascial Compartment Muscles

The muscles are illustrated in Figures 8.64 through 8.70A and summarized in Table 8.6.

Note the following:

- Both the fibularis longus and brevis muscles flex the foot at the ankle joint and evert the foot at the subtalar and transverse tarsal joints. They also play an important role in holding up the lateral longitudinal arch in the foot. In addition, the fibularis longus tendon serves as a tie to the transverse arch of the foot.

Lateral Fascial Compartment Artery

Numerous branches from the **fibular artery** (see Fig. 8.54), which lies in the posterior compartment of the leg, pierce the posterior fascial septum and supply the fibular muscles.

Lateral Fascial Compartment Nerve

The **superficial fibular (peroneal) nerve** is one of the terminal branches of the common fibular (peroneal) nerve (see Fig. 8.43). It arises in the substance of the fibularis longus muscle on the lateral side of the neck of the fibula (see Figs. 8.66 to 8.68). It descends between the fibularis longus and brevis muscles and becomes cutaneous in the lower part of the leg (see Figs. 8.65 and 8.68).

Branches

- **Muscular** branches to the lateral compartment (fibularis longus and brevis) (see Fig. 8.66).
- **Cutaneous:** Medial and lateral branches distribute to the skin on the lower part of the front of the leg and the dorsum of the foot. In addition, branches supply the dorsal surfaces of the skin of all the toes, except the adjacent sides of the first and second toes and the lateral side of the little toe.

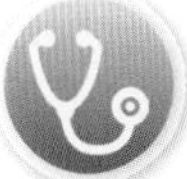

Clinical Notes

Tenosynovitis and Dislocation of Fibularis Longus and Brevis Tendons

Tenosynovitis (inflammation of the synovial sheaths) can affect the tendon sheaths of the fibularis longus and brevis muscles as they pass posterior to the lateral malleolus. Treatment consists of immobilization, heat, and physiotherapy. Tendon dislocation can occur when the tendons of fibularis longus and brevis dislocate forward from behind the lateral malleolus. For this condition to occur, the superior fibular retinaculum must be torn. It usually occurs in older children and is caused by trauma.

Posterior Fascial Compartment Contents

The **deep transverse fascia of the leg** is a septum that divides the muscles of the posterior compartment into **superficial** and **deep groups** (see Fig. 8.64).

- **Superficial group of muscles:** Gastrocnemius, plantaris, and soleus
- **Deep group of muscles:** Popliteus, flexor digitorum longus, flexor hallucis longus, and tibialis posterior
- **Blood supply:** Posterior tibial artery
- **Nerve supply:** Tibial nerve

Posterior Fascial Compartment Muscles: Superficial Group

The muscles are illustrated in Figures 8.64 and 8.72 and summarized in Table 8.7.

Note the following:

- Together, the soleus and gastrocnemius act as powerful plantar flexors of the ankle joint. They provide the main forward propulsive force in locomotion by using the foot as a lever and raising the heel off the ground.

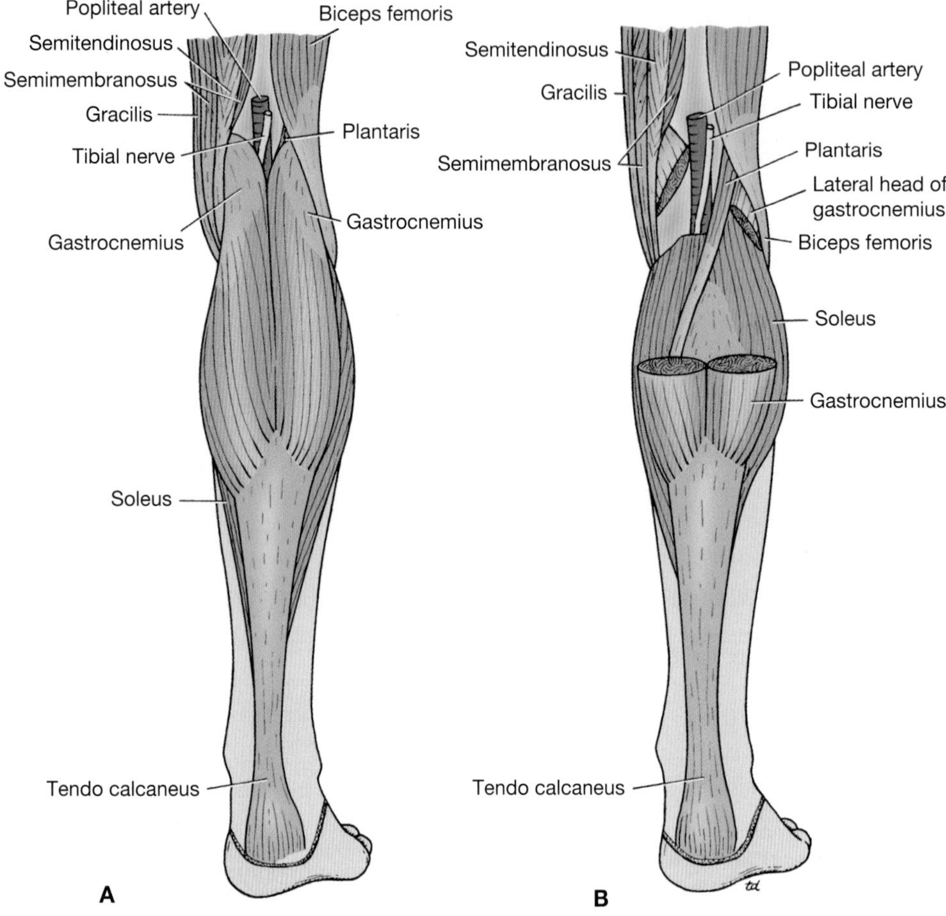

Figure 8.72 Superficial aspect **(A)** of the posterior compartment of the leg. In **(B)** part of the gastrocnemius has been removed.

- The gastrocnemius and soleus insert into the calcaneum together via the common **tendo calcaneus** (**Achilles tendon**). Because this arrangement produces a functionally three-headed muscle in the calf, they are sometimes referred to as the **triceps surae** muscles.

Posterior Fascial Compartment Muscles: Deep Group

The muscles are shown in Figures 8.63, 8.64, 8.69, and 8.70B and summarized in Table 8.7.

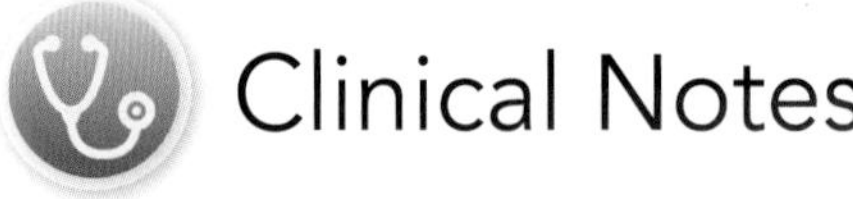

Clinical Notes

Gastrocnemius and Soleus Muscle Tears

Tearing of the gastrocnemius or soleus muscles produces severe localized pain over the damaged muscle. Swelling may be present.

Ruptured Tendo Calcaneus

Rupture of the tendo calcaneus is a common sport-related injury. The rupture occurs at its narrowest part, about 2 in. (5 cm) above its insertion. A sudden, sharp pain is felt, with immediate disability. The gastrocnemius and soleus muscles retract proximally, leaving a palpable gap in the tendon. It is impossible for the patient to actively plantar flex the foot. The tendon should be sutured as soon as possible, and the leg immobilized with the ankle joint plantar flexed and the knee joint flexed.

Plantaris Tendon Rupture

Rupture of the plantaris tendon is rare, although tearing of the fibers of the soleus or partial tearing of the tendo calcaneus is frequently diagnosed as such a rupture.

Plantaris Tendon and Autografts

The plantaris muscle, which is often missing, can be used for tendon autografts in repairing severed flexor tendons to the fingers. The tendon of the palmaris longus muscle can also be used for this purpose.

Table 8.7 Muscles of Posterior Fascial Compartment of Leg

MUSCLE	ORIGIN	INSERTION	NERVE SUPPLY	NERVE ROOT[a]	ACTION
Superficial Group					
Gastrocnemius	Lateral head from lateral condyle of femur and medial head from above medial condyle	Via tendo calcaneus into posterior surface of calcaneum	Tibial nerve	**S1**, S2	Plantar flexes foot at ankle joint; flexes knee joint
Plantaris	Lateral supracondylar ridge of femur	Posterior surface of calcaneum	Tibial nerve	**S1**, S2	Plantar flexes foot at ankle joint; flexes knee joint
Soleus	Shafts of tibia and fibula	Via tendo calcaneus into posterior surface of calcaneum	Tibial nerve	S1, **S2**	Together with gastrocnemius and plantaris is powerful plantar flexor of ankle joint; provides main propulsive force in walking and running
Deep Group					
Popliteus	Lateral surface of lateral condyle of femur	Posterior surface of shaft of tibia above soleal line	Tibial nerve	L4, L5; S1	Flexes leg at knee joint; unlocks knee joint by lateral rotation of femur on tibia and slackens ligaments of joint
Flexor digitorum longus	Posterior surface of shaft of tibia	Bases of distal phalanges of lateral four toes	Tibial nerve	**S2**, S3	Flexes distal phalanges of lateral four toes; plantar flexes foot at ankle joint; supports medial and lateral longitudinal arches of foot
Flexor hallucis longus	Posterior surface of shaft of fibula	Base of distal phalanx of great toe	Tibial nerve	**S2**, S3	Flexes distal phalanx of great toe; plantar flexes foot at ankle joint; supports medial longitudinal arch of foot
Tibialis posterior	Posterior surface of shafts of tibia and fibula and interosseous membrane	Tuberosity of navicular bone and other neighboring bones	Tibial nerve	L4, L5	Plantar flexes foot at ankle joint; inverts foot at subtalar and transverse tarsal joints; supports medial longitudinal arch of foot

[a]The predominant nerve root supply is in bold.

Note the following:

- The popliteus muscle arises inside the capsule of the knee joint and inserts into the upper part of the posterior surface of the tibia. The tendon separates the lateral ligament of the knee joint from the lateral meniscus so that the meniscus is not tethered to the ligament and is freer to move and adapt to the surfaces of the condyle of the femur and the tibia.
- The popliteus muscle is responsible for "unlocking" the knee joint.

Posterior Fascial Compartment Artery

The **posterior tibial artery** is one of the terminal branches of the popliteal artery (see Fig. 8.54). It begins at the level of the lower border of the popliteus muscle and passes downward deep to the gastrocnemius and soleus and the deep transverse fascia of the leg (see Figs. 8.62 to 8.64). It lies on the posterior surface of the tibialis posterior muscle above and on the posterior surface of the tibia below. In the lower part of the leg, the artery is covered only by skin and fascia. The artery passes behind the medial malleolus deep to the flexor retinaculum and terminates by dividing into medial and lateral plantar arteries (see Fig. 8.70B).

Branches

- **Fibular artery**, which is a large artery that arises close to the origin of the posterior tibial artery (see Figs. 8.54 and 8.62 to 8.64). It descends behind the fibula, either within the substance of the flexor hallucis longus muscle or posterior to it. The fibular artery gives off numerous **muscular branches** and a **nutrient artery** to the fibula and ends by taking part in the

anastomosis around the ankle joint (see Fig. 8.70A). A **perforating branch** pierces the interosseous membrane to reach the lower part of the front of the leg.
- **Muscular branches** are distributed to muscles in the posterior compartment of the leg.
- **Nutrient artery to the tibia**.
- **Anastomotic branches,** which join other arteries around the ankle joint.
- **Medial and lateral plantar arteries**, which enter the sole of the foot.
- **Venae comitantes** of the posterior tibial artery join those of the anterior tibial artery in the popliteal fossa to form the popliteal vein.

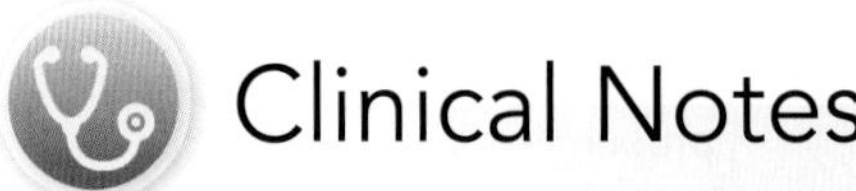

Deep Vein Thrombosis and Long-Distance Air Travel

Passengers who sit immobile for hours on long-distance travels (eg, airline flights) are prone to deep vein thrombosis in the legs. Thrombosis of the veins of the soleus muscle gives rise to mild pain or tightness in the calf and calf muscle tenderness. However, deep vein thrombosis can also occur with no signs or symptoms. If the thrombus become dislodged, it passes rapidly to the heart and lungs, causing pulmonary embolism, which is often fatal. Preventative measures include stretching the legs every hour to improve the venous circulation.

Posterior Fascial Compartment Nerve

The **tibial nerve** is the larger terminal branch of the sciatic nerve in the lower third of the back of the thigh (see Fig. 8.44). It descends through the popliteal fossa and passes deep to the gastrocnemius and soleus muscles (see Figs. 8.61 to 8.64 and 8.72). It lies on the posterior surface of the tibialis posterior and, lower down the leg, on the posterior surface of the tibia. The nerve accompanies the posterior tibial artery and lies at first on its medial side, then crosses posterior to it, and finally lies on its lateral side. The nerve, with the artery, passes behind the medial malleolus, between the tendons of the flexor digitorum longus and the flexor hallucis longus (see Fig. 8.70B). It is covered here by the flexor retinaculum and divides into the medial and lateral plantar nerves.

Leg Branches (Below Popliteal Fossa)

- **Muscular branches** to the posterior compartment (gastrocnemius, soleus, plantaris, flexor digitorum longus, flexor hallucis longus, and tibialis posterior) (see Fig. 8.44).
- **Cutaneous branch:** The **medial calcaneal branch** supplies the skin over the medial surface of the heel (see Fig. 8.70B).
- **Articular branch** to the ankle joint.
- **Medial and lateral plantar nerves:** The terminal branches of the tibial nerve (see Fig. 8.70B).

ANKLE

The ankle is the transition zone between the leg and the foot. Structures passing between the leg and foot do so in an organized pattern that ensures optimal function.

Anterior Aspect

Structures crossing the anterior aspect of the ankle do so anterior to the malleoli and in relation to the extensor retinacula.

Structures That Pass Superficial to Extensor Retinacula from Medial to Lateral

See Figures 8.65 and 8.69.

- Saphenous nerve and great saphenous vein (in front of the medial malleolus)
- Superficial fibular (peroneal) nerve (medial and lateral branches)

Structures That Pass Deep to or through Extensor Retinacula from Medial to Lateral

See Figures 8.65, 8.66, and 8.69.

- Tibialis anterior tendon
- Extensor hallucis longus tendon
- Anterior tibial artery with venae comitantes
- Deep fibular (peroneal) nerve
- Extensor digitorum longus tendons
- Fibularis tertius

As each of the above tendons passes beneath or through the extensor retinacula, a synovial sheath surrounds it. The tendons of extensor digitorum longus and the fibularis tertius share a common synovial sheath.

Structures That Pass Immediately Anterior to Medial Malleolus

See Figures 8.69 and 8.73.

- Great saphenous vein
- Saphenous nerve

Posterior Aspect

Structures crossing the posterior aspect of the ankle do so posterior to the malleoli and in relation to the flexor retinacula.

Structures That Pass behind Medial Malleolus Deep to Flexor Retinaculum from Medial to Lateral

See Figures 8.69 and 8.70.

- Tibialis posterior tendon
- Flexor digitorum longus tendon
- Posterior tibial artery with venae comitantes
- Tibial nerve
- Flexor hallucis longus tendon

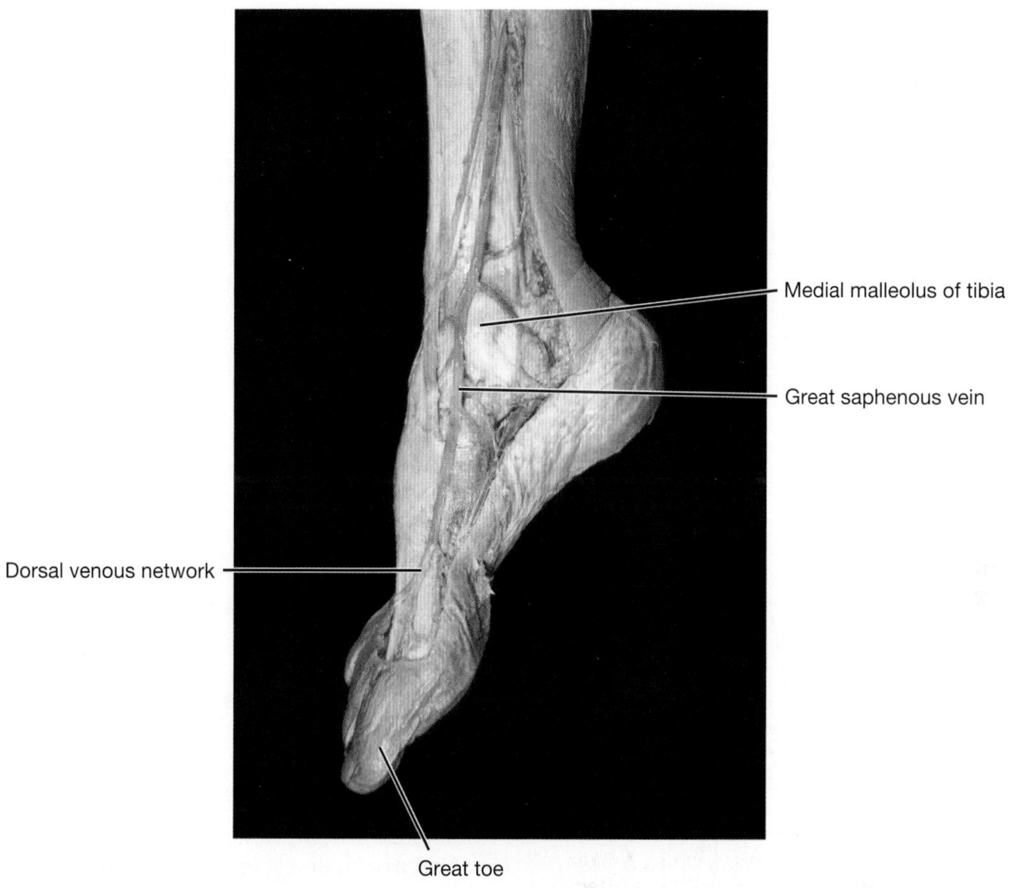

Figure 8.73 Dissection of the right ankle region showing the origin of the great saphenous vein from the dorsal venous arch. Note that the great saphenous vein ascends in front of the medial malleolus of the tibia.

As each of these tendons passes beneath the flexor retinaculum, a synovial sheath surrounds it.

Structures That Pass behind Lateral Malleolus Superficial to Superior Fibular Retinaculum

See Figures 8.68 and 8.69.

- Sural nerve
- Small saphenous vein

Structures That Pass behind Lateral Malleolus Deep to Superior Fibular Retinaculum

See Figures 8.69 and 8.70.

The fibularis longus and brevis tendons share a common synovial sheath. More distally, beneath the inferior fibular retinaculum, they have separate sheaths.

Structures That Lie Directly behind the Ankle

Fat and the large tendo calcaneus lie behind the ankle (see Fig. 8.69).

FOOT

The foot supports the body weight and provides leverage for walking and running. It is unique in that it is constructed in the form of arches, which enable it to adapt its shape to uneven surfaces. It also serves as a resilient spring to absorb shocks, such as in jumping.

In anatomical terms, the foot is the **pes**. The top of the foot is the **dorsum** of the foot (or **superior aspect**). The bottom of the foot is the **sole** or **plantar side** or **ventral side** (or **inferior aspect**). The great toe ("big toe") is **digit #1** or the **hallux**.

Sole

The skin of the sole is thick and hairless. It is firmly bound down to the underlying deep fascia by numerous fibrous bands. The skin shows a few flexure creases at the sites of skin movement. Sweat glands are present in large numbers.

Cutaneous Nerves

See Figure 8.74; see also Figure 8.36.

- **Medial calcaneal branch** of the tibial nerve, which innervates the medial side of the heel
- Branches from the **medial plantar nerve**, which innervate the medial two thirds of the sole
- Branches from the **lateral plantar nerve**, which innervate the lateral third of the sole

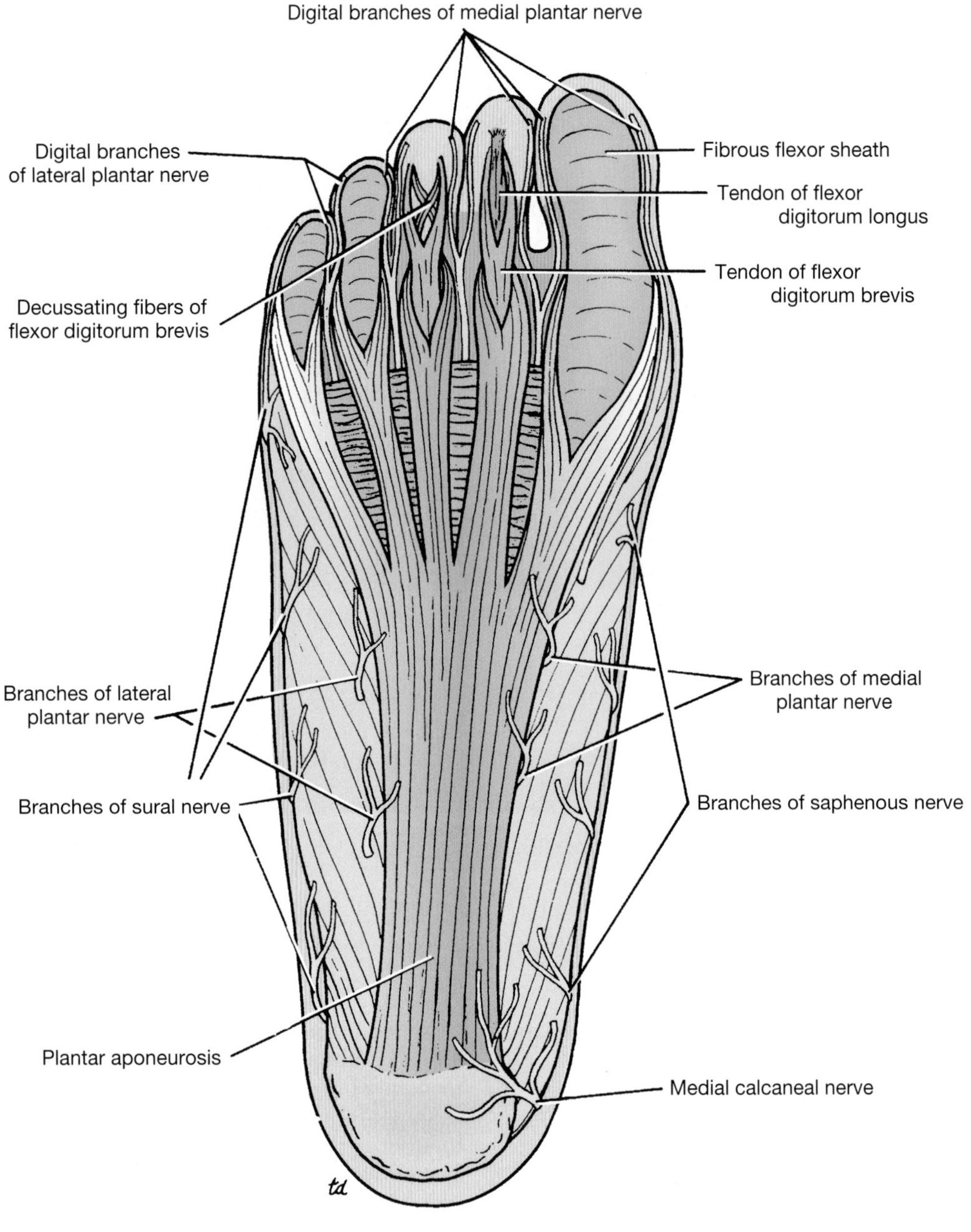

Figure 8.74 Plantar aponeurosis and cutaneous nerves of the sole of the right foot.

Deep Fascia

The **plantar aponeurosis** is a triangular thickening of the deep fascia that protects the underlying nerves, blood vessels, and muscles (see Fig. 8.74). Its apex is attached to the medial and lateral tubercles of the calcaneum. The base of the aponeurosis divides into five slips that pass into the toes.

Sole Muscles

The muscles of the sole are conveniently described in four layers from superficial to deep.

- **First layer:** Abductor hallucis, flexor digitorum brevis, abductor digiti minimi

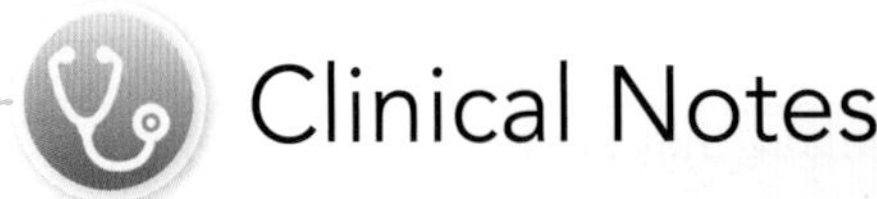

Plantar Fasciitis

Plantar fasciitis, which occurs in individuals who do a great deal of standing or walking, causes pain and tenderness of the sole. The cause may be repeated minor trauma. Repeated attacks of this condition induce ossification in the posterior attachment of the aponeurosis, forming a **calcaneal spur**.

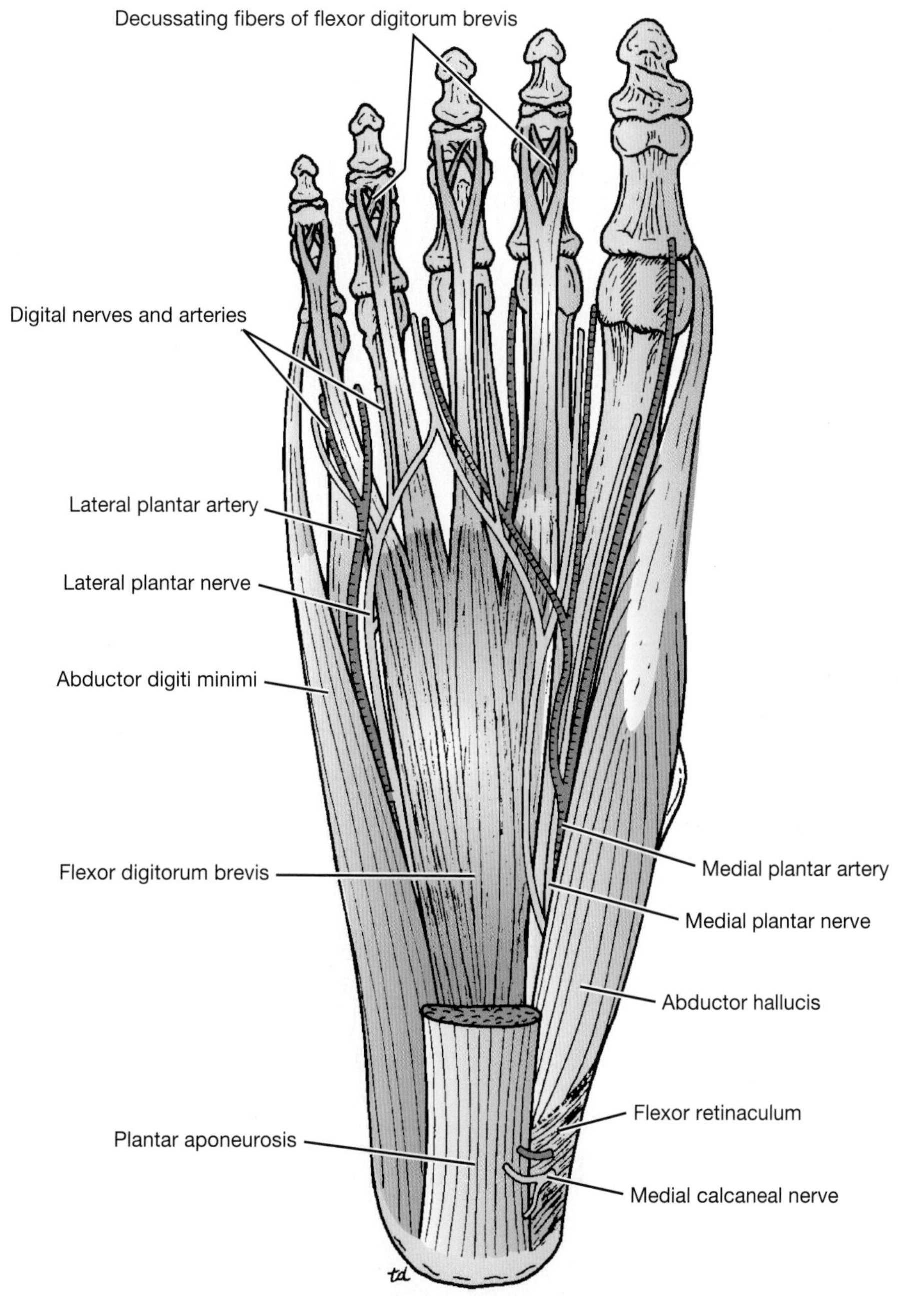

Figure 8.75 First layer of the plantar muscles of the right foot. Medial and lateral plantar arteries and nerves are also shown.

- **Second layer:** Quadratus plantae, lumbricals, flexor digitorum longus tendon, flexor hallucis longus tendon
- **Third layer:** Flexor hallucis brevis, adductor hallucis, flexor digiti minimi brevis
- **Fourth layer:** Interossei, fibularis longus tendon, tibialis posterior tendon

Unlike the small muscles of the hand, the muscles of the sole have few delicate functions and are chiefly concerned with supporting the arches of the foot. Although their names suggest control of individual toes, this function is rarely used in most people.

The muscles of the sole are illustrated in Figures 8.75 through 8.79 and summarized in Table 8.8.

Long Tendons of the Sole

Several muscles that originate in the posterior and lateral compartments of the leg send long tendons into the sole to their points of insertion. The general pattern is similar to that in the anterior aspect of the forearm and hand.

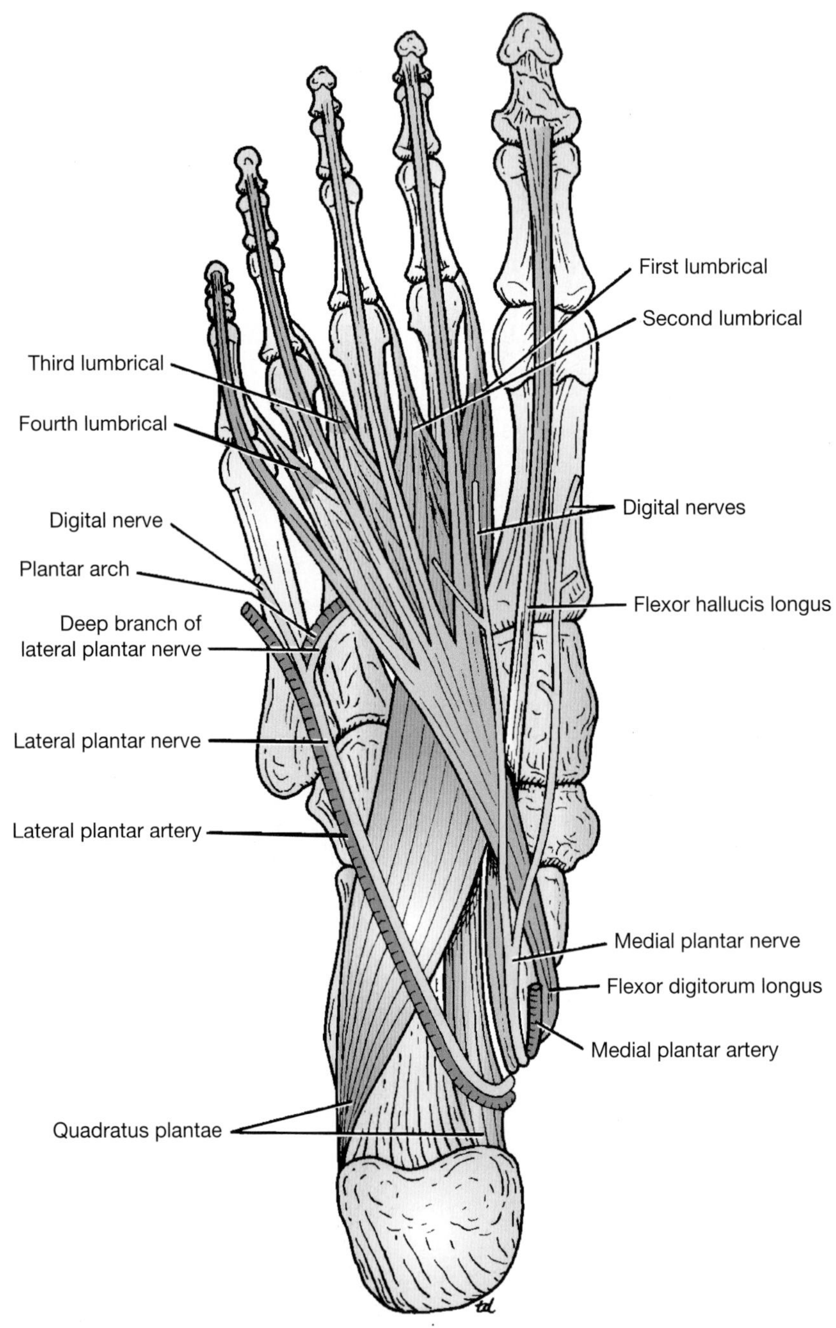

Figure 8.76 Second layer of the plantar muscles of the right foot. Medial and lateral plantar arteries and nerves are also shown.

Flexor Digitorum Longus Tendon

The flexor digitorum longus tendon enters the sole by passing behind the medial malleolus deep to the flexor retinaculum (see Figs. 8.70B, 8.76, and 8.77). It passes forward across the medial surface of the sustentaculum tali and then crosses the tendon of flexor hallucis longus, from which it receives a strong tendinous connection (called a "slip"). Here, it receives the insertion of the quadratus plantae muscle on its lateral border. The tendon next divides into its four tendons of insertion, which pass forward, giving origin to the lumbrical muscles. The tendons then enter the fibrous sheaths of the lateral four toes (see Fig. 8.74). Each tendon perforates the corresponding tendon of flexor digitorum brevis and passes on to insert into the base of the distal phalanx. This arrangement is similar to that for the flexor digitorum profundus in the hand.

Flexor Hallucis Longus Tendon

The flexor hallucis longus tendon enters the sole by passing behind the medial malleolus deep to the flexor retinaculum (see Figs. 8.70B, 8.76, and 8.77). It runs forward

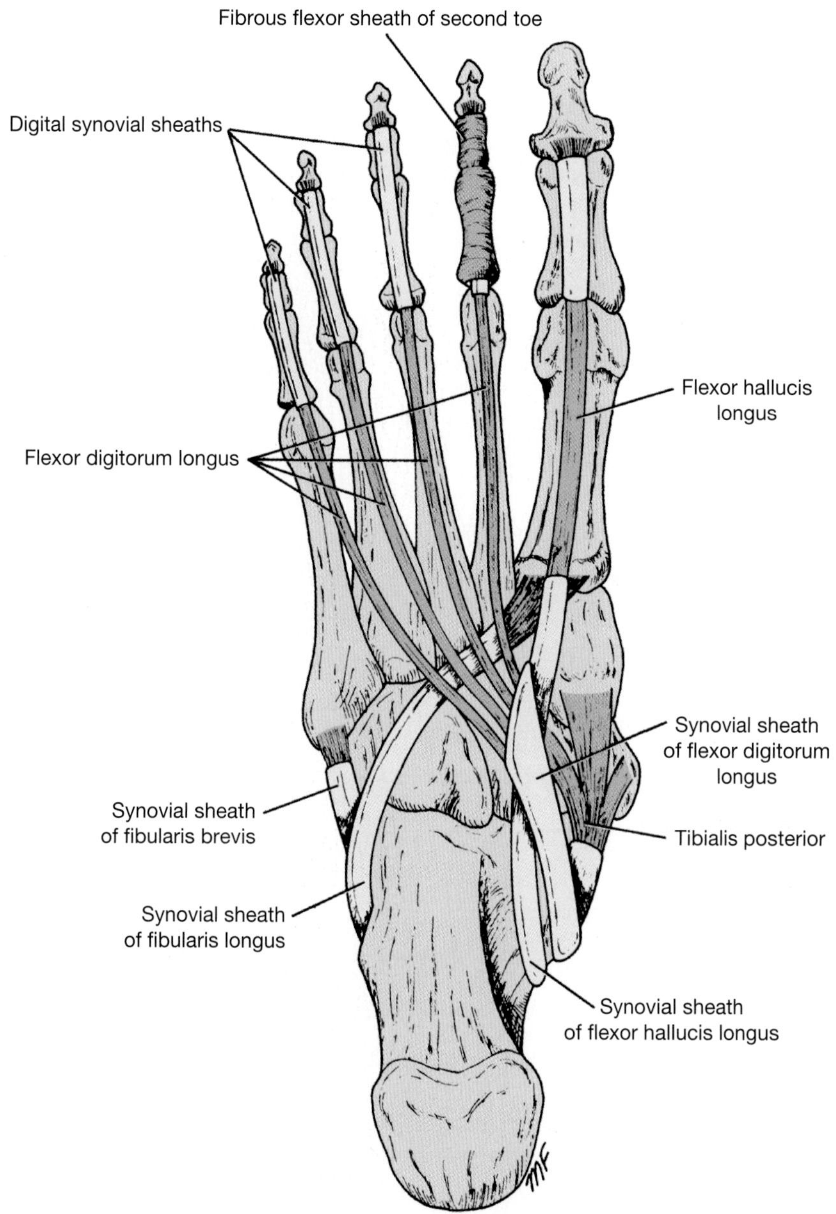

Figure 8.77 Synovial sheaths of the tendons seen on the sole of the right foot.

under the sustentaculum tali and crosses deep to the flexor digitorum longus tendon, to which it gives a strong connection. It then enters the fibrous sheath of the great toe and inserts into the base of the distal phalanx.

FIBROUS FLEXOR SHEATHS

The inferior surface of each toe, from the head of the metatarsal bone to the base of the distal phalanx, is provided with a strong fibrous sheath, which is attached to the sides of the phalanges (see Fig. 8.74). The arrangement is similar to that found in the fingers. The fibrous sheath, together with the inferior surfaces of the phalanges and the interphalangeal joints, forms a blind tunnel in which lie the flexor tendons of the toe (see Fig. 8.77).

SYNOVIAL FLEXOR SHEATHS

Synovial sheaths surround the tendons of the flexor hallucis longus and the flexor digitorum longus (see Figs. 8.70B and 8.77).

Fibularis Longus Tendon

The fibularis longus tendon enters the foot from behind the lateral malleolus and runs obliquely across the sole to insert into the base of the first metatarsal bone and the adjacent part of the medial cuneiform (see Figs. 8.77 and 8.79). The tendon grooves the inferior surface of the cuboid where it is held in position by the **long plantar ligament** and is surrounded by a synovial sheath (see Fig. 8.77).

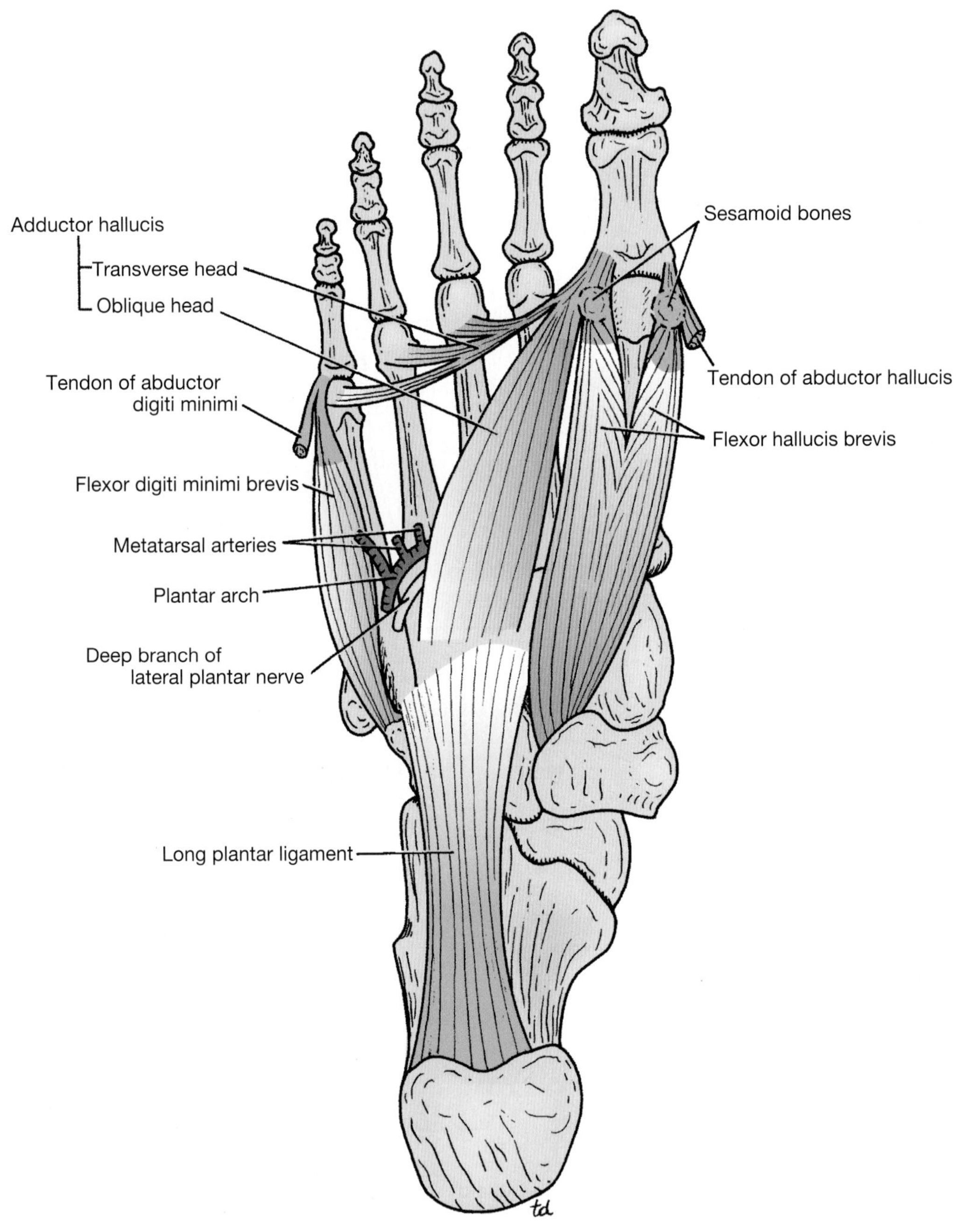

Figure 8.78 Third layer of the plantar muscles of the right foot. The deep branch of the lateral plantar nerve and the plantar arterial arch are also shown.

Tibialis Posterior Tendon

The tibialis posterior tendon (see Fig. 8.79) enters the foot from behind the medial malleolus. It passes deep to the flexor retinaculum and runs downward and forward above the sustentaculum tali to insert mainly into the tuberosity of the navicular. Small tendinous slips pass to the cuboid and the cuneiforms and to the bases of the second, third, and fourth metatarsals. A synovial sheath surrounds the tendon (see Fig. 8.77).

Sole Arteries

The **posterior tibial artery** passes behind the medial malleolus, deep to the flexor retinaculum, and terminates by dividing into the **medial** and **lateral plantar arteries** (see Figs. 8.63 and 8.70B).

Medial Plantar Artery

The medial plantar artery is the smaller of the terminal branches of the posterior tibial artery. It arises deep to the flexor retinaculum and passes forward deep to

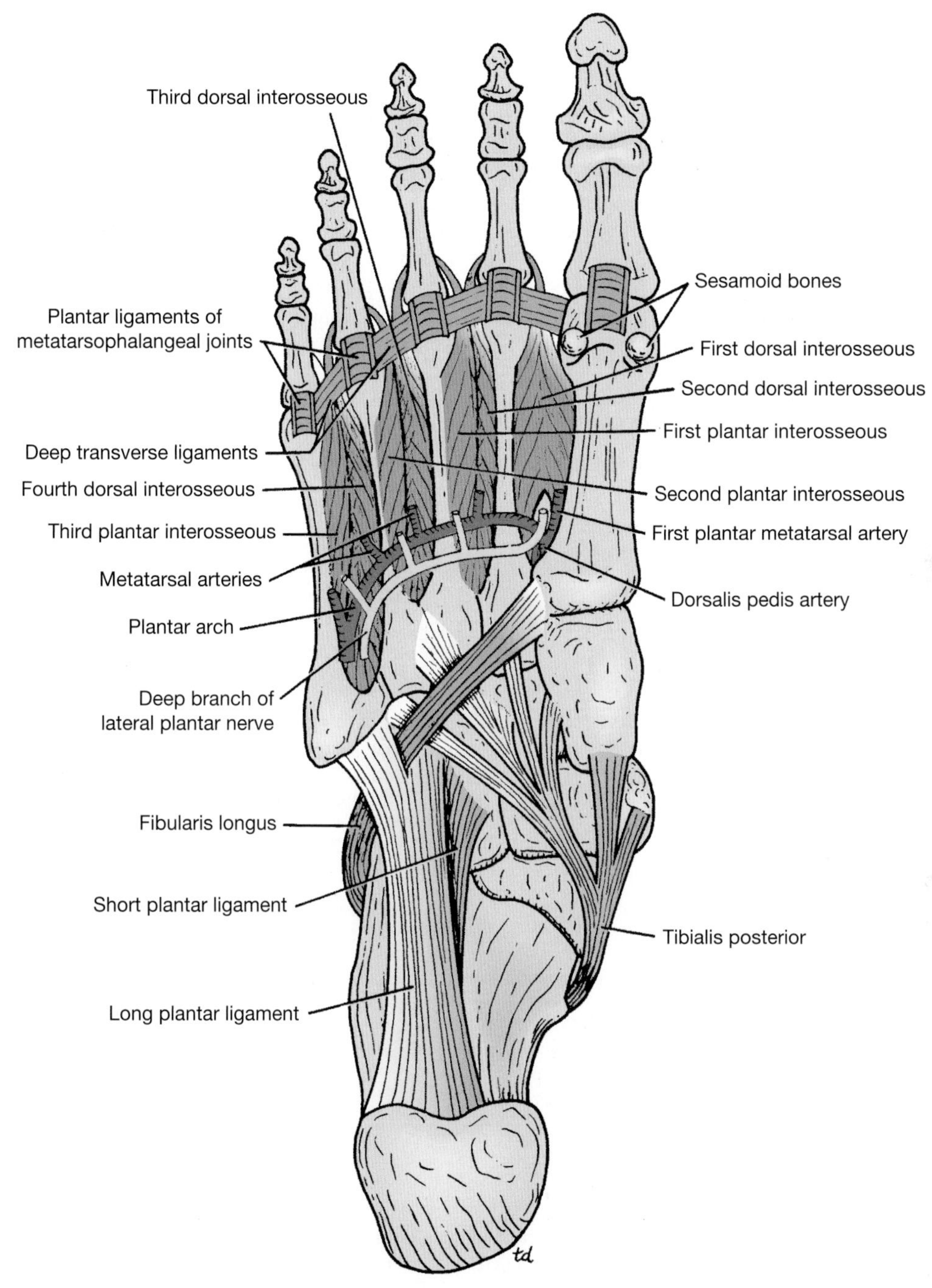

Figure 8.79 Fourth layer of the plantar muscles of the right foot. The deep branch of the lateral plantar nerve and the plantar arterial arch are also shown. Note the deep transverse ligaments.

the abductor hallucis muscle (see Fig. 8.70B). It ends by supplying the medial side of the great toe (see Fig. 8.75). It gives off numerous muscular, cutaneous, and articular branches along its course.

Lateral Plantar Artery

The lateral plantar artery is the larger of the terminal branches of the posterior tibial artery. It arises deep to the flexor retinaculum and passes forward deep to the abductor hallucis and the flexor digitorum brevis (see Figs. 8.70B, 8.75, and 8.76). On reaching the base of the fifth metatarsal bone, the artery curves medially to form the **plantar arch** (see Figs. 8.76, 8.78, and 8.79). At the proximal end of the first intermetatarsal space, it anastomoses with the **deep plantar artery**, which is a branch of the dorsalis pedis artery (see Fig. 8.79). The lateral plantar artery gives off numerous muscular, cutaneous, and articular branches along its course. The

Table 8.8 Sole Muscles

MUSCLE	ORIGIN	INSERTION	NERVE SUPPLY	NERVE ROOT[a]	ACTION
First Layer					
Abductor hallucis	Medial tuberosity of calcaneum and flexor retinaculum	Base of proximal phalanx of great toe	Medial plantar nerve	S2, **S3**	Flexes and abducts great toe; braces medial longitudinal arch
Flexor digitorum brevis	Medial tubercle of calcaneum	Four tendons to four lateral toes—inserted into borders of middle phalanx; tendons perforated by those of flexor digitorum longus	Medial plantar nerve	S2, **S3**	Flexes lateral four toes; braces medial and lateral longitudinal arches
Abductor digiti minimi	Medial and lateral tubercles of calcaneum	Base of proximal phalanx of fifth toe	Lateral plantar nerve	S2, **S3**	Flexes and abducts fifth toe; braces lateral longitudinal arch
Second Layer					
Quadratus plantae	Medial and lateral sides of calcaneum	Tendon of flexor digitorum longus	Lateral plantar nerve	S2, **S3**	Assists flexor digitorum longus in flexing lateral four toes
Lumbricals (4)	Tendons of flexor digitorum longus	Dorsal extensor expansion; bases of proximal phalanges of lateral four toes	First lumbrical: medial plantar nerve; remainder: lateral plantar nerve	S2, **S3**	Extends toes at interphalangeal joints
Flexor digitorum longus tendon	See Table 8.7				
Flexor hallucis longus tendon	See Table 8.7				
Third Layer					
Flexor hallucis brevis	Cuboid, lateral cuneiform, tibialis posterior insertion	Medial tendon into medial side of base of proximal phalanx of great toe; lateral tendon into lateral side of base of proximal phalanx of great toe	Medial plantar nerve	S2, **S3**	Flexes metatarsophalangeal joint of great toe; supports medial longitudinal arch
Adductor hallucis	Oblique head bases of second, third, and fourth metatarsal bones; transverse head from plantar ligaments	Lateral side of base of proximal phalanx of great toe	Deep branch lateral plantar nerve	S2, **S3**	Flexes metatarsophalangeal joint of great toe; holds together metatarsal bones
Flexor digiti minimi brevis	Base of fifth metatarsal bone	Lateral side of base of proximal phalanx of little toe	Lateral plantar nerve	S2, **S3**	Flexes metatarsophalangeal joint of little toe

Table 8.8 Sole Muscles (*Continued*)

MUSCLE	ORIGIN	INSERTION	NERVE SUPPLY	NERVE ROOT[a]	ACTION
Fourth Layer					
Interossei					
Dorsal (4)	Adjacent sides of metatarsal bones	Bases of proximal phalanges—first: medial side of second toe; remainder: lateral sides of second, third, and fourth toes—also dorsal extensor expansion	Lateral plantar nerve	S2, **S3**	Abduction of toes; flexes metatarsophalangeal joints and extends interphalangeal joints
Plantar (3)	Inferior surfaces of third, fourth, and fifth metatarsal bones	Medial side of bases of proximal phalanges of lateral three toes	Lateral plantar nerve	S2, **S3**	Adduction of toes; flexes metatarsophalangeal joints and extends interphalangeal joints
Fibularis longus tendon	See Table 8.6				
Tibialis posterior tendon	See Table 8.7				

[a]The predominant nerve root supply is in bold.

plantar arch gives off **plantar metatarsal arteries** to the toes (see Fig. 8.79).

Sole Veins

Medial and **lateral plantar veins** accompany the corresponding arteries. They unite behind the medial malleolus to form the posterior tibial venae comitantes.

Sole Nerves

The **tibial nerve** passes behind the medial malleolus, deep to the flexor retinaculum, and terminates by dividing into the **medial** and **lateral plantar nerves** (see Figs. 8.44, 8.63, and 8.70B).

Medial Plantar Nerve

The medial plantar nerve is a terminal branch of the tibial nerve (see Fig. 8.44). It arises deep to the flexor retinaculum (see Fig. 8.63) and runs forward deep to the abductor hallucis, with the medial plantar artery (see Figs. 8.75 and 8.76). It comes to lie in the interval between the abductor hallucis and the flexor digitorum brevis.

BRANCHES

- **Muscular branches** to the abductor hallucis, the flexor digitorum brevis, the flexor hallucis brevis, and the first lumbrical muscle (see Fig. 8.44).
- **Cutaneous branches: Plantar digital nerves** run to the sides of the medial three and a half toes (see Figs. 8.74 and 8.75). The nerves extend onto the dorsum and supply the nail beds and the tips of the toes.

Note the similar distributions of the medial plantar nerve and the median nerve in the palm of the hand.

Lateral Plantar Nerve

The lateral plantar nerve is a terminal branch of the tibial nerve (see Fig. 8.44). It arises deep to the flexor retinaculum (see Fig. 8.63) and runs forward deep to the abductor hallucis and the flexor digitorum brevis, in company with the lateral plantar artery (see Figs. 8.75 and 8.76). On reaching the base of the fifth metatarsal bone, it divides into **superficial** and **deep branches**.

BRANCHES

- **From the main trunk:** Muscular branches to the quadratus plantae and abductor digiti minimi; cutaneous branches to the skin of the lateral part of the sole.
- **From the superficial terminal branch:** Muscular branches to the flexor digiti minimi and the interosseous muscles of the fourth intermetatarsal space. **Plantar digital branches** pass to the sides of the lateral one and a half toes. The nerves extend onto the dorsum and supply the nail beds and tips of the toes.
- **From the deep terminal branch** (see Fig. 8.79): This branch curves medially with the lateral plantar artery and supplies the adductor hallucis; second, third and fourth lumbricals; and all the interossei, except those in the fourth intermetatarsal space (see superficial branch above).

Note the similar distributions of the lateral plantar nerve and the ulnar nerve in the palm of the hand.

Dorsum

The skin on the dorsum is thin, hairy, and freely mobile on the underlying tendons and bones. This is much like the condition in the dorsum of the hand.

Cutaneous Nerves

The sensory nerve supply to the skin on the dorsum is derived from the superficial fibular (peroneal) nerve, assisted mainly by the deep fibular (peroneal), saphenous, and sural nerves (see Figs. 8.36, 8.37, 8.43, and 8.56).

- The **superficial fibular (peroneal) nerve** emerges from between the fibularis brevis and the extensor digitorum longus muscle in the lower part of the leg. It divides into **medial** and **lateral cutaneous branches** that supply the skin on the dorsum of the foot, the medial side of the great toe, and the adjacent sides of the second, third, fourth and fifth toes.
- The **deep fibular (peroneal) nerve** supplies the skin of the adjacent sides of the big and second toes.
- The **saphenous nerve** passes onto the dorsum of the foot in front of the medial malleolus. It supplies the skin along the medial side of the foot as far forward as the head of the first metatarsal bone.
- The **sural nerve** enters the foot behind the lateral malleolus and supplies the skin along the lateral margin of the foot and the lateral side of the little toe.
- The **medial and lateral plantar nerves** supply the nail beds and the skin covering the dorsal surfaces of the terminal phalanges (see above).

Dorsal Venous Arch (or Network)

The greater part of the blood from the whole foot drains into the **dorsal venous arch** via digital veins and communicating veins from the sole, which pass through the interosseous spaces.

The dorsal venous arch lies in the subcutaneous tissue over the heads of the metatarsal bones (see Figs. 8.46, 8.67, 8.68, and 8.73). It drains on the medial side into the **great saphenous vein** and on the lateral side into the **small saphenous vein**. The great saphenous vein leaves the dorsum of the foot by ascending into the leg in front of the medial malleolus. The small saphenous vein ascends into the leg behind the lateral malleolus.

Dorsum Muscles

The **extensor digitorum brevis** is the sole intrinsic muscle on the dorsum of the foot. It is shown in Figures 8.65, 8.68, and 8.80 and summarized in Table 8.9. The muscle sends a long tendon to the great toe (effectively an extensor hallucis brevis) but does not run to the fifth digit.

Long Extensor Tendon Insertion

The tendon of extensor digitorum longus passes deep to the superior extensor retinaculum and through the inferior extensor retinaculum, in company with the fibularis tertius muscle (see Fig. 8.80). The tendon divides into four, which fan out over the dorsum of the foot and pass to the lateral four toes. Opposite the metatarsophalangeal joints of the second, third, and fourth toes, each tendon is joined on its lateral side by a tendon of extensor digitorum brevis.

On the dorsal surface of each toe, the extensor tendon joins the fascial expansion called the **extensor (dorsal) expansion**. Near the proximal interphalangeal joint, the extensor expansion splits into three parts: a central part, which is inserted into the base of the middle phalanx, and two lateral parts, which converge to insert into the base of the distal phalanx. The extensor expansion, as in the fingers, receives the tendons of insertion of the interosseous and lumbrical muscles.

Synovial Sheath of Tendon of Extensor Digitorum Longus

A common synovial sheath surrounds the extensor digitorum longus and fibularis tertius tendons as they pass beneath the extensor retinacula (see Fig. 8.80). The sheath extends proximally for a short distance above the malleoli and distally to the level of the base of the fifth metatarsal bone.

Dorsum Arterial Supply

The **dorsalis pedis artery (dorsal artery of the foot)** is the continuation of the anterior tibial artery and supplies the dorsum of the foot (see Figs. 8.54, 8.65, 8.66, and 8.80). It begins in front of the ankle joint at an imaginary line connecting the malleoli. It is superficial in position and is crossed by the inferior extensor retinaculum and the first tendon of extensor digitorum brevis (see Fig. 8.80). On its lateral side lie the terminal part of the deep fibular (peroneal) nerve and the extensor digitorum longus tendons. On the medial side lies the tendon of extensor hallucis longus. Its pulsations can easily be felt in this location. The vessel terminates by joining the lateral plantar artery and completing the **plantar arch** (see Figs. 8.79 and 8.80).

Branches

- **Lateral tarsal artery** crosses the dorsum of the foot just below the ankle joint (see Fig. 8.80).
- **Arcuate artery** runs laterally deep to the extensor tendons opposite the bases of the metatarsal bones (Fig. 8.80). It gives off metatarsal branches to the toes.
- **First dorsal metatarsal** artery supplies both sides of the great toe.
- **Deep plantar artery:** this terminal branch of the dorsalis pedis artery dives into the sole between the two heads of the first dorsal interosseous muscle. It anastomoses with the end of the **lateral plantar artery** to complete the **plantar arterial arch** (see Figs. 8.79 and 8.80).

Dorsum Nerve Supply

The **deep fibular (peroneal) nerve** enters the dorsum by passing deep to the extensor retinacula on the lateral side of the dorsalis pedis artery (see Figs. 8.43, 8.65, 8.66, and 8.80). It divides into terminal, medial, and lateral branches. The medial branch supplies the skin of the adjacent sides of the big and second toes (see Fig. 8.80). The lateral branch supplies the extensor digitorum brevis muscle. Both terminal branches give articular branches to the joints of the foot.

The cutaneous innervation of the dorsum of the foot is described earlier in this section.

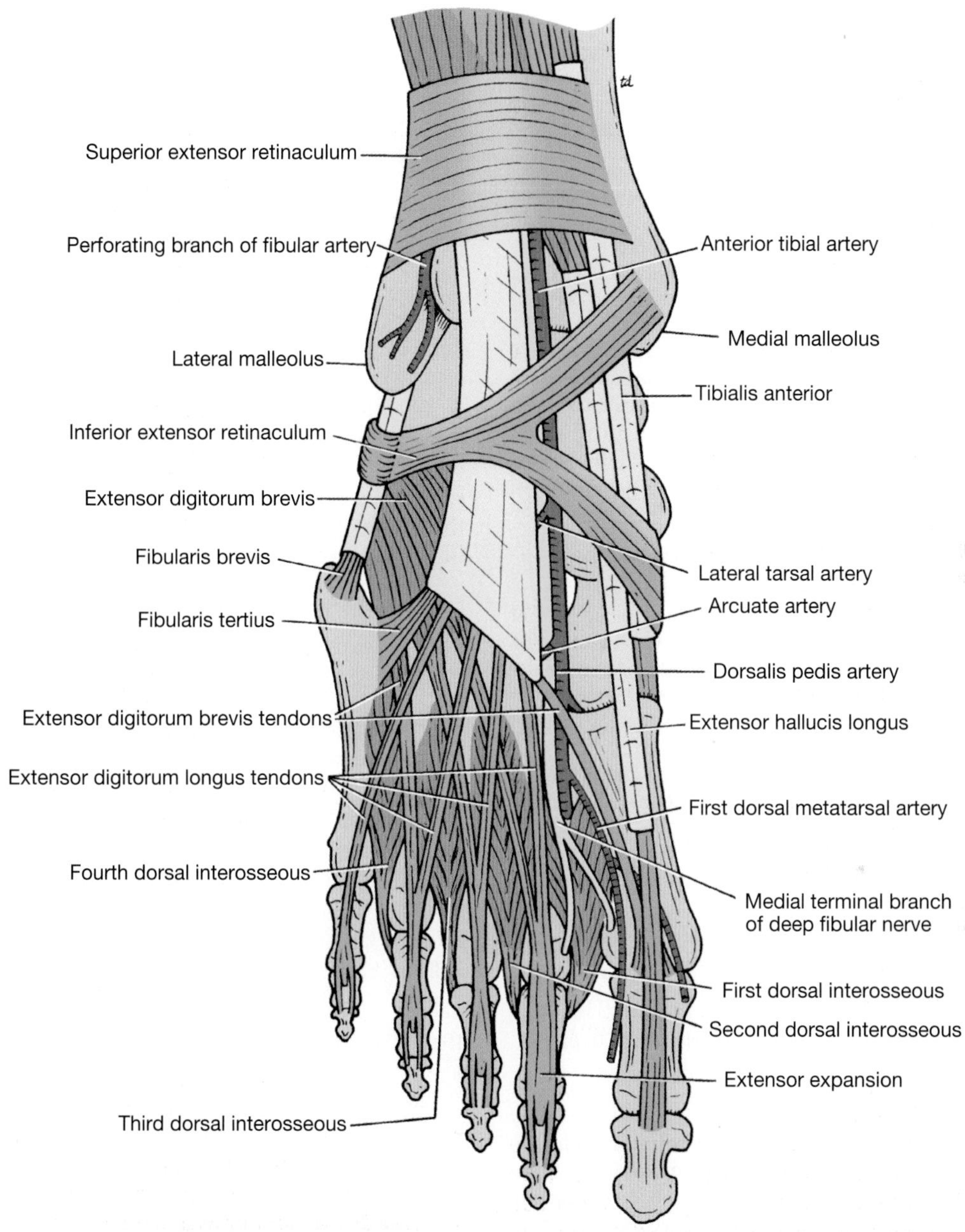

Figure 8.80 Structures in the dorsal aspect of the right foot.

Table 8.9 Dorsum Muscle

MUSCLE	ORIGIN	INSERTION	NERVE SUPPLY	NERVE ROOT	ACTION
Extensor digitorum brevis	Anterior part of upper surface of the calcaneum and from the inferior extensor retinaculum	By four tendons into the proximal phalanx of great toe and long extensor tendons to second, third, and fourth toes	Deep fibular nerve	S1, S2	Extends toes

Embryology Notes

Lower Limb Development

The limb buds appear during week 6 of development as the result of a localized proliferation of the somatopleuric mesenchyme. This causes the overlying ectoderm to bulge from the trunk as two pairs of flattened paddles. The leg buds develop after the arm buds and arise at the level of the L2 to L5 and S1 to S3 segments.

The flattened limb buds have a cephalic **preaxial border** and a caudal **postaxial border**. As the limb buds elongate, the anterior rami of the L2 through S1 nerves innervate the mesenchyme along the preaxial border, and the S1 to S3 sacral nerves supply that of the postaxial border. Later, the mesenchymal masses divide into anterior and posterior groups, and the nerve trunks entering the base of each limb also divide into anterior and posterior divisions. As development continues and the limbs further elongate, their attachment to the trunk moves caudally. At the same time, the mesenchyme within the limbs differentiates into individual muscles that migrate within each limb. Because of these two factors, the anterior rami of the spinal nerves become arranged near the base of the limb into the complicated lumbosacral plexus.

It is interesting to note that the dermatomal pattern in the lower limb appears to be more complicated than that of the upper limb (see Chapter 1). This can be explained embryologically, because during fetal development, the lower limb bud undergoes medial rotation as it grows out from the trunk. This results in the great toe coming to lie on the medial side of the foot and accounts for the spiraling pattern of the dermatomes.

Ectromelia

Ectromelia is a partial absence of a lower limb (Fig. 8.81). The condition in the upper limb is described in Chapter 3.

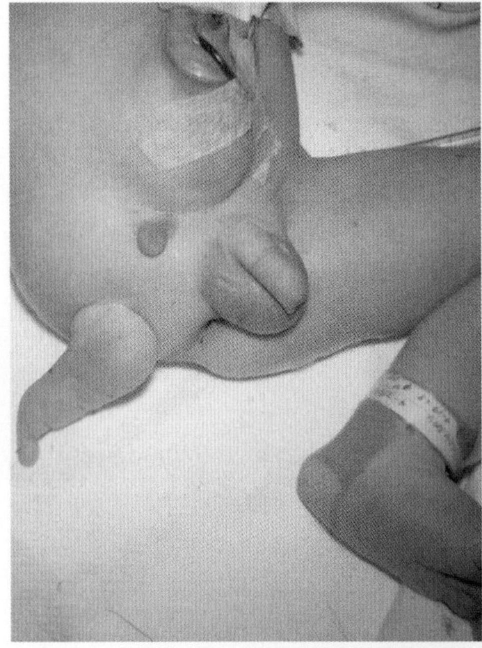

Figure 8.81 Ectromelia. (Courtesy of G. Avery.)

Congenital Hip Dislocation

Congenital dislocation of the hip is 10 times more common in female children and is particularly common in northern Italy (Fig. 8.82). Three possible causes have been suggested:

- **Generalized joint laxity:** Excessive laxity of the ligaments of the hip joint may predispose to this condition.
- **Breech position:** The flexed hip and extended knees of the breech position may alter the normal pressure of the head of the femur on the acetabulum, and this may result in a failure of the upper part of the acetabulum to develop adequately.
- **Shallow acetabulum:** If the acetabulum is poorly developed, the upper lip offers an insufficient shelf under which the head of the femur can lodge. The condition of shallow acetabulum tends to run in families.

Congenital dislocation of the hip should be diagnosed at birth and is treated by splinting the joint in the position of abduction.

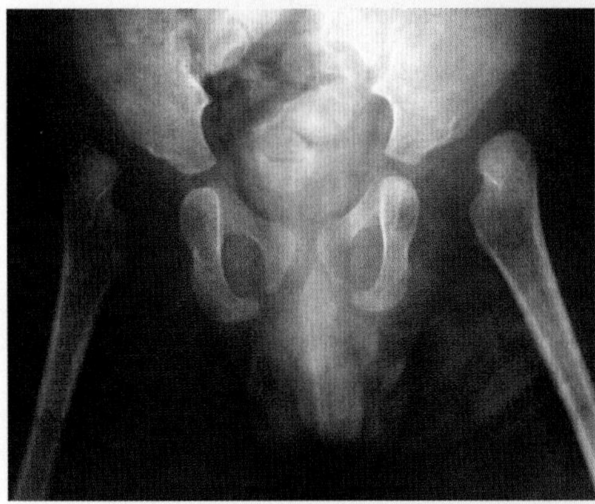

Figure 8.82 Radiograph of bilateral congenital dislocation of the hip showing that the femoral heads are not within the shallow acetabular fossae. (Courtesy of J. Adams.)

Genu Recurvatum

Hyperextension of the knee joint is found in babies who have had a breech presentation with extended legs. No treatment is required because the legs return to normal within a few weeks.

Talipes

Talipes (**clubfoot**) often is caused by abnormal position or restricted movement of the fetus in utero. A small number of cases may be caused by muscle paralysis associated with spina bifida. The different types are named according to the position of the foot. **Talipes calcaneovalgus** is a form of clubfoot in which the foot is dorsiflexed at the ankle joint and everted at the midtarsal joints. In **talipes equinovarus**, the foot is plantar flexed at the ankle joint and inverted at the midtarsal joints (Fig. 8.83). The conditions may be unilateral or bilateral, and they require orthopedic treatment.

Metatarsus Varus

Metatarsus varus is a common condition in which the forefoot is adducted on the rear part of the foot. Correction may be accomplished by manipulation followed by splinting.

Overriding Toes

Overriding toes most commonly involve the fourth and fifth toes. The fourth toe is depressed and overridden by the fifth toe. This may be corrected by the application of splints.

Curly Toes

Curly toes most often affect the fourth and fifth toes; the condition commonly runs in families. The affected toe lies flexed under its medial neighbor. In mild cases, there is no treatment; in severe cases, the flexor digitorum longus tendon is transplanted into the extensor tendon.

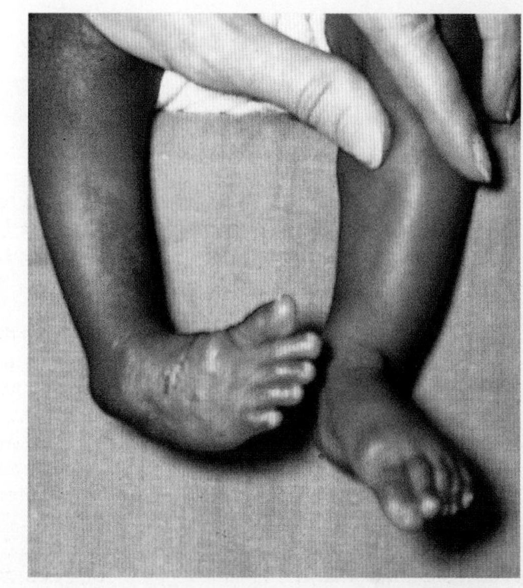

Figure 8.83 Talipes equinovarus. (Courtesy of J. Adams.)

SURFACE ANATOMY

An adequate physical examination of the lower limb of a patient requires a sound knowledge of the surface anatomy of the region. The following information should be verified on the living body.

Gluteal Region

The **iliac crests** are easily palpable along their entire length (Figs. 8.84 and 8.85). Each crest ends in front at the **anterosuperior iliac spine** and behind at the **posterosuperior iliac spine**; the latter lies beneath a skin dimple at the level of the S2 vertebra and the middle of the sacroiliac joint. The **iliac tubercle** is a prominence felt on the outer surface of the iliac crest about 2 in. (5 cm) posterior to the anterosuperior iliac spine.

The **ischial tuberosity** can be palpated in the lower part of the buttock. In the standing position, the tuberosity is covered by the gluteus maximus. In the sitting position, the ischial tuberosity emerges from beneath the lower border of the gluteus maximus and supports the weight of the body. In this position, only a bursa and a pad of fat separate the tuberosity from the skin.

The **greater trochanter** of the femur can be felt on the lateral surface of the thigh and moves beneath the examining finger as the hip joint is flexed and extended. Note that, in the normal hip joint, the upper border of the greater trochanter lies on a line connecting the anterosuperior iliac spine to the ischial tuberosity.

The **spinous processes of the sacrum** are fused with each other to form the **median sacral crest**. The crest can be felt beneath the skin in the upper part of the cleft between the buttocks.

The **tip of the coccyx** can be palpated beneath the skin in the cleft between the buttocks about 1 in. (2.5 cm) behind the anus. The **anterior surface of the coccyx** can be palpated with a gloved finger in the anal canal.

The **fold of the buttock** is most prominent in the standing position. Note that its lower border does not correspond to the lower border of the gluteus maximus muscle.

The **sciatic nerve** in the buttock lies under cover of the gluteus maximus muscle. As it curves laterally and downward, it is situated at first midway between the posterosuperior iliac spine and the ischial tuberosity and, lower down, midway between the tip of the greater trochanter and the ischial tuberosity.

Inguinal Region

The **inguinal ligament** lies beneath the skin fold in the groin and can be felt along its length. It attaches laterally to the anterosuperior iliac spine and medially to the pubic tubercle (Fig. 8.86; see also Fig. 8.85C).

The **symphysis pubis** is a cartilaginous joint that lies in the midline between the bodies of the pubic bones. The upper margin of the symphysis pubis and the bodies of the pubic bones can be felt on palpation through the lower part of the anterior abdominal wall.

The **pubic tubercle** can be felt on the upper border of the pubis. Attached to it is the medial end of the inguinal ligament. The tubercle is easily palpated in the male

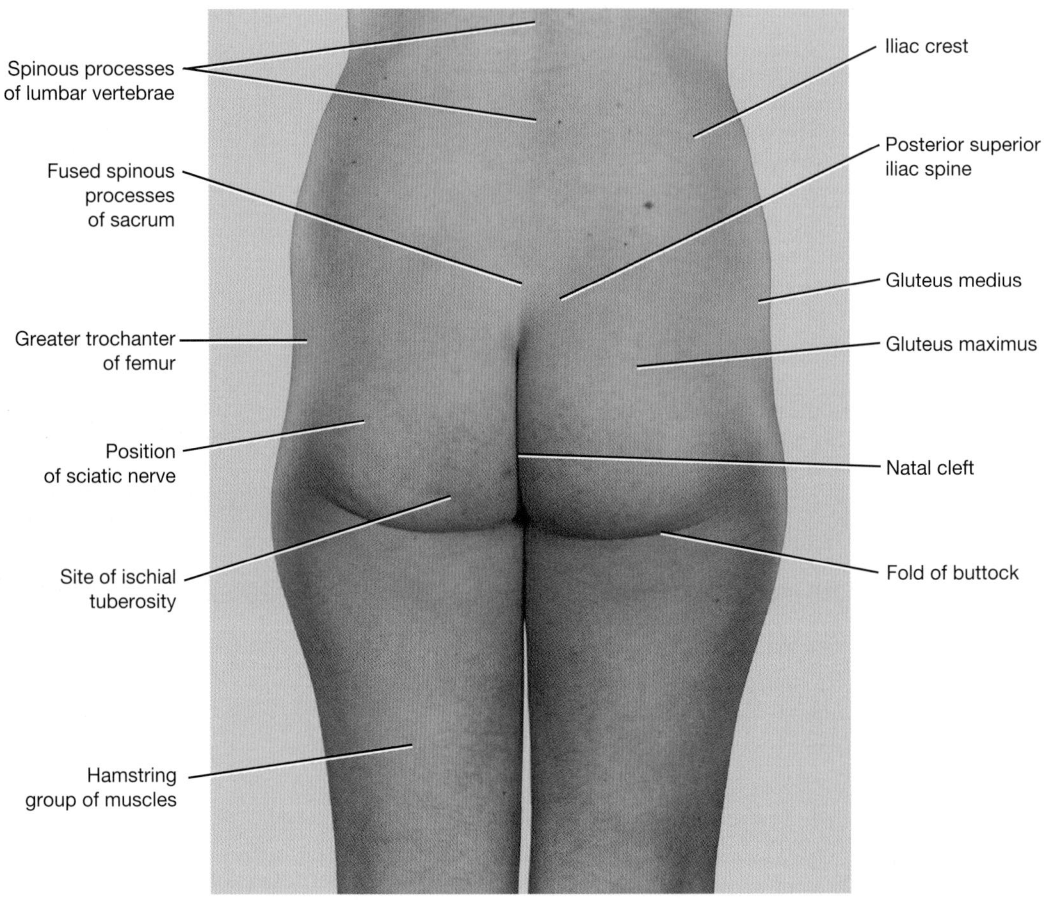

Figure 8.84 Gluteal region and the posterior aspect of the thigh of a young adult female, showing the surface projections of major underlying structures.

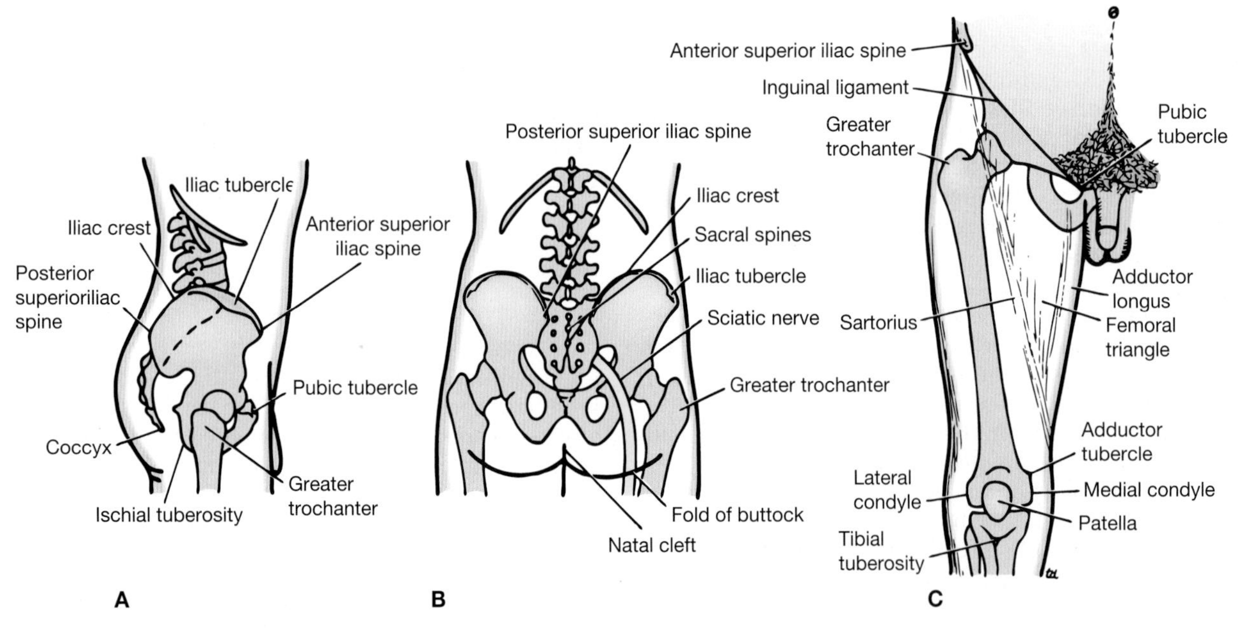

Figure 8.85 Surface markings in the gluteal region and the front of the thigh. **A.** Lateral view. **B.** Posterior view. **C.** Anterior view.

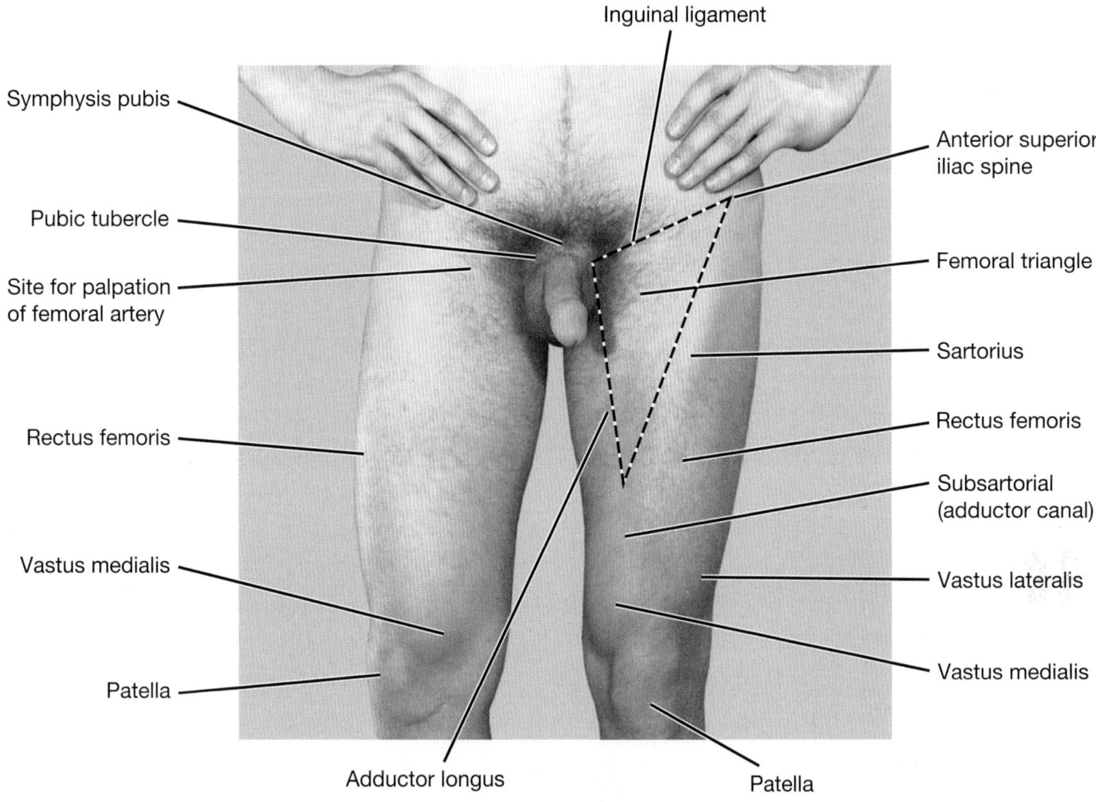

Figure 8.86 Anterior aspect of the thigh of a young adult male. The *broken lines* indicate the boundaries of the femoral triangle. The right leg is laterally rotated at the hip joint.

by invaginating the scrotum with the examining finger. In the female, it can be palpated through the lateral margin of the labium majus.

The **pubic crest** is the ridge of bone on the upper surface of the body of the pubis, medial to the pubic tubercle (see Figs. 8.1 and 8.2).

Femoral Triangle

The femoral triangle is a depression below the fold of the groin in the upper part of the thigh (see Figs. 8.85C and 8.86). In a thin, muscular patient, the boundaries of the triangle can be identified when the thigh is flexed, abducted, and laterally rotated. The inguinal ligament forms the **base** of the triangle, the lateral border of the sartorius muscle forms the **lateral wall**, and the medial border of the adductor longus muscle forms the **medial wall**.

The **horizontal group of superficial inguinal lymph nodes** can be palpated in the superficial fascia just below and parallel to the inguinal ligament (see Fig. 8.38).

The **femoral artery** enters the thigh deep to the inguinal ligament (see Fig. 8.48) at the midpoint of a line joining the symphysis pubis to the anterosuperior iliac spine, where its pulsations are easily felt (see Fig. 8.86).

The **femoral vein** leaves the thigh by passing deep to the inguinal ligament medial to the pulsating femoral artery (see Fig. 8.48).

The lower opening of the **femoral canal** lies below and lateral to the pubic tubercle (see Figs. 8.38 and 8.48).

The **femoral nerve** enters the thigh behind the midpoint of the inguinal ligament, that is, lateral to the pulsating femoral artery.

The **great saphenous vein** pierces the saphenous opening in the deep fascia (fascia lata) of the thigh and joins the femoral vein 1.5 in. (4 cm) below and lateral to the pubic tubercle (see Figs. 8.38 and 8.46).

Adductor Canal

The **adductor (subsartorial) canal** lies in the middle third of the thigh, immediately distal to the apex of the femoral triangle (see Fig. 8.86). It is an intermuscular cleft situated deep to the sartorius muscle and is bounded laterally by the vastus medialis muscle and posteriorly by the adductor longus and magnus muscles. It contains the femoral vessels and the saphenous nerve.

Knee Region

The **patella** and the **ligamentum patellae** can be easily palpated in front of the knee (Fig. 8.87). The ligamentum patellae can be traced downward to its attachment to the **tuberosity of the tibia**.

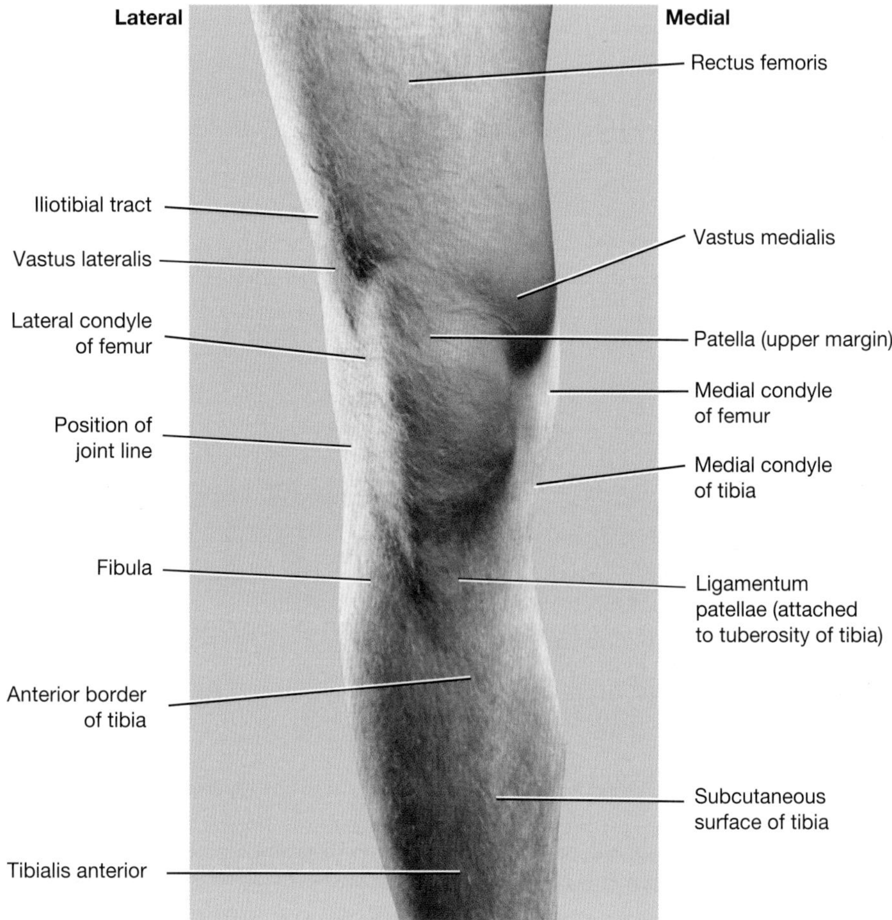

Figure 8.87 Anterior aspect of the right knee of a young adult male, showing the surface projections of major underlying structures.

The **condyles** of the femur and tibia can be recognized on the sides of the knee, and the **joint line** can be identified between them.

The bandlike **medial collateral ligament** and the rounded **lateral collateral ligament** can be palpated on the sides of the joint line; they can be followed above and below to their bony attachments. Because the ligaments cover the joint line, the joint line cannot be palpated at the sites of the collateral ligaments.

The **menisci** are in the interval between the femoral and tibial condyles. Although not recognizable, the outer edges of the medial and lateral menisci can be palpated on the joint line between the ligamentum patellae and the medial and lateral collateral ligaments, respectively.

The tendon of the **biceps femoris** can be felt as a rounded structure on the lateral aspect of the knee and can be traced down to the head of the fibula.

The **common fibular (peroneal) nerve** can be rolled beneath the examining finger on the medial side of the tendon of the biceps femoris, just below the head of the fibula (Fig. 8.88). The nerve descends and passes forward around the lateral side of the bone.

The **adductor tubercle** can be palpated on the medial aspect of the femur just above the medial condyle; the hamstring part of the adductor magnus can be felt passing to it.

Behind the knee joint is a diamond-shaped skin depression called **the popliteal fossa**. When the knee is flexed, the deep fascia, which roofs over the fossa, is relaxed and the boundaries are easily defined. Its upper part is bounded laterally by the tendon of the biceps femoris muscle and medially by the tendons of the semimembranosus and semitendinosus muscles. Its lower part is bounded on each side by one of the heads of the gastrocnemius muscle.

The **popliteal artery** can be felt by gentle palpation in the depths of the popliteal fossa, provided that the deep fascia is fully relaxed by passively flexing the knee joint.

Tibia

The medial surface and anterior border of the tibia are subcutaneous and can be felt throughout their length (see Figs. 8.87 and 8.88).

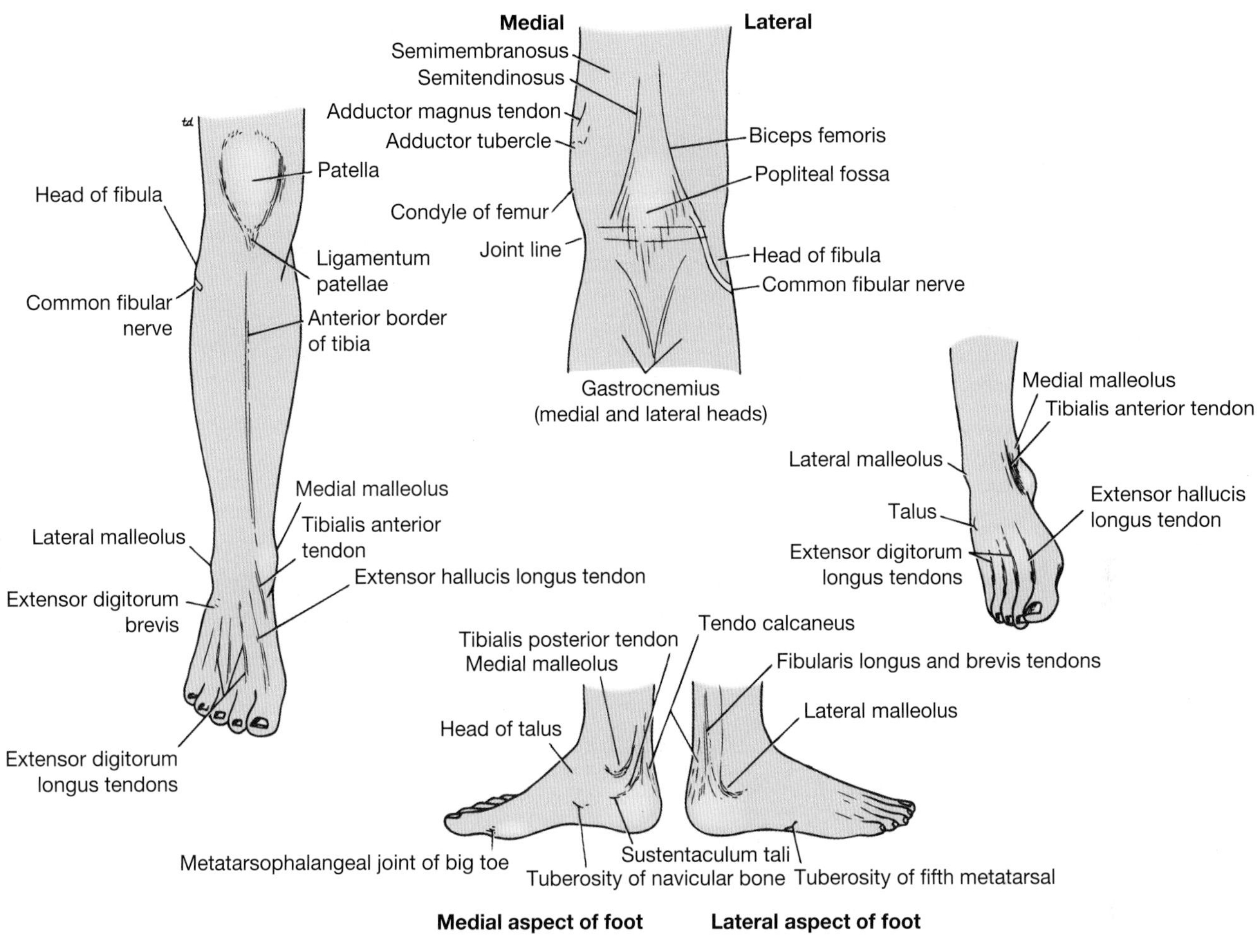

Figure 8.88 Surface markings in the popliteal fossa, front of the leg, and the foot.

Ankle Region and Foot

The fibula is subcutaneous in the ankle region and can be followed downward to form the **lateral malleolus** (Figs. 8.89 and 8.90). The tip of the **medial malleolus** of the tibia lies about 0.5 in. (1.3 cm) proximal to the level of the tip of the lateral malleolus (Figs. 8.89 and 8.90; see also Fig. 8.88).

The following structures, in the order named, lie in the interval behind the medial malleolus and the medial surface of the calcaneum: the **tendon of tibialis posterior**, **tendon of flexor digitorum longus**, **posterior tibial vessels**, **posterior tibial nerve**, and the **tendon of flexor hallucis longus**. The pulsations of the posterior tibial artery can be felt halfway between the medial malleolus and the heel (see Fig. 8.90B). The tendons of **fibularis brevis and longus** are behind the lateral malleolus (see Figs. 8.88 to 8.90).

On the anterior surface of the ankle joint, the **tendon of tibialis anterior** can be seen when the foot is dorsiflexed and inverted. The **tendon of extensor hallucis longus** lies lateral to it and can be made to stand out by extending the great toe. Lateral to the extensor hallucis longus lie the **tendons of extensor digitorum longus** and **fibularis tertius**. The pulsations of the **dorsalis pedis artery** can be felt between the tendons of extensor hallucis longus and extensor digitorum longus, midway between the two malleoli on the front of the ankle.

On the posterior surface of the ankle joint, the **calcaneum** forms the prominence of the heel. Above the heel is the **tendo calcaneus** (**Achilles tendon**).

On the dorsum of the foot, the **head of the talus** can be palpated just in front of the malleoli. The **tendons of extensor digitorum longus** and **extensor hallucis longus** can be made prominent by dorsiflexing the toes.

The **dorsal venous arch** or plexus can be seen on the dorsal surface of the foot proximal to the toes (see Figs. 8.46, 8.89, and 8.90). The **great saphenous vein** leaves the medial part of the plexus and passes upward in front of the medial malleolus. The **small saphenous vein** drains the lateral part of the plexus and passes up behind the lateral malleolus.

On the lateral aspect of the foot, the **tendon of fibularis brevis** passes forward to its insertion on the prominent **tuberosity on the base of the fifth metatarsal**

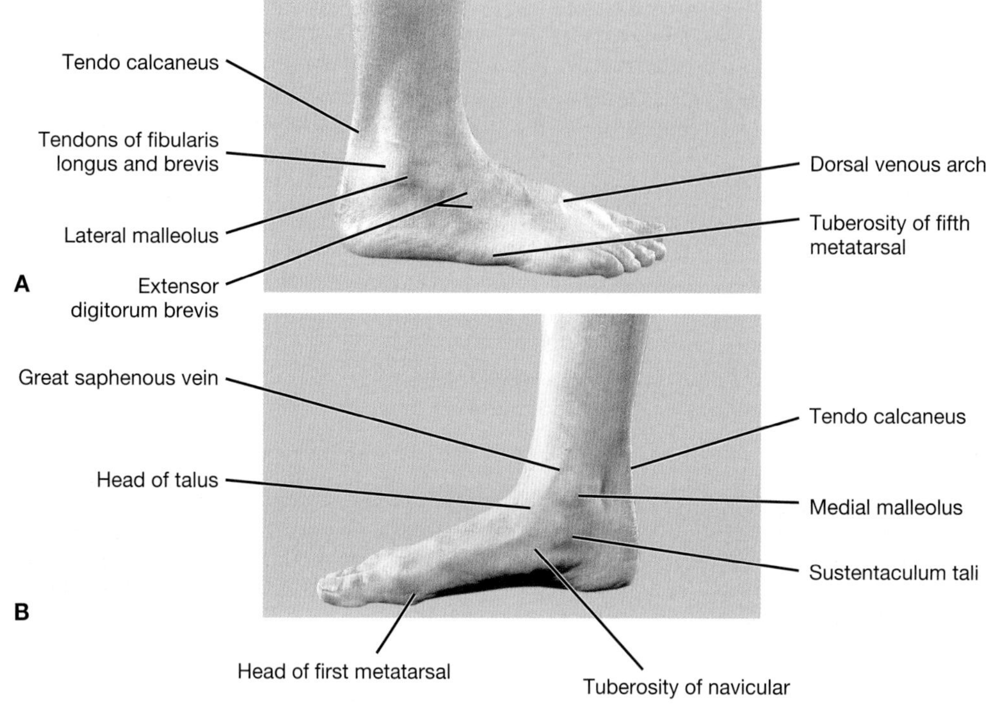

Figure 8.89 Lateral aspect **(A)** and medial aspect **(B)** of the right ankle of a young adult female showing the surface projections of major underlying structures.

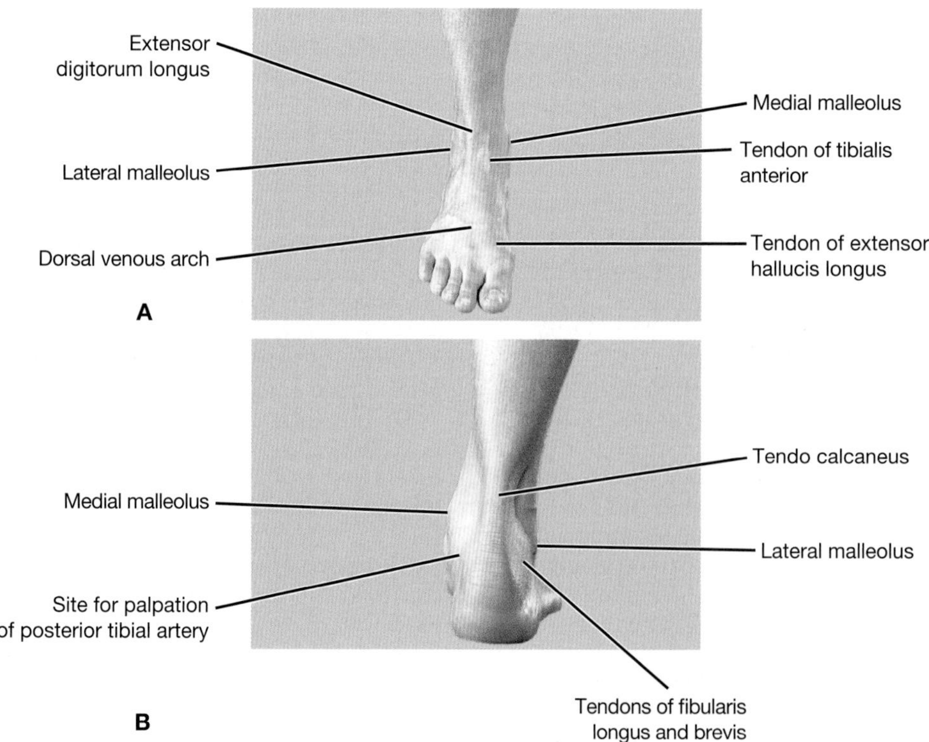

Figure 8.90 Anterior aspect **(A)** and posterior aspect **(B)** of the right foot and ankle of a young adult female showing the surface projections of major underlying structures.

bone. Below that, the **tendon of fibularis longus** passes forward to enter the groove on the under aspect of the cuboid bone.

On the medial aspect of the foot, the **sustentaculum tali** can be palpated about 1 in. (2.5 cm) below the tip of the medial malleolus (see Fig. 8.89). The **tendon of tibialis posterior** lies immediately above the sustentaculum tali; the **tendon of flexor digitorum longus** crosses its medial surface; and the **tendon of flexor hallucis longus** winds around its lower surface.

In front of the sustentaculum tali, the **tuberosity of the navicular bone** can be seen and palpated. It receives the main part of the tendon of insertion of the tibialis posterior muscle.

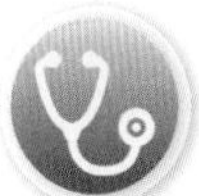

Clinical Notes on Lower Limb Arteries

Arterial Palpation

The **femoral artery** enters the thigh deep to the inguinal ligament at a point midway between the anterosuperior iliac spine and the symphysis pubis (see Fig. 8.86). The artery is easily palpated here because it can be pressed backward against the pectineus muscle and the superior ramus of the pubis.

The **popliteal artery** can be felt by gentle palpation in the depths of the popliteal space provided that the deep fascia is fully relaxed by passively flexing the knee joint (see Fig. 8.61).

The **dorsalis pedis** artery is palpable between the tendons of extensor hallucis longus and extensor digitorum longus, midway between the medial and lateral malleoli on the front of the ankle (see Fig. 8.66).

The **posterior tibial artery** passes behind the medial malleolus and beneath the flexor retinaculum. It lies between the tendons of flexor digitorum longus and flexor hallucis longus. The pulsations of the artery can be felt midway between the medial malleolus and the heel (see Figs. 8.70 and 8.90).

Note that the dorsalis pedis artery is sometimes absent and is replaced by a large perforating branch of the fibular artery. Also, the fibular artery may be larger than normal and replace the posterior tibial artery in the lower part of the leg.

Collateral Circulation

If the arterial supply to the leg is occluded, necrosis or gangrene will follow unless an adequate bypass to the obstruction is present—that is, a collateral circulation. Sudden occlusion of the femoral artery by ligature or embolism, for example, is usually followed by gangrene. However, gradual occlusion such as occurs in atherosclerosis is less likely to be followed by necrosis because the collateral blood vessels have time to dilate fully. The collateral circulation for the proximal part of the femoral artery is through the **cruciate** and **trochanteric anastomoses**. For the femoral artery in the adductor canal, it is through the **perforating branches** of the profunda femoris artery and the **articular** and **muscular branches** of the femoral and popliteal arteries.

Traumatic Injury

Injury to the large femoral artery can cause rapid exsanguination. Unlike in the upper extremity, arterial injuries of the lower limb do not have a good prognosis. The collateral circulations around the hip and knee joints, although present, are not as adequate as those around the shoulder and elbow. Damage to a neighboring large vein can further complicate the situation and causes further impairment of the circulation to the distal part of the limb.

Arterial Occlusive Leg Disease

Arterial occlusive disease of the leg is common in men. Ischemia of the muscles produces a cramplike pain with exercise. If the femoral artery is obstructed, the supply of blood to the calf muscles is inadequate, and the patient is forced to stop walking after a limited distance because of the intensity of the pain. With rest, the oxygen depletion corrects, and the pain disappears. However, on resumption of walking, the pain recurs. This condition is known as **intermittent claudication**.

Sympathetic Innervation of Arteries

Sympathetic innervation of the arteries to the leg is derived from the T10 to T12 and L1 to L2/3 segments of the spinal cord. The preganglionic fibers pass to the lower thoracic and upper lumbar ganglia via white rami. The fibers synapse in the lumbar and sacral ganglia, and the postganglionic fibers reach the blood vessels via branches of the lumbar and sacral plexuses. The femoral artery receives its sympathetic fibers from the femoral and obturator nerves. The more distal arteries receive their postganglionic fibers via the common fibular and tibial nerves.

Lumbar Sympathectomy and Occlusive Arterial Disease

Lumbar sympathectomy may be advocated as a form of treatment for occlusive arterial disease of the lower limb to increase blood flow through the collateral circulation. Preganglionic sympathectomy is performed by removing the L1 to L3 ganglia and the intervening parts of the sympathetic trunk.

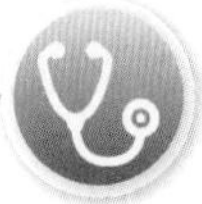

Clinical Notes on Lower Limb Nerves

Tendon Reflexes

Most skeletal muscles receive multisegmental innervation from two to four segments of the spinal cord. Eliciting simple tendon reflexes in the patient can assess the condition of the following spinal segments.

- **Patellar tendon reflex (knee jerk):** L2 to L4 (extension of the knee joint on tapping the patellar ligament)
- **Achilles tendon reflex (ankle jerk):** S1 and S2 (plantar flexion of the ankle joint on tapping the Achilles tendon)

Femoral Nerve Injury

The femoral nerve (L2 to L4) enters the thigh deep to the inguinal ligament, at a point midway between the anterosuperior iliac spine and the pubic tubercle; it lies about a fingerbreadth lateral to the femoral pulse. About 2 in. (5 cm) below the inguinal ligament, the nerve splits into its terminal branches (see Fig. 8.56).

The femoral nerve can get injured in stab or gunshot wounds, but a complete division of the nerve is rare. The following clinical features are present when the nerve is completely divided:

- **Motor:** The quadriceps femoris muscle is paralyzed, and the knee cannot extend. In walking, this is compensated for to some extent by use of the adductor muscles.
- **Sensory:** Skin sensation is lost over the anterior and medial sides of the thigh, over the medial side of the lower part of the leg, and along the medial border of the foot as far as the ball of the great toe; the saphenous nerve normally supplies this area.

Sciatic Nerve Injury

The sciatic nerve (L4 to S3) curves laterally and downward through the gluteal region, situated at first midway between the posterosuperior iliac spine and the ischial tuberosity, and lower down, midway between the tip of the greater trochanter and the ischial tuberosity. The nerve then passes downward in the midline on the posterior aspect of the thigh and divides into the common fibular (peroneal) and tibial nerves, at a variable site above the popliteal fossa (see Figs. 8.43 and 8.44).

Trauma

Penetrating wounds, fractures of the pelvis, and dislocations of the hip joint sometimes injure the sciatic nerve. It is most frequently injured by badly placed intramuscular injections in the gluteal region. To avoid this injury, injections into the gluteus maximus or the gluteus medius should be made well forward in the upper outer quadrant of the buttock. Most nerve lesions are incomplete, and, in 90% of injuries, the common fibular part of the nerve is the most affected. This can probably be explained by the fact that the common fibular nerve fibers lie most superficially in the sciatic nerve. The following clinical features are present:

- **Motor:** The hamstring muscles are paralyzed, but weak flexion of the knee is possible because of the action of the sartorius (femoral nerve) and gracilis (obturator nerve). All the muscles below the knee are paralyzed, and the weight of the foot causes it to assume the plantar-flexed position, or **footdrop** (Fig. 8.91).
- **Sensory:** Sensation is lost below the knee, except for a narrow area down the medial side of the lower part of the leg and along the medial border of the foot as far as the ball of the great toe, which is supplied by the saphenous nerve (femoral nerve).

The result of operative repair of a sciatic nerve injury is poor. It is rare for active movement to return to the small muscles of the foot, and sensory recovery is rarely complete. Loss of sensation in the sole makes the development of trophic ulcers inevitable.

Sciatica

Sciatica is the condition in which patients have pain along the sensory distribution of the sciatic nerve. Thus, the pain is experienced in the posterior aspect of the thigh, the posterior and lateral sides of the leg, and the lateral part of the foot. Sciatica can be caused by prolapse of an intervertebral disc, with pressure on one or more roots of the lower lumbar and sacral spinal nerves, pressure on the sacral plexus or sciatic nerve by an intrapelvic tumor, or inflammation of the sciatic nerve or its terminal branches.

Common Fibular Nerve Injury

The common fibular nerve (see Fig. 8.43) is in an exposed position as it leaves the popliteal fossa and winds around the neck of the fibula to enter the fibularis longus muscle.

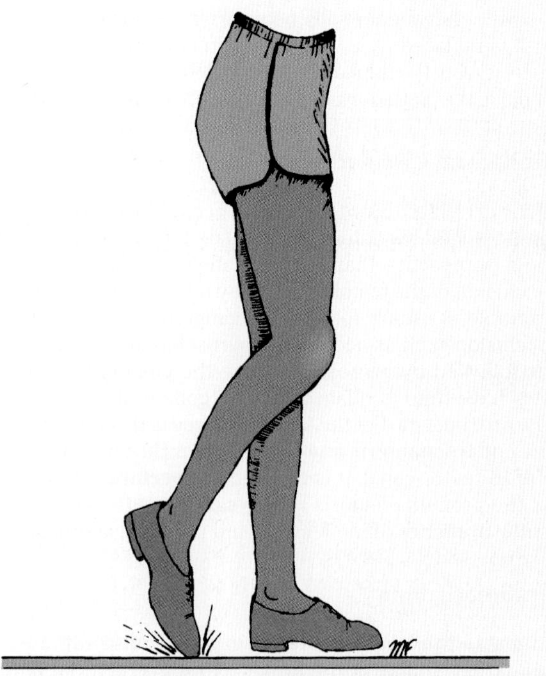

Figure 8.91 Footdrop. With this condition, the individual catches their toes on the ground when walking.

It is commonly injured in fractures of the neck of the fibula and by pressure from casts or splints. The following clinical features are present:

- **Motor**: The muscles of the anterior and lateral compartments of the leg are paralyzed, namely, the tibialis anterior, extensor digitorum longus and brevis, fibularis tertius, extensor hallucis longus (supplied by the deep fibular nerve), and the fibularis longus and brevis (supplied by the superficial fibular nerve). As a result, the opposing muscles, the plantar flexors of the ankle joint and the invertors of the subtalar and transverse tarsal joints, cause the foot to be plantar flexed (footdrop) and inverted, an attitude referred to as **equinovarus** (see Fig. 8.91).
- **Sensory**: Loss of sensation occurs down the anterior and lateral sides of the leg and dorsum of the foot and toes, including the medial side of the great toe. The lateral border of the foot and the lateral side of the little toe are virtually unaffected (sural nerve, mainly formed from the tibial nerve). The medial border of the foot as far as the ball of the great toe is completely unaffected (saphenous nerve, a branch of the femoral nerve).

When the injury occurs distal to the site of origin of the lateral cutaneous nerve of the calf, the loss of sensation is confined to the area of the foot and toes.

Tibial Nerve Injury

The tibial nerve (see Fig. 8.44) leaves the popliteal fossa by passing deep to the gastrocnemius and soleus muscles. Because of its deep and protected position, it is rarely injured. Complete division results in the following clinical features:

- **Motor:** All the muscles in the back of the leg and the sole of the foot are paralyzed. The opposing muscles dorsiflex the foot at the ankle joint and evert the foot at the subtalar and transverse tarsal joints, a position referred to as **calcaneovalgus.**
- **Sensory:** Sensation is lost on the sole; later, trophic ulcers develop.

Obturator Nerve Injury

The obturator nerve (L2 to L4) enters the thigh as anterior and posterior divisions through the upper part of the obturator foramen. The anterior division descends in front of the obturator externus and the adductor brevis, deep to the floor of the femoral triangle. The posterior division descends behind the adductor brevis and in front of the adductor magnus (see Fig. 8.57).

It is injured (rarely) in penetrating wounds, in anterior dislocations of the hip joint, or in abdominal hernia through the obturator foramen. The fetal head may press it on during parturition. The following clinical features occur:

- **Motor:** All the adductor muscles are paralyzed except the hamstring part of the adductor magnus, which is supplied by the sciatic nerve.
- **Sensory:** The cutaneous sensory loss is minimal on the medial aspect of the thigh.

Clinical Case Discussion

The attending physician diagnosed paralysis of the common fibular nerve secondary to blunt trauma to the lateral side of the left fibula. The radiographic examination ruled out the possibility of fracture of the neck of the fibula.

To make this diagnosis, the physician must be cognizant of the detailed anatomy of the course of the common fibular nerve as it winds around the outer side of the neck of the fibula. Knowledge of the distribution of the branches of this nerve enabled them to eliminate other nerve injuries, such as lesions of the superficial or deep fibular nerves. Moreover, they could assess the degree of nerve damage by testing the strength of the various muscles supplied by this nerve and conducting suitable tests to assess the sensory deficits.

Key Concepts

Osteology

- The bones of the lower limb are the os coxae (hip bone), femur, patella, tibia, fibula, tarsal bones, metatarsal bones, and phalanges. The general arrangement of the bones is very similar to that in the upper limb.
- The paired os coxae (plus the sacrum) form the pelvic girdle. Individual os coxae underlie the buttock. The femur forms the thigh. The tibia and fibula form the leg. The tarsal bones (calcaneum, talus, navicular, cuboid, and cuneiforms) form the ankle. The metatarsal bones and the phalanges form the foot and digits.
- Bony features are functionally significant in the context of muscle/ligament attachments and movement deficits resulting from fracture (eg, the quadriceps femoris muscles attach to the tibial tuberosity).
- Several bony features have significant relations with key neurovascular structures that must be considered in the case of bone fractures (eg, common fibular nerve with the neck of the fibula).

Joints

- The hip joint is a synovial, multiaxial, ball-and-socket articulation between the acetabulum and the head of the femur. The cavity of the acetabulum is deepened by the acetabular labrum. The main capsular ligaments are the iliofemoral, pubofemoral, and ischiofemoral ligaments. The ligament of the head of the femur attaches the fovea capitis of the femur to the acetabulum.
- The contralateral gluteus medius and minimus muscles prevent the hip from sinking when the foot is raised during gait. Failure to do so results in a positive Trendelenburg sign (dipping gait).
- Damage to the retinacular arteries of the hip joint and/or the artery to the head of the femur because of the fracture of the neck of the femur or other hip trauma may result in avascular necrosis of the femoral head.
- The knee joint is a synovial, modified hinge articulation between the femoral condyles, patella, and tibial condyles. The major supporting ligaments are the medial and lateral collateral ligaments and the anterior and posterior cruciate ligaments. Paired cartilages, the medial and lateral menisci, attach to the tibial condyles. Multiple bursae are related to the knee.
- The popliteus muscle unlocks the knee from the fully extended position by laterally rotating the femur on the tibia, which permits flexion of the knee.
- The collateral and cruciate ligaments and the menisci are commonly injured. Medial collateral ligament damage often accompanies trauma to the anterior cruciate ligament and/or the medial meniscus. Excessive anteroposterior movement of the tibia against the femur indicates a positive drawer sign and suggests rupture of one of the cruciate ligaments.
- The ankle joint is a synovial hinge articulation between the lower end of the tibia, the two malleoli, and the body of the talus. The major ligaments are the medial (deltoid) ligament and the lateral ligament, which mainly resist eversion and inversion, respectively.
- The tarsal joints are a group of synovial articulations between the tarsal bones.
- Standard plane film radiology provides excellent imaging of bony anatomy. Magnetic resonance imaging (MRI) is useful to demonstrate the soft tissues around the bones.

Foot as Functional Unit

- The foot contains three arches that provide mechanical stability during locomotion and standing posture: medial longitudinal arch, lateral longitudinal arch, and transverse arch.
- The shapes and fits of the bones, the intrinsic ligaments of the foot, and the tone of the muscles maintain the integrity of the arches. Depression of the medial longitudinal arch results in pes planus (flatfoot).

Gluteal Region

- The iliotibial tract/band (ITB) is a thickened band of deep fascia extending from the lateral aspect of the gluteal region to the lateral condyle of the tibia. The tensor fasciae latae and gluteus maximus muscles attach into the ITB.
- The sacrotuberous and sacrospinous ligaments stabilize the sacroiliac joint and aid in forming the greater and lesser sciatic foramina. These foramina are passageways for several structures to pass between the pelvic cavity, gluteal region, and perineum. Notable structures include the piriformis muscle, sciatic nerve, pudendal nerve, internal pudendal vessels, and tendon of the obturator internus muscle.
- The gluteal muscles include the gluteus maximus, gluteus medius, gluteus minimus, tensor fasciae latae, piriformis, obturator internus, superior and inferior gemelli, and quadratus femoris. Muscle actions are largely focused on extension, abduction, and lateral rotation of the hip.
- The sciatic nerve runs down the center of the gluteal region into the thigh and must be considered when administering intragluteal injections. It consists of the tibial and common fibular nerves bound together by fascia. The pudendal nerve has a small but important gluteal segment where it loops around the ischial spine.
- The superior and inferior gluteal arteries are the primary vessels supplying the gluteal region. Both contribute to major collateral networks (trochanteric and cruciate anastomoses) around the hip.

Thigh

- The great and small saphenous veins are extensive superficial vessels that drain much of the lower limb. The great saphenous vein ascends the medial aspect of the limb, pierces the deep fascia of the anterior thigh, and empties into the femoral vein in the femoral triangle. It also receives tributaries from the lower abdominal wall and perineum.
- The inguinal lymph nodes are in the thigh and are divided into superficial and deep groups. They receive drainage from the lower limb, lower anterior abdominal wall, perineum, and lower back.
- The deep fascia (fascia lata) of the lower limb tightly invests the thigh. Deep running septa divide the thigh into three compartments (anterior, medial, posterior), each having its own complement of muscles, nerves, and arteries.

- The anterior compartment of the thigh contains the sartorius, pectineus, iliopsoas, and quadriceps femoris (rectus femoris, vastus lateralis, vastus medialis, vastus intermedius) muscles. The quadriceps group attaches to the tibial tuberosity via the patellar ligament. The femoral artery and its branches and the femoral nerve supply this compartment. The femoral artery is the main arterial supply to the lower limb.
- The femoral triangle is a triangular depression on the anterior thigh. It contains the femoral vessels, femoral nerve, and inguinal lymph nodes. A femoral hernia emerges into the femoral triangle.
- The medial compartment contains the gracilis, adductor longus, adductor brevis, adductor magnus, and obturator externus muscles. The profunda femoris and obturator arteries are the vascular channels. The obturator nerve supplies most of the compartment. The tibial nerve supplies part of the adductor magnus muscle.
- The posterior compartment contains the hamstring muscles: biceps femoris, semitendinosus, semimembranosus, and a small part of the adductor magnus (hamstring portion). The profunda femoris artery is the main vascular supply. The tibial nerve supplies most of the posterior compartment. The common fibular nerve innervates only the short head of the biceps

Popliteal Fossa

- The popliteal fossa is a diamond-shaped intermuscular space situated at the back of the knee. Its major contents are the popliteus muscle, popliteal vessels, termination of the small saphenous vein, common fibular and tibial nerves, and popliteal lymph nodes.
- The popliteus muscle acts to flex the knee and to unlock the knee joint during locomotion.
- The popliteal artery is the continuation of the femoral artery. Multiple genicular arteries form an extensive anastomotic network around the knee. It ends by dividing into anterior and posterior tibial arteries.
- The tibial and common fibular nerves pass through the fossa as they descend into the leg. The common fibular nerve has a close relation to the head and neck of the fibula, where it is readily injured.

Leg

- The deep fascia of the leg forms the compartments of the leg and also forms a series of retinacula that aid the mechanical efficiency of the muscles of the leg.
- The small saphenous vein runs up the middle of the back of the leg and then dives into the popliteal fossa to join the popliteal vein.
- Septa from the deep fascia of the leg plus the interosseous membrane divide the leg into three compartments: anterior, lateral, and posterior.
- The anterior compartment contains the tibialis anterior, extensor digitorum longus, fibularis tertius, and extensor hallucis longus muscles. The anterior tibial vessels are the vascular channels, and the deep fibular nerve supplies the muscles.
- The lateral compartment contains the fibularis longus and brevis muscles. Branches of the fibular artery and the superficial fibular nerve supply the compartment.
- The posterior compartment consists of two parts: the superficial posterior compartment and deep posterior compartment. The superficial group includes the gastrocnemius, soleus, and plantaris muscles. The deep group includes the popliteus, flexor digitorum longus, flexor hallucis longus, and tibialis posterior muscles. The posterior tibial vessels and the tibial nerve supply the entire posterior compartment.
- Damage to the common fibular, superficial fibular, or deep fibular nerves results in varying degrees of footdrop, in which the toes drag on the ground while walking.

Ankle

- Structures crossing the ankle and passing between the leg and foot do so either anterior or posterior to the medial and lateral malleoli.
- Major structures crossing anterior to the malleoli include the great saphenous vein, saphenous nerve, superficial and deep fibular nerves, anterior tibial vessels, and long tendons of the muscles in the anterior compartment of the leg.
- Major structures crossing posterior to the malleoli include the posterior tibial vessels, tibial nerve, sural nerve, small saphenous vein, and tendons of the muscles in the posterior and lateral compartments of the leg.

Foot

- The plantar aponeurosis is a thickening of the deep fascia in the sole.
- The muscles of the sole are described in four layers from superficial to deep. The first layer contains the abductor hallucis, flexor digitorum brevis, and abductor digiti minimi. The second layer includes the quadratus plantae, lumbricals, flexor digitorum longus tendon, and flexor hallucis longus tendon. The third layer consists of the flexor hallucis brevis, adductor hallucis, and flexor digiti minimi brevis. The fourth layer contains the interossei, fibularis longus tendon, and tibialis posterior tendon.
- The posterior tibial artery passes behind the medial malleolus and terminates by dividing into the medial and lateral plantar arteries, which supply the sole. The lateral plantar artery forms the plantar arterial arch, which supplies the digits and anastomoses with the deep plantar artery from the dorsum.

- The tibial nerve passes behind the medial malleolus and terminates by dividing into the medial and lateral plantar nerves, which supply the sole.
- The superficial fibular nerve is the main cutaneous nerve to the dorsum. The deep fibular nerve supplies a small zone between the first two digits. The saphenous nerve supplies the skin along the medial side of the foot, whereas the sural nerve supplies the lateral margin of the foot.
- The greater part of the blood from the whole foot drains into the dorsal venous arch. This drains on the medial side into the great saphenous vein and on the lateral side into the small saphenous vein. The great saphenous vein leaves the dorsum of the foot by ascending into the leg in front of the medial malleolus. The small saphenous vein ascends into the leg behind the lateral malleolus.
- The extensor digitorum brevis is the sole intrinsic muscle on the dorsum.
- The dorsalis pedis artery is the continuation of the anterior tibial artery and supplies the dorsum. Its pulsations can easily be felt.

Surface Anatomy

- Numerous bony and soft tissue structures of the lower limb are visible and palpable in a surface anatomy examination.

9 Head and Neck

A 58-year-old female woke up one morning finding the right side of her face feeling "peculiar and heavy." On looking in the mirror, she saw the corner of her mouth on the right side was drooping, and her right lower eyelid seemed lower than the left. When she attempted to smile, the right side of her face remained immobile and masklike. While eating her breakfast, she noticed her food tended to stick on the inside of her right cheek and liquid dribbled out the corner of her mouth. On taking her dog for a walk, she found she could not whistle for his return to her side; her lips just would not pucker. On examination, the woman's primary care physician found paralysis of the muscles of the entire right side of the face. Also, this patient talked with a slightly slurred speech and her blood pressure was very high.

See the Clinical Case Discussion at the end of this chapter for further insight.

CHAPTER OUTLINE

LEARNING OBJECTIVES

The purpose of this chapter is to examine the anatomy of the head and neck in the context of normal functional organization and common clinical conditions.

Osteology

1. Identify the bones of the skull, hyoid, and cervical spine, and their major features, in dry osteology specimens and in standard medical imaging. Describe the functional aspects of these structures.
2. Identify the components of the temporomandibular joint. Describe the mechanisms of opening and closing the jaws.
3. Identify the muscles of mastication, their attachments, sources of innervation, and major actions in chewing.

Scalp and Face

1. Describe the boundaries and structure of the scalp.
2. Identify the major muscles of facial expression, their actions, and their innervation.
3. Describe the innervation of the face and scalp. Predict the deficit expected following injury to each of the major nerve branches.
4. Trace the flow of blood through the face and scalp.
5. Trace the pattern of lymph drainage from the scalp and face.

Interior of the Skull

1. Identify the cranial fossae, the major bony components and boundaries of each, and the major contents of each.
2. Identify the meninges surrounding the brain and the folds of dura mater that subdivide the cranium. Explain the functional/clinical significance of this arrangement. Describe the innervation of the dura mater.
3. Trace the flow of blood into the cranial cavity, indicating the major anastomoses and collateral routes. Describe the formation of the cerebral arterial circle and explain its functional and clinical significance.
4. Identify the dural venous sinuses, indicating their relations to the cranial meninges. Trace the communications of the venous sinuses with the extracranial venous system and explain the functional/clinical significance of this arrangement.
5. Explain the anatomical basis for epidural, subdural, and subarachnoid cranial hemorrhages.
6. Identify each of the cranial nerves (CNs) as it leaves the cranial cavity. Indicate the relationships of each nerve to particular cranial fossae, to the folds of dura mater, and to venous sinuses along its course. Also indicate the foramina used in exiting the cranium, and any major accompanying structures (eg, blood vessels).
7. Identify the major components of the brain and their functional significance.

Orbit and Eye

1. Identify the bony elements of the orbit. Indicate the major structures surrounding the orbit, and the position of the eyeball relative to the orbit.
2. Identify the extraocular muscles, their actions, and their nerve supply. Predict the functional deficit resulting from damage to each muscle. Describe the method of clinical testing of the individual extraocular muscles and their nerves.
3. Identify the major nerves of the orbit, their functional components, their main branches, and their destinations. Predict the functional deficit resulting from damage to each nerve.
4. Trace the flow of blood into and out of the orbit and orbital structures.

5. Identify the main components of the eyelids. Describe the mechanics of movement of the eyelids.
6. Identify the components of the lacrimal apparatus. Trace the pathway a tear takes from the lacrimal gland to the inferior nasal meatus.
7. Follow the course of autonomic nervous supply to orbital structures, indicating the pre- and postganglionic sources of innervation. Differentiate sympathetic and parasympathetic functions.

Temporal, Infratemporal, and Pterygopalatine Regions

1. Define the temporal, infratemporal, and pterygopalatine fossae. Identify the major structures contained in each region.
2. Trace the flow of blood through the maxillary and superficial temporal arteries and their major branches. Identify the regions supplied and the anastomoses between branches.
3. Identify, and trace the courses of, the nerves that traverse the above fossae. Identify the functional components of each nerve, their sources, and their areas of termination.

Neck

1. Describe the arrangement and functions of the superficial and deep cervical fascia with respect to the organization of the neck.
2. Identify the triangles of the neck and their boundaries and major contents.
3. Identify the muscles in the neck, including their attachments, innervation, and major actions.
4. Describe the vascular supply and drainage of the neck.
5. Describe the lymphatic drainage of the neck.

Vascular and Lymphatic Organization

1. Trace the flow of blood through the carotid arterial tract. Note the regions supplied by each of the major branches, the relationship of the branches to surrounding structures, and anastomoses between branches. Describe the locations and functions of the carotid sinus and carotid body.
2. Trace the flow of blood through the subclavian artery and its major branches. Note the regions supplied by each branch, the relationship of the branches to surrounding structures, and anastomoses between the branches.
3. Identify the primary intracranial and extracranial veins. Trace the flow of blood through the jugular system of veins, noting the regions drained by each of the tributaries and interconnections between the major veins.
4. Trace the routes of lymphatic drainage in the head and neck. Indicate the major aggregations of lymph nodes and their relations to neighboring structures. Differentiate the patterns in the right and left sides.

Neural Organization

1. Identify the 12 pairs of CNs. Identify the functional component(s) contained within and/or conveyed by each nerve. Trace the course of each CN from its origin at the base of the brain to its destination(s). Indicate the avenue(s) taken in exiting the skull and the peripheral relations of each nerve. Predict the functional deficit(s) expected from a lesion of each nerve.
2. Describe the formation of the cervical and brachial plexuses of nerves, noting the spinal segments of origin, relations to surrounding cervical structures, and distribution of peripheral branches. Note the formation, relations, and distributions of the phrenic nerve and the ansa cervicalis.
3. Identify the sources of autonomic innervation to the head. Trace the pathways of preganglionic and postganglionic autonomic neurons in the head from their origins to their final destinations. Indicate specific synapse points. Describe the primary functions governed by each autonomic component in the head.

Ear

1. Identify the boundaries and contents of the external, middle, and internal ear. Describe the relations of each part of the ear apparatus to its neighboring structures. Describe the innervation of the region.
2. Relate the structures of the ear to the mechanics of hearing and equilibrium.

Digestive System

1. Define the boundaries and subdivisions of the oral cavity, pharynx, and esophagus. Describe the main relations of each to its surrounding structures.
2. Identify the muscles of the oral cavity, palate, auditory tube, pharynx, and esophagus and their attachments, actions, and innervation.
3. Identify the extrinsic and intrinsic muscles of the tongue. Describe the sensory and motor nerve supply to the tongue. Predict the deficit expected to follow an injury to each nerve.

4. Describe the mechanism of swallowing. Note the sequence of events, the muscles responsible for each event, and the nerves controlling each event.
5. Describe the location, innervation, lymphatic drainage, secretory drainage, and general relationships of the parotid, submandibular, and sublingual salivary glands. Describe the clinical significance of the relationship between the parotid gland, its duct, and the extracranial distribution of the facial nerve.
6. Describe the pattern of innervation of the oropharyngeal region and esophagus. Identify the source, region supplied, and the functional components of each nerve.
7. Trace the arterial supply to and venous drainage of the oropharyngeal region and esophagus. Identify the major blood vessels, their territories, and any significant anastomoses.
8. Describe the location, lymphatic drainage, and general relationships of the oropharyngeal tonsils.

Respiratory System

1. Identify the components, boundaries, and relations of the nose, paranasal sinuses, larynx, and trachea.
2. Identify the drainage routes of each of the paranasal sinuses. Describe the relationship of each sinus to the surrounding oral, orbital, and cranial cavities.
3. Describe the pattern of innervation of the respiratory system in the head and neck.
4. Trace the arterial supply to and venous drainage from the components of the respiratory system.
5. Trace the lymph drainage from the respiratory components.
6. Identify the major morphological features of the larynx.
7. Identify the extrinsic and intrinsic muscles of the larynx. Determine the actions of these muscles and their roles in sound production.
8. Trace the courses of the neurovascular supply of the larynx. Predict the functional consequences of damage to the different nerves constituting this innervation.

Endocrine System

1. Identify the pituitary, pineal, thyroid, and parathyroid glands.
2. Describe the relations of the endocrine organs to surrounding structures.
3. Trace the vascular, lymph, and nervous supply of the endocrine organs.
4. Briefly describe the primary functions of the endocrine organs.

Radiographic and Surface Anatomy

1. Identify the major structures in the head and neck that are visible in standard medical imaging.
2. Identify the major structures that are palpable and/or have notable surface projections in a basic physical examination of the head and neck.

OVERVIEW

The head and neck region of the body contains many important structures compressed into a relatively small area. The skull, with the enclosed brain and meninges, forms most of the head. The special senses (eye, ear, olfactory area, taste receptors) lie within the skull bones or in the cavities bounded by them. The brain gives rise to 12 pairs of CNs (CNs), which leave the brain and pass through foramina and fissures in the skull. All the CNs are distributed to structures in the head and neck, except CN X (vagus), which also supplies structures in the chest and abdomen. The digestive and respiratory systems begin in the head and traverse the neck to reach the thorax and abdomen. Additionally, key endocrine organs are located in the head and neck.

Head injuries from blunt trauma and penetrating missiles are associated with high mortality and severe disability. Headaches are usually caused by nonserious conditions such as sinusitis or neuralgia; however, they can represent the earliest manifestations of a life-threatening disease.

Facial, scalp, and mouth injuries are commonly encountered in practice and vary in seriousness from a small skin laceration to major maxillofacial trauma. Even an untreated boil on the side of the nose can be life threatening. Facial paralysis and unequal pupils may indicate the existence of a serious neurologic deficit.

Many vital structures are present in the neck. Injuries or pressure on the larynx or trachea can compromise the airway. Swellings can indicate the existence of a tumor of the thyroid gland or the presence of a malignant secondary lesion in a lymph node.

Clearly, many signs and symptoms related to the region of the head and neck are determined by the anatomic arrangement of the various structures. This chapter reviews the basic anatomy of this complicated region and highlights the clinical relevance of the structures considered. It specifically excludes detailed consideration of the brain, which is best covered in a neurobiology text (see Splittgerber, R. *Snell's Clinical Neuroanatomy*, 9e, Wolters Kluwer, Baltimore; 2025).

OSTEOLOGY

The skeleton of the head and neck includes the skull, middle ear ossicles, hyoid bone, and cervical vertebrae. This section describes the skull and hyoid. The ear ossicles are described later, in the section on the middle ear. The cervical vertebrae are covered in Chapter 2 along with the rest of the vertebral column.

The anatomical position of the skull is such that the lower margins of the orbits and the upper margins of the external acoustic meatuses are in the same horizontal plane. This **orbitomeatal ("Frankfurt") plane** corresponds closely with a natural horizontal cranial plane.

The skull is composed of several separate bones united at immobile joints called **sutures**. The connective tissue between the bones forms **sutural ligaments**. The mandible is an exception to this rule, as it is united to the skull by the mobile, synovial **temporomandibular joints (TMJs)**.

The bones of the skull are organized into a **cranial skeleton** that surrounds the brain and a **facial skeleton**. The **cranial cavity** is the space containing the brain. The skull **vault (calvarium)** is the upper part of the cranium and forms the roof and side walls of the cranial cavity. The **base** of the skull is the lowest part of the cranium and forms the floor of the cranial cavity (Figs. 9.1 to 9.3).

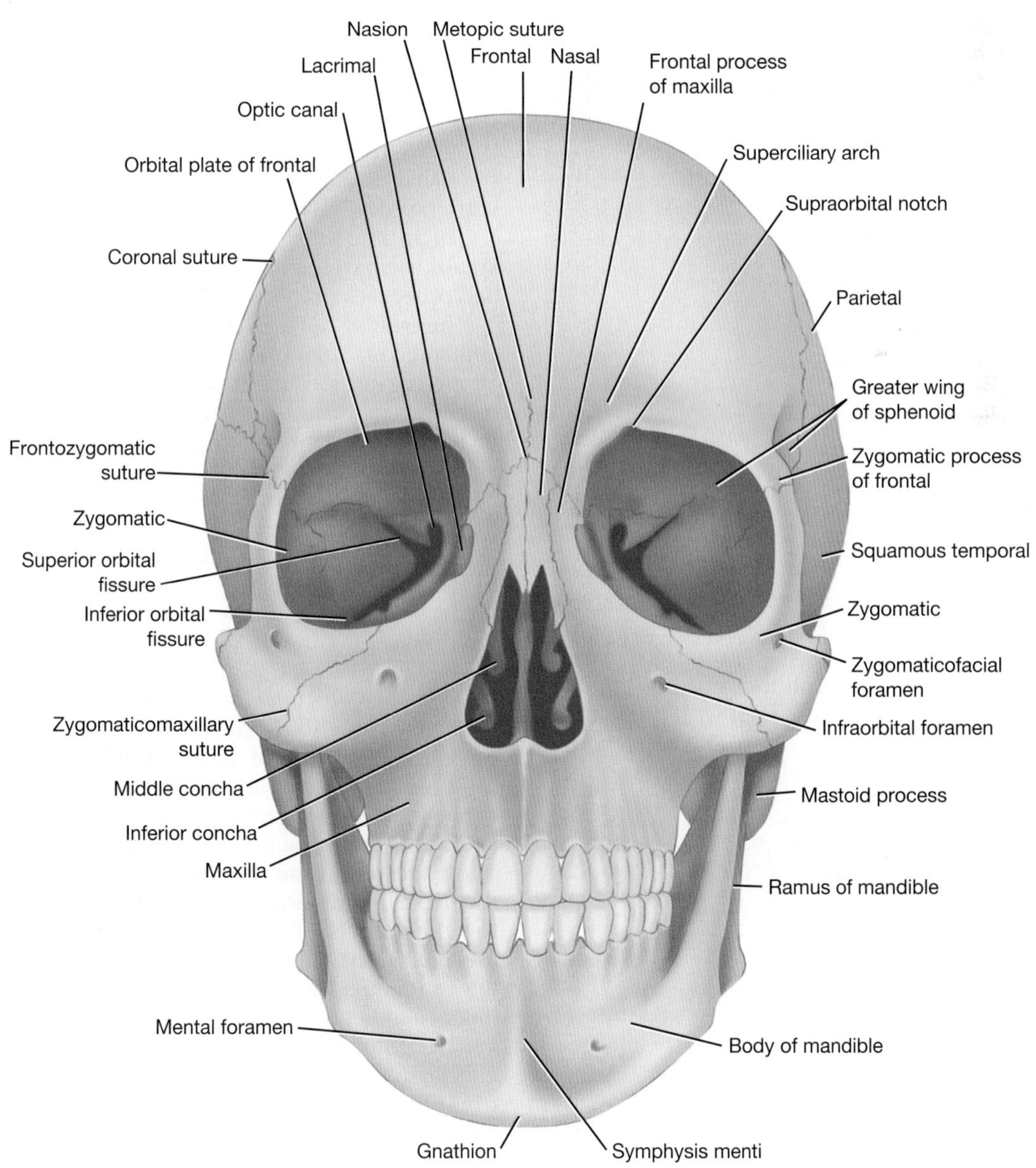

Figure 9.1 Bones of the anterior aspect of the skull.

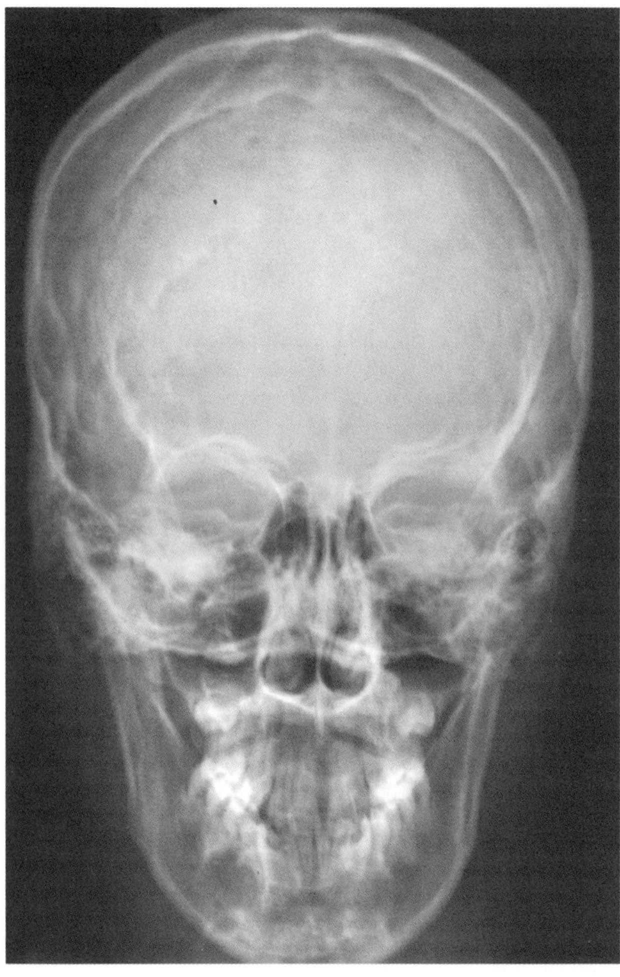

Figure 9.2 Posteroanterior radiograph of the skull.

The relatively flat bones of the vault (frontal, parietals, and part of the occipital) are composed of **external** and **internal tables** of compact bone separated by a layer of spongy bone called the **diploë** (Fig. 9.4). The internal table is thinner and more brittle than the external table. The bones are covered with periosteum on both the outer and inner surfaces. The bones of the vault form via **membranous ossification**, whereas the bones of the cranial base and the facial skeleton form via **endochondral ossification**.

The cranium consists of the following bones, two of which are paired (Figs. 9.5 to 9.8):

- Frontal bone: 1
- Parietal bones: 2
- Occipital bone: 1
- Temporal bones: 2
- Sphenoid bone: 1
- Ethmoid bone: 1

The facial skeleton consists of the following, two of which are single:

- Zygomatic bones: 2
- Maxillae: 2
- Nasal bones: 2
- Lacrimal bones: 2
- Vomer: 1
- Palatine bones: 2
- Inferior conchae: 2
- Mandible: 1

Adult Skull

Biomedical students do not need a comprehensive knowledge of the detailed structure of each individual skull bone. However, it is essential to have sufficient detail to understand clinically relevant applications. Students should be familiar with the skull as a whole and should have a dried skull available for reference as they read the following description.

Anterior View

The **frontal bone**, or forehead bone, curves downward to make the upper margins of the orbits (see Figs. 9.1 to 9.3). The **superciliary arches** are on either side, and the **supraorbital notch** (or **supraorbital foramen**) is at or near the orbital rim. Medially, the frontal bone articulates with the frontal processes of the maxillae and with the nasal bones. Laterally, the frontal bone articulates with the zygomatic bone.

The **orbital margins** are bounded by the frontal bone superiorly, zygomatic bone laterally, maxilla inferiorly, and processes of the maxilla and frontal bone medially.

The frontal bone contains two hollow spaces lined with mucous membrane, the **frontal air sinuses**, just above the orbital margins. These and the other paranasal sinuses (maxillary, ethmoid, sphenoid) communicate with the nose and serve to lighten the facial skeleton and act as voice resonators.

The two **nasal bones** form the bridge of the nose. Their lower borders, with the maxillae, make the **anterior nasal aperture**. The nasal cavity is divided into two by the bony **nasal septum**, which is largely formed by the **vomer** and also by the **perpendicular plate of the ethmoid**. The **superior** and **middle conchae** are shelves of bone that project into the nasal cavity from the ethmoid on each side. The **inferior conchae** are separate bones.

The two **maxillae** form the upper jaw, anterior part of the hard palate, part of the lateral walls of the nasal cavities, and part of the floors of the orbital cavities. The two bones meet in the midline at the **intermaxillary suture** and form the lower margin of the nasal aperture. The **infraorbital foramen** perforates the maxilla below the orbit. The **alveolar process** projects downward and, together with the fellow of the opposite side, forms the **alveolar arch**, which carries the upper teeth. Each maxilla contains a large, pyramid-shaped cavity lined with mucous membrane, the **maxillary sinus**.

The **zygomatic bone** forms the prominence of the cheek and part of the lateral wall and floor of the orbital cavity. Medially, it articulates with the maxilla, and laterally, it articulates with the zygomatic process of the temporal bone to form the **zygomatic arch**. The zygomatic bone is perforated by two foramina for the zygomaticofacial and zygomaticotemporal nerves.

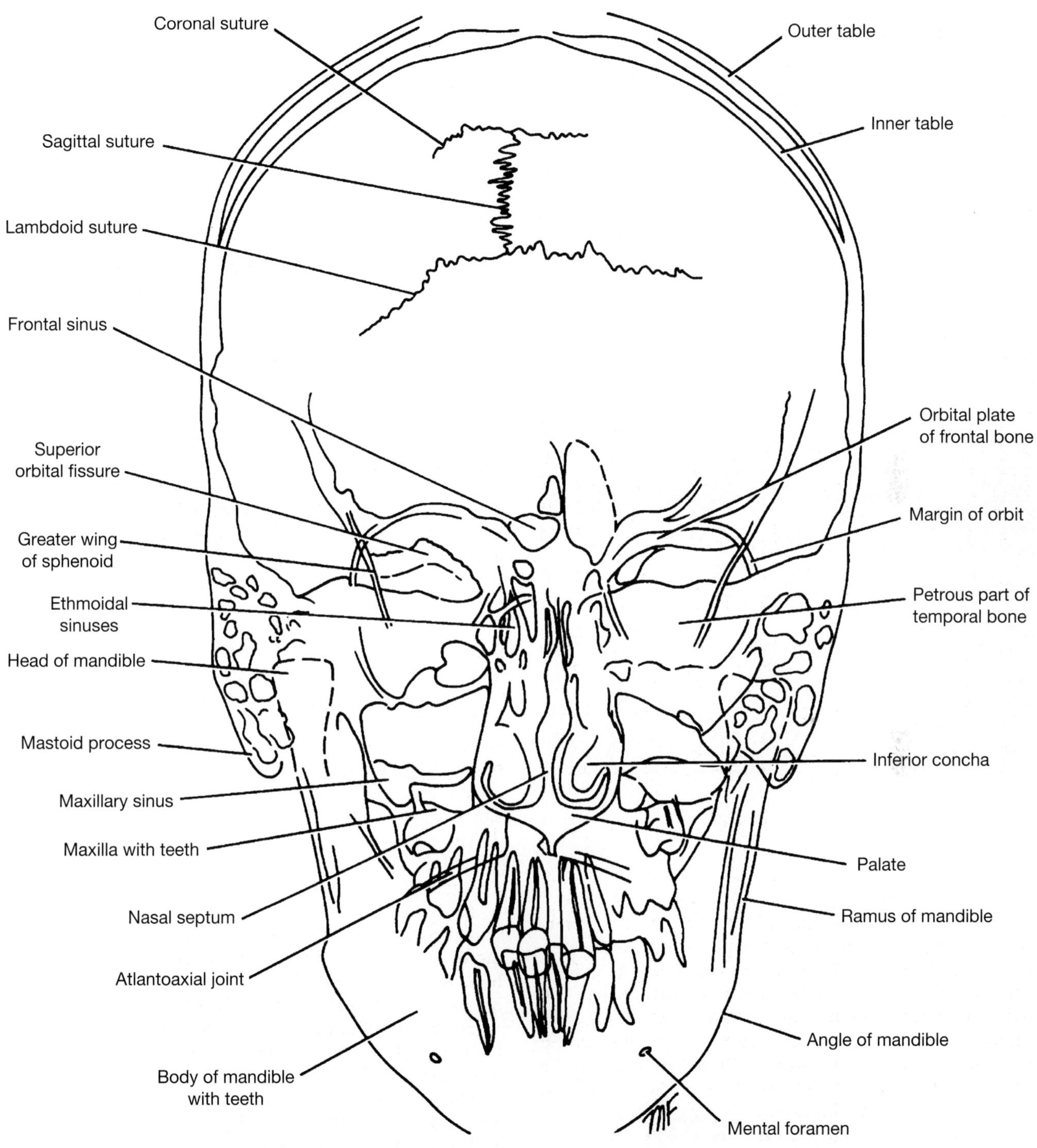

Figure 9.3 Main features that can be seen in the posteroanterior radiograph of the skull in Figure 9.2.

The **mandible**, or lower jaw, consists of a horizontal body and two vertical rami (see Mandible).

Lateral View

The **frontal bone** forms the anterior part of the side of the skull and articulates with the parietal bone at the **coronal suture** (see Figs. 9.5 to 9.7).

The **parietal bones** form the sides and roof of the cranium and articulate with each other in the midline at the **sagittal suture**. They articulate with the occipital bone behind, at the **lambdoid suture**.

The **squamous part of the occipital bone**, parts of the **temporal bone** (namely, the **squamous**; **tympanic**; and **mastoid**, **styloid**, and **zygomatic processes**), and the **greater wing of the sphenoid** complete the skull at the

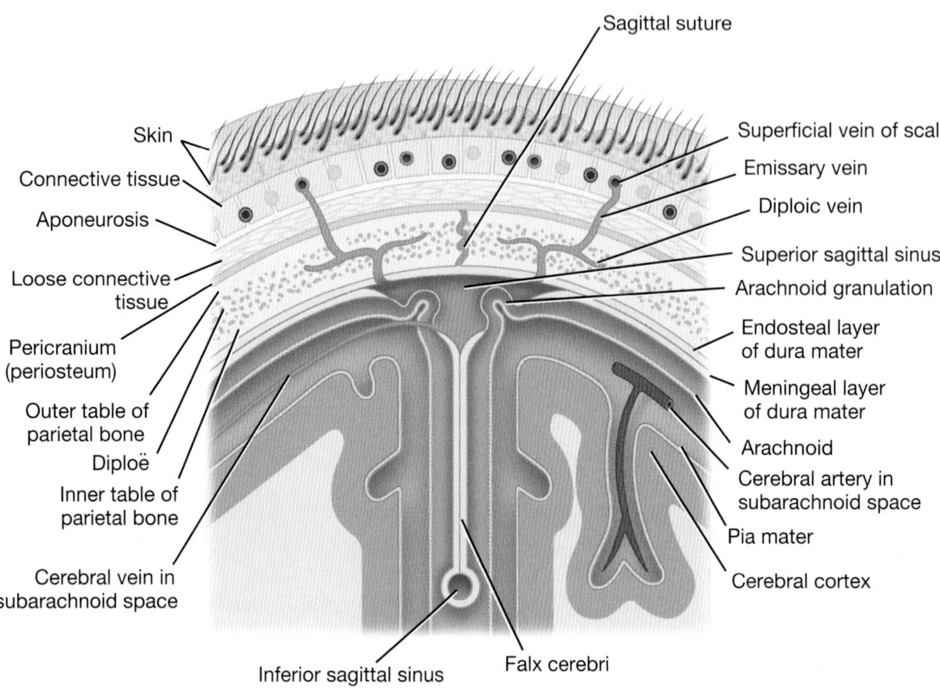

Figure 9.4 Coronal section of the upper part of the head showing the structure of the cranial vault bones, layers of the scalp, sagittal suture, falx cerebri, superior and inferior sagittal venous sinuses, arachnoid granulations, emissary veins, and the relation of cerebral blood vessels to the subarachnoid space.

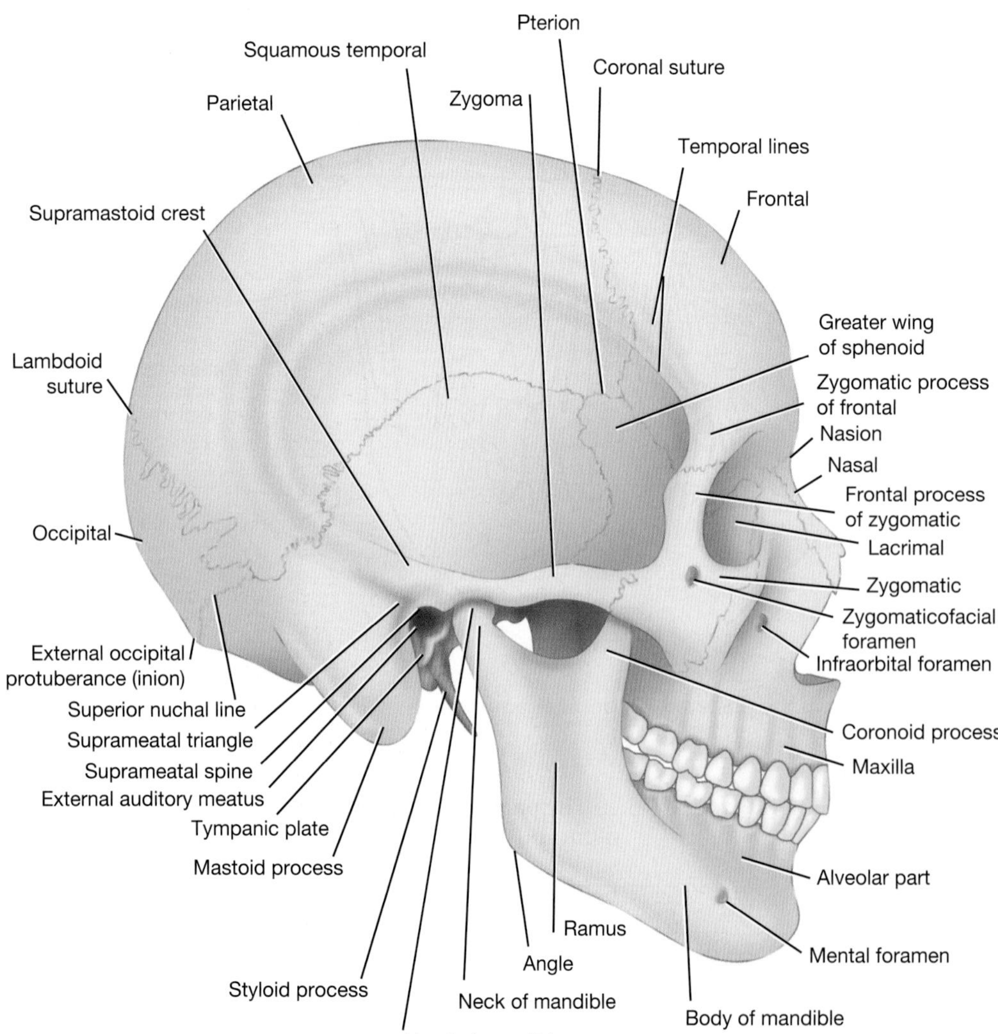

Figure 9.5 Bones of the lateral aspect of the skull.

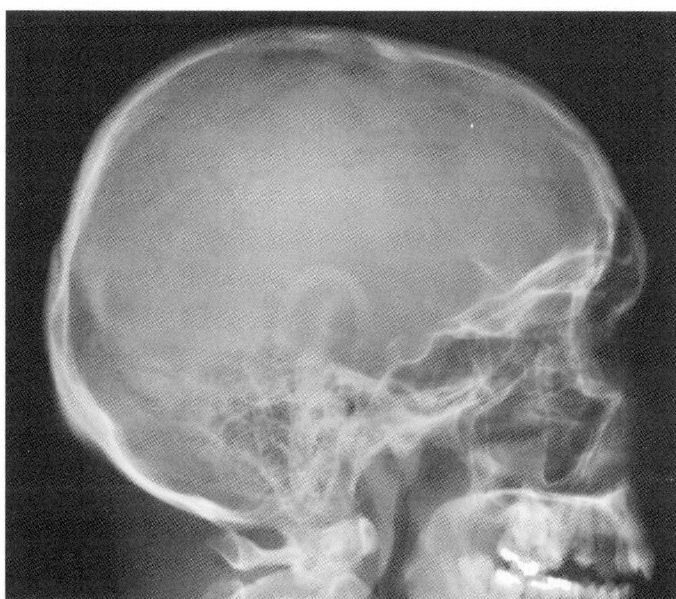

Figure 9.6 Lateral radiograph of the skull.

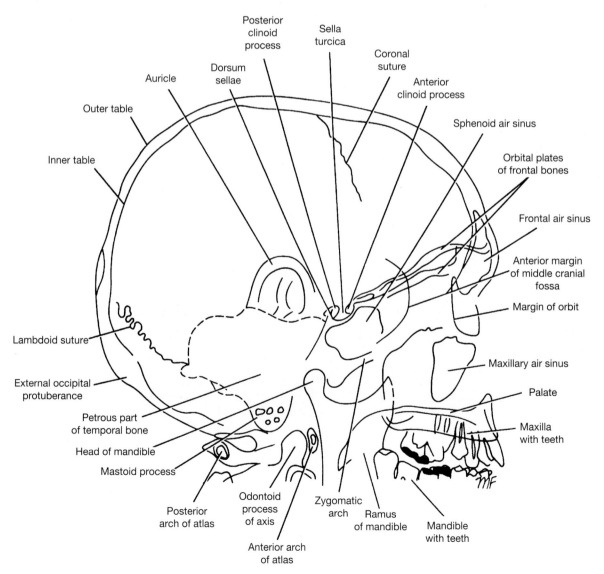

Figure 9.7 Main features that can be seen in the lateral radiograph of the skull in Figure 9.6.

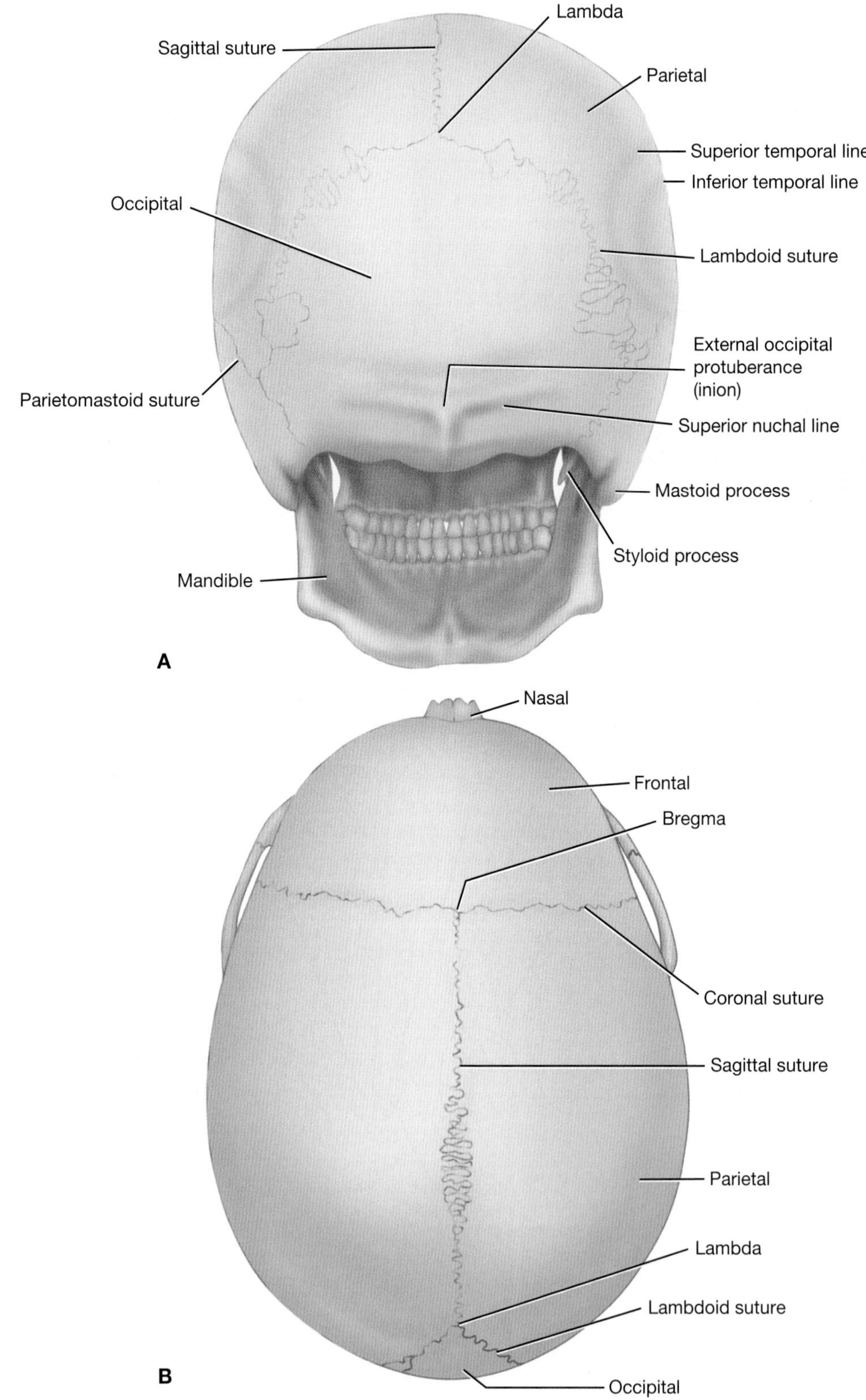

Figure 9.8 Bones of the skull viewed from the posterior **(A)** and superior **(B)** aspects.

side. Note the position of the **external auditory meatus**. The **ramus** and **body of the mandible** lie inferiorly.

Note that the thinnest part of the lateral wall of the skull is where the anteroinferior corner of the parietal bone articulates with the greater wing of the sphenoid. This point is referred to as the **pterion**. Clinically, the pterion is an important area because it overlies the **anterior division of the middle meningeal artery and vein**.

Identify the **superior** and **inferior temporal lines**, which begin as a single line from the posterior margin of the zygomatic process of the frontal bone and diverge as they arch backward. The **temporal fossa** lies below the inferior temporal line.

The **infratemporal fossa** lies below the **infratemporal crest** on the greater wing of the sphenoid. The **pterygomaxillary fissure** is a vertical opening that lies within the fossa between the pterygoid process of the sphenoid bone and back of the maxilla. It leads medially into the **pterygopalatine fossa**.

The **inferior orbital fissure** is a horizontal opening between the greater wing of the sphenoid bone and the maxilla. It leads forward into the orbit.

The **pterygopalatine fossa** is a small space behind and below the orbital cavity (see Pterygopalatine Fossa). It communicates laterally with the infratemporal fossa through the pterygomaxillary fissure, medially with the nasal cavity through the **sphenopalatine foramen**, superiorly with the cranial cavity through the **foramen rotundum**, and anteriorly with the orbit through the **inferior orbital fissure**.

Posterior View

The posterior parts of the two parietal bones with the intervening **sagittal suture** are located superiorly (see Fig. 9.8A). Inferiorly, the parietal bones articulate with the **squamous part of the occipital bone** at the **lambdoid suture**. The occipital bone articulates with the temporal bone on each side. A roughened elevation, the **external occipital protuberance**, lies in the midline of the occipital bone and gives attachment to muscles and the ligamentum nuchae. The **superior nuchal lines** extend laterally toward the temporal bone on either side of the protuberance.

Superior View

Anteriorly, the frontal bone articulates with the two parietal bones at the **coronal (frontal) suture** (see Fig. 9.8B). Occasionally, the two halves of the frontal bone fail to fuse completely, leaving a small midline **metopic suture** (see Fig. 9.1). Posteriorly, the two parietal bones articulate in the midline at the **sagittal suture**.

Inferior View

The anteroinferior part of the skull is formed by the **hard palate**, which is composed of the **palatal processes of the maxillae** and the **horizontal plates (palatal processes) of the palatine bones** (Fig. 9.9). The incisive foramen is in the anterior midline, and the **greater** and **lesser palatine foramina** lay posterolaterally.

The **choanae (posterior nasal apertures)** are above the posterior edge of the hard palate. These are separated from each other by the posterior margin of the **vomer** and are bounded laterally by the **medial pterygoid plates** of the sphenoid bone. The inferior end of the medial pterygoid plate is prolonged as a curved spike of bone, the **pterygoid hamulus**.

The large **foramen ovale** and small **foramen spinosum** pierce the greater wing of the sphenoid posterolateral to the **lateral pterygoid plate**. The **spine of the sphenoid** is posterolateral to the foramen spinosum.

A groove for the cartilaginous part of the **auditory tube** lies behind the spine of the sphenoid, in the interval between the greater wing of the sphenoid and the petrous part of the temporal bone. This groove leads into the opening of the bony part of the tube.

The **mandibular fossa** of the temporal bone and the **articular tubercle** form the upper articular surfaces for the **TMJ**. The **squamotympanic fissure** separates the mandibular fossa from the tympanic plate posteriorly. The chorda tympani nerve exits the tympanic cavity through the medial end of this fissure.

The **styloid process** of the temporal bone projects downward and forward from its inferior aspect. The opening of the **carotid canal** is on the inferior surface of the petrous part of the temporal bone.

The medial end of the petrous part of the temporal bone is irregular and, together with the basilar part of the occipital bone and the greater wing of the sphenoid, forms the **foramen lacerum**. During life, the foramen lacerum is mostly closed with fibrous tissue, and only a few small structures pass through this foramen from the cranial cavity to the exterior (see Middle Cranial Fossa).

The **tympanic plate**, a part of the temporal bone, is C-shaped on section and forms the bony part of the **external auditory meatus**. While examining this region, identify the **suprameatal crest** on the lateral surface of the squamous part of the temporal bone, the **suprameatal triangle**, and the **suprameatal spine**.

The **stylomastoid foramen** sits in the interval between the styloid and mastoid processes. Medial to the styloid process, the petrous part of the temporal bone has a deep notch, which, together with a shallower notch on the occipital bone, forms the **jugular foramen**.

The sphenoid bone and the **basilar part of the occipital bone** are behind the posterior nasal apertures and in front of the foramen magnum. The **pharyngeal tubercle** is a small midline prominence on the undersurface of the basilar part of the occipital bone.

The **occipital condyles** are large, rounded prominences on either side of the **foramen magnum**. They articulate with the superior aspect of the lateral mass of the C1 vertebra, the atlas. The **hypoglossal canal** for transmission of the hypoglossal nerve is anterosuperior to the occipital condyle.

The **external occipital protuberance** is a midline elevation posterior to the foramen magnum. The **superior nuchal lines** curve laterally from each side.

Cranial Cavity

The cranial cavity contains the brain and its surrounding meninges, portions of the CNs, arteries, veins, and venous sinuses.

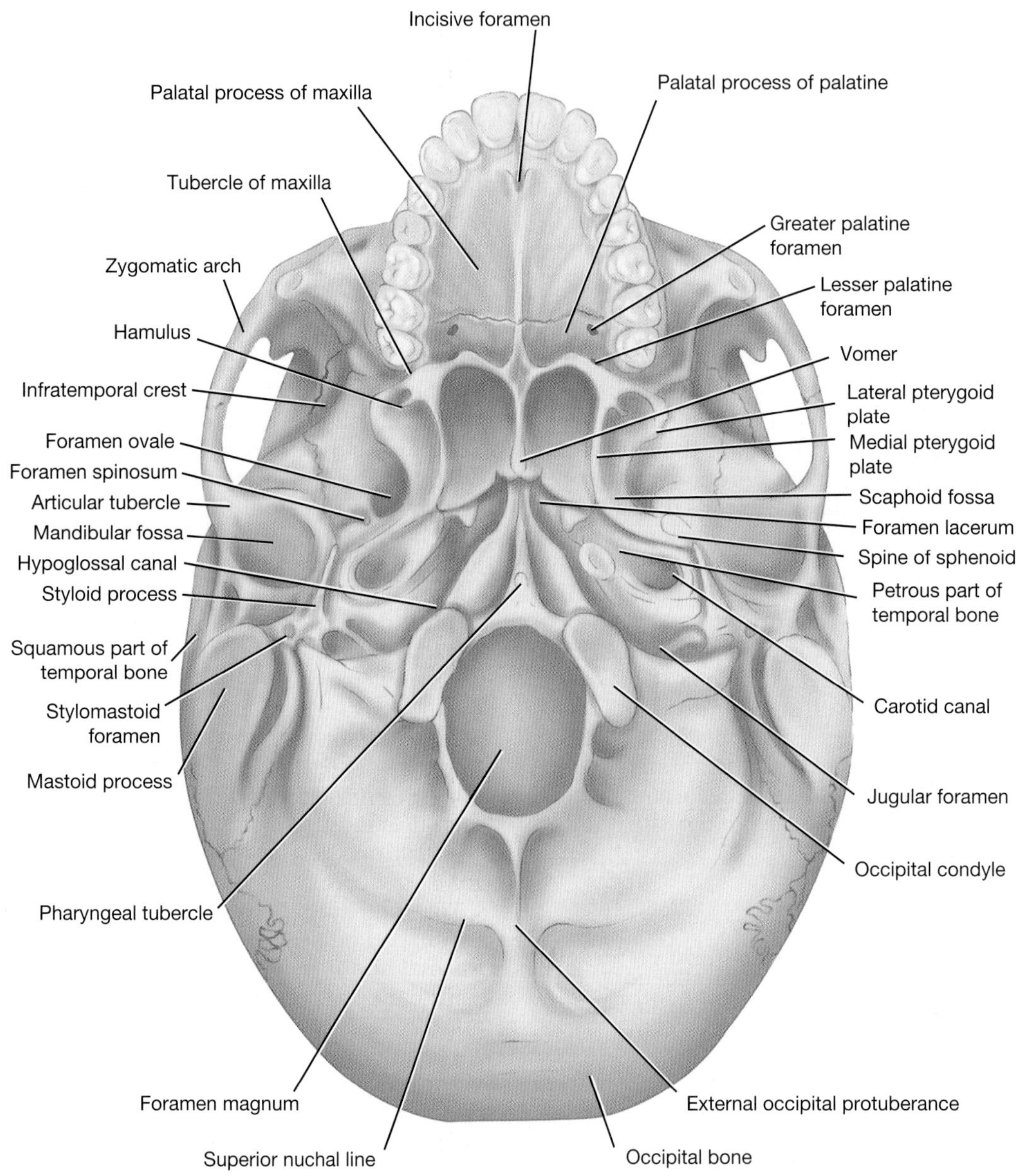

Figure 9.9 Inferior surface of the base of the skull.

Vault of the Skull

The internal surface of the vault shows the coronal, sagittal, and lambdoid sutures. A shallow sagittal groove that lodges the **superior sagittal sinus** runs in the midline. On each side of the groove are several small **granular pits**, which lodge the **lateral lacunae** and **arachnoid granulations** (see Arachnoid Mater). Several narrow grooves are present for the anterior and posterior divisions of the **middle meningeal vessels** as they pass up the side of the skull from the foramen spinosum to the vault.

Base of the Skull

The interior of the base of the skull is divided into three **cranial fossae**: **anterior**, **middle**, and **posterior** (Fig. 9.10). The anterior cranial fossa is separated from the middle cranial fossa by the **lesser wing of the sphenoid**. The middle cranial fossa is separated from the posterior cranial fossa by the **petrous part of the temporal bone**.

ANTERIOR CRANIAL FOSSA

The anterior cranial fossa lodges the frontal lobes of the cerebral hemispheres. It is bounded anteriorly by the inner surface of the frontal bone (see Fig. 9.10). Its posterior boundary is the sharp lesser wing of the sphenoid, which articulates laterally with the frontal bone and meets the anteroinferior angle of the parietal bone at the pterion. The medial end of the lesser wing of the sphenoid forms the **anterior clinoid process** on each side, which gives attachment to the **tentorium cerebelli**. The median part of the anterior cranial fossa is limited posteriorly by the **groove for the optic chiasm**.

The ridged orbital plates of the frontal bone form the lateral floor of the fossa, and the **cribriform plate** of the

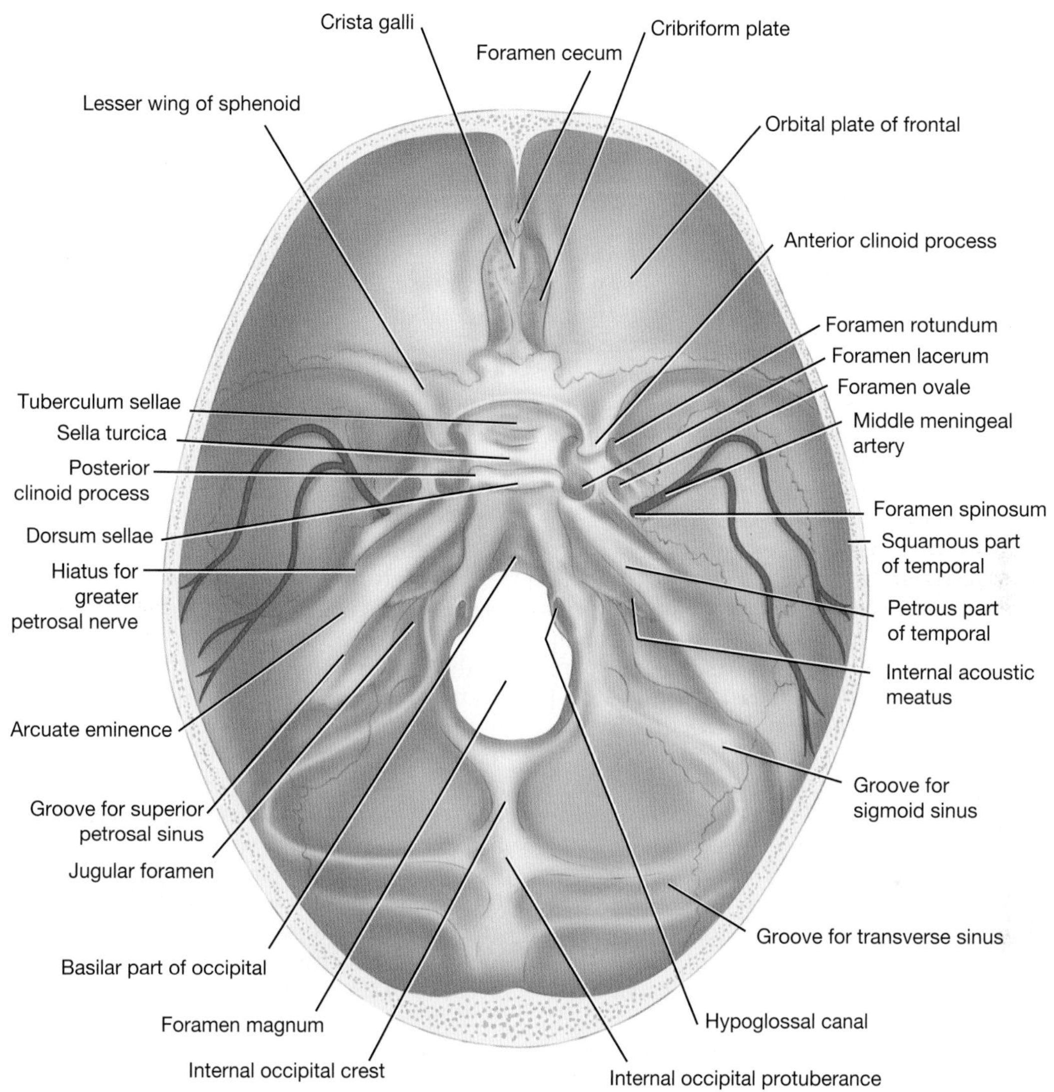

Figure 9.10 Internal surface of the base of the skull. Note the course of the middle meningeal artery and its anterior branch.

ethmoid forms the floor medially. The **crista galli** is a sharp upward projection of the ethmoid bone in the midline for the attachment of the **falx cerebri**. Alongside the crista galli is a narrow slit in the cribriform plate for the passage of the **anterior ethmoidal nerve** into the nasal cavity. The upper surface of the cribriform plate supports the olfactory bulbs, and the small perforations in the cribriform plate permit passage of the olfactory nerves.

MIDDLE CRANIAL FOSSA

The middle cranial fossa consists of a small median part and expanded lateral parts (see Fig. 9.10). The **body of the sphenoid** forms the median raised part, and the expanded lateral parts form concavities on either side, which lodge the temporal lobes of the cerebral hemispheres.

It is bounded anteriorly by the lesser wings of the sphenoid and posteriorly by the superior borders of the petrous parts of the temporal bones. Laterally lie the squamous parts of the temporal bones, greater wings of the sphenoid, and the parietal bones.

The greater wing of the sphenoid and the squamous and petrous parts of the temporal bone form the floor of each lateral part of the middle cranial fossa.

The sphenoid bone resembles a butterfly having a centrally placed **body** with **greater** and **lesser wings** outstretched on each side. The body of the sphenoid contains the **sphenoid air sinuses**, which are lined with mucous membrane and communicate with the nasal cavity.

Anteriorly, the **optic canal** transmits the optic nerve and the ophthalmic artery, a branch of the internal carotid artery, to the orbit. The **superior orbital fissure**, a large slit-like opening between the lesser and the greater wings of the sphenoid, transmits the lacrimal, frontal, trochlear, oculomotor, nasociliary, and abducens nerves, together with the superior ophthalmic vein. The sphenoparietal venous sinus runs medially along the posterior border of the lesser wing of the sphenoid and drains into the cavernous sinus.

The **foramen rotundum**, which is situated behind the medial end of the superior orbital fissure, perforates the greater wing of the sphenoid, and transmits the maxillary nerve from the trigeminal ganglion to the pterygopalatine fossa.

The **foramen ovale** lies posterolateral to the foramen rotundum. It perforates the greater wing of the sphenoid and transmits the large sensory root and small motor root of the mandibular nerve to the infratemporal fossa; the lesser petrosal nerve also passes through it.

The small **foramen spinosum** lays posterolateral to the foramen ovale and also perforates the greater wing of the sphenoid. The foramen transmits the middle meningeal artery from the infratemporal fossa into the cranial cavity. The artery then runs forward and laterally in a groove on the upper surface of the squamous part of the temporal bone and the greater wing of the sphenoid. After a short distance, the artery divides into anterior and posterior branches. The anterior branch passes forward and upward to the pterion. Here, the bone is deeply grooved or tunneled by the artery for a short distance before it runs backward and upward on the parietal bone. Here, the artery may be damaged after a blow to the side of the head. The posterior branch passes backward and upward across the squamous part of the temporal bone to reach the parietal bone.

The large, relatively long (about 1 cm), and irregularly shaped **foramen lacerum** lies between the apex of the petrous part of the temporal bone and the hypophyseal fossa of the sphenoid bone. In life, the inferior opening of the foramen is largely closed by a cartilage plug and fibrous tissue. Only small blood vessels (meningeal branches of the ascending pharyngeal artery, emissary veins from the cavernous sinus) pass through the entire vertical extent of the foramen lacerum.

Notice the foramen lacerum and carotid canal have separate openings in the exterior base of the skull (Fig. 9.11). However, only the foramen lacerum opens into the interior base of the skull (see Fig. 9.10). This often-confusing relationship occurs because the **carotid canal** opens into the posterior side of the foramen lacerum above its closed inferior opening. The internal carotid artery (plus its accompanying sympathetic nerve plexus) enters the upper aspect of the foramen lacerum through the carotid canal and immediately turns upward to exit the foramen at the side of the body of the sphenoid bone. Therefore, the internal carotid artery does not completely traverse the foramen lacerum. The artery next turns forward into the cavernous sinus, through which the vessel crosses.

The trigeminal ganglion makes an impression on the apex of the petrous part of the temporal bone, lateral to the foramen lacerum. Two grooves for nerves are on the anterior surface of the petrous bone. The larger medial groove is for the **greater petrosal nerve**, a branch of the facial nerve. The smaller lateral groove is for the **lesser petrosal nerve**, a branch of the tympanic plexus. The lesser petrosal nerve passes forward into the foramen ovale. The greater petrosal nerve enters the upper opening of the foramen lacerum under the trigeminal ganglion and joins the **deep petrosal nerve** (sympathetic fibers from the internal carotid plexus) within the foramen lacerum to form the **nerve of the pterygoid canal**. This nerve crosses the foramen lacerum and enters the **pterygoid canal** at the anterior lip of the foramen lacerum. Therefore, these nerves run horizontally across the diameter of the foramen lacerum rather than vertically through it.

The abducens nerve bends sharply forward across the apex of the petrous bone, medial to the trigeminal ganglion. Here, it leaves the posterior cranial fossa and enters the cavernous sinus.

The **arcuate eminence** is a rounded eminence on the anterior surface of the petrous bone and is caused by the underlying superior semicircular canal.

The **tegmen tympani**, a thin plate of bone, is a forward extension of the petrous part of the temporal bone and adjoins the squamous part of the bone. From behind forward, it forms the roof of the mastoid antrum, tympanic cavity, and the auditory tube. This thin plate of bone is the only major barrier that separates infection in the tympanic cavity from the temporal lobe of the cerebral hemisphere (see Tympanic Cavity).

The body of the sphenoid bone forms the median part of the middle cranial fossa. In front is the **sulcus chiasmatis**, which is related to the optic chiasm and leads laterally to the **optic canal** on each side. Posterior to the sulcus is an elevation, the **tuberculum sellae**. Behind the elevation is a deep depression, the **hypophyseal fossa**, which lodges the pituitary gland. A square plate of bone, the **dorsum sellae**, bounds the fossa posteriorly. The superior angles of the dorsum sellae have two tubercles, the **posterior clinoid processes**, which give attachment to the fixed margin of the tentorium cerebelli. The sulcus chiasmatis, tuberculum sellae, hypophyseal fossa, dorsum sellae, and anterior and posterior clinoid processes collectively form a complex structure termed the **sella turcica**, so named because of its resemblance to an ancient ornate saddle (*sella turcica* is Latin for "Turkish saddle").

The cavernous sinus is directly related to the side of the body of the sphenoid (see Venous [Dural] Blood Sinuses).

POSTERIOR CRANIAL FOSSA

The posterior cranial fossa is deep and lodges the parts of the hindbrain, namely, the cerebellum, pons, and medulla oblongata. Anteriorly, the **superior border of the petrous part of the temporal bone** bounds the fossa. The posterior boundary is the internal surface of the **squamous part of the occipital bone** (see Fig. 9.10). The floor of the posterior fossa is formed by the **basilar**, **condylar**, and **squamous parts of the occipital bone** and the **mastoid part of the temporal bone**.

The roof of the fossa is formed by a fold of dura, the **tentorium cerebelli**, which intervenes between the cerebellum below and the occipital lobes of the cerebral hemispheres above (see Dura Mater).

The **foramen magnum** (see Fig. 9.10) occupies the central area of the floor and transmits the medulla oblongata and its surrounding meninges, the ascending spinal parts of the accessory nerves, and the two vertebral arteries.

The **hypoglossal canal** is situated above the anterolateral boundary of the foramen magnum and transmits the hypoglossal nerve.

The **jugular foramen** lies between the lower border of the petrous part of the temporal bone and the condylar

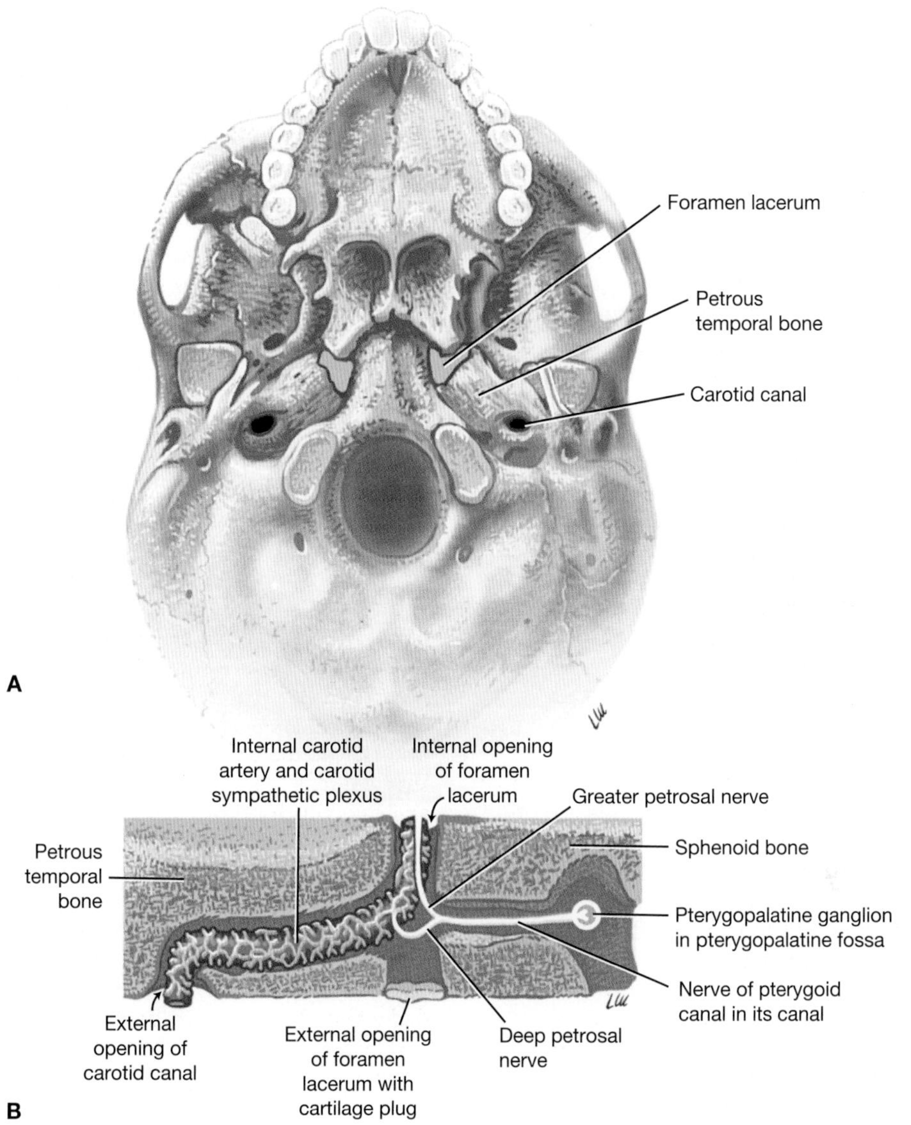

Figure 9.11 **A.** External base of the skull. Note the carotid canal and foramen lacerum are separate openings in this aspect. **B.** Schematic of the internal relations of the carotid canal and foramen lacerum. Note the carotid canal merges into the foramen lacerum. Therefore, the internal carotid artery traverses the entire carotid canal but only the upper part of the foramen lacerum.

part of the occipital bone. It transmits the following structures in anteroposterior sequence: the inferior petrosal sinus; CNs IX, X, and XI; and the large sigmoid sinus. The inferior petrosal sinus descends in the groove on the lower border of the petrous part of the temporal bone to reach the foramen. The sigmoid sinus turns down through the foramen to become the internal jugular vein.

The **internal acoustic meatus** pierces the posterior surface of the petrous part of the temporal bone. It transmits the vestibulocochlear nerve, motor and sensory roots of the facial nerve, and labyrinthine vessels of the inner ear.

The **internal occipital crest** runs upward in the midline posteriorly from the foramen magnum to the internal occipital protuberance. The small falx cerebelli attaches to this crest over the occipital sinus.

A wide **groove for the transverse sinus** lays on each side of the internal occipital protuberance. This groove sweeps around on either side, on the internal surface of the occipital bone, to reach the posteroinferior angle or corner of the parietal bone. The groove next passes onto the mastoid part of the temporal bone; here, the transverse sinus becomes the sigmoid sinus. The superior petrosal sinus runs backward along the upper border of the petrous bone in a narrow groove and drains into the sigmoid sinus. As the sigmoid sinus descends to the jugular foramen, it deeply grooves the back of the petrous bone and the mastoid part of the temporal bone. Here, it lies directly posterior to the mastoid antrum.

Table 9.1 provides a summary of the major openings in the base of the skull and the structures that pass through them.

Table 9.1 Major Openings in the Base of the Skull and Structures Passing Through Them

OPENING IN THE SKULL	BONE OF THE SKULL	STRUCTURES TRANSMITTED
Anterior Cranial Fossa		
Perforations in cribriform plate	Ethmoid	Olfactory nerves
Middle Cranial Fossa		
Optic canal	Lesser wing of sphenoid	Optic nerve; ophthalmic artery
Superior orbital fissure	Between lesser and greater wings of sphenoid	Oculomotor, trochlear, nasociliary, frontal, lacrimal, and abducens nerves; superior ophthalmic vein
Foramen rotundum	Greater wing of sphenoid	Maxillary division of the trigeminal nerve
Foramen ovale	Greater wing of sphenoid	Mandibular division of the trigeminal nerve; accessory meningeal artery; lesser petrosal nerve; emissary veins
Foramen spinosum	Greater wing of sphenoid	Middle meningeal artery
Carotid canal + upper foramen lacerum	Between petrous part of temporal and sphenoid	Internal carotid artery; sympathetic nerve plexus
Foramen lacerum	Between petrous part of temporal and sphenoid	Meningeal branches of ascending pharyngeal artery; emissary veins from cavernous sinus
Posterior Cranial Fossa		
Foramen magnum	Occipital	Medulla oblongata, spinal part of accessory nerve; right and left vertebral arteries
Hypoglossal canal	Occipital	Hypoglossal nerve; meningeal branch of ascending pharyngeal artery
Jugular foramen	Between petrous part of temporal and condylar part of occipital	Glossopharyngeal, vagus, and accessory nerves; sigmoid sinus becomes internal jugular vein
Internal acoustic meatus	Petrous part of temporal	Facial and vestibulocochlear nerves; labyrinthine vessels

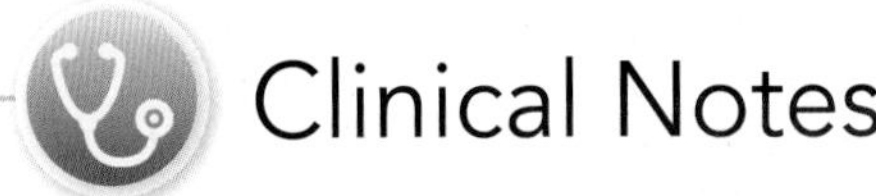

Skull Fractures

Fractures of the skull are common in the adult but much less so in the young child. In the infant skull, the bones are more resilient, and fibrous sutural ligaments separate them. In the adult, the inner table of the skull is particularly brittle. Moreover, the sutural ligaments begin to ossify during middle age.

The type of fracture that occurs in the skull depends on the age of the patient, the severity of the blow, and the area of skull receiving the trauma. The adult skull may be likened to an eggshell in that it possesses a certain limited resilience beyond which it splinters. A severe, localized blow produces a local indentation, often accompanied by splintering of the bone. Blows to the vault often result in a series of linear fractures, which radiate out through the thin areas of bone. The petrous parts of the temporal bones and the occipital crests strongly reinforce the base of the skull and tend to deflect linear fractures.

In the young child, the skull may be likened to a table tennis ball in that a localized blow produces a depression without splintering. This common type of circumscribed lesion is referred to as a **"pond" fracture**.

Anterior Cranial Fossa Fractures

The cribriform plate of the ethmoid bone may be damaged in fractures of the anterior cranial fossa. This usually results in tearing of the overlying meninges and underlying mucoperiosteum. The patient will have bleeding from the nose (**epistaxis**) and leakage of cerebrospinal fluid (CSF) into the nose (**cerebrospinal rhinorrhea**). Fractures involving the orbital plate of the frontal bone result in hemorrhage beneath the conjunctiva and into the orbital cavity, causing **exophthalmos**. The frontal air sinus may be involved, with hemorrhage into the nose.

Middle Cranial Fossa Fractures

Fractures of the middle cranial fossa are common because this is the weakest part of the base of the skull. Anatomically, this weakness is caused by the presence of numerous foramina and canals in this region. The cavities of the middle ear and the sphenoid air sinuses are particularly vulnerable. Leakage of CSF and blood from the external auditory meatus is common. CNs VII and VIII may be involved as they pass through the petrous part of the temporal bone. CNs III, IV, and VI may be damaged if the lateral wall of the cavernous sinus is torn. Blood and CSF may leak into the sphenoid air sinuses and then into the nose.

Posterior Cranial Fossa Fractures

In fractures of the posterior cranial fossa, blood may escape into the nape of the neck deep to the postvertebral muscles. Some days later, it tracks between the muscles and appears in the posterior triangle, close to the mastoid process. The mucous membrane of the roof of the nasopharynx may be torn, and blood may escape there. In fractures involving the jugular foramen, CNs IX, X, and XI may be damaged. The strong bony walls of the hypoglossal canal usually protect CN XII from injury.

Facial Bone Fractures

The developing bones of a child's face are more pliable than an adult's, and fractures may be incomplete or greenstick. In adults, the presence of well-developed, air-filled sinuses and the mucoperiosteal surfaces of the alveolar parts of the upper and lower jaws means that most facial fractures will be open fractures, susceptible to infection and requiring antibiotic therapy.

Anatomy of Common Facial Fractures

Vehicle accidents, blows to the face, and falls are common causes of facial fractures. Fortunately, the upper part of the skull is developed from membrane (whereas the remainder is developed from cartilage). Therefore, this part of the skull in children is relatively flexible and can absorb considerable force without resulting in a fracture.

Signs of fractures of the facial bones include deformity, ocular displacement, and abnormal movement accompanied by crepitation and malocclusion of the teeth. Anesthesia or paresthesia of the facial skin will follow fracture of bones through which branches of the trigeminal nerve pass to the skin.

The muscles of the face are thin and weak and cause little displacement of the bone fragments (eg, prolonged fixation is not needed once a fracture of the maxilla has been reduced). However, in the case of the mandible, the strong muscles of mastication can create considerable displacement, requiring long periods of fixation.

The most common facial fractures involve the nasal bones, followed by the zygomatic bone and then the mandible. Enormous force is required to fracture the maxillary bones and the supraorbital ridges of the frontal bones.

Nasal Fractures

Because of the prominence of the nose, fractures of the nasal bones are the most common facial fractures. Because the bones are lined with mucoperiosteum, the fracture is considered open; the overlying skin may also be lacerated. Although most are simple fractures and are reduced under local anesthesia, some are associated with severe injuries to the nasal septum and require careful treatment under general anesthesia.

Maxillofacial Fractures

Maxillofacial fractures usually occur as the result of massive facial trauma. There is extensive facial swelling, midface mobility of the underlying bone on palpation, malocclusion of the teeth with anterior open bite, and possibly leakage of CSF (**cerebrospinal rhinorrhea**) secondary to fracture of the cribriform plate of the ethmoid bone. Double vision (**diplopia**) may be present, owing to orbital wall damage. Involvement of the infraorbital nerve with anesthesia or paresthesia of the skin of the cheek and upper gum may occur in fractures of the body of the maxilla. Nose bleeding may also occur in maxillary fractures. Blood enters the maxillary air sinus and then leaks into the nasal cavity.

The sites of the fractures are classified as Le Fort type I, II, or III. These fractures are summarized in Figure 9.12.

Blowout Fractures of the Maxilla

A severe blow to the orbit (as from a baseball) may cause the contents of the orbital cavity to explode downward through the floor of the orbit into the maxillary sinus. Damage to the infraorbital nerve may occur, resulting in altered sensation in the skin of the cheek, upper lip, and gum.

Zygoma or Zygomatic Arch Fractures

A blow to the side of the face can fracture the zygoma or zygomatic arch. Although it can occur as an isolated fracture, as from a blow from a clenched fist, it may be associated with multiple other fractures of the face, as often seen in vehicle accidents.

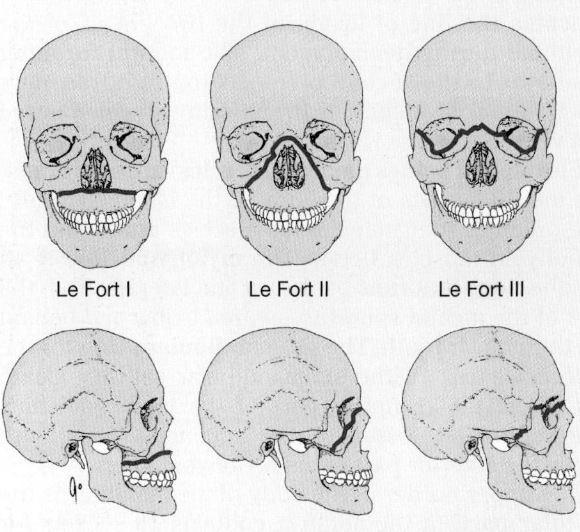

Figure 9.12 Le Fort classification of maxillofacial fractures. The *red line* denotes the fracture line.

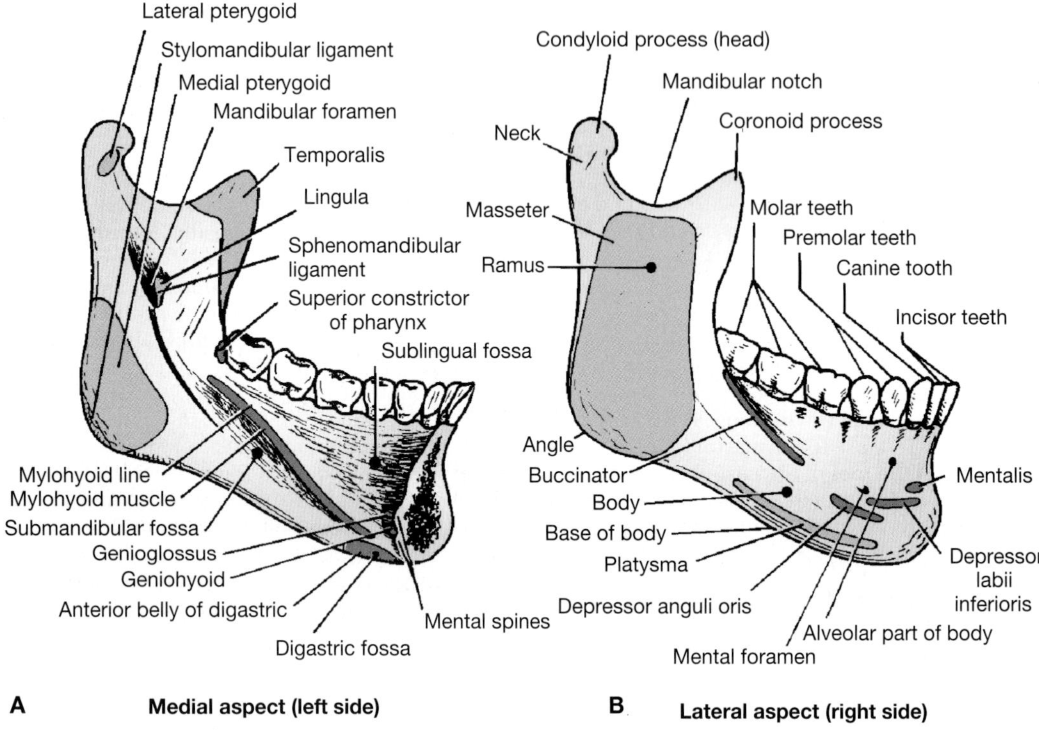

Figure 9.13 Mandible, from the medial **(A)** and lateral **(B)** aspects.

Mandible

The mandible (lower jaw) is the largest and strongest bone of the face. It articulates with the skull at the **temporomandibular joint** (see Fig. 9.5). The mandible consists of a more horizontal, horseshoe-shaped **body** and a pair of vertical **rami**. The body of the mandible meets the ramus on each side at the **angle** of the mandible (Fig. 9.13).

The **symphysis menti** is a faint ridge on the external midline surface of the body of the mandible. This indicates the line of fusion of the two halves of the mandible during development. The **mental foramen** is inferior to the second premolar tooth; it transmits the terminal branches of the inferior alveolar nerve and vessels.

The **mental spines (genial tubercles)** are on the midline medial surface of the body of the mandible; these give origin to the genioglossus muscles above and the geniohyoid muscles below. The **mylohyoid line** is an oblique ridge that runs backward and laterally from the area of the mental spines to an area below and behind the third molar tooth. The **submandibular fossa**, for the superficial part of the submandibular salivary gland, lies below the posterior part of the mylohyoid line. The **sublingual fossa**, for the sublingual gland, lies above the anterior part of the mylohyoid line.

The upper border of the body of the mandible is the **alveolar part**; in the adult, it contains 16 sockets for the roots of the teeth. The **base** is the lower border of the body of the mandible. The **digastric fossa** is a small, roughened depression on the base, on either side of the symphysis menti. The anterior bellies of the digastric muscles attach in these fossae.

The ramus of the mandible has an anterior **coronoid process** and a posterior **condyloid process (head)**. A short **neck** is inferior to the head. The **mandibular notch** separates the coronoid and condyloid processes. The temporalis muscle attaches onto the anterior and medial aspects of the coronoid process.

Markings for the attachment of the masseter muscle appear on the lateral surface of the ramus. The **mandibular foramen** is on the medial surface. This transmits the inferior alveolar nerve and vessels. The **lingula** is a projection in front of the mandibular foramen for the attachment of the sphenomandibular ligament (Fig. 9.14; see also Fig. 9.13). The foramen leads into the **mandibular canal**, which opens on the lateral surface of the body of the mandible at the **mental foramen**. The **incisive canal** is the forward continuation of the mandibular canal beyond the mental foramen and below the incisor teeth.

The attachment sites of the major muscles and ligaments of the mandible are shown in Figure 9.13.

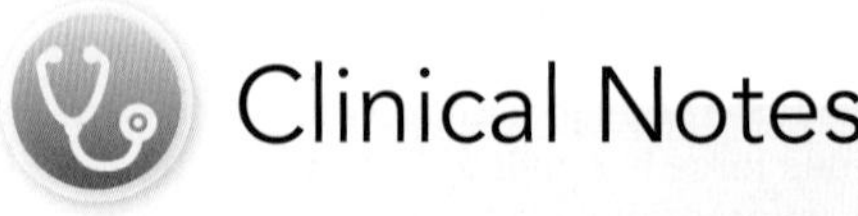

Mandible Fractures

The mandible is horseshoe shaped and forms part of a bony ring with the two temporomandibular joints and the base of the skull. Traumatic impact is transmitted around the ring, causing a single fracture or multiple fractures of the mandible, often far removed from the point of impact.

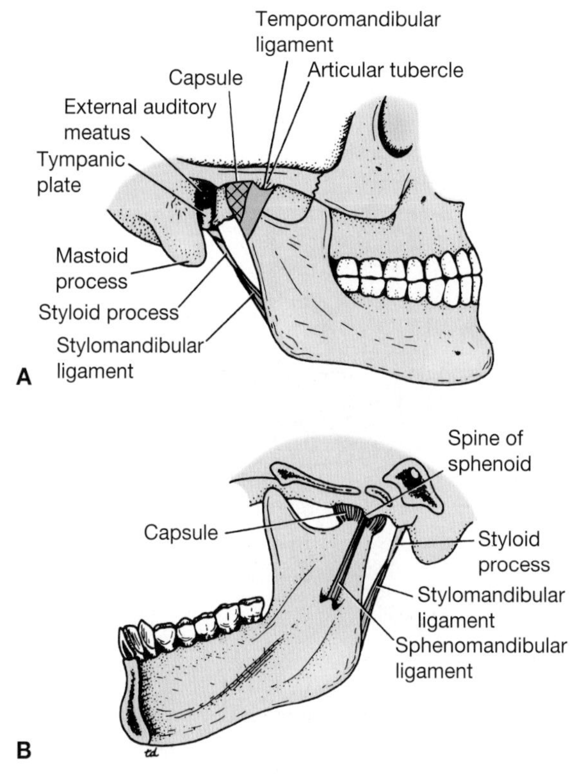

Figure 9.14 Temporomandibular joint as seen from the lateral **(A)** and medial **(B)** aspects.

Temporomandibular Joint

The **TMJ** is the synovial articulation between the **articular tubercle** and the anterior portion of the **mandibular fossa** of the temporal bone above and the **head** (**condyloid process**) of the mandible below (Figs. 9.15 and 9.16; see also Fig. 9.14). The **capsule** surrounds the joint and is attached above to the articular tubercle and the margins of the mandibular fossa and below to the neck of the mandible.

Ligaments

The **lateral temporomandibular ligament** strengthens the lateral aspect of the capsule, and its fibers run downward and backward from the tubercle on the root of the zygoma to the lateral surface of the neck of the mandible (see Fig. 9.14). This ligament limits the movement of the mandible in a posterior direction and thus protects the external auditory meatus.

The **sphenomandibular ligament** lies on the medial side of the joint. It is a thin band attached above to the spine of the sphenoid bone and below to the lingula of the mandibular foramen. It represents the remains of the first pharyngeal arch in this region.

The **stylomandibular ligament** lies behind and medial to the joint and some distance from it. It is merely a band of thickened deep cervical fascia that extends from the apex of the styloid process to the angle of the mandible.

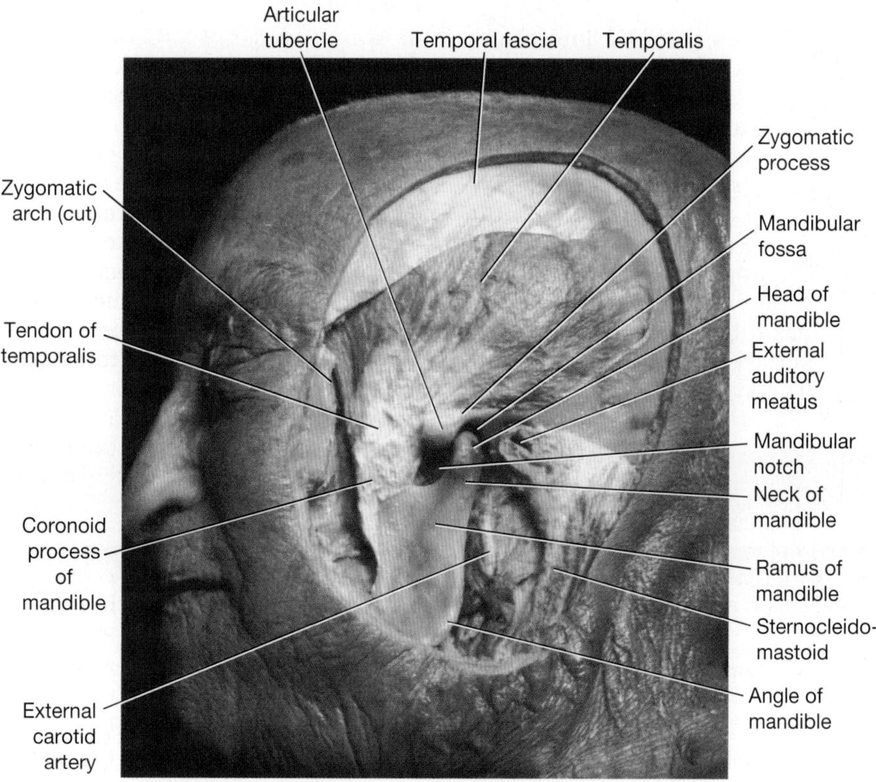

Figure 9.15 Dissection of the left temporomandibular joint. The capsule and lateral temporomandibular ligament have been removed to reveal the interior of the joint. Note the articular tubercle and mandibular fossa of the temporal bone and the head of the mandible. The articular disc is present within the joint cavity on the upper surface of the head of the mandible.

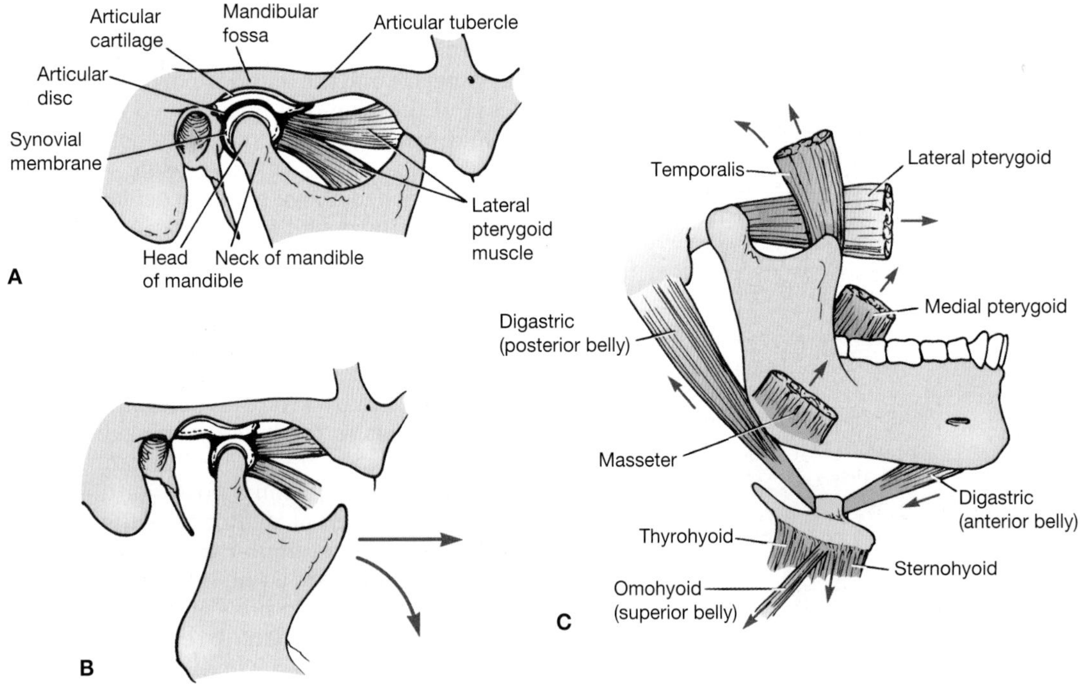

Figure 9.16 Temporomandibular joint with the mouth closed **(A)** and with the mouth open **(B)**. Note the position of the head of the mandible and articular disc in relation to the articular tubercle in each case. **C.** The attachments of the muscles of mastication to the mandible. The *arrows* indicate the direction of their actions.

Articular Disc

A fibrocartilage **articular disc** intervenes between the bony surfaces and divides the TMJ into upper and lower compartments (see Fig. 9.16). The disc is an oval plate that attaches circumferentially to the capsule. It is also attached in front to the tendon of the lateral pterygoid muscle and by fibrous bands to the head of the mandible. These bands ensure that the disc moves forward and backward with the head of the mandible during protraction and retraction of the mandible. The upper surface of the disc is concave-convex from anterior to posterior to fit the shape of the articular tubercle and the mandibular fossa; the lower surface is concave to fit the head of the mandible. The synovial membrane lines the capsule in both the upper and lower cavities of the joint.

Nerve Supply

Auriculotemporal and masseteric branches of the mandibular nerve

Movements

The mandible can be depressed, elevated, protruded, and retracted. Rotation also occurs, as in chewing. In the position of rest, the teeth of the upper and lower jaws are slightly apart. On closure of the jaws, the teeth come into contact (**occlusion**).

The muscles of mastication are summarized in Table 9.2 and Figure 9.16.

Table 9.2 Mastication Muscles

MUSCLE	ORIGIN	INSERTION	NERVE SUPPLY	ACTION
Masseter	Zygomatic arch	Lateral surface of ramus of mandible	Mandibular division of the trigeminal nerve	Elevates the mandible to occlude teeth
Temporalis	Floor of temporal fossa	Coronoid process of the mandible	Mandibular division of the trigeminal nerve	Anterior and superior fibers elevate mandible; posterior fibers retract mandible
Lateral pterygoid (two heads)	Greater wing of the sphenoid and lateral pterygoid plate	Neck of mandible and articular disc	Mandibular division of the trigeminal nerve	Pulls neck of mandible forward (protraction)
Medial pterygoid (two heads)	Tuberosity of maxilla and lateral pterygoid plate	Medial surface of angle of mandible	Mandibular division of the trigeminal nerve	Elevates mandible

MANDIBLE DEPRESSION

As the mouth is opened, the head of the mandible rotates on the undersurface of the articular disc around a horizontal axis. To prevent the angle of the jaw impinging unnecessarily on the parotid gland and the sternocleidomastoid muscle, the mandible is pulled forward (protracted). This is accomplished by the contraction of the lateral pterygoid muscle, which pulls forward the neck of the mandible and the articular disc so that the latter moves onto the articular tubercle (see Fig. 9.16). The forward movement of the disc is limited by the tension of the fibroelastic tissue, which tethers the disc to the temporal bone posteriorly.

Depression of the mandible is brought about by contraction of the digastric, geniohyoid, and mylohyoid muscles. The lateral pterygoids play an important role by pulling the mandible forward.

MANDIBLE ELEVATION

The movements in depression of the mandible are reversed. First, the head of the mandible and the disc move backward, and then the head rotates on the lower surface of the disc.

Elevation of the mandible is brought about by contraction of the temporalis, the masseter, and the medial pterygoids. The head of the mandible is pulled backward by the posterior fibers of the temporalis. The articular disc is pulled backward by the fibroelastic tissue, which tethers the disc to the temporal bone posteriorly.

MANDIBLE PROTRUSION

The articular disc is pulled forward onto the anterior tubercle, carrying the head of the mandible with it. All movement thus takes place in the upper cavity of the joint. In protrusion, the lower teeth are drawn forward over the upper teeth, which is brought about by contraction of the lateral pterygoid muscles of both sides, assisted by both medial pterygoids.

MANDIBLE RETRACTION

The articular disc and the head of the mandible are pulled backward into the mandibular fossa. Retraction is brought about by contraction of the posterior fibers of the temporalis.

LATERAL CHEWING MOVEMENTS

Alternately protruding and retracting the mandible on each side produces lateral motions. For this to take place, a certain amount of rotation occurs, and the muscles responsible on both sides work alternately and not in unison.

Important Temporomandibular Joint Relations

- **Anteriorly:** Mandibular notch (see Fig. 9.13) and the masseteric nerve and artery
- **Posteriorly:** Tympanic plate of the external auditory meatus (see Fig. 9.14A) and the glenoid process of the parotid gland
- **Laterally:** Parotid gland, fascia, and skin
- **Medially:** Maxillary artery and vein and auriculotemporal nerve

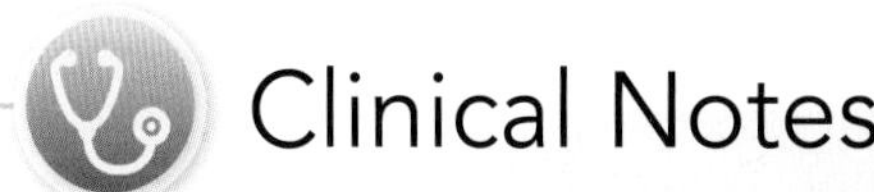

Clinical Significance of the Temporomandibular Joint

The temporomandibular joint (TMJ) lies immediately in front of the external auditory meatus. The great strength of the lateral temporomandibular ligament prevents the head of the mandible from passing backward and fracturing the tympanic plate when a severe blow falls on the chin.

The articular disc of the TMJ may become partially detached from the capsule, and this results in its movement becoming noisy and producing an audible click during movements at the joint.

Temporomandibular Joint Dislocation

Dislocation sometimes occurs when the mandible is depressed. In this movement, the head of the mandible and the articular disc both move forward until they reach the summit of the articular tubercle. In this position, the joint is unstable, and a minor blow on the chin or a sudden contraction of the lateral pterygoid muscles, as in yawning, may be sufficient to pull the disc forward beyond the summit. In bilateral cases, the mouth is fixed in an open position, and both heads of the mandible lie in front of the articular tubercles. Pressing the gloved thumbs downward on the lower molar teeth and pushing the jaw backward easily achieve reduction of the dislocation. The downward pressure overcomes the tension of the temporalis and masseter muscles, and the backward pressure overcomes the spasm of the lateral pterygoid muscles.

Neonatal Skull

The newborn skull, compared with the adult skull, has a disproportionately large cranium relative to the face (Fig. 9.17). The neonatal face to cranium size ratio is approximately 1:8, whereas the adult face to cranium ratio is approximately 1:1. Growth of the oral apparatus (upper and lower jaws, teeth, muscles of mastication, and tongue) and respiratory system (nasal cavities and paranasal sinuses) during childhood results in a great increase in length of the face.

The bones of the skull are smooth and unilaminar, as they have no diploë. Most of the skull bones are ossified at birth, but the process is incomplete, and the bones are mobile on each other, being connected by fibrous tissue or cartilage. The bones of the vault are not closely knit at sutures, as in the adult, but are separated by unossified membranous intervals called **fontanelles** ("soft spots"). Clinically, the anterior and posterior fontanelles are most important and are easily examined in the midline of the vault.

The **anterior (bregmatic) fontanelle** is diamond shaped and lies between the two halves of the frontal bone in front and the two parietal bones behind. The fibrous membrane forming the floor of the anterior fontanelle ossifies and closes by age 18 months. The **posterior (lambdoid) fontanelle** is triangular and lies between the two parietal bones in front and the occipital

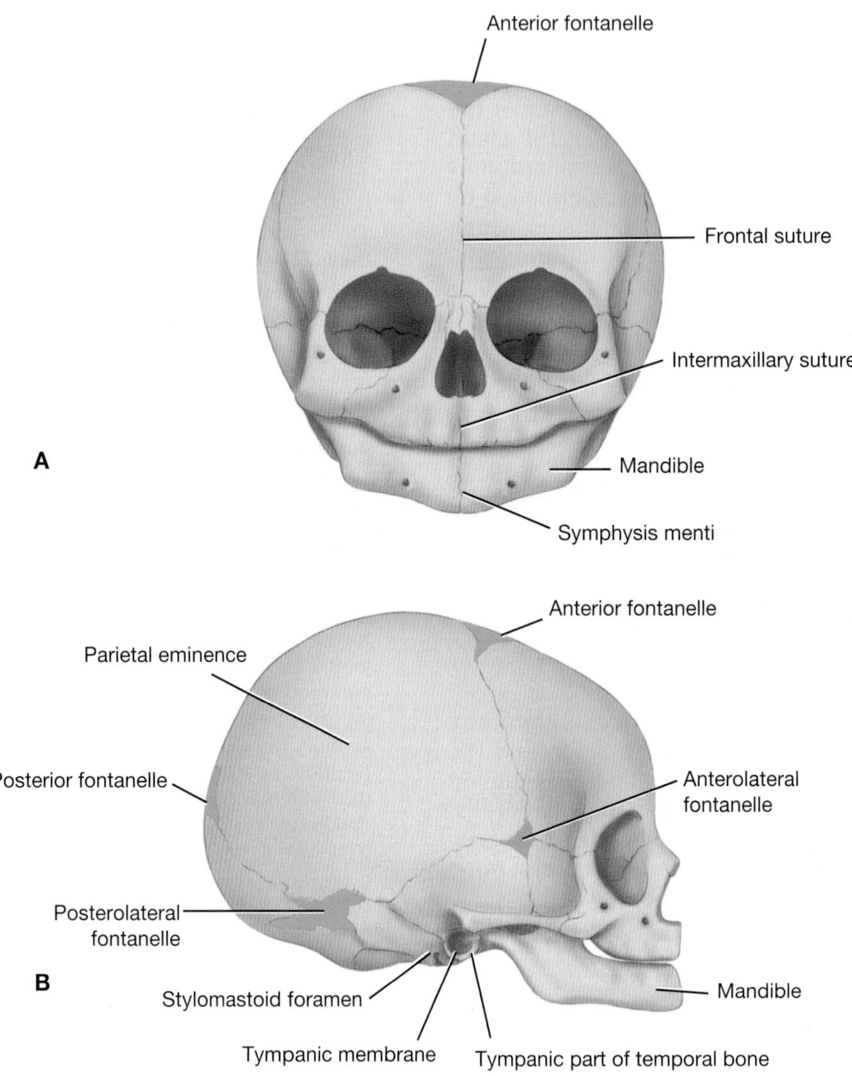

Figure 9.17 Neonatal skull as seen from the anterior **(A)** and lateral **(B)** aspects.

bone behind. This fontanelle usually closes by age 12 months. Two smaller fontanelles are located on each side of the skull. The **anterolateral (sphenoidal) fontanelle** is at the junction of the frontal, parietal, squamous temporal, and greater wing of the sphenoid bones. The **posterolateral (mastoidal) fontanelle** is at the junction of the temporal, parietal, and occipital bones.

The **tympanic part of the temporal bone** is merely a C-shaped ring at birth, compared with a C-shaped curved plate in the adult. Thus, the external auditory meatus is almost entirely cartilaginous in the newborn, and the **tympanic membrane** (eardrum) is nearer the surface. Although the tympanic membrane is nearly as large as in the adult, it faces more inferiorly. During childhood, the tympanic plate grows laterally, forming the bony part of the meatus, and the tympanic membrane comes to face more directly laterally.

The **mastoid process** is not present at birth and develops later in response to the pull of the sternocleidomastoid muscle when the child moves their head.

At birth, the **mastoid antrum** lies about 3 mm deep to the floor of the suprameatal triangle. As growth of the skull continues, the lateral bony wall thickens so that at puberty the antrum may lie as much as 15 mm from the surface.

Two separate right and left **dentary bones**, joined by a midline symphyseal joint, form the lower jaw at birth. The two dentaries fuse at the **symphysis menti** by age 12 months and form the single mandible.

The **angle of the mandible** is obtuse at birth. The head is level with the upper margin of the body, and the coronoid process lies at a superior level to the head. The angle assumes the adult shape after eruption of the permanent teeth, and the head and neck grow so that the head comes to lie higher than the coronoid process.

The size of the mandible reduces when the teeth are lost, such as in old age. As the alveolar part of the bone becomes smaller, the ramus becomes oblique in position so that the head is bent posteriorly.

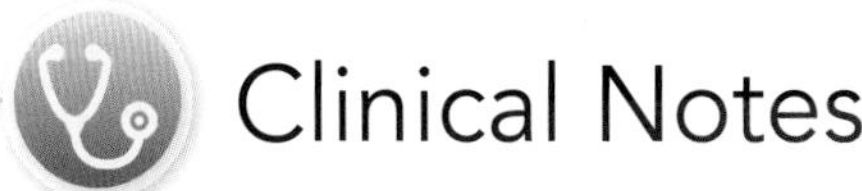

Clinical Notes

Frontal Bone

The frontal bone forms initially as two elements separated by a midline **frontal suture** (see Fig. 9.17A). At birth, the frontal bones are paired. These begin to fuse in the second year, and the frontal suture usually is obliterated by age 8 years. However, a small remnant of the frontal suture may persist as a **metopic suture** in as many as 7% to 8% of people (see Fig. 9.1). Much less often, most, or all of the suture may remain (Fig. 9.18). A clinician must be careful not to mistake a persistent metopic suture as a fracture in medical imaging.

Fontanelles

Palpation of the fontanelles enables the physician to determine the progress of growth in the surrounding bones, the degree of hydration of the infant (eg, if the fontanelles are depressed below the surface, the child is dehydrated), and the state of the intracranial pressure (a bulging fontanelle indicates raised intracranial pressure).

Samples of cerebrospinal fluid can be obtained by passing a long needle obliquely through the anterior fontanelle into the subarachnoid space or even into the lateral ventricle.

Clinically, it is usually not possible to palpate the anterior fontanelle after 18 months, because the frontal and parietal bones have enlarged to close the gap.

Tympanic Membrane

At birth, the tympanic membrane faces more downward and less laterally than in maturity. When examined with the otoscope, it lies more obliquely in the infant than in the adult.

Forceps Delivery and the Facial Nerve

The mastoid process is not developed in the neonate, and the facial nerve is relatively exposed and close to the surface as it emerges from the stylomastoid foramen. Thus, forceps used in a difficult delivery can damage the nerve.

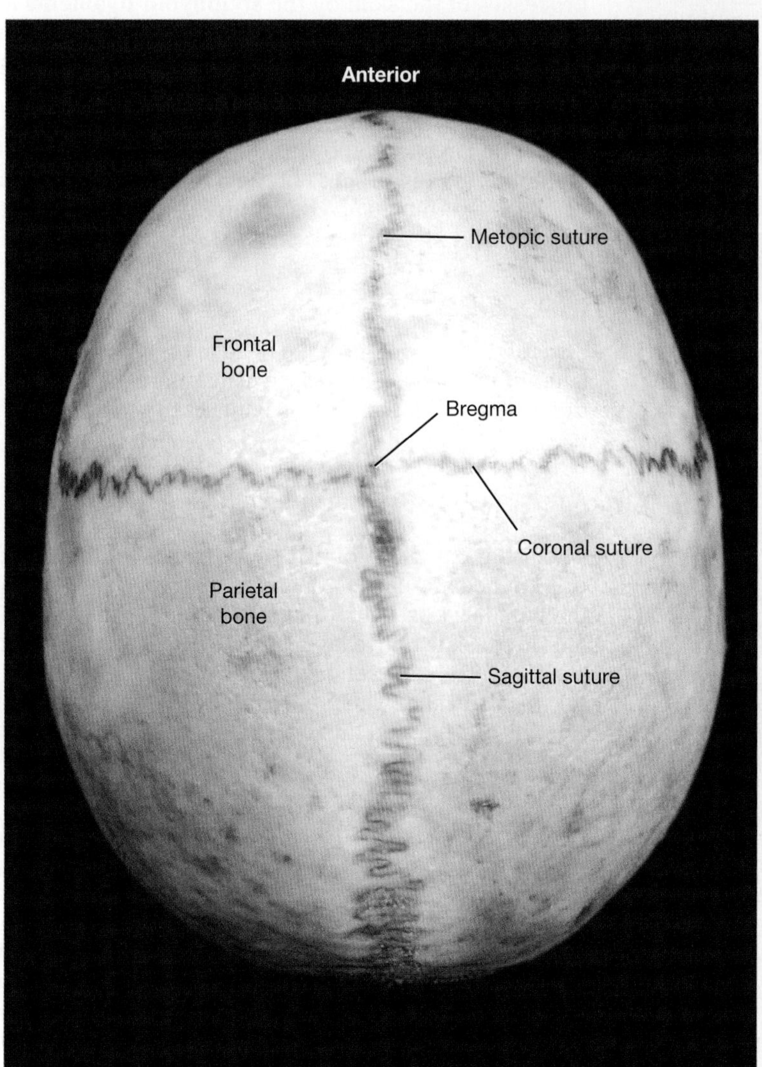

Figure 9.18 Persistent metopic (frontal) suture in the cranium of an adult male.

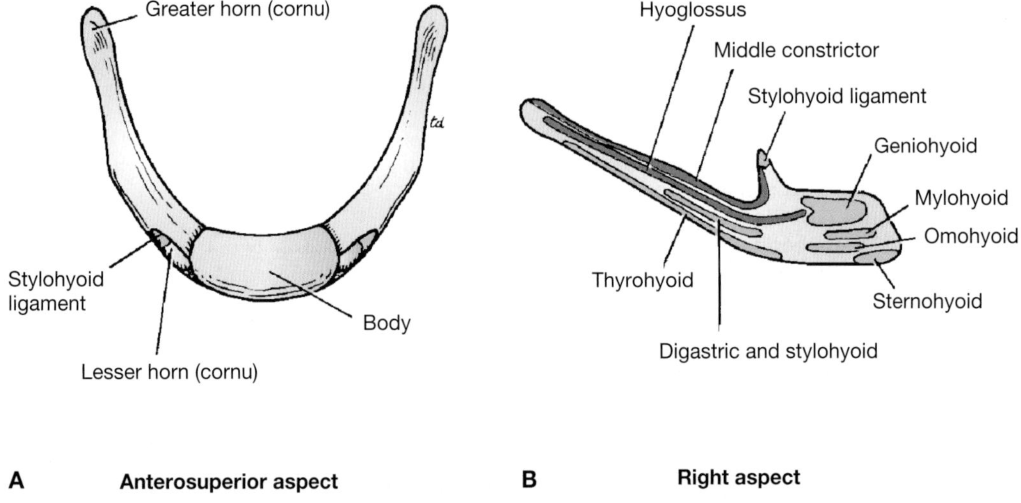

Figure 9.19 Hyoid bone from the anterosuperior **(A)** and right **(B)** aspects.

Hyoid Bone

The hyoid bone is a mobile single bone in the midline of the neck below the mandible and above the thyroid cartilage of the larynx. It does not articulate with any other bones. The hyoid bone is U shaped and consists of a central **body** and paired **greater cornua (horns)** and **lesser cornua** (Fig. 9.19). It attaches to the styloid processes of the skull by the **stylohyoid ligaments** and to the thyroid cartilage by the **thyrohyoid membrane**. The stylohyoid ligaments may ossify to greater or lesser degrees.

The hyoid bone forms a base for the tongue and is suspended in position by muscles that connect it to the mandible, styloid process of the temporal bone, thyroid cartilage, sternum, and the scapula. The major muscles that attach to the hyoid bone are shown in Figure 9.19.

Landmark Points

Several distinct points in the head are reliable landmarks used in cranial references, measurements, and orientation for imaging. These are summarized in Table 9.3.

Table 9.3 Craniometric Landmark Points

LANDMARK POINT	LOCATION
Nasion	Midline depression at the root of the nose, at the junction of the nasofrontal sutures (Fig. 9.140)
Bregma	Midline point at the junction of the coronal and sagittal sutures; this marks the anterior fontanelle in the neonatal skull
Vertex	Highest point on the skull in the sagittal plane (Fig. 9.140)
Inion	External occipital protuberance (Fig. 9.140)
Lambda	Midline point at the junction of the sagittal and lambdoidal sutures; this marks the posterior fontanelle in the neonatal skull
Pterion	Point where the greater wing of the sphenoid meets the anteroinferior angle of the parietal bone; this marks the anterior branch of the middle meningeal artery and the anterolateral fontanelle in the neonatal skull (Fig. 9.140)
Basion	Anterior midpoint of the foramen magnum
Gnathion	Most anteroinferior, median point of the mandible; that is, the midline point of the chin

SCALP

The scalp extends from the superciliary arches anteriorly to the external occipital protuberance and superior nuchal lines posteriorly and to the temporal lines laterally. It consists of five layers (see Fig. 9.4). Conveniently, the first letters of each layer together spell **SCALP**, making recall easier. The first three layers are intimately bound together and move as a unit.

- **S**kin. This is thick and hair bearing and contains numerous sebaceous glands.
- **C**onnective tissue beneath the skin. This is a dense fibrofatty layer containing fibrous septa that unite the skin to the underlying epicranial aponeurosis. This layer contains numerous blood vessels. The arteries are derived from both the external and internal carotid arteries, and free anastomoses occur between them.
- **A**poneurosis (epicranial). This is a thin, tendinous sheet that unites the occipital and frontal bellies of the occipitofrontalis muscle (see Muscles and Fig. 9.20). The lateral margins of the aponeurosis are

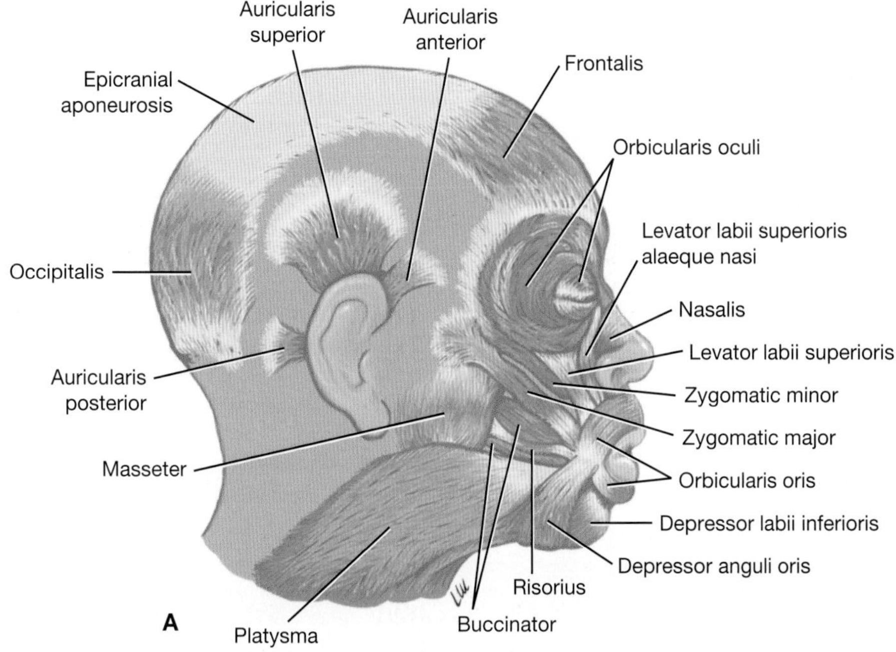

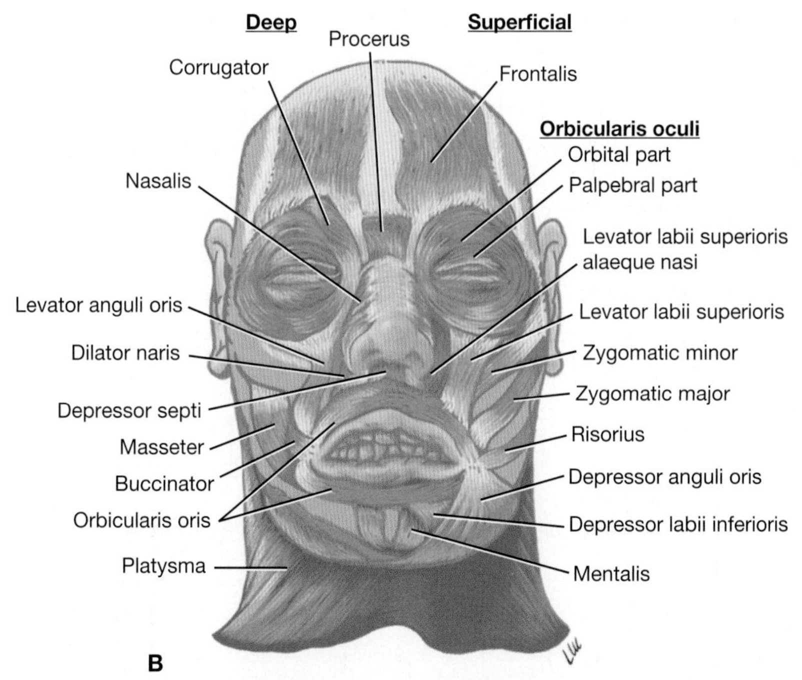

Figure 9.20 Muscles of the scalp and of facial expression from the lateral **(A)** and anterior **(B)** aspects.

attached to the temporal fascia. The **subaponeurotic space** is the potential space deep to the epicranial aponeurosis. It is limited in front and behind by the origins of the occipitofrontalis muscle, and it extends laterally as far as the attachment of the aponeurosis to the temporal fascia.

- **L**oose areolar tissue. This occupies the subaponeurotic space (see Fig. 9.4) and loosely connects the epicranial aponeurosis to the periosteum of the skull (the pericranium). This is the plane of movement of the scalp, that is, when the scalp moves, the first three layers (SCA) slide along this layer relative to the underlying periosteum. The areolar tissue contains a few small arteries, but it also contains some important emissary veins. The **emissary veins** are valveless and connect the superficial veins of the scalp with the diploic veins of the skull bones and with the intracranial venous sinuses.

- **P**ericranium. The pericranium is the periosteum covering the outer surface of the skull bones. The pericranium is continuous with the periosteum on the inner surface of the skull bones (**endosteum**) at the sutures between the individual skull bones.

Muscles

The **occipitofrontalis** (**epicranius**) is the sole skeletal muscle in the scalp (see Fig. 9.20). It is summarized in Table 9.4. The muscle consists of paired frontal and occipital bellies connected by the expansive epicranial aponeurosis. This muscle is responsible for movement of the scalp. Note that when this muscle contracts, the first three layers of the scalp (SCA) move together as a unit. The loose areolar tissue of the fourth layer of the scalp allows the aponeurosis to move on the pericranium. The frontal bellies of the occipitofrontalis can raise the eyebrows in expressions of surprise or horror.

Sensory Nerve Supply

The main trunks of the sensory nerves lie in the dense connective tissue layer (the "C" layer) of the scalp. The nerves are arranged in two main groups: (1) branches of the trigeminal nerve located anterior to the ear and (2) branches of cervical spinal nerves located posterior to the ear (Fig. 9.21). Moving laterally from the anterior midline, the following nerves are present.

Table 9.4 Scalp and Face Muscles

MUSCLE	ORIGIN	INSERTION	NERVE SUPPLY	ACTION
Scalp Muscle				
Occipitofrontalis Occipital belly Frontal belly	Highest nuchal line of occipital bone Skin and superficial fascia of eyebrows	Epicranial aponeurosis	Facial nerve	Moves scalp on skull and raises eyebrows
Facial Expression Muscles				
Orbicularis oculi Palpebral part Orbital part	Medial palpebral ligament Medial palpebral ligament and adjoining bone	Lateral palpebral raphe Loops return to origin	Facial nerve	Closes eyelids and dilates lacrimal sac Throws skin around orbit into folds to protect eyeball
Corrugator supercilii	Superciliary arch	Skin of eyebrow	Facial nerve	Vertical wrinkles of forehead, as in frowning
Compressor nasi	Frontal process of maxilla	Aponeurosis of the bridge of the nose	Facial nerve	Compresses mobile nasal cartilages
Dilator naris	Maxilla	Ala of the nose	Facial nerve	Widens nasal aperture
Procerus	Nasal bone	Skin between eyebrows	Facial nerve	Wrinkles in the skin of the nose
Orbicularis oris	Maxilla, mandible, and skin	Encircles oral orifice	Facial nerve	Compresses lips together
Lip Dilator Muscles				
Levator labii superioris alaeque nasi Levator labii superioris Zygomaticus minor Zygomaticus major Levator anguli oris Risorius Depressor anguli oris Depressor labii inferioris Mentalis	Arise from bones and fascia around oral aperture and insert into substance of lips		Facial nerve	Separate lips
Buccinator	Outer surface of alveolar margins of maxilla and mandible and pterygomandibular ligament		Facial nerve	Compresses cheeks and lips against teeth
Platysma	See Table 9.6			

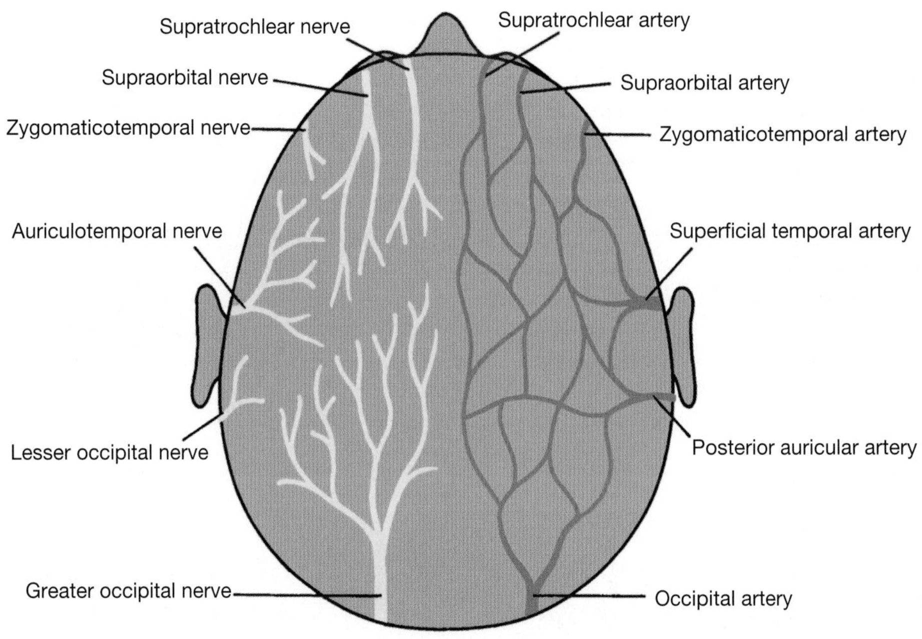

Figure 9.21 Superior view of the sensory nerve supply and arterial supply to the scalp.

Trigeminal branches:

- **Supratrochlear nerve**, a branch of the ophthalmic division of the trigeminal nerve, winds around the superior orbital margin and supplies the scalp. It passes backward close to the median plane and reaches nearly as far as the vertex of the skull.
- **Supraorbital nerve**, a branch of the ophthalmic division of the trigeminal nerve, winds around the superior orbital margin and ascends over the forehead. It supplies the scalp as far backward as the vertex.
- **Zygomaticotemporal nerve**, a branch of the maxillary division of the trigeminal nerve, supplies the scalp over the temple.
- **Auriculotemporal nerve**, a branch of the mandibular division of the trigeminal nerve, ascends over the side of the head from in front of the auricle. Its terminal branches supply the skin over the temporal region.

Cervical spinal nerve branches:

- **Lesser occipital nerve (C2)**, a branch of the cervical plexus, ascends along the posterior edge of the sternocleidomastoid muscle and supplies the scalp over the lateral part of the occipital region and the skin over the medial surface of the auricle.
- **Greater occipital nerve**, a branch of the posterior ramus of the C2 nerve, ascends over the back of the scalp and supplies the skin as far forward as the vertex of the skull.

Arterial Supply

The scalp has a rich blood supply to nourish the hair follicles; for this reason, the smallest cut bleeds profusely. As with the cutaneous nerves, the arteries run through the dense connective tissue layer (the "C" layer) of the scalp, typically follow the nerves, and form an extensive, freely anastomosing network. Moving laterally from the anterior midline, the following arteries are present (see Fig. 9.21):

- **Supratrochlear** and the **supraorbital arteries**, branches of the ophthalmic artery (a branch of the internal carotid artery), ascend over the forehead in company with the supratrochlear and supraorbital nerves.
- **Superficial temporal artery**, the smaller terminal branch of the external carotid artery, ascends in front of the auricle in company with the auriculotemporal nerve. It divides into anterior and posterior branches, which supply the skin over the frontal and temporal regions.
- **Posterior auricular artery**, a branch of the external carotid artery, ascends behind the auricle to supply the scalp above and behind the auricle.
- **Occipital artery**, a branch of the external carotid artery, ascends from the apex of the posterior triangle in company with the greater occipital nerve and pierces the trapezius muscle to reach the scalp. It supplies the skin over the back of the scalp and reaches as high as the vertex of the skull.

Venous Drainage

The **supratrochlear** and **supraorbital veins** unite at the medial margin of the orbit to form the **facial vein** (Fig. 9.22).

The **superficial temporal vein** unites with the **maxillary vein** in the substance of the parotid gland to form the **retromandibular vein**.

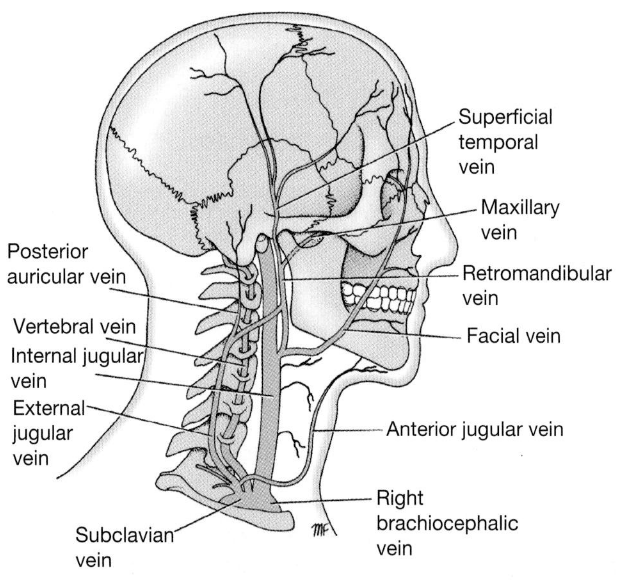

Figure 9.22 Main veins of the head and neck.

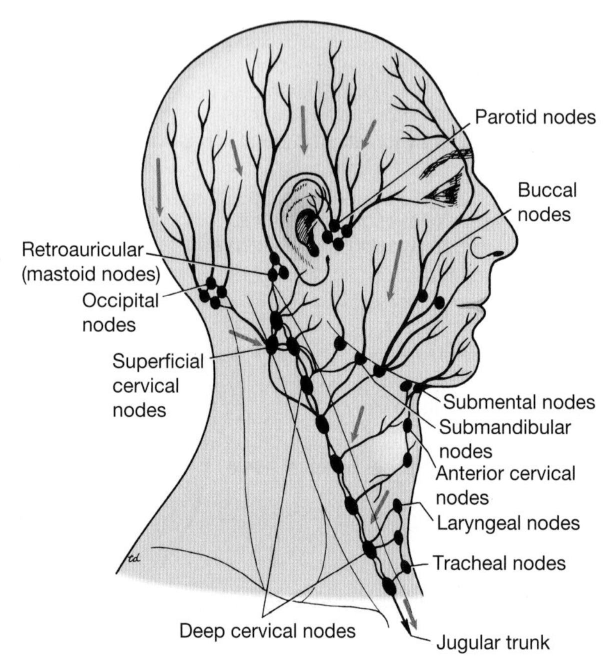

Figure 9.23 Lymph drainage of the head and neck.

The **posterior auricular vein** unites with the **posterior division of the retromandibular vein**, just below the parotid gland, to form the **external jugular vein**.

The **occipital vein** drains into the **suboccipital venous plexus**, which lies beneath the floor of the upper part of the posterior triangle; the plexus in turn drains into the vertebral veins or the internal jugular vein.

The veins of the scalp freely anastomose with one another and are connected to the diploic veins of the skull bones and the intracranial venous sinuses by valveless emissary veins (see Fig. 9.4).

Lymph Drainage

Lymph vessels in the anterior part of the scalp and forehead drain into the **submandibular lymph nodes** (Fig. 9.23). Drainage from the lateral part of the scalp above the ear is into the **superficial parotid (preauricular) nodes**. Lymph vessels in the part of the scalp above and behind the ear drain into the **mastoid nodes**. Vessels in the back of the scalp drain into the **occipital nodes**.

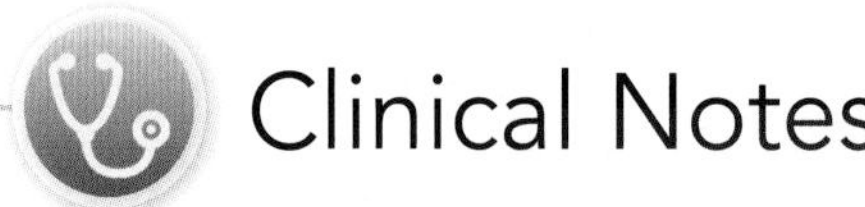

Clinical Notes

Clinical Significance of the Scalp Structure

It is important to realize that the skin, subcutaneous tissue, and the epicranial aponeurosis (scalp layers SCA) are closely united to one another and are separated from the periosteum by loose areolar tissue. The skin of the scalp has numerous sebaceous glands, with ducts prone to infection and damage by repeated hair treatment (eg, combing and brushing). For this reason, **sebaceous cysts** of the scalp are common.

Scalp Lacerations

The scalp has a profuse blood supply to nourish the hair follicles. Even a small laceration of the scalp can cause severe blood loss. It is often difficult to stop the bleeding of a scalp wound because the arterial walls are attached to fibrous septa in the subcutaneous tissue (C layer) and are unable to contract or retract to allow blood clotting to take place. Local pressure applied to the scalp is the only satisfactory method of stopping the bleeding (see Life-Threatening Scalp Hemorrhage).

It is common for large areas of the scalp to be cut off the head as a person is projected forward through the windshield in automobile accidents. Because of the profuse blood supply, it is often possible to replace large areas of scalp that are only hanging to the skull by a narrow pedicle. Appropriate vascular suturing reduces the chance of necrosis.

The tension of the epicranial aponeurosis, produced by the tone of the occipitofrontalis muscles, is important in all deep wounds of the scalp. If the aponeurosis has been divided, the wound will gape open. For satisfactory healing to take place, the opening in the aponeurosis must be closed with sutures.

Often, a wound caused by a blunt object such as a baseball bat closely resembles an incised wound. This is because the scalp is split against the unyielding skull and the pull of the occipitofrontalis muscles causes a gaping wound. This anatomic fact may be of considerable forensic importance.

Life-Threatening Scalp Hemorrhage

Note that all the superficial arteries supplying the scalp ascend from the face and the neck. Thus, in an emergency situation, encircle the head just above the ears and eyebrows with a tie, shoelaces, or even a piece of string and tie it tight. Then, insert a pen, pencil, or stick into the loop and rotate it so that the tourniquet exerts pressure on the arteries.

Scalp Infections

Infections of the scalp tend to remain localized and are usually painful because of the abundant fibrous tissue in the subcutaneous layer.

Occasionally, an infection of the scalp spreads by the emissary veins, which are valveless, to the skull bones, causing **osteomyelitis**. Infected blood in the diploic veins may travel by the emissary veins farther into the venous sinuses and produce **venous sinus thrombosis**.

Blood or pus may collect in the potential space deep to the epicranial aponeurosis (the L layer of the scalp). It tends to spread over the skull, being limited in front by the orbital margin, behind by the nuchal lines, and laterally by the temporal lines. On the other hand, subperiosteal blood or pus is limited to one bone because of the attachment of the periosteum to the sutural ligaments.

FACE

The face is the area from the superciliary arches superiorly to the lower margin of the mandible inferiorly and to the auricles laterally. It contains the orbits, nose, mouth, and ears and therefore houses the interfaces for vision, respiration, olfaction, taste, food processing, vocalization, and hearing between the internal and external environments. Further, the face is critical for individual identity, and facial expression is a highly evolved means of nonvocal communication.

Facial Skeleton

The bones that form the front of the skull are shown in Figure 9.24 (see also Anterior View and Lateral View, earlier in the chapter). The superior orbital margins and the area above them are formed by the **frontal bone**, which contains the frontal air sinuses. The lateral orbital margin is formed by the **zygomatic bone**, and the inferior orbital margin is formed by the zygomatic bone and the **maxilla**. The medial orbital margin is formed above by the maxillary process of the frontal bone and below by the frontal process of the maxilla.

The root of the nose is formed by the **nasal bones**, which articulate below with the maxilla and above with the frontal bones. Anteriorly, upper and lower plates of hyaline cartilage and small cartilages of the ala nasi complete the nose.

The important central bone of the middle third of the face is the maxilla, containing its teeth and the maxillary air sinus. The bone of the lower third of the face is the mandible, with its teeth.

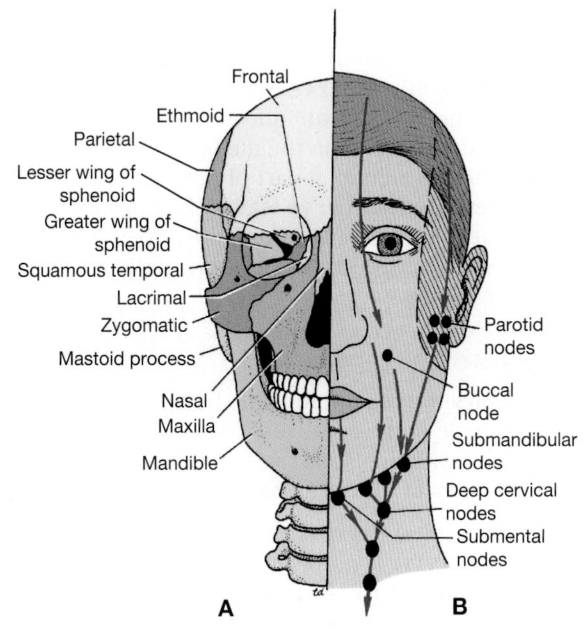

Figure 9.24 **A.** Bones of the front of the skull. **B.** Lymph drainage of the face.

Skin

The skin of the face has numerous sweat and sebaceous glands. It is connected to the underlying bones by loose connective tissue, where the muscles of facial expression are embedded. There is no deep fascia in the face.

Wrinkle lines of the face result from the repeated folding of the skin perpendicular to the long axis of the underlying contracting muscles, coupled with the loss of youthful skin elasticity. Surgical scars of the face are less conspicuous if they follow the wrinkle lines.

Sensory Nerves

The skin of the face is supplied by branches of the three divisions of the trigeminal nerve, except for the small area over the angle of the mandible and the parotid gland (Figs. 9.25A and 9.26), which is supplied by the **great auricular nerve** (C2 and C3). The overlap of the three divisions of the trigeminal nerve is slight compared with the considerable overlap of dermatomes of the trunk and limbs. The **ophthalmic nerve** supplies the region developed from the frontonasal process, the **maxillary nerve** serves the region developed from the maxillary process of the first pharyngeal arch, and the **mandibular nerve** serves the region developed from the mandibular process of the first pharyngeal arch. These nerves not only supply the skin of the face

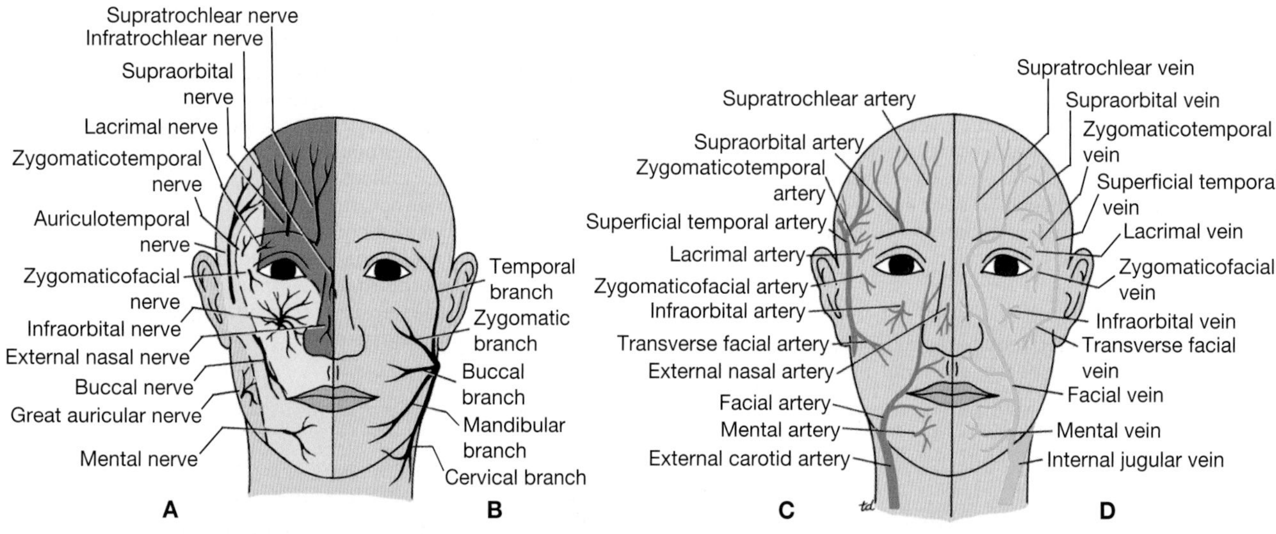

Figure 9.25 **A.** Sensory nerve supply to the skin of the face. **B.** Branches of the facial nerve to muscles of facial expression. **C.** Arterial supply of the face. **D.** Venous drainage of the face.

but also supply proprioceptive fibers to the underlying muscles of facial expression. Additionally, they are the sensory nerve supply to the mouth, teeth, nasal cavities, and paranasal air sinuses.

Ophthalmic Nerve

The ophthalmic nerve supplies the skin of the forehead, upper eyelid, conjunctiva, and the side of the nose down to and including the tip. Five branches of the nerve pass to the skin.

- The **lacrimal nerve** supplies the skin and conjunctiva of the lateral part of the upper eyelid.
- The **supraorbital nerve** winds around the upper margin of the orbit at the **supraorbital notch/supraorbital foramen**. It divides into branches that supply the skin and conjunctiva on the central part of the upper eyelid; it also supplies the skin of the forehead.
- The **supratrochlear nerve** winds around the upper margin of the orbit medial to the supraorbital nerve. It divides into branches that supply the skin and conjunctiva on the medial part of the upper eyelid and the skin over the lower part of the forehead, close to the median plane.
- The **infratrochlear nerve** leaves the orbit below the pulley of the superior oblique muscle. It supplies the skin and conjunctiva on the medial part of the upper eyelid and the adjoining part of the side of the nose.
- The **external nasal nerve** leaves the nose by emerging between the nasal bone and the upper nasal cartilage. It supplies the skin on the side of the nose down as far as the tip.

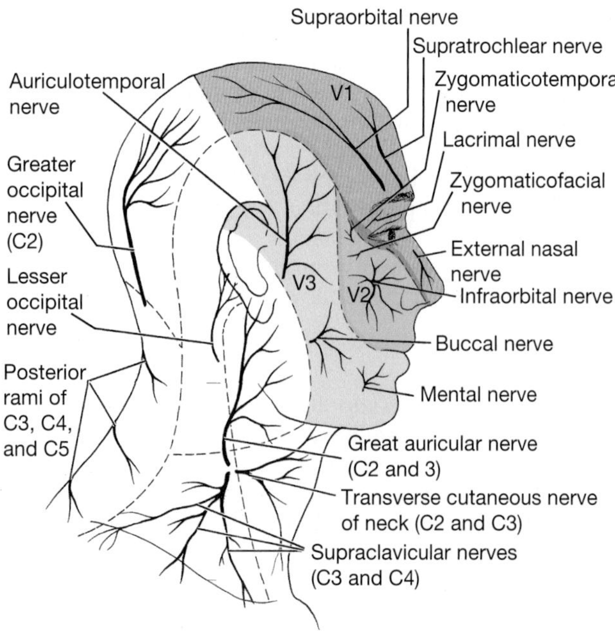

Figure 9.26 Sensory nerve supply to skin of the head and neck. Note that the skin over the angle of the jaw is supplied by the great auricular nerve (C2 and C3) and not by branches of the trigeminal nerve.

Maxillary Nerve

The maxillary nerve supplies the skin on the posterior part of the side of the nose, the lower eyelid, the cheek, the upper lip, and the lateral side of the orbital opening. Three branches of the nerve pass to the skin.

- The **infraorbital nerve** is a direct continuation of the maxillary nerve. It enters the orbit and appears on the face through the **infraorbital foramen**. It immediately divides into numerous small branches, which radiate out from the foramen and supply the skin of the lower eyelid and cheek, side of the nose, and the upper lip.

- The **zygomaticofacial nerve** passes onto the face through a small foramen on the lateral side of the zygomatic bone. It supplies the skin over the prominence of the cheek.
- The **zygomaticotemporal nerve** emerges in the temporal fossa through a small foramen on the posterior surface of the zygomatic bone. It supplies the skin over the temple.

Mandibular Nerve

The mandibular nerve supplies the skin of the lower lip, the lower part of the face, the temporal region, and part of the auricle. It then passes upward to the side of the scalp. Three branches of the nerve pass to the skin.

- The **mental nerve** emerges from the **mental foramen** of the mandible and supplies the skin of the lower lip and chin.
- The **buccal nerve** emerges from beneath the anterior border of the masseter muscle and supplies the skin over a small area of the cheek.
- The **auriculotemporal nerve** ascends from the upper border of the parotid gland between the superficial temporal vessels and the auricle. It supplies the skin of the auricle, external auditory meatus, outer surface of the tympanic membrane, and the skin of the scalp above the auricle.

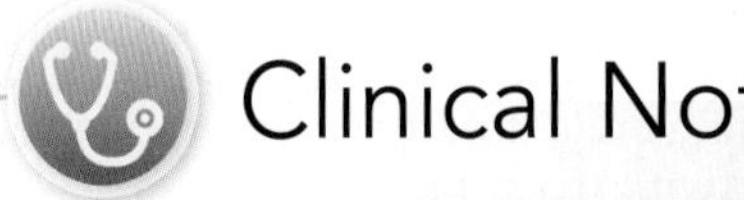

Clinical Notes

Trigeminal Neuralgia

The facial skin receives its sensory nerve supply primarily from the three divisions of the trigeminal nerve. Trigeminal neuralgia (**tic douloureux**) is a relatively common (often idiopathic) condition in which the patient experiences sudden attacks of excruciating pain in the distribution of the mandibular or maxillary division, with the ophthalmic division usually escaping. A clinician should be able to map out accurately the distribution of each of the divisions of the trigeminal nerve on a patient's face.

Arterial Supply

The face receives a rich blood supply from two main vessels, the **facial** and **superficial temporal arteries**, which are supplemented by several small arteries that accompany the sensory nerves of the face (see Fig. 9.25C).

The **facial artery** arises from the external carotid artery in the upper neck (see Head and Neck Arteries later in this chapter). It arches upward and over the submandibular salivary gland and curves around the inferior margin of the body of the mandible at the anterior border of the masseter muscle. Its **pulse can be easily felt here** (see Surface Anatomy, Masseter Muscle). It next runs upward in a tortuous course toward the angle of the mouth and is covered by the platysma and the risorius muscles. It then ascends deep to the zygomaticus muscles and the levator labii superioris muscle and runs along the side of the nose to the medial angle of the eye, where it anastomoses with the terminal branches of the **ophthalmic artery** (see Fig. 9.25C).

Branches

- The **submental artery** arises from the facial artery at the lower border of the body of the mandible. It supplies the skin of the chin and lower lip.
- The **inferior labial artery** arises near the angle of the mouth. It runs medially in the lower lip and anastomoses with its corresponding artery of the opposite side.
- The **superior labial artery** arises near the angle of the mouth. It runs medially in the upper lip and gives branches to the septum and ala of the nose.
- The **lateral nasal artery** arises from the facial artery alongside the nose. It supplies the skin on the side and dorsum of the nose.
- The **angular artery** is the terminal part of the facial artery. It runs in the narrow gap between the side of the nose and the medial canthus of the eye.

The **superficial temporal artery**, the smaller terminal branch of the external carotid artery, commences in the parotid gland. It ascends in front of the auricle to supply the scalp.

Branches

- The **transverse facial artery** arises within the parotid gland. It runs forward across the cheek just above the parotid duct and below the zygomatic arch.
- The **anterior** (**frontal**) and **posterior** (**temporal**) **branches** are the terminal branches of the superficial temporal artery. They distribute across the temporal fossa.

The **supraorbital**, **supratrochlear**, **infraorbital**, and **mental arteries** are small vessels that accompany the like-named cutaneous nerves of the face.

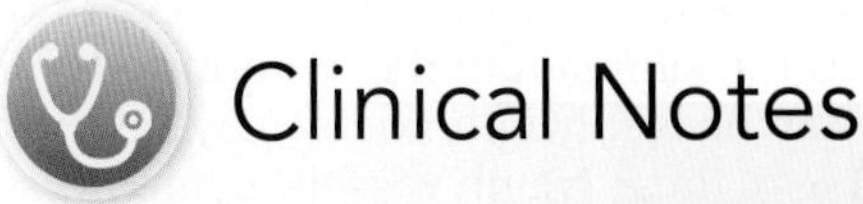

Clinical Notes

Blood Supply of the Facial Skin

The blood supply to the skin of the face is profuse, so that it is rare in plastic surgery for skin flaps to necrose in this region.

Facial Arteries and Taking the Patient's Pulse

The superficial temporal artery, as it crosses the zygomatic arch in front of the ear, and the facial artery, as it winds around the lower margin of the mandible level with the anterior border of the masseter, are commonly used by the anesthetist to take the patient's pulse.

Venous Drainage

The **facial vein** is formed at the medial angle of the eye by the union of the **supraorbital** and **supratrochlear veins** (see Fig. 9.25D). It connects to the **superior ophthalmic vein** directly through the supraorbital vein. The facial vein connects to the **cavernous sinus** by way of the superior ophthalmic vein (see Venous (Dural) Blood Sinuses). This anastomosis is of great clinical importance because it provides a pathway for the spread of infection from the face to the cavernous sinus. The facial vein descends behind the facial artery to the lower margin of the body of the mandible. It crosses superficial to the submandibular gland and is joined by the **anterior division of the retromandibular vein**. The facial vein ends by draining into the **internal jugular vein**.

The facial vein receives tributaries that correspond to the branches of the facial artery. It joins the **pterygoid venous plexus** by the deep facial vein and the cavernous sinus by the superior ophthalmic vein. The **transverse facial vein** joins the superficial temporal vein within the parotid gland.

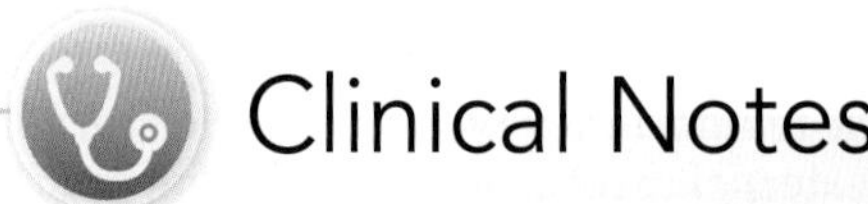

Facial Infections and Cavernous Sinus Thrombosis

The area of facial skin bounded by the nose, the eye, and the upper lip is a potentially dangerous zone in which to have an infection. For example, a boil in this region can cause thrombosis of the facial vein, with spread of organisms through the superior ophthalmic veins to the cavernous sinus. The resulting cavernous sinus thrombosis may be fatal unless adequately treated. For this reason, this area is often referred to the **danger triangle of the face**.

Lymph Drainage

Lymph from the forehead and the anterior part of the face drains into the **submandibular lymph nodes** (see Fig. 9.24B). A few buccal lymph nodes may be present along the course of these lymph vessels. Lymph vessels that end in the **parotid lymph nodes** drain the lateral part of the face, including the lateral parts of the eyelids. The central part of the lower lip and the skin of the chin drain into the **submental lymph nodes**.

Facial Muscles (Muscles of Facial Expression; Mimetic Muscles)

The facial muscles are the skeletal muscles embedded in the superficial fascia of the face (see Fig. 9.20). They should not be confused with the masticatory muscles (eg, masseter and temporalis, which are located in the face) or with the smooth arrector pili muscles that attach onto hair follicles. The facial muscles are integumentary muscles. Most arise from the bones of the skull, and all insert into the skin or other facial muscles.

The primary biological role of the facial muscles is to regulate (constrict or dilate) the facial orifices (ie, the orbits, nostrils, mouth, and ears). Because of these actions, the facial muscles must be considered as accessory muscles of vision, olfaction, respiration, feeding, speech, and hearing. Facial expression is a secondary byproduct of the fine control of the facial orifices, and facial expressions are essentially orifice displays (think about what you are doing when you smile, frown, wink, glare, etc.).

The facial muscles are subject to great individual variability in size, shape, thickness, strength, and general degree of development. Therefore, their actions are individually variable and diverse, especially in their subtler uses. All the facial muscles develop from the **second pharyngeal arch** and are supplied by the **facial nerve**.

The eyelids, nostrils, lips, and auricles guard the facial orifices. The facial muscles are organized around these structures and are summarized in Table 9.4. The auricular muscles that operate the external ear are essentially a group of vestigial muscles in humans.

Eyelid Muscles

The **orbicularis oculi** is the sphincter muscle of the eyelids, whereas the **occipitofrontalis** is a dilator muscle. The **corrugator** and **procerus** also act on the orbit. The **levator palpebrae superioris** also elevates the upper eyelid but is generally considered an extraocular muscle and is described with the orbit.

Nostril Muscles

The **nasalis** (**compressor naris**) and **depressor septi** are the sphincter muscles, and the **dilator naris** and **levator labii superioris alaeque nasi** are the dilator muscles.

Lip and Cheek Muscles

The **orbicularis oris** is the primary sphincter muscle of the lips and has a complex structure. Some of the fibers arise near the midline from the maxilla above and the mandible below. Other fibers arise from the deep surface of the skin and pass obliquely to the mucous membrane lining the inner surface of the lips. Many of the fibers are derived from the buccinator muscle.

A series of small muscles that radiate out from the lips make up the dilator muscles. Their action is to separate the lips; this movement is usually accompanied by opening of the jaws. The muscles arise from the bones and fascia around the oral aperture and converge to be inserted into the substance of the lips. Traced from the side of the nose to the angle of the mouth and then below the oral aperture, the muscles are named as follows:

- Levator labii superioris alaeque nasi (this also dilates the nostril)
- Levator labii superioris
- Zygomaticus minor (an inconstant muscle that often is part of the orbicularis oculi)

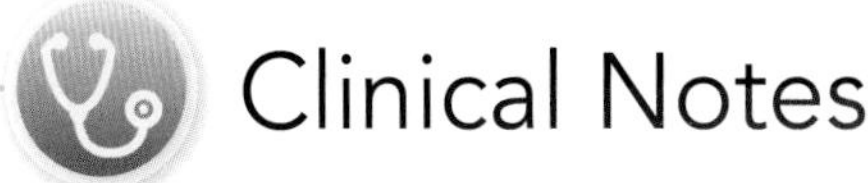

Clinical Notes

Facial Muscle Paralysis

The facial muscles are innervated by the facial nerve. Damage to the facial nerve in the internal acoustic meatus (by a tumor), in the middle ear (by infection or surgery), in the facial nerve canal (perineuritis, Bell palsy), or in the parotid gland (by a tumor) or caused by lacerations of the face causes distortion of the face. Inability to close the eyelids, drooping of the lower eyelid, and sagging of the angle of the mouth on the affected side are characteristic sequelae. The patient has an expressionless, masklike side of the face and commonly dribbles from the corner of the mouth when attempting to eat or drink. This is essentially a lower motor neuron lesion. An upper motor neuron lesion (involvement of the pyramidal tracts) will leave the upper part of the face normal because the neurons supplying this part of the face receive corticobulbar fibers from both cerebral cortices.

- Zygomaticus major
- Levator anguli oris (deep to the zygomatic muscles)
- Risorius
- Buccinator
- Depressor anguli oris
- Depressor labii inferioris
- Mentalis

The **buccinator** muscle originates from the outer surface of the alveolar margins of the maxilla and mandible opposite the molar teeth and from the pterygomandibular ligament. The muscle fibers pass forward, forming the muscle layer of the cheek, and the parotid duct pierces the muscle. At the angle of the mouth, the central fibers decussate, those from below entering the upper lip and those from above entering the lower lip; the highest and lowest fibers continue into the upper and lower lips, respectively, without intersecting. The buccinator muscle thus blends with and forms part of the orbicularis oris muscle. The decussation of the buccinator fibers causes a small indentation in the cheek of some individuals when the buccinator contracts. This appears as a "dimple" and is highly variable in form. The buccinator is a significant muscle in food processing in that it compresses the cheeks and lips against the teeth, thus positioning food for efficient chewing. The compression action also is important in producing sucking and so is critical in nursing neonates. Cheek compression is also important in producing blowing actions, such as in blowing a horn.

Facial Nerve

The facial nerve divides into its five terminal branches as it runs forward within the substance of the parotid salivary gland (see Fig. 9.25B).

- The **temporal branch** emerges from the upper border of the gland and supplies the anterior and superior auricular muscles, frontal belly of the occipitofrontalis, orbicularis oculi, and the corrugator supercilii.
- The **zygomatic branch** emerges from the anterior border of the gland and supplies the orbicularis oculi.
- The **buccal branch** emerges from the anterior border of the gland below the parotid duct and supplies the buccinator muscle and the muscles of the upper lip and nostril.
- The **mandibular branch** emerges from the anterior border of the gland and supplies the muscles of the lower lip.
- The **cervical branch** emerges from the lower border of the gland and passes forward in the neck below the mandible to supply the platysma muscle; it may cross the lower margin of the body of the mandible to supply the depressor anguli oris muscle.

The facial nerve is the nerve of the second pharyngeal arch and supplies all the muscles of facial expression. It does not supply the skin, but its branches communicate with branches of the trigeminal nerve. Proprioceptive nerve fibers of the facial muscles are believed to leave the facial nerve in these communicating branches and pass to the central nervous system via the trigeminal nerve.

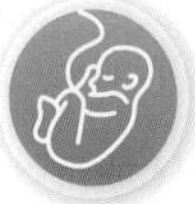

Embryology Notes

Face Development

Early in development, the face of the embryo is represented by an area bounded cranially by the neural plate, caudally by the pericardium and the mandibular process of the first pharyngeal arch, and laterally by the maxillary process of the first pharyngeal arch on each side (Fig. 9.27). A depression in the ectoderm termed the **stomodeum** is in the center of this area. The **buccopharyngeal membrane** is in the floor of the stomodeum. By week 4, the buccopharyngeal membrane breaks down so that the stomodeum communicates with the foregut.

Further development of the face depends on the coming together and fusion of several important processes, namely, the **frontonasal**, **maxillary**, and **mandibular processes**. The frontonasal process begins as a proliferation of mesenchyme

(continued)

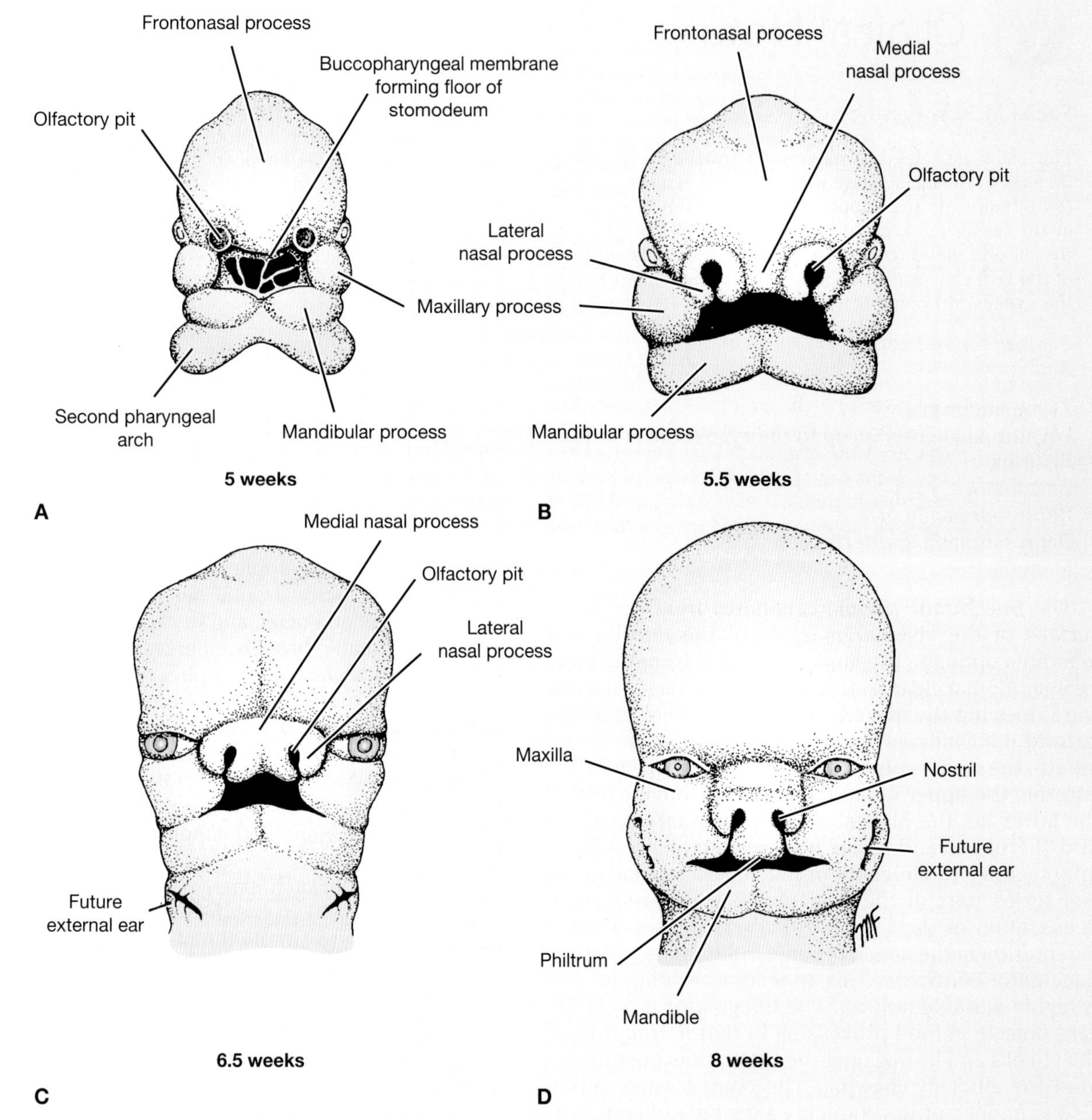

Figure 9.27 Progressive stages **(A–D)** in the development of the face.

on the ventral surface of the developing brain, and this grows toward the stomodeum. Meanwhile, the maxillary process grows out from the upper end of each first arch and passes medially, forming the lower border of the developing orbit. The mandibular processes of the first arches now approach one another in the midline below the stomodeum and fuse to form the lower jaw and lower lip.

The **olfactory pits** appear as depressions in the lower edge of the advancing frontonasal process, dividing it into paired **medial** and **lateral nasal processes**. With further development, the maxillary processes grow medially and fuse with the lateral nasal processes and with the medial nasal process. The medial nasal process forms the **philtrum** of the upper lip and the **premaxilla**. The maxillary processes extend medially, forming the upper jaw and the cheek, and finally bury the premaxilla and fuse in the midline. The various processes that ultimately form the face unite during month 2 of development.

The **upper lip** is formed by the medial growth of the maxillary processes of the first pharyngeal arch on each side. Ultimately, the maxillary processes meet in the midline and fuse with each other and with the medial nasal process. Thus, the lateral parts of the upper lip are formed from the maxillary processes and the medial part, or philtrum, from the medial nasal process, with contributions from the maxillary processes.

The **lower lip** is formed from the mandibular process of the first pharyngeal arch on each side. These processes grow medially below the stomodeum and fuse in the midline to form the entire lower lip.

Each lip separates from its respective gum as the result of the appearance of a linear thickening of ectoderm, the **labiogingival lamina**, which grows down into the underlying mesenchyme and later degenerates. A deep groove thus forms between the lips and the gums. In the midline, a short area of the labiogingival lamina remains and tethers each lip to the gum, thus forming the **frenulum**.

At first, the **mouth** has a broad opening, but later, this diminishes in extent because of fusion of the lips at the lateral angles.

Sensory Nerve Supply to the Skin of the Developing Face

The area of skin overlying the frontonasal process and its derivatives receives its sensory nerve supply from the ophthalmic division of the trigeminal nerve, whereas the maxillary division of the trigeminal nerve supplies the area of skin overlying the maxillary process. The mandibular division of the trigeminal nerve supplies the area of skin overlying the mandibular process.

Muscles of the Developing Face (Muscles of Facial Expression)

The muscles of the face are derived from the mesenchyme of the second pharyngeal arch. The nerve supply of these muscles is the nerve of the second pharyngeal arch—namely, CN VII.

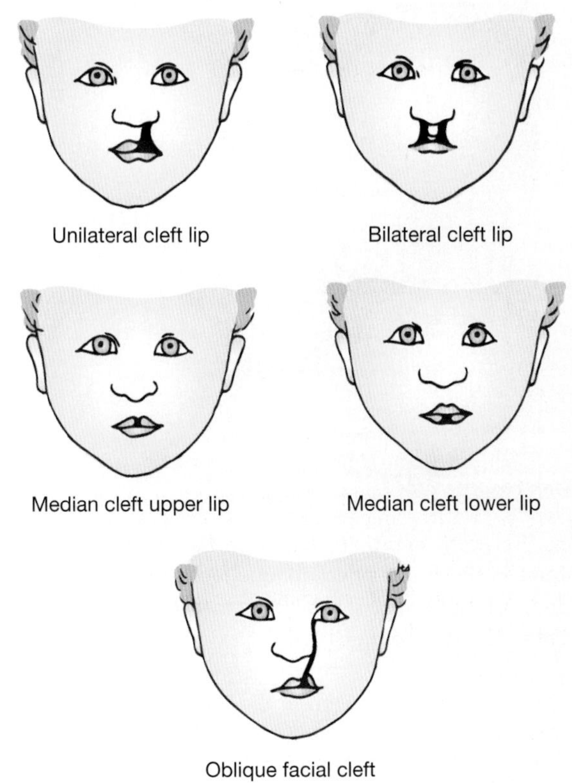

Figure 9.28 Various forms of cleft lip.

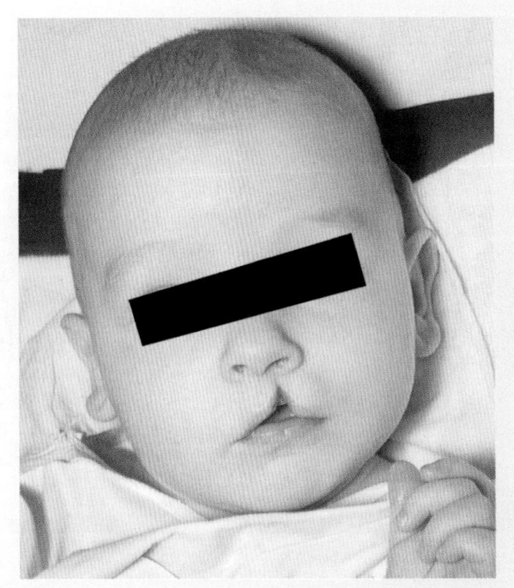

Figure 9.29 Unilateral cleft upper lip. (Courtesy of R. Chase.)

Cleft Upper Lip

Cleft upper lip may be confined to the lip or may be associated with a cleft palate. The anomaly is usually **unilateral cleft lip** and is caused by a failure of the maxillary process to fuse with the medial nasal process (Figs. 9.28 and 9.29). **Bilateral cleft lip** is caused by a failure of both maxillary processes to fuse with the medial nasal process, which then remains as a central flap of tissue (Figs. 9.30 and 9.31; see also Fig. 9.28). **Median cleft upper lip** is very rare and is caused by the failure of the rounded swellings of the medial nasal process to fuse in the midline (see Figs. 9.28 and 9.31B).

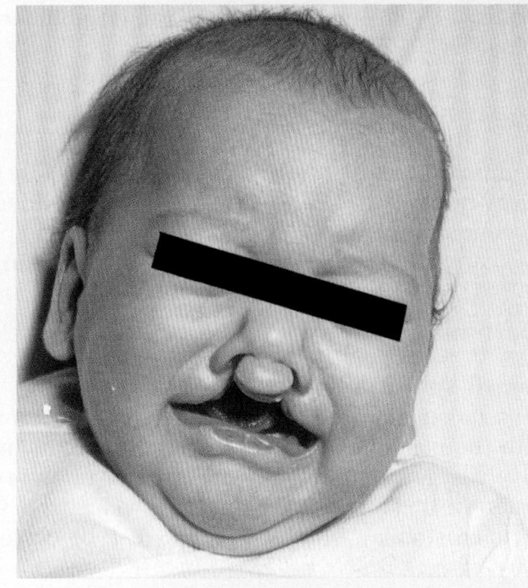

Figure 9.30 Bilateral cleft upper lip and palate. (Courtesy of R. Chase.)

(continued)

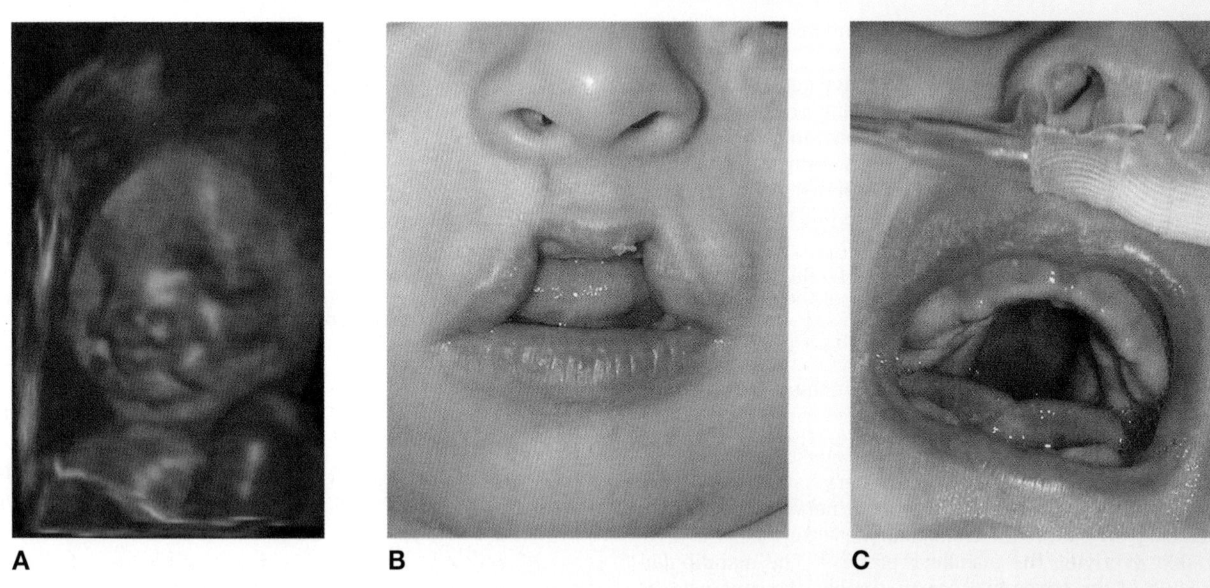

Figure 9.31 Cleft lip and palate. **A.** Three-dimensional ultrasound reveals bilateral cleft lip at 22 weeks of gestation. (Courtesy of Dr. B. Benacerraf.) **B.** An infant with median cleft upper lip. **C.** An infant with cleft palate. (**B** and **C**, from Sadler, T. W., *Langman's Medical Embryology*, 14th ed. Wolters Kluwer, 2019.)

Oblique Facial Cleft

Oblique facial cleft is a rare condition in which the cleft lip on one side extends to the medial margin of the orbit (Fig. 9.32; see also Fig. 9.28). This is caused by the failure of the maxillary process to fuse with the lateral and medial nasal processes.

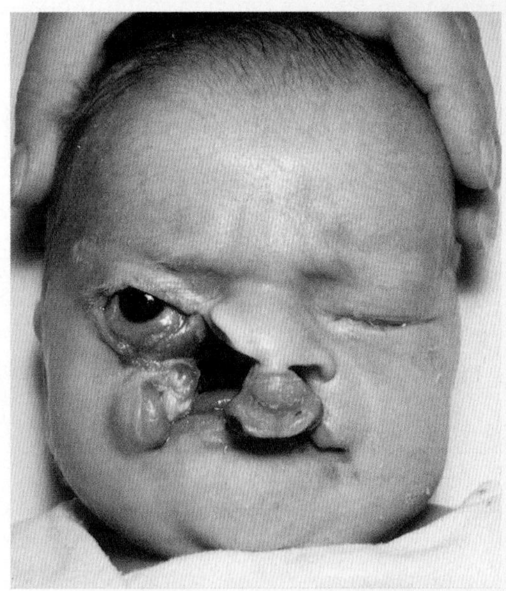

Figure 9.32 Right-sided oblique facial cleft and left-sided cleft upper lip. There also is total bilateral cleft palate. (Courtesy of R. Chase.)

Cleft Lower Lip

Cleft lower lip is a rare condition. The cleft is exactly central and is caused by incomplete fusion of the mandibular processes (see Fig. 9.28).

Treatment of Isolated Cleft Lip

The condition of isolated cleft lip usually is treated by plastic surgery no later than 2 months after birth, provided the infant's condition permits. The surgeon strives to approximate the vermilion border and to form a normal-looking lip.

Macrostomia and Microstomia

The normal size of the mouth shows considerable individual variation. Rarely, incomplete fusion of the maxillary with the mandibular processes occurs, producing an excessively large mouth (macrostomia). Very rarely, excessive fusion of these processes occurs, producing a small mouth (microstomia). These conditions can be corrected surgically.

INTERIOR OF THE SKULL

The skeletal features of the interior of the skull are described earlier in this chapter. This section reviews the meninges and the brain.

Meninges

Three membranes (**meninges**) surround and protect the brain in the skull. From superficial to deep, these are the **dura mater**, **arachnoid mater**, and **pia mater**. They are mostly continuous with the spinal meninges that surround the spinal cord in the vertebral column (see Chapter 2).

Dura Mater

The dura mater is conventionally described as two layers: endosteal and meningeal layers (see Fig. 9.4). These are closely united except along certain lines, where they separate to form venous sinuses.

The **endosteal layer** is the periosteum (endosteum) covering the inner surface of the skull bones. It does **not** extend through the foramen magnum to become continuous with the dura mater of the spinal cord. It does become continuous with the periosteum on the outside of the skull bones around the margins of all the foramina in the skull. It is also continuous with the sutural ligaments at the sutures. It is most strongly adherent to the bones over the base of the skull.

The **meningeal layer** is the dura mater proper. It is a dense, strong, fibrous membrane covering the brain and is continuous through the foramen magnum with the dura mater of the spinal cord. It provides tubular sheaths for the CNs as they pass through the foramina in the skull. Outside the skull, the sheaths fuse with the epineurium of the nerves.

Four septa (falx cerebri, falx cerebelli, tentorium cerebelli, and diaphragma sellae) extend inward from the meningeal layer and divide the cranial cavity into freely communicating spaces lodging major subdivisions of the brain. The septa stabilize the position of the brain by restricting its rotatory displacement during movement of the head.

The **falx cerebri** is a large, sickle-shaped fold (*falx* is Latin for "sickle") of dura mater that lies in the midline between the two cerebral hemispheres (Figs. 9.33 to 9.35; see also Fig. 9.4). Its narrow anterior end attaches to the internal frontal crest and the crista galli. Its broad posterior part blends in the midline with the upper surface of the tentorium cerebelli. The superior sagittal sinus runs in its upper fixed margin, the inferior sagittal sinus runs in its lower concave free margin, and the straight sinus runs along its attachment to the tentorium cerebelli.

The **falx cerebelli** is a small, midline, sickle-shaped fold of dura mater that attaches to the internal occipital crest and projects forward between the two cerebellar hemispheres. Its posterior fixed margin contains the occipital sinus.

The **tentorium cerebelli** is a crescent-shaped fold of dura mater that roofs over the posterior cranial fossa (*tentori* is Latin for "a tent") (Figs. 9.36 and 9.37; see also Figs. 9.33 to 9.35). It covers the upper surface of the cerebellum and supports the occipital lobes of the cerebral hemispheres. An anterior gap, the **tentorial notch**, allows for passage of the midbrain, thus producing an inner free border and an outer attached or fixed border. The **fixed border** attaches to the posterior clinoid processes, the superior borders of the petrous bones, and the margins of the grooves for the transverse sinuses on the occipital bone. The **free border** runs forward at its two ends, crosses the attached border, and fixes to the anterior clinoid process on each side. At the point where the two borders cross, CNs III and IV pass forward to enter the lateral wall of the cavernous sinus (Fig. 9.38).

Close to the apex of the petrous part of the temporal bone, the lower layer of the tentorium pouches forward beneath the superior petrosal sinus to form a recess for the trigeminal nerve and the trigeminal ganglion (see Fig. 9.37).

The falx cerebri and the falx cerebelli attach to the upper and lower surfaces of the tentorium, respectively. The straight sinus runs along the tentorial attachment to the falx cerebri, the superior petrosal sinus runs along its attachment to the petrous bone, and the transverse sinus passes along its attachment to the occipital bone (see Figs. 9.34 to 9.36).

The **diaphragma sellae** is a small circular fold of dura mater that forms the roof for the sella turcica (Fig. 9.39; see also Figs. 9.34, 9.36, and 9.38). A small opening in its center allows passage of the stalk of the pituitary gland.

Dural Nerve Supply

Branches of the trigeminal, vagus, and first three cervical nerves and branches from the sympathetic system pass to the dura. The dura has a rich sensory supply and is very sensitive to stretching, which produces the sensation of headache. Stimulation of the sensory endings of the trigeminal nerve **above the level of the tentorium cerebelli** produces referred pain to an area of skin on the same side of the head. Stimulation of the dural endings **below the level of the tentorium** produces referred pain to the back of the neck and back of the scalp along the distribution of the greater occipital nerve.

Dural Arterial Supply

Numerous arteries from the internal carotid, maxillary, ascending pharyngeal, occipital, and vertebral arteries supply the dura mater. From a clinical standpoint, the most important is the middle meningeal artery, which is commonly damaged in head injuries.

The **middle meningeal artery** arises from the maxillary artery in the infratemporal fossa. It enters the cranial cavity through the foramen spinosum to lie between the meningeal and endosteal layers of dura. It then runs forward and laterally in a groove on the upper surface of the squamous part of the temporal bone (see Fig. 9.10). The **anterior (frontal) branch** deeply grooves or tunnels the anteroinferior angle of the parietal bone, and its course corresponds roughly to the line of the underlying precentral gyrus of the brain. The **posterior**

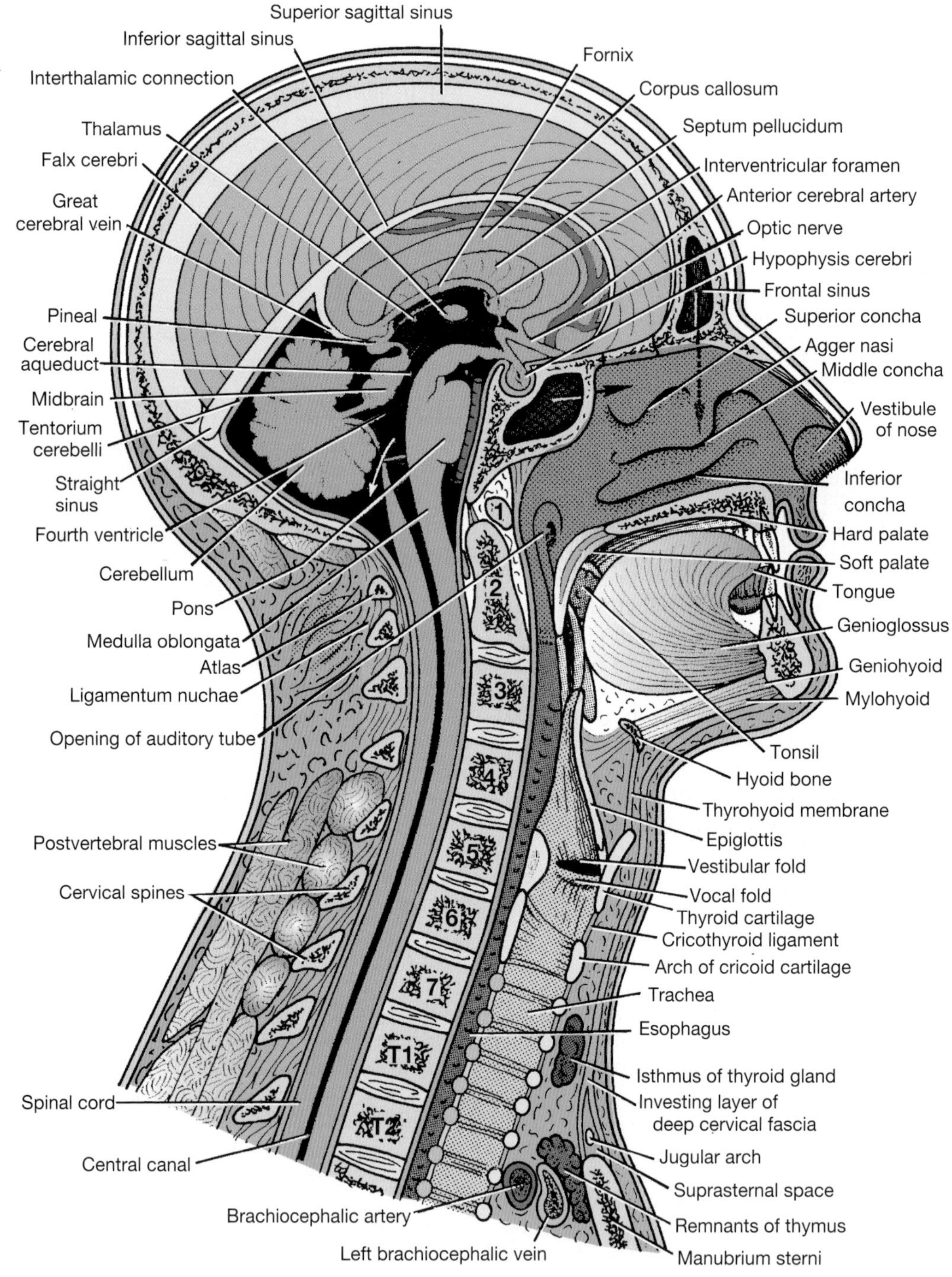

Figure 9.33 Sagittal section of the head and neck.

(parietal) branch curves backward and supplies the posterior part of the dura mater.

Dural Venous Drainage

The meningeal veins lie in the endosteal layer of dura. The **middle meningeal vein** follows the branches of the middle meningeal artery and drains into the pterygoid venous plexus or the sphenoparietal sinus. The veins lie lateral to the arteries.

Arachnoid Mater

The arachnoid mater is a delicate, impermeable membrane covering the brain and lying between the pia mater internally and the dura mater externally (see Fig. 9.4). It intimately adheres to the deep side of the dura and is separated from the pia mater by the **subarachnoid space**, which is filled with **cerebrospinal fluid (CSF)**.

The arachnoid bridges over the sulci on the surface of the brain, and in certain situations, the arachnoid

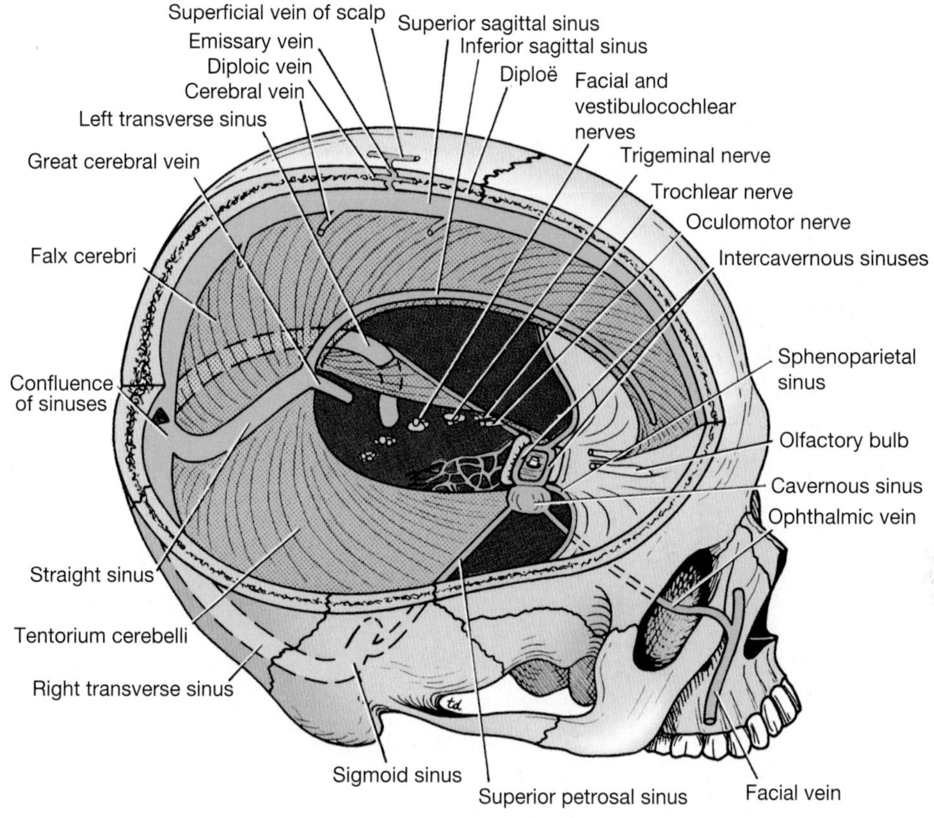

Figure 9.34 Interior of the skull showing the dura mater and its contained venous sinuses. Note the connections of the veins of the scalp and the facial vein with the venous sinuses.

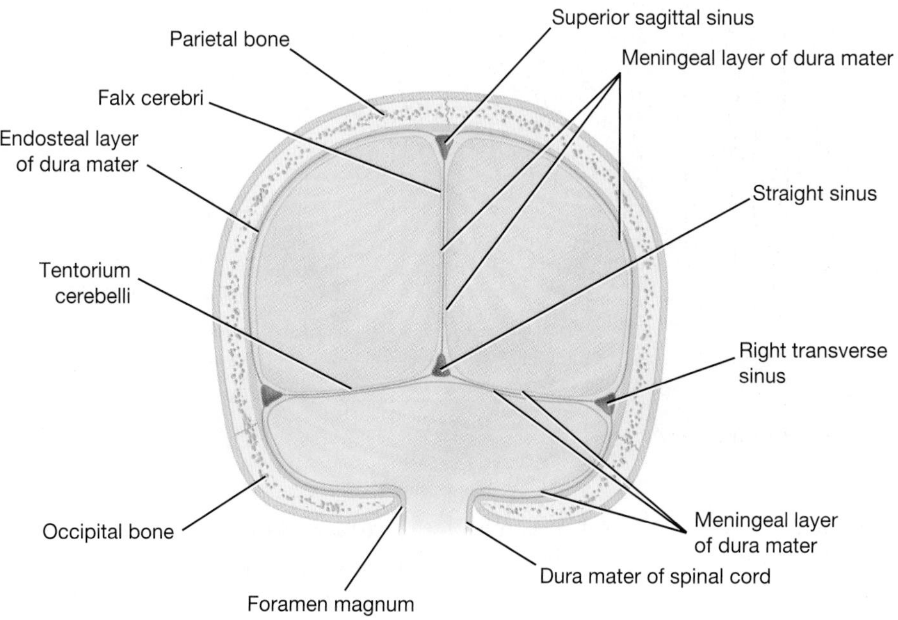

Figure 9.35 Falx cerebri and tentorium cerebelli. Note the separations between the endosteal and meningeal layers of the dura mater that create dural blood sinuses.

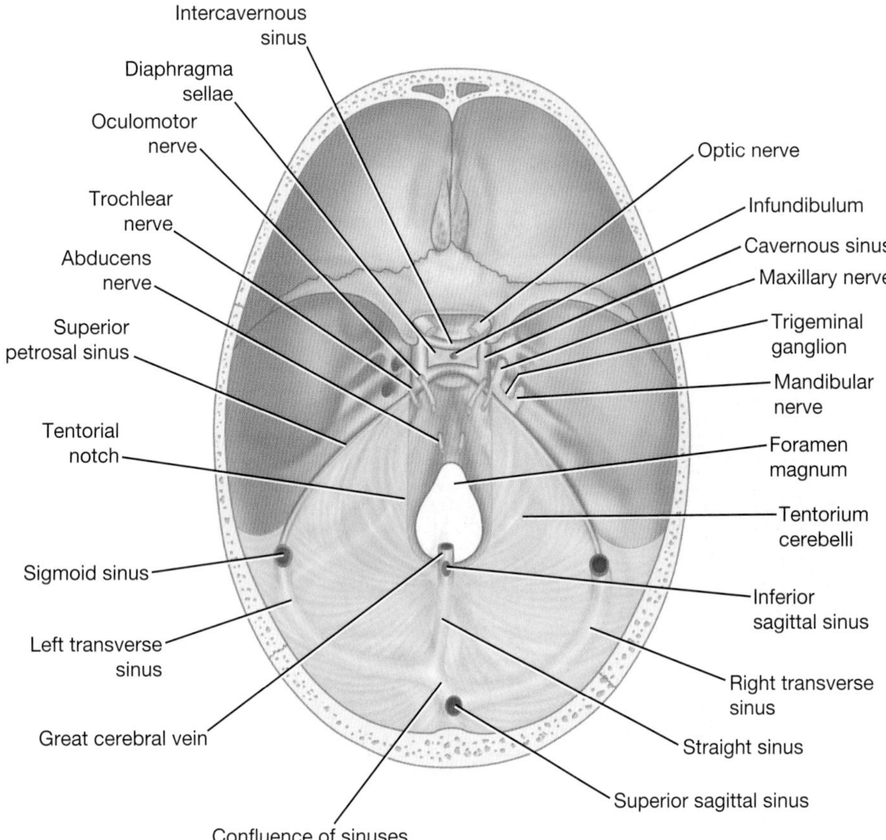

Figure 9.36 Interior base of the skull from above showing the diaphragma sellae and tentorium cerebelli. Note the positions of the dural sinuses and cranial nerves.

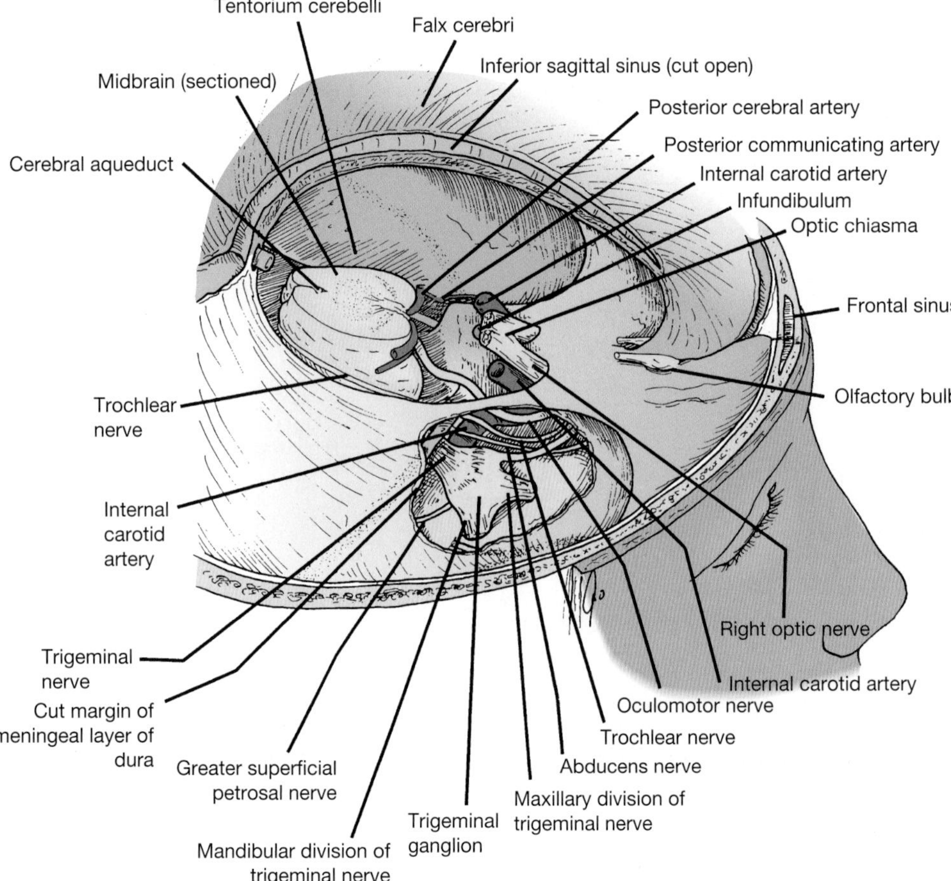

Figure 9.37 Oblique view of the interior of the skull showing the falx cerebri, tentorium cerebelli, brainstem, and trigeminal ganglion.

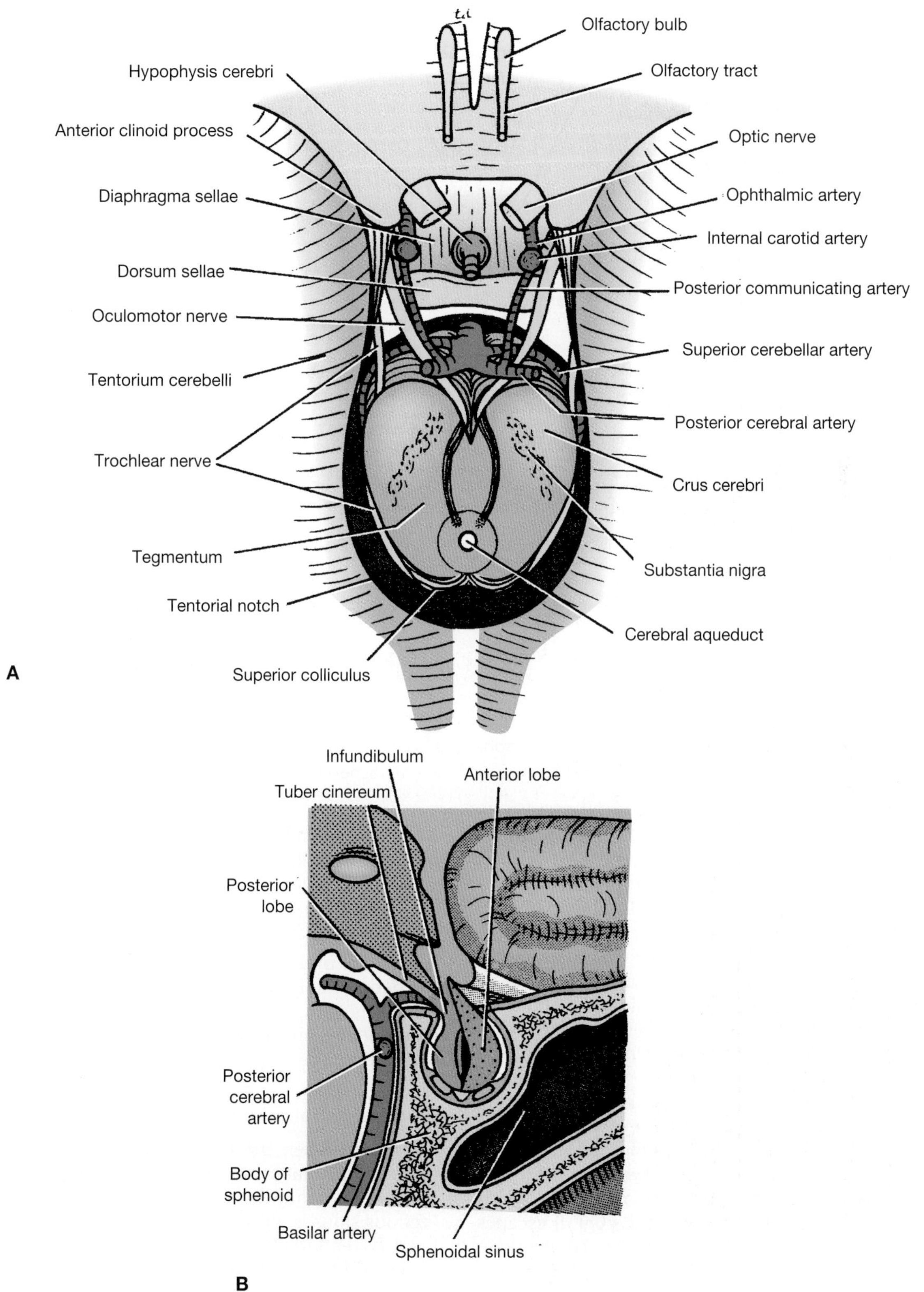

Figure 9.38 **A.** Superior view of the sella turcica. The forebrain has been removed, leaving the midbrain, diaphragma sellae, hypophysis cerebri, and internal carotid arteries in position. **B.** Sagittal section through the sella turcica showing the hypophysis cerebri.

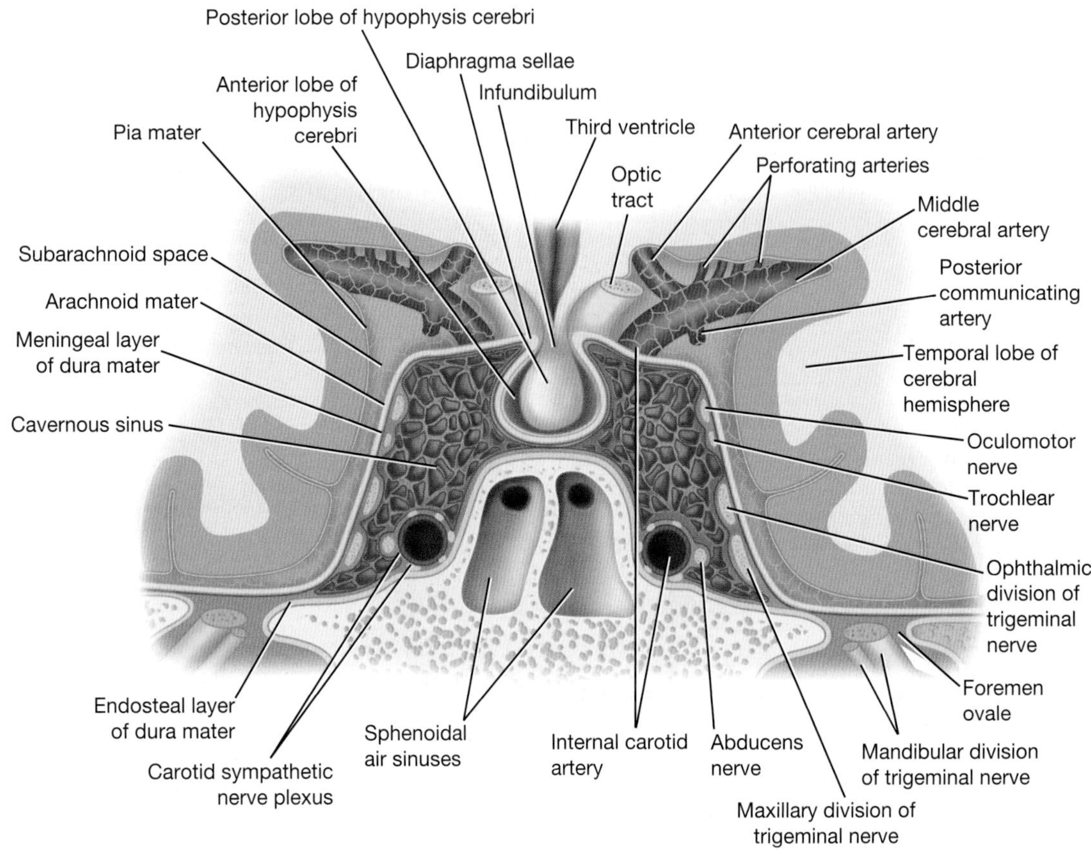

Figure 9.39 Coronal section through the body of the sphenoid bone showing the hypophysis cerebri and the cavernous sinuses. Note the positions of the internal carotid arteries and the cranial nerves.

and pia are widely separated to form the **subarachnoid cisternae**.

In certain areas, the arachnoid projects into the venous sinuses to form **arachnoid villi**. The arachnoid villi are most numerous along the superior sagittal sinus. Aggregations of arachnoid villi are referred to as **arachnoid granulations** (see Fig. 9.4). Arachnoid villi serve as sites where the CSF diffuses into the bloodstream.

The arachnoid fuses with the epineurium of the CNs at their point of exit from the skull. In the case of the optic nerve, the arachnoid forms a sheath for the nerve that extends into the orbital cavity through the optic canal and fuses with the sclera of the eyeball (see Optic Nerve [CN I]). Thus, the subarachnoid space extends around the optic nerve as far as the eyeball.

The **choroid plexuses** within the lateral, third, and fourth ventricles of the brain produce the CSF. It escapes from the ventricular system of the brain through the three foramina in the roof of the fourth ventricle and so enters the subarachnoid space. It now circulates both upward over the surfaces of the cerebral hemispheres and downward around the spinal cord. The spinal subarachnoid space extends down as far as the S2 vertebra (see Chapter 2). Eventually, the fluid enters the bloodstream by passing into the arachnoid villi and diffusing through their walls.

In addition to removing waste products associated with neuronal activity, CSF provides a fluid medium in which the brain floats. This mechanism effectively protects the brain from trauma.

Pia Mater

The pia mater is a vascular membrane that closely invests the brain, covering the gyri and descending into the deepest sulci (see Fig. 9.4). It extends over the CNs and fuses with their epineurium. The cerebral arteries entering the substance of the brain carry a sheath of pia with them.

Venous (Dural) Blood Sinuses

As noted earlier, the endosteal and meningeal layers of the dura mater are inseparable, except in certain places where they do separate to form venous channels (venous sinuses; dural sinuses) (see Fig. 9.4). These are lined by endothelium; their walls are thick and composed of fibrous tissue; they have no muscular tissue and **no valves**. They receive tributaries from the brain, the diploë of the skull, the orbit, and the internal ear.

All blood from the brain drains into the dural sinuses and then out of the cranium via true veins. Most of the blood from the brain drains to the **internal jugular veins**.

The **superior sagittal sinus** lies in the upper fixed border of the falx cerebri (see Figs. 9.33 and 9.34). It runs backward and becomes continuous with the confluence of sinuses and the right transverse sinus. The sinus communicates on each side with the **venous lacunae**. Numerous arachnoid villi and granulations project into the lacunae (see Fig. 9.4). The superior sagittal sinus receives the superior cerebral veins.

The **inferior sagittal sinus** lies in the free lower margin of the falx cerebri (see Figs. 9.4, 9.33, and 9.34). It runs backward and joins the great cerebral vein to form the straight sinus. It receives cerebral veins from the medial surface of the cerebral hemispheres.

The **straight sinus** lies at the junction of the falx cerebri with the tentorium cerebelli (see Figs. 9.33 to 9.36). The union of the inferior sagittal sinus with the great cerebral vein forms the straight sinus, which drains into the confluence of sinuses and left transverse sinus.

The **confluence of sinuses** overlies the internal occipital protuberance (see Figs. 9.34 to 9.36). This is a point of convergence where the superior sagittal and straight sinuses join together. The confluence gives rise to the transverse sinuses.

The **right transverse sinus** originates from the confluence of sinuses as a continuation of the superior sagittal sinus; the **left transverse sinus** comes off the confluence and is usually a continuation of the straight sinus (see Figs. 9.34 and 9.36). Each sinus lies in the lateral attached margin of the tentorium cerebelli, and they end on each side by becoming the sigmoid sinus.

The **sigmoid sinuses** are direct continuations of the transverse sinuses. Each sinus turns downward behind the mastoid antrum of the temporal bone and then leaves the skull through the jugular foramen to become the **internal jugular vein**.

The **occipital sinus** lies in the attached margin of the falx cerebelli. It communicates with the vertebral veins through the foramen magnum and with the transverse sinuses.

Each **cavernous sinus** lies on the lateral side of the body of the sphenoid bone (see Figs. 9.34, 9.36, and 9.39). Anteriorly, the sinus receives the superior ophthalmic vein and the central vein of the retina. The sinus drains posteriorly into the transverse sinus through the **superior petrosal sinus** and into the sigmoid sinus through the **inferior petrosal sinus. Intercavernous sinuses** connect the two cavernous sinuses through the sella turcica. The cavernous sinus also drains into the **basilar sinus plexus**, which drains through the foramen magnum and connects to the vertebral venous plexuses. Further, the cavernous sinus has several emissary vein connections through the floor of the middle cranial fossa into the pterygoid and pharyngeal venous plexuses in the infratemporal fossa.

Important Structures Associated with the Cavernous Sinuses

- The internal carotid artery and the abducens nerve (CN VI), which travel through it.
- In the lateral wall, CNs III and IV and the ophthalmic and maxillary divisions of CN V.
- The pituitary gland, which lies medially in the sella turcica.
- The veins of the face, which are connected with the cavernous sinus via the facial vein and superior ophthalmic vein, are an important route for the spread of infection from the face.
- The superior and inferior petrosal sinuses, which run along the upper and lower borders of the petrous part of the temporal bone.

Pituitary Gland (Hypophysis Cerebri)

The pituitary gland is a small, oval organ attached to the undersurface of the brain by the **infundibulum** (see Figs. 9.33, 9.36, 9.38, and 9.39). The gland is well protected by virtue of its location in the sella turcica of the sphenoid bone. The pituitary gland is vital to life and is fully described later in this chapter.

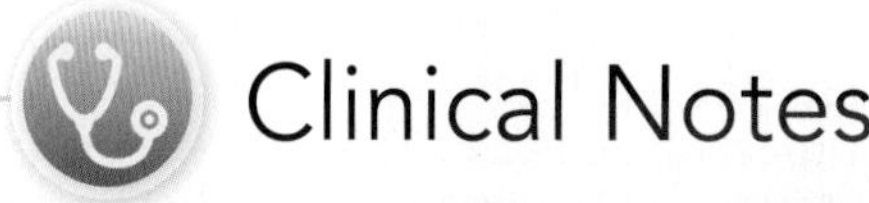

Clinical Notes

Intracranial Hemorrhage

Intracranial hemorrhage may result from trauma or cerebral vascular lesions. Four varieties are considered here: extradural, subdural, subarachnoid, and cerebral.

Extradural (epidural) hemorrhage results from injuries to the meningeal arteries or veins (Fig. 9.40). The most common artery to be damaged is the **anterior division of the middle meningeal artery**. A comparatively minor blow to the side of the head, resulting in fracture of the skull in the region of the **pterion** (anteroinferior portion of the parietal bone), may sever the artery. The arterial or venous injury is especially liable to occur if the vessels enter a bony canal in this region. Bleeding occurs and dissects the dura from the internal surface of the skull. Intracranial pressure rises, and the enlarging blood clot exerts local pressure on the underlying motor area in the precentral gyrus. Blood may also pass outward through the fracture line to form a soft swelling under the temporalis muscle. The torn artery or vein must be ligated or plugged to stop the hemorrhage.

Subdural hemorrhage results from tearing of the **superior cerebral veins** at their point of entrance into the superior sagittal sinus (see Fig. 9.40). The cause is usually a blow on the front or the back of the head, causing excessive anteroposterior displacement of the brain within the skull.

This condition, which is much more common than middle meningeal hemorrhage, can be produced by a sudden minor blow. Once the vein is torn, blood under low pressure begins to separate the dura–arachnoid cell layers and accumulates in the potential space between the dura and the arachnoid. In about half the cases, the condition is bilateral.

Acute and chronic forms of the clinical condition occur, depending on the speed of accumulation of fluid. For example, if the patient starts to vomit, the venous pressure rises as a result of a rise in the intrathoracic pressure. Under these circumstances, the subdural blood clot increases

(continued)

rapidly in size and produces acute symptoms. In the chronic form, over a course of several months, the small blood clot attracts fluid by osmosis so that a hemorrhagic cyst is formed, which gradually expands and produces pressure symptoms. In both forms, the blood clot must be removed through burr holes in the skull.

Subarachnoid hemorrhage results from leakage or rupture of a congenital aneurysm on the **cerebral arterial circle** (of Willis) or, less commonly, from an angioma. The symptoms, which are sudden in onset, include severe headache, stiffness of the neck, and loss of consciousness. The diagnosis is established by withdrawing heavily blood-stained cerebrospinal fluid through a lumbar puncture (see Chapter 2).

Rupture of the thin-walled lenticulostriate artery, a branch of the middle cerebral artery, generally causes **cerebral hemorrhage**. The hemorrhage involves the vital corticobulbar and corticospinal fibers in the internal capsule and produces hemiplegia on the opposite side of the body. The patient immediately loses consciousness, and the paralysis is evident when consciousness is regained.

Intracranial Hemorrhage in the Infant

Intracranial hemorrhage in the infant may occur during birth and may result from excessive molding of the head. Bleeding may occur from the cerebral veins or the venous sinuses. Excessive anteroposterior compression of the head often tears the anterior attachment of the falx cerebri from the tentorium cerebelli. Bleeding then takes place from the great cerebral veins, the straight sinus, or the inferior sagittal sinus.

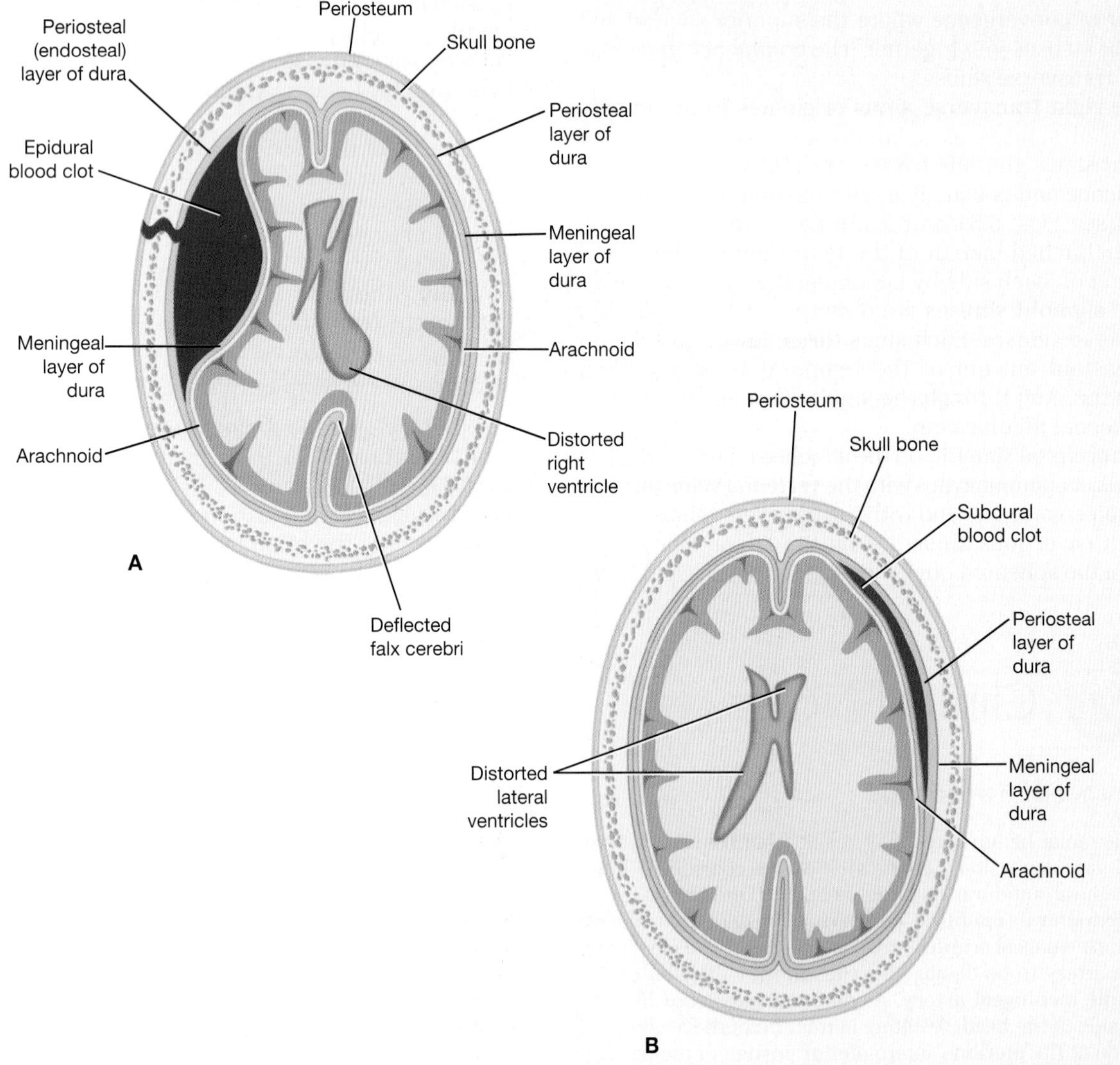

Figure 9.40 Diagrammatic representations of epidural and subdural hemorrhages. **A.** Epidural hemorrhage from the middle meningeal artery on the left side. The hematoma is lens shaped and occupies the space between the endosteal layer of dura (periosteum of the skull) and the meningeal layer of dura (true dura). **B.** Subdural hemorrhage from the cerebral veins at the site of entrance into the venous sinus on the right side. The hematoma is crescent shaped and occupies the space between the meningeal layer of dura and the arachnoid.

Brain

The brain is that part of the central nervous system that lies inside the cranial cavity (see Nervous System in Chapter 1). It is continuous with the spinal cord through the foramen magnum. Consult a textbook of neurobiology for a detailed description of the structure of the brain. The following account describes only the major parts of the brain.

Major Parts of the Brain		Cavities of the Brain
Forebrain	Cerebrum	Right and left lateral ventricles
	Diencephalon	Third ventricle
Midbrain		Cerebral aqueduct
Hindbrain	Pons Medulla oblongata Cerebellum	Fourth ventricle and central canal

Cerebrum

The cerebrum is the largest part of the brain and consists of two **cerebral hemispheres** connected by a mass of white matter called the **corpus callosum** (see Fig. 9.33). Each hemisphere extends from the frontal to the occipital bones and lies in the anterior and middle cranial fossae and, posteriorly, above the tentorium cerebelli. The hemispheres are separated by a deep cleft, the **longitudinal fissure**, into which projects the **falx cerebri**.

The surface layer of each hemisphere is called the **cortex** and is composed of gray matter (see Fig. 9.4). The cerebral cortex is thrown into folds, or **gyri**, separated by fissures, or **sulci**. This architecture greatly increases the surface area of the cortex. Several of the large sulci conveniently subdivide the surface of each hemisphere into lobes. The lobes are named for the cranial bones that overlie them (Fig. 9.41).

The **frontal lobe** is situated in front of the **central sulcus** and above the **lateral sulcus**. The **parietal lobe** is situated behind the central sulcus and above the lateral sulcus.

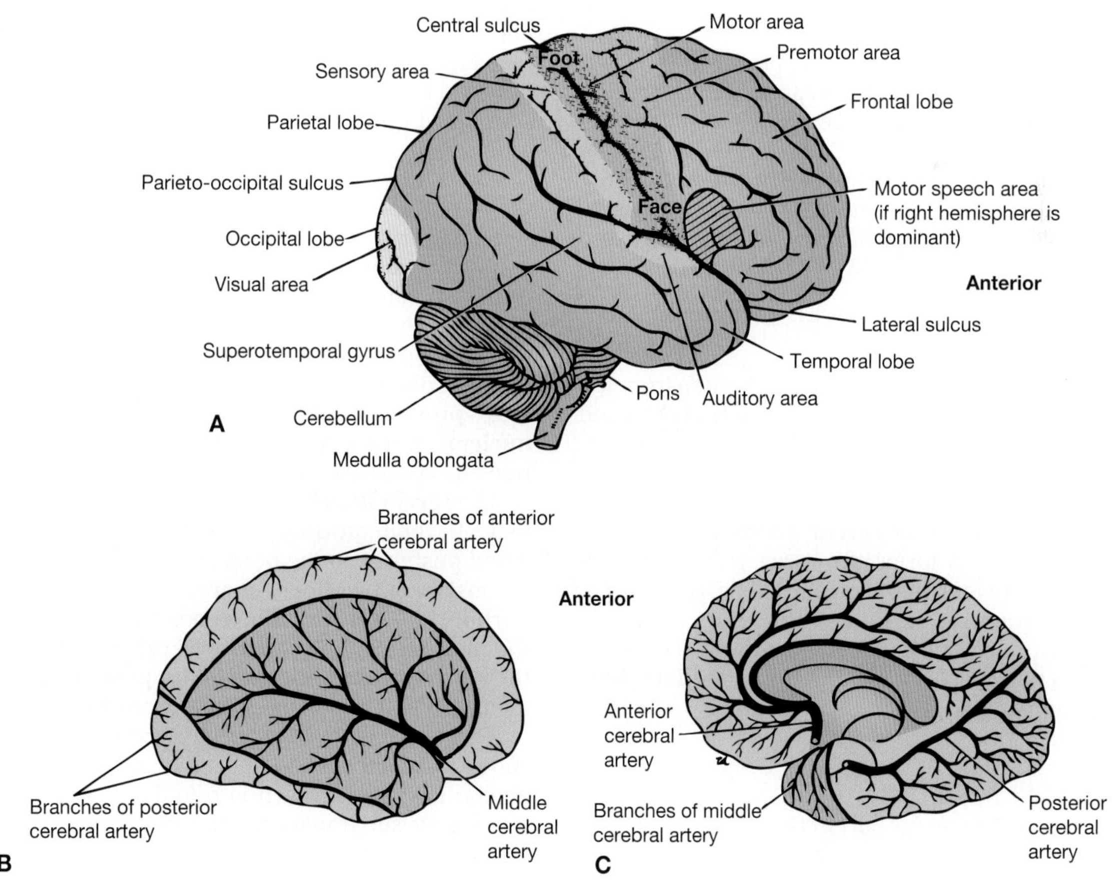

Figure 9.41 **A.** Right side of the brain showing some important localized areas of cerebral function. Note that the motor speech area is most commonly located in the left rather than the right cerebral hemisphere. **B.** Lateral surface of the cerebral hemisphere showing areas supplied by the cerebral arteries. In this and the next figure, the anterior cerebral artery supplies areas colored in *blue*, the middle cerebral artery those colored in *red*, and the posterior cerebral artery those colored in *green*. **C.** Medial surface of the cerebral hemisphere showing the areas supplied by the cerebral arteries.

The **occipital lobe** lies below the **parietooccipital sulcus**. The **temporal lobe** is situated below the lateral sulcus.

The **precentral gyrus** lies immediately anterior to the central sulcus and is known as the **motor area**. The large motor nerve cells in this area control voluntary movements on the opposite side of the body. Most nerve fibers cross over to the opposite side in the medulla oblongata as they descend to the spinal cord. The body is represented in an inverted position in the motor area, with the nerve cells controlling the movements of the feet located in the upper part and those controlling the movements of the face and hands in the lower part.

The **postcentral gyrus** lies immediately posterior to the central sulcus and is known as the **sensory area**. The small nerve cells in this area receive and interpret sensations of pain, temperature, touch, and pressure from the opposite side of the body.

The **superior temporal gyrus** lies immediately below the lateral sulcus. The middle of this gyrus is concerned with the reception and interpretation of sound and is known as the **auditory area**.

The **Broca area**, or the **motor speech area**, lies just above the lateral sulcus. It controls the movements employed in speech. It is dominant in the left hemisphere in right-handed persons and in the right hemisphere in left-handed persons.

The **visual area** is situated on the posterior pole and medial aspect of the cerebral hemisphere in the region of the **calcarine sulcus**. It is the receiving area for visual impressions.

The **lateral ventricle** is the cavity present within each cerebral hemisphere. The lateral ventricles communicate with the third ventricle through the **interventricular foramina** (see Fig. 9.33).

Diencephalon

The diencephalon is almost completely hidden from the surface of the brain. It consists of a dorsal **thalamus** and a ventral **hypothalamus** (see Fig. 9.33). The thalamus is a large mass of gray matter that lies on either side of the **third ventricle**. It is the great relay station on the afferent sensory pathway to the cerebral cortex.

The hypothalamus forms the lower part of the lateral wall and floor of the third ventricle. The following structures are found in the floor of the third ventricle in anteroposterior sequence: the **optic chiasm** (Fig. 9.42), **tuber cinereum** and **infundibulum**, **mammillary bodies**, and the **posterior perforated substance**.

Midbrain

The midbrain is the narrow part of the brain that passes through the tentorial notch and connects the forebrain to the hindbrain (see Fig. 9.33).

The midbrain comprises two lateral halves called the **cerebral peduncles**. Each peduncle is divided into an anterior part, the **crus cerebri**, and a posterior part, the **tegmentum**, by a pigmented band of gray matter, the **substantia nigra** (see Fig. 9.38A). The narrow cavity of the midbrain is the **cerebral aqueduct**, which connects the third and fourth ventricles. The **tectum** is the part of the midbrain posterior to the cerebral aqueduct; it has four small surface swellings, namely, the two **superior** and two **inferior colliculi**. The colliculi are deeply placed between the cerebellum and the cerebral hemispheres.

The **pineal body** is a small glandular structure that lies between the superior colliculi (see Fig. 9.33). It is attached by a stalk to the region of the posterior wall of the third ventricle. The pineal commonly calcifies in middle age, and thus, it can be visualized on radiographs.

Hindbrain

The **pons** is situated on the anterior surface of the cerebellum below the midbrain and above the medulla oblongata (see Fig. 9.33). It is composed mainly of nerve fibers, which connect the two halves of the cerebellum. It also contains ascending and descending fibers connecting the forebrain, the midbrain, and the spinal cord. Some of the nerve cells within the pons serve as relay stations, whereas others form CN nuclei.

The **medulla oblongata** is conical in shape and connects the pons above to the spinal cord below. A **median fissure** is present on the anterior surface of the medulla, and on each side of this is a swelling called the **pyramid** (see Fig. 9.42). The pyramids are composed of bundles of nerve fibers that originate in large nerve cells in the precentral gyrus of the cerebral cortex. The pyramids taper below; here, most of the descending fibers cross over to the opposite side, forming the **decussation of the pyramids**.

Posterior to the pyramids are the **olives**, which are oval elevations produced by the underlying **olivary nuclei**. Behind the olives are the **inferior cerebellar peduncles**, which connect the medulla to the cerebellum.

On the posterior surface of the inferior part of the medulla oblongata are the **gracile** and **cuneate tubercles**, produced by the medially placed underlying **nucleus gracilis** and the laterally placed underlying **nucleus cuneatus**.

The **cerebellum** lies within the posterior cranial fossa beneath the tentorium cerebelli (see Fig. 9.33). It is situated posterior to the pons and the medulla oblongata. It consists of two **hemispheres** connected by a median portion, the **vermis**. The cerebellum is connected to the midbrain by the **superior cerebellar peduncles**, to the pons by the **middle cerebellar peduncles**, and to the medulla by the **inferior cerebellar peduncles**.

The surface layer of each cerebellar hemisphere, called the **cortex**, is composed of gray matter. The cerebellar cortex is thrown into folds, or **folia**, separated by closely set **transverse fissures**. Certain masses of gray matter are found in the interior of the cerebellum, embedded in the white matter; the largest of these is known as the **dentate nucleus**.

The cerebellum plays an important role in the control of muscle tone and the coordination of muscle movement on the same side of the body.

The cavity of the hindbrain is the **fourth ventricle**. This is bounded in front by the pons and the medulla

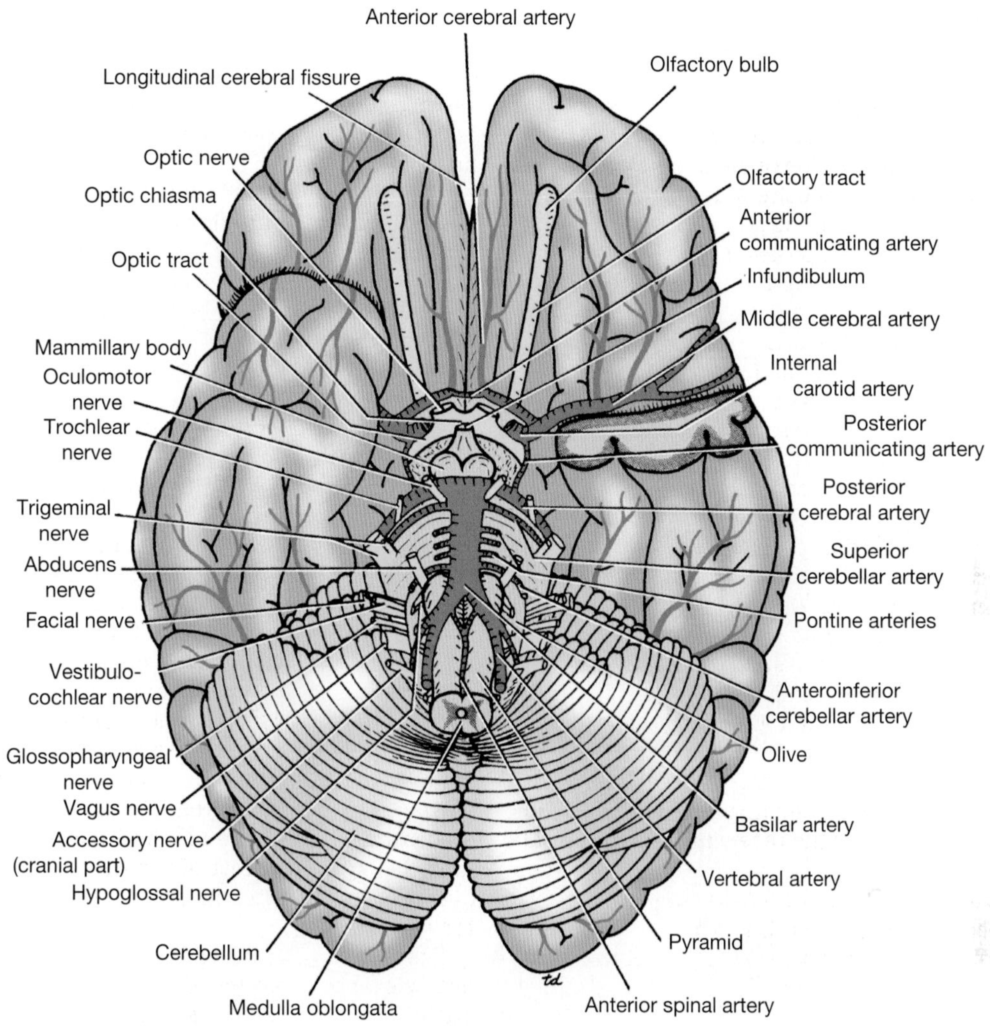

Figure 9.42 Arteries and cranial nerves seen on the inferior surface of the brain. The anterior pole of the left temporal lobe has been removed to show the course of the middle cerebral artery.

oblongata and behind by the **superior** and **inferior medullary vela** and the cerebellum. The fourth ventricle is connected above to the third ventricle by the **cerebral aqueduct**, and below, it is continuous with the central canal of the spinal cord. It communicates with the subarachnoid space through three openings in the lower part of the roof: a median and two lateral openings.

Ventricles

The ventricles of the brain consist of the two **lateral ventricles**, the **third ventricle**, and the **fourth ventricle**. The two lateral ventricles communicate with the third ventricle through the **interventricular foramina** (see Fig. 9.33). The third ventricle communicates with the fourth ventricle by the **cerebral aqueduct**. The fourth ventricle, in turn, is continuous with the narrow **central canal of the spinal cord** and, through the three foramina in its roof, with the subarachnoid space. The ventricles are filled with CSF, which is produced by the **choroid plexuses** of each ventricle. The detailed anatomy of the brain, including the size and shape of the cerebral ventricles can be visualized clinically using computed tomography (CT) scans and magnetic resonance imaging (MRI) (Figs. 9.43 to 9.45).

Blood Supply of the Brain

The two **internal carotid** and two **vertebral arteries** supply blood to the brain (see Fig. 9.42). The four arteries anastomose on the inferior surface of the brain and form the **cerebral arterial circle** (circle of Willis; circulus arteriosus). Three pairs of cerebral arteries branch off the circle and supply the cerebrum (Figs. 9.46 to 9.49; see also Figs. 9.41 and 9.42).

The veins of the brain have no muscular tissue in their thin walls, and they possess no valves. They emerge from the brain and drain into the cranial venous sinuses (see Fig. 9.4). Cerebral and cerebellar veins and veins of the brainstem are present. The **great cerebral vein** is formed by the union of the two **internal cerebral veins** and drains into the **straight sinus** (see Fig. 9.34).

(text continue on page 669)

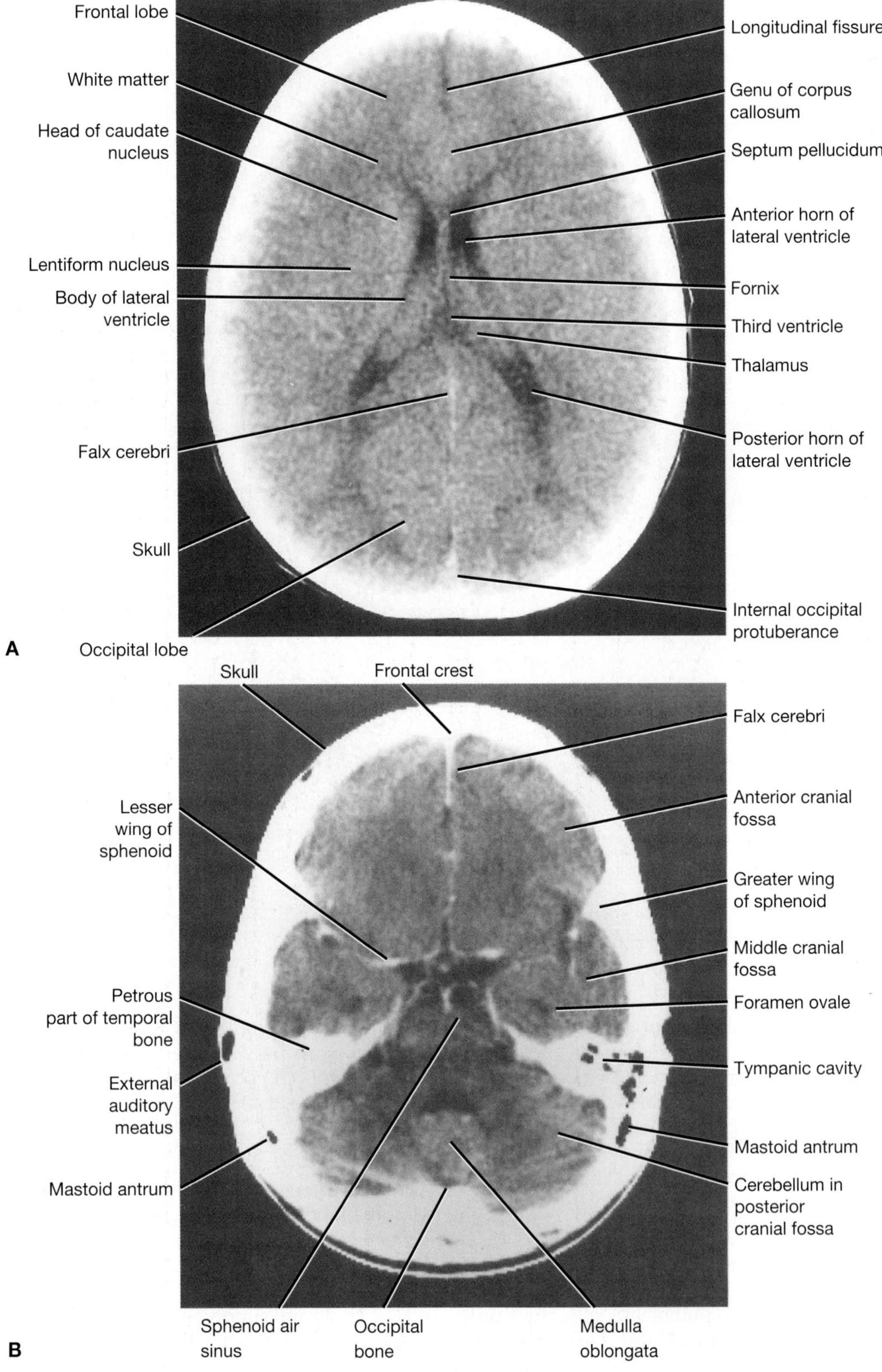

Figure 9.43 Axial (horizontal) CT scans of the skull. **A.** The skull bones, the brain, and the different parts of the lateral ventricles. **B.** A scan made at a lower level showing the three cranial fossae.

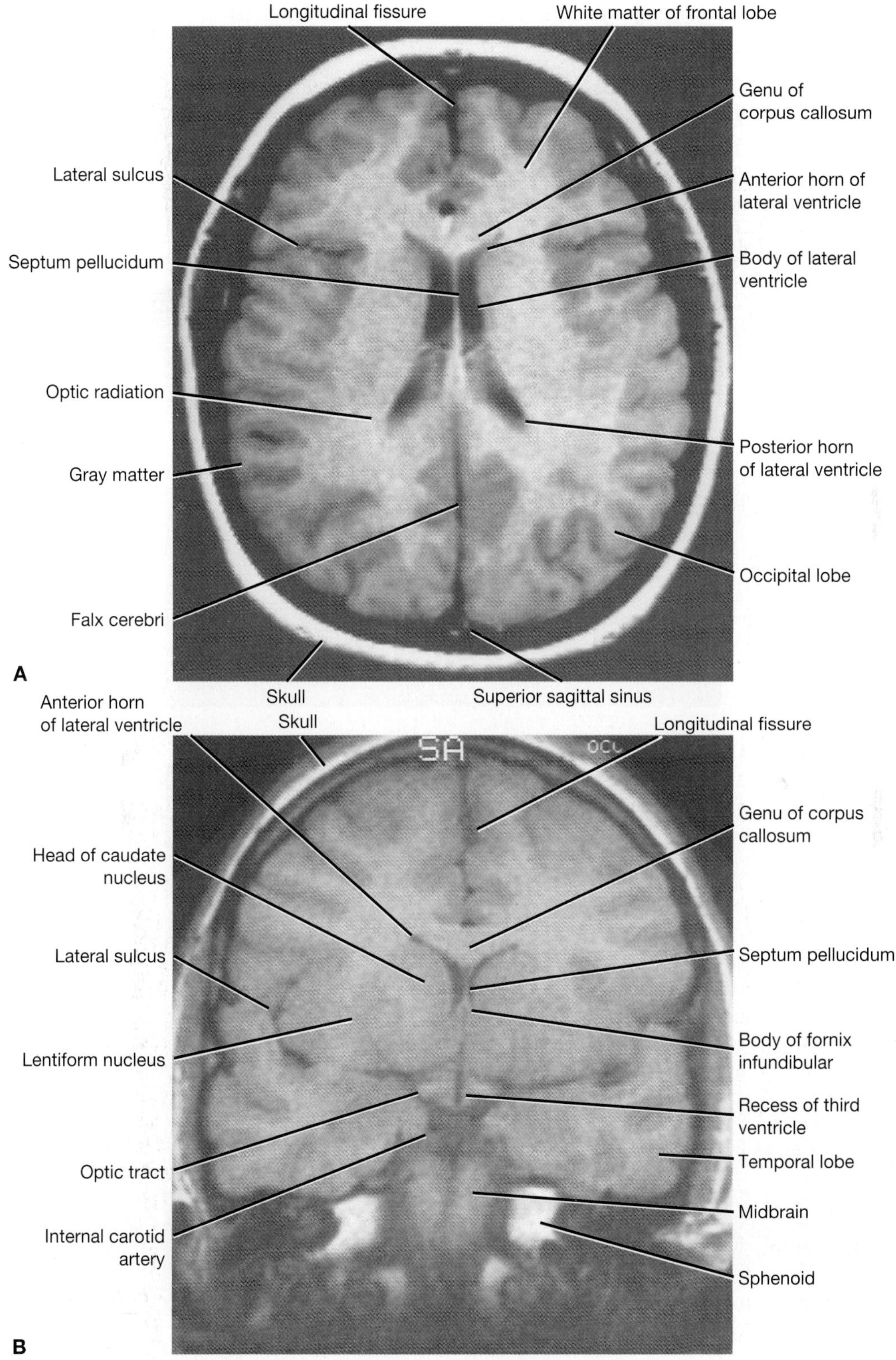

Figure 9.44 MRI of the skull. **A.** Axial image of the brain showing the different parts of the lateral ventricle and the lateral sulcus of the cerebral hemisphere. **B.** Coronal image through the frontal lobe of the brain showing the anterior horn of the lateral ventricle. Note the improved contrast between the gray and white matter compared with the CT scans seen in Figure 9.43.

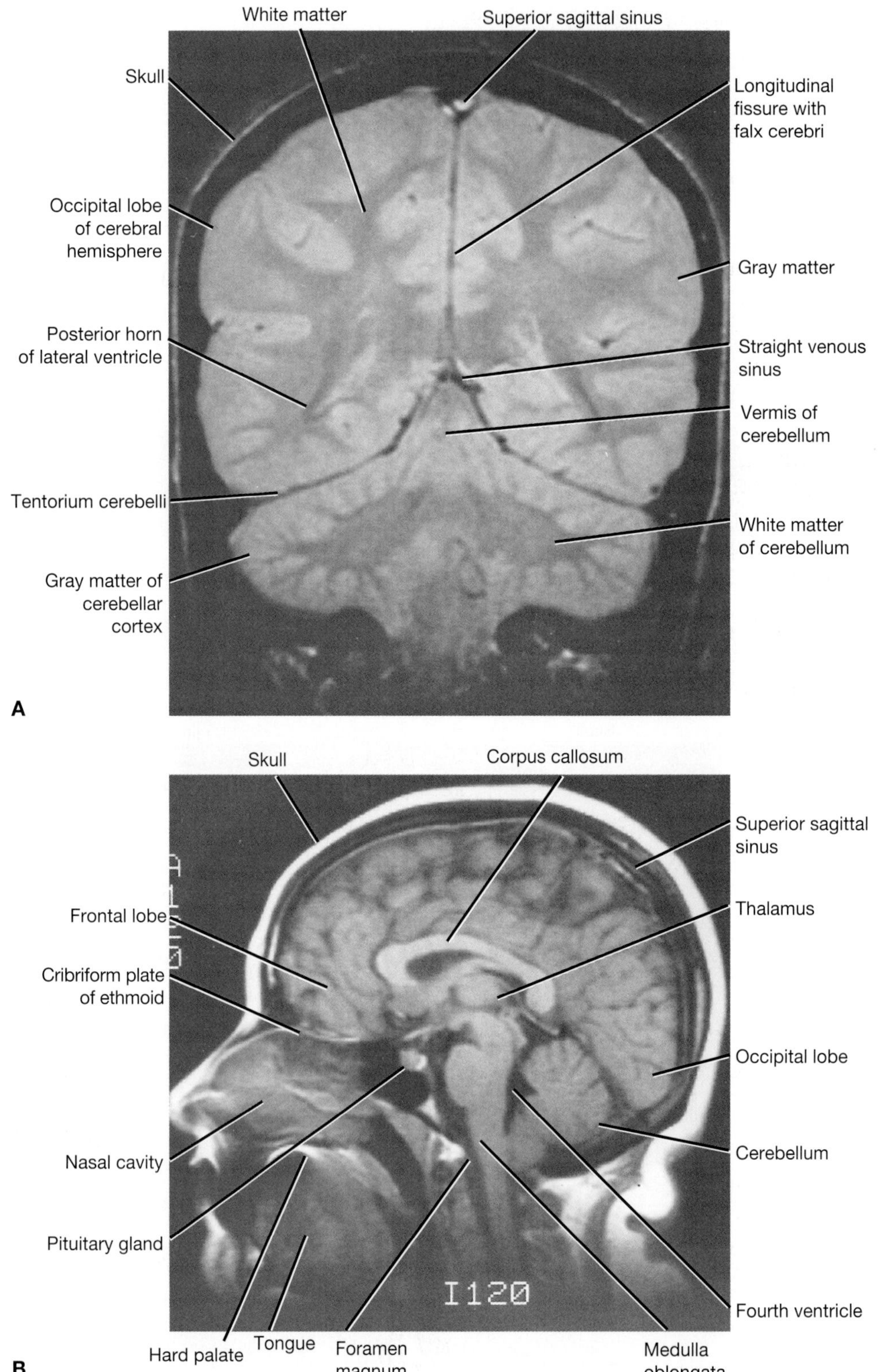

Figure 9.45 MRIs of the head. **A.** Coronal image through the occipital lobes of the brain showing the posterior horn of the lateral ventricle and the cerebellum. **B.** Sagittal image showing the different parts of the brain and the nasal and oral cavities.

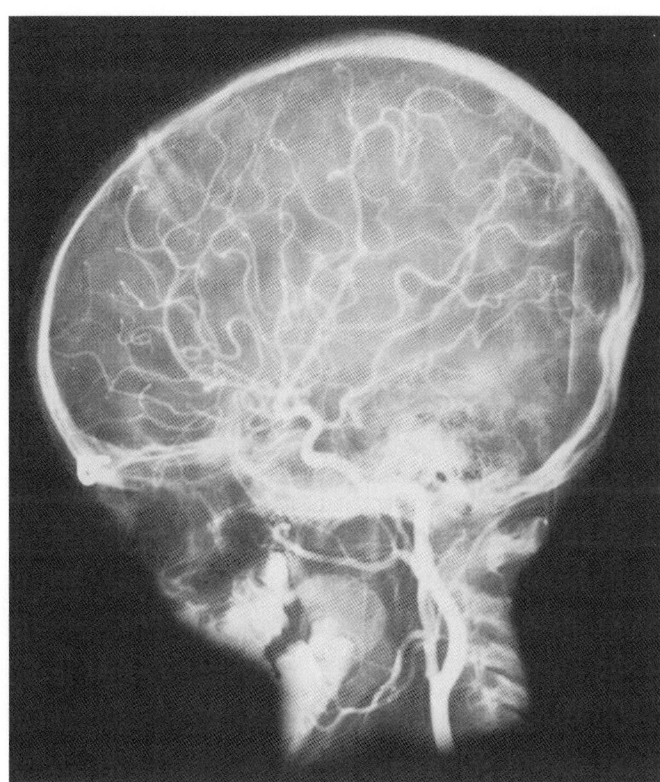

Figure 9.46 Lateral internal carotid arteriogram.

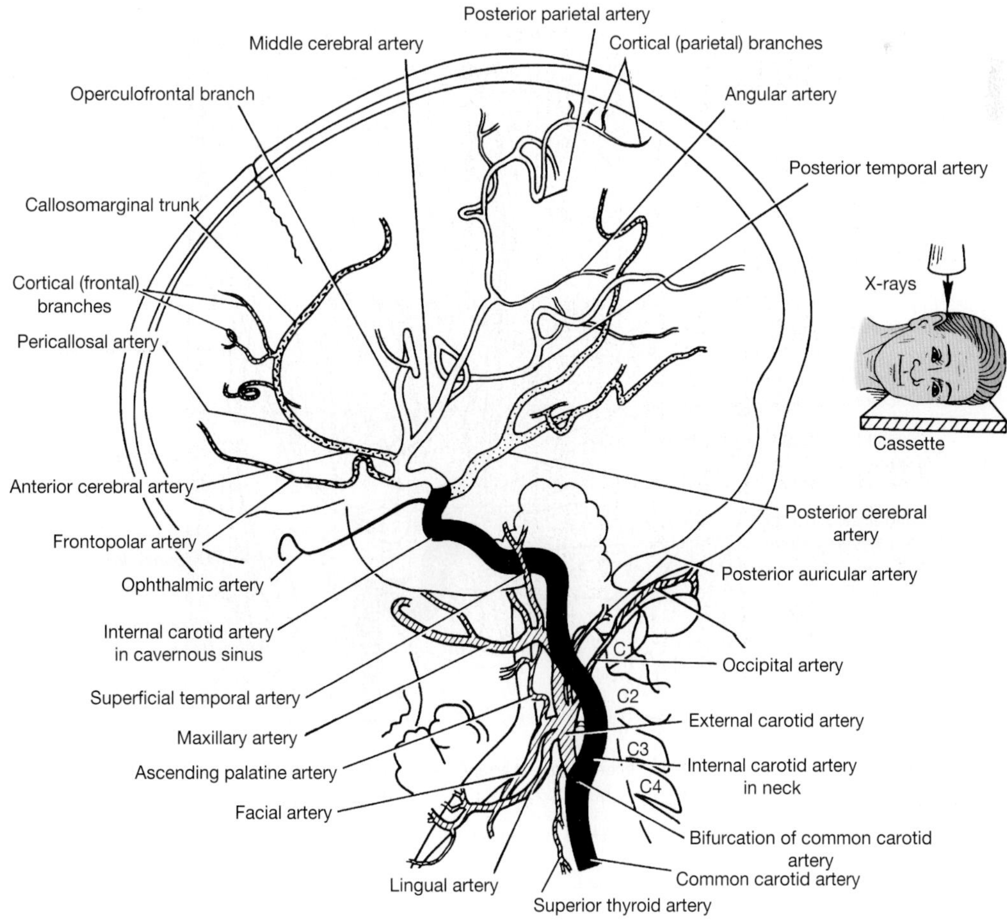

Figure 9.47 Main features that can be seen in the arteriogram in Figure 9.46.

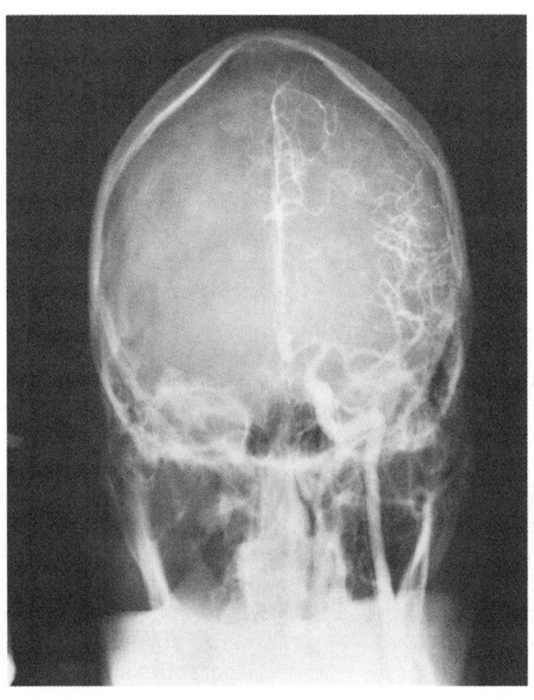

Figure 9.48 Anteroposterior internal carotid arteriogram.

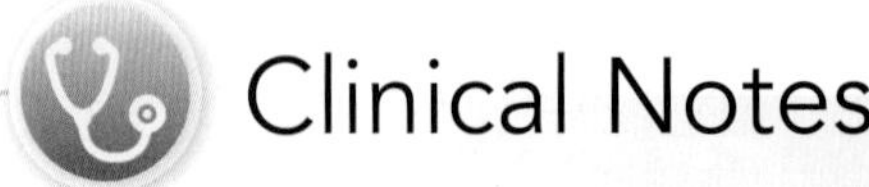

Brain Injuries

Direct injuries of the brain are produced by displacement and distortion of the neuronal tissues at the moment of impact. The brain may be likened to a log soaked with water floating submerged in water. The brain is floating in the cerebrospinal fluid in the subarachnoid space and is capable of a certain amount of anteroposterior movement, which is limited by the attachment of the superior cerebral veins to the superior sagittal sinus. Lateral displacement of the brain is limited by the falx cerebri. The tentorium cerebelli and the falx cerebelli also restrict displacement of the brain.

Blows on the front or back of the head lead to anteroposterior displacement of the brain, which may produce severe cerebral damage, stretching and distortion of the brainstem, and stretching and even tearing of the commissures of the brain. The terms **concussion**, **contusion**, and **laceration** are used clinically to describe the degrees of brain injury.

Blows on the side of the head produce less cerebral displacement, and the direct injuries to the brain consequently tend to be less severe.

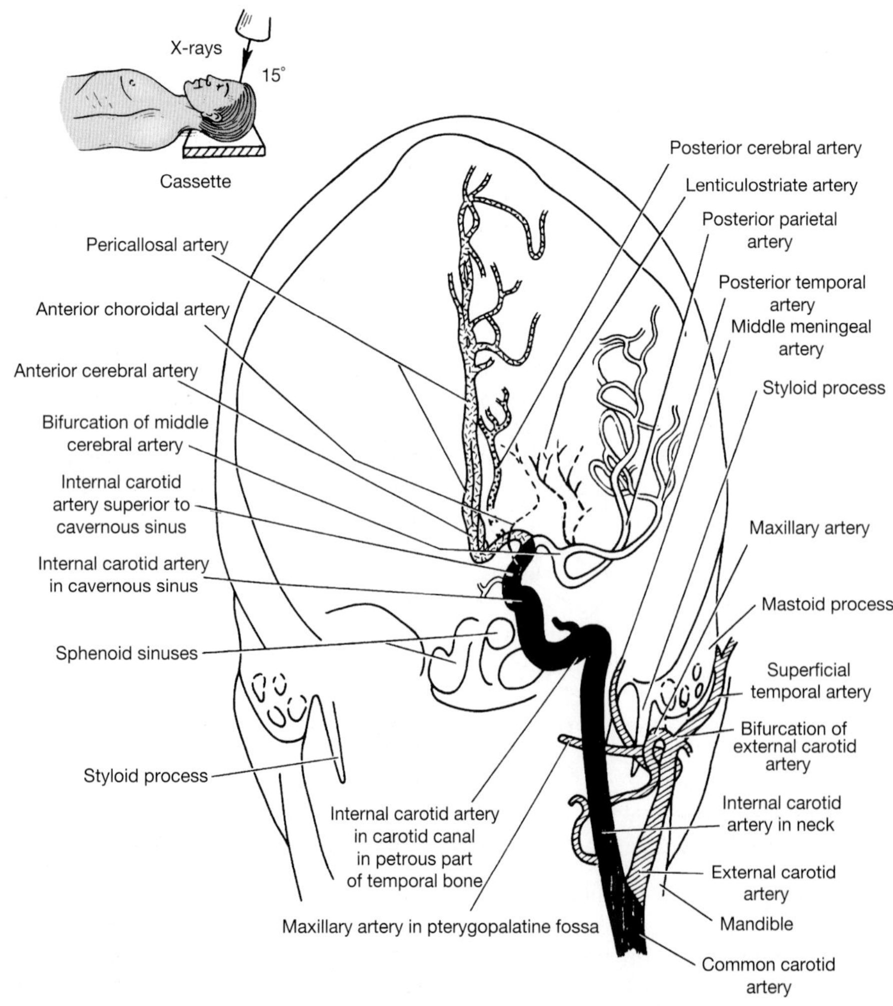

Figure 9.49 Main features that can be seen in the arteriogram in Figure 9.48.

Cranial Nerves in the Cranial Cavity

Twelve pairs of CNs branch off the base of the brain and upper spinal cord (see Fig. 9.42):

I. Olfactory (sensory)
II. Optic (sensory)
III. Oculomotor (motor)
IV. Trochlear (motor)
V. Trigeminal (mixed)
VI. Abducens (motor)
VII. Facial (mixed)
VIII. Vestibulocochlear (sensory)
IX. Glossopharyngeal (mixed)
X. Vagus (mixed)
XI. Accessory (motor)
XII. Hypoglossal (motor)

The nerves pass through foramina and fissures in the base of the skull to emerge from the cranial cavity. All are distributed in the head and neck except the vagus, which also supplies structures in the thorax and abdomen. The olfactory (CN I), optic (CN II), and vestibulocochlear (CN VIII) nerves are entirely sensory. The oculomotor (CN III), trochlear (CN IV), abducens (CN VI), accessory (CN XI), and hypoglossal (CN XII) nerves are entirely motor. The remaining nerves are mixed. The CNs are described in detail later in this chapter (see CRANIAL NERVES).

ORBIT AND EYE

The orbits are a pair of bony cavities in the face that contain the eyeballs; their associated muscles, nerves, vessels, and fat; and most of the lacrimal apparatus. Two thin, movable folds, the eyelids, guard the orbital opening.

Eyelids

The eyelids protect the eye from injury and excessive light. The upper eyelid is larger and more mobile than the lower, and they meet each other at the **medial** and **lateral angles** (Fig. 9.50). The **palpebral fissure** is the elliptical opening between the eyelids and is the entrance into the **conjunctival sac**. When the eye is closed, the upper eyelid completely covers the cornea of the eye. When the eye is open and looking straight ahead, the upper lid just covers the upper margin of the cornea. The lower lid lies just below the cornea when the eye is open and rises only slightly when the eye is closed.

The superficial surface of the eyelids is covered by skin, and the deep surface is covered by a mucous membrane called the **conjunctiva**. The **eyelashes** are short, curved hairs on the free edges of the eyelids. They are arranged in double or triple rows at the mucocutaneous junction. The **sebaceous glands** open directly into the eyelash follicles. The **ciliary glands** are modified sweat glands that open separately between adjacent lashes. The **tarsal glands** are long, modified sebaceous glands that pour their oily secretion onto the margin of the lid; their openings lie behind the eyelashes. This oily material prevents the overflow of tears and helps make the closed eyelids airtight.

The more rounded medial angle is separated from the eyeball by a small space, the **lacus lacrimalis**, in the center of which is a small, reddish yellow elevation, the **caruncula lacrimalis** (Fig. 9.51; see also Fig. 9.50). A reddish semilunar fold, called the **plica semilunaris**, lies on the lateral side of the caruncle.

A small elevation, the **papilla lacrimalis**, is present near the medial angle of the eye. On the summit of the papilla is a small hole, the **punctum lacrimale**, which leads into the **canaliculus lacrimalis**. The papilla lacrimalis projects into the lacus, and the punctum and canaliculus carry tears down into the nose (see Lacrimal Apparatus).

The **conjunctiva** is a thin mucous membrane that lines the eyelids and is reflected at the **superior** and **inferior fornices** onto the anterior surface of the eyeball (see Fig. 9.50). Its epithelium is continuous with that of the cornea. The ducts of the lacrimal gland pierce the upper lateral part of the superior fornix (see below). The conjunctiva thus forms a potential space, the **conjunctival sac**, which is open at the palpebral fissure. The **subtarsal sulcus** is a groove on the deep side of the eyelid that runs close to and parallel with the margin of the lid. The sulcus tends to trap small foreign particles introduced into the conjunctival sac and is thus clinically important.

The **orbital septum** is a fibrous sheet that forms the framework of the eyelids. This is attached to the periosteum at the orbital margins. The orbital septum is thickened at the margins of the lids to form the **superior** and **inferior tarsal plates**. The **lateral palpebral ligament** is a band that connects the lateral ends of the tarsal plates to a bony tubercle just within the orbital margin. The **medial palpebral ligament** attaches the medial ends of the plates to the crest of the lacrimal bone. The tarsal glands are embedded in the posterior surface of the tarsal plates.

The superficial surface of the tarsal plates and the orbital septum are covered by the **palpebral fibers of the orbicularis oculi muscle**. The aponeurosis of insertion of the **levator palpebrae superioris** muscle pierces the orbital septum to reach the anterior surface of the superior tarsal plate and the skin. A thin smooth muscle band, the **superior tarsal muscle**, underlies the levator.

Eyelid Movements

The actions of the eyelid muscles are most pronounced at the upper eyelid. Thus, "opening the eye" generally describes the action of elevating (lifting) the upper eyelid. Conversely, "closing the eye" denotes depressing (lowering) the upper eyelid.

The position of the eyelids at rest depends on the tone of the **orbicularis oculi**, **levator palpebrae superioris**, and **superior tarsal** muscles and the position of the eyeball. The eyelids are closed by the contraction of the orbicularis oculi and the relaxation of

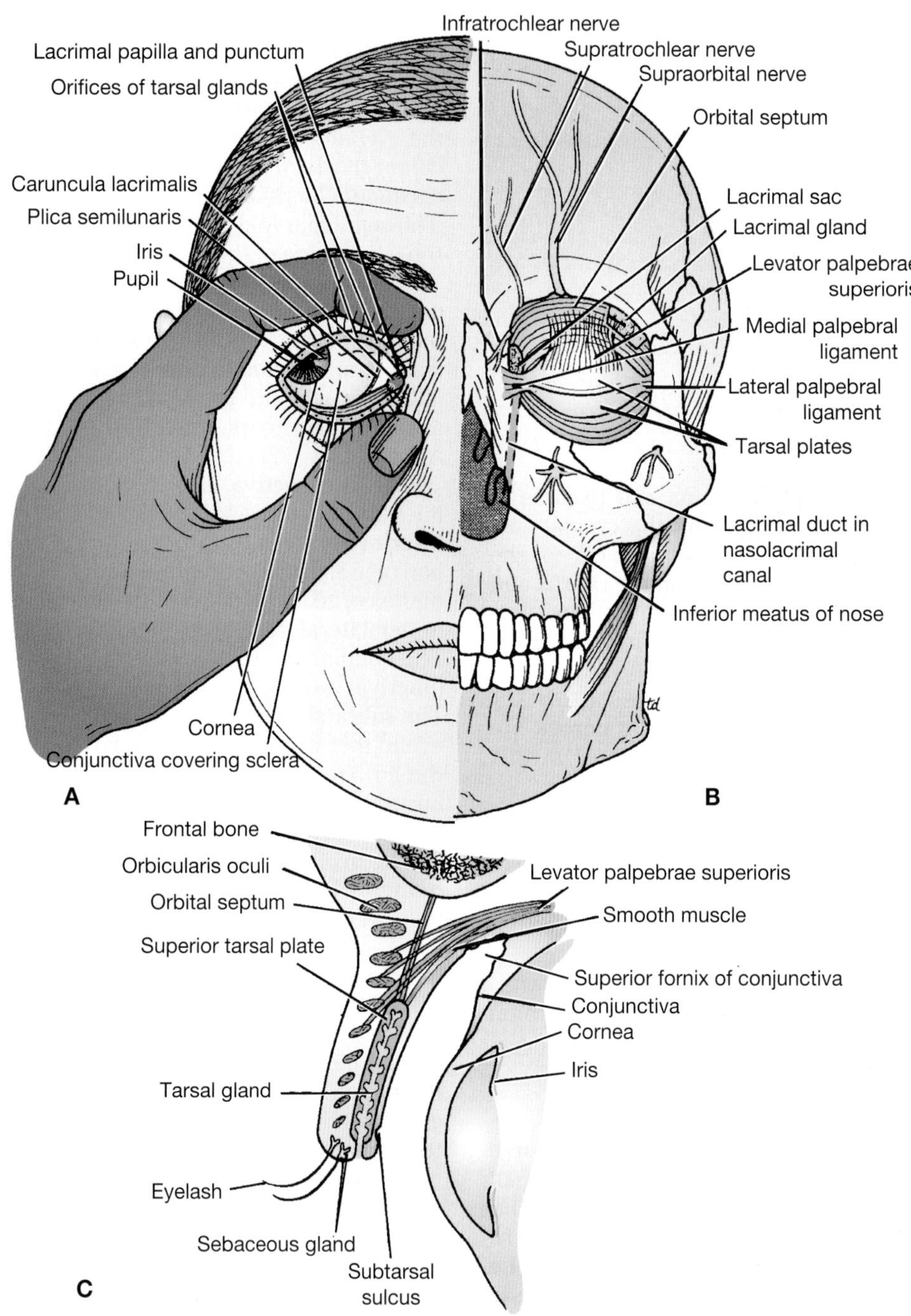

Figure 9.50 **A.** Anterior view of the right eye, with the eyelids separated to show the openings of the tarsal glands, plica semilunaris, caruncula lacrimalis, and puncta lacrimalis. **B.** Left eye, showing the superior and inferior tarsal plates and the lacrimal gland, sac, and duct. Note that a small window has been cut in the orbital septum to show the underlying lacrimal gland and fat (*yellow*). **C.** Sagittal section through the upper eyelid and the superior fornix of the conjunctiva. Note the presence of smooth muscle in the levator palpebrae superioris. This is usually identified as the superior tarsal muscle.

the levator palpebrae superioris and superior tarsal muscles. The eye is opened by the levator palpebrae superioris and/or superior tarsal raising the upper lid. On looking upward, the levator palpebrae superioris contracts, and the upper lid moves with the eyeball. On looking downward, both lids move, the upper lid continues to cover the upper part of the cornea, and the lower lid is pulled downward slightly by the conjunctiva, which is attached to the sclera and the lower lid.

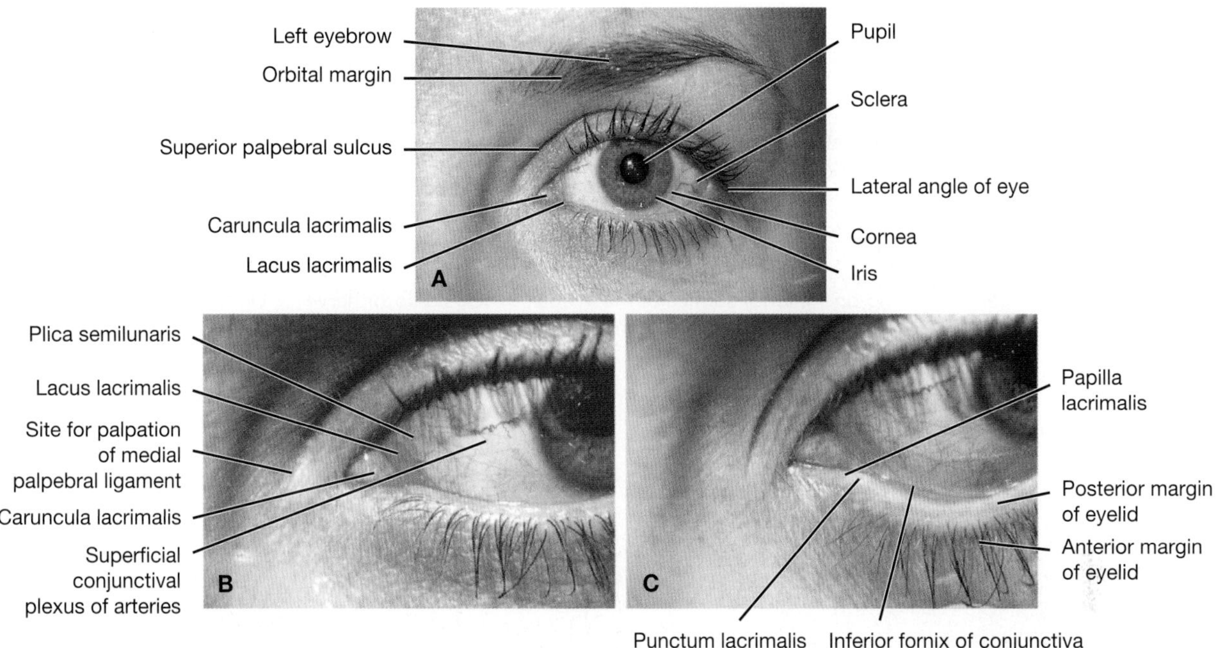

Figure 9.51 Left eye of an adult female. **A.** The names of structures seen in the examination of the eye. **B.** An enlarged view of the medial angle between the eyelids. **C.** The lower eyelid pulled downward and slightly everted to reveal the punctum lacrimalis.

The muscles of the eyelids are summarized in Table 9.5.

Lacrimal Apparatus

The lacrimal apparatus consists of the structures that secrete and collect tears, that is, the lacrimal gland and the lacrimal ducts. Proper function of this system is critical in ensuring the cornea remains moist.

Lacrimal Gland

The lacrimal gland consists of a large **orbital part** and a small **palpebral part**, which are continuous with each other around the lateral edge of the aponeurosis of the levator palpebrae superioris. The gland is situated above the eyeball in the upper anterolateral part of the orbit posterior to the orbital septum (see Fig. 9.50). The gland opens into the lateral part of the superior fornix of the conjunctiva by ~12 ducts.

The **parasympathetic secretomotor nerve supply** is derived from the lacrimal nucleus of the **facial nerve**. The preganglionic fibers reach the pterygopalatine ganglion via the nervus intermedius and its **great petrosal branch** and via the nerve of the pterygoid canal. The postganglionic fibers leave the ganglion and join the maxillary nerve. They then pass into its zygomatic branch and the zygomaticotemporal nerve. They reach the lacrimal gland within the **lacrimal nerve**.

The **sympathetic postganglionic nerve supply** is from the internal carotid plexus and travels in the **deep petrosal nerve**, the nerve of the pterygoid canal, the maxillary nerve, the zygomatic nerve, the zygomaticotemporal nerve, and finally the lacrimal nerve.

Lacrimal Ducts

Tears secreted from the lacrimal gland circulate across the cornea and accumulate in the **lacus lacrimalis**. From here, the tears enter the **canaliculi lacrimales** through the **puncta lacrimalis**. The canaliculi lacrimales pass medially and open into the **lacrimal sac** (see Fig. 9.50), which lies in the lacrimal groove behind the medial palpebral ligament and is the upper blind end of the nasolacrimal duct.

The **nasolacrimal duct** is about 0.5 in. (1.3 cm) long and emerges from the lower end of the lacrimal sac. The duct descends downward, backward, and laterally in a bony canal and opens into the **inferior nasal meatus** in the inferior lateral wall of the nasal passage. A fold of mucous membrane, the **lacrimal fold**, guards the opening. This prevents air from being forced up the duct into the lacrimal sac on blowing the nose.

Orbit

The orbit is a pyramidal cavity with its base anterior and its apex posterior (Fig. 9.52). Parts of three bones form the **orbital margin**, which circumscribes the base:

- **Superior margin:** frontal bone
- **Lateral margin:** processes of the frontal and zygomatic bones
- **Inferior margin:** zygomatic bone and the maxilla
- **Medial margin:** processes of the maxilla and the frontal bone

Table 9.5 Eyeball and Eyelid Muscles

MUSCLE	ORIGIN	INSERTION	NERVE SUPPLY	ACTION
Eyeball Extrinsic Muscles (Striated Skeletal Muscle)				
Superior rectus	Tendinous ring on posterior wall of orbital cavity	Superior surface of eyeball just posterior to corneoscleral junction	Oculomotor nerve (CN III)	Raises the cornea upward and medially
Inferior rectus	Tendinous ring on posterior wall of orbital cavity	Inferior surface of the eyeball just posterior to corneoscleral junction	Oculomotor nerve (CN III)	Depresses the cornea downward and medially
Medial rectus	Tendinous ring on posterior wall of orbital cavity	Medial surface of eyeball just posterior to corneoscleral junction	Oculomotor nerve (CN III)	Rotates eyeball so that the cornea looks medially
Lateral rectus	Tendinous ring on posterior wall of orbital cavity	Lateral surface of eyeball just posterior to corneoscleral junction	Abducens nerve (CN VI)	Rotates eyeball so that the cornea looks laterally
Superior oblique	Posterior wall of orbital cavity	Passes through pulley and is attached to superior surface of eyeball beneath superior rectus	Trochlear nerve (CN IV)	Rotates eyeball so that the cornea looks downward and laterally
Inferior oblique	Floor of orbital cavity	Lateral surface of eyeball deep to lateral rectus	Oculomotor nerve (CN III)	Rotates eyeball so that cornea looks upward and laterally
Eyeball Intrinsic Muscles (Smooth Muscle)				
Sphincter pupillae of the iris			Parasympathetic via oculomotor nerve	Constricts the pupil
Dilator pupillae of the iris			Sympathetic	Dilates the pupil
Ciliary muscle			Parasympathetic via oculomotor nerve	Controls shape of lens; in accommodation, it makes lens more globular
Eyelid Muscles				
Orbicularis oculi (see Table 9.4)				
Levator palpebrae superioris	Back of orbital cavity	Anterior surface and upper margin of superior tarsal plate	Striated muscle oculomotor nerve, smooth muscle (sympathetic)	Raises upper lid

CN = cranial nerve.

The orbital margins lead back to four **orbital walls** that are composed of multiple elements:

- **Roof (superior wall):** Formed by the orbital plate of the frontal bone and the lesser wing of the sphenoid. These separate the orbital cavity from the anterior cranial fossa and the frontal lobe of the cerebral hemisphere.
- **Lateral wall:** Formed by the zygomatic bone and the greater wing of the sphenoid.
- **Floor (inferior wall):** Formed largely by the orbital plate of the maxilla (which separates the orbital cavity from the maxillary sinus) and to a smaller degree by the zygomatic and palatine bones.
- **Medial wall:** Formed anteroposteriorly by the frontal process of the maxilla, the lacrimal bone, the orbital plate of the ethmoid (which separates the orbital cavity from the ethmoid sinuses), and the body of the sphenoid.

Openings into the Orbital Cavity

Several openings connect the orbit with immediately neighboring areas and convey multiple neurovascular structures (see Fig. 9.52).

- **Orbital opening:** This is the large anterior opening that forms the base of the orbit and communicates directly with the face. About one sixth of the eyeball protrudes through the base and is exposed; the walls of the orbit protect the remainder.
- **Supraorbital notch** (often a **supraorbital foramen):** Situated in the frontal bone, on the superior orbital margin. It transmits the supraorbital nerve and blood vessels.

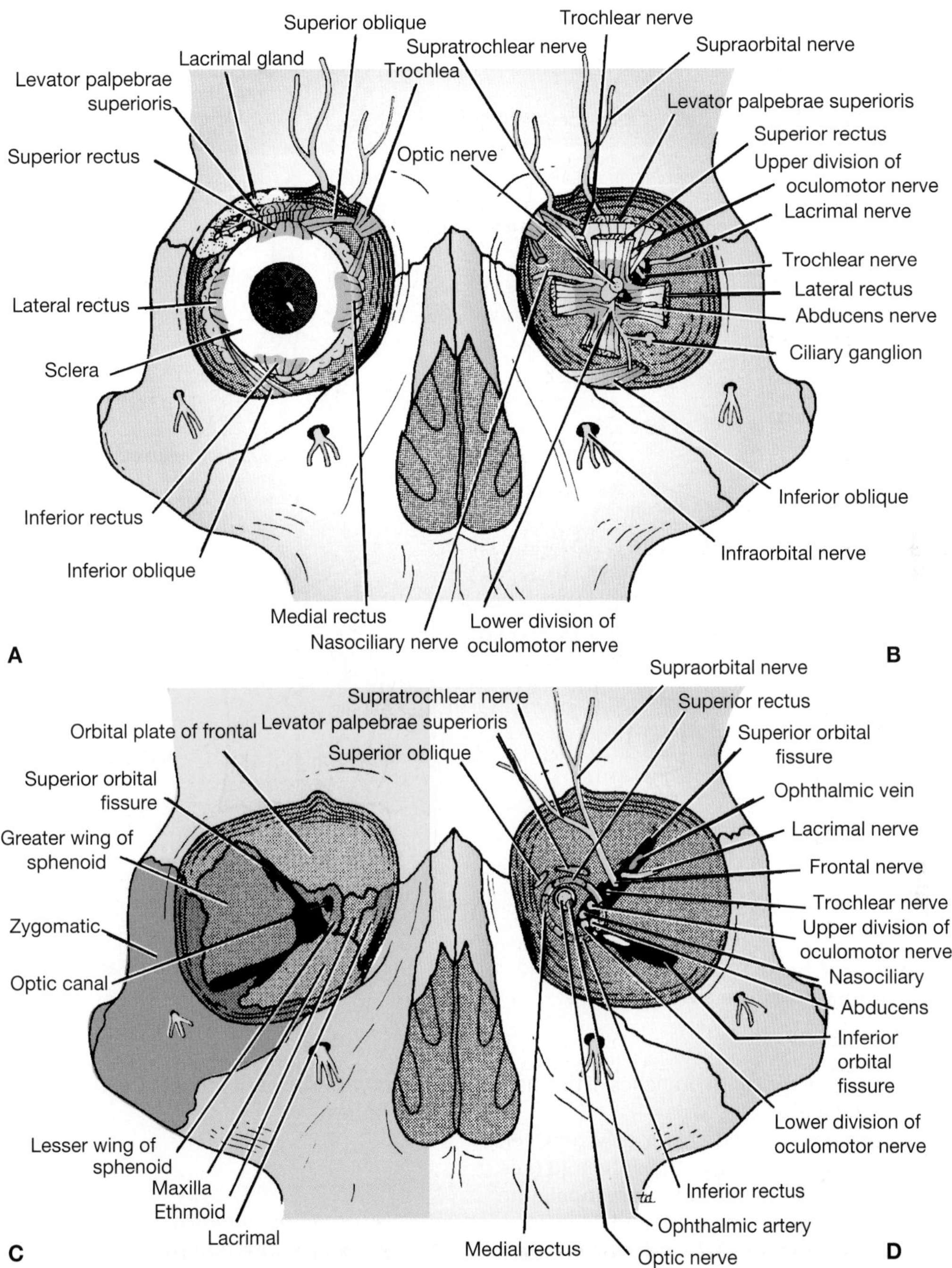

Figure 9.52 **A.** Right eyeball exposed from in front. **B.** Muscles and nerves of the left orbit as seen from in front. **C.** Bones forming the walls of the right orbit. **D.** The optic canal and the superior and inferior orbital fissures on the left side.

- **Infraorbital groove and canal:** Situated on the floor of the orbit in the orbital plate of the maxilla (Fig. 9.53). They transmit the infraorbital nerve (a continuation of the maxillary nerve) and blood vessels.
- **Nasolacrimal canal:** Located anteriorly on the medial wall, in the lacrimal bone. It transmits the nasolacrimal duct and communicates with the inferior meatus of the nose (see Fig. 9.50).
- **Anterior and posterior ethmoidal foramina:** Two small openings on the medial wall, typically in the ethmoid bone. These transmit the anterior and posterior ethmoid nerves (both branches of the ophthalmic nerve), respectively.
- **Zygomaticotemporal and zygomaticofacial foramina:** Two small openings on the lateral wall, usually in the zygomatic bone. These convey the zygomaticotemporal

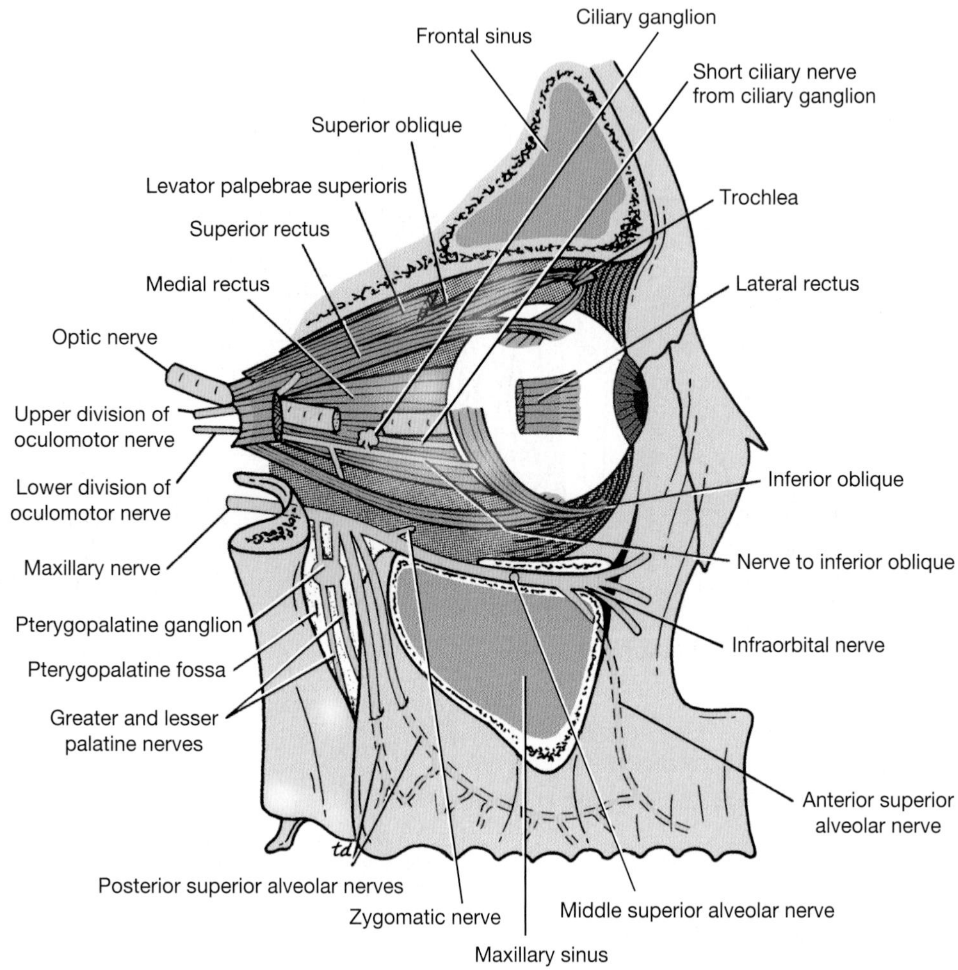

Figure 9.53 Muscles and nerves of the right orbit viewed from the lateral side. The maxillary nerve and the pterygopalatine ganglion in the pterygopalatine fossa are also shown.

and zygomaticofacial nerves (both branches of the maxillary nerve), respectively.

- **Inferior orbital fissure:** Located posteriorly, between the maxilla and the greater wing of the sphenoid (see Fig. 9.52); it communicates with the pterygopalatine fossa. It transmits the maxillary nerve and its infraorbital and zygomatic branches, the inferior ophthalmic vein, and sympathetic nerves.
- **Superior orbital fissure:** Located posteriorly, between the greater and lesser wings of the sphenoid; it communicates with the middle cranial fossa. It transmits the oculomotor, trochlear, ophthalmic, and abducens nerves and the superior ophthalmic vein.
- **Optic canal:** Located posteriorly, in the lesser wing of the sphenoid, at the apex of the orbit; it communicates with the middle cranial fossa. It transmits the optic nerve and the ophthalmic artery.

Orbital Fascia

The orbital fascia is the periosteum of the bones that form the walls of the orbit. It is loosely attached to the bones and is continuous through the foramina and fissures with the periosteum covering the outer surfaces of the bones.

Nerves

Six CNs (optic, oculomotor, trochlear, trigeminal, abducens, and facial) plus additional autonomic components supply the orbit.

Optic Nerve (CN I)

The optic nerve enters the orbit from the middle cranial fossa by passing through the optic canal (Fig. 9.54; see also Figs. 9.52 and 9.53). It is accompanied by the ophthalmic artery, which lies on its lower lateral side. Sheaths of pia mater, arachnoid mater, and dura mater surround the nerve (see Eye Structure). It runs forward and laterally within the cone of the recti muscles and pierces the sclera at a point medial to the posterior pole of the eyeball. Here, the meninges fuse with the sclera so that the subarachnoid space with its contained CSF extends forward from the middle cranial fossa, around the optic nerve, and through the optic canal, as far as

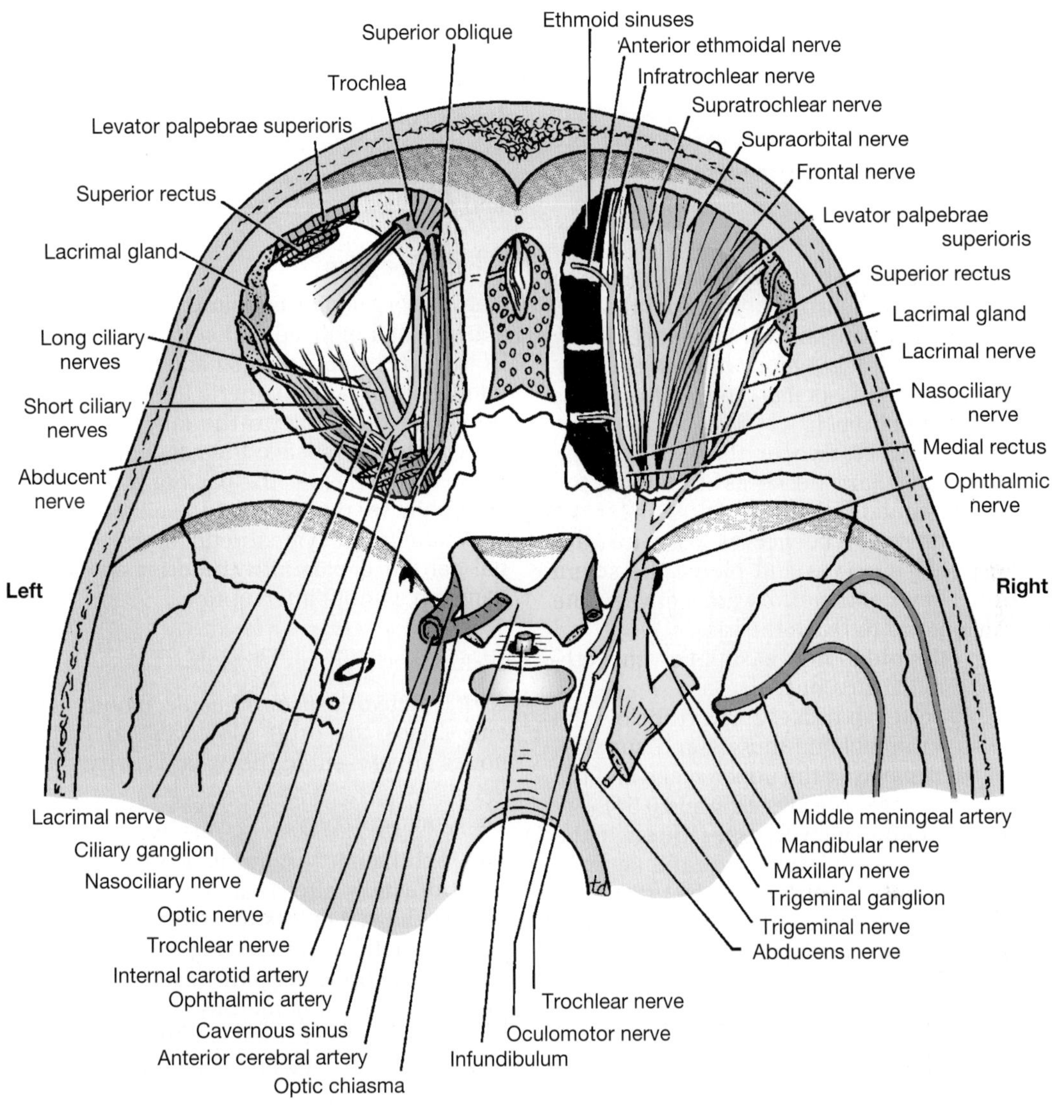

Figure 9.54 Right and left orbital cavities viewed from above. The roof of the orbit, formed by the orbital plate of the frontal bone, has been removed from both sides. On the left side, the levator palpebrae superioris and the superior rectus muscles have also been removed to expose the underlying structures.

the eyeball. Thus, a rise in CSF pressure within the cranial cavity is transmitted to the back of the eyeball.

Oculomotor Nerve (CN III)

The oculomotor nerve divides into two parts, a superior and an inferior ramus, as it enters the orbit through the lower part of the superior orbital fissure (see Figs. 9.52 and 9.53). The **superior ramus** supplies the superior rectus muscle, then pierces it, and supplies the levator palpebrae superioris muscle. The **inferior ramus** supplies the inferior rectus, medial rectus, and the inferior oblique muscles. The nerve to the inferior oblique gives off a branch that passes to the **ciliary ganglion** (see Fig. 9.53) and carries parasympathetic fibers to the sphincter pupillae and the ciliary muscle (see below).

Trochlear Nerve (CN IV)

The trochlear nerve enters the orbit through the upper part of the superior orbital fissure (see Fig. 9.52). It runs forward and supplies the superior oblique muscle (see Fig. 9.54).

Trigeminal Nerve (CN V)

The ophthalmic division of the trigeminal nerve passes through the superior orbital fissure and immediately divides into three branches. From medial to lateral, these are the nasociliary, frontal, and lacrimal nerves (see Fig. 9.54). The maxillary division of the trigeminal nerve crosses the inferior orbital fissure and gives off the infraorbital nerve, which enters the infraorbital canal in the floor of the orbit (see Fig. 9.53).

Nasociliary Nerve

The nasociliary nerve enters the orbit through the lower part of the superior orbital fissure. It crosses above the optic nerve, runs forward along the upper margin of the medial rectus muscle, and ends by dividing into the **anterior ethmoidal** and **infratrochlear nerves** (see Fig. 9.54).

BRANCHES

- The **communicating branch to the ciliary ganglion** is a sensory nerve. The sensory fibers from the eyeball pass to the ciliary ganglion via the **short ciliary nerves**, pass through the ganglion without interruption, and then join the nasociliary nerve by means of the communicating branch.
- The **long ciliary nerves**, two or three in number, arise from the nasociliary nerve as it crosses the optic nerve. They contain sympathetic fibers for the dilator pupillae muscle. The nerves pass forward with the short ciliary nerves and pierce the sclera of the eyeball. They continue forward between the sclera and the choroid to reach the iris.
- The **posterior ethmoidal nerve** supplies the ethmoidal and sphenoidal air sinuses.
- The **infratrochlear nerve** passes forward below the pulley of the superior oblique muscle and supplies the skin of the medial part of the upper eyelid and the adjacent part of the nose (see Figs. 9.50 and 9.54).
- The **anterior ethmoidal nerve** passes through the anterior ethmoidal foramen and enters the anterior cranial fossa on the upper surface of the cribriform plate of the ethmoid (see Fig. 9.54). It enters the nasal cavity through a slit like opening alongside the crista galli. After supplying an area of mucous membrane, it appears on the face as the **external nasal branch** at the lower border of the nasal bone and supplies the skin of the nose down as far as the tip.

Frontal Nerve

The frontal nerve enters the orbit through the upper part of the superior orbital fissure and passes forward on the upper surface of the levator palpebrae superioris beneath the roof of the orbit (see Fig. 9.54). It divides into the **supratrochlear** and **supraorbital nerves** that wind around the upper margin of the orbital cavity to supply the skin of the forehead; the supraorbital nerve also supplies the mucous membrane of the frontal air sinus.

Lacrimal Nerve

The lacrimal nerve enters the orbit through the upper part of the superior orbital fissure and passes forward along the upper border of the lateral rectus muscle. It joins a branch of the zygomaticotemporal nerve, which later leaves it to enter the lacrimal gland (parasympathetic secretomotor fibers). The lacrimal nerve ends by supplying the skin of the lateral part of the upper lid.

Abducens Nerve (CN VI)

The abducens nerve enters the orbit through the lower part of the superior orbital fissure (see Fig. 9.52). It supplies the lateral rectus muscle.

Facial Nerve (CN VII)

The facial nerve does not enter the orbit. However, its temporal and zygomatic branches supply the orbicularis oculi muscle and other facial muscles that influence the eyelids. Also, it initiates the parasympathetic pathway that eventually connects to the lacrimal nerve and supplies secretomotor fibers to the lacrimal gland.

Ciliary Ganglion

The ciliary ganglion is a parasympathetic ganglion about the size of a pinhead and situated in the posterior part of the orbit (see Figs. 9.53 and 9.54). It receives its preganglionic parasympathetic fibers from the oculomotor nerve via the nerve to the inferior oblique. The postganglionic fibers leave the ganglion in the short ciliary nerves, which enter the back of the eyeball and supply the sphincter pupillae and the ciliary muscle.

A number of sympathetic fibers pass from the internal carotid plexus into the orbit and run through the ganglion without interruption.

Blood and Lymph Vessels

A rich network of ophthalmic blood vessels supplies and drains the orbit. However, no lymph vessels or nodes are present in the orbital cavity.

Ophthalmic Artery

The ophthalmic artery is a branch of the **internal carotid artery** after that vessel emerges from the cavernous sinus. It enters the orbit through the optic canal with the optic nerve (see Fig. 9.54). It runs forward and crosses the optic nerve to reach the medial wall of the orbit. It gives off numerous branches that accompany the nerves in the orbital cavity. The ophthalmic artery forms a notable **facial anastomosis** with the angular artery (the terminal end of the facial artery) and the frontal branch of the superficial temporal artery.

Branches

- The **central artery of the retina** is a small branch that pierces the meningeal sheaths of the optic nerve to gain entrance to the nerve (see Eye Structure). It runs in the substance of the optic nerve and enters the eyeball at the center of the optic disc. Here, it divides into branches, which may be studied in a patient through an ophthalmoscope. The central artery is the end artery to the retina.
- The **muscular branches**.
- The **ciliary arteries** supply the eyeball; they are divided into anterior and posterior groups. The former group enters the eyeball near the corneoscleral junction; the latter group enters near the optic nerve.
- The **lacrimal artery** to the lacrimal gland.
- The **supratrochlear** and **supraorbital arteries** are distributed to the skin of the forehead.

Ophthalmic Veins

Two main ophthalmic veins, superior and inferior, pass through the orbit. The **superior ophthalmic vein** forms from the union of the supraorbital and supratrochlear veins draining the forehead. It communicates with the facial vein at the medial angle of the eye (see Fig. 9.34). The **inferior ophthalmic vein** communicates through the inferior orbital fissure with the pterygoid venous plexus. Both ophthalmic veins pass posteriorly through the superior orbital fissure and drain into the **cavernous sinus**.

Eyeball Movements

A **fascial sheath (bulbar fascia)** surrounds the eyeball from the optic nerve to the corneoscleral junction and separates the eyeball from the fat that fills much of the orbit (see Eye Structure). This allows the eyeball to effectively float in the orbital fat and provides it with a socket for free movement.

The tendons of the extraocular muscles perforate the fascial sheath, which reflects onto each of them as a tubular sheath. The sheaths for the tendons of the medial and lateral recti attach to the medial and lateral walls of the orbit by triangular ligaments called the **medial** and **lateral check ligaments.** Do not confuse the check ligaments with the medial and lateral palpebral ligaments of the eyelids.

The lower part of the fascial sheath, which passes beneath the eyeball and connects the check ligaments, is thickened and serves to suspend the eyeball; it is called the **suspensory ligament of the eye**. Thus, the eye is suspended from the medial and lateral walls of the orbit, as if in a hammock.

The **orbitalis muscle** (muscle of Müller) is a thin layer of smooth muscle that bridges the inferior orbital fissure. Sympathetic nerves supply it. Its function is uncertain. However, it may assist in suspending the eyeball and posturing it in its normal forward position in the orbit.

The net mechanical effect of this architecture is that the eyeball can move freely, smoothly, and extremely quickly ("in the twinkling of an eye") to very fine or very large degrees.

Movement Terminology

The center of the cornea or the center of the pupil is used as the anatomic "anterior pole" of the eye. All movements of the eye are related to the direction of the movement of the anterior pole as it rotates on any one of three axes (horizontal, vertical, and sagittal) (Figs. 9.55 and 9.56). **Elevation/depression** is rotation about the transverse (horizontal) axis, so that the pupil moves upward (elevation) or downward (depression). **Abduction/adduction** is rotation about the vertical axis,

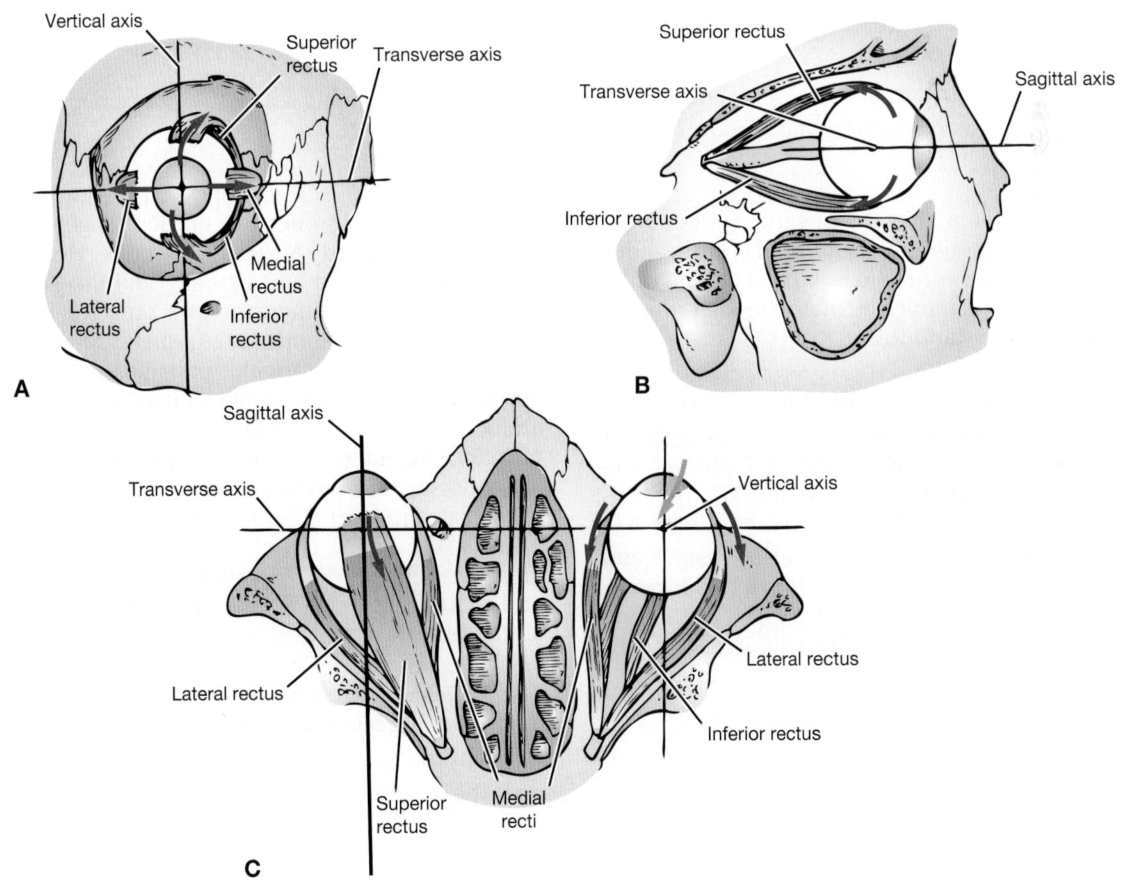

Figure 9.55 Anterior **(A)**, lateral **(B)**, and superior **(C)** views of the orbit showing the actions of the four recti muscles in producing movements of the eyeball.

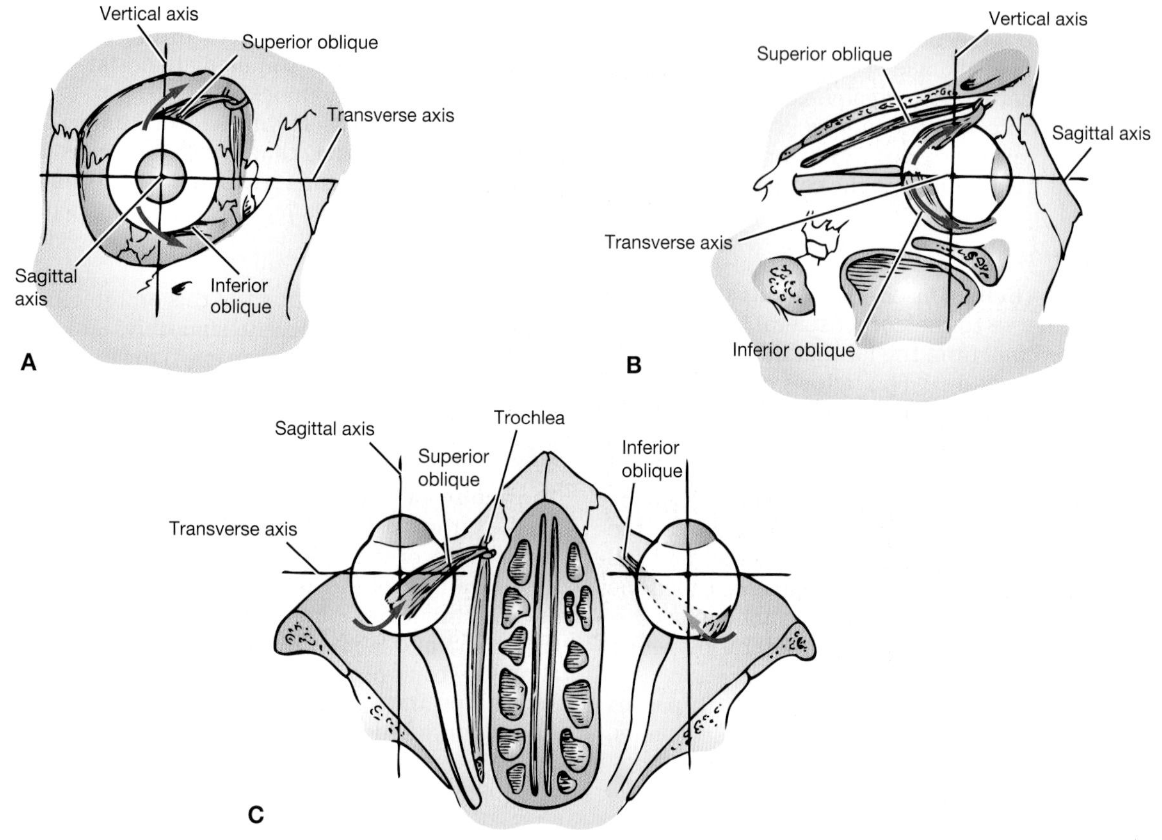

Figure 9.56 Anterior **(A)**, lateral **(B)**, and superior **(C)** views of the orbit showing the actions of the superior and inferior oblique muscles in producing movements of the eyeball.

so that the pupil turns medially inward (adduction) or laterally outward (abduction). **Rotation** is turning about the sagittal (anteroposterior) axis, so that a point on the upper rim of the pupil moves medially (medial rotation) or laterally (lateral rotation).

Extrinsic Ocular (Extraocular) Muscles

Six skeletal muscles (**superior**, **inferior**, **medial**, and **lateral rectus** and **superior** and **inferior oblique**) run from the bony walls of the orbit to insertions on the exterior of the eyeball (Fig. 9.57; see also Figs. 9.52, 9.55, and 9.56). The four rectus muscles arise from a **common tendinous ring** surrounding the optic foramen. The superior oblique arises nearby. Only the inferior oblique originates from the anterior floor of the orbit. Details of the extraocular muscles are summarized in Table 9.5.

Because the superior and the inferior recti are inserted on the medial side of the vertical axis of the eyeball, they raise and depress the pupil, respectively, but also rotate it medially (see Fig. 9.55). For the superior rectus muscle to raise the pupil directly upward, the inferior oblique muscle must assist; for the inferior rectus to depress the pupil directly downward, the superior oblique muscle must assist (see Figs. 9.55 and 9.56). Note that the tendon of the superior oblique muscle passes through a fibrocartilaginous pulley (**trochlea**) attached to the frontal bone. Here, the tendon turns backward and laterally and inserts into the sclera beneath the superior rectus muscle.

Three CNs (oculomotor, trochlear, and abducens) control the six extraocular muscles. The trochlear nerve supplies only the superior oblique muscle. The abducens nerve innervates only the lateral rectus muscle. The oculomotor nerve governs all the remaining muscles. A convenient way to recall this motor organization is with the chemical formula $SO_4(LR_6)_3$. That is, CN IV (4) (trochlear) supplies the superior oblique (SO), CN VI (6) (abducens) supplies the lateral rectus (LR), and CN III (3) (oculomotor) supplies all the others.

Clinical Testing for Actions of Superior and Inferior Recti and Superior and Inferior Oblique Muscles

Because the actions of the superior and inferior recti and the superior and inferior oblique muscles are complicated when a patient is asked to look vertically upward or vertically downward, the physician tests the eye movements where the single action of each muscle predominates (Fig. 9.58).

The origins of the superior and inferior recti are situated about 23° medial to their insertions; therefore,

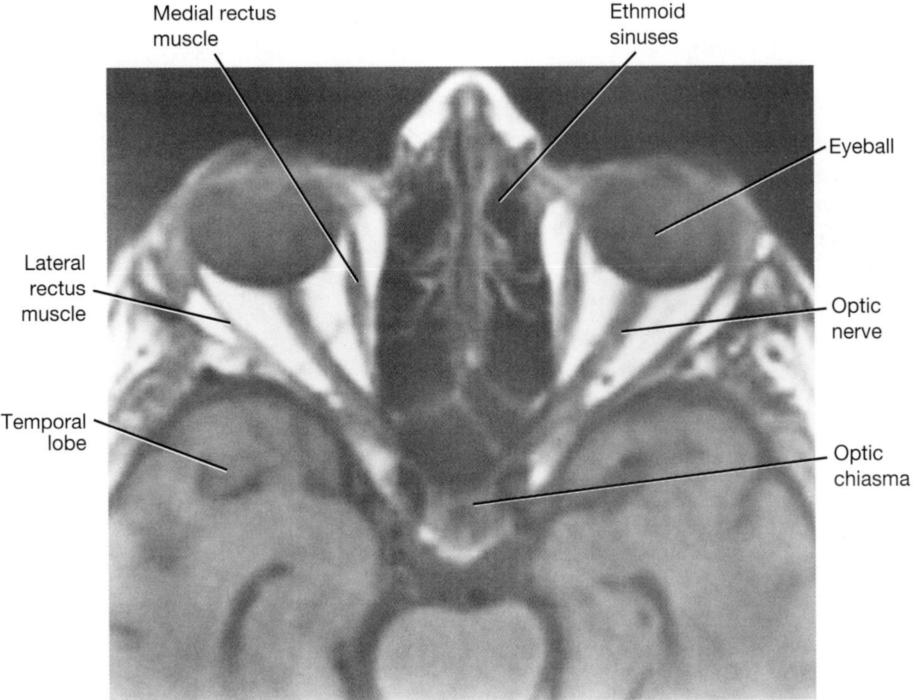

Figure 9.57 Axial (horizontal) MRI showing the contents of the orbital and the cranial cavities. Note that the eyeballs, the optic nerves, the optic chiasma, and the extraocular muscles can be identified.

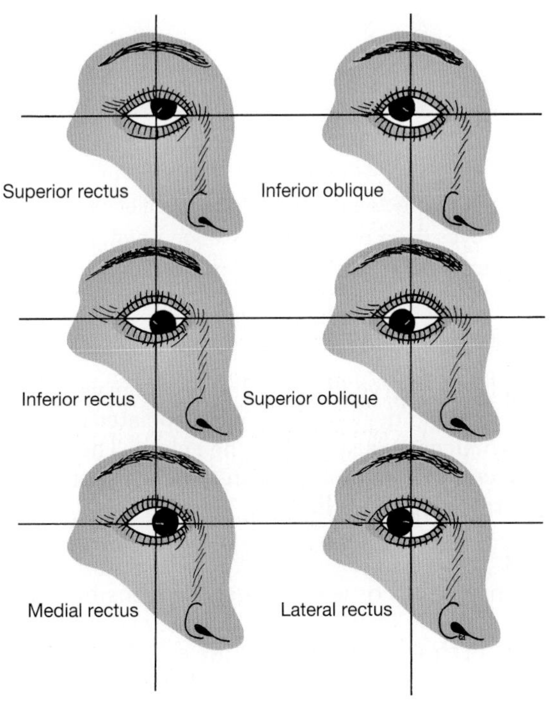

Figure 9.58 Actions of the four recti and two oblique muscles of the right orbit, assuming that each muscle is acting alone. The position of the pupil in relation to the vertical and horizontal planes should be noted in each case. The actions of the superior and inferior recti and the oblique muscles in the living intact eye are tested clinically, as described in the text.

when the patient is asked to turn the pupil laterally (abduct), these muscles are placed in the optimum position to raise (superior rectus) or lower (inferior rectus) the pupil.

The superior and inferior oblique muscles can be tested using the same rationale. The pulley of the superior oblique and the origin of the inferior oblique muscles lie medial and anterior to their insertions. The clinician tests the action of these muscles by asking the patient first to look medially (adduct), thus placing these muscles in the optimum position to lower (superior oblique) or raise (inferior oblique) the pupil. In other words, when you ask a patient to look medially and downward at the tip of their nose, you are testing the superior oblique at its best position. Conversely, by asking the patient to look medially and upward, you are testing the inferior oblique at its best position.

Because the lateral and medial recti are simply placed relative to the eyeball, asking the patient to turn their pupil directly laterally tests the lateral rectus, and turning the pupil directly medially tests the medial rectus.

The cardinal positions of the eyes and the actions of the recti and oblique muscles are shown in Figure 9.59.

Intrinsic Ocular Muscles

Three smooth muscles (**dilator pupillae**, **sphincter pupillae**, and **ciliary muscle**) occupy the eyeball. However, none of these acts to move the eyeball. The intrinsic muscles are discussed later in this chapter.

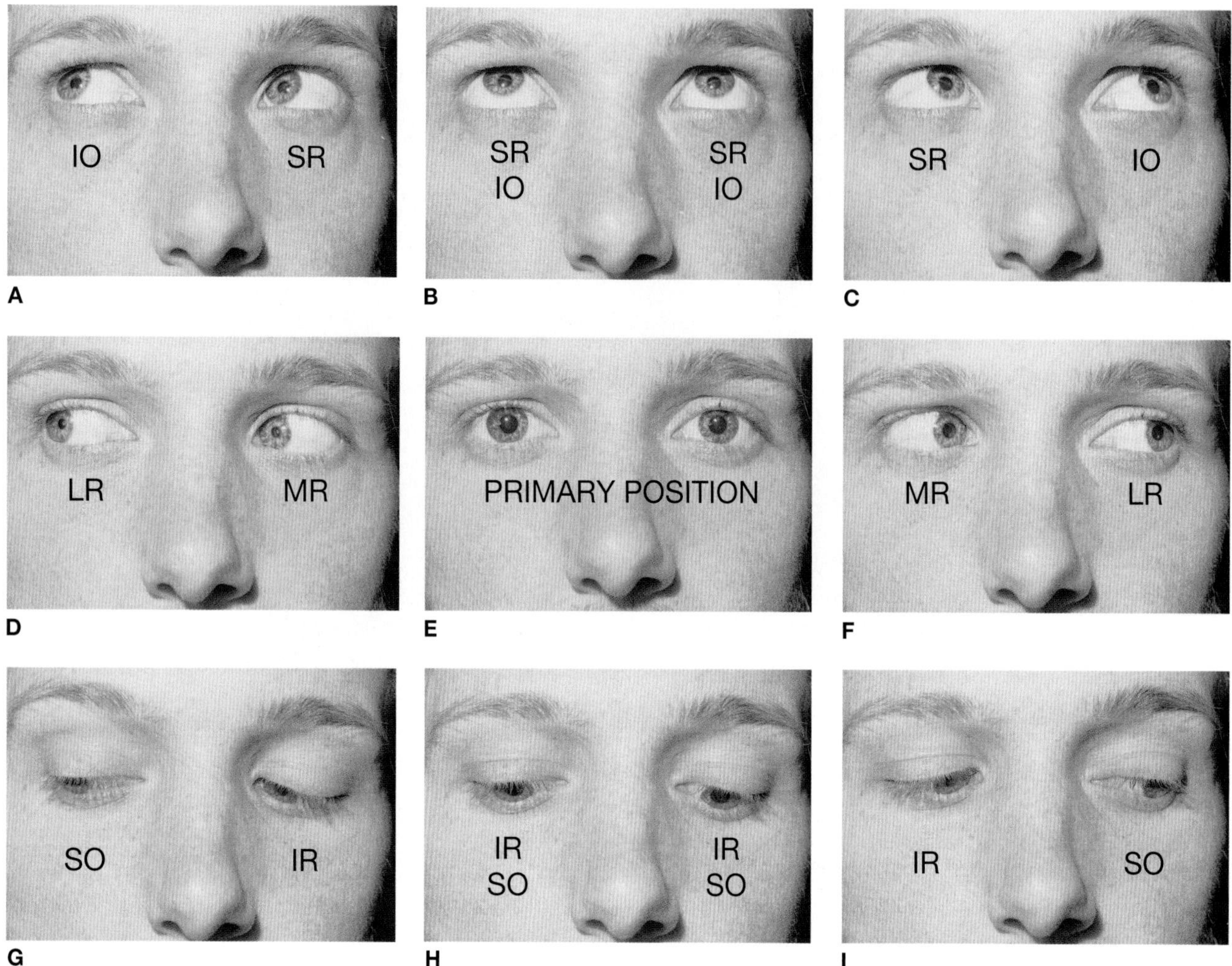

Figure 9.59 Cardinal positions of the right and left eyes and the actions of the recti and the oblique muscles principally responsible for the movements of the eyes. **E.** Primary position, with the eyes fixed on a distant fixation point. All movements begin from the primary position. For example, in frame **D** (looking to the right), the LR is primarily responsible for the right eye moving laterally, whereas the MR is the prime mover for the left eye moving medially. IO, inferior oblique; IR, inferior rectus; LR, lateral rectus; MR, medial rectus; SO, superior oblique; SR, superior rectus.

Eye Structure

The eyeball consists of **three coats** or layers (Fig. 9.60). From external to internal, these are (1) the external **fibrous coat**, (2) middle **vascular coat**, and (3) inner **nervous coat**. The eyeball contains three major supportive/refractive media: **aqueous humor**, **vitreous body**, and the **lens**.

Fibrous Coat

The external, protective fibrous coat is made up of a posterior opaque part, the **sclera**, and an anterior transparent part, the **cornea**.

Sclera

The opaque sclera is composed of dense fibrous tissue and is white. The optic nerve pierces the sclera posteriorly, and the nerve's dural sheath fuses with the sclera. The **lamina cribrosa** is the area of the sclera that is pierced by the nerve fibers of the optic nerve. The ciliary arteries and nerves and their associated veins, the **venae vorticosae**, also pierce the sclera. The sclera is directly continuous in front with the cornea at the corneoscleral junction, or **limbus**.

Cornea

The transparent cornea is largely responsible for the refraction of the light entering the eye and is the most important refractive medium of the eye. This refractive power occurs on the anterior surface of the cornea, where the refractive index of the cornea differs greatly from that of the air. The film of tears secreted from the lacrimal gland is critical in maintaining the normal environment for the corneal epithelial cells. The cornea is in contact with the aqueous humor posteriorly.

Blood supply. The cornea is avascular and devoid of lymphatic drainage. It is nourished by diffusion from the aqueous humor and from the capillaries at its edge.

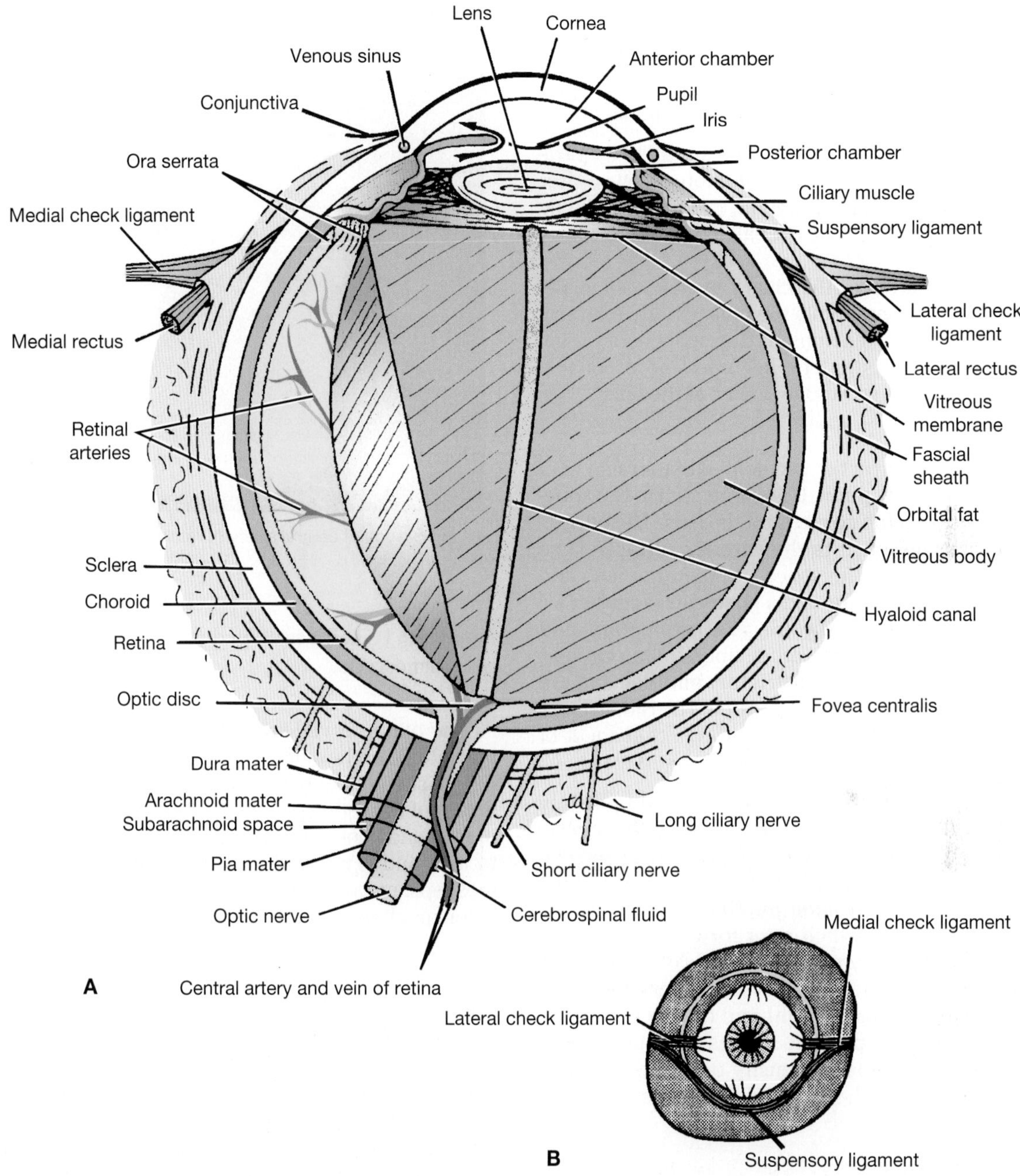

Figure 9.60 **A.** Horizontal section through the eyeball and the optic nerve. Note that the central artery and vein of the retina cross the subarachnoid space to reach the optic nerve. **B.** Check ligaments and suspensory ligament of the eyeball.

Nerve supply. Long ciliary nerves from the ophthalmic division of the trigeminal nerve

Vascular Pigmented Coat

The middle vascular pigmented coat consists, from behind forward, of the **choroid**, the **ciliary body**, and the **iris**.

Choroid

The choroid is composed of an **outer pigmented layer** and an **inner**, **highly vascular layer**.

Ciliary Body

The ciliary body is continuous posteriorly with the choroid, and anteriorly, it lies behind the peripheral margin of the iris. It is composed of the ciliary ring, ciliary processes, and the ciliary muscle.

The **ciliary ring** is the posterior part of the body; its surface has shallow grooves, the **ciliary striae**.

The **ciliary processes** are radially arranged folds, or ridges, to the posterior surfaces of which are connected the **suspensory ligaments of the lens**.

The **ciliary muscle** is composed of meridional and circular fibers of smooth muscle. The meridional fibers run backward from the region of the corneoscleral junction to the ciliary processes. The circular fibers are fewer in number and lie internal to the meridional fibers.

- **Nerve supply:** The ciliary muscle is supplied by parasympathetic fibers from the oculomotor nerve. After synapsing in the ciliary ganglion, the postganglionic fibers pass forward to the eyeball in the short ciliary nerves.
- **Action:** Contraction of the ciliary muscle, especially the meridional fibers, pulls the ciliary body forward. This relieves the tension in the suspensory ligaments, and the elastic lens becomes more convex. This increases the refractive power of the lens.

Iris and Pupil

The **iris** is a thin, contractile, pigmented diaphragm with a central aperture, the **pupil**. It is suspended in the aqueous humor between the cornea and the lens. The periphery of the iris is attached to the anterior surface of the ciliary body. It divides the space between the lens and the cornea into an **anterior** and a **posterior chamber**.

The muscle fibers of the iris are involuntary and consist of circular and radiating fibers. The circular fibers form the **sphincter (constrictor) pupillae** and are arranged around the margin of the pupil. The radial fibers form the **dilator pupillae** and consist of a thin sheet of radial fibers that lie close to the posterior surface.

- **Nerve supply:** The **sphincter pupillae** is supplied by parasympathetic fibers from the oculomotor nerve. After synapsing in the ciliary ganglion, the postganglionic fibers pass forward to the eyeball in the short ciliary nerves. The **dilator pupillae** is supplied by sympathetic fibers, which pass forward to the eyeball in the long ciliary nerves.
- **Action:** The sphincter pupillae constricts the pupil in the presence of bright light and during accommodation. The dilator pupillae dilates the pupil in the presence of light of low intensity or in the presence of excessive sympathetic activity such as occurs in fright.

Nervous Coat

The inner nervous (sensory) coat consists of the **retina**. The retina consists of an **outer pigmented layer** and an **inner nervous layer**. Its outer surface is in contact with the choroid, and its inner surface is in contact with the vitreous body. The posterior three quarters of the retina is the receptor organ. Its anterior edge forms a wavy ring, the **ora serrata**, where the nervous tissues end. The anterior part of the retina is nonreceptive and consists of pigment cells, with a deeper layer of columnar epithelium. This anterior part of the retina covers the ciliary processes and the back of the iris.

At the center of the posterior part of the retina is an oval, yellowish area, the **macula lutea**, which is the area of the retina for the most distinct vision. It has a central depression, the **fovea centralis** (Fig. 9.61; see also Fig. 9.60).

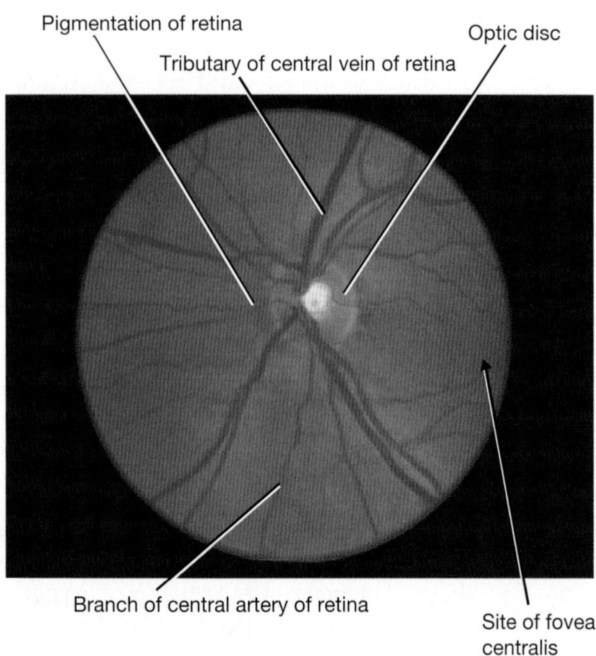

Figure 9.61 Left ocular fundus as seen with an ophthalmoscope.

The optic nerve leaves the retina about 3 mm to the medial side of the macula lutea by the optic disc. The **optic disc** is slightly depressed at its center, where the **central artery of the retina** pierces it. There is a complete absence of rods and cones at the optic disc, so that it is insensitive to light and is referred to as the **blind spot**. On ophthalmoscopic examination, the optic disc appears pale pink in color, much paler than the surrounding retina.

Aqueous Humor

The aqueous humor is a clear fluid that fills the anterior and posterior chambers of the eyeball (see Fig. 9.60). It is believed to be a secretion from the ciliary processes, from which it enters the posterior chamber. It then flows into the anterior chamber through the pupil and is drained away through the spaces at the iridocorneal angle into the **canal of Schlemm**. Obstruction to the draining of the aqueous humor results in a rise in intraocular pressure called **glaucoma**. This can produce degenerative changes in the retina, with consequent blindness.

The function of the aqueous humor is to support the wall of the eyeball by exerting internal pressure and thus maintaining its optical shape. It also nourishes the cornea and the lens and removes the products of metabolism; these functions are important because the cornea and the lens do not possess a blood supply.

Vitreous Body

The vitreous body is a transparent gel that fills the eyeball behind the lens. The **hyaloid canal** is a narrow channel that runs through the vitreous body from the optic disc to the posterior surface of the lens. In the fetus, it is filled by the **hyaloid artery**, which disappears before birth.

The function of the vitreous body is to contribute slightly to the magnifying power of the eye. It supports the posterior surface of the lens and assists in holding the neural part of the retina against the pigmented part of the retina.

Lens

The lens is a transparent, biconvex structure enclosed in a transparent capsule. It is situated behind the iris and in front of the vitreous body and is encircled by the ciliary processes.

The lens consists of an elastic **capsule**, which envelops the structure; a **cuboidal epithelium**, which is confined to the anterior surface of the lens; and **lens fibers**, which are formed from the cuboidal epithelium at the equator of the lens. The lens fibers make up the bulk of the lens.

The elastic lens capsule is under tension, causing the lens constantly to endeavor to assume a globular rather than a disc shape. The equatorial region, or circumference, of the lens attaches to the ciliary processes of the ciliary body by the **suspensory ligament**. The pull of the radiating fibers of the suspensory ligament tends to keep the elastic lens flattened so that the eye can be focused on distant objects.

Eye Accommodation

To accommodate the eye for visualizing close objects, the ciliary muscle contracts and pulls the ciliary body forward and inward so that the radiating fibers of the suspensory ligament are relaxed. This allows the elastic lens to assume a more globular shape.

With advancing age, the lens becomes denser and less elastic; as a result, the ability to accommodate decreases (**presbyopia**). This disability can be overcome using an additional lens (eg, glasses or contact lenses) to assist the eye in focusing on nearby objects.

Pupil Constriction during Eye Accommodation

To ensure that the light rays pass through the central part of the lens so spherical aberration is diminished during accommodation for near objects, the sphincter pupillae muscle contracts so the pupil becomes smaller.

Eye Convergence during Lens Accommodation

In humans, the retinae of both eyes focus on only one set of objects (single binocular vision). When an object moves from a distance toward an individual, the eyes converge so that a single object, not two, is seen. Convergence of the eyes results from the coordinated contraction of the medial rectus muscles.

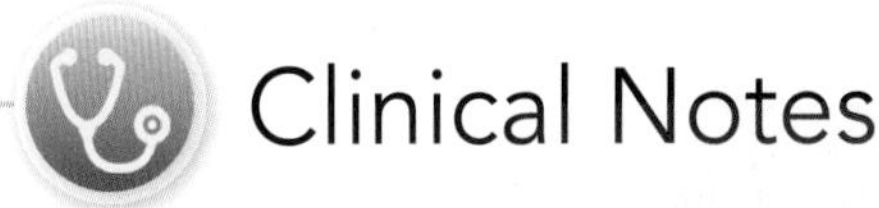

Clinical Notes

Eye Trauma

Although the eyeball is well protected by the surrounding bony orbit, it is protected anteriorly only from large objects, such as tennis balls, which tend to strike the orbital margin but not the globe. The bony orbit provides no protection from small objects, such as golf balls, which can cause severe damage to the eye. Careful examination of the eyeball relative to the orbital margins shows that it is least protected from the lateral side.

Blowout fractures of the orbital floor involving the maxillary sinus commonly occur as a result of blunt force to the face. If the force is applied to the eye, the orbital fat explodes inferiorly into the maxillary sinus, fracturing the orbital floor. Blowout fractures can cause displacement of the eyeball, with resulting symptoms of double vision (**diplopia**). The fracture can also injure the infraorbital nerve, producing loss of sensation of the skin of the cheek and the gum on that side. Entrapment of the inferior rectus muscle in the fracture may limit upward gaze.

Strabismus

Many cases of strabismus are nonparalytic and are caused by an imbalance in the action of opposing muscles. This type of strabismus is known as **concomitant strabismus** and is common in infancy.

Pupillary Reflexes

The pupillary reflexes—that is, the reaction of the pupils to light and accommodation—depend on the integrity of nervous pathways. In the **direct light reflex**, the normal pupil reflexively contracts when a light is shone into the patient's eye. The nervous impulses pass from the retina along the optic nerve to the optic chiasma and then along the optic tract. Before reaching the lateral geniculate body, the fibers concerned with this reflex leave the tract and pass to the oculomotor nuclei on both sides via the pretectal nuclei. From the parasympathetic part of the nucleus, efferent fibers leave the midbrain in the oculomotor nerve and reach the ciliary ganglion via the nerve to the inferior oblique. Postganglionic fibers pass to the constrictor pupillae muscles via the short ciliary nerves.

Shining the light in one eye and noting the contraction of the pupil in the opposite eye tests the **consensual light reflex**. This reflex is possible because the afferent pathway just described travels to the parasympathetic nuclei of both oculomotor nerves.

The **accommodation reflex** is the contraction of the pupil that occurs when a person suddenly focuses on a near object after having focused on a distant object. The nerve impulses pass from the retina via the optic nerve, optic chiasma, optic tract, lateral geniculate body, optic radiation, and the cerebral cortex of the occipital lobe of the brain. The visual cortex is connected to the eye field of the frontal cortex. From here, efferent pathways pass to the parasympathetic nucleus of the oculomotor nerve. From there, the efferent impulses reach the constrictor pupillae via the oculomotor nerve, ciliary ganglion, and the short ciliary nerves.

TEMPORAL, INFRATEMPORAL, AND PTERYGOPALATINE FOSSAE

The temporal, infratemporal, and pterygopalatine fossae are adjoining regions that form a continuous, progressively deepening pathway from the superficial lateral to deep lateral aspects of the head. The importance of these regions is that they serve as (1) attachment sites for the muscles of mastication (therefore, the morphology of the region determines much about the lines of action of the muscles) and (2) distribution centers for major neurovascular networks. The main contents of these fossae include:

- **Major muscles of mastication** (see Mandible, discussed earlier)
- **Superficial temporal artery**
- **Maxillary artery**
- **Pterygoid venous plexus**
- **Maxillary nerve**
- **Mandibular nerve**
- **Chorda tympani nerve**
- **Otic ganglion**
- **Pterygopalatine ganglion**

Temporal Fossa

This is a roughly oval area on the superficial lateral side of the head (Fig. 9.62; see also Fig. 9.5). Its major contents are the **temporalis muscle** and the terminal distribution of the **superficial temporal artery**.

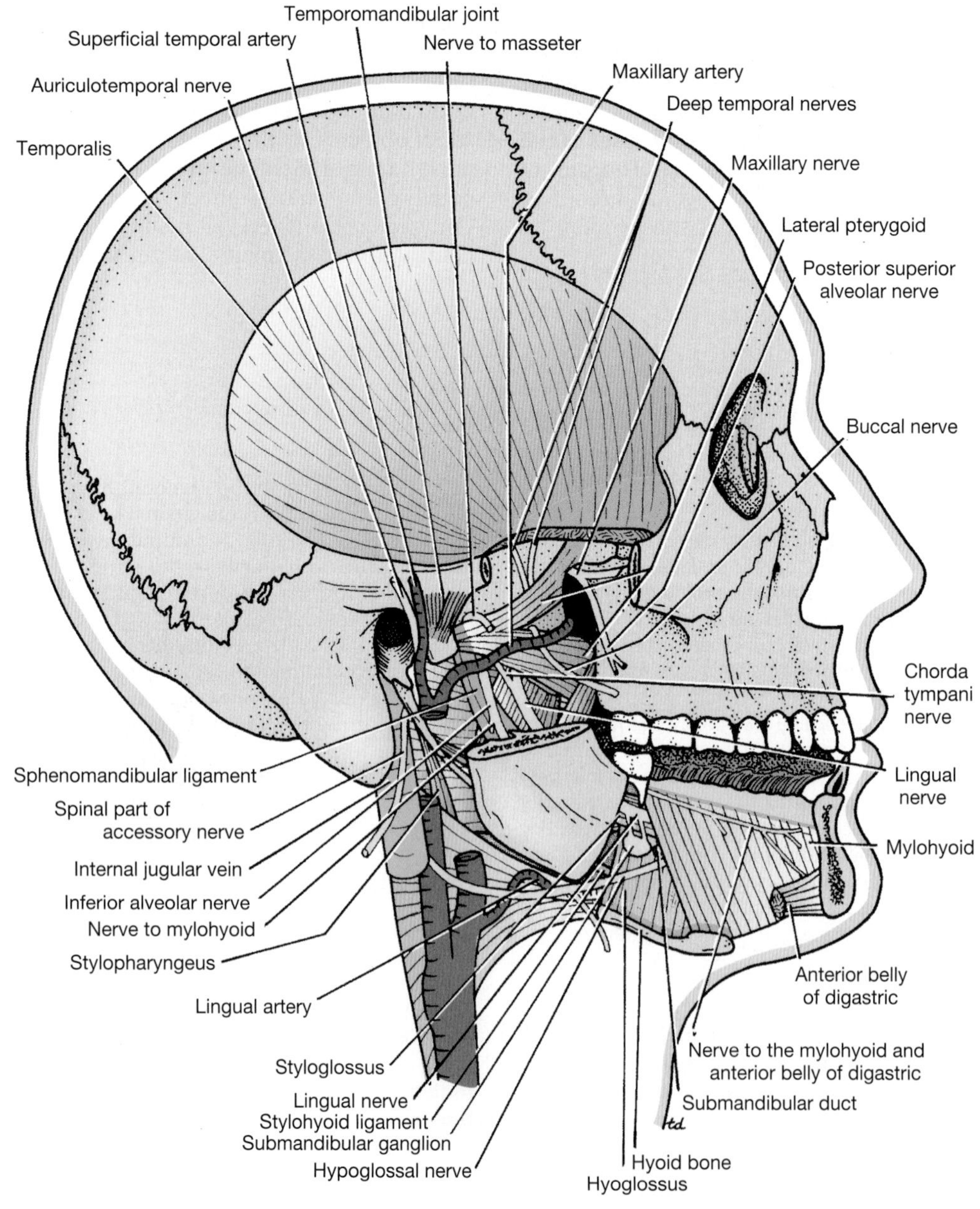

Figure 9.62 Temporal, infratemporal, and submandibular regions. Parts of the zygomatic arch, the ramus, and the body of the mandible have been removed to display deeper structures.

Boundaries

- **Anterior:** Frontal process of the zygomatic bone
- **Superior:** Temporal lines on the frontal and parietal bones
- **Posterior:** Posterior root of the zygomatic arch
- **Inferior:** Infratemporal crest
- **Lateral:** Zygomatic arch

Primary Communications

- **Orbit** via the inferior orbital fissure
- **Infratemporal fossa** deep to the zygomatic arch

Infratemporal Fossa

This is an irregularly shaped area located inferior and medial to the zygomatic arch, between the ramus of the mandible and the pharynx (Fig. 9.63; see also Fig. 9.62). Its major contents are the **medial** and **lateral pterygoid muscles**, **maxillary artery**, **pterygoid venous plexus**, **mandibular nerve**, **chorda tympani nerve**, and **otic ganglion**.

Boundaries

- **Anterior:** Posterior (infratemporal) surface of the maxilla

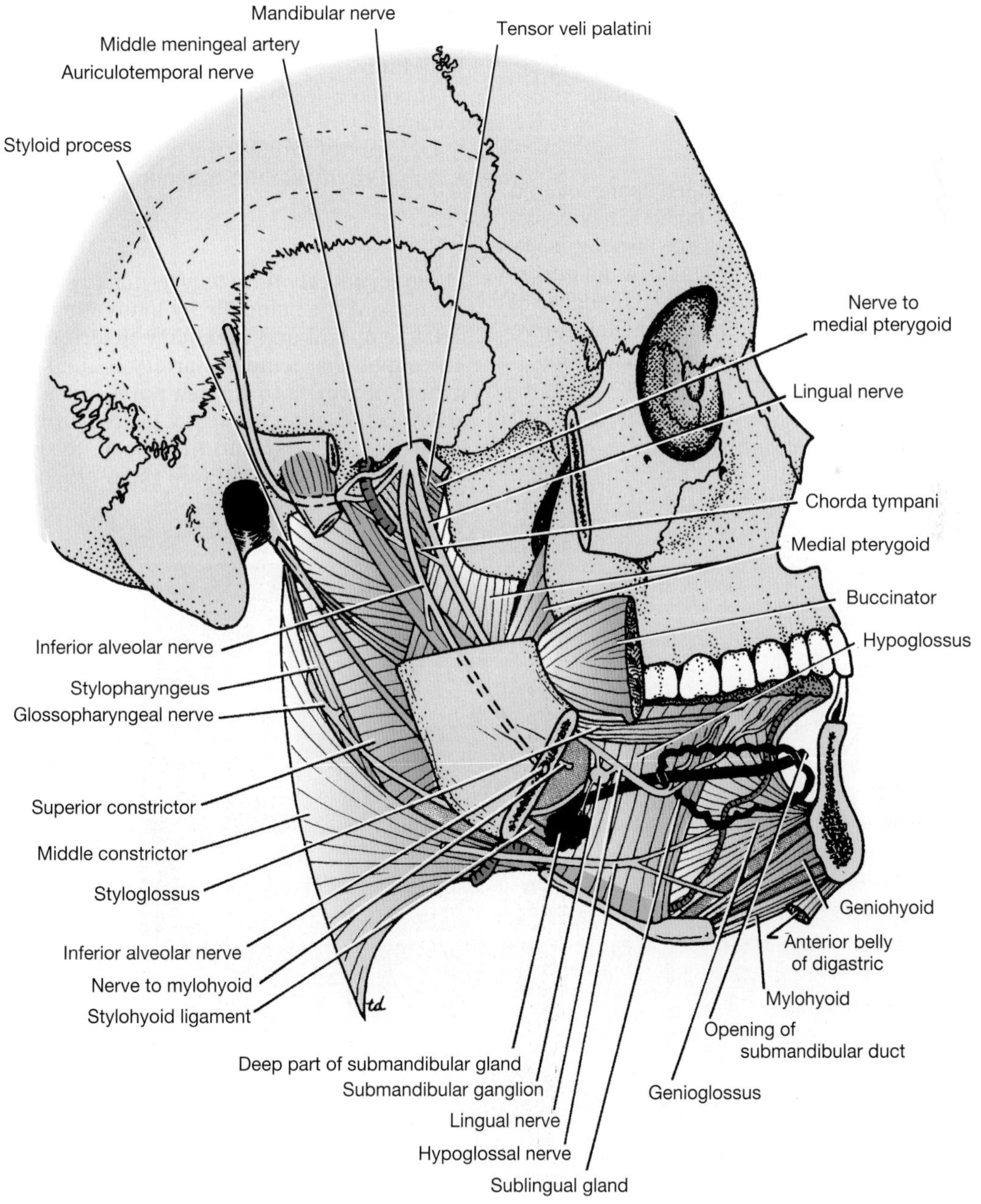

Figure 9.63 Infratemporal and submandibular regions. Parts of the zygomatic arch, the ramus, and the body of the mandible have been removed. Mylohyoid and lateral pterygoid muscles have also been removed to display deeper structures. The outline of the sublingual gland is shown as a *solid black wavy line*.

- **Posterior:** Mandibular fossa, styloid process, spine of the sphenoid bone
- **Superior:** Infratemporal crest
- **Inferior:** Alveolar border of the maxilla
- **Medial:** Lateral pterygoid plate
- **Lateral:** Zygomatic arch and ramus of the mandible

Primary Communications

- **Temporal fossa** deep to the zygomatic arch
- **Cranial cavity** via the foramen ovale and foramen spinosum
- **Tympanic cavity** via the petrotympanic fissure
- **Maxillary teeth and sinus** through the posterior superior alveolar foramina
- **Orbit** by way of the inferior orbital fissure
- **Pterygopalatine fossa** via the pterygomaxillary fissure
- **Submandibular region** deep to the mandible

Pterygopalatine Fossa

This is a small, roughly pyramidal-shaped space located in the deep lateral aspect of the head, immediately posterior and inferior to the orbit (Fig. 9.64: see also Fig. 9.53). Despite its small size, this fossa is a significant neurovascular hub. Its major contents are the terminal branches of the **maxillary artery**, **maxillary nerve branches**, **nerve of the pterygoid canal**, and **pterygopalatine ganglion**.

Boundaries

- **Anterior:** Posterior (infratemporal) surface of the maxilla
- **Posterior:** Base of the pterygoid process of the sphenoid bone
- **Superior:** Apex of the orbit
- **Inferior:** Inferior margin of the pterygomaxillary fissure
- **Medial:** Posterolateral wall of the nasal cavity (perpendicular plate of the palatine bone)
- **Lateral:** Pterygomaxillary fissure

Primary Communications

- **Infratemporal fossa** via the pterygomaxillary fissure
- **Cranial cavity** through the foramen rotundum
- **External base of the skull** through the pterygoid canal
- **Nasopharynx** via the pharyngeal canal
- **Orbit** by way of the inferior orbital fissure
- **Maxillary teeth and sinus** through the infraorbital canal
- **Oral cavity** through the pterygopalatine canal
- **Nasal cavity** via the sphenopalatine foramen

Arteries

The **external carotid artery** terminates at approximately the neck of the mandible by bifurcating into the **superficial temporal** and **maxillary arteries** (see Fig. 9.62). The superficial temporal artery is the smaller branch; it runs upward into the temporal fossa. The maxillary artery is the larger branch; it passes forward across the infratemporal fossa and then deep, through the pterygomaxillary fissure, and into the pterygopalatine fossa.

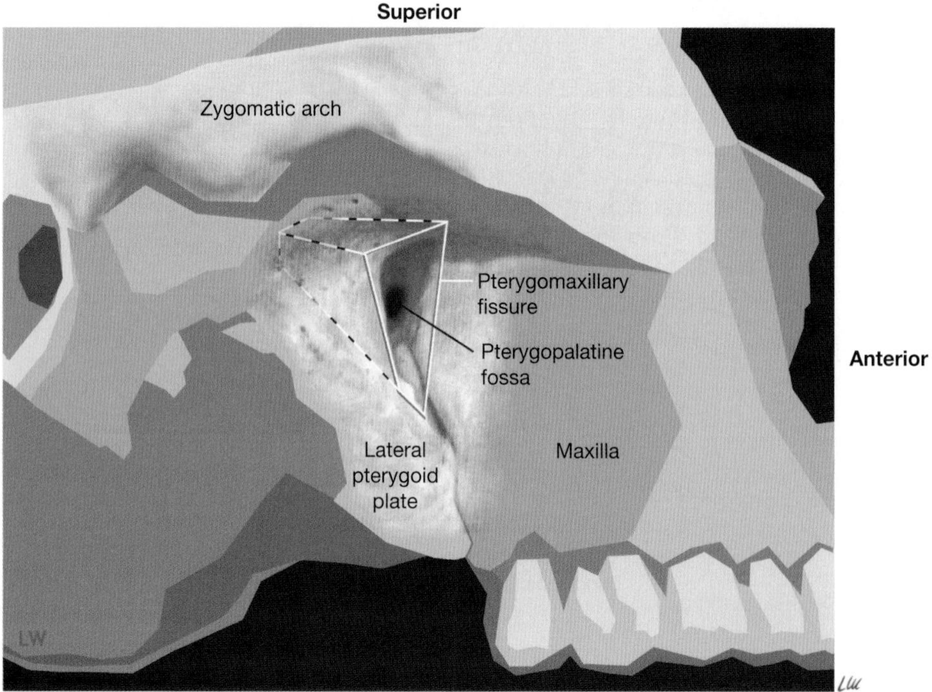

Figure 9.64 Schematic showing the pterygopalatine fossa. Think of the pterygomaxillary fissure as the doorway into a room (the pterygopalatine fossa). The fissure is lateral (superficial) to the fossa. The *solid lines* are the frame of the doorway (ie, the fissure). The *dashed lines* mark the walls of the room (ie, the fossa) extending medially.

The major arterial branches are listed here for organizational purposes. See Head and Neck Arteries for further details.

Branches of the Superficial Temporal Artery

- **Transverse facial artery**
- **Anterior (frontal) branch**
- **Posterior (parietal) branch**

Branches of the Maxillary Artery

Branches in the infratemporal fossa include the following:

- **Small branches to the external auditory meatus and tympanic membrane**
- **Middle meningeal artery**
- **Inferior alveolar artery**
- **Muscular branches to the muscles of mastication**
- **Posterior superior alveolar artery**

Branches in the pterygopalatine fossa include the following:

- **Descending palatine artery**
- **Pharyngeal branch**
- **Artery of the pterygoid canal**
- **Infraorbital artery**
- **Sphenopalatine artery**

Nerves

The **maxillary nerve**, a division of the trigeminal nerve, runs through the foramen rotundum and enters the pterygopalatine fossa (see Fig. 9.53). From here, it sends numerous sensory branches across a wide distribution in the cranium, midface, nasal cavity, oral cavity, and nasopharynx.

The **mandibular nerve**, another division of the trigeminal nerve, passes through the foramen ovale and enters the deep upper aspect of the infratemporal fossa (see Figs. 9.62 and 9.63). It immediately sends many motor and sensory branches to the cranium, infratemporal fossa, temporal fossa, lower jaw, oral cavity, and lower face.

The major nerve branches are listed here for organizational purposes. See Cranial Nerves and Autonomic Nervous System for further details.

Maxillary Nerve Branches

- **Middle meningeal nerve**
- **Ganglionic branches to the pterygopalatine ganglion**
- **Zygomatic nerve**
- **Posterior superior alveolar nerve**
- **Infraorbital nerve**
- **Greater and lesser palatine nerves**
- **Nasopalatine nerve**
- **Pharyngeal nerve**

Mandibular Nerve Branches

- **Meningeal (spinous) nerve**
- **Motor branches to the muscles of mastication, tensor veli palatini, and tensor tympani**
- **Buccal nerve**
- **Lingual nerve**
- **Inferior alveolar nerve**
- **Auriculotemporal nerve**

The **nerve of the pterygoid canal** is a composite of the **greater petrosal nerve** (parasympathetic branch of the facial nerve) and the **deep petrosal nerve** (sympathetic bundle from the carotid plexus). It joins the **pterygopalatine ganglion** and distributes postganglionic fibers along the branches of the maxillary nerve (see Fig. 9.11).

The **lesser petrosal nerve** is a parasympathetic component of the glossopharyngeal nerve. It runs from the middle ear into the infratemporal fossa, where it joins the **otic ganglion**. Postganglionic fibers then join the **auriculotemporal branch** of the mandibular nerve. The lesser petrosal nerve provides the secretomotor fibers to the **parotid gland**.

The **chorda tympani nerve** is a branch of the facial nerve; it carries parasympathetic and taste fibers. The chorda tympani joins the **lingual branch** of the mandibular nerve deep in the infratemporal fossa and distributes its fibers into the oral floor through the lingual nerve (see Fig. 9.63).

NECK

The neck is the region of the body that lies between the lower margin of the mandible above and the suprasternal notch and the upper border of the clavicle below. The cervical part of the vertebral column, which is convex forward and supports the skull, forms the bony longitudinal axis of the neck. The hyoid bone moves relatively freely and anchors the tongue. A mass of extensor muscles lies posterior to the vertebrae, and a smaller group of flexor muscles sits anteriorly (Fig. 9.65). Parts of the respiratory system (larynx and trachea) run through the anterior central region of the neck, and parts of the alimentary system (pharynx and esophagus) pass through the posterior central region. At the sides of these structures are the vertically running carotid arteries, internal jugular veins, vagus nerve, and deep cervical lymph nodes.

Skin and Superficial Fascia

The natural lines of cleavage of the skin are constant and run almost horizontally around the neck. This is important clinically because an incision along a cleavage line will heal as a narrow scar, whereas one that crosses the lines will heal as a wide or heaped-up scar. The superficial fascia of the neck forms a thin layer that encloses the cutaneous nerves, the platysma muscle, the superficial veins, and the superficial lymph nodes.

Cutaneous Nerves

The **posterior rami of the C2 to C5 nerves** supply the skin overlying the trapezius muscle on the back of the

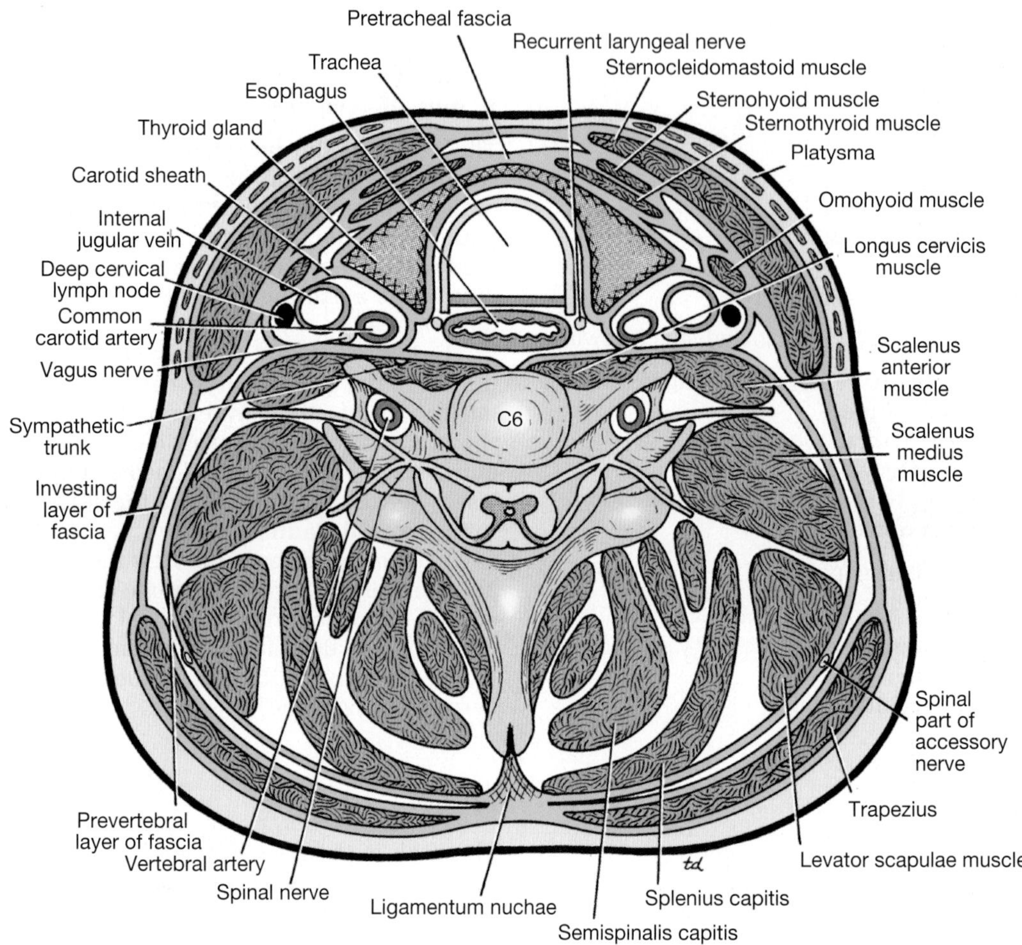

Figure 9.65 Cross section of the neck at the level of the C6 vertebra.

neck and the back of the scalp as high as the vertex (see Fig. 9.26). The **greater occipital nerve** is a branch of the posterior ramus of the C2 nerve. The C1 nerve has no cutaneous branch.

The skin of the front and sides of the neck is supplied by anterior rami of the C2 to C4 nerves through branches of the **cervical plexus**. The branches emerge from beneath the posterior border of the sternocleidomastoid muscle.

The **lesser occipital nerve** (C2) hooks around the accessory nerve and ascends along the posterior border of the sternocleidomastoid (SCM) muscle to supply the skin over the lateral part of the occipital region and the medial surface of the auricle.

The **great auricular nerve** (C2 and C3) ascends across the SCM muscle and divides into branches that supply the skin over the angle of the mandible, on the parotid gland, and on both surfaces of the auricle.

The **transverse cutaneous nerve** (C2 and C3) emerges from behind the middle of the posterior border of the SCM muscle. It passes forward across that muscle and divides into branches that supply the skin on the anterior and lateral surfaces of the neck, from the body of the mandible to the sternum.

The **supraclavicular nerves** (C3 and C4) emerge from beneath the posterior border of the SCM muscle and descend across the side of the neck. They pass onto the chest wall and shoulder region and down to the level of rib 2. The medial supraclavicular nerve crosses the medial end of the clavicle and supplies the skin as far as the median plane. The intermediate supraclavicular nerve crosses the middle of the clavicle and supplies the skin of the chest wall. The lateral supraclavicular nerve crosses the lateral end of the clavicle and supplies the skin over the shoulder and the upper half of the deltoid muscle; this nerve also supplies the posterior aspect of the shoulder as far down as the spine of the scapula.

Platysma

The platysma is a thin, broad, clinically important muscular sheet embedded in the superficial fascia (Fig. 9.66; see also Fig. 9.20). It is summarized in Table 9.6. Although located mainly in the neck, the platysma acts on the skin of the mouth. It is one of the facial muscles derived from the first pharyngeal arch and innervated by the facial nerve.

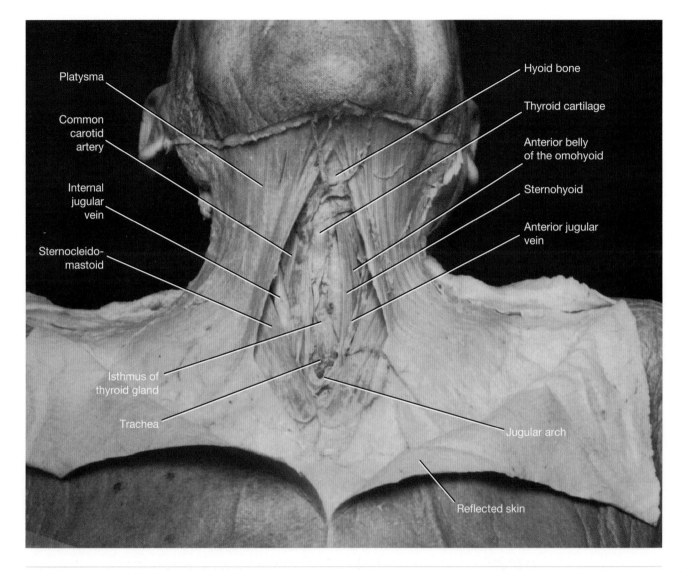

Platysma
Common carotid artery
Internal jugular vein
Sternocleido-mastoid
Isthmus of thyroid gland
Trachea
Hyoid bone
Thyroid cartilage
Anterior belly of the omohyoid
Sternohyoid
Anterior jugular vein
Jugular arch
Reflected skin

Figure 9.66 Dissection of the anterior aspect of the neck showing the platysma muscles and the lower ends of the sternocleidomastoid muscles on both sides. The skin has been reflected downward.

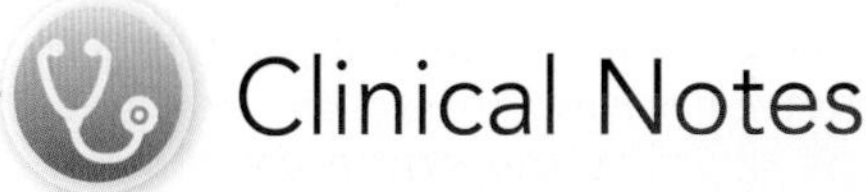

Clinical Notes

Clinical Identification of the Platysma

The platysma can be seen as a thin sheet of muscle just beneath the skin by having the patient clench their jaws firmly. The muscle extends from the body of the mandible downward over the clavicle onto the anterior chest wall.

Platysma Tone and Neck Incisions

In lacerations or surgical incisions in the neck, it is very important that the subcutaneous layer with the platysma be carefully sutured, because the tone of the platysma can pull on the scar tissue, resulting in broad, unsightly scars.

Platysma Innervation and Mouth Distortion

The **cervical branch of the facial nerve** (see Fig. 9.25) innervates the platysma muscle. This nerve emerges from the lower end of the parotid gland and travels forward to the platysma; it then sometimes crosses the lower border of the mandible to supply the depressor anguli oris muscle. Thus, skin lacerations over the mandible or upper part of the neck that affect the platysma may distort the shape of the mouth.

Table 9.6 Neck Muscles

MUSCLE	ORIGIN	INSERTION	NERVE SUPPLY	ACTION
Platysma	Deep fascia over pectoralis major and deltoid	Body of the mandible and angle of the mouth	Facial nerve cervical branch	Depresses the mandible and angle of the mouth
Sternocleidomastoid	Manubrium sterni and medial third of the clavicle	Mastoid process of the temporal bone and occipital bone	Spinal part of accessory nerve and C2 and C3	Two muscles acting together extend the head and flex the neck; one muscle rotates the head to the opposite side
Digastric, posterior belly	Digastric notch on the mastoid process of the temporal bone	Intermediate tendon (held to hyoid by fascial sling)	Facial nerve	Depresses the mandible or elevates hyoid bone
Digastric, anterior belly	Digastric fossa on the body of the mandible	Intermediate tendon (held to hyoid by fascial sling)	Nerve to mylohyoid	
Stylohyoid	Styloid process	Body of hyoid bone	Facial nerve	Elevates hyoid bone
Mylohyoid	Mylohyoid line of body of the mandible	Body of hyoid bone and fibrous raphe	Inferior alveolar nerve	Elevates floor of the mouth and hyoid bone or depresses the mandible
Geniohyoid	Inferior mental spine of the mandible	Body of hyoid bone	C1 nerve	Elevates hyoid bone or depresses mandible
Sternohyoid	Manubrium sterni and clavicle	Body of hyoid bone	Ansa cervicalis; C1 to C3	Depresses hyoid bone
Sternothyroid	Manubrium sterni	Oblique line on lamina of thyroid cartilage	Ansa cervicalis; C1 to C3	Depresses the larynx
Thyrohyoid	Oblique line on lamina of thyroid cartilage	Lower border of body of hyoid bone	C1 nerve	Depresses hyoid bone or elevates the larynx
Omohyoid, inferior belly	Upper margin of scapula and suprascapular ligament	Intermediate tendon (held to clavicle and rib 1 by fascial sling)	Ansa cervicalis; C1 to C3	Depresses hyoid bone
Omohyoid, superior belly	Intermediate tendon (held to clavicle and rib 1 by fascial sling)	Lower border of body of hyoid bone		
Scalenus anterior	Transverse processes of C3 to C6 vertebrae	Rib 1	C4 to C6	Elevates rib 1; laterally flexes and rotates cervical part of the vertebral column
Scalenus medius	Transverse processes of C1 to C6 vertebrae	Rib 1	Anterior rami of cervical nerves	Elevates rib 1; laterally flexes and rotates cervical part of the vertebral column
Scalenus posterior	Transverse processes of C5 to C7 vertebrae	Rib 2	Anterior rami of cervical nerves	Elevates rib 2; laterally flexes and rotates cervical part of the vertebral column

External Jugular Vein

The external jugular vein begins just behind the angle of the mandible by the union of the **posterior auricular vein** with the **posterior division of the retromandibular vein** (Fig. 9.67). It descends obliquely across the SCM muscle and, just above the clavicle in the posterior triangle, pierces the deep fascia and drains into the subclavian vein. It varies considerably in size, and its course extends from the angle of the mandible to the middle of the clavicle.

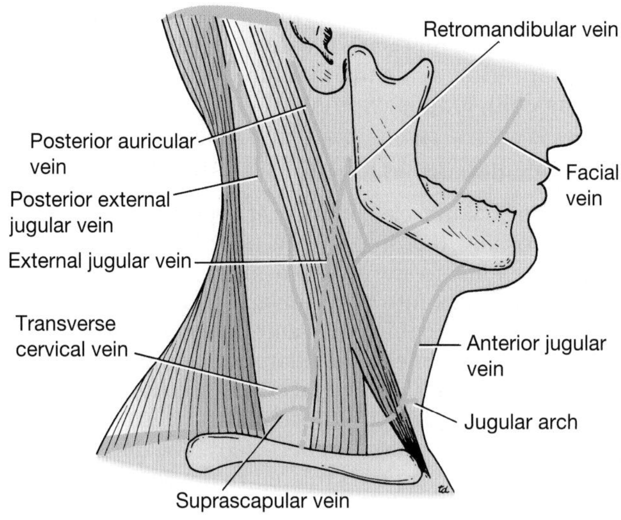

Figure 9.67 Major superficial veins of the face and neck.

Tributaries

The external jugular vein has the following tributaries (see Fig. 9.67):

- **Posterior auricular vein**
- **Posterior division of the retromandibular vein**
- **Posterior external jugular vein**: a small vein that drains the posterior part of the scalp and neck and joins the external jugular vein about halfway along its course
- **Transverse cervical vein**
- **Suprascapular vein**
- **Anterior jugular vein**

The anterior jugular vein begins just below the chin, by the union of several small veins. It runs down the neck close to the midline. Just above the suprasternal notch, the veins of the two sides unite by a transverse trunk called the **jugular arch**. The vein then turns sharply laterally and passes deep to the sternocleidomastoid muscle to drain into the external jugular vein.

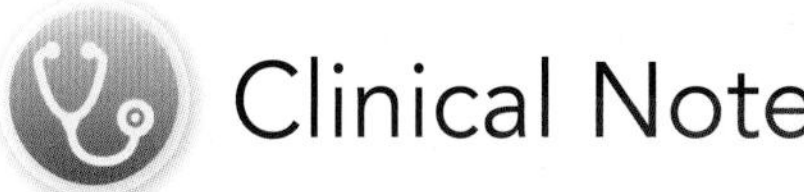

Clinical Notes

External Jugular Vein Visibility

The external jugular vein is less obvious in children and females because their subcutaneous tissue tends to be thicker than the tissue of adult males. In obese individuals, the vein may be difficult to identify even when they are asked to hold their breath, which impedes the venous return to the right side of the heart and distends the vein.

The superficial veins of the neck tend to be enlarged and often tortuous in professional singers because of prolonged periods of raised intrathoracic pressure.

External Jugular Vein as a Venous Manometer

The external jugular vein serves as a useful venous manometer. Normally, when the patient is lying at a horizontal angle of 30°, the level of the blood in the external jugular veins reaches about one third of the way up the neck. As the patient sits up, the blood level falls until it is no longer visible behind the clavicle.

External Jugular Vein Catheterization

The external jugular vein can be used for catheterization, but the presence of valves or tortuosity may make the passage of the catheter difficult. Because the right external jugular vein is in the most direct line with the superior vena cava, it is the one most used (Fig. 9.68). The vein is catheterized about halfway between the level of the cricoid cartilage and the clavicle. The passage of the catheter should be performed during inspiration when the valves are open.

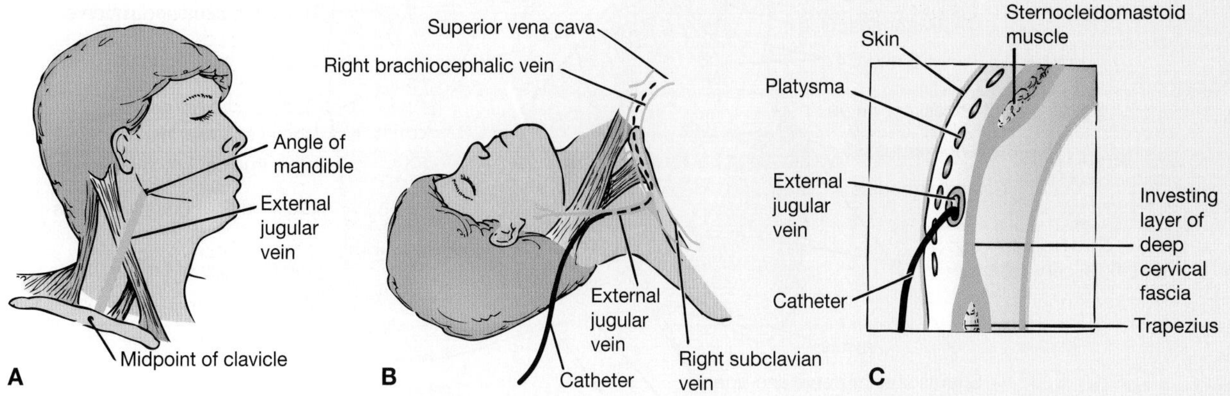

Figure 9.68 Catheterization of the right external jugular vein. **A.** Surface marking of the vein. **B.** Site of catheterization. Note how the external jugular vein joins the subclavian vein at a right angle. **C.** Cross section of the neck showing the relationships of the external jugular vein as it crosses the posterior triangle of the neck.

Superficial Lymph Nodes

The **superficial cervical lymph nodes** lie along the external jugular vein superficial to the SCM muscle (see Fig. 9.23). They receive lymph vessels from the occipital and mastoid lymph nodes and drain into the **deep cervical lymph nodes**.

Neck Muscles

The muscles of the neck are summarized in Table 9.6 and illustrated in Figures 9.66 and 9.69 to 9.72. The SCM muscle and the muscles anterior to it, plus the inferior belly of the omohyoid, are elongated bands and are collectively referred to as the **strap muscles** of the neck. Those superior to the hyoid bone are the **suprahyoid** muscles (anterior and posterior bellies of the digastric, mylohyoid, geniohyoid, genioglossus, stylohyoid); those inferior are the **infrahyoid** muscles (omohyoid, sternohyoid, sternothyroid, thyrohyoid). Others are the **deep neck** muscles (scalenus anterior, scalenus medius, scalenus posterior, longus colli, longus capitis).

Sternocleidomastoid Muscle

When the SCM muscle contracts, it appears as an oblique band crossing the side of the neck from the sternoclavicular joint to the mastoid process of the skull. It divides the neck into **anterior** and **posterior triangles** (see Figs. 9.70 and 9.71). The anterior border covers the carotid arteries, internal jugular vein, and the deep cervical lymph nodes; it also overlaps the thyroid gland. Skin, fascia, the platysma muscle, and the external jugular vein cover the muscle superficially. The deep surface of the posterior border is related to the cervical plexus of nerves, the phrenic nerve, and the upper part of the brachial plexus.

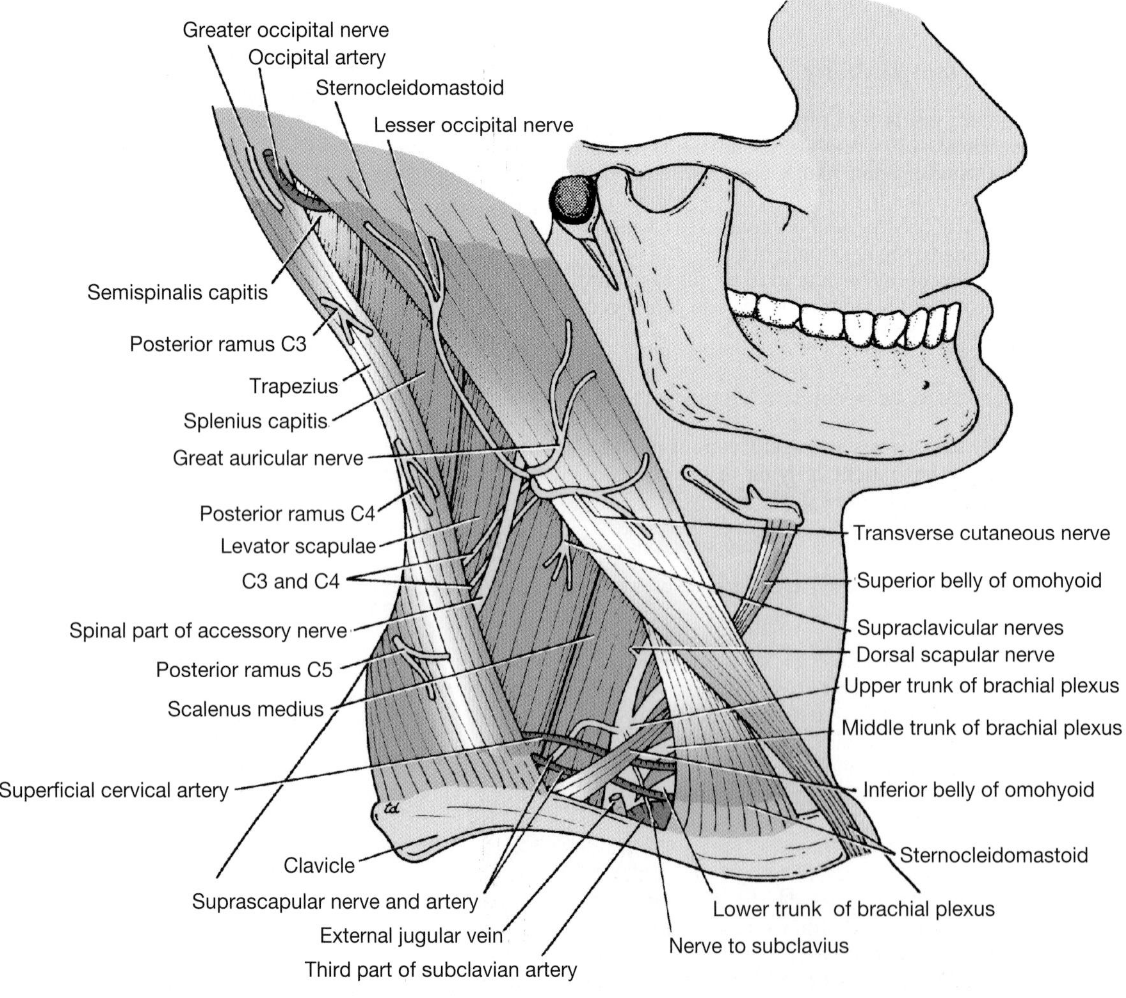

Figure 9.69 Posterior triangle of the neck.

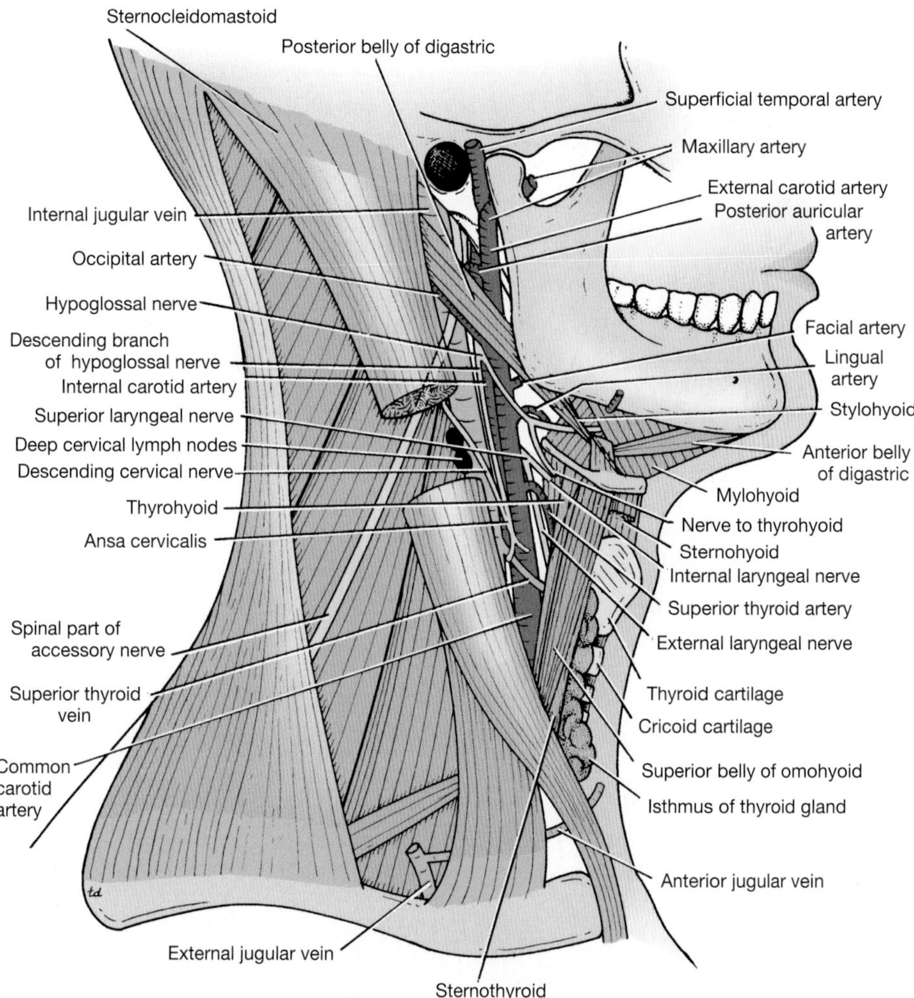

Figure 9.70 Anterior and posterior triangles of the neck.

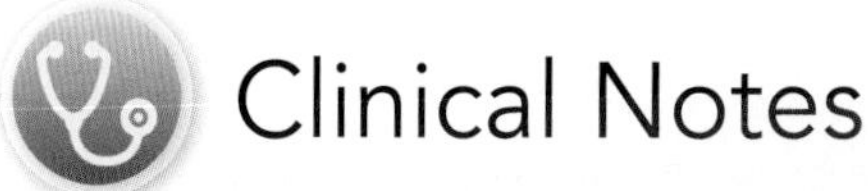

Clinical Notes

Sternocleidomastoid Muscle and Protection from Trauma

The sternocleidomastoid (SCM) muscle, a strong, thick muscle crossing the side of the neck, protects the underlying soft structures from blunt trauma. Suicide attempts by cutting one's throat often fail because the individual first extends the neck before making several horizontal cuts with a knife. Extension of the cervical part of the vertebral column and extension of the head at the atlanto-occipital joint cause the carotid sheath with its contained large blood vessels to slide posteriorly beneath the SCM muscle. To achieve the desired result with the head and neck fully extended, some individuals must make several attempts and only succeed when the larynx and the greater part of the SCM muscles have been severed. The common sites for the wounds are immediately above and below the hyoid bone.

Congenital Torticollis

Most cases of congenital torticollis are a result of excessive stretching of the SCM muscle during a difficult labor. Hemorrhage occurs into the muscle and may be detected as a small, rounded "tumor" during the early weeks after birth. Later, this becomes invaded by fibrous tissue, which contracts and shortens the muscle. The mastoid process is thus pulled down toward the sternoclavicular joint of the same side, the cervical spine is flexed, and the face looks upward to the opposite side. If left untreated, asymmetrical growth changes occur in the face, and the cervical vertebrae may become wedge shaped.

Spasmodic Torticollis

Spasmodic torticollis, which results from repeated chronic contractions of the SCM and trapezius muscles, is usually psychogenic in origin. Section of the spinal part of the accessory nerve may be necessary in severe cases.

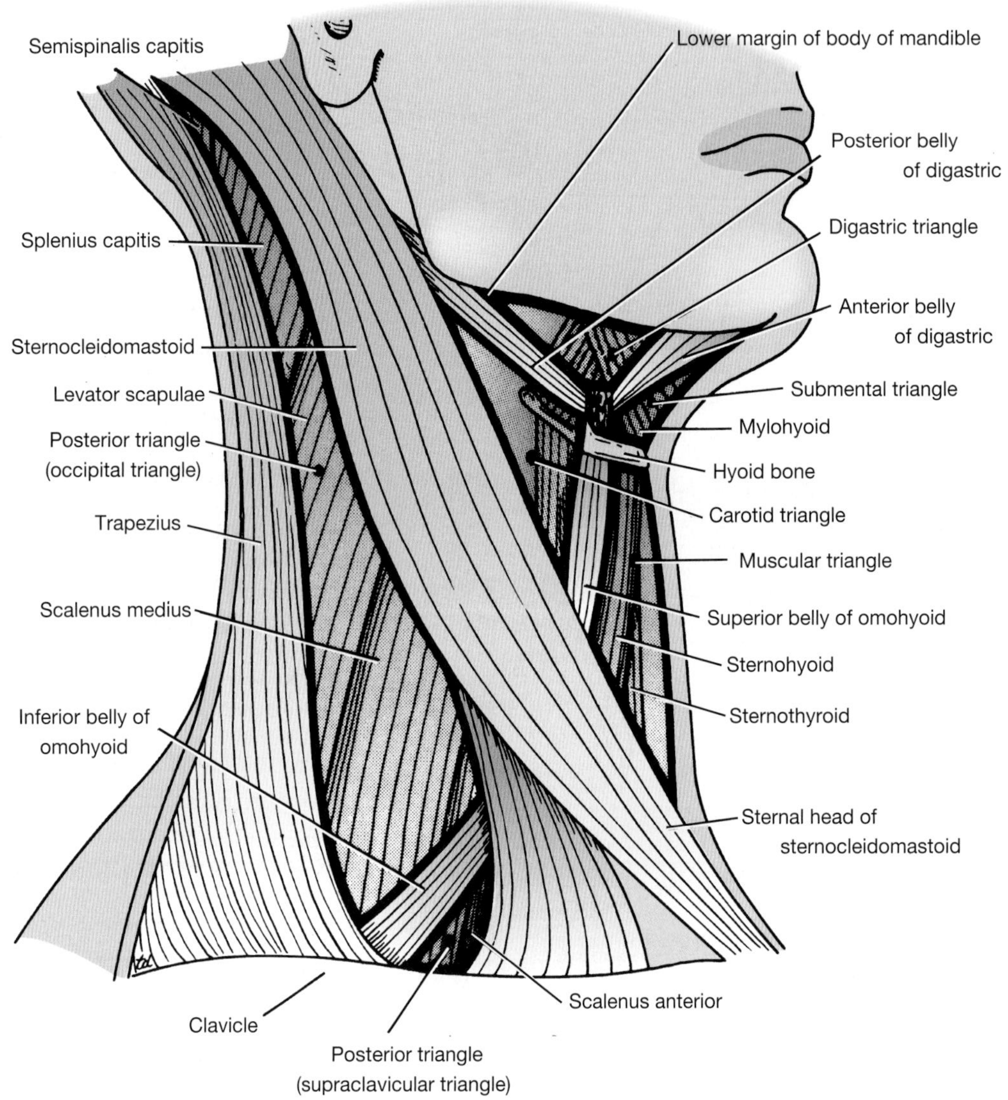

Figure 9.71 Muscular contents of the triangles of the neck.

Scalenus Anterior Muscle

The scalenus anterior muscle is a key structure in understanding the root of the neck (see Figs. 9.65 and 9.72). It is deeply placed, and it descends almost vertically from the vertebral column to rib 1.

Important Relations

- **Anteriorly:** Related to the carotid arteries, the vagus nerve, the internal jugular vein, and the deep cervical lymph nodes. The transverse cervical and suprascapular arteries and the prevertebral layer of deep cervical fascia bind the **phrenic nerve** to the anterior surface of the muscle (see Fig. 9.72).
- **Posteriorly:** Related to the cervical pleura, the origin of the brachial plexus, and the second part of the subclavian artery. The scalenus medius muscle lies behind the scalenus anterior muscle.
- **Medially:** Related to the vertebral artery and vein and the sympathetic trunk. On the left side, the medial border is related to the thoracic duct.
- **Laterally:** Related to the emerging branches of the cervical plexus, the roots of the brachial plexus, and the third part of the subclavian artery.

The adjacent edges of the scalenus anterior and medius muscles and rib 1 form a triangular gap, the **interscalene triangle**. The **subclavian artery** and the **roots of the brachial plexus** pass through the triangle. Narrowing of the interscalene triangle (eg, owing to extra muscle slips or a cervical rib) may compress its neurovascular contents, resulting in ischemia and/or nerve dysfunction in the upper limb. Structures passing outside the triangle (subclavian vein, transverse cervical artery, suprascapular artery, and phrenic nerve) are spared this danger.

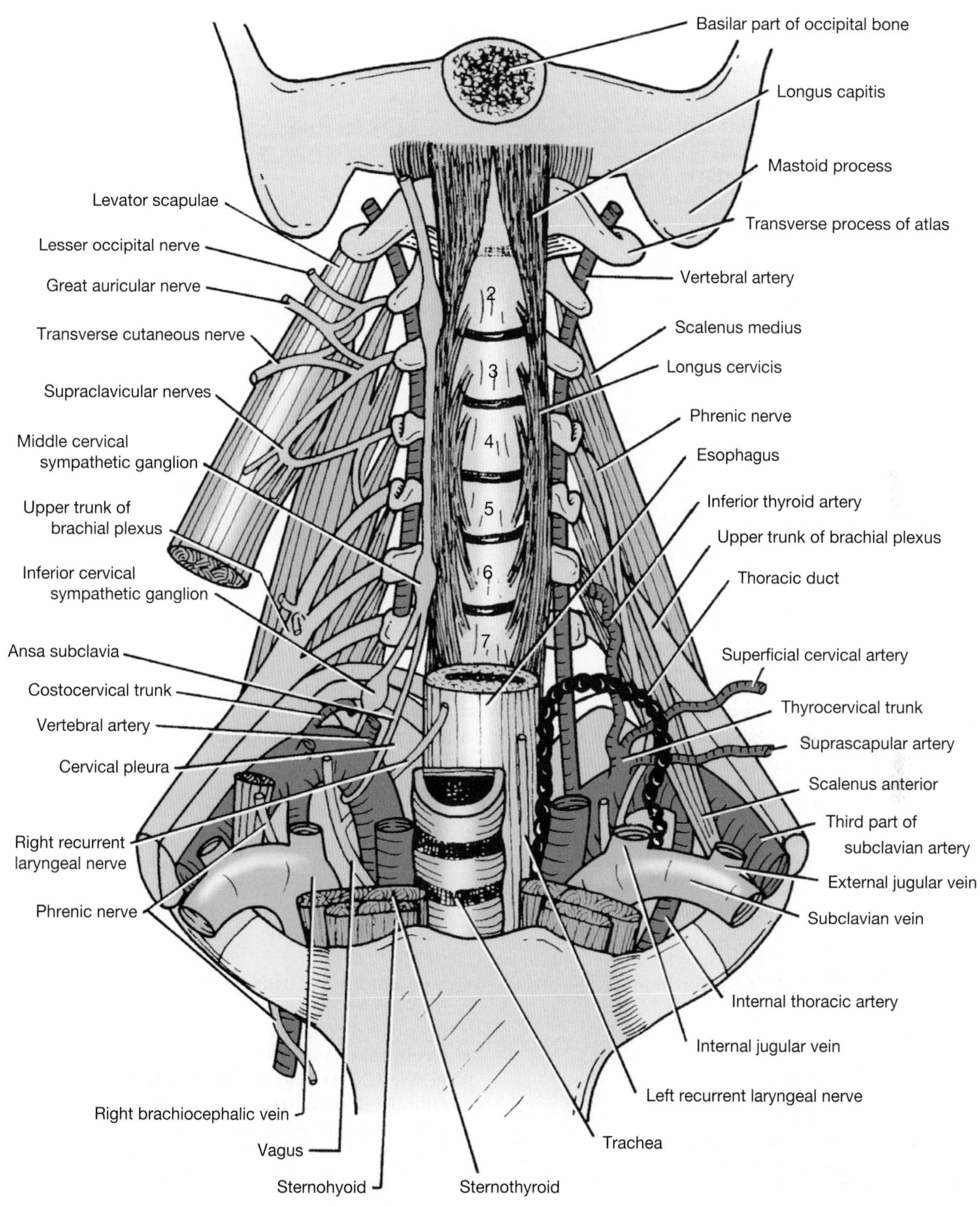

Figure 9.72 Prevertebral region and the root of the neck.

Neck Triangles

The strap muscles divide the neck into several triangular spaces that are useful in organizing the contents of the neck. The SCM muscle divides the neck into large **anterior** and **posterior triangles** (Figs. 9.73 and 9.74). Each of these contains smaller triangular spaces.

Anterior Triangle

The boundaries are the SCM muscle, midline of the neck, and lower margin of the body of the mandible.

Subdivisions and boundaries:

- **Muscular (omotracheal) triangle:** Anterior midline, anterior edge of SCM, superior belly of the omohyoid

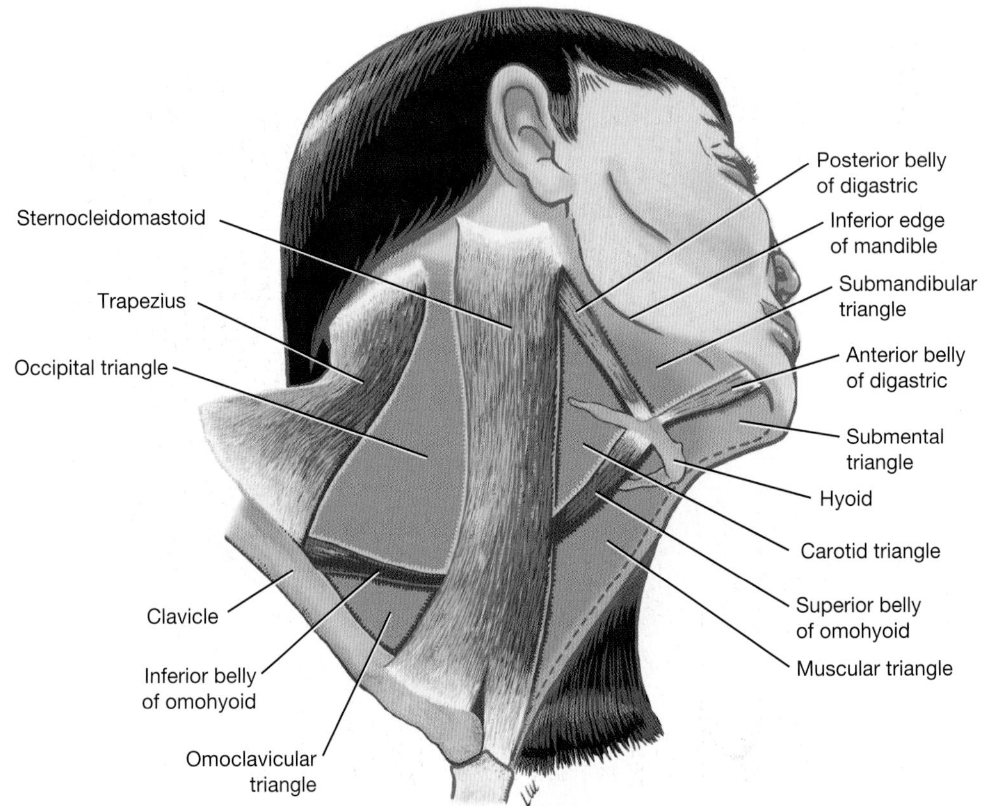

Figure 9.73 Triangles of the neck and their boundaries in posterolateral view. The four triangles anterior to the sternocleidomastoid (submandibular, submental, muscular, and carotid) constitute the anterior triangle of the neck. The two triangles posterior to the sternocleidomastoid (occipital and omoclavicular) form the posterior triangle of the neck.

- **Carotid triangle:** Superior belly of the omohyoid, anterior edge of SCM, posterior belly of digastric
- **Submental triangle:** Anterior midline, hyoid bone, anterior belly of digastric
- **Submandibular (digastric) triangle:** Lower margin of body of the mandible, anterior belly of digastric, posterior belly of digastric

Posterior Triangle

The boundaries are the SCM muscle, trapezius muscle, and the clavicle.

Subdivisions and boundaries:

- **Occipital triangle:** Sternocleidomastoid, trapezius, inferior belly of omohyoid
- **Omoclavicular (subclavian) triangle:** Sternocleidomastoid, inferior belly of omohyoid, clavicle

Major Triangle Contents

- **Muscular triangle:** Sternohyoid and sternothyroid muscles; larynx; thyroid and parathyroid glands (see Fig. 9.70)
- **Carotid triangle:** Carotid sheath containing common carotid artery, internal jugular vein, and vagus nerve (CN X); external and internal carotid arteries; spinal accessory nerve (CN XI); hypoglossal nerve (CN XII) and superior limb of ansa cervicalis; cervical plexus branches; deep cervical lymph nodes
- **Submental triangle:** Submental lymph nodes; anterior jugular vein
- **Submandibular triangle:** Submandibular gland; submandibular lymph nodes; hypoglossal nerve (CN XII); mylohyoid nerve
- **Occipital triangle:** Occipital artery, spinal accessory nerve (CN XI), brachial plexus (trunks) (see Fig. 9.69)
- **Omoclavicular triangle:** Subclavian artery (third part); suprascapular artery

Deep Cervical Fascia

The deep cervical fascia supports the muscles, the vessels, and the viscera of the neck (see Fig. 9.65). In certain areas, it is condensed to form well-defined, fibrous sheets called the **investing layer**, **pretracheal layer**, and **prevertebral layer**. It is also condensed to form the **carotid sheath** and the **axillary sheath**.

Investing Layer (Investing Deep Fascia)

The investing layer is a thick layer that encircles the neck. It splits to enclose the trapezius and SCM muscles.

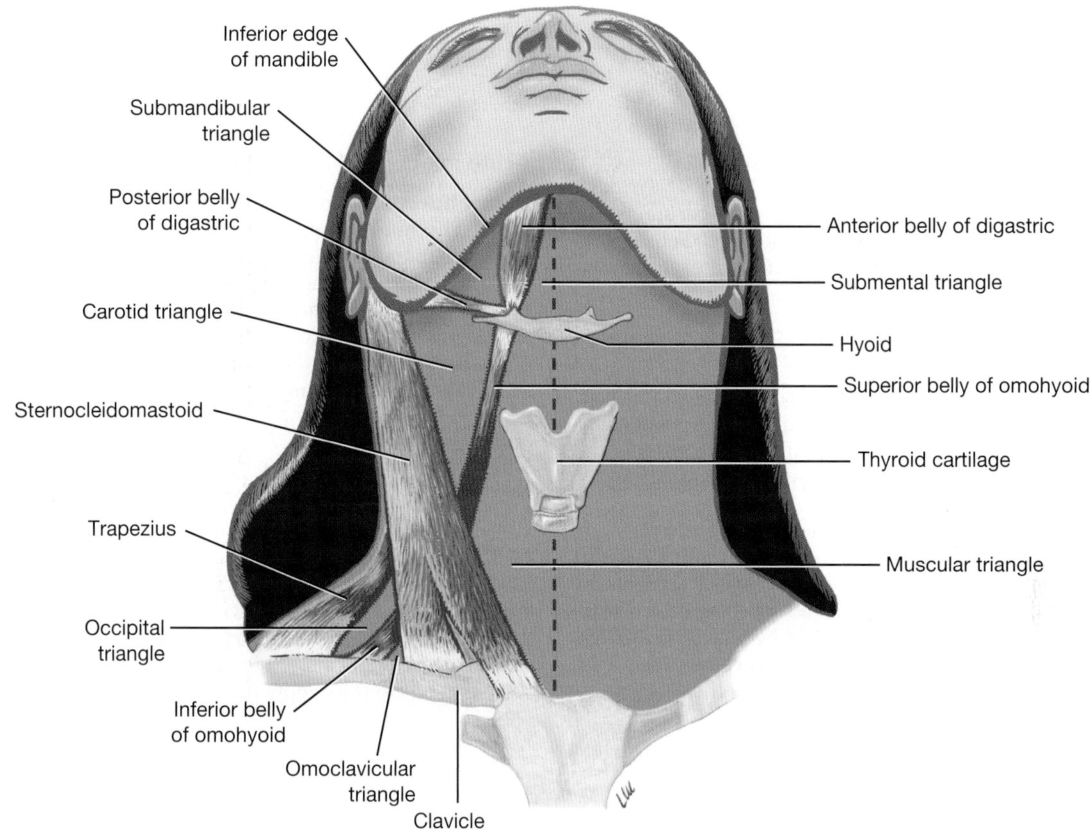

Figure 9.74 Triangles of the neck and their boundaries in anterior view. The four triangles anterior to the sternocleidomastoid (submandibular, submental, muscular, and carotid) constitute the anterior triangle of the neck. The two triangles posterior to the sternocleidomastoid (occipital and omoclavicular) form the posterior triangle of the neck.

Pretracheal Layer (Pretracheal Fascia; Thyroid Capsule)

The pretracheal layer is a thin layer that is attached above to the laryngeal cartilages. It surrounds the thyroid and the parathyroid glands, forming a sheath for them, and encloses the infrahyoid muscles.

Prevertebral Layer (Prevertebral Fascia)

The prevertebral layer is a thick layer that passes like a septum across the neck behind the pharynx and the esophagus and in front of the prevertebral muscles and the vertebral column. It forms the fascial floor of the posterior triangle, and it extends laterally over rib 1 into the axilla to form the important axillary sheath.

Carotid Sheath

The carotid sheath is a local condensation of the prevertebral, pretracheal, and investing layers of the deep fascia that surround the common and internal carotid arteries, internal jugular vein, vagus nerve, and deep cervical lymph nodes.

Axillary Sheath

All the anterior rami of the cervical nerves that emerge in the interval between the scalenus anterior and scalenus medius muscles lie at first deep to the prevertebral fascia. As the subclavian artery and the brachial plexus emerge in the interscalene triangle, they carry with them a sheath of the fascia, which extends into the axilla and is called the axillary sheath.

Cervical Ligaments

- **Stylohyoid ligament:** Connects the styloid process to the lesser cornu of the hyoid bone
- **Stylomandibular ligament:** Connects the styloid process to the angle of the mandible (see Fig. 9.14)
- **Sphenomandibular ligament:** Connects the spine of the sphenoid bone to the lingula of the mandible (see Fig. 9.14)
- **Pterygomandibular ligament (raphe):** Connects the hamular process of the medial pterygoid plate to the posterior end of the mylohyoid line of the mandible. It gives attachment to the superior constrictor and the buccinator muscles

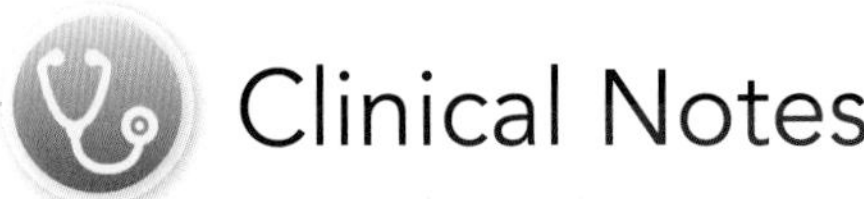

Clinical Notes

Clinical Significance of Neck Deep Fascia

As previously described, the deep fascia in certain areas forms distinct sheets called the **investing**, **pretracheal**, and **prevertebral** layers. These fascial layers are easily recognizable by the surgeon at operation.

Fascial Spaces

Between the denser layers of deep fascia in the neck, loose connective tissue forms potential spaces that are clinically important. Among the more important spaces are the **visceral**, **retropharyngeal**, **submandibular**, and **masticatory** spaces (Fig. 9.75).

The deep fascia and the fascial spaces are important because organisms originating in the mouth, teeth, pharynx, and esophagus can spread among the fascial planes and spaces and the tough fascia can determine the direction of spread of infection and the path taken by pus. It is possible for blood, pus, or air in the retropharyngeal space to spread downward into the superior mediastinum of the thorax.

Acute Infection of Neck Fascial Spaces

Dental infections most commonly involve the lower molar teeth. The infection spreads medially from the mandible into the submandibular and masticatory spaces and pushes the tongue forward and upward. Further spread downward may involve the visceral space and lead to edema of the vocal cords and airway obstruction.

Ludwig angina is an acute infection of the submandibular fascial space and is commonly secondary to dental infection.

Chronic Infection of Neck Fascial Spaces

Tuberculous infection of the deep cervical lymph nodes can result in liquefaction and destruction of one or more of the nodes. The investing layer of the deep fascia at first limits the pus. Later, this becomes eroded at one point, and the pus passes into the less restricted superficial fascia. A dumbbell or collar-stud abscess is now present. The clinician is aware of the superficial abscess but must not forget the existence of the deeply placed abscess.

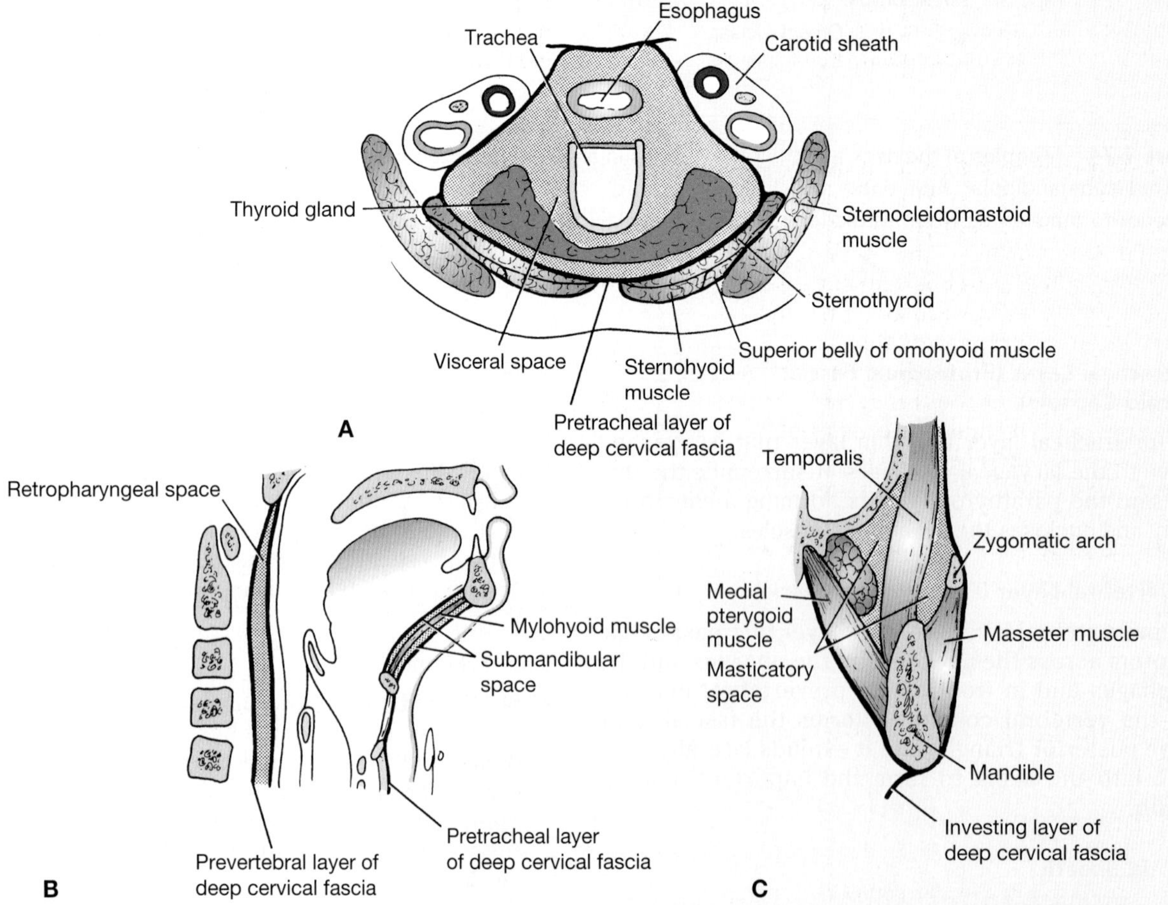

Figure 9.75 **A.** Cross section of the neck showing the visceral space. **B.** Sagittal section of the neck showing the positions of the retropharyngeal and submandibular spaces. **C.** Vertical section of the body of the mandible close to the angle showing the masticatory space.

Root of the Neck

The root of the neck is the area immediately above the inlet into the thorax (see Fig. 9.72). The scalenus anterior muscle is a key structure to understanding the root of the neck and was described earlier. The subclavian blood vessels and the thoracic duct are notable structures in this region.

Subclavian Artery

The **right subclavian artery** arises from the brachiocephalic artery, behind the right sternoclavicular joint. It passes upward and laterally as a gentle curve behind the scalenus anterior muscle, and at the outer border of rib 1, it becomes the axillary artery. The **left subclavian artery** arises from the arch of the aorta in the thorax. It ascends to the root of the neck and then arches laterally in a manner similar to that of the right subclavian artery. Further details are provided in Subclavian System.

Subclavian Vein

The subclavian vein begins at the outer border of rib 1 as a continuation of the axillary vein. At the medial border of the scalenus anterior, it joins the internal jugular vein to form the brachiocephalic vein.

Thoracic Duct

The thoracic duct begins in the abdomen at the upper end of the **cisterna chyli** (see Chapter 4). It enters the thorax through the aortic opening in the diaphragm and ascends through the posterior mediastinum, inclining gradually to the left. In the superior mediastinum, it passes upward along the left margin of the esophagus. At the root of the neck, it continues to ascend along the left margin of the esophagus until it reaches the level of the transverse process of the C7 vertebra. Here, it bends laterally behind the carotid sheath. At the medial border of the scalenus anterior, it turns downward and drains into the beginning of the left brachiocephalic vein. However, it may end in the terminal part of the subclavian or internal jugular veins.

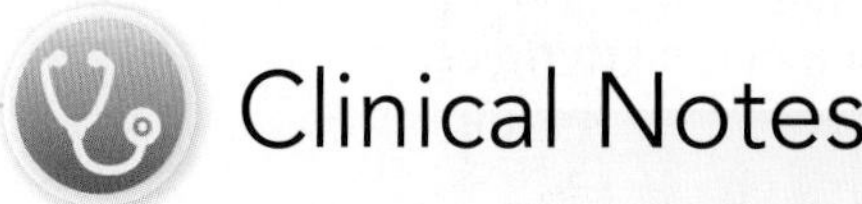

Clinical Notes

Pleura and Lung Injuries in the Root of the Neck

The **cervical dome of the pleura** and the **apex of the lung** extend up into the root of the neck on each side (see Fig. 9.72). Covered by the **suprapleural membrane**, they lie behind the subclavian artery. Thus, a penetrating wound above the medial end of the clavicle may involve the apex of the lung.

HEAD AND NECK ARTERIES

Two arterial tracts supply blood to the head and neck: (1) the **carotid system** and (2) the **subclavian system** (Fig. 9.76). The carotid system delivers blood to the upper neck and the head. The subclavian system provides blood to the lower neck, deep neck, inside of the cranium, shoulder, upper limb, and thorax.

Carotid System

The carotid system begins with the paired common carotid arteries, each of which has a different origin in the root of the neck or the chest (see Chapter 4 and Fig. 4.63).

Common Carotid Artery

The right common carotid artery arises from the brachiocephalic artery behind the right sternoclavicular joint (see Figs. 4.63, 9.72, and 9.76). The left artery arises from the arch of the aorta in the superior mediastinum. The common carotid artery runs upward through the neck within the **carotid sheath** (closely related to the internal jugular vein and vagus nerve), under cover of the anterior border of the SCM muscle, from the sternoclavicular joint to the **upper border of the thyroid cartilage**. Here (in the carotid triangle of the neck), it divides into the external and internal carotid arteries (Fig. 9.77; see also Fig. 9.70). The common carotid has no branches, except its two terminal branches.

Carotid Sinus

At its point of division, the terminal part of the common carotid artery (or the beginning of the internal carotid

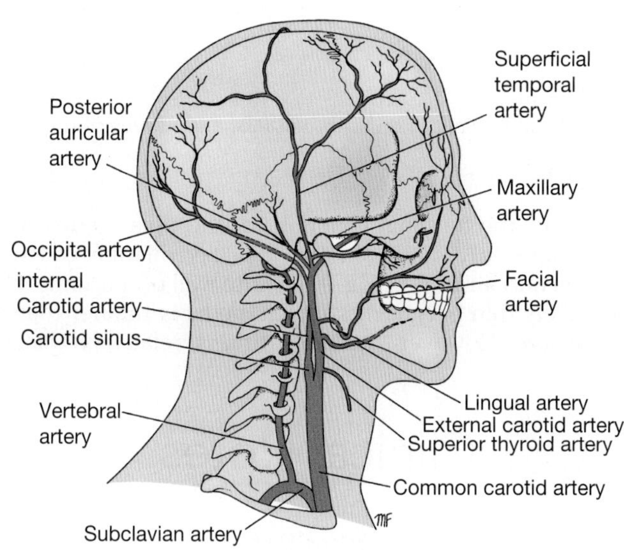

Figure 9.76 Main arteries of the head and neck. Note that for clarity, the thyrocervical trunk, costocervical trunk, and the internal thoracic artery (branches of the subclavian artery) are not shown.

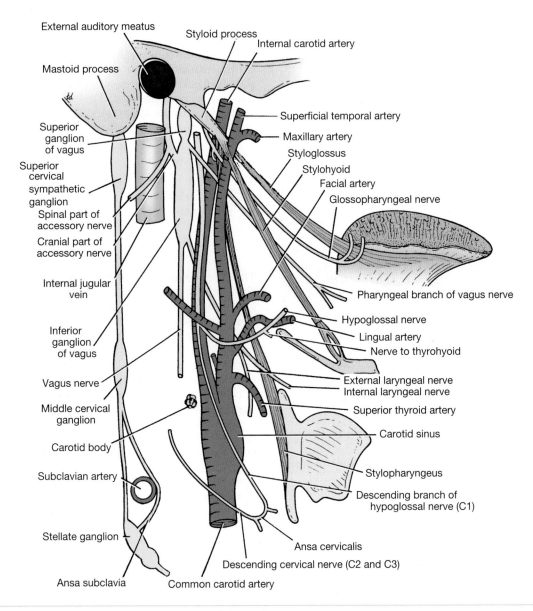

Figure 9.77 Styloid muscles, vessels, and nerves of the neck.

artery or the terminal common carotid plus the origin of the internal carotid) shows a localized dilation, called the **carotid sinus** (see Fig. 9.77). The wall of the sinus is relatively thin because its tunica media is thinner than elsewhere. However, the adventitia is relatively thick and contains numerous nerve endings derived from the **glossopharyngeal nerve**. The carotid sinus serves as a reflex pressoreceptor (baroreceptor) mechanism: a rise in blood pressure causes a reduction of the heart rate and vasodilation of the arterioles.

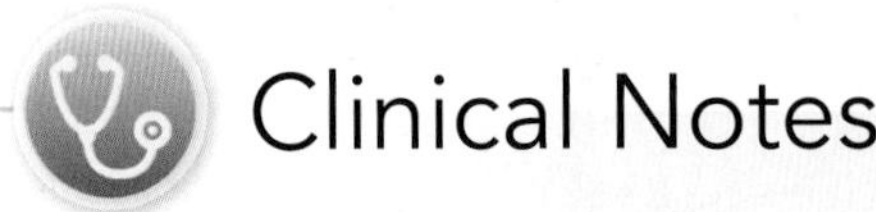

Clinical Notes

Carotid Sinus Hypersensitivity

In cases of carotid sinus hypersensitivity, external pressure on one or both carotid sinuses can cause excessive slowing of the heart rate, a fall in blood pressure, and cerebral ischemia with fainting (**syncope**).

Carotid Body

The carotid body is a small structure that lies posterior to the point of bifurcation of the common carotid artery or in the angle of the bifurcation (see Fig. 9.77). It is innervated by the glossopharyngeal nerve (and possibly supplemented by the vagus nerve). The carotid body is a chemoreceptor, being sensitive to excess carbon dioxide and reduced oxygen tension in the blood. Such a stimulus reflexively produces a rise in blood pressure and heart rate and an increase in respiratory movements.

Common Carotid Artery Relations

- **Anterolaterally:** Skin, fascia, SCM, the sternohyoid, sternothyroid, and superior belly of the omohyoid (see Fig. 9.70)
- **Posteriorly:** Transverse processes of the C4 to C7 vertebrae, prevertebral muscles, and the sympathetic trunk (see Fig. 9.72); vertebral vessels in the lower part of the neck
- **Medially:** The larynx and pharynx and, below these, the trachea and esophagus (see Fig. 9.65); lobe of the thyroid gland also lies medially
- **Laterally:** Internal jugular vein and, posterolaterally, the vagus nerve

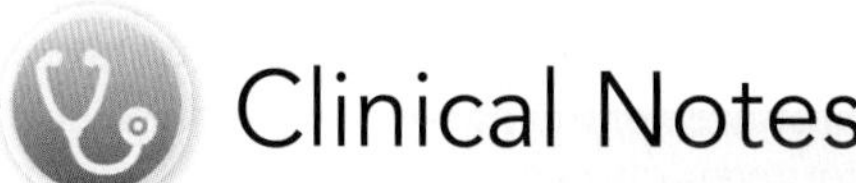

Clinical Notes

Taking the Carotid Pulse

The bifurcation of the common carotid artery into the internal and external carotid arteries can be easily palpated just beneath the anterior border of the sternocleidomastoid muscle at the level of the superior border of the thyroid cartilage. This is a convenient site to take the **carotid pulse (neck pulse)**.

External Carotid Artery

The external carotid artery is one of the terminal branches of the common carotid artery (see Figs. 9.76 and 9.77). It supplies structures in the neck, face, and scalp; it also supplies the tongue and the maxilla. The artery begins at the level of the upper border of the thyroid cartilage and terminates in the substance of the parotid gland posterior to the neck of the mandible by dividing into the **superficial temporal** and **maxillary arteries**.

Close to its origin, the artery emerges from under cover of the SCM muscle, where its pulsations can be felt. At first, it lies medial to the internal carotid artery, but as it ascends in the neck, it passes backward and lateral to it.

External Carotid Artery Relations

- **Anterolaterally**: The anterior border of the sternocleidomastoid overlaps the beginning of the artery. Above this level, the artery is comparatively superficial, being covered by skin and fascia. The hypoglossal nerve, the posterior belly of the digastric muscle, and the stylohyoid muscle cross over it (see Fig. 9.70). The facial nerve crosses it within the parotid gland (see Parotid Gland). The internal jugular vein first lies lateral to the artery and then posterior to it.
- **Medially**: The wall of the pharynx and the internal carotid artery. The stylopharyngeus muscle, glossopharyngeal nerve, and the pharyngeal branch of the vagus pass between the external and internal carotid arteries (see Fig. 9.77). See Parotid Gland for the relations of the external carotid artery in the parotid gland.

External Carotid Artery Branches

- **Superior thyroid artery:** Curves downward to the upper pole of the thyroid gland (see Figs. 9.70, 9.76, and 9.77). It gives off the **superior laryngeal artery** (which pierces the thyrohyoid membrane) and descends in company with the **external laryngeal nerve**, which supplies the cricothyroid muscle.
- **Ascending pharyngeal artery:** Ascends vertically along and supplies the pharyngeal wall.
- **Lingual artery:** Loops upward and forward and supplies the tongue.
- **Facial artery:** Loops upward close to the outer surface of the pharynx and the tonsil. It runs deep to the submandibular salivary gland and emerges and bends around the lower border of the mandible. It then ascends into the face close to the anterior border of the masseter muscle. The artery continues upward around the lateral corner of the mouth and terminates at the medial angle of the eye. Branches of the facial artery supply the tonsil (via the **tonsillar branch**), the submandibular salivary gland, and the muscles and the skin of the face. The lingual and facial arteries commonly arise from a common trunk, which is termed the **linguofacial trunk**.
- **Occipital artery:** Supplies the back of the scalp.
- **Posterior auricular artery:** Supplies the auricle and the scalp.
- **Superficial temporal artery:** The smaller terminal branch of the external carotid artery ascends over the zygomatic arch, where it may be palpated just in front of the auricle. It accompanies the auriculotemporal nerve and supplies the scalp.
- **Maxillary artery:** This larger terminal branch of the external carotid artery runs forward deep to the neck of the mandible. It proceeds across the infratemporal fossa and enters the pterygopalatine fossa of the skull. Branches supply the upper and the lower jaws, the muscles of mastication, the nose, the palate, and the meninges inside the skull.

The **middle meningeal artery** branches off the maxillary artery, enters the skull through the foramen spinosum, runs laterally, and divides into anterior and posterior branches (see Fig. 9.54; see also Surface Anatomy). The anterior branch is important because it lies close to the motor area of the cerebral cortex of the brain. Accompanied by its vein, it grooves (or tunnels) across the pterion of the skull, where it is prone to damage after a blow to the head.

Internal Carotid Artery

The internal carotid artery begins at the bifurcation of the common carotid artery at the level of the upper border of the thyroid cartilage (see Figs. 9.70 and 9.77). It supplies the brain, eye, forehead, and part of the nose. The artery ascends in the neck embedded in the carotid sheath with the internal jugular vein and vagus nerve.

At first, it lies superficially; it then passes deep to the parotid salivary gland.

The internal carotid artery leaves the neck by passing into the cranial cavity through the **carotid canal** in the petrous part of the temporal bone. It then passes upward and forward in the **cavernous venous sinus** (without communicating with it). The artery then leaves the sinus and passes upward again medial to the anterior clinoid process of the sphenoid bone. The internal carotid artery then inclines backward, lateral to the optic chiasma, and terminates by dividing into the **anterior** and the **middle cerebral arteries** (see Fig. 9.42).

Internal Carotid Artery Neck Relations

- **Anterolaterally:** Below the digastric lie the skin, fascia, anterior border of the SCM, and the hypoglossal nerve (see Fig. 9.70). Above the digastric lie the stylohyoid muscle, stylopharyngeus muscle, glossopharyngeal nerve, pharyngeal branch of the vagus, parotid gland, and the external carotid artery (see Fig. 9.77).
- **Posteriorly:** Sympathetic trunk, the longus capitis muscle, and the transverse processes of the C1 to C3 vertebrae.
- **Medially:** Pharyngeal wall and the superior laryngeal nerve.
- **Laterally:** Internal jugular vein and the vagus nerve.

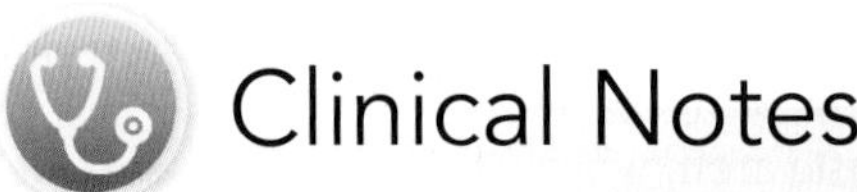

Internal Carotid Artery Arteriosclerosis

Extensive arteriosclerosis of the internal carotid artery in the neck can cause visual impairment or blindness in the eye on the side of the lesion because of insufficient blood flow through the retinal artery. Motor paralysis and sensory loss may also occur on the opposite side of the body because of insufficient blood flow through the middle cerebral artery.

Internal Carotid Artery Branches

Although branches do not exist in the neck, many important branches are given off in the cranial cavity.

Ophthalmic artery: Arising from the internal carotid artery as it emerges from the cavernous sinus (see Figs. 9.38 and 9.54), it passes forward into the orbital cavity through the optic canal and distributes throughout the orbit. It gives off the **central artery of the retina**, which enters the optic nerve and runs forward to enter the eyeball. The central artery is an end artery and the only blood supply to the retina.

Posterior communicating artery: This artery runs posteriorly to join the posterior cerebral artery (see Fig. 9.42).

Anterior cerebral artery: This is a terminal branch of the internal carotid artery. It passes forward between the cerebral hemispheres and then winds around the corpus callosum of the brain to supply the medial and the superolateral surfaces of the cerebral hemisphere. It is joined to the artery of the opposite side by the **anterior communicating artery**.

Middle cerebral artery: This is the larger terminal branch of the internal carotid artery, and it runs laterally in the lateral cerebral sulcus of the brain. It supplies the entire lateral surface of the cerebral hemisphere except the narrow strip along the superolateral margin (which is supplied by the anterior cerebral artery) and the occipital pole and inferolateral surface of the hemisphere (both of which are supplied by the posterior cerebral artery). The middle cerebral artery thus supplies all the motor area of the cerebral cortex except the leg area. It also gives off central branches that supply central masses of gray matter and the internal capsule of the brain.

Cerebral arterial circle (circle of Willis): The cerebral arterial circle is a roughly circular network of arteries ringing the sella turcica at the base of the brain. It is formed by anastomoses between branches of the two internal carotid arteries and the two vertebral arteries (see Fig. 9.42). The internal carotid contributes the **anterior communicating**, **anterior cerebral**, **middle cerebral**, and **posterior communicating arteries** to the network. The vertebral arteries merge to form a single **basilar artery**, which divides into the **posterior cerebral arteries**. These anastomose with the posterior communicating arteries to complete the circle. Cortical and central branches arise from the circle and supply the brain.

Subclavian System

The subclavian system consists of the paired subclavian arteries and their branches. As with the common carotid arteries, the subclavian arteries have different origins on the right and left sides (see Chapter 4).

Subclavian Artery

The **right subclavian artery** arises from the brachiocephalic artery, behind the right sternoclavicular joint (see Figs. 4.63, 9.72, and 9.76). It arches upward and laterally over the pleura and through the interscalene triangle between the scalenus anterior and medius muscles. At the outer border of rib 1, it becomes the **axillary artery**.

The **left subclavian artery** arises from the arch of the aorta in the thorax. It ascends to the root of the neck and then arches laterally in a manner similar to that of the right subclavian artery.

The scalenus anterior muscle passes anterior to the artery on each side and divides it into three parts.

First Part of the Subclavian Artery

The first part of the subclavian artery extends from the origin of the subclavian artery to the medial border of the scalenus anterior muscle (see Fig. 9.72). This part gives off the **vertebral artery**, **thyrocervical trunk**, and the **internal thoracic artery**.

The **vertebral artery** ascends in the neck through the foramina in the transverse processes of the upper six cervical vertebrae, giving off spinal and muscular branches along its way. It passes medially above the posterior arch of the atlas and then ascends through the foramen magnum into the skull. On reaching the anterior surface of the medulla oblongata of the brain at the level of the lower border of the pons, it joins the vessel of the opposite side to form the **basilar artery**.

The basilar artery (see Fig. 9.42) ascends in a groove on the anterior surface of the pons. It gives off branches to the pons, cerebellum, and internal ear. It finally divides into the two **posterior cerebral arteries**.

On each side, the posterior cerebral artery curves laterally and backward around the midbrain. Cortical branches supply the inferolateral surfaces of the temporal lobe and the visual cortex on the lateral and the medial surfaces of the occipital lobe.

The **thyrocervical trunk** is a short trunk that gives off three terminal branches: inferior thyroid artery, transverse cervical artery, and suprascapular artery (see Fig. 9.72).

The **inferior thyroid artery** ascends to the posterior surface of the thyroid gland, where it is closely related to the recurrent laryngeal nerve. It supplies the thyroid and the inferior parathyroid glands.

The **transverse cervical artery** is a small branch that crosses the brachial plexus and runs to the trapezius muscle.

The **suprascapular artery** runs laterally over the brachial plexus and follows the suprascapular nerve onto the back of the scapula.

The **internal thoracic artery** descends into the thorax behind costal cartilage 1 and in front of the pleura. It descends vertically one fingerbreadth lateral to the sternum. In the sixth intercostal space, it divides into the superior epigastric and the musculophrenic arteries.

Second Part of the Subclavian Artery

The second part of the subclavian artery lies behind the scalenus anterior muscle, within the interscalene triangle.

The **costocervical trunk** is the only branch off the second part. It runs backward over the dome of the pleura and divides into the **superior intercostal artery**, which supplies the first and the second intercostal spaces, and the **deep cervical artery**, which supplies the deep muscles of the neck.

Third Part of the Subclavian Artery

The third part of the subclavian artery extends from the lateral border of the scalenus anterior muscle across the posterior triangle of the neck to the lateral border of rib 1, where it becomes the axillary artery. Here, in the root of the neck, it is closely related to the nerves of the brachial plexus.

The third part of the subclavian artery usually has no branches. Occasionally, however, the transverse cervical artery, the suprascapular artery, or both arise from this part.

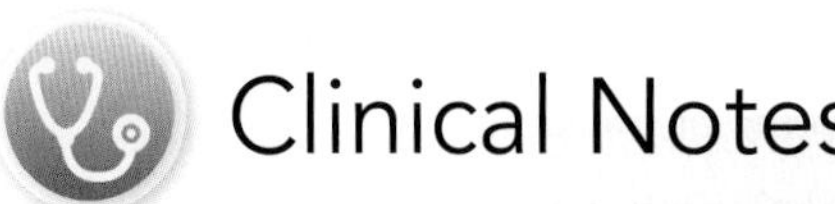

Palpation and Compression of the Subclavian Artery in Patients with Upper Limb Hemorrhage

In severe traumatic accidents to the upper limb involving laceration of the brachial or axillary arteries, remember that exerting strong pressure downward and backward on the third part of the subclavian artery can stop the hemorrhage. The use of a blunt object to exert the pressure is of great help, and the artery is compressed against the upper surface of rib 1.

HEAD AND NECK VEINS

The veins of the head and neck are organized in two groups: **intracranial veins** inside the cranium and **extracranial** veins outside the skull.

Intracranial Veins

These are the veins of the brain, dural venous sinuses, diploic veins, and emissary veins.

Brain Veins

The veins of the brain are thin walled and have no valves. They consist of the cerebral veins, the cerebellar veins, and the veins of the brainstem, all of which drain into the neighboring dural venous sinuses.

Dural Venous Sinuses

The dural sinuses are situated between the endosteal and the meningeal layer of the dura mater (see Fig. 9.4). They have thick, fibrous walls but possess no valves. They receive tributaries from the brain, skull bones, orbit, and internal ear. The dural sinuses include the superior and inferior sagittal sinuses, straight sinus, transverse sinuses, sigmoid sinuses, occipital sinus, cavernous sinuses, and superior and inferior petrosal sinuses. All these sinuses are described earlier in this chapter.

Diploic Veins

The diploic veins occupy channels within the bones of the vault of the skull.

Emissary Veins

The emissary veins are valveless veins that pass through the skull bones. They connect the dural sinuses to the extracranial veins. While the direction of venous flow through emissary veins is usually from intracranial to extracranial vessels, the absence of valves in the emissary veins creates the potential for reverse flow. Thus, the emissary veins are important potential routes for the spread of infection from the exterior into the cranial cavity.

Extracranial Veins

These are the veins of the scalp, face, and neck.

Facial Vein

The facial vein is formed at the medial angle of the eye by the union of the **supraorbital** and **supratrochlear veins** (see Fig. 9.22). It is connected with the cavernous sinus through the **superior ophthalmic vein**. The facial vein descends down the face with the facial artery and passes around the lateral side of the mouth. It then crosses the mandible, is joined by the **anterior division of the retromandibular vein**, and drains into the **internal jugular vein**.

Superficial Temporal Vein

The superficial temporal vein is formed on the side of the scalp. It follows the superficial temporal artery and the auriculotemporal nerve and enters the parotid salivary gland, where it joins the **maxillary vein** to form the **retromandibular vein**.

Maxillary Vein

The maxillary vein is formed in the infratemporal fossa from the **pterygoid venous plexus**. The maxillary vein joins the superficial temporal vein to form the retromandibular vein.

Retromandibular Vein

The retromandibular vein is formed by the union of the **superficial temporal** and the **maxillary veins**. On leaving the parotid salivary gland, it divides into an **anterior branch**, which joins the facial vein, and a **posterior branch**, which joins the **posterior auricular vein** to form the **external jugular vein**.

External Jugular Vein

The external jugular vein is formed behind the angle of the jaw by the union of the **posterior auricular vein** with the **posterior division of the retromandibular vein**. It descends across the SCM muscle and deep to the platysma muscle and drains into the **subclavian vein** behind the middle of the clavicle.

Tributaries

- **Posterior external jugular vein** from the back of the scalp
- **Transverse cervical vein** from the skin and the fascia over the posterior triangle
- **Suprascapular vein** from the back of the scapula
- **Anterior jugular vein**

Anterior Jugular Vein

The anterior jugular vein descends in the front of the neck close to the midline. Just above the sternum, it is joined to the opposite vein by the **jugular arch**. The anterior jugular vein joins the **external jugular vein** deep to the sternocleidomastoid muscle.

Internal Jugular Vein

The internal jugular vein is a large vein that receives blood from the brain, scalp, face, and neck. It starts as a continuation of the **sigmoid sinus** and leaves the skull through the **jugular foramen**. It then descends through the neck in the carotid sheath lateral to the vagus nerve and the internal and common carotid arteries. It ends by joining the **subclavian vein** behind the medial end of the clavicle to form the **brachiocephalic vein**. Throughout its course, it is closely related to the **deep cervical lymph nodes**.

The vein has a dilation at its upper end called the **superior bulb** and another near its termination called the **inferior bulb**. A bicuspid valve is situated directly above the inferior bulb.

Internal Jugular Vein Relations

- **Anterolaterally:** The skin, fascia, SCM, and parotid salivary gland. Its lower part is covered by the sternothyroid, sternohyoid, and omohyoid muscles, which intervene between the vein and the SCM (see Fig. 9.70). Higher up, it is crossed by the stylohyoid, posterior belly of the digastric, and the spinal part of the accessory nerve. The chain of deep cervical lymph nodes runs alongside the vein.
- **Posteriorly:** The transverse processes of the cervical vertebrae, levator scapulae, scalenus medius, scalenus anterior, cervical plexus, phrenic nerve, thyrocervical trunk, vertebral vein, and the first part of the subclavian artery (see Fig. 9.72). On the left side, it passes in front of the thoracic duct.
- **Medially:** Above lie the internal carotid artery and CNs IX to XII. Below lie the common carotid artery and the vagus nerve.

Internal Jugular Vein Tributaries

- **Inferior petrosal sinus**
- **Facial vein**
- **Pharyngeal veins**
- **Lingual vein**
- **Superior thyroid vein**
- **Middle thyroid vein**

Subclavian Vein

The subclavian vein is a continuation of the **axillary vein** at the outer border of rib 1 (see Fig. 9.72). It joins the **internal jugular vein** to form the **brachiocephalic vein**, and it receives the external jugular vein. In addition, it often receives the **thoracic duct** on the left side and the right lymphatic duct on the right.

Relations

- **Anteriorly:** Clavicle
- **Posteriorly:** Scalenus anterior muscle and the phrenic nerve
- **Inferiorly:** Upper surface of rib 1

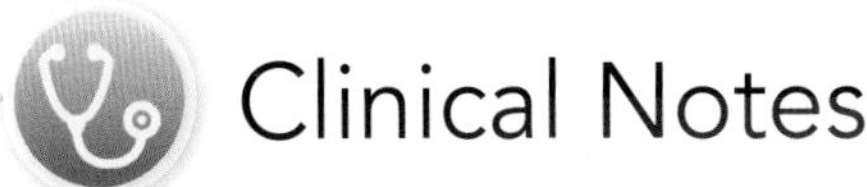

Clinical Notes

Internal Jugular Vein Penetrating Wounds

The hemorrhage of low-pressure venous blood into the loose connective tissue beneath the investing layer of deep cervical fascia may present as a large, slowly expanding hematoma. Air embolism is a serious complication of a lacerated wall of the internal jugular vein. Because the wall of this large vein contains little smooth muscle, its injury is not followed by contraction and retraction (as occurs with arterial injuries). Moreover, the adventitia of the vein wall is attached to the deep fascia of the carotid sheath, which hinders collapse of the vein. Blind clamping of the vein is prohibited because the vagus and hypoglossal nerves are in the vicinity.

Internal Jugular Vein Catheterization

The internal jugular vein is remarkably constant in position. It descends through the neck from a point halfway between the tip of the mastoid process and the angle of the jaw to the sternoclavicular joint. Above, the anterior border of the SCM muscle overlaps it, and below, this muscle covers it laterally. Just above the sternoclavicular joint, the vein lies beneath a skin depression (**lesser supraclavicular fossa**) between the sternal and clavicular heads of the SCM muscle and the clavicle. In the posterior approach, the tip of the needle and the catheter are introduced into the vein about two fingerbreadths above the clavicle at the posterior border of the SCM muscle (Fig. 9.78). In the anterior approach, with the patient's head turned to the opposite side, the lesser supraclavicular fossa is identified. A shallow skin depression usually overlies the triangle. The needle and catheter are inserted into the vein at the apex of the triangle in a caudal direction.

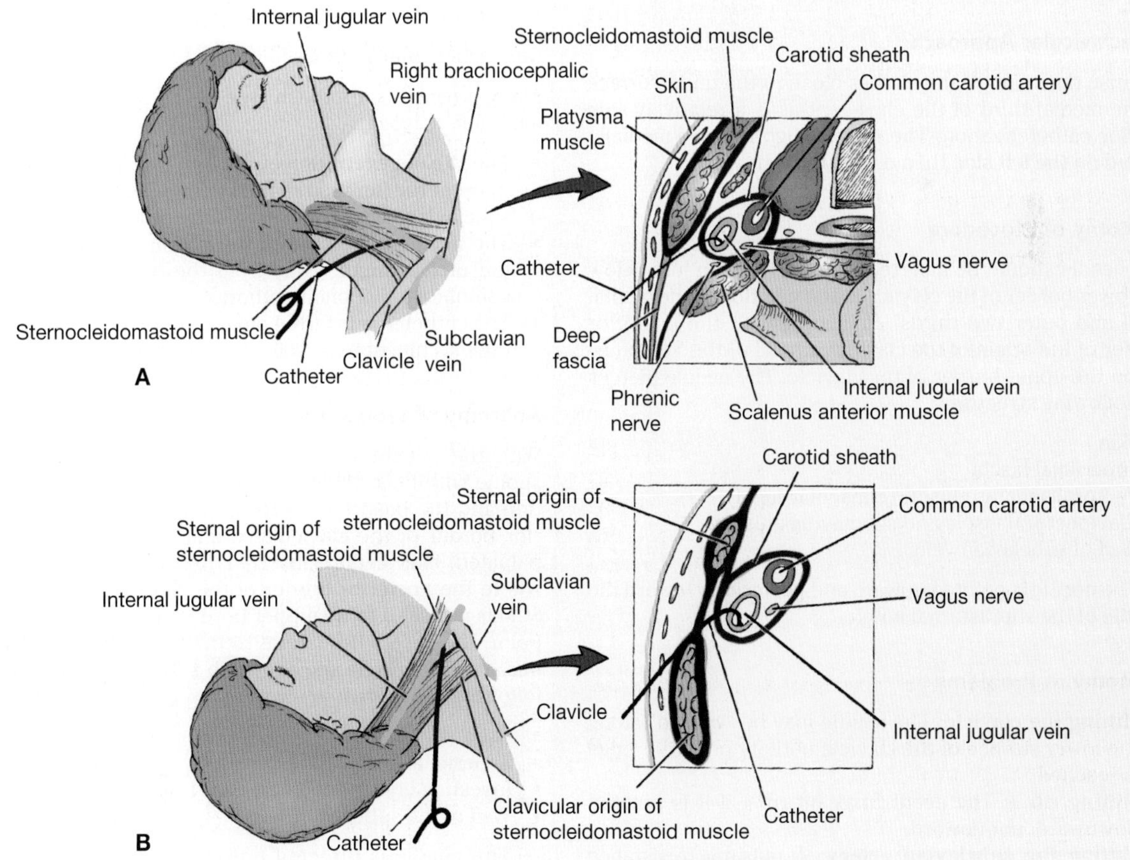

Figure 9.78 Catheterization of the right internal jugular vein. **A.** Posterior approach. Note the position of the catheter relative to the sternocleidomastoid muscle and the common carotid artery. **B.** Anterior approach. Note that the catheter is inserted into the vein close to the apex of the triangle formed by the sternal and clavicular heads of the sternocleidomastoid muscle and the clavicle.

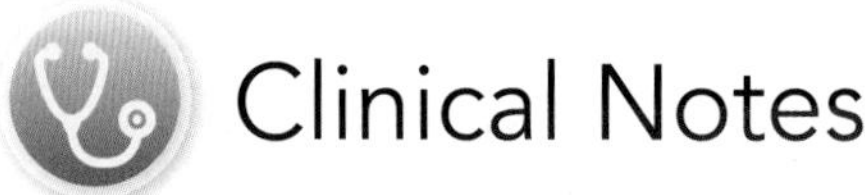

Subclavian Vein Thrombosis

Spontaneous thrombosis of the subclavian and/or axillary veins occasionally occurs after excessive and unaccustomed use of the arm at the shoulder joint. The close relationship of these veins to rib 1 and the clavicle and the possibility of repeated minor trauma from these structures are probably factors in its development.

Secondary thrombosis of subclavian and/or axillary veins is a common complication of an indwelling venous catheter. Rarely, the condition may follow a radical mastectomy with a block dissection of the lymph nodes of the axilla. Persistent pain, heaviness, and edema of the upper limb, especially after exercise, are complications of this condition.

Anatomy of Subclavian Vein Catheterization

The subclavian vein is in the lower anterior corner of the posterior triangle of the neck (Fig. 9.79), where it lies immediately posterior to the medial third of the clavicle.

Infraclavicular Approach

Because the subclavian vein lies close to the undersurface of the medial third of the clavicle, this is a relatively safe site for catheterization. The vein is slightly more medially placed on the left side than on the right side.

Anatomy of Procedure

The needle should be inserted through the skin just below the lower border of the clavicle at the junction of the medial third and outer two thirds, coinciding with the posterior border of the origin of the clavicular head of the SCM muscle on the upper border of the clavicle. The needle pierces the following structures:

- Skin
- Superficial fascia
- Pectoralis major muscle (clavicular head)
- Clavipectoral fascia and subclavius muscle
- Wall of subclavian vein

The needle is pointed upward and posteriorly toward the middle of the suprasternal notch.

Anatomy of Problems

- **Hitting the clavicle:** The needle may be "walked" along the lower surface of the clavicle until its posterior edge is reached.
- **Hitting rib 1:** The needle may hit rib 1 if it is pointed downward, not upward.
- **Hitting the subclavian artery:** A pulsatile resistance and bright red blood flow indicate that the needle has passed posterior to the scalenus anterior muscle and perforated the subclavian artery.

Anatomy of Complications

Refer to Figure 9.79.

- **Pneumothorax:** The needle may pierce the cervical dome of the pleura, permitting air to enter the pleural cavity. This complication is more common in children, in whom the pleural reflection is higher than in adults.
- **Hemothorax:** The catheter may pierce the posterior wall of the subclavian vein and the pleura.
- **Subclavian artery puncture:** The needle pierces the wall of the artery during its insertion.
- **Internal thoracic artery injury:** Hemorrhage may occur into the superior mediastinum.
- **Diaphragmatic paralysis:** This occurs when the needle damages the phrenic nerve.

Procedure in Children

The needle pierces the skin in the deltopectoral groove about 2 cm from the clavicle. The catheter is tunneled beneath the skin to enter the subclavian vein at the point where the clavicle and rib 1 cross. The more oblique approach in children minimizes the possibility of entering the subclavian artery.

Supraclavicular Approach

Many prefer this approach (see Fig. 9.79) for the following anatomic reasons:

- The site of penetration of the vein wall is larger, because it lies at the junction of the internal jugular vein and the subclavian vein, which makes the procedure easier.
- The needle is pointed downward and medially toward the mediastinum, away from the pleura, avoiding the complication of pneumothorax.
- The catheter is inserted along a more direct course into the brachiocephalic vein and superior vena cava.

Anatomy of Procedure

With the patient in the Trendelenburg position (patient supine with head tilted downward) or simple supine position and the head turned to the opposite side, the posterior border of the clavicular origin of the SCM muscle is palpated. The needle is inserted through the skin at the site where the posterior border of the clavicular origin of the SCM is attached to the upper border of the clavicle. At this point, the needle lies lateral to the lateral border of scalenus anterior muscle and above rib 1. The needle pierces the following structures:

- Skin
- Superficial fascia and platysma
- Investing layer of deep cervical fascia
- Wall of the subclavian vein

The needle is directed downward in the direction of the opposite nipple. The needle enters the junction of the internal jugular vein and the subclavian vein. It is important that the operator understands that the pleura is not being penetrated and that it is possible for the needle to lie in a zone between the chest wall and the cervical dome of the parietal pleura but outside the pleural space (cavity).

Anatomic Complications

The following complications may occur as the result of damage to neighboring anatomic structures:

- **Diaphragm paralysis:** This is caused by injury to the phrenic nerve as it descends posterior to the internal jugular vein on the surface of the scalenus anterior muscle.
- **Pneumothorax or hemothorax:** This is caused by damage to the pleura and/or internal thoracic artery by the needle passing posteriorly and downward.
- **Brachial plexus injury:** The needle passing posteriorly into the roots or trunks of the plexus causes this.

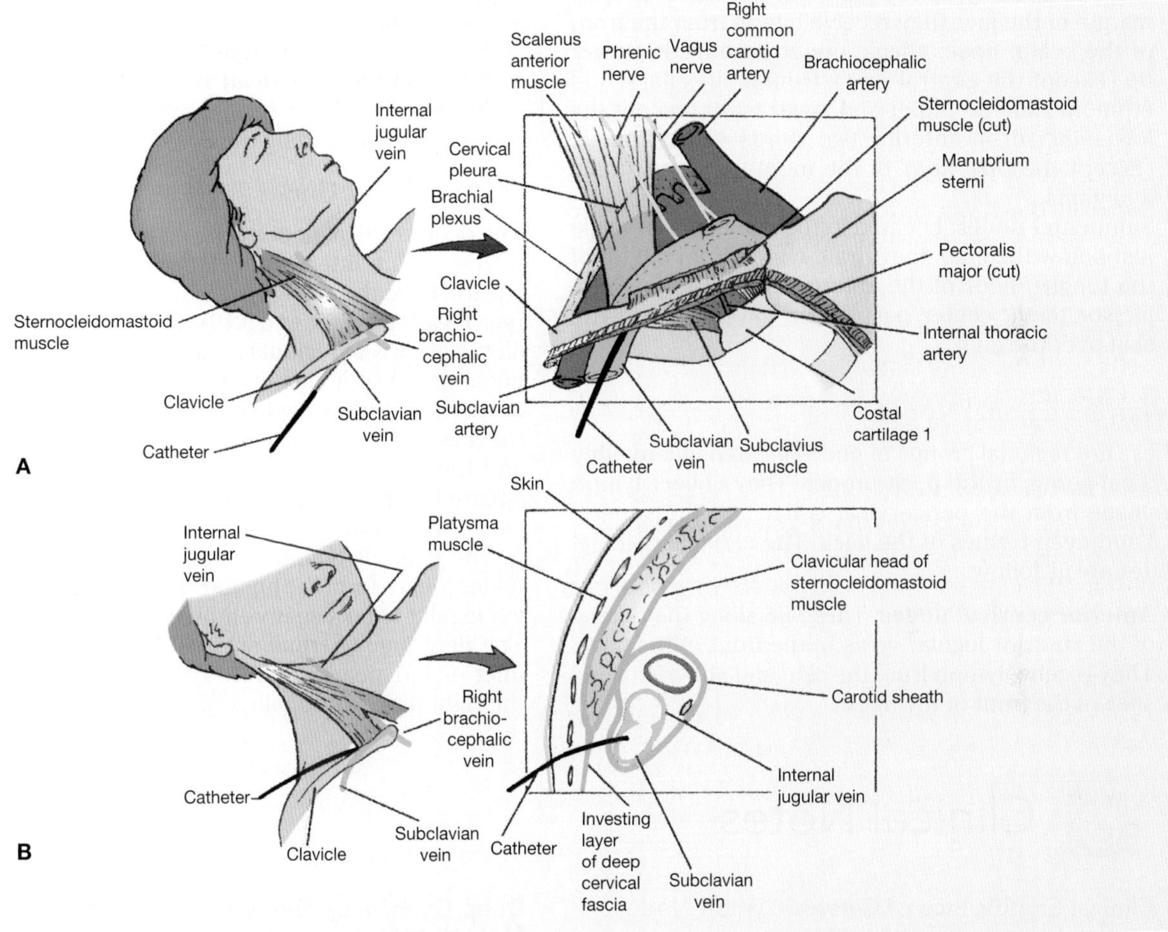

Figure 9.79 Subclavian vein catheterization. **A.** Infraclavicular approach. Note the many important anatomic structures located in this region. **B.** Supraclavicular approach. The catheter enters the subclavian vein close to its junction with the internal jugular vein to form the brachiocephalic vein.

HEAD AND NECK LYMPH DRAINAGE

The lymph nodes of the head and neck are arranged in three groups: (1) a **pericervical collar** that extends from below the chin to the back of the head, (2) a **regional cervical group** located in the neck proper, and (3) a **deep terminal group** that is embedded in the carotid sheath in the neck (see Figs. 9.23 and 9.70).

Pericervical Collar Nodes

The pericervical collar is a series of several regional groups of nodes arranged roughly in a ring around approximately the junction of the head and neck. The superficial tissues of the head drain into appropriately placed groups in the collar or directly into the superficial cervical nodes. Basically, the tissues drain into the nodal group located most closely. Lymph vessels and nodes do not occur in the cranial cavity or orbit. The pericervical nodes are arranged as follows:

- **Occipital nodes:** Located over the occipital bone on the back of the skull, they receive lymph from the back of the scalp.
- **Mastoid (retroauricular) nodes:** Located behind the ear over the mastoid process, they receive lymph from the scalp above the ear, auricle, and external auditory meatus.

- **Parotid nodes:** Located on or within the parotid salivary gland, they receive lymph from the scalp above the parotid gland, eyelids, parotid gland, auricle, and external auditory meatus.
- **Buccal (facial) nodes:** One or two nodes lie in the cheek over the buccinator muscle. They drain lymph that ultimately passes into the submandibular nodes.
- **Submandibular nodes:** Located superficial to the submandibular salivary gland just below the lower margin of the jaw, they receive lymph from the front of the scalp; nose; cheek; upper lip and the lower lip (except the central part); frontal, maxillary, and ethmoid sinuses; upper and lower teeth (except the lower incisors); anterior two thirds of the tongue (except the tip); floor of the mouth and vestibule; and gums.
- **Submental nodes:** Located in the submental triangle just below the chin, they drain lymph from the tip of the tongue, floor of the anterior part of the mouth, incisor teeth, center part of the lower lip, and the skin over the chin.

Cervical Regional Nodes

These are regional groups of nodes located in a roughly vertical series in the neck proper. They collect lymph drainage from the pericervical collar and the superficial and deep tissues of the neck. The cervical regional nodes are as follows:

- **Anterior cervical nodes:** These lie along the course of the anterior jugular veins in the front of the neck. They receive lymph from the skin and superficial tissues of the front of the neck.
- **Superficial cervical nodes:** These lie along the course of the external jugular vein on the side of the neck. They drain lymph from the skin over the angle of the jaw, the skin over the lower part of the parotid gland, and the lobe of the ear.
- **Retropharyngeal nodes:** These lie behind the pharynx and in front of the vertebral column. They receive lymph from the nasopharynx, auditory tube, and vertebral column.
- **Laryngeal nodes:** These lie in front of the larynx. They receive lymph from the larynx.
- **Tracheal (paratracheal) nodes:** These lie alongside the trachea. They receive lymph from neighboring structures, including the thyroid gland.

Deep Cervical Nodes

The deep cervical nodes form a vertical chain along the course of the internal jugular vein, within the carotid sheath, from the base of the skull to the root of the neck (see Figs. 9.23, 9.65, and 9.70). They receive lymph from all the groups of regional nodes and as such are the terminal group of nodes in the neck. The **jugulodigastric node**, which is located below and behind the angle of the jaw, is mainly concerned with drainage of the tonsil and the tongue. The **jugulo-omohyoid node**, which is situated close to the omohyoid muscle, is mainly associated with drainage of the tongue.

The efferent lymph vessels from the deep cervical nodes join to form the **jugular trunks** (see Fig. 9.23). The left jugular trunk usually empties into the **thoracic duct**. The right jugular trunk drains into the **right lymphatic duct** or independently into the region of formation of the right brachiocephalic vein.

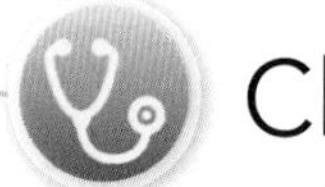

Clinical Notes

Clinical Significance of Cervical Lymph Nodes

The lymph drainage of an organ or region is of great clinical importance. Examination of a patient may reveal an enlarged lymph node. It is the clinician's responsibility to determine the cause and be knowledgeable about the area of the body that drains its lymph into a particular node. For example, an enlarged submandibular node can be caused by a pathologic condition in the scalp, face, maxillary sinus, or the tongue. An infected tooth of the upper or lower jaw may be responsible. Often, a clinician has to search systematically the various areas known to drain into a node to discover the cause.

Deep Cervical Lymph Node Examination

Lymph nodes in the neck should be examined from behind the patient. The examination is made easier by asking the patient to flex the neck slightly to reduce the tension of the muscles. The groups of nodes should be examined in a definite order to avoid omitting any. If enlarged lymph nodes are identified, possible sites of infection or neoplastic growth should be examined, including the face, scalp, tongue, mouth, tonsil, and pharynx.

Deep Cervical Lymph Node Carcinoma Metastases

In the head and neck, all the lymph ultimately drains into the deep cervical group of nodes. Secondary carcinomatous deposits in these nodes are common. The primary growth may be easy to find. On the other hand, at certain anatomic sites, the primary growth may be small and overlooked, for example, in the larynx, pharynx, cervical part of the esophagus, and external auditory meatus. The bronchi, breast, and stomach are sometimes the site of the primary tumor. In these cases, the secondary growth has spread far beyond the local lymph nodes.

When cervical metastases occur, the surgeon usually decides to perform a **block dissection** of the cervical nodes. This procedure involves the removal en bloc of the internal jugular vein, the fascia, lymph nodes, and submandibular salivary gland. The aim of the operation is removal of all the lymph tissues on the affected side of the neck. The carotid arteries and the vagus nerve are carefully preserved. It is often necessary to sacrifice the hypoglossal and vagus nerves, which may be involved in the cancerous deposits. In patients with bilateral spread, a bilateral block dissection may be necessary. An interval of 3 to 4 weeks is necessary before removing the second internal jugular vein.

CRANIAL NERVES

Twelve pairs of CNs branch off the brain and upper spinal cord and pass through the cranial foramina (see Fig. 9.42; see also Cranial Nerves in the Cranial Cavity, discussed earlier). These nerves are identified by name and/or Roman numerals with the abbreviation CN (cranial nerve). For example, CN I is cranial nerve one, the olfactory nerve. The components of the CNs, their functions, and the openings in the skull through which the nerves leave the cranial cavity are summarized in Table 9.7.

Olfactory Nerves (CN I)

The olfactory nerves arise from **olfactory receptor nerve cells** in the olfactory mucous membrane. The olfactory mucous membrane is situated in the upper part of the nasal cavity above the level of the superior concha (Fig. 9.80A). Bundles of these olfactory nerve fibers pass through the openings of the cribriform plate of the ethmoid bone to enter the **olfactory bulb** in the cranial cavity. The olfactory bulb is connected to the olfactory area of the cerebral cortex by the **olfactory tract** (see Fig. 9.42).

Optic Nerve (CN II)

The optic nerve is composed of the axons of the cells of the **ganglionic layer of the retina**. The optic nerve emerges from the back of the eyeball and leaves the orbital cavity through the optic canal to enter the cranial cavity (see Fig. 9.80B). The optic nerve then unites with the optic nerve of the opposite side to form the **optic chiasma**.

In the chiasma, the fibers from the medial half of each retina cross the midline and enter the optic tract of the opposite side, whereas the fibers from the lateral half of each retina pass posteriorly in the optic tract of the same side. Most of the fibers of the optic tract terminate by synapsing with nerve cells in the lateral geniculate body. A few fibers pass to the pretectal nucleus and the superior colliculus and are concerned with light reflexes.

The axons of the nerve cells of the lateral geniculate body pass posteriorly as the optic radiation and terminate in the visual cortex of the cerebral hemisphere.

Oculomotor Nerve (CN III)

The oculomotor nerve emerges on the anterior surface of the midbrain (Figs. 9.42 and 9.81A). It passes forward between the posterior cerebral and superior cerebellar arteries. It then continues into the middle cranial fossa in the lateral wall of the cavernous sinus (see Fig. 9.39). Here, it divides into a superior ramus and an inferior ramus, which enter the orbital cavity through the superior orbital fissure (see Fig. 9.52).

The oculomotor nerve supplies the following:

- **Extrinsic eye muscles.** Somatic motor fibers supply the levator palpebrae superioris, superior rectus, medial rectus, inferior rectus, and inferior oblique (see Fig. 9.81A).
- **Intrinsic eye muscles.** The parasympathetic component of the oculomotor nerve supplies the constrictor pupillae of the iris and the ciliary muscles. These fibers synapse in the **ciliary ganglion** and reach the eyeball in the **short ciliary nerves** (see Fig. 9.53).

The oculomotor nerve is entirely motor (both somatic and visceral motor). It is responsible for lifting the upper eyelid; turning the eye upward, downward, and medially; constricting the pupil; and accommodation of the eye.

Trochlear Nerve (CN IV)

The trochlear nerve is the slenderest CN. Having crossed the nerve of the opposite side, it leaves the posterior surface of the midbrain (Fig. 9.81B). It then passes forward through the middle cranial fossa in the lateral wall of the cavernous sinus and enters the orbit through the superior orbital fissure (see Figs. 9.39 and 9.52).

The trochlear nerve supplies only the **superior oblique muscle** of the eyeball (an extrinsic muscle) (see Fig. 9.54). The nerve is entirely motor and assists in turning the eye downward and laterally.

Trigeminal Nerve (CN V)

The trigeminal nerve is the largest CN in the head (the vagus nerve has an extensive postcranial territory) (Fig. 9.82A). It leaves the anterior aspect of the pons as a small motor root and a large sensory root (see Fig. 9.42), and it passes forward, out of the posterior cranial fossa, to reach the apex of the petrous part of the temporal bone in the middle cranial fossa. Here, the large sensory root expands to form the trigeminal ganglion (see Figs. 9.54 and 9.82A). The ganglion lies within a pouch of dura mater called the **trigeminal cave**. The motor root of the trigeminal nerve is situated below the sensory ganglion and is completely separated from it. The **ophthalmic (V1)**, **maxillary (V2)**, and **mandibular (V3) nerves** arise from the anterior border of the ganglion.

Ophthalmic Nerve (V1)

The ophthalmic nerve is purely sensory (see Fig. 9.26). It runs forward in the lateral wall of the cavernous sinus in the middle cranial fossa (see Fig. 9.39) and divides into three branches, the **lacrimal**, **frontal**, and **nasociliary nerves**, which enter the orbital cavity through the superior orbital fissure (see Figs. 9.52, 9.54, and 9.82A).

Branches

The **lacrimal nerve** runs forward on the upper border of the lateral rectus muscle (see Fig. 9.54). The zygomaticotemporal branch of the maxillary nerve, which contains the parasympathetic secretomotor fibers to the lacrimal gland, joins it. The lacrimal nerve then enters the lacrimal gland and gives branches to the conjunctiva and the skin of the upper eyelid.

Table 9.7 Cranial Nerves

NERVE	COMPONENTS	FUNCTION	OPENING IN THE SKULL
I. Olfactory	Sensory	Smell	Openings in cribriform plate of ethmoid
II. Optic	Sensory	Vision	Optic canal
III. Oculomotor	Motor	Lifts upper eyelid; turns eyeball upward, downward, and medially; constricts pupil; accommodates eye	Superior orbital fissure
IV. Trochlear	Motor	Assists in turning eyeball downward and laterally	Superior orbital fissure
V. Trigeminal			
Ophthalmic division	Sensory	Cornea, skin of forehead, scalp, eyelids, and nose; also mucous membrane of paranasal sinuses and nasal cavity	Superior orbital fissure
Maxillary division	Sensory	Skin of face over the maxilla and the upper lip, teeth of the upper jaw, mucous membrane of the nose, the maxillary air sinus, and palate	Foramen rotundum
Mandibular division	Motor	Muscles of mastication, mylohyoid, anterior belly of digastric, tensor veli palatini, and tensor tympani	Foramen ovale
	Sensory	Skin of cheek; skin over mandible, lower lip, and side of head; teeth of lower jaw and temporomandibular joint; mucous membrane of the mouth and anterior two thirds of the tongue	
VI. Abducens	Motor	Lateral rectus muscle: turns eyeball laterally	Superior orbital fissure
VII. Facial	Motor	Muscles of the face, cheek, and scalp; stapedius muscle of the middle ear; stylohyoid; and posterior belly of digastric	Internal acoustic meatus, facial canal, stylomastoid foramen
	Sensory	Taste from anterior two thirds of the tongue, floor of mouth, and palate	
	Secretomotor parasympathetic	Submandibular and sublingual salivary glands, lacrimal gland, and glands of the nose and palate	Petrotympanic fissure; hiatus of facial canal, foramen lacerum, pterygoid canal
VIII. Vestibulocochlear			
Vestibular	Sensory	Position and movement of the head	Internal acoustic meatus
Cochlear	Sensory	Hearing	
IX. Glossopharyngeal	Motor	Stylopharyngeus muscle: assists swallowing	Jugular foramen
	Secretomotor parasympathetic	Parotid salivary gland	Jugular foramen
	Sensory	General sensation and taste from posterior third of the tongue and pharynx; carotid sinus and carotid body	Jugular foramen
X. Vagus	Motor	Constrictor muscles of the pharynx and intrinsic muscles of the larynx; involuntary muscle of trachea and bronchi, heart, alimentary tract from pharynx to splenic flexure of colon; liver and pancreas	Jugular foramen
	Sensory	Taste from epiglottis and vallecula and afferent fibers from structures named above	
XI. Accessory			
Cranial root	Motor	Muscles of the soft palate, pharynx, and larynx	Jugular foramen
Spinal root	Motor	Sternocleidomastoid and trapezius muscles	Foramen magnum, jugular foramen
XII. Hypoglossal	Motor	Muscles of the tongue controlling its shape and movement (except palatoglossus)	Hypoglossal canal

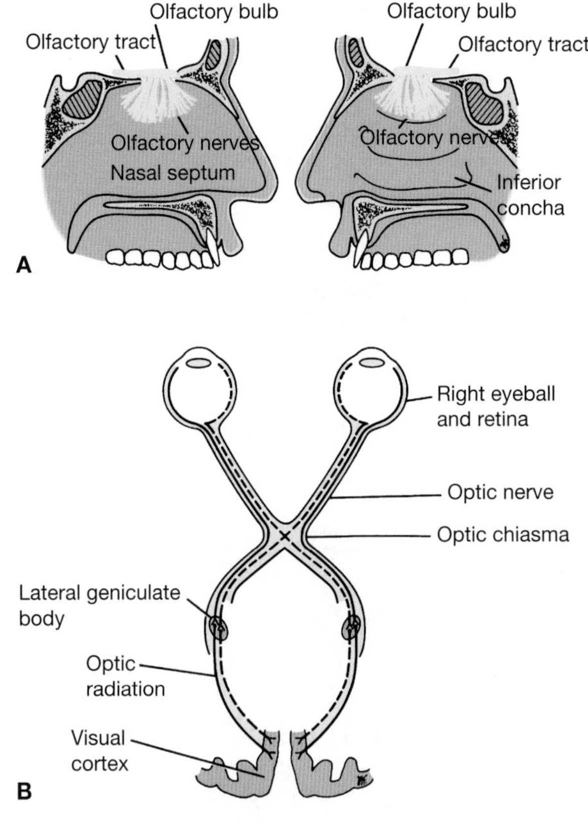

Figure 9.80 **A.** Distribution of the olfactory nerves on the nasal septum and the lateral wall of the nose. **B.** The optic nerve and its connections.

The **frontal nerve** runs forward on the upper surface of the levator palpebrae superioris muscle and divides into the **supraorbital** and **supratrochlear nerves**. These nerves leave the orbital cavity and supply the frontal air sinus and the skin of the forehead and the scalp.

The **nasociliary nerve** crosses the optic nerve, runs forward on the upper border of the medial rectus muscle, and continues as the **anterior ethmoid nerve** through the anterior ethmoidal foramen to enter the cranial cavity. It then descends through a slit at the side of the crista galli to enter the nasal cavity. It gives off two **internal nasal br**anches, and it then supplies the skin of the tip of the nose with the **external nasal nerve**. Its branches include the following:

- **Sensory fibers** to the ciliary ganglion
- **Long ciliary nerves** that contain sympathetic fibers to the dilator pupillae muscle and sensory fibers to the cornea
- **Infratrochlear nerve** that supplies the skin of the eyelids
- **Posterior ethmoidal nerve** that is sensory to the ethmoid and sphenoid sinuses

Maxillary Nerve (V2)

The maxillary nerve is purely sensory (see Fig. 9.26). It arises from the trigeminal ganglion in the middle cranial fossa, passes forward in the lateral wall of the cavernous sinus, and leaves the skull through the foramen rotundum (see Figs. 9.39 and 9.54). It then enters the pterygopalatine fossa, where it divides into several branches (see Fig. 9.53).

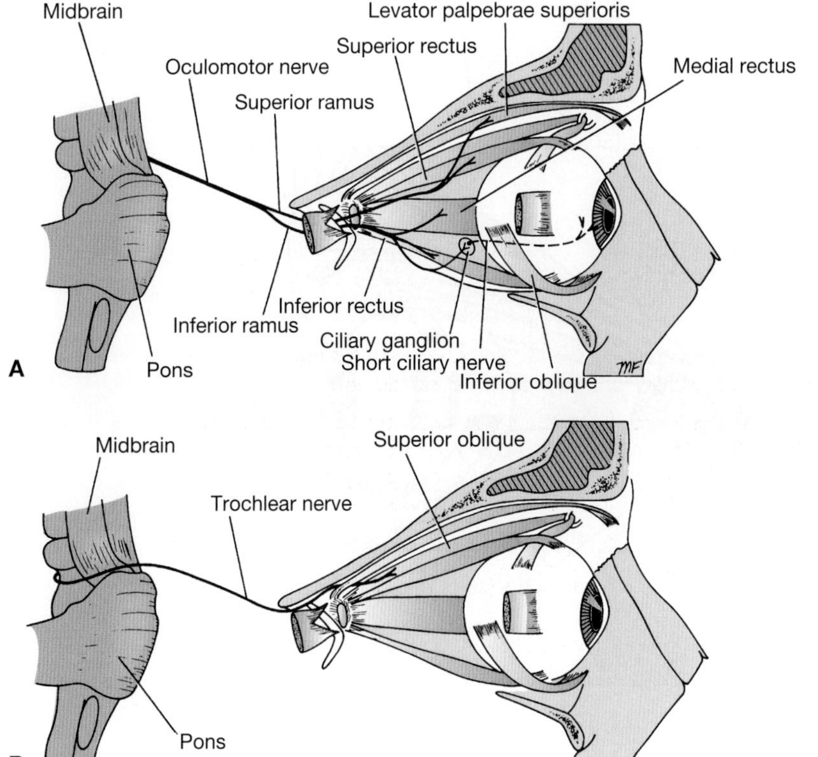

Figure 9.81 **A.** Origin and distribution of the oculomotor nerve. **B.** Origin and distribution of the trochlear nerve.

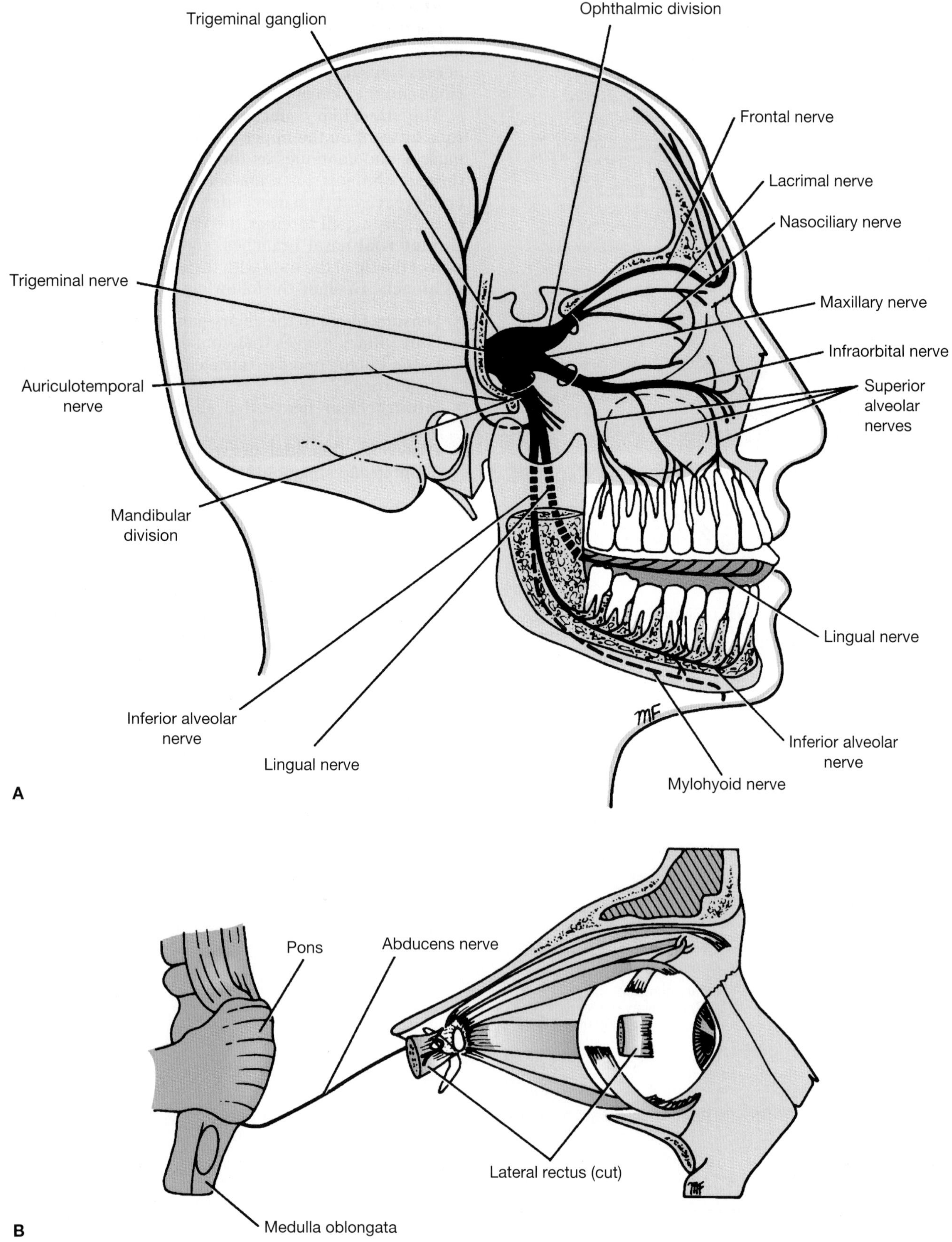

Figure 9.82 **A.** Distribution of the trigeminal nerve. **B.** Origin and distribution of the abducens nerve.

Branches

- **Meningeal branches** (**middle meningeal nerve**) to the dura mater lining the middle cranial fossa.
- **Zygomatic branch**, which divides into the **zygomaticotemporal** and the **zygomaticofacial nerves** that supply the skin of the face. The zygomaticotemporal branch gives parasympathetic secretomotor fibers to the lacrimal gland via the lacrimal nerve.
- **Infraorbital nerve** is the main continuation of the maxillary nerve into the infraorbital groove. As it proceeds forward, it gives off the **middle superior alveolar** and **anterior superior alveolar nerves** to the maxillary sinus, the upper teeth and gums, and the cheek. Finally, it emerges on the face through the infraorbital foramen and gives sensory fibers to the skin of the face and the side of the nose.
- **Ganglionic branches**, which are two short nerves that suspend the **pterygopalatine ganglion** in the pterygopalatine fossa. They contain sensory fibers that have passed through the ganglion from the nose, palate, and pharynx. They also contain postganglionic parasympathetic fibers that are going to the lacrimal gland.
- **Posterior superior alveolar nerve**, which supplies the maxillary sinus as well as the upper molar teeth and adjoining parts of the gum and the cheek.

Pterygopalatine Ganglion

The pterygopalatine ganglion is a **parasympathetic ganglion**, which is suspended from the maxillary nerve in the pterygopalatine fossa. It is secretomotor to the lacrimal and nasal glands. Its branches also convey somatic sensory fibers into the maxillary nerve.

- **Orbital branches**, which enter the orbit through the inferior orbital fissure
- **Greater and lesser palatine nerves**, which descend through the pterygopalatine canal and exit through the greater and lesser palatine foramina, respectively, to supply the palate, the tonsil, and the nasal cavity
- **Pharyngeal nerve**, which supplies the roof of the nasopharynx
- **Nasopalatine nerve**, which passes through the sphenopalatine foramen and courses across the nasal septum to the incisive foramen and the anterior hard palate

Mandibular Nerve (V3)

The mandibular nerve is both motor and sensory. The sensory root leaves the trigeminal ganglion and passes out of the skull through the foramen ovale to enter the infratemporal fossa. The motor root of the trigeminal nerve also leaves the skull through the foramen ovale and joins the sensory root to form the trunk of the mandibular nerve, which then divides into a small anterior and a large posterior division (see Fig. 9.63; also Figs. 9.54, 9.62, and 9.82A).

Mandibular Nerve Main Trunk Branches

- **Meningeal branch (spinous nerve)**. This is the major nerve to the dura mater; it follows the middle meningeal artery.
- **Nerve to the medial pterygoid muscle**, which supplies both the medial pterygoid and the tensor veli palatini muscles.

Mandibular Nerve Anterior Division Branches

- **Masseteric nerve** to the masseter muscle
- **Deep temporal nerves** to the temporalis muscle
- **Nerve to the lateral pterygoid muscle**
- **Buccal nerve** to the skin and the mucous membrane of the cheek. The buccal nerve does not supply the buccinator muscle (which is supplied by the facial nerve), and it is the only sensory branch of the anterior division of the mandibular nerve.

Mandibular Nerve Posterior Division Branches

- **Auriculotemporal nerve**, which supplies the skin of the auricle, the external auditory meatus, the TMJ, and the scalp. This nerve also conveys postganglionic parasympathetic secretomotor fibers from the **otic ganglion** to the parotid salivary gland.
- **Lingual nerve**, which descends in front of the inferior alveolar nerve and enters the mouth. It then runs forward on the side of the tongue and crosses the submandibular duct. The **chorda tympani nerve** (branch of the facial nerve) joins the lingual nerve deep in the infratemporal fossa. The lingual nerve fibers carry general sensation from the mucous membrane of the anterior two thirds of the tongue and the floor of the mouth. The chorda tympani fibers carry taste from the anterior two thirds of the tongue and also give off preganglionic parasympathetic secretomotor fibers to the submandibular ganglion.
- **Inferior alveolar nerve**, which enters the mandibular foramen and canal to supply the teeth of the lower jaw and emerges through the mental foramen (**mental nerve**) to supply the skin of the chin. Before entering the canal, it gives off the **mylohyoid nerve**, which supplies the mylohyoid muscle and the anterior belly of the digastric muscle.
- **Communicating branch**, which frequently runs from the inferior alveolar nerve to the lingual nerve.

The branches of the posterior division of the mandibular nerve are sensory (except the nerve to the mylohyoid muscle).

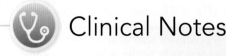

Lingual Nerve Injury

The lingual nerve passes forward into the submandibular region from the infratemporal fossa by running beneath the origin of the superior constrictor muscle, which is attached to the posterior border of the mylohyoid line on the mandible. Here, it is closely related to the last molar tooth and is liable to be damaged in cases of difficult extraction of an impacted third molar.

Otic Ganglion

The otic ganglion is a **parasympathetic ganglion** located medial to the mandibular nerve just below the skull; it adheres to the nerve to the medial pterygoid muscle. The preganglionic fibers originate in the **glossopharyngeal nerve**, and reach the ganglion via the **lesser petrosal nerve** (see Glossopharyngeal Nerve [CN IX]). The postganglionic secretomotor fibers reach the parotid salivary gland via the **auriculotemporal nerve**.

Submandibular Ganglion

The submandibular ganglion is a **parasympathetic ganglion** that lies deep to the submandibular salivary gland and is attached to the lingual nerve by small connecting branches (see Figs. 9.62 and 9.63). Preganglionic parasympathetic fibers reach the ganglion from the facial nerve via the **chorda tympani** and the **lingual nerves**. Postganglionic secretomotor fibers pass to the submandibular and the sublingual salivary glands.

The trigeminal nerve is thus the main sensory nerve of the head and innervates the muscles of mastication. It also tenses the soft palate and the tympanic membrane.

Abducens Nerve (CN VI)

This small nerve emerges from the anterior surface of the hindbrain between the pons and the medulla oblongata (see Figs. 9.42 and 9.82B). It passes forward with the internal carotid artery through the cavernous sinus in the middle cranial fossa and enters the orbit through the superior orbital fissure (see Figs. 9.39 and 9.52). The abducens nerve supplies the **lateral rectus muscle** (see Figs. 9.54 and 9.82B) and is therefore responsible for turning the eye laterally.

Facial Nerve (CN VII)

The facial nerve has a motor root and a sensory root **(nervus intermedius)** (Fig. 9.83). The nerve emerges on the anterior surface of the hindbrain between the pons and the medulla oblongata (see Fig. 9.42). The roots pass laterally in the posterior cranial fossa with the vestibulocochlear nerve and enter the internal acoustic meatus in the petrous part of the temporal bone. At the bottom of the meatus, the nerve enters the facial canal that runs laterally through the inner ear. On reaching the medial wall of the middle ear (tympanic cavity), the nerve swells to form the sensory **geniculate ganglion** (Fig. 9.83B; see also Middle Ear). The nerve then bends sharply backward above the promontory and, at the posterior wall of the middle ear, bends down on the medial side of the aditus of the mastoid antrum. The nerve descends behind the pyramid and emerges from the temporal bone through the stylomastoid foramen. The facial nerve now passes forward through the parotid gland to its distribution across the face (Fig. 9.83A).

Important Branches

- **Greater petrosal nerve** arises from the nerve at the geniculate ganglion (see Fig. 9.83B). It contains preganglionic parasympathetic fibers that synapse in the **pterygopalatine ganglion**. The postganglionic fibers are secretomotor to the lacrimal gland and the glands of the nose and the palate. The greater petrosal nerve may also contain taste fibers from the palate.
- **Nerve to stapedius** supplies the stapedius muscle in the middle ear.
- **Chorda tympani nerve** arises from the facial nerve in the facial canal in the posterior wall of the middle ear. It runs forward over the medial surface of the upper part of the tympanic membrane, leaves the middle ear through the petrotympanic fissure, and enters the infratemporal fossa, where it joins the **lingual nerve**. The chorda tympani contains **preganglionic parasympathetic secretomotor fibers** to the submandibular and the sublingual salivary glands. It also contains **taste fibers** from the anterior two thirds of the tongue and floor of the mouth.
- **Posterior auricular nerve** is a small **mixed branch** given off by the facial nerve as it emerges from the stylomastoid foramen; it supplies the back of the auricle, external auditory meatus, tympanic membrane, and posterior auricular muscle. Small **muscular branches** to the posterior belly of digastric and the stylohyoid muscles emerge in the same way (see Fig. 9.83A).
- **Five terminal branches to the muscles of facial expression**. These are the **temporal**, **zygomatic buccal**, **mandibular**, and **cervical branches**.

The facial nerve lies within the parotid salivary gland (see Parotid Gland) after leaving the stylomastoid foramen and is located between the superficial and the deep parts of the gland. Here, it gives off the terminal branches that emerge from the anterior border of the gland and pass to the muscles of the face and the scalp. The buccal branch supplies the buccinator muscle, and the cervical branch supplies the platysma.

The facial nerve thus controls facial expression, salivation, and lacrimation; it is a pathway for taste sensation from the anterior part of the tongue and floor of the mouth and from the palate; it also affects hearing.

Vestibulocochlear Nerve (CN VIII)

The vestibulocochlear nerve is a sensory nerve that consists of two sets of fibers: **vestibular** and **cochlear**. They leave the anterior surface of the brain between the pons and the medulla oblongata (Fig. 9.84A; see also Fig. 9.42). They cross the posterior cranial fossa and enter the internal acoustic meatus with the facial nerve.

Vestibular Fibers

The vestibular fibers are the central processes of the nerve cells of the **vestibular ganglion** situated in the internal acoustic meatus (see Fig. 9.84A). The vestibular fibers originate from the vestibule and the semicircular

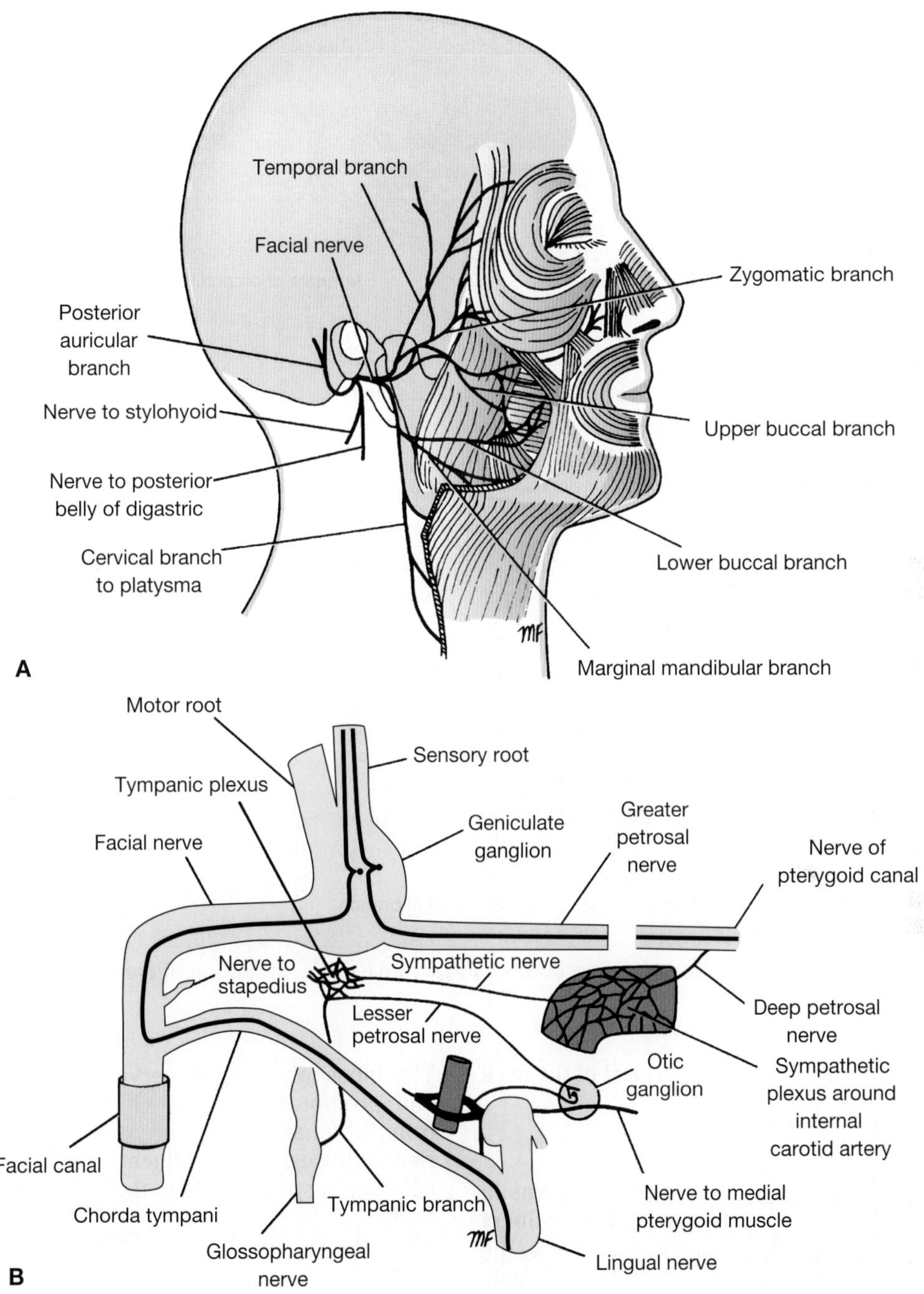

Figure 9.83 **A.** Distribution of the facial nerve. **B.** Branches of the facial nerve within the petrous part of the temporal bone; the taste fibers are shown in *black*. The glossopharyngeal nerve is also shown.

canals; therefore, they are concerned with the sense of position and with movement of the head.

Cochlear Fibers

The cochlear fibers are the central processes of the nerve cells of the **spiral ganglion of the cochlea** (see Fig. 9.84A). The cochlear fibers originate in the **spiral organ of Corti** and are therefore concerned with hearing.

Glossopharyngeal Nerve (CN IX)

The glossopharyngeal nerve is a mixed motor and sensory nerve. It emerges from the anterior surface of the medulla oblongata between the olive and the inferior cerebellar peduncle (see Figs. 9.42 and 9.84B). It passes laterally in the posterior cranial fossa and leaves the skull by passing through the jugular foramen. The **superior** and **inferior sensory ganglia** are located on the nerve as it passes through the foramen. The glossopharyngeal

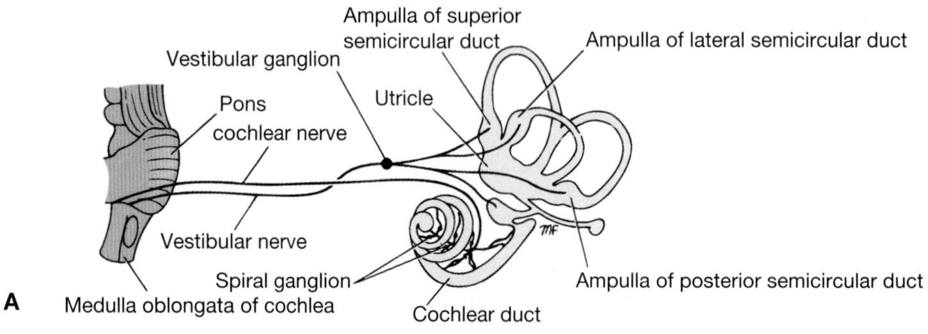

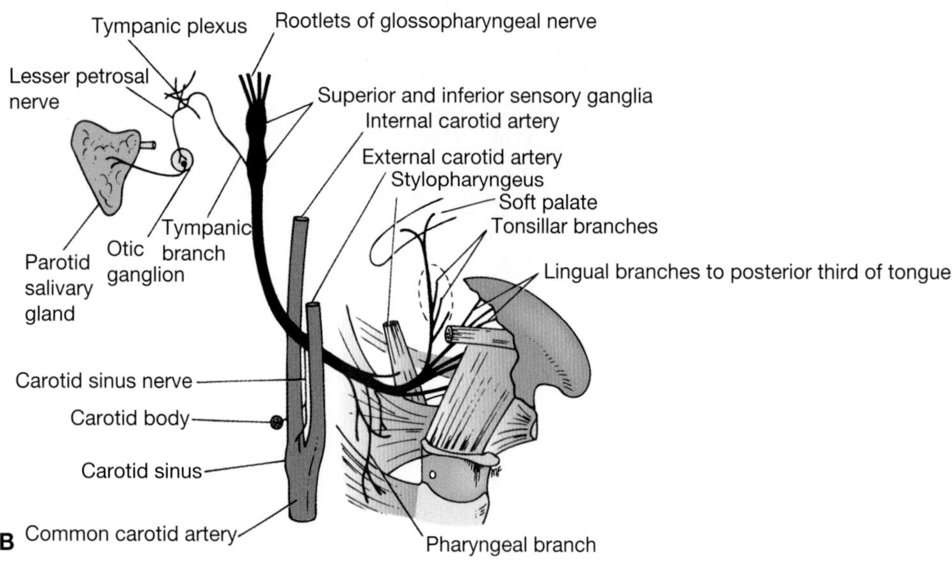

Figure 9.84 **A.** Origin and distribution of the vestibulocochlear nerve. **B.** Distribution of the glossopharyngeal nerve.

nerve then descends through the upper part of the neck to the back of the tongue.

Important Branches

- **Tympanic nerve** passes to the **tympanic plexus** in the middle ear. Preganglionic parasympathetic fibers for the parotid salivary gland leave the plexus as the **lesser petrosal nerve**; they synapse in the **otic ganglion**. Postganglionic fibers attach to the auriculotemporal nerve (a branch of V3) and follow that to the parotid gland.
- **Carotid nerve** contains sensory fibers from the **carotid sinus** (pressoreceptor mechanism for the regulation of blood pressure) and the **carotid body** (chemoreceptor mechanism for the regulation of heart rate and respiration).
- **Nerve to the stylopharyngeus muscle**. This is the sole muscle supplied by the glossopharyngeal nerve.
- **Pharyngeal branches** run to the **pharyngeal plexus** and also receive branches from the vagus nerve and the sympathetic trunk.
- **Lingual branch** carries general sensory and taste fibers from the mucous membrane of the posterior third of the tongue (including the vallate papillae).

The glossopharyngeal nerve thus assists swallowing and promotes salivation. It also conducts sensation from the pharynx and the back of the tongue and carries impulses, which influence the arterial blood pressure and respiration, from the carotid sinus and carotid body.

Vagus Nerve (CN X)

The vagus nerve is composed of motor and sensory fibers and has the most extensive distribution of all the CNs. It emerges from the anterior surface of the medulla oblongata between the olive and the inferior cerebellar peduncle (see Fig. 9.42). The nerve passes laterally through the posterior cranial fossa and leaves the skull through the jugular foramen. The vagus nerve has both **superior** and **inferior sensory ganglia** (Fig. 9.85). Below the inferior ganglion, the **cranial root of the accessory nerve** joins the vagus nerve and distributes mainly in its pharyngeal and recurrent laryngeal branches.

The vagus nerve descends through the neck alongside the carotid arteries and internal jugular vein within the carotid sheath (see Fig. 9.65). It passes through the mediastinum of the thorax, passing behind the root of

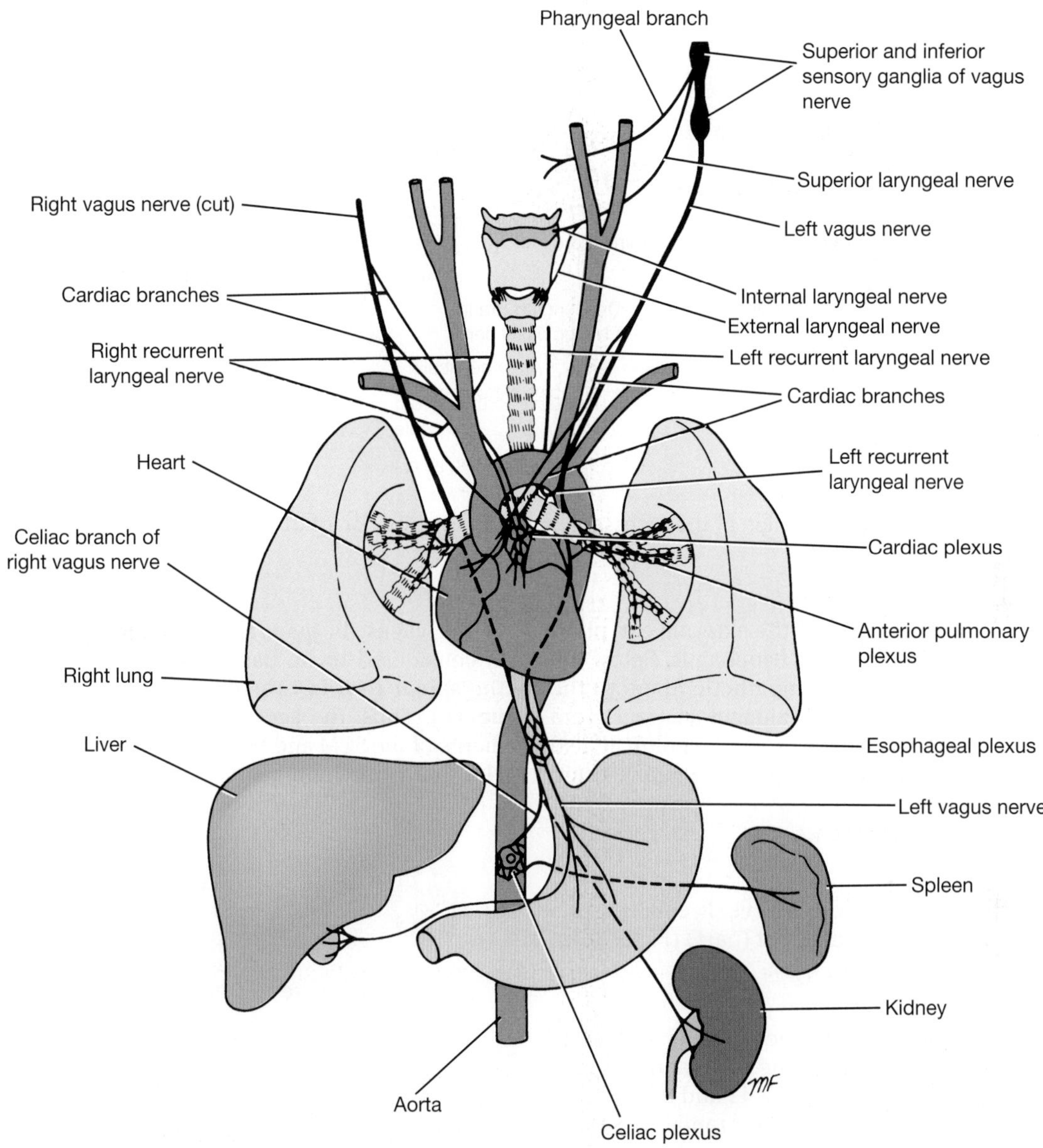

Figure 9.85 Distribution of the vagus nerve.

the lung, and enters the abdomen through the esophageal opening in the diaphragm (see Fig. 9.85).

Important Branches in the Head and Neck

- **Auricular branch** supplies the pinna, external auditory meatus, and tympanic membrane.
- **Pharyngeal branch** contains nerve fibers from the **cranial part of the accessory nerve**. This branch joins the **pharyngeal plexus** and supplies all the muscles of the pharynx (except the stylopharyngeus) and of the soft palate (except the tensor veli palatini).
- **Superior laryngeal nerve** divides into the internal and the external laryngeal nerves. The **internal laryngeal nerve** is sensory to the mucous membrane of the piriform fossa and the larynx down as far as the vocal cords. The **external laryngeal nerve** is motor and is located close to the superior thyroid artery; it supplies the cricothyroid muscle.
- **Recurrent laryngeal nerve** hooks around the **first part of the subclavian artery** on the right side and then ascends in the groove between the trachea and the esophagus. On the left side, the nerve hooks around the **arch of the aorta** and then ascends into the neck between the trachea and the esophagus. The nerve is closely related to the inferior thyroid artery, and it supplies all the muscles of the larynx (except the cricothyroid muscle), the mucous membrane of the larynx below the vocal cords, and the mucous membrane of the upper part of the trachea.
- **Cardiac branches** (two or three) arise in the neck, descend into the thorax, and end in the **cardiac plexus**.

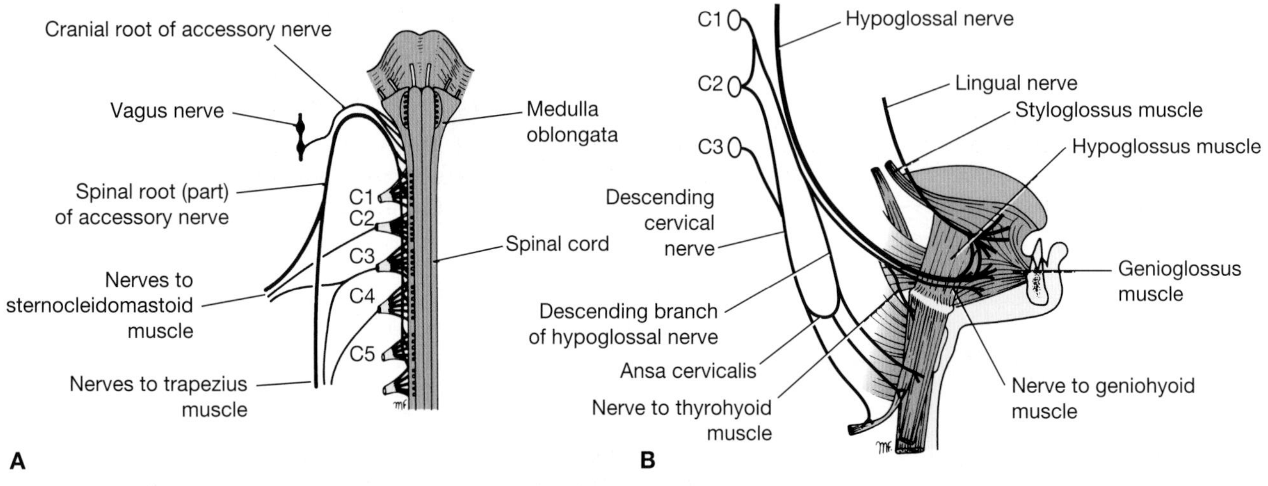

Figure 9.86 **A.** Origin and distribution of the accessory nerve. **B.** Distribution of the hypoglossal nerve.

The vagus nerve thus innervates the external ear, pharynx, larynx, trachea, and cervical esophagus. Below the neck, the vagus supplies parasympathetic fibers to the thoracic viscera and much of the alimentary tract, from the esophagus to the splenic flexure of the colon. It also supplies glands associated with the alimentary tract, such as the liver and pancreas.

Accessory Nerve (CN XI)

The accessory nerve is a motor nerve. It consists of a **cranial root** (part) and a **spinal root** (part) (Fig. 9.86A).

Cranial Root

The cranial root emerges from the anterior surface of the medulla oblongata between the olive and the inferior cerebellar peduncle (see Figs. 9.42 and 9.86A). The nerve runs laterally in the posterior cranial fossa and joins the spinal root.

Spinal Root

The spinal root arises from nerve cells in the anterior gray column (horn) of the C1 to C5 segments of the spinal cord (see Fig. 9.86A). The nerve ascends alongside the spinal cord and enters the skull through the foramen magnum. It then turns laterally to join the cranial root.

The two roots unite and leave the skull through the jugular foramen. The roots then separate: the **cranial root** joins the **vagus nerve** and is distributed in its branches to the muscles of the soft palate and pharynx (via the pharyngeal plexus) and to the muscles of the larynx (except the cricothyroid muscle). The **spinal root** runs downward and laterally and enters the deep surface of the sternocleidomastoid muscle, which it supplies, and then crosses the posterior triangle of the neck to supply the trapezius muscle (see Fig. 9.70).

The cranial root is considered accessory to the vagus nerve by providing a large part of the motor component of the vagus. In general terminology, the cranial root is considered to be part of the vagus nerve, whereas the **spinal root is considered to be CN XI** (**accessory nerve**). Thus, the accessory nerve controls the movements of the SCM and trapezius muscles, two large muscles in the neck and back.

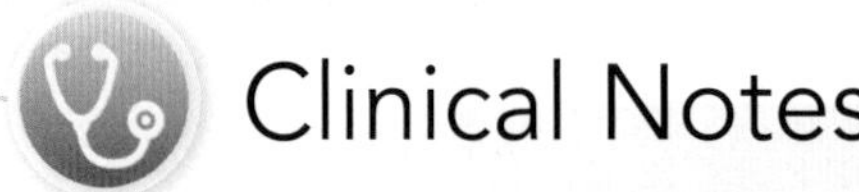

Accessory Nerve Injury

The accessory nerve crosses the posterior triangle of the neck in a relatively superficial position. It can be injured at operation or from penetrating wounds. The trapezius muscle is paralyzed, the muscle shows wasting, and the shoulder drops. The patient will experience difficulty in elevating the arm above the head, having abducted it to a right angle by using the deltoid muscle.

Clinical examination of this nerve involves asking the patient to rotate the head to one side against resistance, causing the sternocleidomastoid of the opposite side to come into action. Then, the patient is asked to shrug the shoulders, causing the trapezius muscles to come into action.

Hypoglossal Nerve (CN XII)

The hypoglossal nerve is a motor nerve. It emerges on the anterior surface of the medulla oblongata between the pyramid and the olive (see Fig. 9.42), crosses the posterior cranial fossa, and leaves the skull through the hypoglossal canal. The nerve then passes downward and forward in the neck and crosses the internal and external carotid arteries to reach the tongue (Fig. 9.86B). In the upper part of its course, C1 fibers from the cervical plexus join it.

Important Branches

- **Meningeal branch**.
- **Descending branch** (C1 fibers) passes downward and joins the descending cervical nerve (C2 and C3) to form the **ansa cervicalis**. Branches from this loop supply the omohyoid, the sternohyoid, and the sternothyroid muscles.
- **Nerve to the thyrohyoid muscle (C1)**.
- **Muscular branches to all the muscles of the tongue** except the palatoglossus (pharyngeal plexus).
- **Nerve to the geniohyoid muscle (C1)**.

The hypoglossal nerve thus innervates the muscles of the tongue (except the palatoglossus) and therefore controls the shape and movements of the tongue.

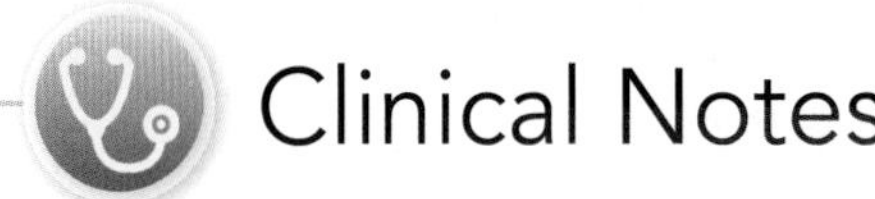

Clinical Notes

Cranial Nerve Clinical Testing

Systematic examination of the 12 CNs is an important part of the examination of every neurologic patient. It may reveal a lesion of a CN nucleus or its central connections, or it may show an interruption of the lower motor neurons.

Testing Olfactory Nerve Integrity

Applying substances with different odors to each nostril in turn can test the olfactory nerve. It should be remembered that food flavors depend on the sense of smell and not on the sense of taste. Fractures of the anterior cranial fossa or cerebral tumors of the frontal lobes may produce lesions of the olfactory nerves, with consequent loss of the sense of smell (**anosmia**).

Testing Optic Nerve Integrity

The optic nerve is evaluated by first asking the patient whether any changes in eyesight have been noted. Using charts with lines of print of varying sizes, then test the acuity of vision. The retinas and optic discs should then be examined with an ophthalmoscope. When examining the optic disc, it should be remembered that the intracranial subarachnoid space extends forward around the optic nerve to the back of the eyeball. The retinal artery and vein run in the optic nerve and cross the subarachnoid space of the nerve sheath a short distance behind the eyeball. A rise in cerebrospinal fluid pressure in the subarachnoid space will compress the thin walls of the retinal vein as it crosses the space, resulting in congestion of the retinal veins, edema of the retina, and bulging of the optic disc (**papilledema**).

The visual fields should then be tested. The patient is asked to gaze straight ahead at a fixed object with the eye under test, the opposite eye being covered. A small object is then moved in an arc around the periphery of the field of vision, and the patient is asked whether they can see the object. It is important not to miss loss or impairment of vision in the central area of the field (**central scotoma**).

Blindness in one half of each visual field is called **hemianopia**. Lesions of the optic tract and optic radiation produce the same hemianopia for both eyes, that is, **homonymous hemianopia. Bitemporal hemianopia** is a loss of the lateral halves of the fields of vision of both eyes (ie, loss of function of the medial half of both retinas). This condition is most commonly produced by a tumor of the pituitary gland exerting pressure on the optic chiasma.

Testing Oculomotor, Trochlear, and Abducens Nerve Integrity

The oculomotor, trochlear, and abducens nerves innervate the muscles that move the eyeball. The oculomotor nerve supplies all the orbital muscles except the superior oblique and the lateral rectus. It also supplies the levator palpebrae superioris and the smooth muscles concerned with accommodation—namely, the sphincter pupillae and the ciliary muscle. The trochlear nerve supplies the superior oblique muscle, and the abducens nerve supplies the lateral rectus.

To examine the ocular muscles, the patient's head is fixed, and they are asked to move the eyes in turn to the left, right, upward, and downward, as far as possible in each direction.

In **complete CN III paralysis**, the eye cannot be moved up, down, or inward. At rest, the eye looks laterally (**external strabismus**) because of the activity of the lateral rectus and downward because of the activity of the superior oblique. The patient sees double (**diplopia**). Drooping of the upper eyelid (**ptosis**) occurs because of paralysis of the levator palpebrae superioris (or possibly the superior tarsal muscle). The pupil is widely dilated and nonreactive to light because of the paralysis of the sphincter pupillae and the unopposed action of the dilator pupillae (supplied by sympathetic fibers). Accommodation of the eye is paralyzed.

In **CN IV paralysis**, the patient complains of double vision on looking straight downward. This is because the superior oblique is paralyzed, and the eye turns medially as the inferior rectus pulls the eye downward.

In **CN VI paralysis**, the patient cannot turn the eyeball laterally. When looking straight ahead, the lateral rectus is paralyzed, and the unopposed medial rectus pulls the eyeball medially, causing **internal strabismus**.

Testing Trigeminal Nerve Integrity

The trigeminal nerve has sensory and motor roots. The sensory root passes to the trigeminal ganglion, from which emerge the ophthalmic (V1), maxillary (V2), and mandibular (V3) divisions. The motor root joins the mandibular division.

(continued)

Sensory function can be tested by using a cotton wisp over each area of the face supplied by the divisions of the trigeminal nerve (see Fig. 9.26).

Asking the patient to clench the teeth can test **motor function**. The masseter and the temporalis muscles, which are innervated by the mandibular division of the trigeminal nerve, can be palpated, and felt to harden as they contract.

Testing Facial Nerve Integrity

The facial nerve supplies the muscles of facial expression; supplies the anterior two thirds of the tongue with taste fibers; and is secretomotor to the lacrimal, submandibular, and sublingual glands.

The anatomic relationship of this nerve to other structures enables a physician to localize lesions of the nerve accurately. If CNs VI and VII were not functioning, this would suggest a lesion within the pons of the brain. If CNs VII and VIII were not functioning, this would suggest a lesion in the internal acoustic meatus. If the patient is excessively sensitive to sound in one ear (**hyperacusis**), the lesion probably involves the nerve to the stapedius. Loss of taste over the anterior two thirds of the tongue implies that the seventh nerve is damaged proximal to the point where it gives off the chorda tympani.

To test the facial nerve, the patient is asked to show their teeth by separating their lips with the teeth clenched and then to close their eyes. Taste on each half of the anterior two thirds of the tongue can be tested with sugar, salt, vinegar, and quinine for the sweet, salt, sour, and bitter sensations, respectively.

It should be remembered that the part of the facial nerve nucleus that controls the muscles of the upper part of the face receives corticobulbar fibers from both cerebral cortices. Therefore, in patients with an **upper motor neuron lesion**, only the muscles of the lower part of the face will be paralyzed. However, in patients with a **lower motor neuron lesion**, all the muscles on the affected side of the face will be paralyzed. The lower eyelid will droop, and the angle of the mouth will sag. Tears will flow over the lower eyelid, and saliva will dribble from the corner of the mouth. The patient will be unable to close the eye and cannot expose their teeth fully on the affected side.

Testing Vestibulocochlear Nerve Integrity

The vestibulocochlear nerve innervates the utricle and saccule, which are sensitive to static changes in equilibrium; semicircular canals, which are sensitive to changes in dynamic equilibrium; and the cochlea, which is sensitive to sound.

Disturbances of vestibular function include dizziness (**vertigo**) and **nystagmus**. The latter is an uncontrollable pendular movement of the eyes. Disturbances of cochlear function reveal themselves as **deafness** and ringing in the ears (**tinnitus**). The patient's ability to hear a voice or a tuning fork should be tested, with each ear tested separately.

Testing Glossopharyngeal Nerve Integrity

The glossopharyngeal nerve supplies the stylopharyngeus muscle and sends secretomotor fibers to the parotid gland. Sensory fibers innervate the posterior one third of the tongue.

The integrity of this nerve may be evaluated by testing the patient's general sensation and that of taste on the posterior third of the tongue.

Testing Vagus Nerve Integrity

The vagus nerve innervates many organs, but the examination of this nerve depends on testing the function of the branches to the pharynx, soft palate, and larynx. Touching the lateral wall of the pharynx with a spatula may test the pharyngeal reflex. This should immediately cause the patient to gag—that is, the pharyngeal muscles will contract.

Asking the patient to say "ah" can test the innervation of the soft palate. Normally, the soft palate rises, and the uvula moves backward in the midline.

All the muscles of the larynx are supplied by the recurrent laryngeal branch of the vagus, except the cricothyroid muscle, which is supplied by the external laryngeal branch of the superior laryngeal branch of the vagus. **Hoarseness** or **absence of the voice** may occur. Laryngoscopic examination may reveal abductor paralysis.

Testing Accessory Nerve Integrity

The accessory nerve supplies the SCM and trapezius muscles. The patient should be asked to rotate the head to one side against resistance, causing the SCM of the opposite side to come into action. Then, the patient should be asked to shrug the shoulders, causing the trapezius muscles to come into action.

Testing Hypoglossal Nerve Integrity

The hypoglossal nerve supplies the muscles of the tongue. The patient is asked to stick out their tongue; if a lesion of the nerve is present, it will be noted that the tongue deviates toward the paralyzed side (see Tongue Movements). This can be explained as follows. One of the genioglossus muscles, which pull the tongue forward, is paralyzed on the affected side. The other, normal genioglossus muscle pulls the unaffected side of the tongue forward, leaving the paralyzed side of the tongue stationary. The result is the tip of the tongue's deviation toward the paralyzed side. In patients with long-standing paralysis, the muscles on the affected side are wasted, and the tongue is wrinkled on that side.

CERVICAL PLEXUS

The **anterior rami of the C1 to C4 nerves** form the cervical plexus. The rami join by connecting branches, which form loops that lie in front of the origins of the levator scapulae and the scalenus medius muscles (see Fig. 9.72). The prevertebral layer of deep cervical fascia covers the plexus in front, and the plexus is related to the internal jugular vein within the carotid sheath. The cervical plexus supplies skin and muscles of the head, neck, and shoulder, plus the diaphragm and other thoracic structures (Table 9.8).

Table 9.8 Cervical Plexus Branches and Their Distribution

BRANCHES	DISTRIBUTION
Cutaneous	
Lesser occipital	Skin of the scalp behind the ear
Great auricular	Skin over the parotid salivary gland, auricle, and angle of jaw
Transverse cervical	Skin over side and front of the neck
Supraclavicular	Skin over the upper part of the chest and shoulder
Muscular	
Segmental branches	Prevertebral muscles, levator scapulae
Ansa cervicalis (C1 to C3)	Omohyoid, sternohyoid, sternothyroid
C1 fibers via the hypoglossal nerve	Thyrohyoid, geniohyoid
Phrenic nerve (C3 to C5)	Motor to diaphragm; Sensory from pericardium, mediastinal parietal pleura, and pleura and peritoneum covering the central diaphragm

Cutaneous Branches

Four cutaneous nerves (lesser occipital, great auricular, transverse cervical, and supraclavicular) branch off the cervical plexus and supply the skin over the lower head and the front and sides of the neck (see Fig. 9.26). These nerves emerge at a common point (**nerve point of the neck**) at the posterior margin of the SCM muscle, at about the midpoint of the muscle, and distribute from there (see Fig. 9.69).

The **lesser occipital nerve** (C2) supplies the back of the scalp and the auricle.

The **great auricular nerve** (C2 and C3) supplies the skin over the angle of the mandible.

The **transverse cervical nerve** (C2 and C3) supplies the skin over the front of the neck.

The **supraclavicular nerves** (C3 and C4) have medial, intermediate, and lateral branches that supply the skin over the shoulder region. These nerves are important clinically, because pain may be referred along them from the phrenic nerve (eg, in gallbladder disease).

Muscular Branches (Neck)

Nerve branches supply the **prevertebral muscles**, **sternocleidomastoid**, **levator scapulae**, and **trapezius**. The cervical plexus branches to the sternocleidomastoid (C2, C3) and trapezius (C3, C4) are proprioceptive.

A **branch from C1** joins the **hypoglossal nerve**. Some of these C1 fibers later leave the hypoglossal as the **descending branch**, which unites with the **descending cervical nerve** (C2 and C3), to form the **ansa cervicalis** (see Figs. 9.77 and 9.86B). The ansa cervicalis supplies the omohyoid, sternohyoid, and sternothyroid muscles. Other C1 fibers within the hypoglossal nerve leave it as the **nerves to the thyrohyoid and geniohyoid**.

Phrenic Nerve

The phrenic nerve arises in the neck from the C3 to C5 nerves of the cervical plexus. It runs vertically downward across the front of the **scalenus anterior** muscle (see Fig. 9.72) and enters the thorax by passing in front of the subclavian artery. Its further course in the thorax is described in Chapter 4 (Thorax).

The phrenic nerve is the only motor nerve supply to the diaphragm. It also carries sensory branches from the pericardium, mediastinal parietal pleura, and the pleura and peritoneum covering the upper and lower surfaces of the central part of the diaphragm (see Table 9.8).

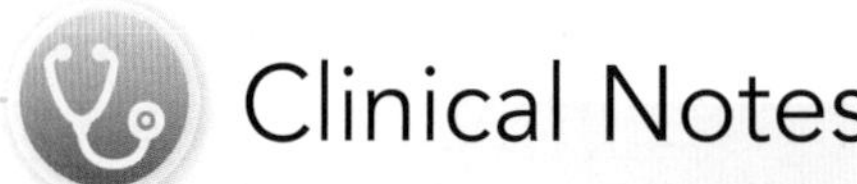

Phrenic Nerve Injury and Diaphragm Paralysis

The phrenic nerve is of considerable clinical importance because it is the sole nerve supply to the muscle of the diaphragm. Each phrenic nerve supplies the corresponding half of the diaphragm.

Penetrating wounds in the neck can injure the phrenic nerve. If that occurs, the paralyzed half of the diaphragm relaxes and is pushed up into the thorax by the positive abdominal pressure. Consequently, the lower lobe of the lung on that side may collapse.

About one third of individuals have an **accessory phrenic nerve**. The root from the C5 nerve may be incorporated in the nerve to the subclavius and may join the main phrenic nerve trunk in the thorax.

BRACHIAL PLEXUS

The brachial plexus forms in the posterior triangle of the neck by the union of the anterior rami of spinal nerves C5 to T1 (Fig. 9.87). This plexus is divided into **roots**, **trunks**, **divisions**, and **cords**. The roots of C5 and C6 unite to form the **upper trunk**, the root of C7 continues as the **middle trunk**, and the roots of C8 and T1 unite to form the **lower trunk**. Each trunk then divides into **anterior** and **posterior divisions**. The anterior divisions of the upper and middle trunks unite to form the **lateral cord**, the anterior division of the lower trunk continues as the **medial cord**, and the posterior divisions of all three trunks join to form the **posterior cord**.

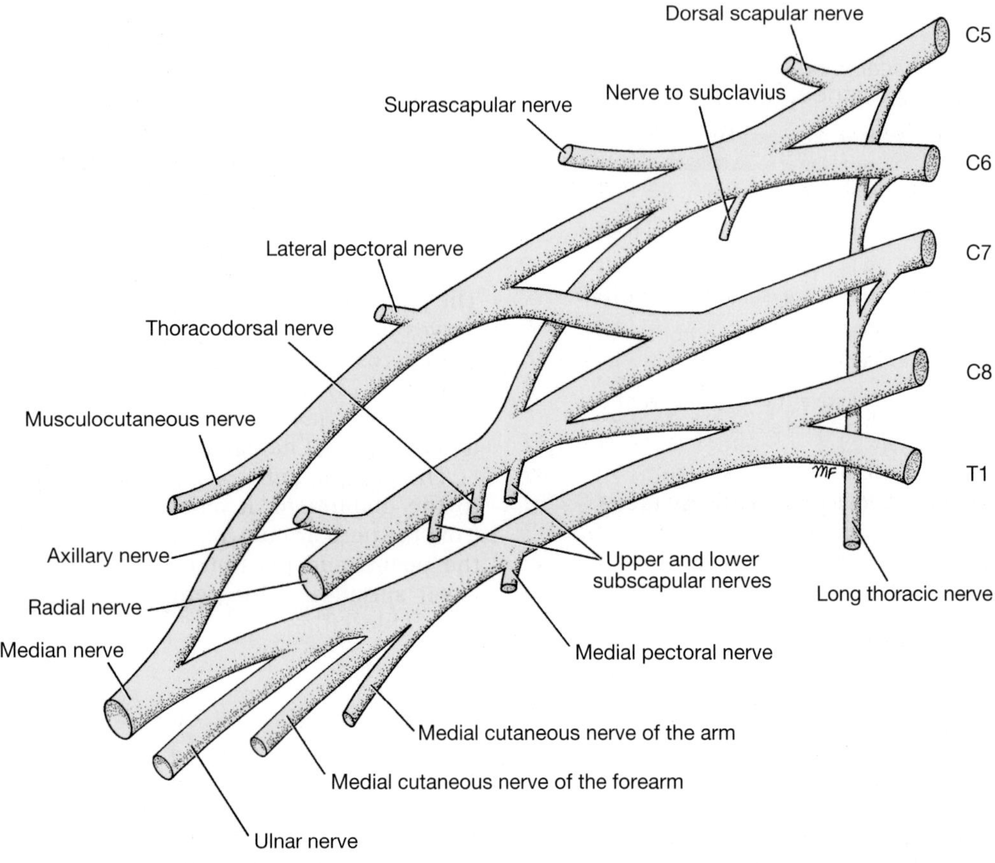

Figure 9.87 Brachial plexus and its branches.

The roots of the brachial plexus enter the base of the neck between the scalenus anterior and the scalenus medius muscles and pass through the **interscalene triangle** (see Fig. 9.72). The trunks and divisions cross the posterior triangle of the neck, and the cords become arranged around the second part of the axillary artery in the axilla. Here, the brachial plexus and the axillary artery and vein are enclosed in the **axillary sheath**. See Chapter 3 (Upper Limb) for a full discussion of the brachial plexus.

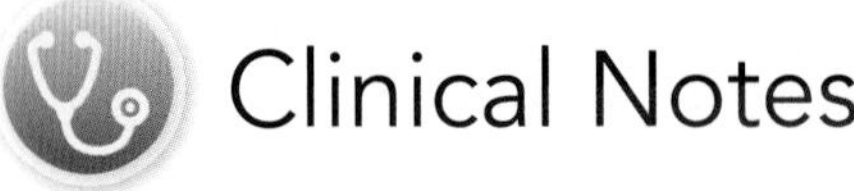

Clinical Notes

Brachial Plexus Injury

The roots and trunks of the brachial plexus occupy the anteroinferior angle of the posterior triangle of the neck. Incomplete lesions can result from stab or bullet wounds, traction, or pressure injuries.

Brachial Plexus Nerve Block

The **axillary sheath**, formed from the prevertebral layer of deep cervical fascia, encloses the brachial plexus and the axillary artery. Closing the distal part of the sheath in the axilla with finger pressure, inserting a syringe needle into the proximal part of the sheath, and then injecting a local anesthetic can easily obtain a brachial plexus nerve block. The anesthetic solution is massaged along the sheath, producing a nerve block. The syringe needle may be inserted into the axillary sheath in the lower part of the posterior triangle of the neck or in the axilla.

Brachial Plexus and Subclavian Artery Compression

At the root of the neck, the brachial plexus and the subclavian artery enter the posterior triangle through the narrow interscalene triangle. In the presence of a cervical rib (see Chapter 4, Thorax), the first thoracic nerve and the subclavian artery are raised and angulated as they pass over the rib. Partial or complete occlusion of the artery causes ischemic muscle pain in the arm, which is worsened by exercise. Rarely, pressure on the first thoracic nerve causes symptoms of pain in the forearm and hand and wasting of the small muscles of the hand.

AUTONOMIC NERVOUS SYSTEM

The craniocervical autonomic nervous system consists of both sympathetic and parasympathetic components. The sympathetic part has a comparatively simple organizational scheme, whereas the parasympathetic part has more components and more complex pathways.

Sympathetic Part

Preganglionic neurons originate in the lateral horn of the T1 to T4 spinal cord segments. Axons enter the **sympathetic trunk** at those levels (via **white rami communicantes**) and ascend through it. The cervical part of the sympathetic trunk extends from the base of the skull down to the neck of rib 1, where it becomes continuous with the thoracic part of the sympathetic trunk. It lies directly behind the internal and common carotid arteries (ie, medial to the vagus nerve) and is embedded in deep fascia between the carotid sheath and the prevertebral layer of deep fascia (see Fig. 9.65).

The sympathetic trunk possesses three ganglia: **superior**, **middle**, and **inferior cervical ganglia** (see Figs. 9.72 and 9.77). Most preganglionic fibers synapse in the cervical ganglia, and **postganglionic fibers** distribute from those.

Superior Cervical Ganglion

The superior cervical ganglion is the cranial end of the sympathetic trunk and lies immediately below the skull. It is the largest of the sympathetic chain ganglia, being formed of the embryonic C1 to C4 sympathetic ganglia primordia. It is located at the level of the C2 vertebra and is embedded in deep fascia between the carotid sheath and the prevertebral fascia over the longus capitis muscle. **All sympathetic fibers in the head are postganglionic fibers that branch off the superior cervical ganglion.**

Branches

- **Vascular branches**. **Arterial branches** pass to the common carotid, external carotid, and vertebral arteries. These branches form plexuses around the arteries (eg, carotid and vertebral plexuses) and distribute along the branches of the arteries. The **internal carotid nerve** accompanies the internal carotid artery into the carotid canal in the temporal bone. It divides into branches around the artery to form the internal carotid plexus. Several sympathetic nerves branch off the vascular plexuses and distribute the nerves further. The **caroticotympanic nerve** comes off the carotid plexus and joins the tympanic plexus in the middle ear. The **deep petrosal nerve** joins the greater petrosal nerve to form the nerve of the pterygoid canal at the base of the skull. The **sympathetic root of the ciliary ganglion** branches off the internal carotid plexus and connects with that ganglion in the orbit. **CN branches** join the oculomotor, trochlear, trigeminal, abducens, and facial nerves.
- **Gray rami communicantes** pass to the anterior rami of the C1 to C4 spinal nerves.
- **Cranial nerve branches** join the glossopharyngeal, vagus, and hypoglossal nerves.
- **Pharyngeal branches** unite with the pharyngeal branches of the glossopharyngeal and vagus nerves to form the pharyngeal plexus.
- The **superior cardiac** nerve descends in the neck and ends in the cardiac plexus in the thorax (see Chapter 4, Thorax).

Middle Cervical Ganglion

The middle cervical ganglion lies at the level of the cricoid cartilage.

Branches

- **Gray rami communicantes** to the anterior rami of the C5 and C6 nerves
- **Thyroid branches**, which pass along the inferior thyroid artery to the thyroid gland
- The **middle cardiac nerve**, which descends in the neck and ends in the cardiac plexus in the thorax

Inferior Cervical Ganglion

The inferior cervical ganglion in most people fuses with the T1 ganglion to form the **stellate ganglion**. It lies in the interval between the transverse process of the C7 vertebra and the neck of the rib 1, behind the vertebral artery.

Two or more nerve bundles represent the part of the sympathetic trunk connecting the middle cervical ganglion to the inferior or stellate ganglion. The most anterior bundle crosses in front of the first part of the subclavian artery and then turns upward behind it. This anterior bundle is referred to as the **ansa subclavia** (see Fig. 9.77).

Branches

- **Gray rami communicantes** to the anterior rami of the C7 and C8 nerves
- **Arterial branches** to the subclavian and vertebral arteries
- The **inferior cardiac nerve**, which descends to join the cardiac plexus in the thorax

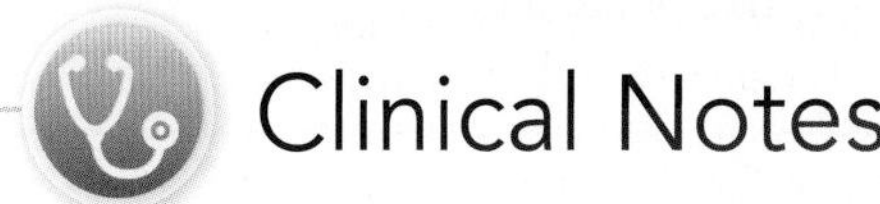

Sympathectomy for Upper Limb Arterial Insufficiency

Sympathetic innervation of the upper limb is as follows: preganglionic fibers leave the spinal cord in the T2 to T8 nerves. On reaching the sympathetic trunk via the white rami, they ascend within the trunk and are relayed in the T2, stellate, and middle cervical ganglia. Postganglionic fibers then join the roots of the brachial plexus as gray rami. Sympathectomy of the upper limb is a relatively common

(continued)

procedure for the treatment of arterial insufficiency. From this information, it is clear that the stellate and T2 ganglia should be removed to block the sympathetic pathway to the arm completely.

Removal of the stellate ganglion also removes the sympathetic nerve supply to the head and neck on that side. This produces not only vasodilation of the skin vessels but also anhidrosis, nasal congestion, and Horner syndrome. For this reason, the stellate ganglion is usually left intact in sympathectomies of the upper limb.

Horner Syndrome

Horner syndrome includes constriction of the pupil (**miosis**), drooping of the upper eyelid (**ptosis**), and lack of sweating plus vasodilation (**anhidrosis**). Depression of the eyeball into the orbital cavity (**enophthalmos**) may occur but is probably more apparent than real. It is caused by an interruption of the sympathetic nerve supply to the head. Pathologic causes include lesions of the brainstem or cervical part of the spinal cord, traumatic injury to the cervical part of the sympathetic trunk, traction of the stellate ganglion caused by a cervical rib, and involvement of the ganglion in cancerous growth, which may interrupt the peripheral part of the sympathetic pathway to the orbit.

Stellate Ganglion Block

A stellate ganglion block is performed by first palpating the large anterior tubercle (carotid tubercle) of the transverse process of the C6 vertebra, which lies about a fingerbreadth lateral to the cricoid cartilage. The carotid sheath and the sternocleidomastoid muscle are pushed laterally, and the needle of the anesthetic syringe is inserted through the skin over the tubercle. Local anesthetic is then injected beneath the prevertebral layer of deep cervical fascia. This procedure effectively blocks the ganglion and its rami communicantes.

Parasympathetic Part

Preganglionic neurons of the cranial outflow of the parasympathetic part of the autonomic nervous system originate in the nuclei of the **oculomotor (CN III)**, **facial (CN VII)**, **glossopharyngeal (CN IX)**, and **vagus (CN X) nerves**. The parasympathetic nucleus of the oculomotor nerve is the **Edinger–Westphal nucleus**, those of the facial nerve are the **lacrimatory** and **superior salivary nuclei**, that of the glossopharyngeal nerve is the **inferior salivary nucleus**, and that of the vagus nerve is the **dorsal nucleus of the vagus**. The axons of these cells are myelinated fibers that emerge from the brain within the CNs.

These preganglionic fibers synapse in peripheral ganglia located close to the viscera they innervate. The cranial parasympathetic ganglia are the **ciliary**, **pterygopalatine**, **submandibular**, and **otic**.

The **oculomotor nerve** projects to the **ciliary ganglion** in the orbit, where synapsing occurs. Postganglionic fibers travel through the **short ciliary nerves** to the sphincter pupillae and ciliary muscle in the eyeball (see Fig. 9.81A). These are active in the **pupillary light reflex** and **accommodation**, respectively.

The **facial nerve** projects to the **pterygopalatine ganglion** in the pterygopalatine fossa and to the **submandibular ganglion** in the oral floor (see Figs. 9.53 and 9.63). The **greater petrosal nerve** (see Fig. 9.83B) runs from the geniculate ganglion of the facial nerve to the pterygopalatine ganglion. Postganglionic fibers then traverse branches of the maxillary and ophthalmic nerves to reach the **lacrimal gland** and **nasal glands**. This is the secretomotor pathway for lacrimation. The **chorda tympani nerve** (see Fig. 9.83B) passes from the facial nerve through the middle ear cavity and into the infratemporal fossa, where it joins the **lingual nerve** (from the mandibular nerve). The lingual nerve sends parasympathetic branches to the **submandibular ganglion**, where synapses occur. Postganglionic fibers run to the **submandibular** and **sublingual salivary glands** and glands in the oral floor.

The **glossopharyngeal nerve** projects to the **otic ganglion** in the infratemporal fossa via its **tympanic** and **lesser petrosal branches** (see Fig. 9.84B). Postganglionic fibers join the **auriculotemporal nerve** (branch of the mandibular nerve) and use that to reach the **parotid salivary gland**.

The **vagus nerve** sends its parasympathetic components into the neck, thorax, and abdomen. It has no cranial parasympathetic projection and does not relate to any of the cranial parasympathetic ganglia. Its preganglionic fibers run to postcranial ganglia or plexuses such as the **cardiac**, **pulmonary**, **myenteric (Auerbach)**, and **mucosal (Meissner) plexus**. The postganglionic fibers are nonmyelinated, and they are short in length.

EAR

The ear consists of three main parts: (1) **external ear**, (2) **middle ear**, and (3) **internal ear**. The external and middle ear structures function for sound conduction and transmission, whereas the internal ear functions for sound perception and equilibrium. The external ear collects airborne vibrational waveforms. The middle ear converts airborne waveforms into solid-borne waveforms and transmits those to the internal ear. The hearing part of the internal ear converts solid-borne waveforms into fluid-borne waveforms, which are translated into sound. The equilibrium part translates fluid dynamics into a sense of balance.

External Ear

The external ear has an auricle and an external auditory meatus. The **auricle (pinna)** has a characteristic shape (Fig. 9.88) and collects air vibrations. It consists of a thin plate of elastic cartilage covered by skin. Its main components are the **helix** (elevated margin of the auricle), **tragus** (projection from the anterior margin of the auricle that extends over the opening of the

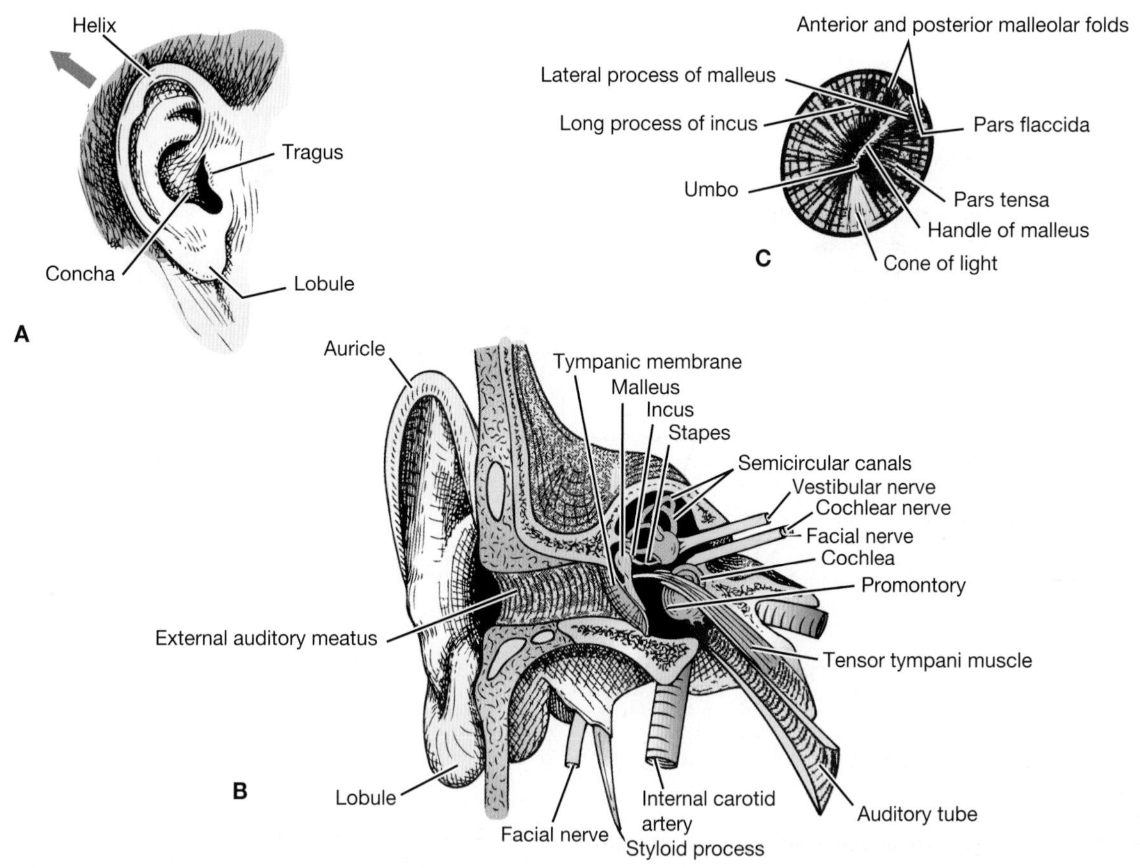

Figure 9.88 **A.** Different parts of the auricle of the external ear. The *arrow* indicates the direction that the auricle should be pulled to straighten the external auditory meatus before insertion of the otoscope in the adult. **B.** Right ear apparatus viewed from in front. **C.** The right tympanic membrane as seen through the otoscope.

external acoustic meatus), **lobule** (**earlobe**, which does not contain cartilage), and **concha** (deepest depression within the auricle that leads into the external meatus). The auricle is an effective sound collecting and localizing device in many mammals. However, that function is highly questionable in humans. The **auricular muscles** (see Fig. 9.20) are essentially vestigial in humans but are variably entertaining to those able to wiggle their ears.

The **external auditory** (**acoustic**) **meatus** is a slender curved tube that leads from the concha of the auricle to the tympanic membrane (Fig. 9.89; see also Fig. 9.88). It conducts sound waves from the auricle to the tympanic membrane.

The outer (lateral) third of the meatus is elastic cartilage. The inner (medial) two thirds is bony and formed by the tympanic plate of the temporal bone. The meatus is lined by skin, and its outer third is provided with **hairs** and **sebaceous** and **ceruminous glands**. The latter are modified sweat glands that secrete a yellowish brown earwax (**cerumen**). The hairs and the wax provide a sticky barrier that prevents the entrance of foreign bodies.

The **lesser occipital** and **great auricular nerves** (branches of the cervical plexus) are the main sensory nerves of the auricle. These are supplemented by small components of the facial and glossopharyngeal nerves. The **auriculotemporal nerve** and the **auricular branch of the vagus nerve** are the primary sensory nerves for the external meatus and the external surface of the tympanic membrane.

The **lymph drainage** is to the superficial parotid, mastoid, and superficial cervical lymph nodes.

Tympanic Membrane

The **tympanic membrane** (**eardrum**) is a thin, fibrous structure that forms the interface between the external and middle ears (see Fig. 9.88). The membrane is obliquely oriented, facing inferiorly, anteriorly, and laterally. It is slightly concave laterally, with a small depression (**umbo**) at the depth of the concavity. The tip of the handle of the malleus produces the umbo. When the membrane is illuminated through an otoscope, the concavity produces a **cone of light**, which is a bright, light-reflecting area that radiates anteriorly and inferiorly from the umbo.

The tympanic membrane is circular and measures about 1 cm in diameter. The circumference is thickened and slotted into a groove in the bone. The groove (**tympanic sulcus**) is deficient superiorly, which forms a notch. From the sides of the notch, two bands, the **anterior** and **posterior malleolar folds**, pass to the lateral

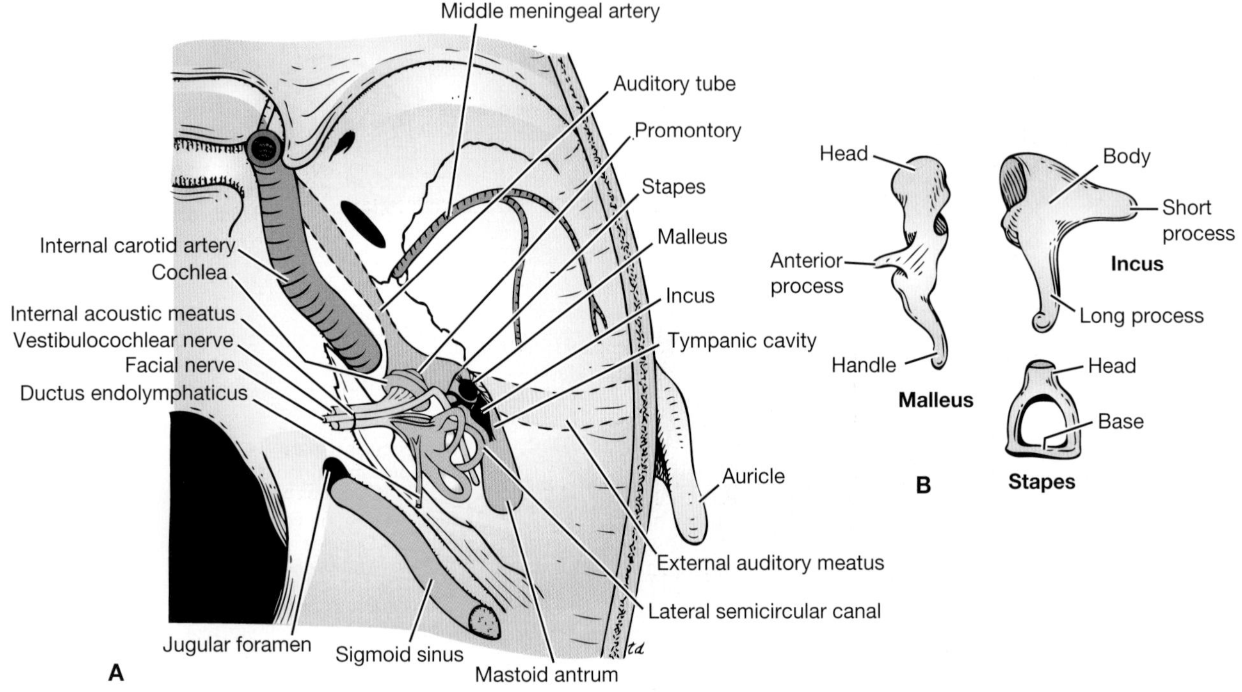

Figure 9.89 **A.** Parts of the right ear in relation to the temporal bone viewed from above. **B.** The auditory ossicles.

process of the malleus. The small triangular area on the tympanic membrane bounded by the folds is slack and called the **pars flaccida**. The remainder of the membrane is tense and called the **pars tensa**. The handle of the malleus is bound to the inner surface of the tympanic membrane by the mucous membrane.

The tympanic membrane is extremely sensitive to pain. The **auriculotemporal nerve** and the **auricular branch of the vagus nerve** innervate its outer surface, and the **tympanic plexus of the glossopharyngeal nerve** supplies its inner aspect.

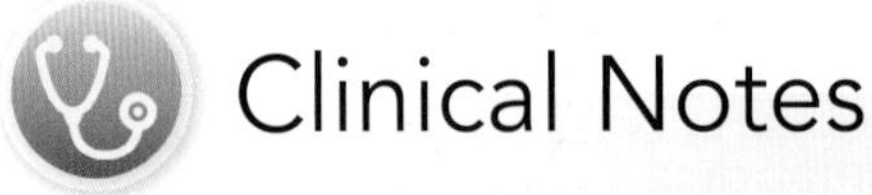

Clinical Notes

Tympanic Membrane Examination

Otoscopic examination of the tympanic membrane is facilitated by first straightening the external auditory meatus by gently pulling the auricle upward and backward in the adult and straight backward or backward and downward in the infant. Normally, the tympanic membrane is pearly gray and concave. In the adult, the external meatus is about 1 in. (2.5 cm) long and is narrowest about 0.2 in. (5 mm) from the tympanic membrane.

Tympanic Membrane Perforation

Perforation of the tympanic membrane (**ruptured eardrum**) has multiple possible causes, such as otitis media, penetration by a foreign object, and excessive pressure. This may result in conduction deafness.

Middle Ear

The middle ear is an air-containing cavity within the petrous part of the temporal bone and is lined with a mucous membrane (see Figs. 9.88 and 9.89). It is a narrow, oblique, slit-like cavity whose long axis lies approximately parallel to the plane of the tympanic membrane. It communicates with the **nasopharynx** anteriorly and with the **mastoid antrum** posteriorly. The middle ear has four main components: (1) tympanic cavity, (2) auditory ossicles and their muscles, (3) auditory tube, and (4) mastoid area.

Tympanic Cavity

The tympanic cavity is the main chamber of the middle ear. It consists of two parts: (1) **tympanic cavity proper** and (2) **epitympanic recess**. The tympanic cavity proper is the area directly medial to the tympanic membrane. The epitympanic recess is the upper portion of the chamber located superior to the tympanic membrane.

Conceptually, think of the tympanic cavity as a six-sided box with a roof (superior wall), floor (inferior wall), anterior wall, posterior wall, medial wall, and lateral wall (Figs. 9.90 and 9.91).

The **roof** is a thin plate of bone, the **tegmen tympani**, which is part of the petrous temporal bone. It separates the epitympanic recess of the tympanic cavity from the dura mater lining the floor of the middle cranial fossa. Fracture of the tegmen tympani may cause CSF to leak into the tympanic cavity.

The **floor (jugular wall)** is a thin plate of bone, which may be partly replaced by fibrous tissue. It separates

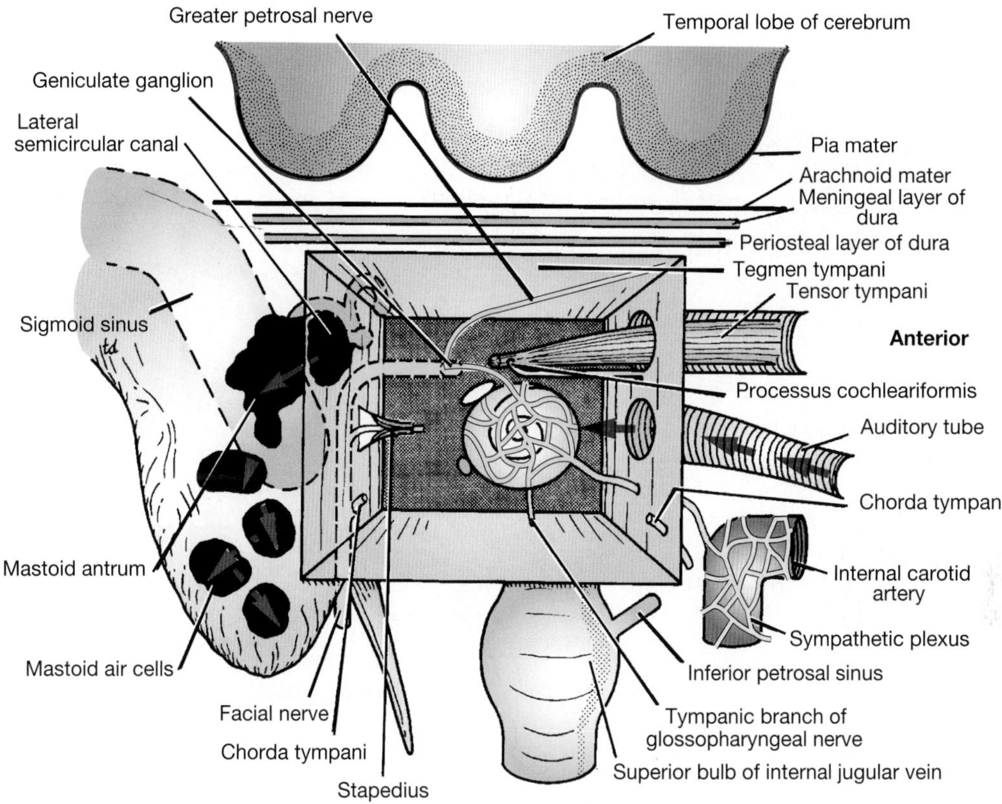

Figure 9.90 Middle ear and its relations.

the tympanic cavity from the **superior bulb of the internal jugular vein**. The **tympanic nerve** (branch of CN IX) pierces the floor to enter the tympanic cavity.

The **anterior (carotid) wall** has two openings in its upper part. The upper, smaller opening conveys the **tensor tympani muscle**. The lower, larger opening leads into the **auditory tube**. The thin, bony septum that separates the canals is prolonged backward on the medial wall, where it forms a shelflike projection. The **carotid canal** (containing the internal carotid artery) lies immediately adjacent to the thin, lower part of the anterior wall, beneath the bony wall of the auditory tube.

The **posterior (mastoid) wall** has a large, irregular opening, the **aditus ad antrum (aditus to the mastoid antrum)**, in its upper part. This opening is the entrance to the cavity (antrum) of the mastoid process and the mastoid air cells. It connects the epitympanic recess to the mastoid antrum. A small, hollow, conical projection, the **pyramid (pyramidal eminence)**, sits below the aditus. The pyramid houses the **stapedius muscle**; the tendon of the stapedius emerges from its apex. The **main stem of the facial nerve** (CN VII) descends within the facial canal immediately adjacent to the posterior wall. This close relationship forms the elevated **prominence of the facial canal** along the posterior wall. A small opening inferior to the pyramid transmits the **chorda tympani nerve** from the facial nerve into the tympanic cavity.

The **medial (labyrinthine) wall** separates the tympanic cavity from the internal ear. Thus, the medial wall of the tympanic cavity is the lateral wall of the internal ear. The greater part of this wall shows a rounded projection, the **promontory**, which results from the underlying first turn of the cochlea (see Figs. 9.89 to 9.91). The **fenestra vestibuli (oval window)**, which is closed by the **footplate of the stapes**, lies above and behind the promontory (see Figs. 9.90 and 9.91). The **fenestra cochleae (foramen tympani, round window)**, which is round and closed by the **secondary tympanic membrane**, sits below the posterior end of the promontory. The **prominence of the facial canal** is an elevation above the oval window formed by the adjacent facial nerve within the facial canal. It appears on both the medial and posterior walls. It runs horizontally above the promontory and oval window and then curves downward on the posterior wall behind the pyramid. The **prominence of the lateral semicircular canal** is an elevation above the prominence of the facial canal that is formed by the lateral semicircular canal. The bony shelf that extends from the anterior wall onto the medial wall supports the **tensor tympani muscle**. Its posterior end is curved upward and forms a pulley, the **processus cochleariformis**, around which the tendon of the tensor tympani bends laterally to reach its insertion on the handle of the malleus.

The **lateral (membranous) wall** is largely formed by the tympanic membrane (see Figs. 9.88 and 9.91A). This wall has a **superior part** formed by the epitympanic recess and an **inferior part** formed by the eardrum.

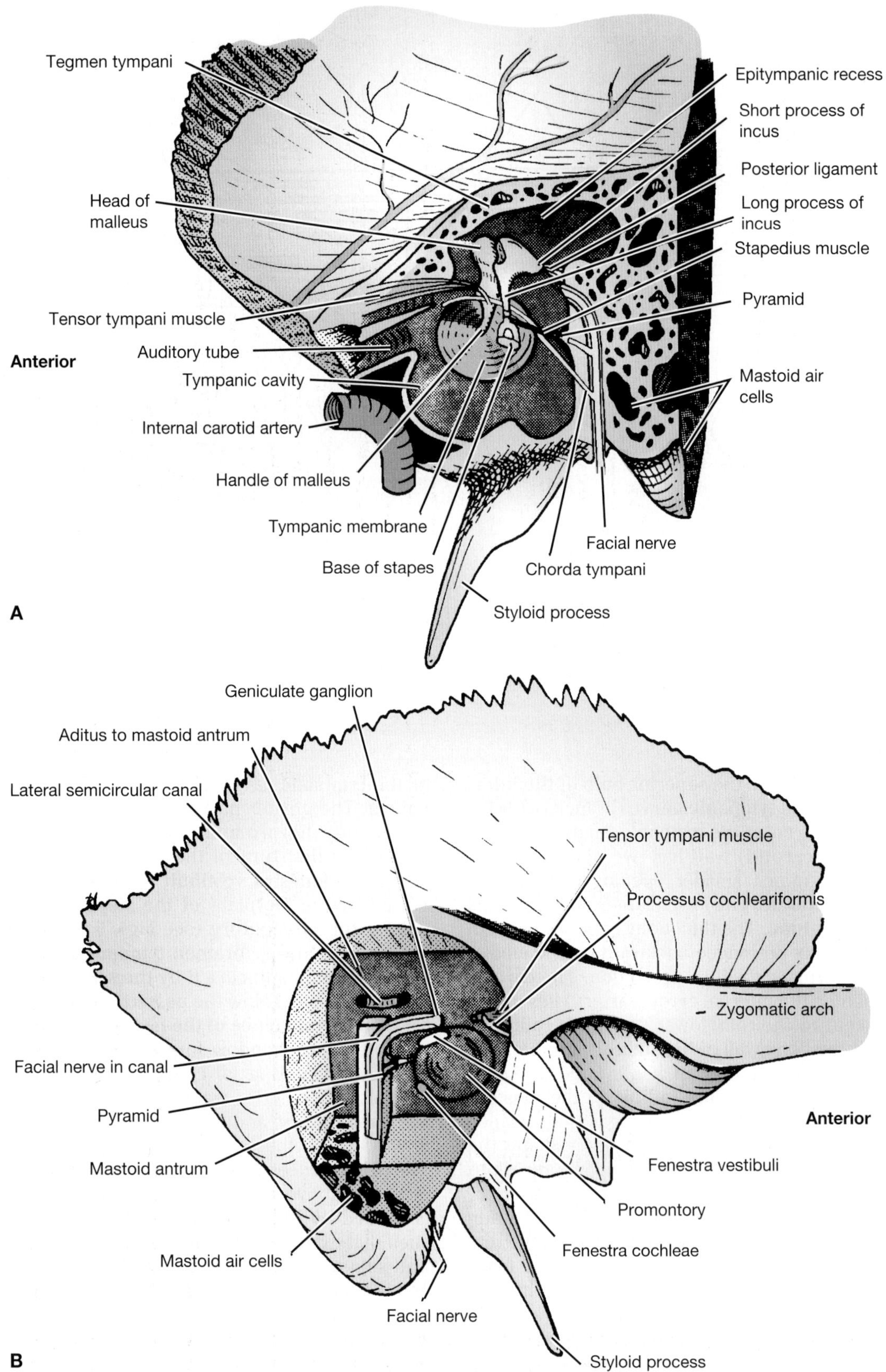

Figure 9.91 **A.** Lateral wall of the right middle ear viewed from the medial side. Note the position of the ossicles and the mastoid antrum. **B.** Medial wall of the right middle ear viewed from the lateral side. Note the position of the facial nerve in its bony canal.

Auditory Ossicles and Associated Muscles

The three auditory ossicles are the malleus, incus, and stapes (see Figs. 9.89 and 9.91). These form a mobile osseous bridge from the tympanic membrane to the oval window. The joints between the ossicles are synovial.

The **malleus** is the largest ossicle and possesses a head, neck, long process (handle), anterior process, and a lateral process. The **head** is rounded and articulates posteriorly with the incus. The **neck** is the constricted part below the head. The **handle** passes downward and backward and is firmly attached to the medial surface of the tympanic membrane. It is visible through the tympanic membrane on otoscopic examination. The **anterior process** is a spicule of bone that connects to the anterior wall of the tympanic cavity by a ligament. The **lateral process** projects laterally and attaches to the anterior and posterior malleolar folds of the tympanic membrane.

The **incus** possesses a large body and two processes. The **body** is rounded and articulates anteriorly with the head of the malleus. The head of the malleus and the body of the incus occupy much of the epitympanic recess. The **long process** descends behind and parallel to the handle of the malleus. Its lower end bends medially and articulates with the head of the stapes. Its shadow on the tympanic membrane can sometimes be recognized on otoscopic examination. The **short process** projects backward and attaches to the posterior wall of the tympanic cavity by a ligament.

The **stapes** has a head, neck, two limbs, and a base. The **head** is small and articulates with the long process of the incus. The **neck** is narrow and receives the insertion of the stapedius muscle. The two **limbs** diverge from the neck and attach to the oval base. The edge of the **base** (**footplate**) attaches to the margin of the oval window by a ring of fibrous tissue, the **annular ligament**.

Two muscles, the **tensor tympani** and the **stapedius**, attach to the ossicles. The stapedius is the smallest skeletal muscle in the human body. Details of the muscles are summarized in Table 9.9.

Auditory Ossicle Movement

The malleus and incus rotate on an anteroposterior axis that runs through the ligament connecting the anterior process of the malleus to the anterior wall of the tympanic cavity, the anterior process of the malleus and the short process of the incus, and the ligament connecting the short process of the incus to the posterior wall of the tympanic cavity (Fig. 9.92).

When the tympanic membrane moves medially, the handle of the malleus also moves medially. The head of the malleus and the body of the incus move laterally. The long process of the incus moves medially with the stapes. The base of the stapes is pushed medially in the fenestra vestibuli, and the motion is communicated to the perilymph in the scala vestibuli of the internal ear. Liquid being incompressible, the perilymph causes an outward bulging of the secondary tympanic membrane in the fenestra cochleae at the lower end of the scala tympani. The above movements are reversed if the tympanic membrane moves laterally. Excessive lateral movements of the head of the malleus cause a temporary separation of the articular surfaces between the malleus and incus so that the base of the stapes is not pulled laterally out of the fenestra vestibuli.

During passage of the vibrations from the tympanic membrane to the perilymph via the small ossicles, the leverage increases at a rate of 1.3:1. Moreover, the area of the tympanic membrane is about 17 times greater than that of the base of the stapes, causing the effective pressure on the perilymph to increase by a total of 22:1.

Auditory Tube

The **auditory** (**pharyngotympanic**) **tube** connects the anterior wall of the tympanic cavity to the nasopharynx (see Figs. 9.88 to 9.90). As the tube descends, it passes over the upper border of the superior constrictor muscle.

The tube functions to equalize air pressure in the middle ear with atmospheric pressure, thus balancing pressure on both sides of the tympanic membrane. This balance allows the eardrum to move easily. The tube also functions as a drainage route for the serous secretions of the mucous membrane lining the middle ear.

The **lateral third** of the auditory tube is bony and the **medial two thirds** is cartilaginous. The entire tube is lined with a **mucous membrane** that is continuous with the epithelium of the tympanic cavity and the nasopharynx. The cartilage part is roughly C shaped. The mucous membrane of the open part of the "C" is normally collapsed and in apposition with the mucous membrane lining the cartilage. Therefore, in order to function, the auditory tube must be actively opened.

Contractions of the **tensor veli palatini** and **levator veli palatini** muscles cause the collapsed mucous membrane to separate from the cartilage wall and open the auditory tube. Because these are muscles of the soft palate, opening of the auditory tube occurs during palatal

Table 9.9 Middle Ear Muscles

MUSCLE	ORIGIN	INSERTION	NERVE SUPPLY	ACTION
Tensor tympani	Wall of auditory tube and wall of its own canal	Handle of malleus	Mandibular division of the trigeminal nerve	Dampens vibrations of tympanic membrane
Stapedius	Pyramid of the middle ear	Neck of stapes	Facial nerve	Dampens vibrations of stapes

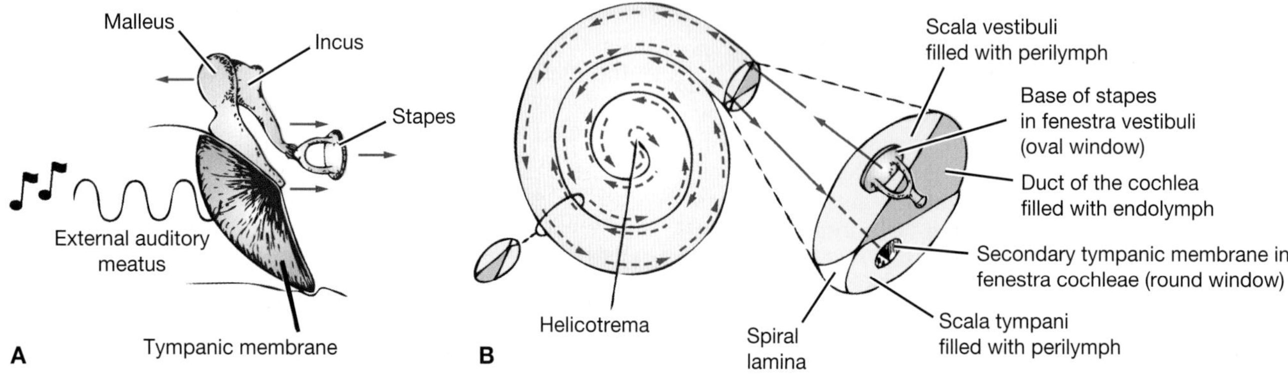

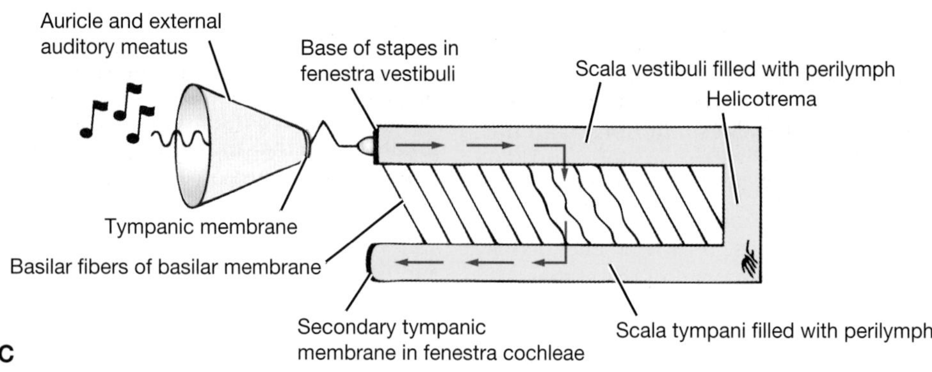

Figure 9.92 **A.** Vibrations of music passing into the external auditory meatus cause the tympanic membrane to move medially; the head of the malleus and incus move laterally, and the long process of the incus, with the stapes, moves laterally. **B.** The medial movement of the base of the stapes in the fenestra vestibuli causes motion (*arrows*) in the perilymph in the scala vestibuli. At the apex of the cochlea (the helicotrema), the compression wave in the perilymph passes down the scala tympani, causing a lateral bulging of the secondary tympanic membrane in the fenestra cochleae. **C.** Movement of the perilymph (*arrows*) after movement of the base of the stapes. Note the position of the basilar fibers of the basilar membrane.

activity, such as during swallowing and yawning. Thus, these are optimal activities for equalizing pressure and draining the middle ear. Think about what you must do in order to "pop" your ears when changing altitude.

Because of the continuity of the mucous membrane from nasopharynx to auditory tube to middle ear, the auditory tube may serve as a route for spread of infection from the nasopharynx to the middle ear.

Mastoid Area

The mastoid area consists of two main parts: (1) mastoid antrum and (2) mastoid air cells (see Figs. 9.90 and 9.91).

The **mastoid antrum** is the main cavity within the mastoid process of the temporal bone. The aditus ad antrum in the posterior wall of the tympanic cavity is the doorway that leads from the epitympanic recess into the antrum.

The relations of the mastoid antrum are important in understanding the spread of infection.

- **Anterior wall:** Related to the tympanic cavity and contains the aditus to the mastoid antrum
- **Posterior wall:** Separates the antrum from the sigmoid venous sinus and the cerebellum
- **Lateral wall:** Forms the floor of the suprameatal triangle and is 1.5 cm thick
- **Medial wall:** Related to the posterior semicircular canal
- **Superior wall:** Thin plate of bone, the tegmen tympani, which is related to the meninges of the middle cranial fossa and the temporal lobe of the brain
- **Inferior wall:** Perforated with holes, through which the antrum communicates with the mastoid air cells

The **mastoid air cells** are a honeycomb-like network of hollow spaces within the mastoid process. They are continuous above with the antrum and are lined with **mucous membrane** that is continuous with that of the antrum and the rest of the middle ear apparatus. Thus, infection may readily spread from the tympanic cavity into the mastoid air cells or vice versa. The mastoid process and air cells are not present at birth. The mastoid process begins to develop during the second year of life, in response to traction from the SCM muscle.

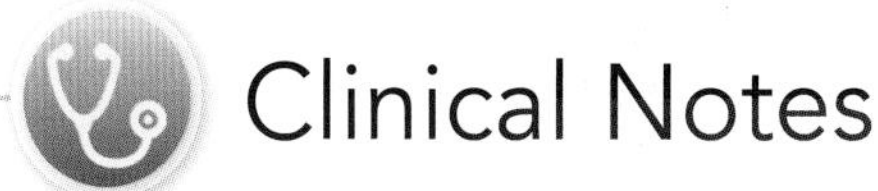

Clinical Notes

Infections and Otitis Media

Otitis media is acute infection of the middle ear. Pathogenic organisms can gain entrance to the middle ear secondary to upper respiratory tract infection by ascending along the common mucous membrane from the nasopharynx into the auditory tube. Inflammation of the mucous membrane may cause obstruction of the auditory tube. Acute infection produces bulging and redness of the tympanic membrane because of the increased pressure and/or fluid accumulation within the tympanic cavity. The outcome may be impaired hearing.

Complications of Otitis Media

Inadequate treatment of otitis media can result in the spread of the infection into the mastoid antrum and the mastoid air cells (**acute mastoiditis**). Acute mastoiditis may be followed by the further spread of pathogens beyond the confines of the middle ear. The meninges and the temporal lobe of the brain lie superiorly. A spread of the infection in this direction could produce **meningitis** and/or a **cerebral abscess** in the temporal lobe. The facial nerve and internal ear lay beyond the medial wall of the middle ear. A spread of the infection in this direction can cause a facial nerve palsy and **labyrinthitis** with **vertigo**. The posterior wall of the mastoid antrum is related to the sigmoid venous sinus. If the infection spreads in this direction, a **thrombosis** in the sigmoid sinus may occur.

Ossicle Disruption

Otosclerosis is abnormal bone formation causing fixation of the footplate of the stapes into the oval window. The resulting limited movement of the stapes may cause a form of conduction deafness. **Hyperacusis** is excessively acute hearing sensitivity because of the paralysis of the stapedius muscle, usually as a result of a facial nerve lesion. In this condition, the normal mobility of the stapes bone is limited, and the chain of ossicles cannot effectively dampen sudden, loud sound.

Nerves

Two CNs, the **facial nerve** (CN VII) and the **glossopharyngeal nerve** (CN IX), have significant relations to the middle ear. Each nerve is described fully earlier in this chapter (see CRANIAL NERVES).

Facial Nerve

The facial nerve enters the facial canal at the bottom of the internal auditory meatus (see Figs. 9.88 and 9.89). The nerve runs laterally above the vestibule of the internal ear until it reaches the medial wall of the middle ear. Here, the nerve expands to form the sensory **geniculate ganglion** (see Figs. 9.90 and 9.91). The nerve then bends sharply backward above the promontory. On arriving at the posterior wall of the middle ear, it curves downward on the medial side of the aditus of the mastoid antrum. It descends in the posterior wall of the middle ear, behind the pyramid, and finally emerges through the stylomastoid foramen at the exterior base of the skull.

IMPORTANT BRANCHES: INTRAPETROUS PART

- The **greater petrosal nerve** arises from the facial nerve at the geniculate ganglion. It contains preganglionic parasympathetic fibers that pass to the pterygopalatine ganglion and are there relayed through the zygomatic and lacrimal nerves to the lacrimal gland; other postganglionic fibers pass through the nasal and palatine nerves to the glands of the mucous membrane of the nose and palate. It may also contain taste fibers from the mucous membrane of the palate. The nerve emerges on the superior surface of the petrous part of the temporal bone, travels forward, and drops into the foramen lacerum. It joins the **deep petrosal nerve** from the sympathetic plexus on the internal carotid artery, and the two form the **nerve of the pterygoid canal** at the anterior lip of the foramen lacerum. This passes forward and enters the pterygopalatine fossa, where it ends in the **pterygopalatine ganglion**.
- The **nerve to the stapedius** arises from the facial nerve as it descends in the facial canal behind the pyramid. It supplies the muscle within the pyramid.
- The **chorda tympani nerve** arises from the facial nerve just inside the stylomastoid foramen. It enters the middle ear close to the posterior border of the tympanic membrane, runs forward across the inner surface of the tympanic membrane, and crosses the root of the handle of the malleus. It lies in the interval between the mucous membrane and the fibrous layers of the tympanic membrane, which explains the naming of the nerve. The nerve leaves the middle ear through the petrotympanic fissure and enters the infratemporal fossa, where it joins the lingual nerve. The chorda tympani contains **taste fibers** from the mucous membrane covering the anterior two thirds of the tongue (not the vallate papillae). The taste fibers are the peripheral processes of the cells in the geniculate ganglion. The nerve also carries **preganglionic parasympathetic secretomotor fibers** that reach the **submandibular ganglion** and are there relayed to the submandibular and sublingual salivary glands.

Glossopharyngeal Nerve

The **tympanic nerve** arises from the glossopharyngeal nerve just below the jugular foramen (see Fig. 9.84B). It passes through the floor of the middle ear and onto the promontory (see Fig. 9.90). Here, it splits into branches, which form the **tympanic plexus**. The tympanic plexus supplies the lining of the middle ear and gives off the **lesser petrosal nerve**, which sends secretomotor fibers to the parotid gland via the otic ganglion. The

caroticotympanic nerve is a sympathetic nerve that branches from the carotid plexus and joins the tympanic nerve in forming the tympanic plexus.

Internal Ear

The internal ear (labyrinth) is situated in the petrous part of the temporal bone, medial to the middle ear (see Fig. 9.89). It consists of the **bony labyrinth**, comprising a series of cavities within the bone, and the **membranous labyrinth**, comprising a series of membranous sacs and ducts contained within the bony labyrinth.

Bony Labyrinth

The bony labyrinth consists of three parts: **vestibule**, **semicircular canals**, and **cochlea** (Fig. 9.93A). These are cavities situated in the substance of a dense bone. They are lined by endosteum and contain a clear fluid, the perilymph, in which is suspended the membranous labyrinth.

The **vestibule**, the central part of the bony labyrinth, lies posterior to the cochlea and anterior to the semicircular canals. In its lateral wall is the **fenestra vestibuli**, which is closed by the base of the stapes and its annular ligament, and the **fenestra cochleae**, which is closed by the secondary tympanic membrane. The **saccule** and **utricle** of the membranous labyrinth are lodged within the vestibule.

The three **semicircular canals—superior**, **posterior**, and **lateral**—open into the posterior part of the vestibule. Each canal has a swelling at one end called the **ampulla**. The canals open into the vestibule by five orifices, one of which is common to two of the canals. The **semicircular ducts** are lodged within the canals.

The **superior semicircular canal** is vertical and placed at right angles to the long axis of the petrous bone. The **posterior canal** is also vertical but is placed parallel with the long axis of the petrous bone. The **lateral canal** is set in a horizontal position, and it lies in the medial wall of the aditus to the mastoid antrum, above the facial nerve canal.

The **cochlea** resembles a snail shell. It opens into the anterior part of the vestibule. Basically, it consists of a central pillar, the **modiolus**, around which a hollow bony tube makes two and a half spiral turns. Each successive turn is of decreasing radius so that the whole structure is conical. The apex faces anterolaterally, and the base faces posteromedially. The first basal turn of the cochlea is responsible for the **promontory** seen on the medial wall of the middle ear.

The modiolus has a broad base, which is situated at the bottom of the internal acoustic meatus. Branches of the cochlear nerve perforate it. A spiral ledge, the **spiral lamina**, winds around the modiolus and projects into the interior of the canal and partially divides it. The **basilar membrane** stretches from the free edge of the spiral lamina to the outer bony wall, thus dividing the cochlear canal into the **scala vestibuli** above and the **scala tympani** below. The **perilymph** within the scala vestibuli is separated from the middle ear by the base of the stapes and the annular ligament at the fenestra vestibuli. The perilymph in the scala tympani is separated from the middle ear by the secondary tympanic membrane at the fenestra cochleae.

Membranous Labyrinth

The membranous labyrinth is lodged within the bony labyrinth (see Fig. 9.93B). It is filled with **endolymph** and surrounded by **perilymph**. It consists of the **utricle** and **saccule**, which are lodged in the bony vestibule; **three semicircular ducts**, which lie within the bony semicircular canals; and the **duct of the cochlea**, which lies within the bony cochlea. All these structures freely communicate with one another.

The **utricle** is the larger of the two vestibular sacs. It is indirectly connected to the saccule and the **ductus endolymphaticus** by the **ductus utriculosaccularis**.

The **saccule** is globular and is connected to the utricle, as described previously. The ductus endolymphaticus, after being joined by the ductus utriculosaccularis, passes on to end in a small blind pouch, the **saccus**

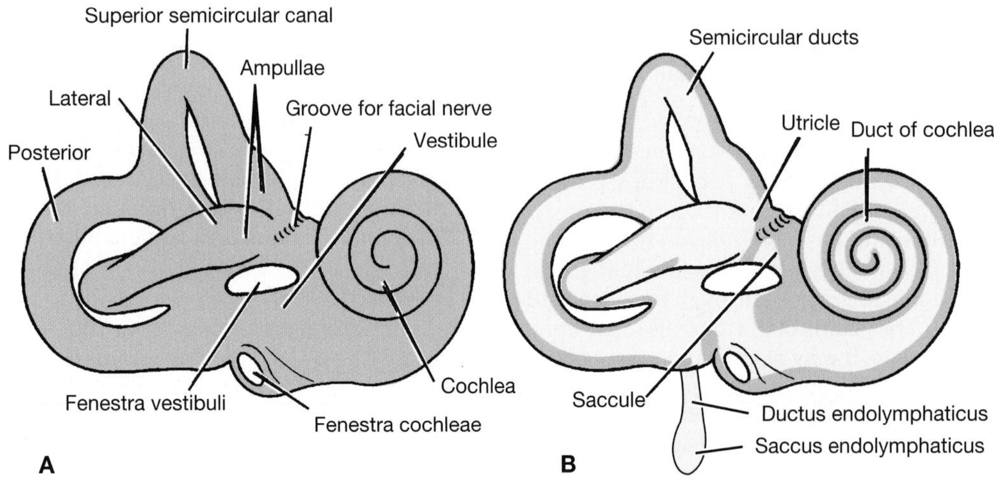

Figure 9.93 Bony **(A)** and membranous **(B)** labyrinths.

endolymphaticus. This lies beneath the dura on the posterior surface of the petrous part of the temporal bone.

Located on the walls of the utricle and saccule are specialized sensory receptors, which are sensitive to the orientation of the head to gravity or other acceleration forces.

The semicircular ducts, although much smaller in diameter than the semicircular canals, have the same configuration. They are arranged at right angles to each other so that all three planes are represented. Whenever the head begins or ceases to move, or whenever a movement of the head accelerates or decelerates, the endolymph in the semicircular ducts changes its speed of movement relative to that of the walls of the semicircular ducts. This change is detected in the sensory receptors in the **ampullae of the semicircular ducts**.

The **duct of the cochlea** is triangular in cross section and is connected to the saccule by the **ductus reuniens**. The highly specialized epithelium that lies on the basilar membrane forms the spiral **organ of Corti** and contains the sensory receptors for hearing. Consult a histology textbook for a detailed description of the spiral organ.

Vestibulocochlear Nerve

The vestibulocochlear nerve (CN VIII) divides into vestibular and cochlear portions at the bottom of the internal acoustic meatus.

The **vestibular nerve** expands to form the **vestibular ganglion**. The branches of the nerve then pierce the lateral end of the internal acoustic meatus and enter the membranous labyrinth, where they supply the utricle, the saccule, and the ampullae of the semicircular ducts.

The **cochlear nerve** divides into branches, which enter the foramina at the base of the modiolus. The sensory ganglion of this nerve takes the form of an elongated **spiral ganglion** that is lodged in a canal winding around the modiolus in the base of the spiral lamina. The peripheral branches of this nerve pass from the ganglion to the **spiral organ of Corti**.

DIGESTIVE SYSTEM

Three major components of the digestive system traverse the head and neck: (1) **oral cavity**, (2) **pharynx**, and (3) **esophagus**.

Oral Cavity

For purposes of description, the oral cavity includes the lips, teeth, tongue, palate, and salivary glands.

Lips

The lips are two fleshy folds that surround the oral orifice (Fig. 9.94). They are covered on the outside by skin and are lined on the inside by mucous membrane. The orbicularis oris muscle and the muscles that radiate from the lips into the face make up the substance of the lips (Fig. 9.95). Also included are the labial blood vessels and nerves, connective tissue, and many small salivary glands. The **philtrum** is the shallow vertical groove seen in the midline on the superficial surface of the upper lip. Median folds of mucous membrane—the **labial frenulae**—connect the inner surface of the lips to the gums.

Oral Cavity

The oral cavity extends from the lips to the pharynx. The paired palatoglossal folds (see Fig. 9.94) form the oropharyngeal isthmus, which is the entrance into the pharynx. The oral cavity has two components: the **vestibule** and the **oral cavity proper**.

Vestibule

The vestibule is a slit-like space that lies between the lips and the cheeks externally and the gums and the teeth internally (see Fig. 9.94A; see also Parotid Gland). It communicates with the exterior through the **oral fissure** between the lips. When the jaws are closed, it communicates with the oral cavity proper behind the third molar tooth on each side. The vestibule is limited above

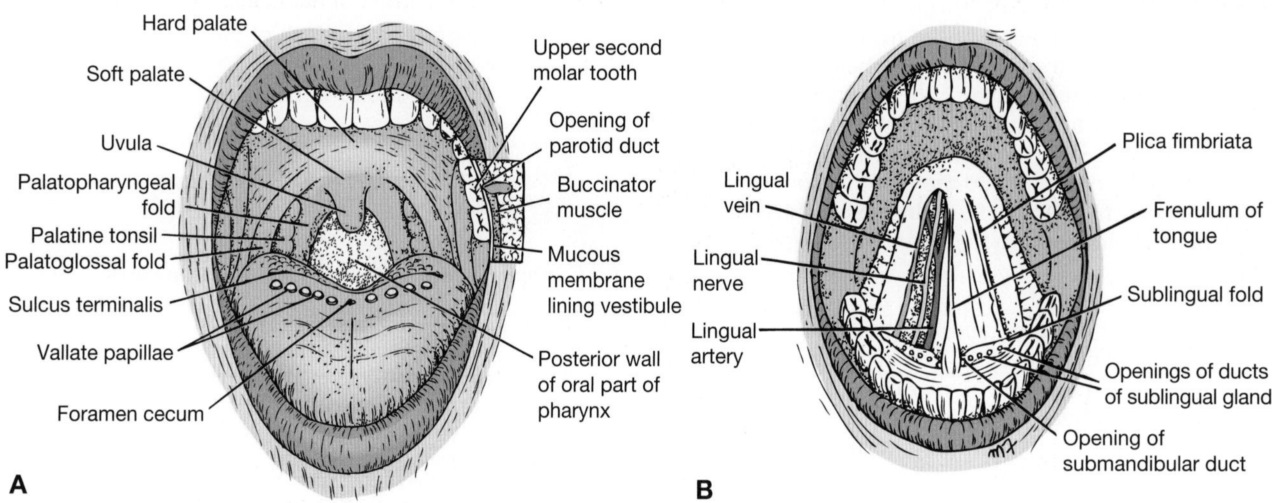

Figure 9.94 A. Oral cavity from in front. The cheek on the left side of the face has been cut away to show the buccinator muscle and the parotid duct. **B.** Undersurface of the tongue from in front.

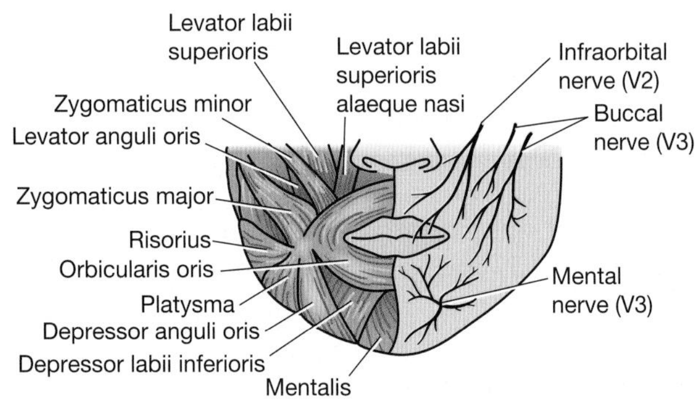

Figure 9.95 Arrangement of the facial muscles around the lips and the sensory nerve supply of the lips.

and below by the reflection of the mucous membrane from the lips and cheeks onto the gums.

The lateral wall of the vestibule is formed by the **cheek**, which is made up by the **buccinator muscle** and lined with **mucous membrane**. The mucous membrane is tethered to the buccinator muscle by elastic fibers in the submucosa that prevent redundant folds of mucous membrane from being bitten between the teeth when the jaws are closed. The mucous membrane of the gingiva, or gum, is strongly attached to the alveolar periosteum. The tone of the buccinator muscle and that of the muscles of the lips keeps the walls of the vestibule in contact with one another. The **duct of the parotid salivary gland** opens on a small papilla into the vestibule opposite the upper second molar tooth.

Oral Cavity Proper

The oral cavity proper has a roof and a floor. The **palate** forms the roof; it consists of the **hard palate** in front and the **soft palate** behind.

The **anterior two thirds of the tongue** and the **reflection of the mucous membrane** from the sides of the tongue to the gum of the mandible largely form the **floor**. A midline fold of mucous membrane, the **frenulum of the tongue**, connects the undersurface of the tongue to the floor of the mouth. Lateral to the frenulum, the mucous membrane forms a fringed fold, the **plica fimbriata**.

The **submandibular duct** of the submandibular gland opens onto the floor of the mouth on the summit of a small papilla on either side of the frenulum of the tongue. The sublingual gland projects up into the mouth, producing a low fold of mucous membrane, the **sublingual fold**. Numerous ducts of the gland open on the summit of the fold.

Oral Cavity Sensory Innervation

- **Roof:** Greater palatine and nasopalatine nerves from the maxillary division of the trigeminal nerve (Fig. 9.96).
- **Floor:** The lingual nerve (general sensation), a branch of the mandibular division of the trigeminal nerve. The taste fibers travel in the chorda tympani nerve, a branch of the facial nerve.
- **Cheek:** The buccal nerve, a branch of the mandibular division of the trigeminal nerve. Note: the buccal branch of the facial nerve innervates the buccinator muscle, whereas the buccal nerve supplies sensory fibers to the cheek.

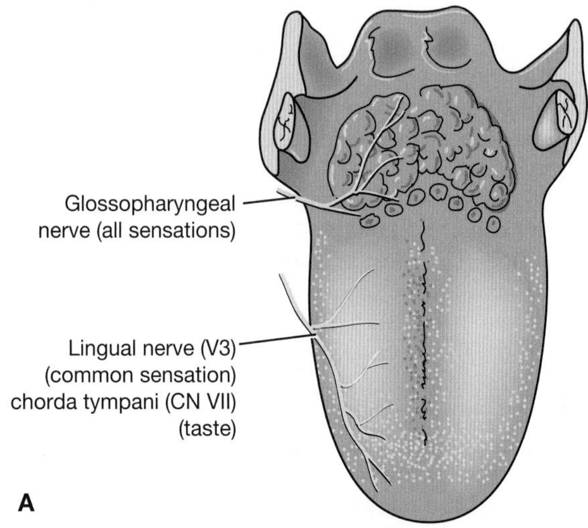

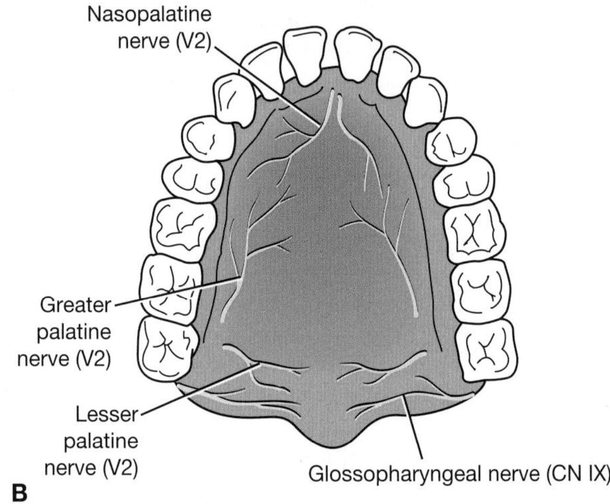

Figure 9.96 **A.** Sensory nerve supply to the mucous membrane of the tongue. **B.** Sensory nerve supply to the mucous membrane of the hard and soft palate; taste fibers run with branches of the maxillary nerve (V2) and join the greater petrosal branch of the facial nerve. CN = cranial nerve.

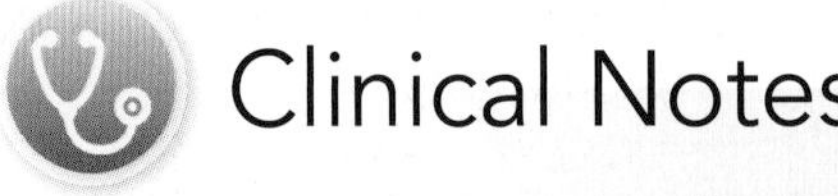

Clinical Significance of Oral Examination

The oral cavity is an area that requires routine physical examination. The clinician must be able to recognize all the structures visible in the mouth and be familiar with the normal variations in the color of the mucous membrane covering underlying structures. The sensory nerve supply and lymph drainage of the cavity should be known. The close relation of the lingual nerve to the lower third molar tooth should be remembered. The close relation of the submandibular duct to the floor of the mouth may enable one to palpate a calculus in cases of periodic swelling of the submandibular salivary gland.

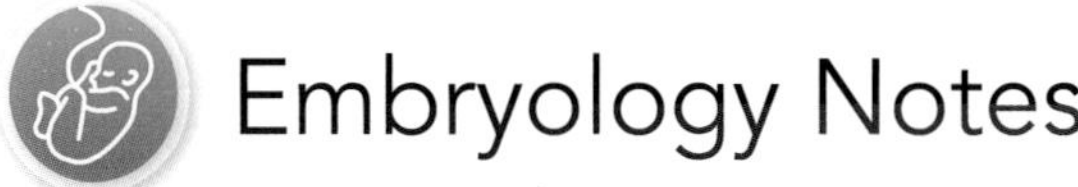

Embryology Notes

Oral Cavity Development

The oral cavity is formed from two sources: a depression from the exterior, the **stomodeum**, which is lined with **ectoderm**, and a part immediately posterior to this, derived from the cephalic end of the foregut and lined with **endoderm**. The **buccopharyngeal membrane** separates these two parts at first, but this breaks down and disappears during week 3 of development (Fig. 9.97). If this membrane were to persist into adult life, it would occupy an imaginary plane extending obliquely from the region of the body of the sphenoid through the soft palate and down to the inner surface of the mandible inferior to the incisor teeth. This means that the structures that are situated in the mouth anterior to this plane are derived from ectoderm. Thus, the epithelium of the hard palate, sides of the mouth, lips, and enamel of the teeth are ectodermal structures. The secretory epithelium and cells lining the ducts of the parotid salivary gland also are derived from ectoderm. On the other hand, the epithelium of the tongue, floor of the mouth, palatoglossal and palatopharyngeal folds, and most of the soft palate are endodermal in origin. The secretory and duct epithelia of the sublingual and submandibular salivary glands also are believed to be of endodermal origin.

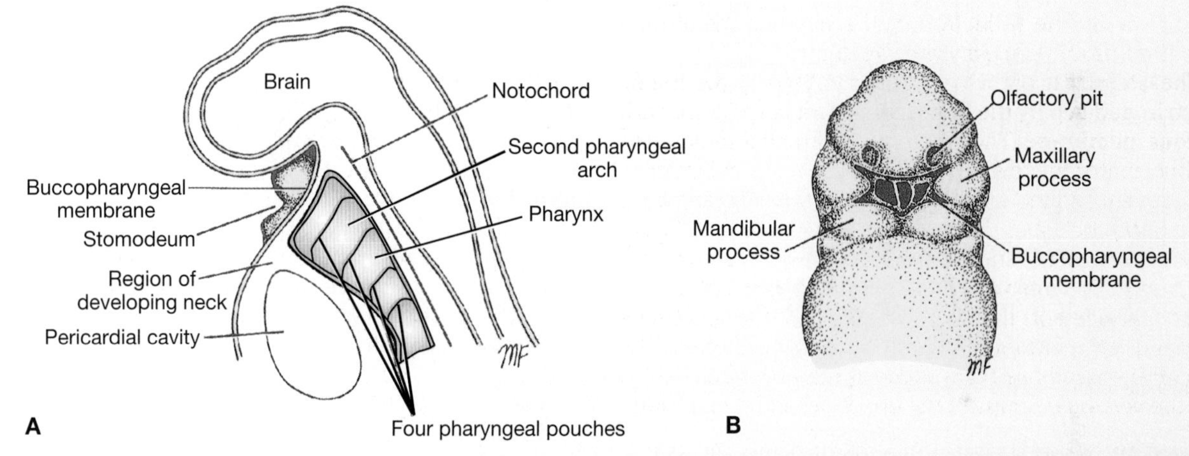

Figure 9.97 **A.** Sagittal section of an embryo showing the position of the buccopharyngeal membrane. **B.** Face of the developing embryo showing the buccopharyngeal membrane breaking down.

Teeth

The teeth are placed in the **alveolar margins** of the maxillae (upper jaw) and mandible (lower jaw). Each tooth occupies its own socket and is anchored in place by **periodontal ligaments** (Fig. 9.98). This fixation constitutes a type of **fibrous joint**.

The four types of teeth are the incisors, canines, premolars, and molars. Each type has an enamel-covered **crown** projecting above the **gingiva** (gum) and a **root** embedded in the alveolae. Consult a histology text for further details regarding the structure of the teeth.

Humans have two successive overlapping generations of teeth. The first teeth (**primary dentition**; **deciduous teeth**; **baby teeth**) appear early in postnatal life and eventually fall out. The **permanent dentition** replaces the primary dentition with a larger number of teeth accommodated for by the growth of the jaws.

The 20 deciduous teeth are 4 incisors, 2 canines, and 4 molars in each jaw. They begin to erupt at about age 6 months and have all erupted by the end of 2 years. The teeth of the lower jaw usually appear before those of the upper jaw (Fig. 9.99).

The 32 permanent teeth are 4 incisors, 2 canines, 4 premolars, and 6 molars in each jaw. They begin to erupt at age 6 years. The last tooth to erupt is the third molar, which may happen between ages 17 and 30 years. The teeth of the lower jaw appear before those of the upper jaw (Fig. 9.100).

Tongue

The tongue is a mass of striated muscle covered with mucous membrane (Fig. 9.101). Muscles attach the tongue to the styloid process and the soft palate above and to the mandible and the hyoid bone below. A **median fibrous septum** divides the tongue into right and left halves.

Lingual Mucous Membrane

A V-shaped sulcus, the **sulcus terminalis**, divides the mucous membrane of the upper surface of the tongue into anterior and posterior parts. The apex of the sulcus projects backward and is marked by a small pit, the **foramen cecum**. The sulcus divides the tongue into the **anterior two thirds** (**oral part; body**) and the **posterior third** (**pharyngeal part; root**). The foramen cecum is an embryologic remnant and marks the site of the upper end of the **thyroglossal duct** (see Thyroid Gland Development).

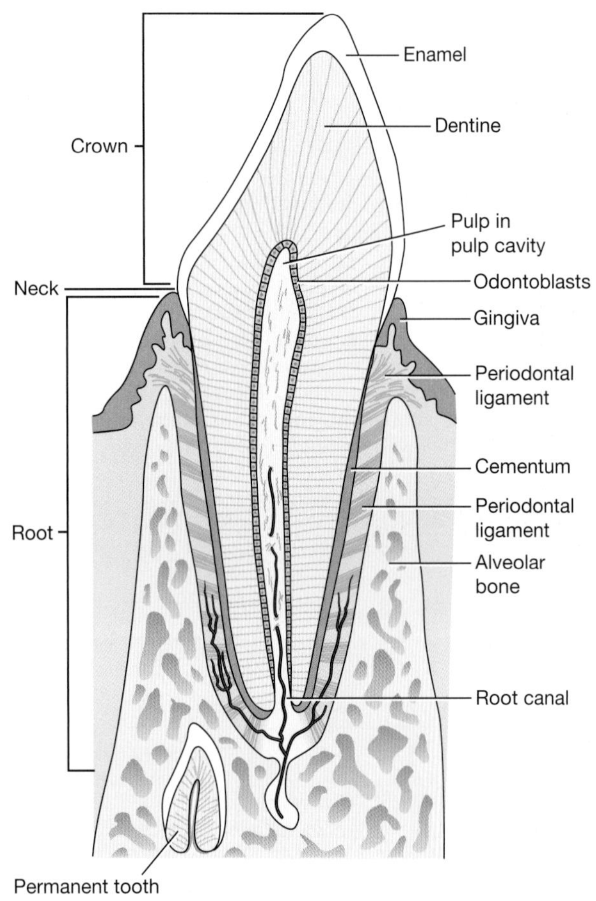

Figure 9.98 Sagittal section through the lower jaw and gum showing an erupted temporary incisor tooth and a developing permanent tooth.

Three types of papillae are present on the upper surface of the anterior two thirds of the tongue: **filiform**, **fungiform**, and **vallate papillae**. The large vallate papillae lie alongside the sulcus terminalis and help identify that structure.

The mucous membrane covering the posterior third of the tongue is devoid of papillae but has an irregular surface, caused by the presence of underlying lymph nodules, the **lingual tonsil**.

The mucous membrane on the inferior surface of the tongue is reflected from the tongue to the floor of the mouth. In the midline anteriorly, the undersurface of the tongue is connected to the floor of the mouth by a fold of mucous membrane, the **lingual frenulum** (see Fig. 9.94B). On the lateral side of the frenulum, the lingual vein can be seen through the mucous membrane. Lateral to the lingual vein, the mucous membrane forms a fringed fold called the **plica fimbriata**.

Tongue Muscles

The tongue has two groups of skeletal muscles: intrinsic and extrinsic. **Intrinsic muscles** are confined to the tongue and are not attached to bone. **Extrinsic muscles** originate outside the tongue; they attach to bones and the soft palate. The tongue muscles are summarized in Table 9.10. Note: the hypoglossal nerve (CN XII) supplies all the tongue muscles, except one, the **palatoglossus** (supplied by vagus fibers in the pharyngeal plexus).

Tongue Movements

- **Protrusion:** Genioglossus muscles on both sides acting together (Fig. 9.102)
- **Retraction:** Styloglossus and hyoglossus muscles on both sides acting together

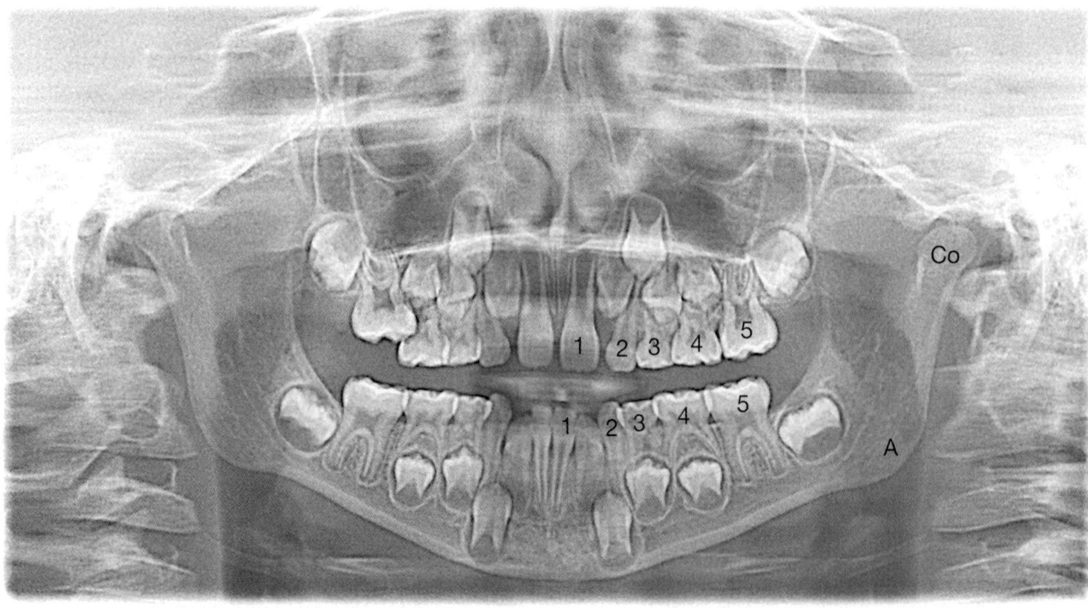

Figure 9.99 Dental panorama of a 7-year-old female showing mixed primary and permanent dentition. 1, permanent central incisor; 2, primary canine; 3, primary 1st molar; 4, primary 2nd molar; 5, permanent 1st molar; A, angle of mandible; Co, condyle. (Courtesy of J. Robinson, DMD.)

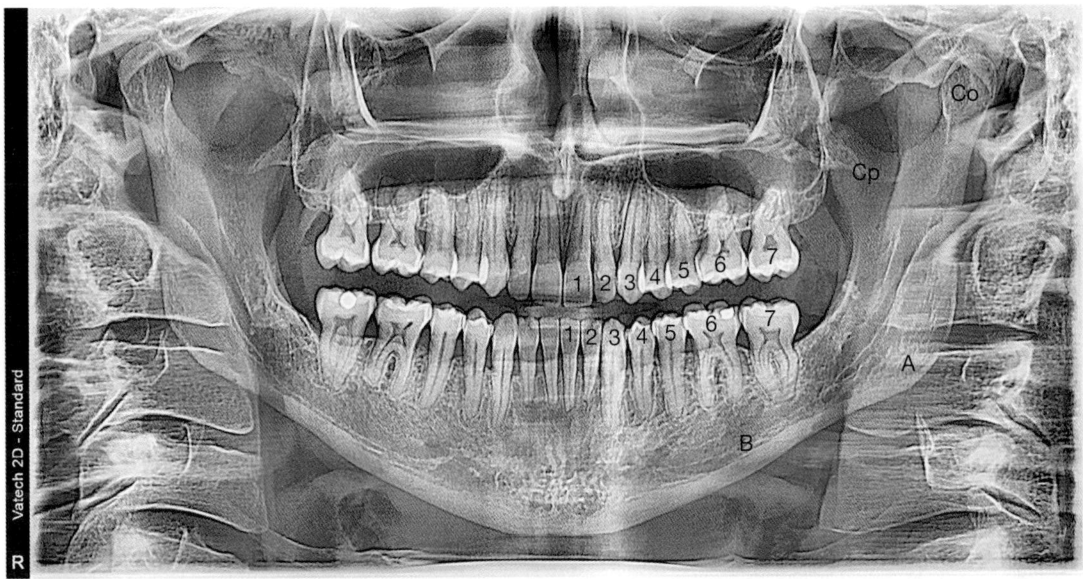

Figure 9.100 Dental panorama of an adult male showing permanent dentition. The third molars have been extracted. 1, central incisor; 2, lateral incisor; 3, canine; 4, 1st premolar; 5, 2nd premolar; 6, 1st molar; 7, 2nd molar; A, angle; B, body, Co, condyle, Cp, coronoid process. (Courtesy of J. Robinson, DMD.)

- **Depression:** Hyoglossus muscles on both sides acting together
- **Retraction and elevation of the posterior third:** Styloglossus and palatoglossus muscles on both sides acting together
- **Shape changes:** Intrinsic muscles

Blood Supply

The lingual artery, tonsillar branch of the facial artery, and the ascending pharyngeal artery supply the tongue. The veins drain into the internal jugular vein.

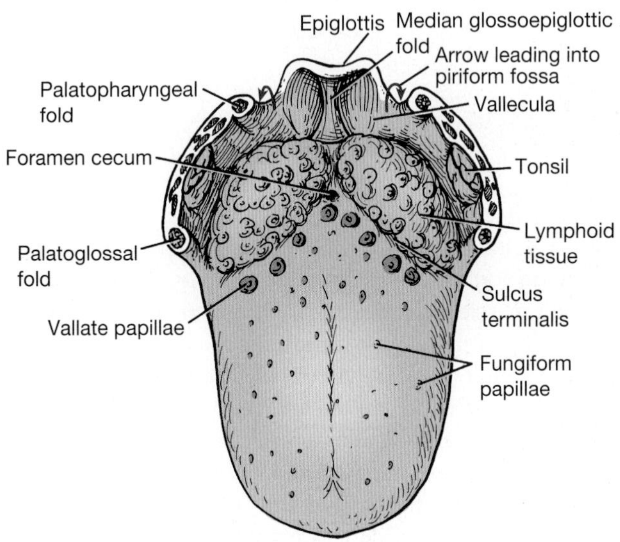

Figure 9.101 Dorsal surface of the tongue showing the palatine and lingual tonsils, the epiglottis, the valleculae, and the entrance into the piriform fossa on each side (*arrows*).

Lymph Drainage

- **Tip:** Submental lymph nodes
- **Sides of the anterior two thirds:** Submandibular and deep cervical lymph nodes
- **Posterior third:** Deep cervical lymph nodes

Sensory Innervation

- **Anterior two thirds:** Lingual nerve branch of the mandibular division of trigeminal nerve (general sensation) and chorda tympani branch of the facial nerve (taste); see Fig. 9.96A
- **Posterior third:** Glossopharyngeal nerve (general sensation and taste)

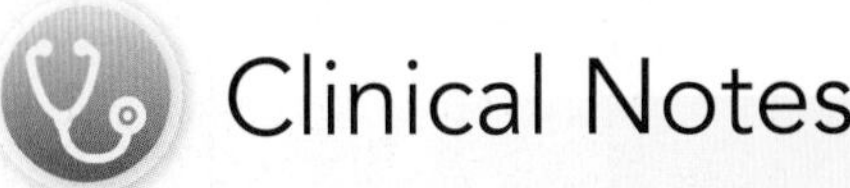

Clinical Notes

Tongue Laceration

The patient's teeth, following a blow on the chin when the tongue is partly protruded from the mouth, often cause a tongue wound. It can also occur when a patient accidentally bites the tongue while eating, during recovery from an anesthetic, or during an epileptic attack. Bleeding is halted by grasping the tongue between the finger and thumb posterior to the laceration, thus occluding the branches of the lingual artery.

Hypoglossal Nerve Testing

Asking the patient to protrude their tongue is a basic test of the function of the hypoglossal nerve (see Fig. 9.102). Deviation of the tip of the tongue indicates lesion of the nerve on the side to which the deviation occurs, that is, the ipsilateral nerve.

Table 9.10 Tongue Muscles

MUSCLE	ORIGIN	INSERTION	NERVE SUPPLY	ACTION
Intrinsic Muscles				
Longitudinal	Median septum and submucosa	Mucous membrane	Hypoglossal nerve	Alters shape of the tongue
Transverse				
Vertical				
Extrinsic Muscles				
Genioglossus	Superior genial spine of the mandible	Blends with other muscles of the tongue	Hypoglossal nerve	Protrudes apex of the tongue through the mouth
Hyoglossus	Body and greater cornu of hyoid bone	Blends with other muscles of the tongue	Hypoglossal nerve	Depresses the tongue
Styloglossus	Styloid process of the temporal bone	Blends with other muscles of the tongue	Hypoglossal nerve	Draws the tongue upward and backward
Palatoglossus	Palatine aponeurosis	Side of the tongue	Vagus nerve (pharyngeal plexus)	Pulls roots of the tongue upward and backward, narrows oropharyngeal isthmus

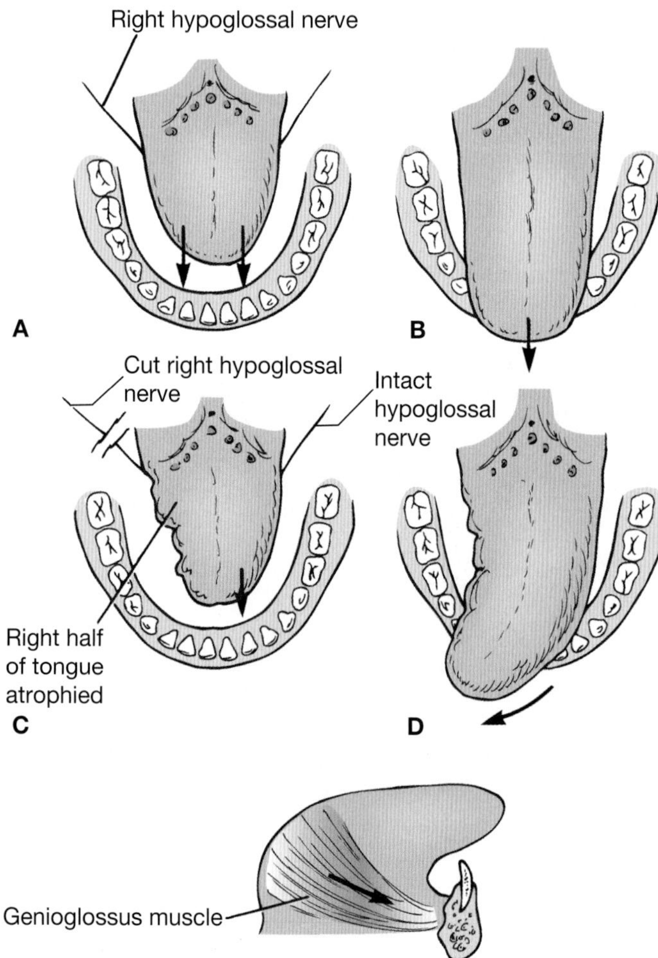

Figure 9.102 Diagrammatic representation of the action of the genioglossus muscles of the tongue. **A.** The right and left muscles contract equally together, and as a result, **(B)** the tip of the tongue is protruded in the midline. **C.** The right hypoglossal nerve (which innervates the genioglossus muscle and the intrinsic tongue muscles on the same side) is cut, and as a result, the right side of the tongue is atrophied and wrinkled. **D.** When the patient is asked to protrude the tongue, the tip points to the side of the nerve lesion. **E.** The attachments and direction of pull of the genioglossus muscle.

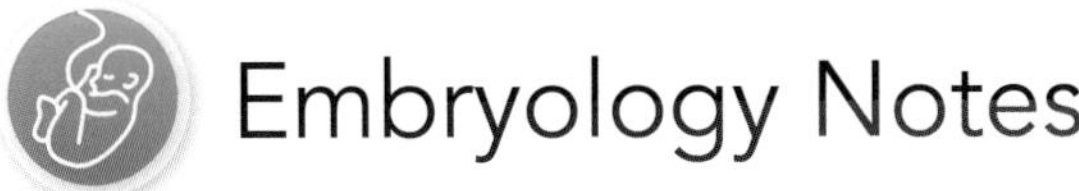

Embryology Notes

Tongue Development

At about week 4, a median swelling (**tuberculum impar**) appears in the endodermal ventral wall or floor of the pharynx (Fig. 9.103). A little later, another swelling, the **lateral lingual swelling** (derived from the anterior end of each first pharyngeal arch), appears on each side of the tuberculum impar. The lateral lingual swellings now enlarge, grow medially, and fuse with each other and the tuberculum impar. The lingual swellings thus form the anterior two thirds (body) of the tongue. Because they are derived from the first pharyngeal arches, the lingual nerve (a branch of

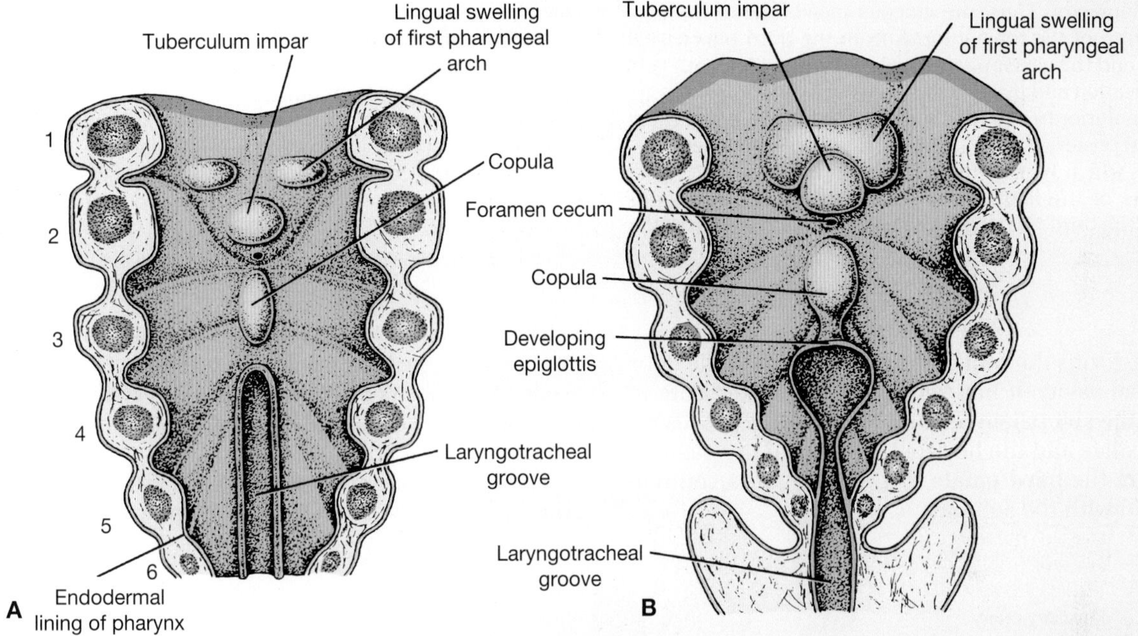

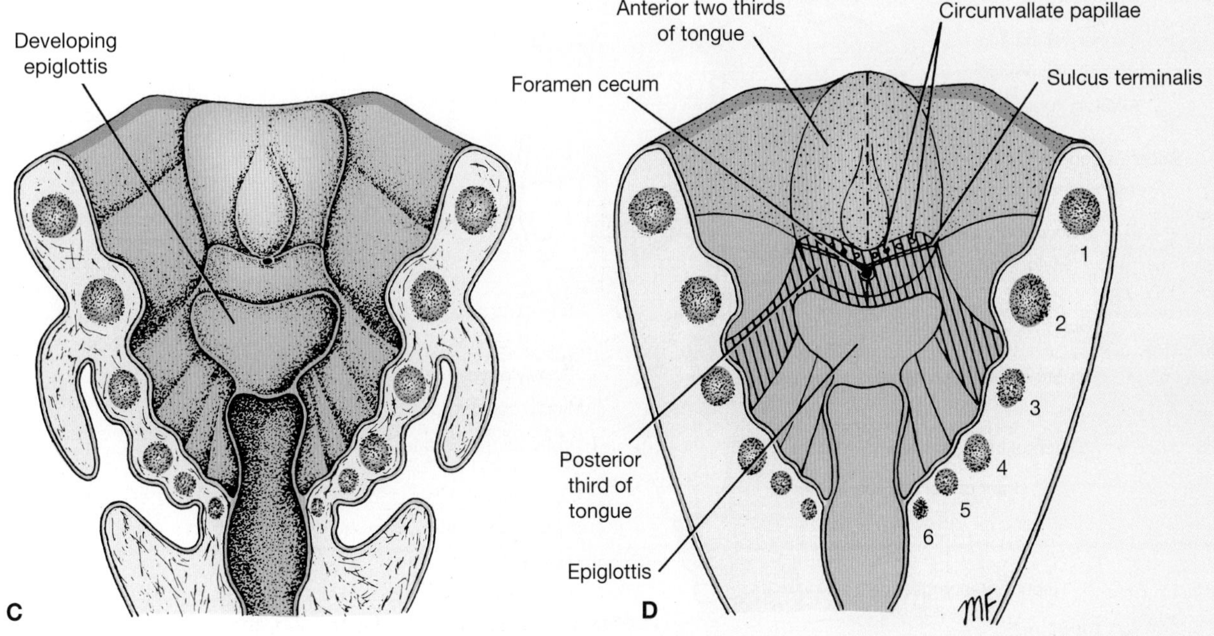

Figure 9.103 Progressive stages **(A–D)** in development of the floor of the pharynx showing formation of the tongue. See text for details.

(continued)

the mandibular nerve) provides general sensation to the lingual swellings. The chorda tympani (from CN VII) also supplies this area and provides taste fibers.

Meanwhile, a second median swelling, the **copula**, appears in the floor of the pharynx behind the tuberculum impar. The copula extends forward on each side of the tuberculum impar and becomes V shaped. At about this time, the anterior ends of the second, third, and fourth pharyngeal arches are entering this region. The anterior ends of the third arch on each side overgrow the other arches and extend into the copula, fusing in the midline. The copula now disappears. Thus, the mucous membrane of the posterior third of the tongue forms from the third pharyngeal arches, and the glossopharyngeal nerve provides both general sensation and taste to this area.

The anterior two thirds (body) of the tongue is separated from the posterior third (root) by a groove, the **sulcus terminalis**, which represents the interval between the lingual swellings of the first pharyngeal arches and the anterior ends of the third pharyngeal arches. Around the edge of the body of the tongue, the endodermal cells proliferate and grow inferiorly into the underlying mesenchyme. Later, these cells degenerate so that this part of the tongue becomes free. Some of the endodermal cells remain in the midline and help form the **frenulum of the tongue**.

Remember that the **circumvallate papillae** are situated on the mucous membrane just anterior to the sulcus terminalis and that their taste buds are innervated by the glossopharyngeal nerve. It is presumed that during development, the mucous membrane of the root of the tongue becomes pulled anteriorly slightly, so that fibers of CN IX cross the sulcus terminalis to supply these taste buds.

Occipital myotomes give rise to the muscles of the tongue. These myotomes first are closely related to the developing hindbrain and later migrate inferiorly and anteriorly around the pharynx and enter the tongue. The migrating myotomes carry with them their innervation (CN XII), and this explains the long curving course taken by the hypoglossal nerve as it passes downward and forward in the carotid triangle of the neck.

Palate

The palate forms the roof of the oral cavity and the floor of the nasal cavity. It has two parts: the hard palate in front and the soft palate behind. The palatine processes of the maxillae and the horizontal plates of the palatine bones form the **hard palate** (Fig. 9.104B). It is continuous behind with the soft palate.

The **soft palate** is a mobile fold attached to the posterior border of the hard palate (Fig. 9.105). Its free posterior border presents a conical projection in the midline called the **uvula**. The soft palate is continuous at the sides with the lateral walls of the pharynx.

The soft palate is composed of mucous membrane, palatine aponeurosis, and muscles. The **mucous membrane**

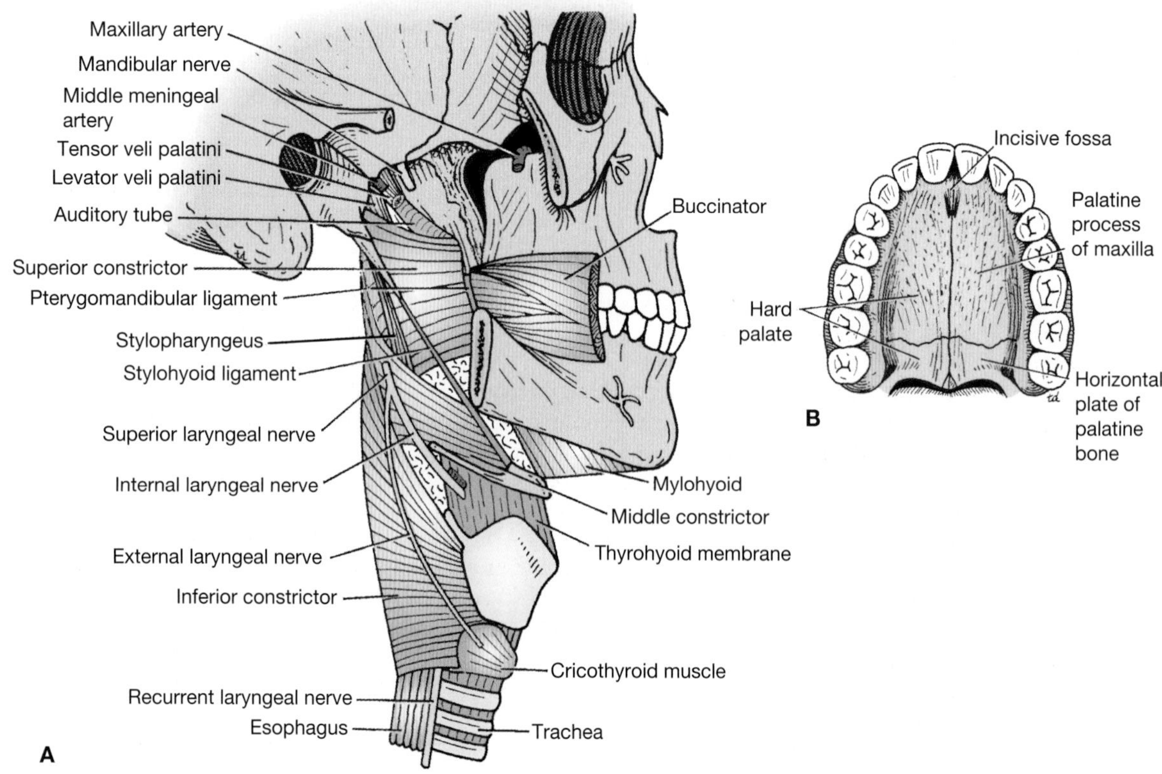

Figure 9.104 **A.** Three constrictor muscles of the pharynx. The superior and recurrent laryngeal nerves are also shown. **B.** Oral view of the hard palate showing its bony composition.

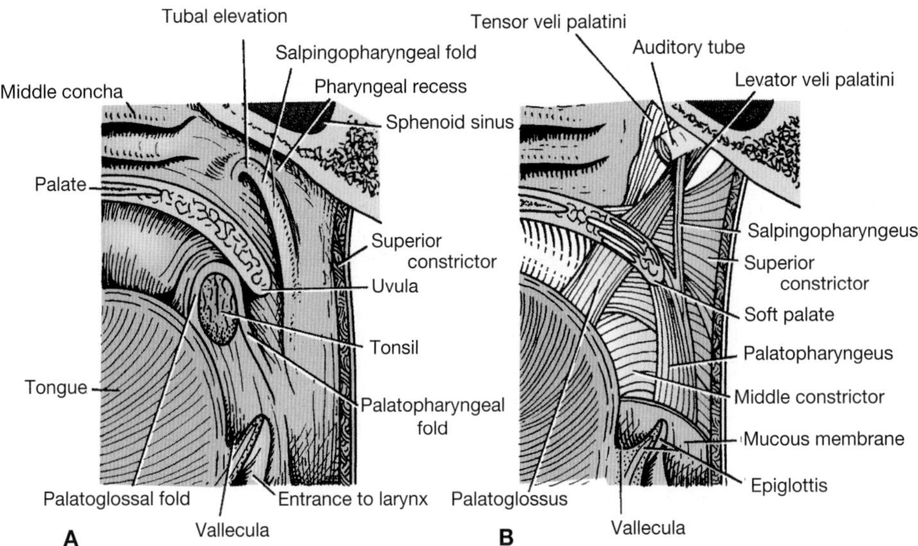

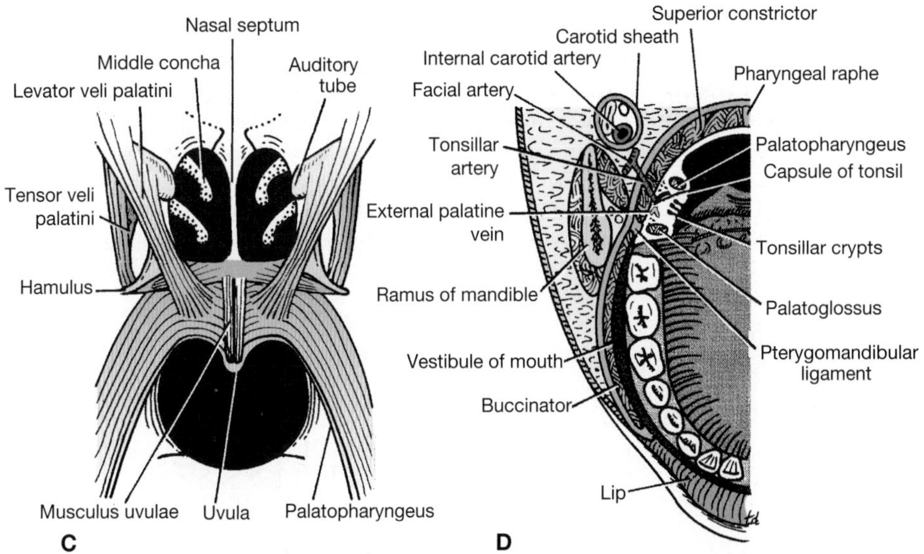

Figure 9.105 **A.** Junction of the nose with the nasopharynx and the mouth with the oropharynx. Note the position of the palatine tonsil and the opening of the auditory tube. **B.** Muscles of the soft palate and the upper part of the pharynx. **C.** Muscles of the soft palate seen from behind. **D.** Horizontal section through the mouth and the oropharynx showing the relations of the palatine tonsil.

covers the upper and lower surfaces of the soft palate. The **palatine aponeurosis** is a fibrous sheet attached to the posterior border of the hard palate. It is the expanded tendon of the tensor veli palatini muscle.

The muscles of the soft palate are the **tensor veli palatini**, **levator veli palatini**, **palatoglossus**, **palatopharyngeus**, and the **musculus uvulae**. These are summarized in Table 9.11. Note: the **vagus nerve** (CN X), via the pharyngeal plexus, supplies all the muscles of the soft palate except one, the **tensor veli palatini** (supplied by the mandibular division of the trigeminal nerve).

The muscle fibers of the tensor veli palatini converge as they descend from their origin to form a narrow tendon, which turns medially around the **pterygoid hamulus**. The tendon, together with the tendon of the opposite side, expands to form the **palatine aponeurosis**, which is most pronounced in the anterior aspect of the soft palate. When the muscles of the two sides contract, the soft palate (especially its more anterior portion) tightens so that it may move upward or downward as a tense sheet.

The tensor and levator palatini muscles also act on the mucous membrane of the auditory tube and so affect function in the middle ear. See Auditory Tube earlier for further details.

Two arches extend off each side of the soft palate. The **palatoglossal arch** is a fold of mucous membrane containing the **palatoglossus muscle**, which extends from the soft palate to the side of the tongue (see Figs. 9.94A and 9.105). The **palatoglossal arch marks where the oral cavity becomes the pharynx**. The **palatopharyngeal arch** is a fold of mucous membrane behind the palatoglossal arch that runs downward and laterally to join the pharyngeal wall. This arch contains the **palatopharyngeus muscle**. The **palatine tonsils**, which are masses of lymphoid tissue, are in the **tonsillar fossa** between the palatoglossal and palatopharyngeal arches (see Fig. 9.105).

Soft Palate Movements

Raising the soft palate closes the **pharyngeal isthmus** (communicating channel between the nasal and oral

Table 9.11 Soft Palate Muscles

MUSCLE	ORIGIN	INSERTION	NERVE SUPPLY	ACTION
Tensor veli palatini	Spine of sphenoid, auditory tube	With muscle of other sides, forms palatine aponeurosis	Nerve to medial pterygoid from mandibular nerve	Tenses soft palate
Levator veli palatini	Petrous part of the temporal bone, auditory tube	Palatine aponeurosis	Pharyngeal plexus (vagus nerve)	Raises soft palate
Palatoglossus	Palatine aponeurosis	Side of the tongue	Pharyngeal plexus (vagus nerve)	Pulls root of the tongue upward and backward, narrows oropharyngeal isthmus
Palatopharyngeus	Palatine aponeurosis	Posterior border of thyroid cartilage	Pharyngeal plexus (vagus nerve)	Elevates wall of the pharynx, pulls palatopharyngeal folds medially
Musculus uvulae	Posterior border of the hard palate	Mucous membrane of the uvula	Pharyngeal plexus (vagus)	Elevates uvula

parts of the pharynx). Closure occurs during the production of explosive consonants in speech and during swallowing.

Bilateral contraction of the levator veli palatini muscles raises the soft palate. At the same time, the upper fibers of the superior constrictor muscle contract and pull the posterior pharyngeal wall forward. The palatopharyngeus muscles on both sides also contract so that the palatopharyngeal arches are pulled medially, like side curtains. Further, the musculus uvulae elevates the uvula, thereby contributing to raising the soft palate. The summative effect is that multiple muscles act as a collective sphincter to close the pharyngeal isthmus.

Sensory Innervation

The **greater** and **lesser palatine nerves** from the maxillary division of the trigeminal nerve enter the palate through the greater and lesser palatine foramina (see Fig. 9.96B). The greater palatine nerve runs forward and mainly supplies the hard palate. The lesser palatine nerve mainly passes posteriorly and supplies the soft palate. The **nasopalatine nerve**, also a branch of the maxillary nerve, enters the front of the hard palate through the incisive foramen. The glossopharyngeal nerve also supplies the soft palate.

Blood Supply

The greater palatine branch of the maxillary artery, ascending palatine branch of the facial artery, and the ascending pharyngeal artery supply the palate.

Palatal Lymph Drainage

Lymph drains to the deep cervical lymph nodes.

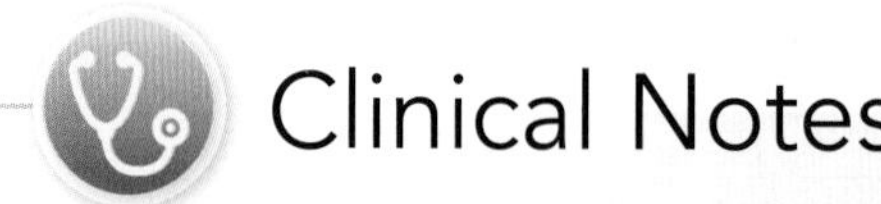

Clinical Notes

Angioedema of the Uvula (Quincke Uvula)

The uvula has a core of voluntary muscle, the **musculus uvulae**, that is attached to the posterior border of the hard palate. Surrounding the muscle is the loose connective tissue of the submucosa that is responsible for the great swelling of this structure secondary to angioedema.

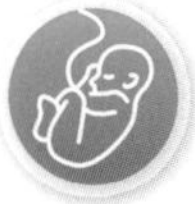

Embryology Notes

Palatal Development

In early fetal life, the nasal and oral cavities are in communication, but later, they become separated by the development of the palate (Fig. 9.106). This process of palatogenesis is critical in establishing the ability to breathe and process food simultaneously, such as during suckling. The medial nasal process forms the **primary palate**, which carries the four incisor teeth. Posterior to the primary palate, the maxillary process on each side sends medially a horizontal plate called the **palatal process**; these plates fuse to form the **secondary palate** and also unite with the primary palate and the developing **nasal septum**. The fusion takes place from the anterior to the posterior region. The primary and secondary palates later will form the **hard palate**. Two folds grow posteriorly from the posterior edge

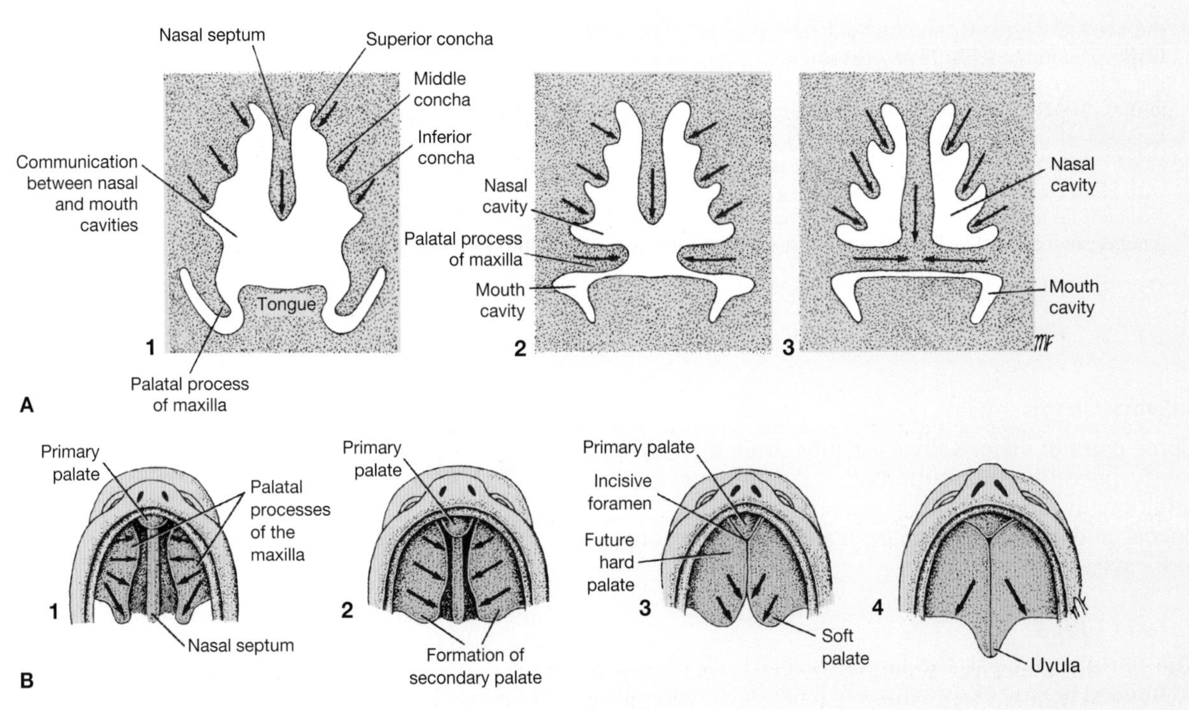

Figure 9.106 **A.** Frontal sections showing the formation of the palate and the nasal septum. **B.** Inferior views showing the different stages in the formation of the palate.

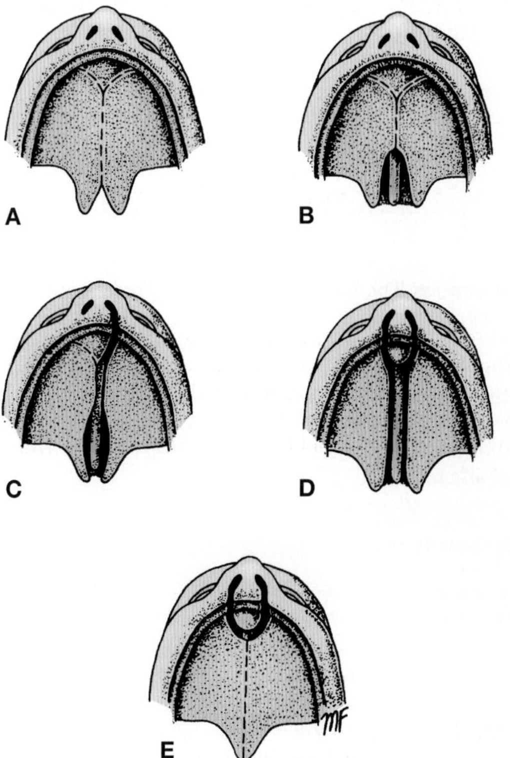

Figure 9.107 Different forms of cleft palate: **(A)** cleft uvula, **(B)** cleft soft and hard palate, **(C)** total unilateral cleft palate and cleft lip, **(D)** total bilateral cleft palate and cleft lip, and **(E)** bilateral cleft lip and jaw.

of the palatal processes to create the **soft palate**, so that the **uvula** is the last structure to form. The union of the two folds of the soft palate occurs during week 8. The two parts of the uvula fuse in the midline during week 11. The interval between the primary palate and secondary palate is represented in the midline by the **incisive foramen**.

Cleft Palate

Different forms of failure of fusion of the facial primordia cause various types of cleft palate, in similar fashion as the formation of facial clefts (Figs. 9.107 and 9.108; see also Figs. 9.27 to 9.31). The first degree of severity is cleft uvula;

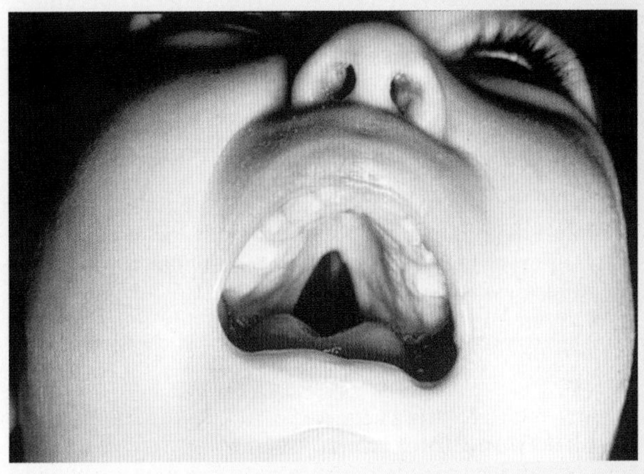

Figure 9.108 Cleft hard and soft palate. (Courtesy of R. Chase.)

(continued)

the second degree is ununited palatal processes. The third degree is ununited palatal processes and a cleft on one side of the primary palate. This type is usually associated with unilateral cleft lip. The fourth degree of severity, which is rare, consists of ununited palatal processes and a cleft on both sides of the primary palate. This type is usually associated with bilateral cleft lip. A rare form may occur in which a bilateral cleft lip and failure of the primary palate to fuse with the palatal processes of the maxilla on each side are present.

An infant born with a severe cleft palate presents a difficult feeding problem, because they are unable to suck efficiently. They often receive some milk in the mouth, which then is regurgitated through the nose or aspirated into the lungs, leading to respiratory infection. For this reason, careful artificial feeding is required until the infant is strong enough to undergo surgery. Plastic surgery usually is recommended early postnatally, before improper speech habits are acquired.

Salivary Glands

Three pairs of major salivary glands drain into the oral cavity: **parotid**, **submandibular**, and **sublingual glands**. Additionally, several minor salivary glands (eg, labial, buccal, and palatal glands) are scattered throughout the oral cavity.

Parotid Gland

The parotid gland is the largest salivary gland and is composed mostly of serous acini. It lies in a deep hollow below the external auditory meatus, behind the ramus of the mandible, and in front of the SCM muscle (Fig. 9.109). The facial nerve divides the gland into **superficial** and **deep lobes**. The **parotid duct** emerges from the anterior border of the gland and passes forward over the lateral surface of the masseter. It pierces the buccinator muscle and enters the vestibule of the mouth upon a small papilla opposite the upper second molar tooth (see Fig. 9.94A). Multiple structures pass through the parotid gland, where they may be affected by the condition of the gland (eg, infection, tumor growth). These include the facial nerve, auriculotemporal nerve, terminal division of the external carotid artery, formation of the retromandibular vein, and parotid lymph nodes (see Fig. 9.109).

NERVE SUPPLY

The **glossopharyngeal nerve** (CN IX) carries preganglionic parasympathetic secretomotor fibers. These pass into the **tympanic nerve** and synapse in the **otic ganglion** (see Fig. 9.84B). Postganglionic fibers attach to the **auriculotemporal nerve** and follow that to the gland.

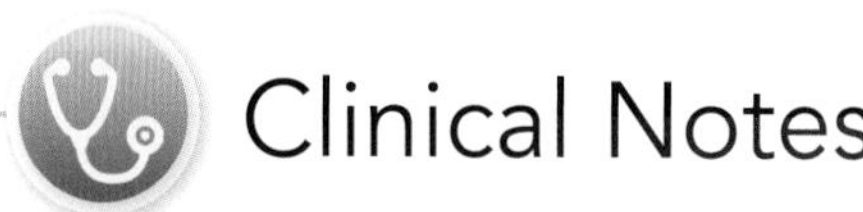

Clinical Notes

Parotid Duct Injury

The parotid duct, which is a comparatively superficial structure on the face, may be damaged in injuries to the face or may be inadvertently cut during surgical operations on the face. The duct is about 2 in. (5 cm) long and passes forward across the masseter about a fingerbreadth below the zygomatic arch.

Parotid Salivary Gland and Facial Nerve Lesions

The parotid salivary gland consists essentially of superficial and deep parts, and the important facial nerve lies in the interval between these parts. A benign parotid neoplasm rarely, if ever, causes facial palsy. However, a malignant tumor of the parotid is usually highly invasive and quickly involves the facial nerve, causing unilateral facial paralysis.

Parotid Gland Infections

The parotid gland may become acutely inflamed as a result of retrograde bacterial infection from the mouth via the parotid duct. The gland may also become infected via the bloodstream, as in mumps. In both cases, the gland is swollen; it is painful because the **fascial capsule** derived from the investing layer of deep cervical fascia is strong and limits the swelling of the gland. The swollen glenoid process, which extends medially behind the temporomandibular joint, is responsible for the pain experienced in acute parotitis when eating.

Frey Syndrome

Frey syndrome (auriculotemporal nerve syndrome) is an interesting complication that sometimes develops after penetrating wounds of the parotid gland. When the patient eats, beads of perspiration appear on the skin covering the parotid. This condition is caused by damage to the **auriculotemporal** and **great auricular nerves**. During the process of healing, the parasympathetic secretomotor fibers in the auriculotemporal nerve grow out and join the distal end of the great auricular nerve. Eventually, these fibers reach the sweat glands in the facial skin. By this means, a stimulus intended for saliva production produces sweat secretion instead.

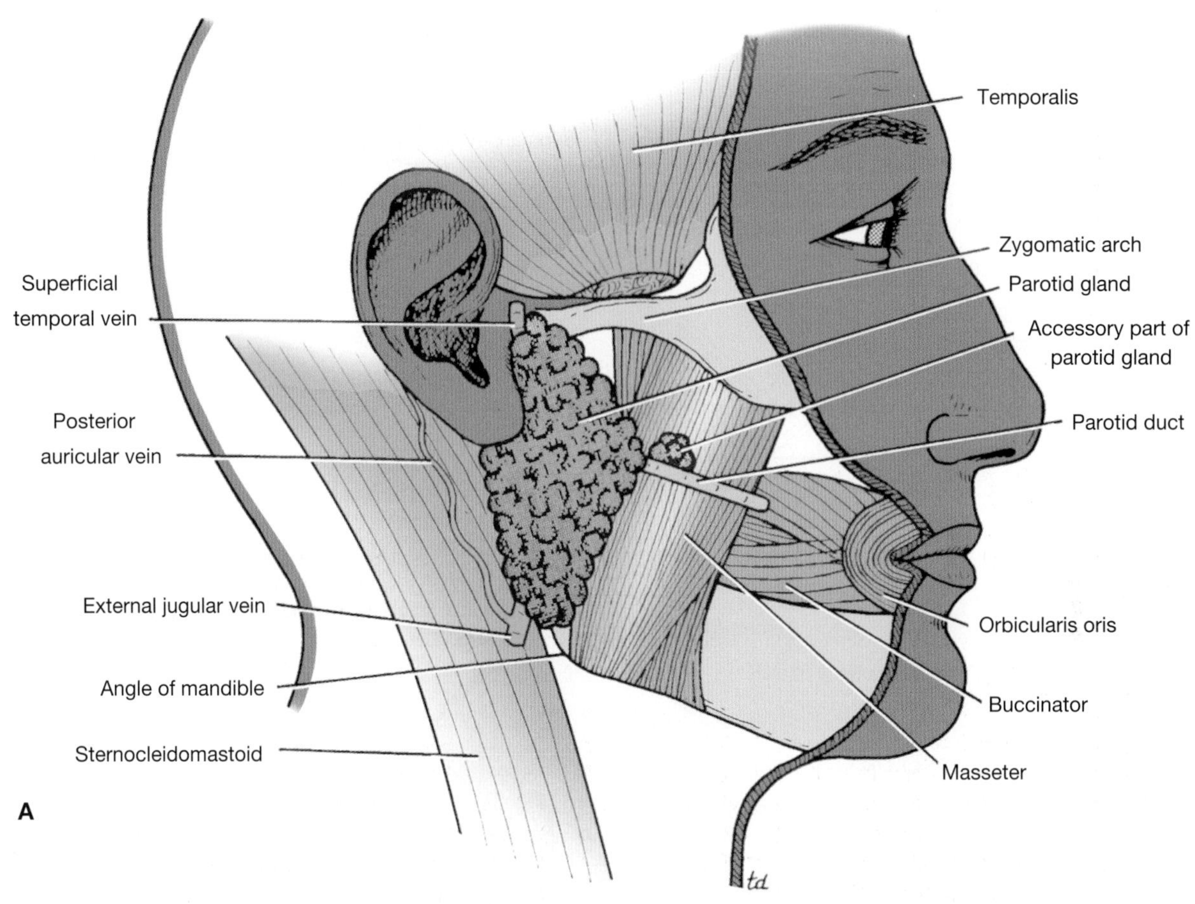

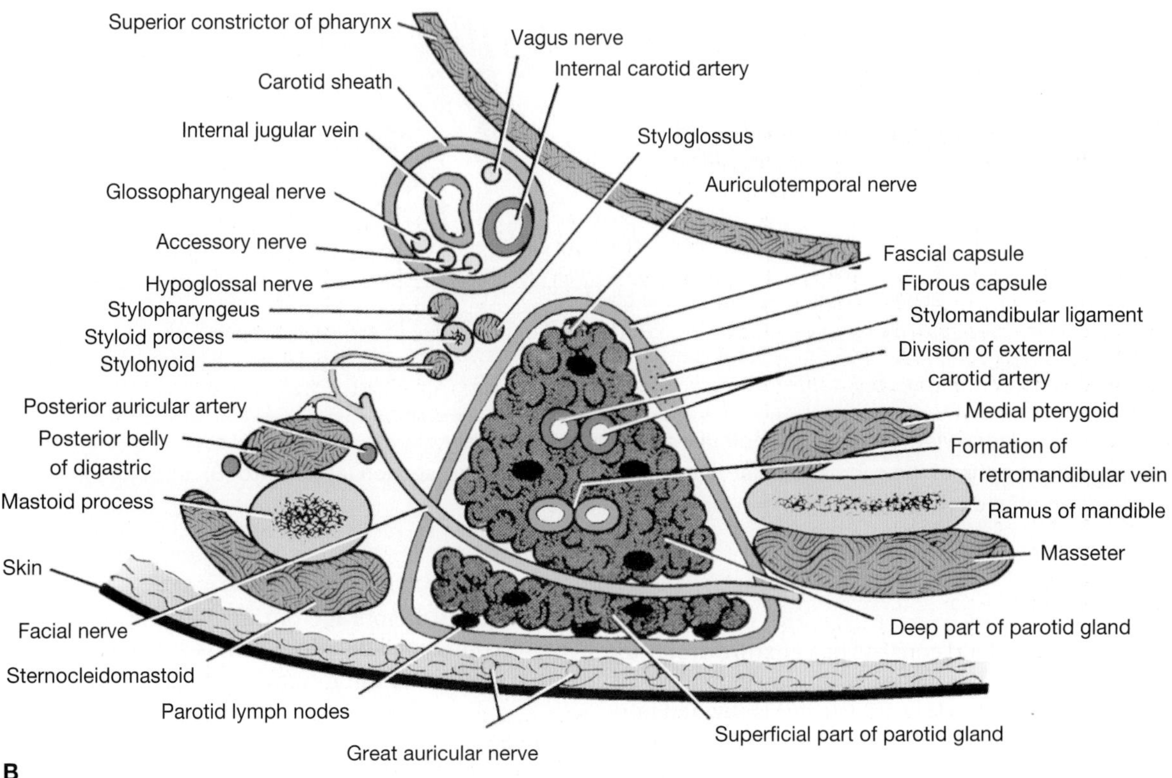

Figure 9.109 Parotid gland and its relations. **A.** Lateral surface of the gland and the course of the parotid duct. **B.** Horizontal section of the parotid gland and adnexa.

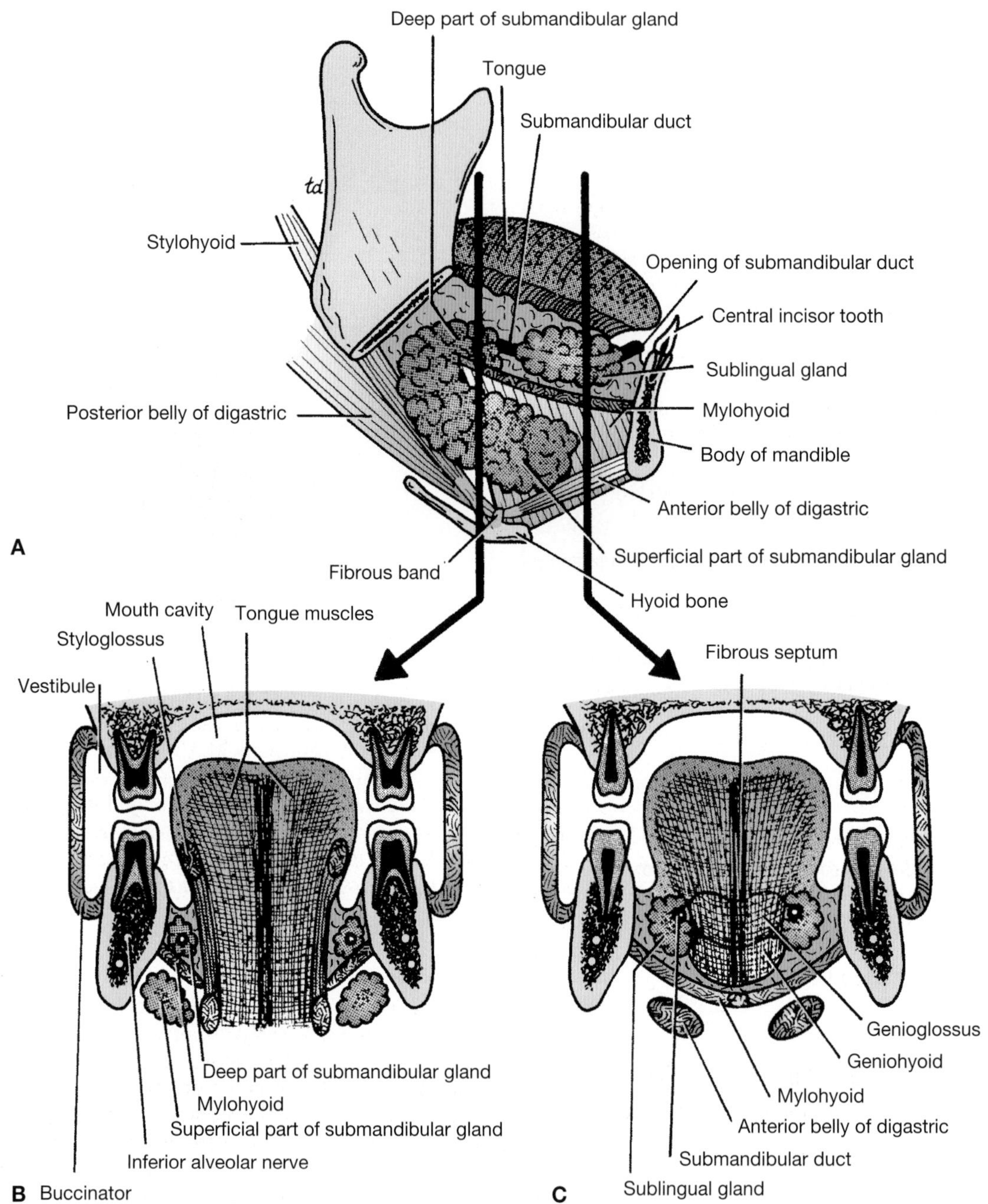

Figure 9.110 **A.** Lateral view of the submandibular and sublingual salivary glands. **B.** Coronal section through the superficial and deep parts of the submandibular salivary glands. **C.** Coronal section (anterior to **B**) through the sublingual salivary glands and the ducts of the submandibular salivary glands.

Submandibular Gland

The submandibular gland consists of a mixture of serous and mucous acini. It lies beneath the lower border of the body of the mandible (Fig. 9.110) and is divided into superficial and deep parts by the mylohyoid muscle. The deep part of the gland lies beneath the mucous membrane of the mouth on the side of the tongue. The **submandibular duct** emerges from the anterior end of the deep part of the gland and runs forward beneath the mucous membrane of the mouth. It opens into the mouth on a small papilla, which is situated at the side of the **frenulum of the tongue** (see Fig. 9.94B).

NERVE SUPPLY

The **facial nerve** (CN VII) provides the parasympathetic secretomotor supply via its **chorda tympani** branch and the **submandibular ganglion** (see Fig. 9.83B). The postganglionic fibers pass directly to the gland.

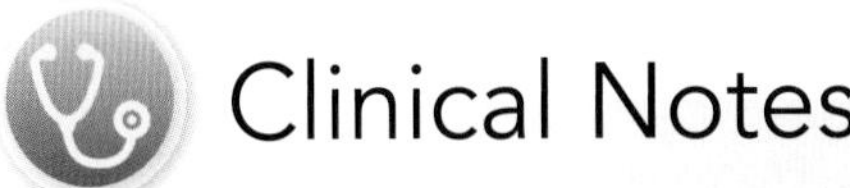

Clinical Notes

Submandibular Salivary Gland: Calculus Formation

The submandibular salivary gland is a common site of calculus formation. This condition is rare in other salivary glands. The presence of a tense swelling below the body of the mandible, which is greatest before or during a meal and is reduced in size or absent between meals, is diagnostic of the condition. Examination of the floor of the mouth will reveal absence of ejection of saliva from the orifice of the duct of the affected gland. Frequently, the stone can be palpated in the duct, which lies below the mucous membrane of the floor of the mouth.

Submandibular Lymph Node Enlargement and Submandibular Salivary Gland Swelling

The submandibular lymph nodes are commonly enlarged as a result of a pathologic condition of the scalp, face, maxillary sinus, or oral cavity. One of the most common causes of painful enlargement of these nodes is acute infection of the teeth. Enlargement of these nodes should not be confused with pathologic swelling of the submandibular salivary gland.

Sublingual Gland

The sublingual gland lies beneath the mucous membrane (**sublingual fold**) of the floor of the mouth, close to the frenulum of the tongue (see Fig. 9.110). It has both serous and mucous acini, with the latter predominating. The **sublingual ducts** (8 to 20 in number) open into the mouth on the summit of the sublingual fold (see Fig. 9.94B).

NERVE SUPPLY

The nerve supply to the sublingual gland is the same as that for the submandibular gland (see above).

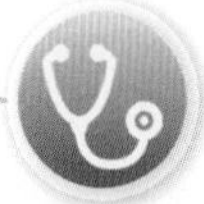

Clinical Notes

Sublingual Salivary Gland and Cyst Formation

The sublingual salivary gland, which lies beneath the sublingual fold of the floor of the mouth, opens into the mouth by numerous small ducts. Blockage of one or more of these ducts is believed to be the cause of cysts under the tongue.

Pharynx

The pharynx is situated behind the nasal cavities, the mouth, and the larynx and aptly consists of three parts: **nasopharynx**, **oropharynx**, and **laryngopharynx** (Fig. 9.111). The pharynx is funnel shaped; its upper, wider end lies under the base of the skull; its lower, narrow end is continuous with the esophagus opposite the C6 vertebra. The pharynx has a musculomembranous wall, which is deficient anteriorly. Here, it is replaced by the posterior openings into the nose (**choanae**), the opening into the mouth, and the inlet of the larynx. The pharynx is also continuous with the tympanic cavity via the auditory tube.

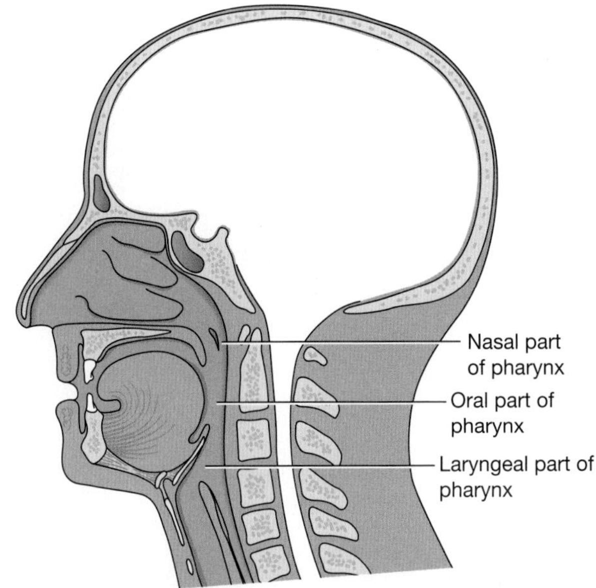

Figure 9.111 Sagittal section through the nose, mouth, pharynx, and larynx to show the subdivisions of the pharynx.

Nasopharynx (Nasal Pharynx)

This lies above the soft palate and behind the nasal cavities. A collection of lymphoid tissue, the **pharyngeal tonsil**, sits in the submucosa of the roof (Fig. 9.112). The **pharyngeal isthmus** is the opening in the floor between the soft palate and the posterior pharyngeal wall. The opening of the auditory tube is on the lateral wall. The elevated ridge that caps the opening is the **tubal elevation** (**torus tubarius**). The **pharyngeal recess** is a depression in the pharyngeal wall behind the tubal elevation. The **salpingopharyngeal fold** is a vertical fold of mucous membrane covering the **salpingopharyngeus muscle**. This extends downward from the tubal elevation, behind the auditory tube.

Oropharynx (Oral Pharynx)

This lies behind the oral cavity. The floor is the posterior one third of the tongue and the interval between the tongue and epiglottis. The **median glossoepiglottic fold** is in the midline (Fig. 9.113; see also Fig. 9.101), and the **lateral glossoepiglottic fold** is to the side. The depression on each side of the median glossoepiglottic fold is the **vallecula**.

The **palatoglossal** and **palatopharyngeal arches** or folds are on the lateral wall (see Fig. 9.112). The

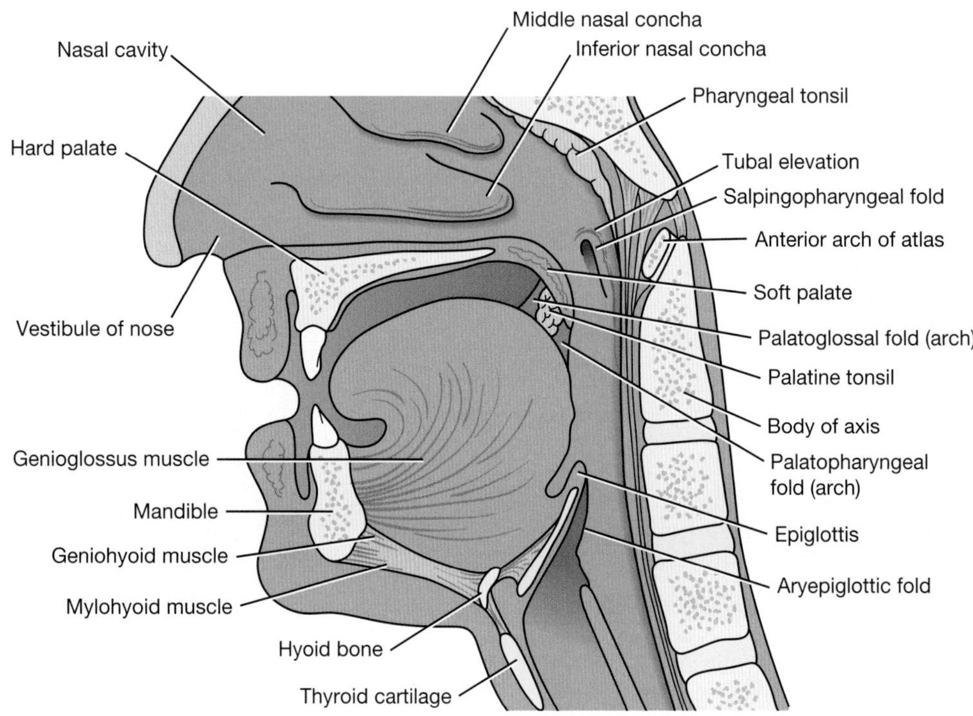

Figure 9.112 Sagittal section of the head and neck, showing the relations of the nasal cavity, mouth, pharynx, and larynx.

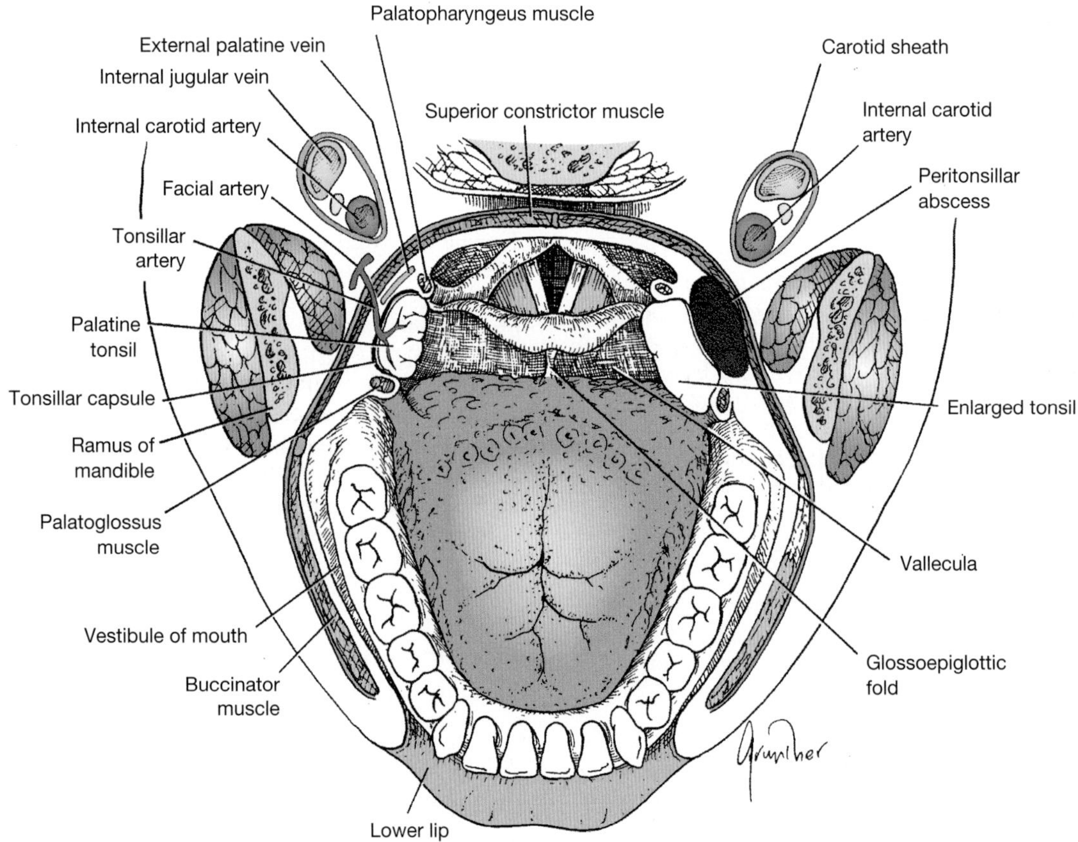

Figure 9.113 Horizontal section through the mouth and the oropharynx. **Left.** Normal palatine tonsil and its relationships. **Right.** Position of a peritonsillar abscess. Note the relationship of the abscess to the superior constrictor muscle and the carotid sheath. The opening into the larynx can also be seen below and behind the tongue.

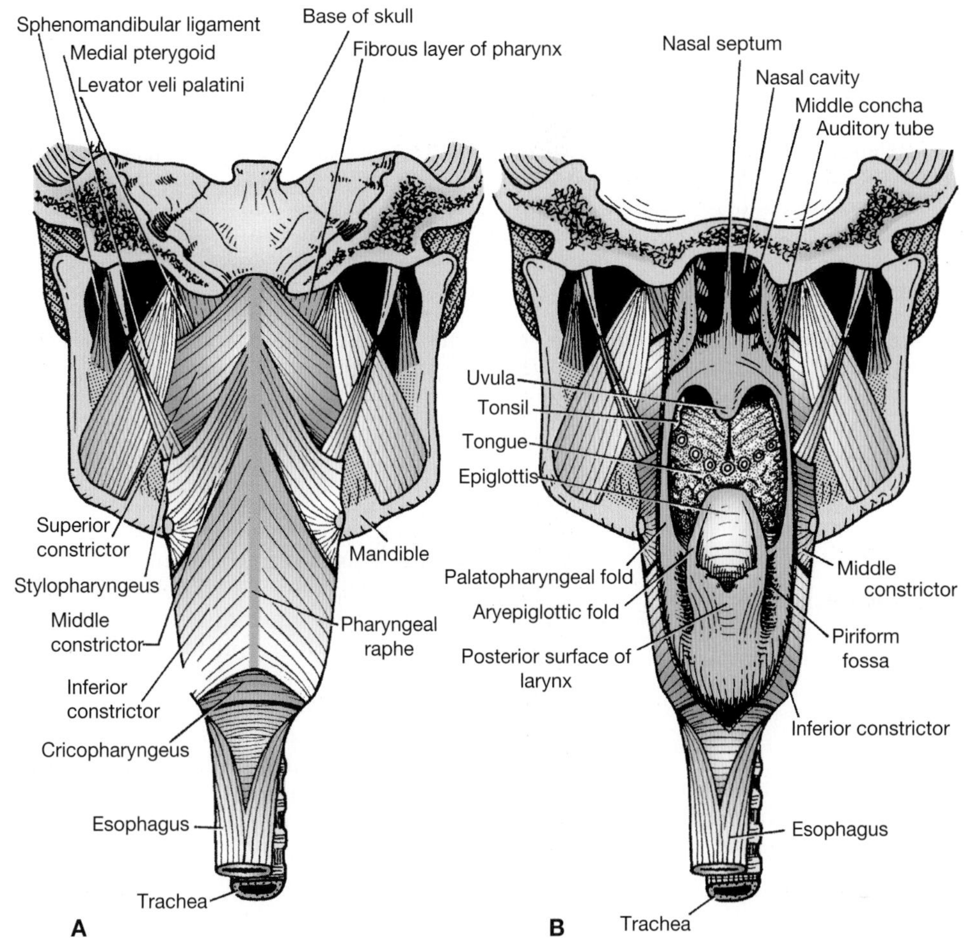

Figure 9.114 Pharynx seen from behind. **A.** Note the three constrictor muscles and the position of the stylopharyngeus muscles. **B.** The greater part of the posterior wall of the pharynx has been removed to display the nasal, oral, and laryngeal parts of the pharynx.

palatoglossal arch is a fold of mucous membrane covering the **palatoglossus muscle**. The interval between the paired palatoglossal arches is called the **oropharyngeal isthmus** and marks the boundary between the mouth and pharynx. The palatopharyngeal arch is a fold of mucous membrane covering the **palatopharyngeus muscle**. The **palatine tonsil** occupies the recess between the palatoglossal and palatopharyngeal arches.

Laryngopharynx (Laryngeal Pharynx)

This lies behind the opening into the larynx. The thyroid cartilage and the thyrohyoid membrane form the lateral wall. The **piriform fossa** is a depression in the mucous membrane on each side of the laryngeal inlet (see Fig. 9.114B). Its medial boundary is the aryepiglottic fold, and its lateral boundary is the thyroid cartilage.

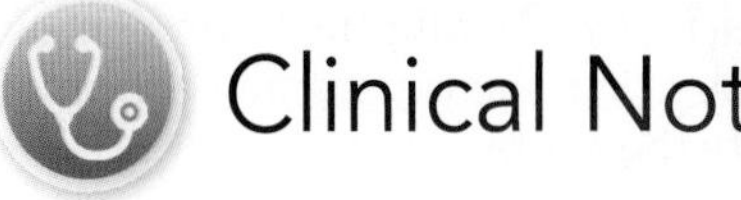

Clinical Notes

Piriform Fossa and Foreign Bodies

The piriform fossa is a recess of mucous membrane situated on either side of the entrance of the larynx. Clinically, it is important because it is a common site for the lodging of sharp ingested bodies such as fish bones. The presence of such a foreign body immediately causes the patient to gag violently. Once the object has become jammed, it is difficult for the patient to remove it without a clinician's assistance.

Pharyngeal Pouch

Examination of the lower part of the posterior surface of the inferior constrictor muscle reveals a potential gap between the upper oblique and the lower horizontal fibers (**cricopharyngeus**). A dimple marks this area in the lining mucous membrane. It is believed that the function of the cricopharyngeus is to prevent air entering into the esophagus. Should the cricopharyngeus fail to relax during

(continued)

swallowing, the internal pharyngeal pressure may rise and force the mucosa and submucosa of the dimple posteriorly, to produce a diverticulum. Once the diverticulum has been formed, it may gradually enlarge and fill with food with each meal. Unable to expand posteriorly because of the vertebral column, it turns downward, usually on the left side. The presence of the pouch filled with food causes difficulty in swallowing (**dysphagia**).

Cervical Tuberculous Osteomyelitis

Pus arising from tuberculosis of the upper cervical vertebrae is limited in front by the prevertebral layer of deep fascia. A midline swelling is formed and bulges forward in the posterior wall of the pharynx. The pus then tracks laterally and downward behind the carotid sheath to reach the posterior triangle. Here, the fascia, which forms a covering to the muscular floor of the triangle, is weaker, and the abscess points behind the sternocleidomastoid. Rarely, the abscess may track downward behind the prevertebral fascia to reach the superior and posterior mediastina in the thorax.

It is important to distinguish this condition from an abscess involving the retropharyngeal lymph nodes. These nodes lie in front of the prevertebral layer of fascia but behind the fascia that covers the outer surface of the constrictor muscles. Such an abscess usually points on the posterior pharyngeal wall and, if untreated, ruptures into the pharyngeal cavity.

Pharyngeal Mucous Membrane Sensory Nerve Supply

- **Nasopharynx:** Maxillary nerve (CN V2)
- **Oropharynx:** Glossopharyngeal nerve (CN IX)
- **Laryngopharynx** (around the entrance into the larynx): Internal laryngeal branch of the vagus nerve (CN X)

Pharyngeal Blood Supply

Ascending pharyngeal artery, tonsillar branches of facial arteries, and branches of the maxillary and lingual arteries supply blood to the pharynx.

Pharyngeal Muscles

The muscles in the wall of the pharynx are the **superior**, **middle**, and **inferior constrictor muscles**, whose fibers run in a somewhat circular direction, and the **stylopharyngeus** and **salpingopharyngeus** muscles, whose fibers run in a somewhat longitudinal direction (see Figs. 9.104A and 9.114).

The three constrictor muscles extend around the pharyngeal wall and insert into a posterior midline fibrous band (**pharyngeal raphe**) that extends from the pharyngeal tubercle on the basilar part of the occipital bone of the skull down to the esophagus (see Fig. 9.114). The three constrictor muscles overlap each other so that the middle constrictor lies on the outside of the lower part of the superior constrictor and the inferior constrictor lies outside the lower part of the middle constrictor.

The lower part of the inferior constrictor, which arises from the cricoid cartilage, is called the **cricopharyngeus muscle**. The fibers of the cricopharyngeus pass horizontally around the lowest and narrowest part of the pharynx and act as a sphincter. The **Killian dehiscence** is the area on the posterior pharyngeal wall between the upper propulsive part of the inferior constrictor and the lower sphincteric part, the cricopharyngeus.

The pharyngeal muscles are summarized in Table 9.12.

Process of Swallowing (Deglutition)

Masticated food is formed into a ball or bolus on the dorsum of the tongue and voluntarily pushed upward and backward against the undersurface of the hard palate. This is brought about by the contraction of the styloglossus muscles on both sides, which pull the root of the tongue upward and backward. The palatoglossus muscles then squeeze the bolus backward into the pharynx. From this point onward, the process of swallowing becomes an involuntary act.

The nasal part of the pharynx is now shut off from the oral part of the pharynx by the elevation of the soft palate, the pulling forward of the posterior wall of the pharynx by the upper fibers of the superior constrictor muscle, and the contraction of the palatopharyngeus muscles. This prevents the passage of food and drink into the nasal cavities.

The larynx and the laryngeal part of the pharynx are pulled upward by the contraction of the stylopharyngeus, salpingopharyngeus, thyrohyoid, and palatopharyngeus muscles. The main part of the larynx is thus elevated to the posterior surface of the epiglottis, and the entrance into the larynx is closed. The laryngeal entrance is made smaller by the approximation of the aryepiglottic folds, and the arytenoid cartilages are pulled forward by the contraction of the aryepiglottic, oblique arytenoid, and thyroarytenoid muscles.

The bolus moves downward over the epiglottis, the closed entrance into the larynx, and reaches the lower part of the pharynx as the result of the successive contraction of the superior, middle, and inferior constrictor muscles. Some of the food slides down the groove on either side of the entrance into the larynx, that is, down through the piriform fossae. Finally, the lower part of the pharyngeal wall (the cricopharyngeus muscle) relaxes, and the bolus enters the esophagus.

Crossing of Food and Air Pathways in the Pharynx

The food (digestive system) and air (respiratory system) pathways cross in the pharynx. This is possible because of the soft palate, which serves as a flap valve. This flap shuts off the mouth from the oropharynx during the process of chewing food so that breathing may continue unaffected. The completely raised soft palate shuts off the nasopharynx from the oropharynx, thus preventing food entering the nasopharynx in swallowing (see

Table 9.12 Pharynx Muscles

MUSCLE	ORIGIN	INSERTION	NERVE SUPPLY	ACTION
Superior constrictor	Medial pterygoid plate, pterygoid hamulus, pterygomandibular ligament, mylohyoid line of the mandible	Pharyngeal tubercle of the occipital bone, raphe in midline posteriorly	Pharyngeal plexus (vagus nerve)	Aids soft palate in closing off nasal pharynx, propels bolus downward
Middle constrictor	Lower part of stylohyoid ligament, lesser and greater cornu of hyoid bone	Pharyngeal raphe	Pharyngeal plexus (vagus nerve)	Propels bolus downward
Inferior constrictor	Lamina of thyroid cartilage, cricoid cartilage	Pharyngeal raphe	Pharyngeal plexus (vagus nerve)	Propels bolus downward
Cricopharyngeus	Lowest fibers of inferior constrictor muscle			Sphincter at lower end of the pharynx
Stylopharyngeus	Styloid process of the temporal bone	Posterior border of the thyroid cartilage	Glossopharyngeal nerve	Elevates the larynx during swallowing
Salpingopharyngeus	Auditory tube	Blends with palatopharyngeus	Pharyngeal plexus (vagus nerve)	Elevates pharynx
Palatopharyngeus	Palatine aponeurosis	Posterior border of the thyroid cartilage	Pharyngeal plexus (vagus nerve)	Elevates wall of the pharynx, pulls palatopharyngeal arch medially

above). When it is desirable to direct the maximum amount of air in and out of the larynx, the soft palate is raised to direct air through the mouth rather than the narrow cavities of the nose. This arrangement permits the expectoration of mucus from the respiratory system through the mouth. It also allows the maximum expiration of air through the mouth, as in playing wind instruments such as the trumpet.

Pharyngeal Lymph Drainage

Lymph drains directly into the deep cervical lymph nodes or indirectly via the retropharyngeal or paratracheal nodes into the deep cervical nodes.

Tonsils

Collections of lymphoid tissue (**tonsils**) of considerable clinical importance are located at the junction of the mouth with the oral part of the pharynx (**palatine** and **lingual tonsils**) and the nose with the nasal part of the pharynx (**pharyngeal tonsil**). The palatine tonsils and the pharyngeal tonsils are the most important.

Palatine Tonsils

The palatine tonsils are two masses of lymphoid tissue, each located in the depression (tonsillar fossa) on the lateral wall of the oropharynx between the palatoglossal and palatopharyngeal arches (see Figs. 9.101 and 9.113). Each tonsil is covered by mucous membrane, and its free medial surface projects into the pharynx. The surface is pitted by numerous small openings that lead into the **tonsillar crypts**.

The tonsil is covered on its lateral surface by a fibrous **tonsillar capsule**. The capsule is separated from the superior constrictor muscle by loose areolar tissue, and the external palatine vein descends from the soft palate in this tissue to join the pharyngeal venous plexus. Lateral to the superior constrictor muscle lie the styloglossus muscle, the loop of the facial artery, and the internal carotid artery.

The tonsil reaches its maximum size during early childhood, but after puberty, it diminishes considerably in size.

BLOOD SUPPLY

Blood supply is from the tonsillar branch of the facial artery. The veins pierce the superior constrictor muscle and join the external palatine, pharyngeal, or facial veins.

TONSIL LYMPH DRAINAGE

The upper deep cervical lymph nodes, just below and behind the angle of the mandible, provide drainage.

Pharyngeal Lymphatic Ring (Waldeyer Throat Ring) of Lymphoid Tissue

The lymphoid tissue that surrounds the opening into the respiratory and digestive systems forms a ring. The palatine tonsils and tubal tonsils (lymphoid tissue around the opening of the auditory tube) form the lateral part of the ring. The pharyngeal tonsil in the roof of the nasopharynx forms the upper part, and the lingual tonsil on the posterior third of the tongue forms the lower part.

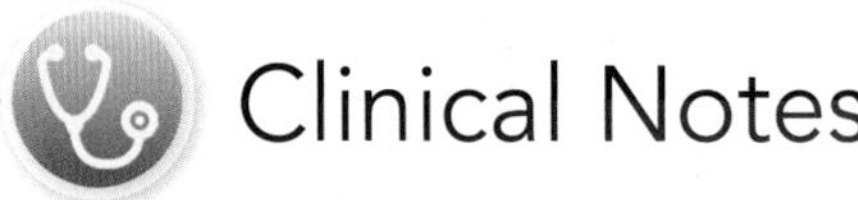

Clinical Notes

Tonsils and Tonsillitis

The palatine tonsils reach their maximum normal size in early childhood. After puberty, together with other lymphoid tissues in the body, they gradually atrophy. The palatine tonsils are a common site of infection, producing the characteristic sore throat and pyrexia. The deep cervical lymph node situated below and behind the angle of the mandible, which drains lymph from this organ, is usually enlarged and tender. Recurrent attacks of tonsillitis are best treated by tonsillectomy. After tonsillectomy, the external palatine vein, which lies lateral to the tonsil, may be the source of troublesome postoperative bleeding.

The pharyngeal tonsil consists of a collection of lymphoid tissue beneath the epithelium of the roof of the nasal part of the pharynx. Like the palatine tonsil, it is largest in early childhood and starts to atrophy after puberty.

Quinsy

A **peritonsillar abscess** (quinsy) is caused by spread of infection from the palatine tonsil to the loose connective tissue outside the capsule (see Fig. 9.113).

Adenoids

Excessive hypertrophy of the lymphoid tissue, usually associated with infection, causes the pharyngeal tonsils to become enlarged; they are then commonly referred to as **adenoids**. Marked hypertrophy blocks the posterior nasal openings and causes the patient to snore loudly at night and to breathe through the open mouth. The close relationship of the infected lymphoid tissue to the auditory tube may be the cause of deafness and recurrent otitis media. Adenoidectomy is the treatment of choice for hypertrophied adenoids with infection.

The nasopharynx, including the pharyngeal tonsil, may be viewed clinically by a mirror passed through the mouth (Fig. 9.115).

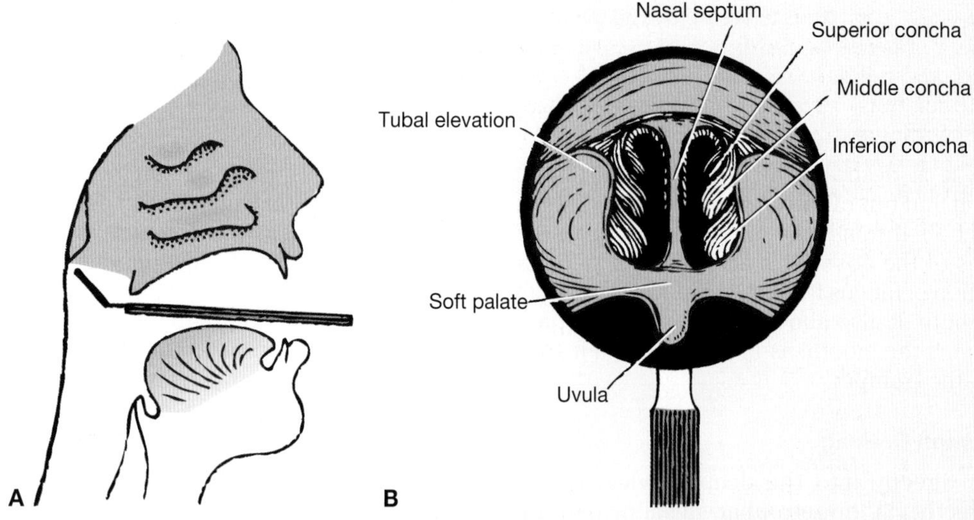

Figure 9.115 **A.** Sagittal section through the nose, mouth, larynx, and pharynx showing the position of the mirror in posterior rhinoscopy. **B.** Structures seen in posterior rhinoscopy.

Esophagus

The esophagus is a muscular tube about 10 in. (25 cm) long, extending from the pharynx to the stomach (see Figs. 9.33 and 9.114). It begins at the level of the cricoid cartilage, opposite the body of the C6 vertebra. It commences in the midline, but as it descends through the neck, it inclines to the left side. Its further course in the thorax is described in Chapter 4.

Relations in the Neck

- **Anteriorly:** Trachea; the recurrent laryngeal nerves ascend one on each side, in the groove between the trachea and the esophagus (see Fig. 9.65).
- **Posteriorly:** Prevertebral layer of deep cervical fascia, longus colli, and the vertebral column.
- **Laterally:** On each side lie the lobe of the thyroid gland and the carotid sheath.

Blood Supply in the Neck

The inferior thyroid arteries supply the esophagus in the neck. The veins drain into the inferior thyroid veins.

Lymph Drainage in the Neck

The lymph vessels drain into the deep cervical lymph nodes.

Nerve Supply in the Neck

The recurrent laryngeal nerves and the sympathetic trunks supply the esophagus in the neck.

RESPIRATORY SYSTEM

Four major components of the respiratory system cross the head and neck: (1) **nose**, (2) **paranasal sinuses**, (3) **larynx**, and (4) **trachea**.

Nose

The nose consists of the **external nose** and the **nasal cavity**. The **nasal septum** divides both of these into right and left halves.

External Nose

The external nose attaches to the forehead by the **root (bridge)** of the nose. It has two elliptical, external orifices called the **nostrils (nares)**, which are separated from each other by the **nasal septum** (Fig. 9.116). The lateral margin, the **ala nasi**, is rounded and mobile.

Several bones and cartilages make up the skeleton of the external nose. The **nasal** bones, **frontal processes of the maxillae**, and the **nasal part of the frontal** bone are the peripheral bony elements. Below the bones, multiple **nasal cartilages** complete the framework. The nasal cartilages are plates of hyaline cartilage that make up the majority of the external nose. The nasal septum contributes to both the external nose and nasal cavity; it consists of bony and cartilage parts.

The **nasalis (compressor naris)**, **dilator naris**, and **levator labii superioris alaeque nasi** are the primary muscles of the external nose. All are facial muscles innervated by the facial nerve (CN VII).

External Nose Blood Supply

Branches of the **ophthalmic** and **maxillary arteries** supply the skin of the external nose. Branches from the **facial artery** supply the skin of the ala and the lower part of the septum.

External Nose Sensory Innervation

The **infratrochlear** and **external nasal** branches of the ophthalmic nerve (CN V1) innervate the bridge and crest of the nose. The **infraorbital branch** of the maxillary nerve (CN V2) supplies the side of the nose.

Nasal Cavity

The nasal cavity extends from the **nostrils** in front to the **posterior nasal apertures (choanae)** behind, where the nose opens into the nasopharynx. The nasal **vestibule** is the area of the nasal cavity lying just inside the nostril (Fig. 9.117). The **atrium** is the entrance to the middle meatus and sits just superior to the vestibule. The nasal septum divides the cavity into right and left halves.

Nasal Cavity Walls

Each half of the nasal cavity has a roof, floor, lateral wall, and medial wall.

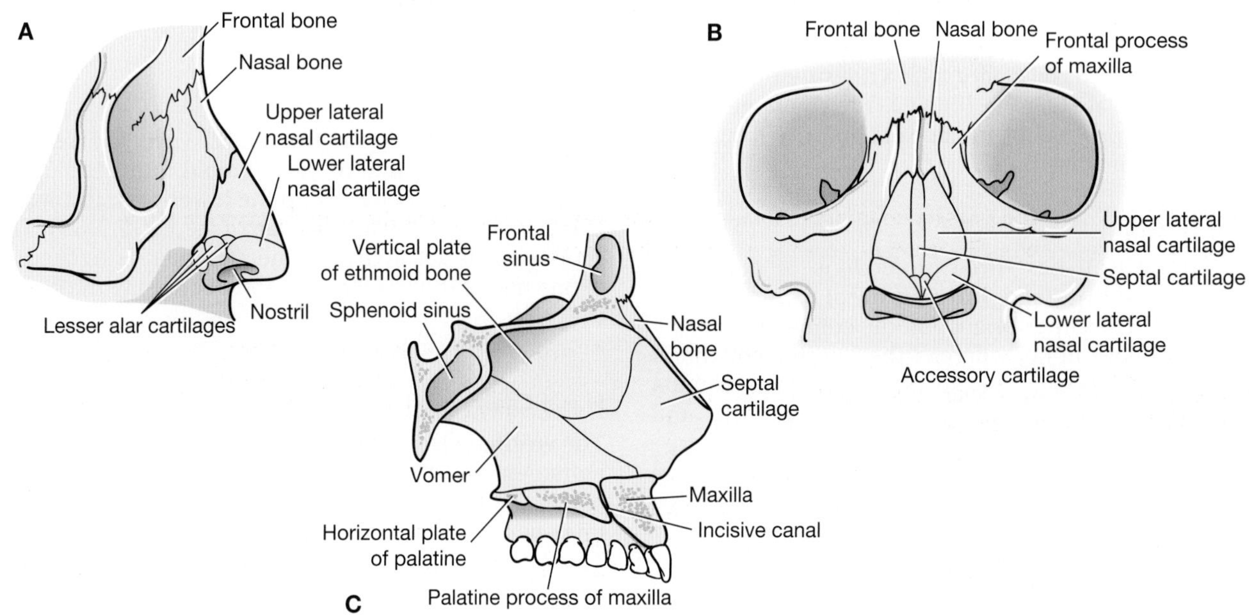

Figure 9.116 External nose and nasal septum. **A.** Lateral view of bony and cartilaginous skeleton of external nose. **B.** Anterior view of bony and cartilaginous skeleton of the external nose. **C.** Bony and cartilaginous skeleton of the nasal septum.

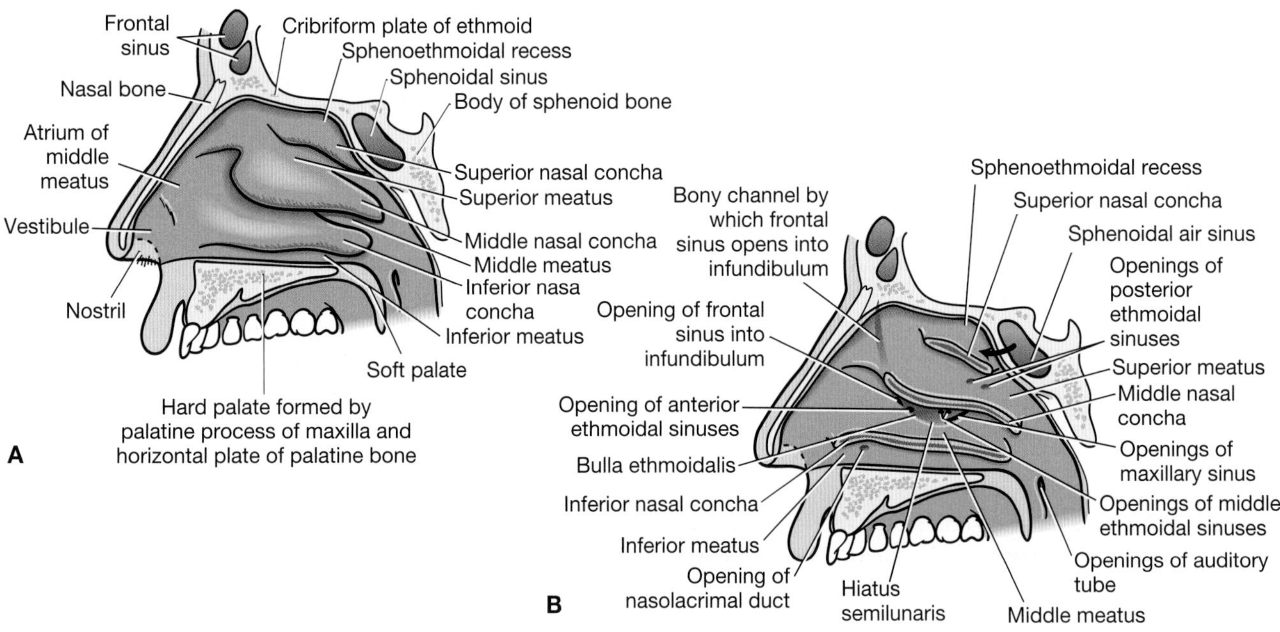

Figure 9.117 **A.** Lateral wall of the right nasal cavity. **B.** Lateral wall of the right nasal cavity; the superior, middle, and inferior conchae have been partially removed to show openings of the paranasal sinuses and the nasolacrimal duct into the meatuses.

Roof (Apex)

The roof is narrow and is formed anteriorly by the nasal and frontal bones (beneath the bridge of the nose), in the middle by the cribriform plate of the ethmoid (located beneath the anterior cranial fossa), and posteriorly by the downward sloping body of the sphenoid.

Floor (Base)

The floor of the nasal cavity is also the superior surface of the hard palate (see Fig. 9.116C). The components are the palatine process of the maxilla and the horizontal plate of the palatine bone.

Lateral Wall

The lateral wall has three projections of bone: the **superior**, **middle**, and **inferior nasal conchae** (see Fig. 9.117). The superior and middle conchae are parts of the ethmoid bone, whereas the inferior concha is an individual bone. The space below each concha is a **meatus**, and so there are **superior**, **middle**, and **inferior meatuses**.

The **sphenoethmoidal recess** is a small area above the superior concha. It receives the opening of the **sphenoid air sinus**.

The **superior meatus** lies below the superior concha. It receives the openings of the **posterior ethmoid sinuses**.

The **middle meatus** lies below the middle concha. It has a rounded swelling called the **bulla ethmoidalis** that is formed by the **middle ethmoidal air sinuses**, which open on its upper border. A curved opening, the **hiatus semilunaris**, lies just below the bulla. The anterior end of the hiatus leads into a funnel-shaped channel called the **infundibulum**, which is continuous with the **frontal sinus**. The maxillary sinus opens into the middle meatus through the hiatus semilunaris.

The **inferior meatus** lies below the inferior concha and receives the opening of the lower end of the **nasolacrimal duct**, which is guarded by a fold of mucous membrane.

Medial Wall

The nasal septum forms the medial wall. The **vertical (perpendicular) plate of the ethmoid** forms the upper portion; the **vomer** makes up the lower part; the **septal cartilage** forms the anterior part (see Fig. 9.116C). The septum rarely lies in the midline, thus increasing the size of one half of the nasal cavity and decreasing the size of the other.

Nasal Cavity Mucous Membrane

The **vestibule** is lined with modified skin and has coarse hairs. A small **olfactory region** above the superior concha is lined with olfactory mucous membrane and contains nerve endings sensitive to the reception of smell. The olfactory area is approximately dime to quarter sized. It includes the roof of the nasal cavity, sphenoethmoidal recess, superior surface of the superior concha, and the superior edge of the nasal septum. The remainder of the nasal cavity (except for the vestibule) is the **respiratory region**; it is lined with a respiratory mucous membrane.

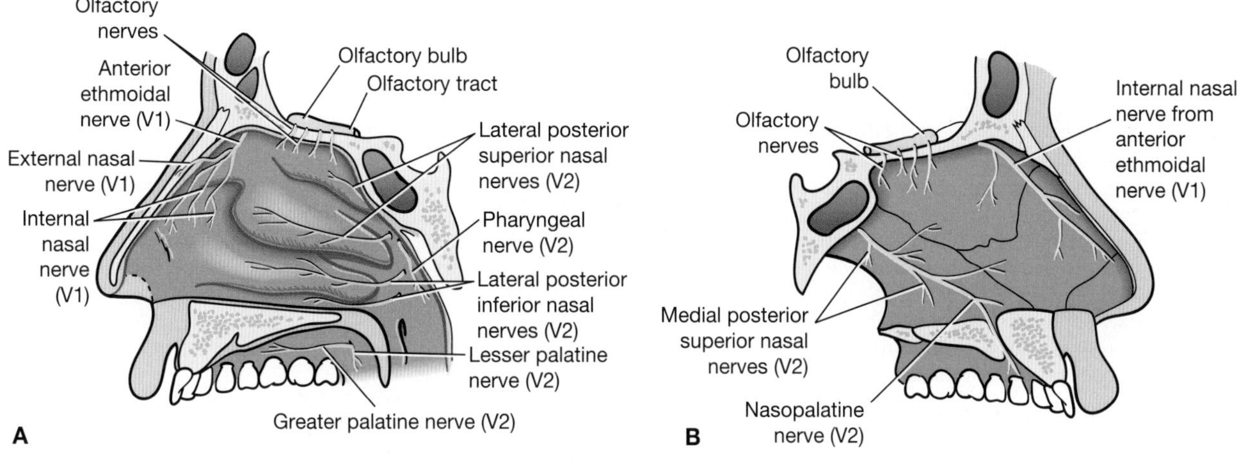

Figure 9.118 **A.** Lateral wall of the nasal cavity showing sensory innervation of the mucous membrane. **B.** The nasal septum showing sensory innervation of mucous membrane.

A large plexus of veins occupies the submucous connective tissue in the respiratory region. The presence of warm blood in the venous plexuses serves to warm the inspired air as it enters the respiratory system. The presence of mucus on the surfaces of the conchae moistens the area and traps foreign particles and organisms in the inspired air, which are then swallowed and destroyed by gastric acid.

Nasal Cavity Nerve Supply

The **olfactory nerves** from the olfactory mucous membrane ascend through the cribriform plate of the ethmoid bone to the olfactory bulbs (Fig. 9.118). The nerves of **general sensation** are branches of the **ophthalmic division (V1)** and the **maxillary division (V2)** of the trigeminal nerve.

Nasal Cavity Blood Supply

The arterial supply to the nasal cavity is from branches of the **maxillary artery**, one of the terminal branches of the external carotid artery (Fig. 9.119). The most important branch is the **sphenopalatine artery**. The sphenopalatine artery anastomoses with the **septal branch of the superior labial branch of the facial artery** in the region of the vestibule. The submucous venous plexus drains into veins that accompany the arteries.

Nasal Cavity Lymph Drainage

The lymph vessels draining the vestibule end in the **submandibular nodes**. The remainder of the nasal cavity drains by vessels that pass to the **upper deep cervical nodes**.

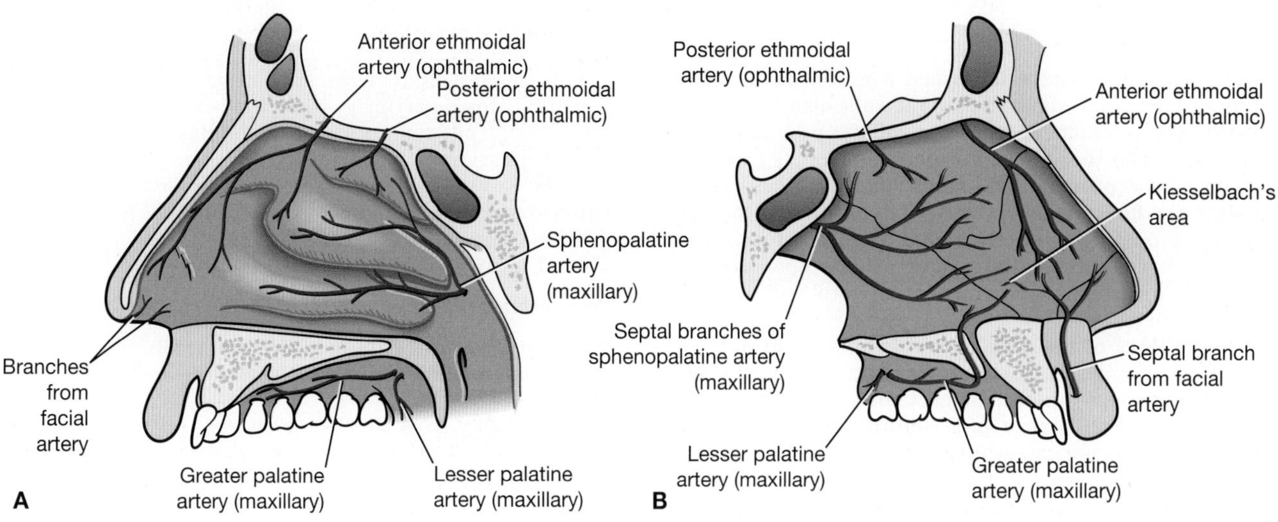

Figure 9.119 **A.** Lateral wall of the nasal cavity showing the arterial supply of the mucous membrane. **B.** The nasal septum showing the arterial supply of the mucous membrane.

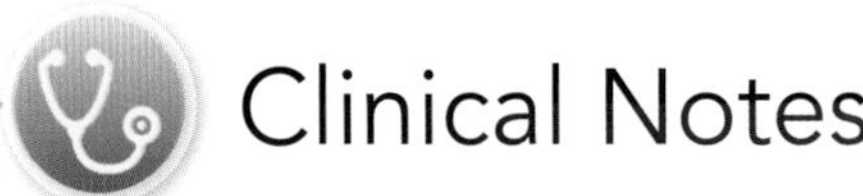

Clinical Notes

Nasal Cavity Examination

Examination of the nasal cavity may be carried out by inserting a speculum through the external nares or by means of a mirror in the pharynx. In the latter case, the choanae and the posterior border of the nasal septum can be visualized (see Fig. 9.115).

The nasal septum is rarely situated directly in the midline. A severely **deviated septum** may interfere with drainage of the nose and the paranasal sinuses.

Nose Trauma

Fractures involving the nasal bones are common. Blows directed from the front may cause one or both nasal bones to be displaced downward and inward. Lateral fractures also occur in which one nasal bone is driven inward and the other outward; the nasal septum is usually involved.

Nasal Cavity Infection

Infection of the nasal cavity can spread in a variety of directions. The paranasal sinuses are especially prone to infection. Organisms may spread via the nasopharynx and the auditory tube to the middle ear. It is possible for organisms to ascend to the meninges of the anterior cranial fossa along the sheaths of the olfactory nerves through the cribriform plate and produce meningitis.

Foreign Bodies in the Nose

Foreign bodies in the nose are common in children. The presence of the nasal septum and the existence of the folded, shelflike conchae make impaction and retention of items such as balloons, peas, and small toys relatively easy.

Nose Bleeding

Epistaxis (chronic profuse bleeding from the nose) is a frequent condition. Common causes include nose picking and degeneration of the nasal septum resulting from chronic use of cocaine. The bleeding may be arterial or venous. Most episodes occur on the anteroinferior portion of the septum and involve the septal branches of the sphenopalatine and facial vessels.

Transnasal Surgery

A convenient surgical path to the pituitary gland is a transnasal approach (see Fig. 9.117). Instruments run across the nasal cavity to its posterior roof at the body of the sphenoid. The surgeon pierces the sphenoid, traverses the sphenoid air sinus, and enters the sella turcica from below.

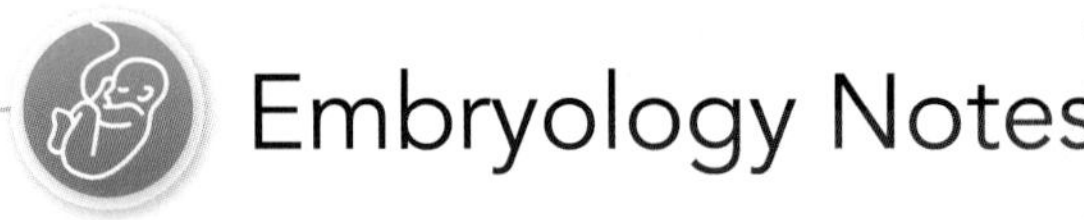

Embryology Notes

Nose Development

The **roof of the nose** is formed from the lateral nasal processes, from which the lateral walls also are formed, with the assistance of the maxillary processes (see Fig. 9.27). The **nose** begins as paired olfactory pits in the frontonasal process. The medial nasal process (medially), the lateral nasal process (laterally), and the maxillary process (inferiorly) bound each olfactory pit. As these processes fuse, the olfactory pits deepen and form well-defined blind sacs, the opening into each of which is the nostril.

The **floor of the nose** at first is very short and consists of the medial nasal process and the anterior part of the maxillary process on each side. At this stage, the floors of the olfactory pits rupture so that the nasal cavities communicate with the developing mouth (see Fig. 9.106). Meanwhile, the nasal septum is forming as a downgrowth from the medial nasal process. Later, the palatal processes of the maxilla grow medially and fuse with each other and with the nasal septum, thus completing the floor of the nose. Each nasal cavity therefore communicates anteriorly with the exterior through the nostril and posteriorly through the choana with the nasopharynx.

In the early stages of development, the nose is a much flattened structure and gains its recognizable form only after facial development is complete.

Median Nasal Furrow

In median nasal furrow, the nasal septum is split, separating the two halves of the nose (Fig. 9.120A).

Lateral Proboscis

In lateral proboscis, a skin-covered process develops, usually with a dimple at its lower end (see Fig. 9.120B).

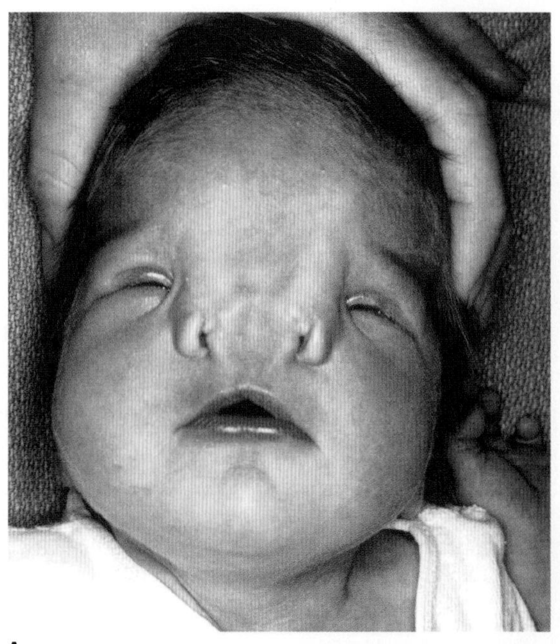

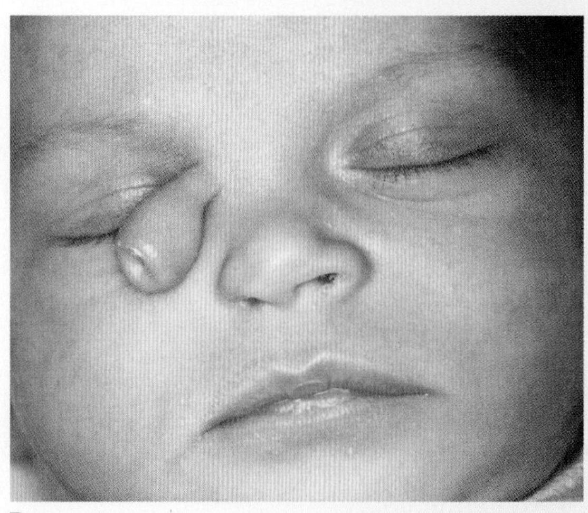

Figure 9.120 **A.** Median nasal furrow in which the nasal septum has completely split, separating the two halves of the nose. Note that a wide furrow separates the external nares. (Courtesy of L. Thompson.) **B.** Lateral proboscis. (Courtesy of R. Chase.)

Paranasal Sinuses

The paranasal sinuses are cavities in the interior of the **maxillary**, **frontal**, **sphenoid**, and **ethmoid bones** (Fig. 9.121). They are lined with mucoperiosteum and filled with air; they communicate with the nasal cavity through relatively small apertures. The sinuses and their openings into the nasal cavity are summarized in Table 9.13.

The paranasal sinuses function to decrease the weight of the skull (by approximately a 7% to 20% factor) and give resonance to the voice. The quality of the voice is markedly changed when the apertures of the sinuses are blocked, or they become filled with fluid.

The mucus produced by the mucous membrane is moved into the nose by ciliary action of the columnar cells. Drainage of the mucus is also achieved by the siphon action created during the blowing of the nose.

Rudiments of the sinuses may appear prenatally. However, most sinuses do not develop until postnatal life. The maxillary and sphenoid sinuses are present in a rudimentary form at birth; they enlarge appreciably after the eighth year and achieve full form in adolescence. Expansion of the paranasal sinuses is one of the factors responsible for the significant postnatal growth of the facial skeleton.

Maxillary Sinus

The maxillary sinus is pyramidal in shape and located within the body of the maxilla behind the skin of the cheek. The floor of the orbit forms the roof, and the floor is related to the roots of the premolars and molar teeth.

Frontal Sinuses

The frontal bone contains the two frontal sinuses. They are separated from each other by a bony septum. Each sinus is roughly triangular, extending upward above the medial end of the eyebrow and backward into the medial part of the roof of the orbit.

Sphenoid Sinuses

The two sphenoidal sinuses lie within the body of the sphenoid bone. A thin bony septum separates the sinuses.

Ethmoid Sinuses

The ethmoid bone houses three pairs of sinuses (**anterior**, **middle**, and **posterior**) between the nose and the orbit. They are separated from the orbit by an extremely thin plate of bone, and infection can readily spread from the sinuses into the orbit.

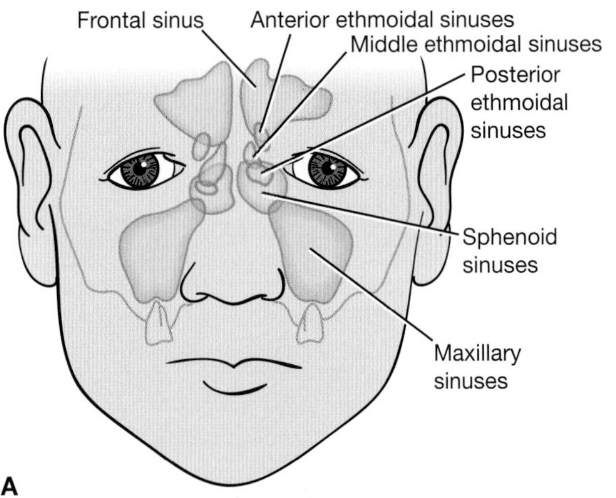

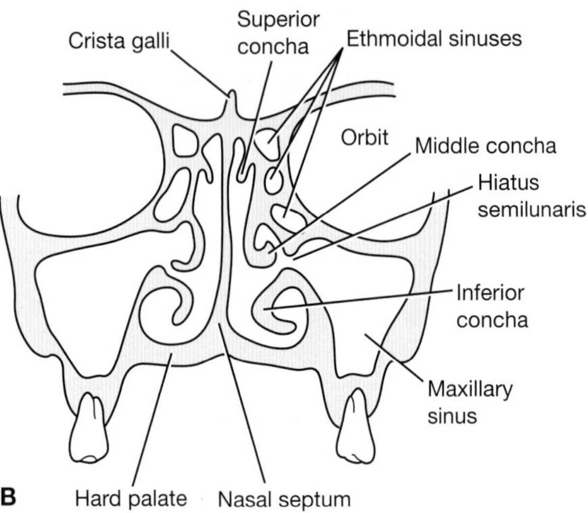

Figure 9.121 **A.** Anterior view showing the position of the paranasal sinuses in relation to the face. **B.** Coronal section through the nasal cavity showing the ethmoidal and maxillary sinuses.

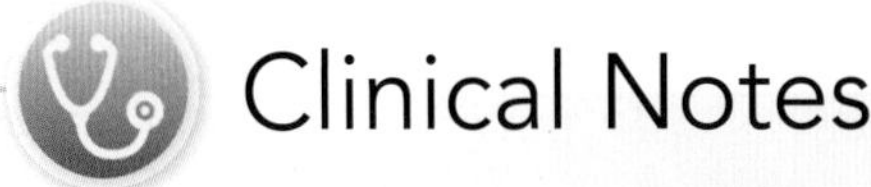

Sinusitis and Paranasal Sinus Examination

Infection of the paranasal sinuses is a common complication of nasal infections. Rarely, the cause of maxillary sinusitis is extension from an apical dental abscess. The frontal, ethmoidal, and maxillary sinuses can be palpated clinically for areas of tenderness. The **frontal sinus** can be examined by pressing the finger upward beneath the medial end of the superior orbital margin. Here, the floor of the frontal sinus is closest to the surface.

The **ethmoid sinuses** can be palpated by pressing the finger medially against the medial wall of the orbit. The **maxillary sinus** can be examined for tenderness by pressing the finger against the anterior wall of the maxilla below the inferior orbital margin; pressure over the infraorbital nerve may reveal increased sensitivity.

Directing the beam of a flashlight either through the roof of the mouth or through the cheek in a darkened room will often enable a clinician to determine whether the maxillary sinus is full of inflammatory fluid rather than air. This method of **transillumination** is simple and effective. Radiologic examination of the sinuses is also most helpful in making a diagnosis. Always compare the clinical findings of each sinus on the two sides of the body.

The supraorbital nerve innervates the frontal sinus and also supplies the skin of the forehead and scalp as far back as the vertex. Therefore, it is not surprising that patients with frontal sinusitis have pain referred over this area. The infraorbital nerve innervates the maxillary sinus, and in this case, pain is referred to the upper jaw, including the teeth.

The frontal sinus drains into the hiatus semilunaris, via the infundibulum, close to the orifice of the maxillary sinus on the lateral wall of the nose. It is thus not unexpected to find that a patient with frontal sinusitis nearly always has a maxillary sinusitis. The maxillary sinus is particularly prone to infection because its drainage orifice through the hiatus semilunaris is badly placed near the roof of the sinus. In other words, the sinus has to fill up with fluid before it can effectively drain with the person in the upright position.

Table 9.13 Paranasal Sinuses and Sites of Drainage into the Nose

SINUS	SITE OF DRAINAGE
Maxillary sinus	Middle meatus through hiatus semilunaris
Frontal sinuses	Middle meatus via infundibulum
Sphenoid sinuses	Sphenoethmoidal recess
Ethmoid sinuses	
Anterior group	Infundibulum and into the middle meatus
Middle group	Middle meatus on or above bulla ethmoidalis
Posterior group	Superior meatus

Larynx

The larynx provides a protective sphincter at the inlet of the air passages and is responsible for voice production. It is situated below the tongue and hyoid bone and between the great blood vessels of the neck and lies at the level of the C4 to C6 vertebrae (see Figs. 9.70 and 9.111). It opens above into the laryngopharynx and is continuous with the trachea below. The larynx is covered in front by the infrahyoid strap muscles and at the sides by the thyroid gland.

The framework of the larynx is formed of cartilages held together by ligaments and membranes, moved by muscles, and lined by mucous membrane.

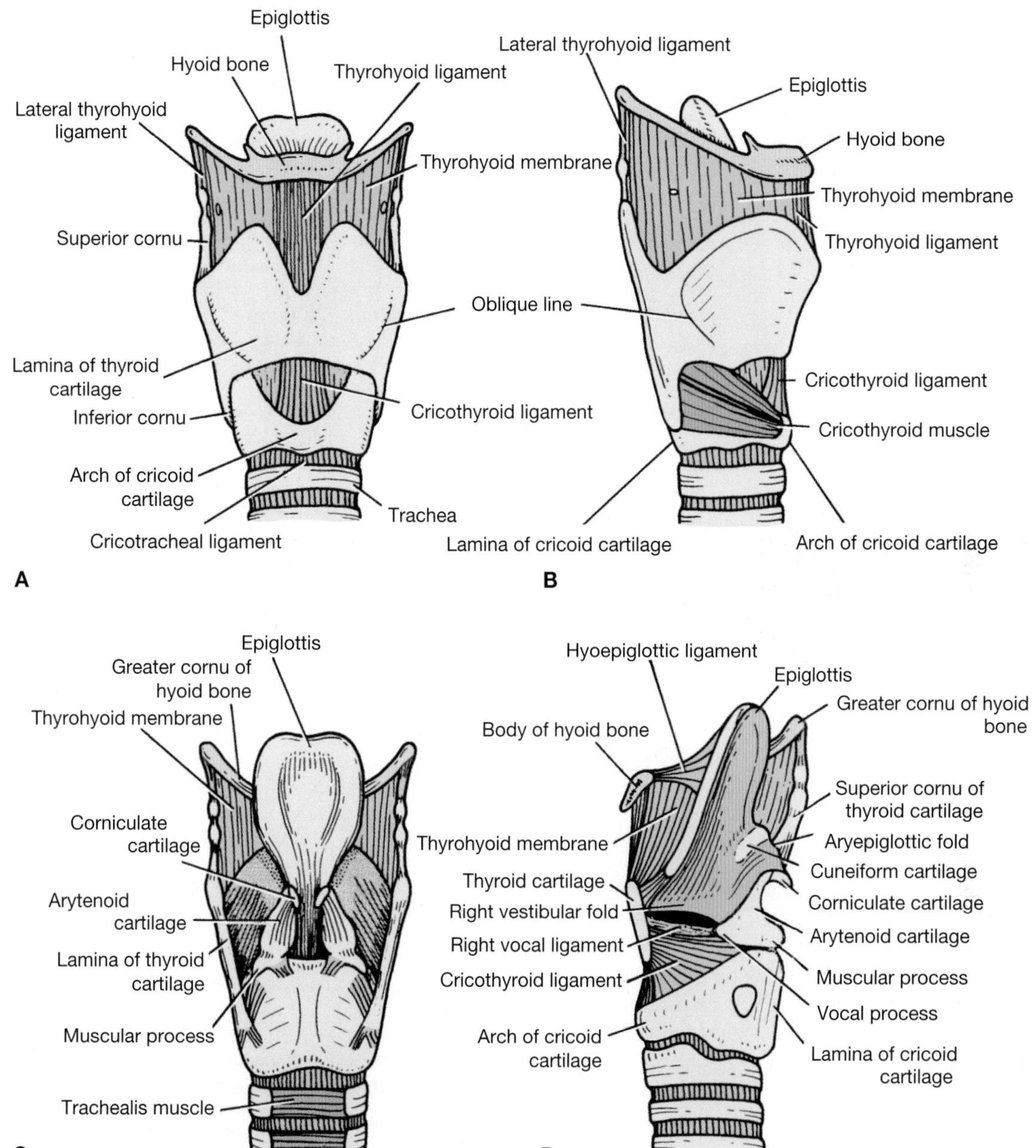

Figure 9.122 Larynx and its ligaments from the front **(A)**, from the lateral aspect **(B)**, and from behind **(C)**. **D.** Lateral view with the left lamina of the thyroid cartilage removed to display the interior of the larynx.

Laryngeal Cartilages

Nine hyaline cartilage elements make up the skeleton of the larynx (Fig. 9.122).

Thyroid cartilage: This is the largest cartilage of the larynx and consists of two **laminae** that meet in the midline in the deep-set **thyroid notch** (**V angle**). The distinct **laryngeal prominence** (**Adam's apple**) projects forward from the apex of the thyroid notch. The posterior border extends upward into a **superior cornu** and downward into an **inferior cornu**. An **oblique line** for the attachment of muscles is on the outer surface of each lamina.

Cricoid cartilage: This cartilage lies below the thyroid cartilage and is shaped like a signet ring, having a broad **lamina** behind and a shallow **arch** in front. It is the only completely circular element in the respiratory tract. The cricoid cartilage has an **articular facet** on each side of the lateral surface for articulation with the inferior cornu of the thyroid cartilage. Posteriorly, the lamina has an articular facet on its upper border on each side for articulation with the arytenoid cartilage.

Arytenoid cartilages: Paired, small, pyramid-shaped arytenoid cartilages located at the back of the larynx

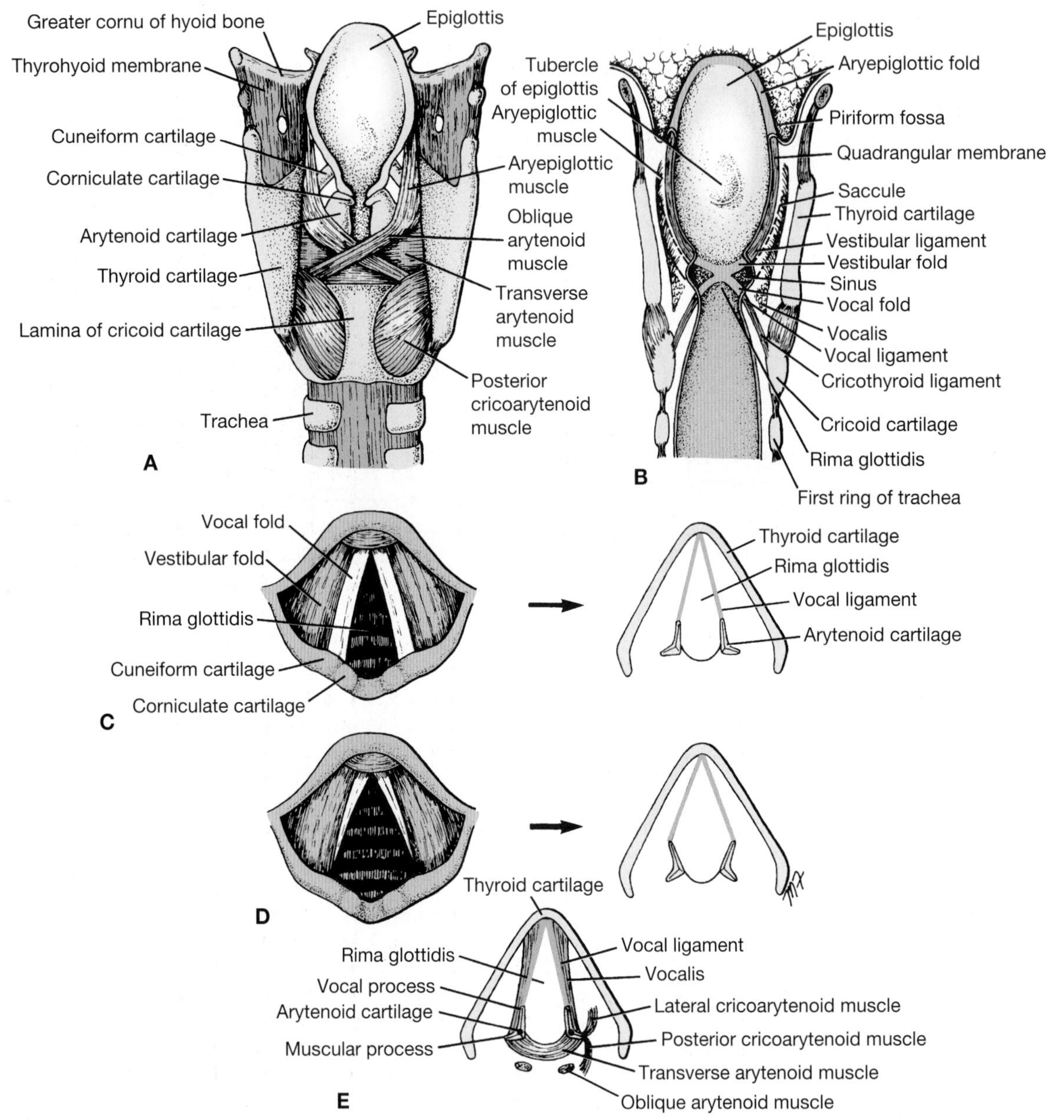

Figure 9.123 **A.** Muscles of the larynx seen from behind. **B.** Coronal section through the larynx. **C.** Rima glottidis partially open as in quiet breathing. **D.** Rima glottidis wide open as in deep breathing. **E.** Muscles that move the vocal ligaments.

articulate with the upper border of the lamina of the cricoid cartilage. Each cartilage has an **apex** above that articulates with the small corniculate cartilage, a **base** below that articulates with the lamina of the cricoid cartilage, and a **vocal process** that projects forward and gives attachment to the vocal ligament. A **muscular process** that projects laterally gives attachment to the posterior and lateral cricoarytenoid muscles.

Corniculate cartilages: Two small, conical-shaped corniculate cartilages articulate with the apices of the arytenoid cartilages. They give attachment to the **aryepiglottic folds** (Fig. 9.123; see also Figs. 9.114B and 9.122).

Cuneiform cartilages: These two small rod-shaped cartilages are in the aryepiglottic folds and serve to strengthen them.

Epiglottic cartilage: This leaf-shaped lamina of elastic cartilage lies behind the root of the tongue (see Figs. 9.122 and 9.123). Its stalk is attached to the inner surface of the thyroid cartilage. The sides of the epiglottis are attached to the arytenoid cartilages by the **aryepiglottic folds** of mucous membrane. The upper edge of the epiglottis is free. The covering of mucous membrane passes forward onto the posterior surface of the tongue as the **median glossoepiglottic fold**; the depression on each side of the fold is the **vallecula** (see Fig. 9.113).

Laterally, the mucous membrane passes onto the wall of the pharynx as the **lateral glossoepiglottic fold**.

Joints

Two pairs of synovial joints exist in the larynx (see Fig. 9.122). The **cricothyroid joint** is between the inferior cornu of the thyroid cartilage and the lateral side of the cricoid cartilage. The **cricoarytenoid joint** is between the base of the arytenoid cartilage and the superior border of the lamina of the cricoid cartilage.

Each joint allows multiaxial movements of rotation and gliding. These movements can occur simultaneously or independently.

Membranes and Ligaments

- **Thyrohyoid membrane:** This connects the upper margin of the thyroid cartilage to the hyoid bone (see Figs. 9.122 and 9.123). It is thickened in the anterior midline to form the **median thyrohyoid ligament**. The superior laryngeal vessels and the internal laryngeal nerve pierce the membrane on each side (see Fig. 9.104).
- **Thyroepiglottic ligament:** This connects the inferior end of the epiglottic cartilage to the posterior median aspect of the thyroid lamina.
- **Cricotracheal ligament:** This connects the cricoid cartilage to the first tracheal ring (see Fig. 9.122).
- **Quadrangular membrane:** This extends between the epiglottis and the arytenoid cartilages (see Fig. 9.123). Its thickened inferior margin forms the **vestibular ligament**, and the vestibular ligaments form the interior of the **vestibular folds**.
- **Cricothyroid ligament:** This interconnects the cricoid, thyroid, and arytenoid cartilages (see Fig. 9.122). The lower margin is attached to the upper border of the arch of the cricoid cartilage. The superior margin of the ligament, instead of being attached to the thyroid cartilage, ascends on the medial surface of the thyroid cartilage. Its upper free margin, composed almost entirely of elastic tissue, forms the important **vocal ligament** on each side. The vocal ligaments form the interior of the **vocal folds (vocal cords)**. The anterior end of each vocal ligament is attached to the inner surface of the lamina of the thyroid cartilage, and the posterior end is attached to the vocal process of the arytenoid cartilage.

Internal Features

The larynx possesses several distinctive features on its internal aspect.

Laryngeal Inlet

The inlet is the opening from the pharynx into the larynx and is formed by the **epiglottis** and the **aryepiglottic folds**. It looks backward and upward into the laryngopharynx (see Fig. 9.114B). The opening is wider in front than behind and is bounded in front by the epiglottis, laterally by the aryepiglottic fold of mucous membrane, and posteriorly by the arytenoid cartilages with the corniculate cartilages. The cuneiform cartilage lies within and strengthens the aryepiglottic fold and produces a small elevation on the upper border.

Piriform Fossa

The piriform fossa is a recess on either side of the inlet. The aryepiglottic fold is the medial boundary, and the thyroid cartilage plus the thyrohyoid membrane are the lateral boundaries.

Vestibular Fold (False Vocal Fold)

The vestibular fold is a **fixed fold** on each side of the larynx (see Figs. 9.122 and 9.123). It is formed by mucous membrane covering the vestibular ligament and is vascular and pink in color.

Vocal Fold (True Vocal Fold)

The vocal fold is a **mobile fold** on each side of the larynx and is concerned with voice production. It is formed by mucous membrane covering the **vocal ligament** and is avascular and white in color. The vocal fold moves with respiration, and its white color is easily seen when viewed with a laryngoscope.

The **rima glottidis** is the aperture between the vocal folds. The **glottis** is the rima plus the vocal folds. The glottis is the narrowest part of the larynx and measures about 2.5 cm from front to back in the male adult and less in the female. In children, the lower part of the larynx within the cricoid cartilage is the narrowest part.

Laryngeal Cavity

The cavity (lumen) of the larynx extends from the inlet to the lower border of the cricoid cartilage, where it is continuous with the cavity (lumen) of the trachea. It is divided into three regions:

- The **vestibule** (upper region) is the area between the inlet and the vestibular folds.
- The **middle region** is the central space (airway) situated between the opposite vestibular folds and vocal folds. The **ventricle** is a lateral recess between the vestibular fold above and the vocal fold below. The **saccule** is a mucous membrane-lined diverticulum that ascends from the ventricle (see Fig. 9.123). Mucous secretion lubricates the vocal fold.
- The **infraglottic cavity** (lower region) is the area between the vocal folds above and the lower border of the cricoid cartilage below.

Laryngeal Muscles

The muscles of the larynx are arranged in two groups: extrinsic and intrinsic. The extrinsic muscles have attachments outside the larynx itself, whereas the intrinsic muscles have both origin and insertion onto laryngeal elements.

Extrinsic Muscles

These muscles move the larynx up (elevation) and down (depression) during swallowing. Note that many are attached to the hyoid bone, which is attached to the thyroid cartilage via the thyrohyoid membrane. Thus, movements of the larynx accompany movements of the hyoid bone. The **suprahyoid muscles** elevate the larynx and the **infrahyoid muscles** depress the larynx.

Elevation: Digastric, stylohyoid, mylohyoid, geniohyoid, stylopharyngeus, salpingopharyngeus, and palatopharyngeus muscles

Depression: Sternothyroid, sternohyoid, and omohyoid muscles

Intrinsic Muscles

The intrinsic muscles of the larynx are summarized in Table 9.14.

Two muscles modify the laryngeal inlet (see Fig. 9.123):

- **Narrowing the inlet:** Oblique arytenoid muscle
- **Widening the inlet:** Thyroepiglottis muscle

Five muscles move the vocal folds (cords):

- **Tensing the vocal cords:** Cricothyroid and vocalis muscles
- **Relaxing the vocal cords:** Thyroarytenoid muscle
- **Adducting the vocal cords:** Lateral cricoarytenoid muscle
- **Abducting the vocal cords:** Posterior cricoarytenoid muscle
- **Approximates the arytenoid cartilages:** Transverse arytenoid muscle

Vocal Fold (Cord) Movement

The movements of the vocal folds depend on the movements of the arytenoid cartilages, which rotate and slide up and down on the sloping shoulder of the superior border of the cricoid cartilage.

The rima glottidis opens by the contraction of the posterior cricoarytenoid, which rotates the arytenoid cartilage and abducts the vocal process. The elastic tissue in the capsules of the cricoarytenoid joints keeps the arytenoid cartilages apart so that the posterior part of the glottis is open.

The rima glottidis closes by contraction of the lateral cricoarytenoid, which rotates the arytenoid cartilage and adducts the vocal process. The posterior part of the glottis is narrowed when the arytenoid cartilages are drawn together by contraction of the transverse arytenoid muscles.

The vocal folds are stretched by contraction of the cricothyroid muscle (Fig. 9.124) and slackened by contraction of the thyroarytenoid muscle (see Fig. 9.123). The vocalis muscle, which is a subpart of the thyroarytenoid, locally tenses the vocal ligament.

VOCAL FOLD MOVEMENT WITH RESPIRATION

On quiet inspiration, the vocal folds abduct and the rima glottidis is triangular in shape with the apex in front. On expiration, the vocal folds adduct, leaving a small gap between them.

Table 9.14 Laryngeal Intrinsic Muscles

MUSCLE	ORIGIN	INSERTION	NERVE SUPPLY	ACTION
Muscles Controlling the Laryngeal Inlet				
Oblique arytenoid	Muscular process of arytenoid cartilage	Apex of opposite arytenoid cartilage	Recurrent laryngeal nerve	Narrows the inlet by bringing the aryepiglottic folds together
Thyroepiglottis	Medial surface of thyroid cartilage	Lateral margin of epiglottis and aryepiglottic fold	Recurrent laryngeal nerve	Widens the inlet by pulling the aryepiglottic folds apart
Muscles Controlling Vocal Fold (Cord) Movement				
Cricothyroid	Side of cricoid cartilage	Lower border and inferior cornu of thyroid cartilage	External laryngeal nerve	Tenses vocal cords
Thyroarytenoid	Inner surface of thyroid cartilage	Arytenoid cartilage	Recurrent laryngeal nerve	Relaxes vocal ligament
Vocalis	Deep fibers of the thyroarytenoid		Recurrent laryngeal nerve	Local tension on vocal ligament
Lateral cricoarytenoid	Upper border of cricoid cartilage	Muscular process of arytenoid cartilage	Recurrent laryngeal nerve	Adducts the vocal cords by rotating arytenoid cartilage
Posterior cricoarytenoid	Back of cricoid cartilage	Muscular process of arytenoid cartilage	Recurrent laryngeal nerve	Abducts the vocal cords by rotating arytenoid cartilage
Transverse arytenoid	Back of arytenoid cartilage	Back of opposite arytenoid cartilage	Recurrent laryngeal nerve	Closes the posterior part of rima glottidis by approximating arytenoid cartilages

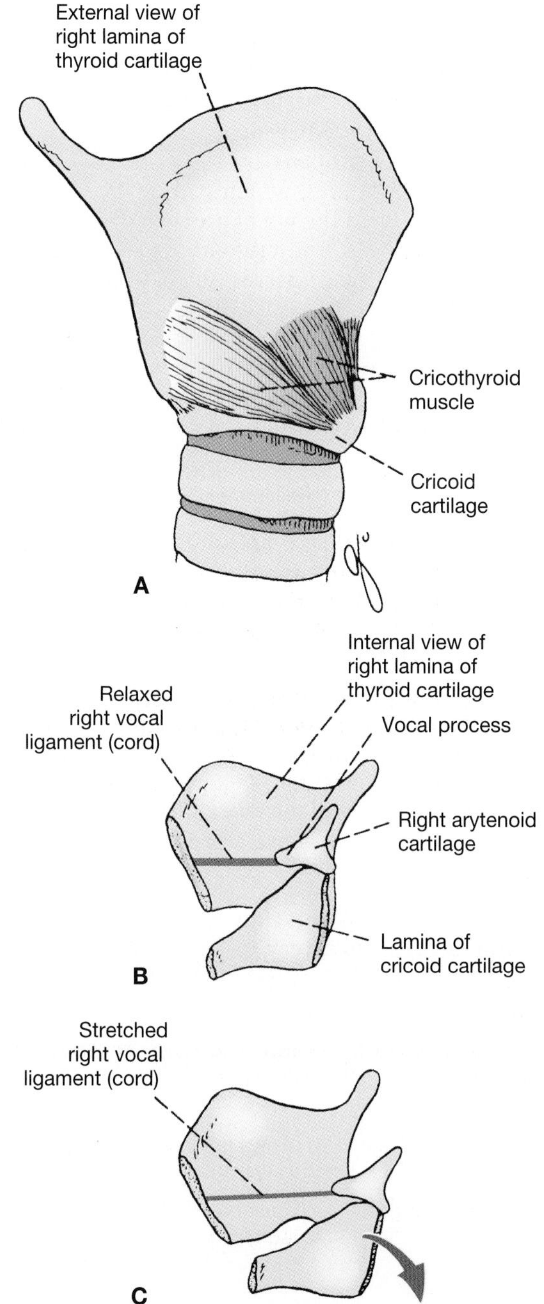

Figure 9.124 Diagrams showing the attachments and actions of the cricothyroid muscle. **A.** Right lateral view of the larynx and the cricothyroid muscle. **B.** Interior view of the larynx showing the relaxed right vocal ligament. **C.** Interior view of the larynx showing the right vocal ligament stretched as a result of the thyroid cartilage tilting forward and the arytenoid cartilage tilting backward by contraction of the cricothyroid muscle.

On deep inspiration, the vocal folds maximally abduct, and the triangular shape of the glottis becomes a diamond shape because of the maximal lateral rotation of the arytenoid cartilages.

LARYNGEAL SPHINCTERIC FUNCTION

Two sphincters exist in the larynx: one at the inlet and another at the rima glottidis.

The **sphincter at the inlet** is used only during swallowing. As the bolus of food is passed backward between the tongue and the hard palate, the larynx is pulled up beneath the back of the tongue. The inlet of the larynx is narrowed by the action of the oblique arytenoid and aryepiglottic muscles. The epiglottis is pushed backward by the tongue and serves as a cap over the laryngeal inlet. The bolus of food, or fluids, then enters the esophagus by passing over the epiglottis or moving down the grooves on either side of the laryngeal inlet, the piriform fossae.

In coughing or sneezing, the **rima glottidis serves as a sphincter**. After inspiration, the vocal folds are adducted, and the muscles of expiration are made to contract strongly. As a result, the intrathoracic pressure rises, and the vocal folds suddenly abduct. The sudden release of the compressed air will often dislodge foreign particles or mucus from the respiratory tract and carry the material up into the pharynx, where the material is either swallowed or expectorated.

In the **Valsalva maneuver**, forced expiration takes place against a closed glottis. In abdominal straining associated with micturition, defecation, and parturition, air is often held temporarily in the respiratory tract by closing the rima glottidis. After deep inspiration, the rima glottidis is closed. The muscles of the anterior abdominal wall now contract, and the upward movement of the diaphragm is prevented by the presence of compressed air within the respiratory tract. After a prolonged effort, the person often releases some of the air by momentarily opening the rima glottidis, producing a grunting sound.

VOICE PRODUCTION IN THE LARYNX

The intermittent release of expired air between the adducted vocal folds results in their vibration and in the production of sound. The **frequency**, or pitch, of the sound is determined by changes in the length and tension of the vocal ligaments. The **quality** of the voice depends on the resonators above the larynx, namely, the pharynx, mouth, and paranasal sinuses. The quality of the voice is controlled by the muscles of the soft plate, tongue, floor of the mouth, cheeks, lips, and jaws. Normal speech depends on the modification of the sound into recognizable consonants and vowels by the use of the tongue, teeth, and lips. Vowel sounds are usually purely oral with the soft palate raised so that the air is channeled through the mouth rather than the nose.

Speech involves the intermittent release of expired air between the adducted vocal folds. Singing a note requires a more prolonged release of the expired air between the adducted vocal folds. In whispering, the vocal folds are adducted, but the arytenoid cartilages are separated; the vibrations are given to a constant stream of expired air that passes through the posterior part of the rima glottidis.

Laryngeal Mucous Membrane

The mucous membrane of the larynx lines the cavity and is covered with ciliated columnar epithelium. On the vocal cords, however, where the mucous membrane is subject to repeated trauma during phonation, the mucous membrane is covered with stratified squamous epithelium.

Laryngeal Nerve Supply

The **vagus nerve** (**CN X**) supplies the entire larynx through its superior and recurrent branches (Fig. 9.125). The **superior laryngeal nerve** divides into **external** and **internal laryngeal nerves** above the larynx. The external laryngeal nerve descends on the exterior of the larynx and extends to the cricothyroid muscle. The internal laryngeal nerve penetrates the lateral aspect of the thyrohyoid membrane (in company with the superior laryngeal artery) and enters the larynx. The **recurrent laryngeal nerve** ascends the neck and becomes the **inferior laryngeal nerve** when it passes the inferior border of the cricoid cartilage and enters the larynx.

Sensory Nerves

- **Above the vocal folds:** Internal laryngeal nerve
- **Below the level of the vocal cords:** Inferior laryngeal nerve

Motor Nerves

- The **external laryngeal nerve** supplies the cricothyroid muscle.
- The **recurrent laryngeal nerve** supplies all the intrinsic muscles of the larynx except the cricothyroid muscle.

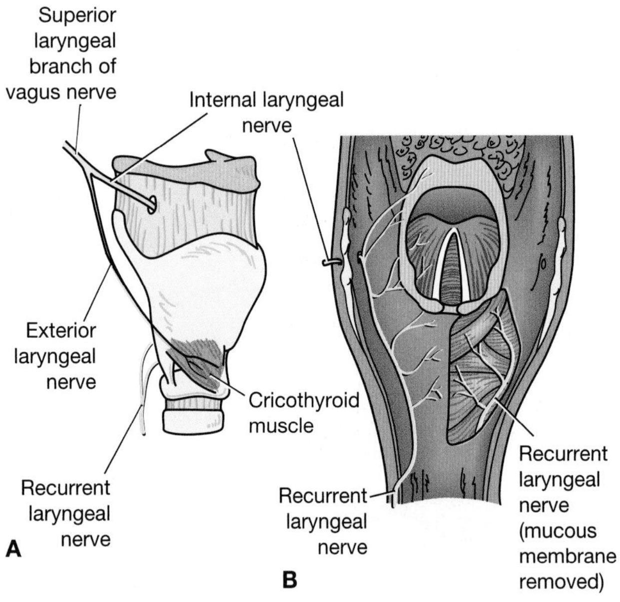

Figure 9.125 **A.** Lateral view of the larynx showing the internal and external laryngeal branches of the superior laryngeal branch of the vagus nerve. **B.** The distribution of the terminal branches of the internal and recurrent laryngeal nerves. The terminal branches of the recurrent laryngeal nerve are named the inferior laryngeal nerve. The larynx is viewed from above and posteriorly.

Laryngeal Blood Supply

- **Upper half of the larynx:** Superior laryngeal branch of the superior thyroid artery
- **Lower half of the larynx:** Inferior laryngeal branch of the inferior thyroid artery

Laryngeal Lymph Drainage

The lymph vessels drain into the **deep cervical** group of nodes.

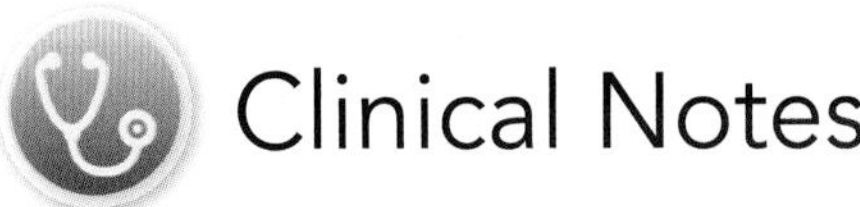

Clinical Notes

Laryngeal Nerve Lesions

The recurrent laryngeal nerves innervate the intrinsic muscles of the larynx, except for the cricothyroid muscle. Both these nerves are vulnerable during operations on the thyroid gland because of the close relationship between them and the arteries of the gland. The left recurrent laryngeal nerve may be involved in a bronchial or esophageal carcinoma or in secondary metastatic deposits in the mediastinal lymph nodes. The right and left recurrent laryngeal nerves may be damaged by malignant involvement of the deep cervical lymph nodes.

Section of the external laryngeal nerve produces weakness of the voice because the cricothyroid muscle is paralyzed, and the vocal fold cannot be tensed (Fig. 9.126A).

Unilateral complete section of the recurrent laryngeal nerve results in the vocal fold on the affected side assuming the position midway between abduction and adduction. It lies just laterally to the midline. Speech is not greatly affected because the other vocal fold compensates to some extent and moves toward the affected vocal fold (see Fig. 9.126B).

Bilateral complete section of the recurrent laryngeal nerve results in both vocal folds assuming the position midway between abduction and adduction. Breathing is impaired because the rima glottidis is partially closed, and speech is lost (see Fig. 9.126C).

Unilateral partial section of the recurrent laryngeal nerve results in a greater degree of paralysis of the abductor muscles than of the adductor muscles. Thus, the affected vocal fold assumes the adducted midline position (see Fig. 9.126D). This assumes that the abductor muscles receive a greater number of nerves than the adductor muscles, and thus, partial damage of the recurrent laryngeal

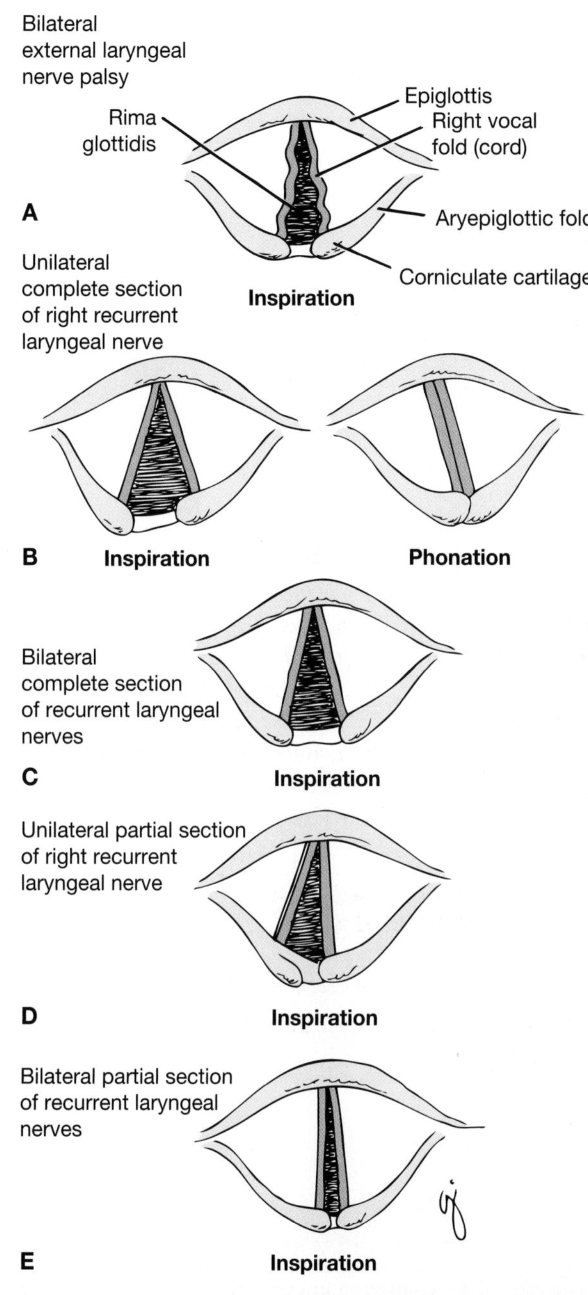

Figure 9.126 Different positions **(A–E)** of the vocal folds (cords) following damage to the external and/or recurrent laryngeal nerves.

nerve results in damage to relatively more nerve fibers to the abductor muscles. Another possibility is that the nerve fibers to the abductor muscles travel in a more exposed position in the recurrent laryngeal nerve and are therefore more prone to damage.

Bilateral partial section of the recurrent laryngeal nerves results in bilateral paralysis of the abductor muscles and the drawing together of the vocal folds (see Fig. 9.126E). Acute breathlessness (**dyspnea**) and **stridor** follow, and cricothyroidotomy or tracheostomy is necessary.

Laryngeal Mucous Membrane Edema

The mucous membrane of the larynx is loosely attached to the underlying structures by submucous connective tissue. However, it is firmly attached to the vocal ligaments in the region of the vocal folds. This fact is of clinical importance in cases of edema of the larynx. The accumulation of tissue fluid causes the mucous membrane above the rima glottidis to swell and encroach on the airway. In severe cases, a cricothyroidotomy or tracheostomy may be necessary.

Laryngeal Mirror and Laryngoscope

The interior of the larynx can be inspected **indirectly** through a laryngeal mirror passed through the open mouth into the oropharynx (Fig. 9.127). A more satisfactory method is the **direct method** using the laryngoscope. The neck is brought forward on a pillow, and the head is fully extended at the atlanto-occipital joints. The illuminated instrument can then be introduced into the larynx over the back of the tongue. The valleculae, piriform fossae, epiglottis, and aryepiglottic folds are clearly seen. The two elevations produced by the corniculate and cuneiform cartilages can be recognized. Within the larynx, the vestibular folds and the vocal folds can be seen. The former are fixed, widely separated, and reddish in color; the latter move with respiration and are white in color. With quiet breathing, the rima glottidis is triangular, with the apex in front. With deep inspiration, the rima glottidis assumes a diamond shape because of the lateral rotation of the arytenoid cartilages. If the patient is asked to breathe deeply, the vocal folds become widely abducted, and the inside of the trachea is visible.

Important Anatomic Axes for Endotracheal Intubation

Three upper airway axes must be brought into alignment if the glottis is to be viewed adequately through a laryngoscope: those of the mouth, pharynx, and trachea (Fig. 9.128).

The following procedures are necessary. First, the head is extended at the atlanto-occipital joints. This brings the axis of the mouth into the correct position. Then, the neck is flexed at cervical vertebrae C4 to C7 by elevating the back of the head off the table, often with the help of a pillow. This brings the axes of the pharynx and the trachea in line with the axis of the mouth.

Anatomy of Vocal Cord Visualization with Laryngoscopy

- The pear-shaped epiglottis attaches by its stalk at its lower end to the interior of the thyroid cartilage (see Fig. 9.123).
- The vocal cords (ligaments) attach at their anterior ends to the thyroid cartilage just below the attachment of the epiglottis.
- Therefore, manipulation of the epiglottis and possibly the thyroid cartilage will greatly assist the operator in visualizing the cords and the glottis.

The patient's head and neck are correctly positioned so that the three axes of the airway are established, and the patient has assumed the "sniffing" position (see Important Anatomic Axes discussed earlier). The laryngoscope is inserted into

(continued)

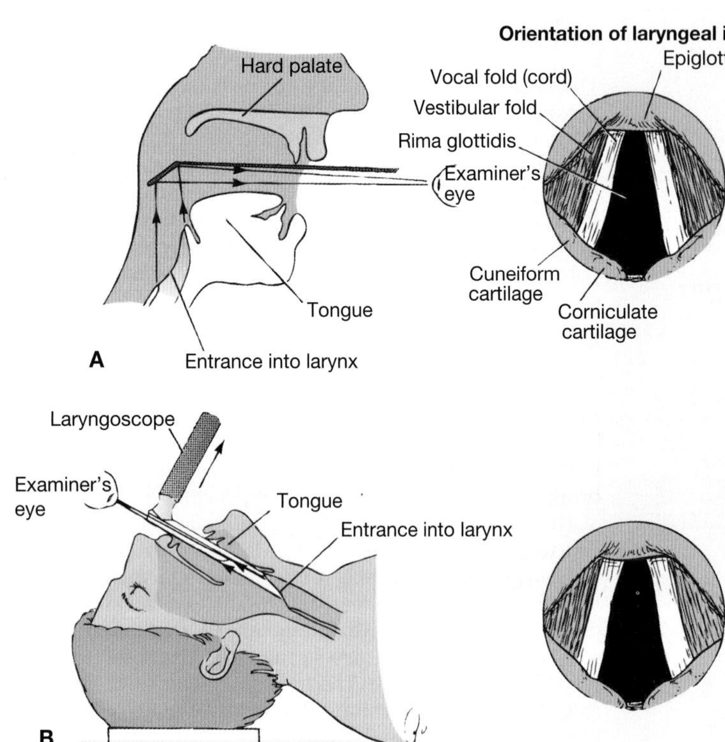

Figure 9.127 Inspection of the vocal folds (cords) indirectly through a laryngeal mirror **(A)** and through a laryngoscope **(B)**. Note the orientation of the structures forming the laryngeal inlet.

the patient's mouth, and the blade is correctly placed alongside the right mandibular molar teeth. The blade can then pass over the tongue and down into the esophagus. The tip of the blade must be fully inserted into the esophagus (so that you know where it is anatomically). The blade should by now have moved toward the midline and followed the anatomic curvature on the posterior surface of the tongue.

The laryngoscopic blade is then gently and slowly withdrawn. The tip of the blade is kept under direct vision at all times and is permitted to rise up out of the esophagus. Remember that the tip of the blade is at first in the esophagus and is, therefore, distal to the level of the vocal cords. Once the blade tip has left the esophagus, it is in the laryngeal part of the pharynx (see Figs. 9.111 and 9.114), and a view of the glottis should immediately be apparent. This is the critical stage. If the glottis is not visualized, then the operator is viewing the posterior surface of the epiglottis.

With the tip of the blade of the laryngoscope applied to the posterior surface of the epiglottis, gently lift up and elevate the epiglottis to expose the glottis. If the glottis is still not in view, grasp the thyroid cartilage (to which the cords and the epiglottis are attached) with the free right hand between finger and thumb and apply firm **B**ackward, **U**pward, **R**ightward **P**ressure (**BURP**). This maneuver realigns the box of the larynx relative to the laryngoscopic blade and the visual axis of the operator, and the glottis should immediately be seen.

Reflex Activity Secondary to Endotracheal Intubation

Stimulation of the mucous membrane of the upper airway during the process of intubation may produce cardiovascular changes such as bradycardia and hypertension. These changes are largely mediated through the branches of the vagus nerves.

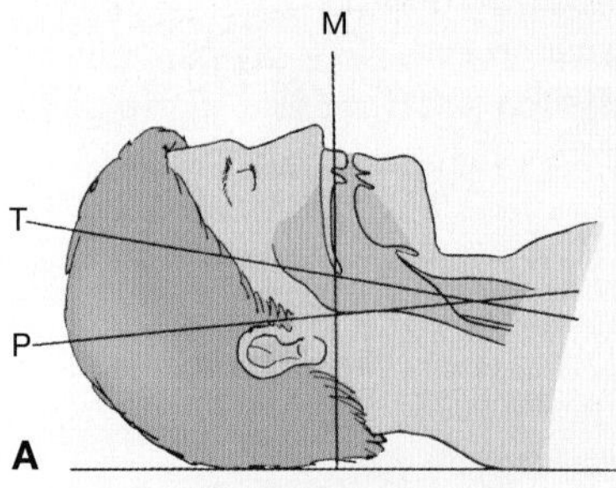

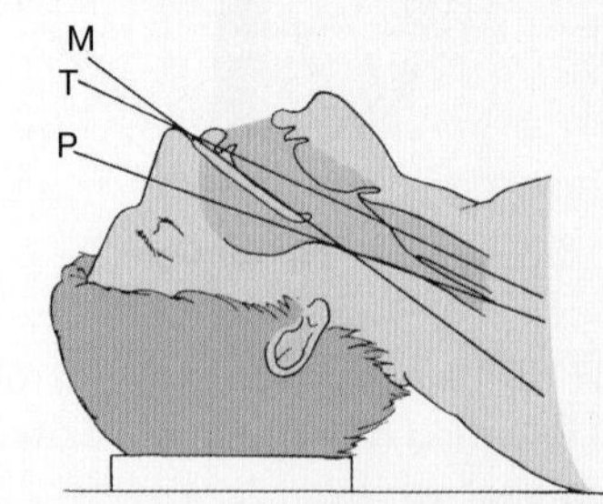

Figure 9.128 Anatomic axes for endotracheal intubation. **A.** With the head in the neutral position, the axis of the mouth (*M*), the axis of the trachea (*T*), and the axis of the pharynx (*P*) are not aligned with one another. **B.** If the head is extended at the atlanto-occipital joints, the axis of the mouth is correctly placed. If the back of the head is raised off the table with a pillow, thus flexing the cervical vertebral column, the axes of the trachea and pharynx are brought in line with the axis of the mouth.

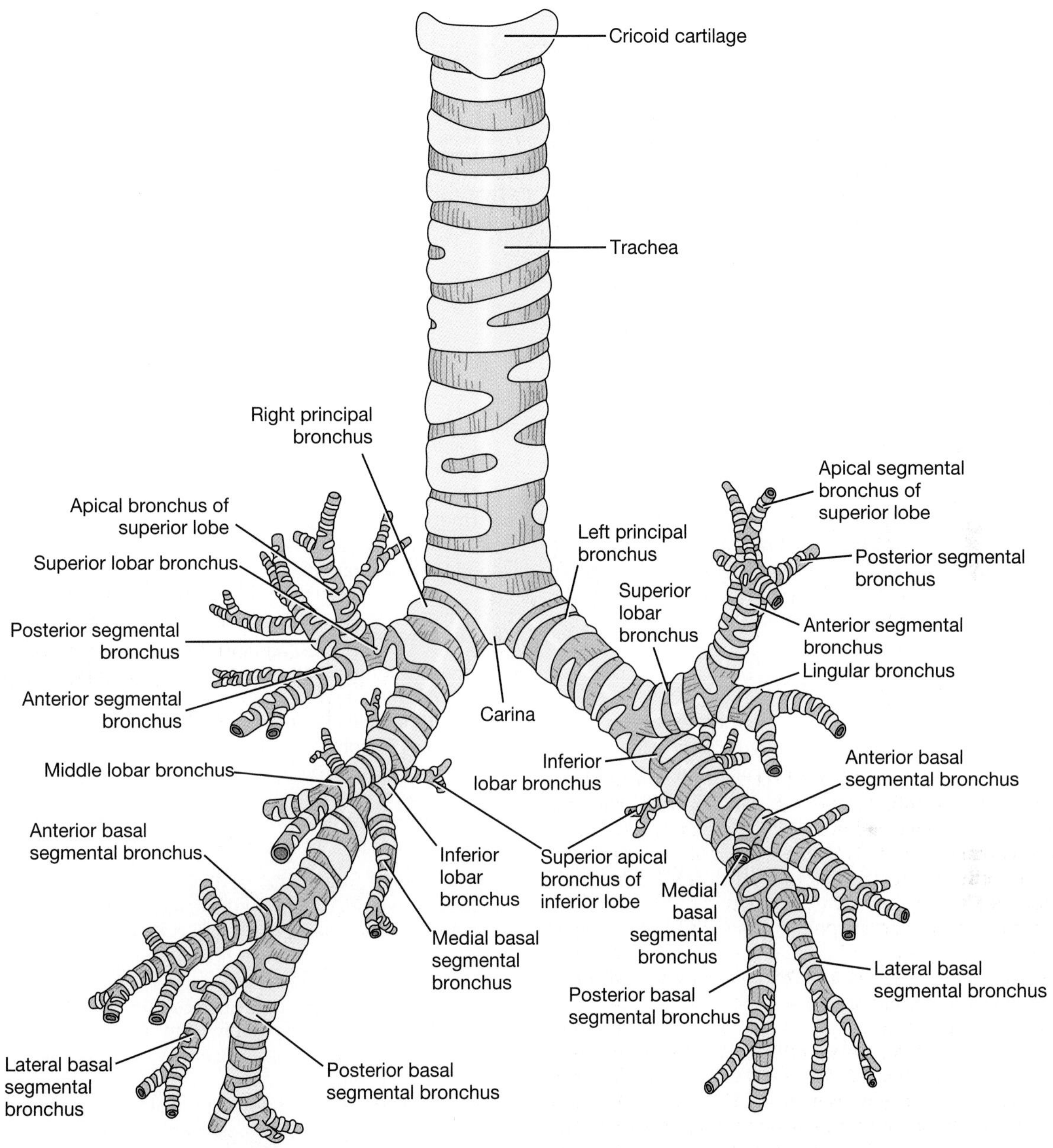

Figure 9.129 Trachea and the bronchi.

Trachea

The trachea is a mobile cartilaginous and membranous tube (Fig. 9.129). It begins as a continuation of the larynx at the lower border of the cricoid cartilage at the level of the C6 vertebra. It descends in the midline of the neck. In the thorax, the trachea ends at the **carina** by dividing into right and left **principal (main) bronchi** at the level of the sternal angle (opposite the disc between the T4 and T5 vertebrae).

The fibroelastic tube is kept patent by the presence of U-shaped cartilaginous bar (rings) of hyaline cartilage embedded in its wall. The posterior free ends of the cartilage are connected by smooth muscle, the **trachealis muscle**.

The mucous membrane of the trachea is lined with pseudostratified ciliated columnar epithelium and contains many goblet cells and tubular mucous glands.

Relations in the Neck

- **Anteriorly:** The skin, fascia, isthmus of the thyroid gland (in front of the second, third, and fourth rings), inferior thyroid vein, jugular arch, thyroidea ima artery (if present), and left brachiocephalic vein in children, overlapped by the sternothyroid and sternohyoid muscles (see Fig. 9.65)

- **Posteriorly:** Right and left recurrent laryngeal nerves and the esophagus
- **Laterally:** Lobes of the thyroid gland and the carotid sheath and contents

Tracheal Nerve Supply

The sensory nerve supply is from direct vagal branches and the **recurrent laryngeal nerves**.

Tracheal Blood Supply

The **inferior thyroid arteries** supply the upper two thirds, and the **bronchial arteries** supply the lower third.

Tracheal Lymph Drainage

Lymph empties into the pretracheal and paratracheal lymph nodes and the deep cervical nodes.

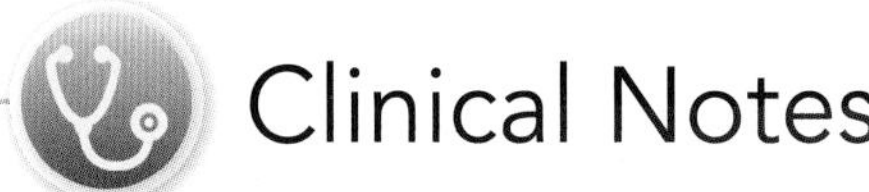

Clinical Notes

Neck Midline Structures

Multiple midline structures in the neck are readily recognizable as one passes an examining finger down the neck from the chin to the suprasternal notch (see Neck Surface Landmarks). An enlarged submental lymph node may be caused by a pathologic condition anywhere between the tip of the tongue and the point of the chin.

Trachea Palpation

The trachea is readily palpable below the larynx. As it descends, it moves deeper and may lie as much as 1.5 in. (4 cm) from the surface at the suprasternal notch. In the adult, it may measure as much as 1 in. (2.5 cm) in diameter, but in a 3-year-old child, it may measure only 0.5 in. in diameter. The trachea is a mobile elastic tube and is easily displaced by the enlargement of adjacent organs or the presence of tumors. Also, a pathologic lesion in the thorax may cause lateral displacement of the cervical part of the trachea.

Compromised Airway

No medical emergency quite produces the urgency and anxiety of the compromised airway. The clinician has to institute almost immediate treatment. All techniques of airway management require a detailed knowledge of anatomy.

Cricothyroidotomy

In cricothyroidotomy, a tube is inserted in the interval between the cricoid cartilage and the thyroid cartilage. A vertical or transverse incision is made in the skin in the interval between the cartilages (Fig. 9.130). The incision is made through the following structures: skin, superficial fascia (beware of the anterior jugular veins, which lie close together on either side of the midline), investing layer of deep cervical fascia, pretracheal fascia (separate the sternohyoid muscles and incise the fascia), and the larynx. The larynx is incised through a horizontal incision through the **cricothyroid ligament** and the tube inserted.

Complications

- **Esophageal perforation:** Because the lower end of the pharynx and the beginning of the esophagus lie directly behind the cricoid cartilage, it is imperative that the scalpel incision through the cricothyroid membrane not be carried too far posteriorly. This is particularly important in young children, in whom the cross diameter of the larynx is so small.
- **Hemorrhage:** The small branches of the superior thyroid artery that occasionally cross the front of the cricothyroid membrane to anastomose with one another should be avoided.

Tracheostomy

Tracheostomy generally is limited to patients with extensive laryngeal damage and infants with severe airway obstruction. Because of the presence of major vascular structures (carotid arteries and internal jugular vein), the thyroid gland, the nerves (recurrent laryngeal branch of vagus and vagus nerve), the pleural cavities, and the esophagus, meticulous attention to anatomic detail has to be observed (Fig. 9.131). The procedure is as follows:

1. The thyroid and cricoid cartilages are identified, and the neck is extended to bring the trachea forward.
2. A vertical midline skin incision is made from the region of the cricothyroid membrane inferiorly toward the suprasternal notch.
3. The incision is carried through the superficial fascia and the fibers of the platysma muscle. The anterior jugular veins in the superficial fascia are avoided by maintaining a midline position.
4. The investing layer of deep cervical fascia is incised.
5. The pretracheal muscles embedded in the pretracheal fascia are split in the midline two fingerbreadths superior to the sternal notch.
6. The tracheal rings are then palpable in the midline, or the isthmus of the thyroid gland is visible. If a hook is placed under the lower border of the cricoid cartilage and traction is applied upward, the slack is taken out of the elastic trachea; this stops it from slipping from side to side.
7. A decision is then made as to whether to enter the trachea through the second ring above the isthmus of the thyroid gland; through the third, fourth, or fifth ring by first dividing the vascular isthmus of the thyroid gland; or through the lower tracheal rings below the thyroid isthmus. At the latter site, the trachea is receding from the surface of the neck, and the pretracheal fascia contains the inferior thyroid veins and possibly the thyroidea ima artery.
8. The **preferred site** is through the second tracheal ring in the midline, with the thyroid isthmus retracted inferiorly. A vertical tracheal incision is made, and the tracheostomy tube is inserted.

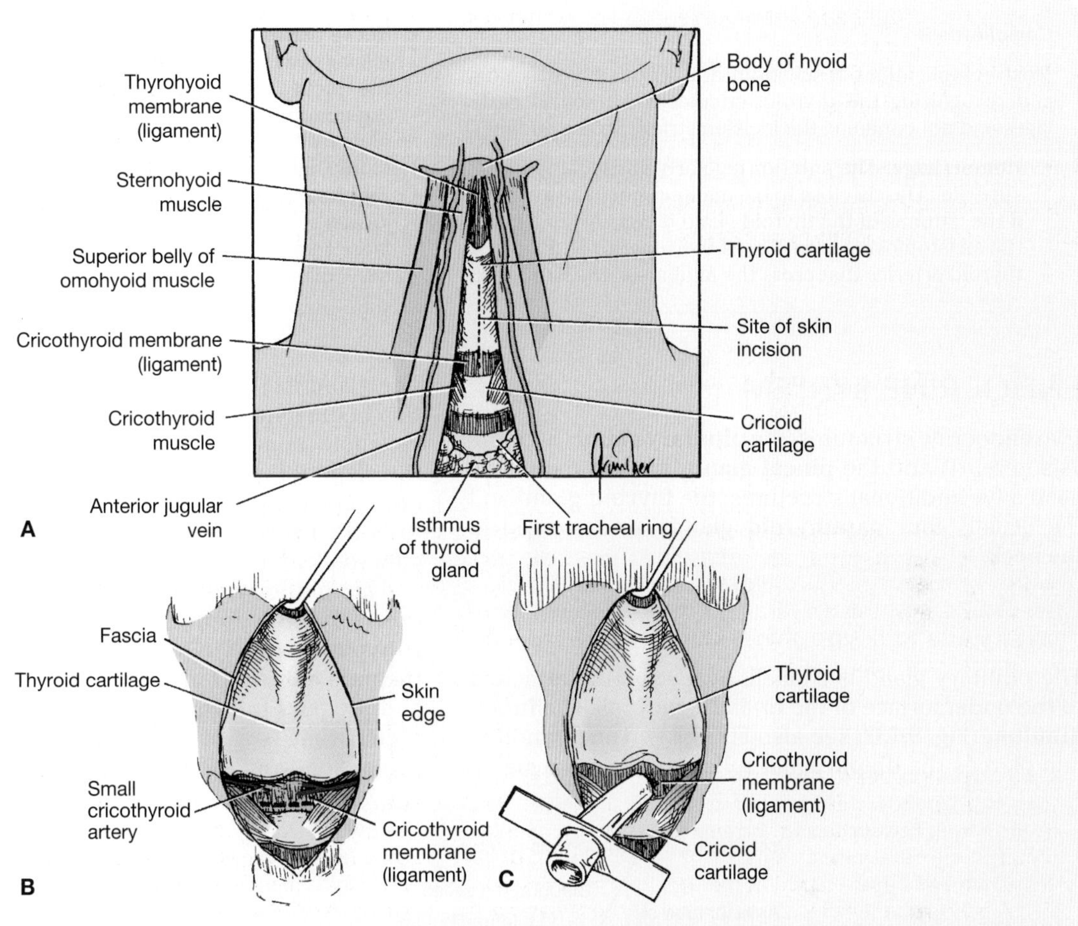

Figure 9.130 Anatomy of cricothyroidotomy. **A.** A vertical incision is made through the skin and superficial and deep cervical fasciae. **B.** The cricothyroid membrane (ligament) is incised through a horizontal incision close to the upper border of the cricoid cartilage. **C.** Insertion of the tube.

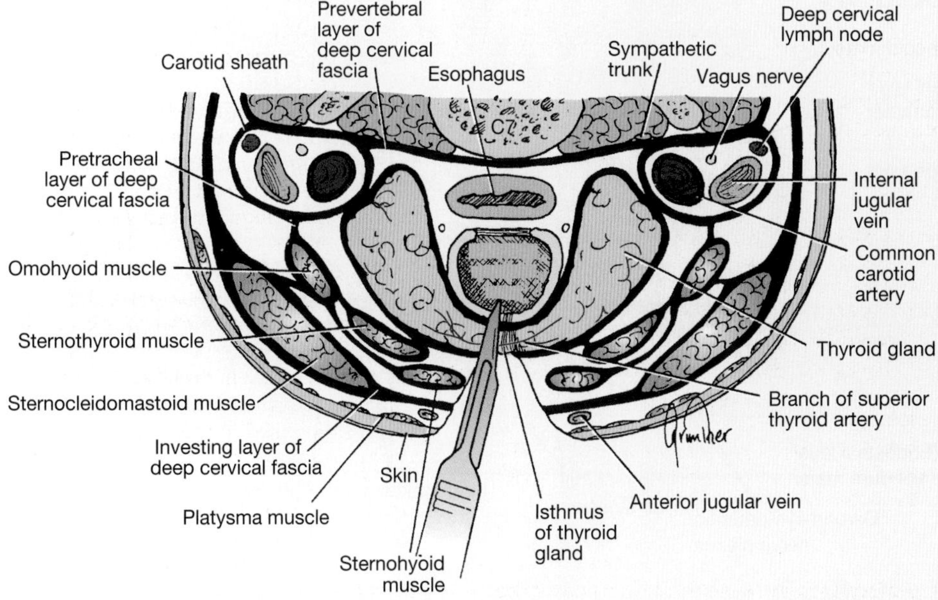

Figure 9.131 Cross section of the neck at the level of the second tracheal ring. A vertical incision is made through the ring, and the tracheostomy tube is inserted.

(continued)

Complications

Most complications result from not adequately palpating and recognizing the thyroid, cricoid, and tracheal cartilages and not confining the incision strictly to the midline.

- **Hemorrhage:** The anterior jugular veins located in the superficial fascia close to the midline should be avoided. If the isthmus of the thyroid gland is transected, secure the anastomosing branches of the superior and inferior thyroid arteries that cross the midline on the isthmus.
- **Nerve paralysis:** The recurrent laryngeal nerves may be damaged as they ascend the neck in the groove between the trachea and the esophagus.
- **Pneumothorax:** The cervical dome of the pleura may be pierced. This is especially common in children because of the high level of the pleura in the neck.
- **Esophageal injury:** Damage to the esophagus, which is located immediately posterior to the trachea, occurs most commonly in infants; it follows penetration of the small diameter trachea by the point of the scalpel blade.

ENDOCRINE SYSTEM

Two endocrine structures, the **pituitary gland** (hypophysis cerebri) and the **pineal gland**, are located in the head. Five additional structures, the **thyroid gland** and the usually four **parathyroid glands**, are situated in the neck.

Pituitary Gland (Hypophysis Cerebri)

The pituitary gland is a small, oval structure attached to the undersurface of the brain by the stalk-like **infundibulum** (Fig. 9.132; see also Fig. 9.33). The infundibulum pierces the **diaphragma sellae** to reach the gland. The gland itself is well protected by virtue of its location in the **hypophyseal fossa** of the **sella turcica** of the sphenoid bone. Because the hormones produced by the gland influence the activities of many other endocrine glands, the hypophysis cerebri is often referred to as the **master endocrine gland**. For this reason, it is vital to life.

The pituitary gland has two lobes: an **anterior lobe** (**adenohypophysis**) and a **posterior lobe** (**neurohypophysis**). The anterior lobe is subdivided into the **pars anterior** (sometimes called the **pars distalis**) and the **pars intermedia**, which may be separated by a cleft that is a remnant of an embryonic pouch. A projection from the pars anterior, the **pars tuberalis**,

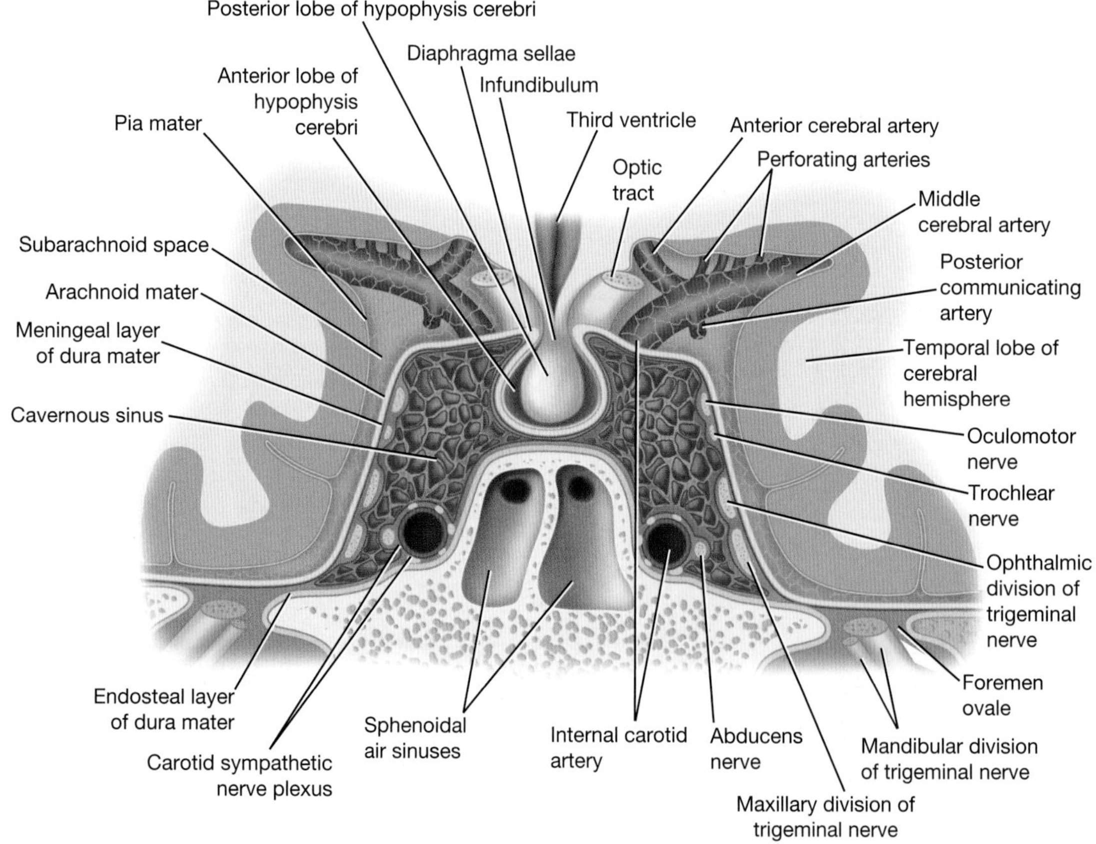

Figure 9.132 Coronal section through the body of the sphenoid bone, showing the pituitary gland and the cavernous sinuses. Note the position of the pituitary within the sella turcica.

extends up along the anterior and lateral surfaces of the pituitary stalk.

Relations

- **Anterior:** Sphenoid sinus (see Fig. 9.33).
- **Posterior:** Dorsum sellae, the basilar artery, and the pons.
- **Superior:** Diaphragma sellae has a central aperture that allows the passage of the infundibulum and separates the anterior lobe from the optic chiasma (see Fig. 9.132).
- **Inferior:** Body of the sphenoid, with its sphenoid air sinuses.
- **Lateral:** Cavernous sinus and its contents.

Blood Supply

The **superior** and **inferior hypophyseal arteries**, branches of the internal carotid artery, supply the pituitary. The veins drain into the **intercavernous sinuses**.

Pituitary Gland Functions

The pituitary gland influences the activities of many other endocrine glands. The pituitary gland is itself controlled by the hypothalamus, and the activities of the hypothalamus are modified by the information received along numerous nervous afferent pathways from different parts of the central nervous system and by the plasma levels of the circulating electrolytes and hormones.

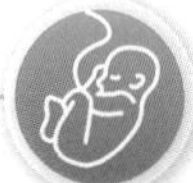

Embryology Notes

Pituitary Gland Development

The pituitary gland develops from **two sources**: a small ectodermal diverticulum (Rathke pouch), which grows superiorly from the roof of the stomodeum immediately anterior to the buccopharyngeal membrane, and a small ectodermal diverticulum (the **infundibulum**), which grows inferiorly from the floor of the diencephalon of the brain (Fig. 9.133).

During month 2 of development, the Rathke pouch meets the anterior surface of the infundibulum, and its connection with the oral epithelium elongates, narrows, and finally disappears. The Rathke pouch now is a vesicle that flattens itself around the anterior and lateral surfaces of the infundibulum. The cells of the anterior wall of the vesicle proliferate and form the **pars anterior** of the pituitary. A cellular extension from the vesicle's upper part grows superiorly and around the stalk of the infundibulum, forming the **pars tuberalis**. The cells of the posterior wall of the vesicle never develop extensively; they form the **pars intermedia**. Some of the cells later migrate anteriorly into the pars anterior. The cavity of the vesicle is reduced to a narrow cleft, which may disappear completely. Meanwhile, the infundibulum differentiates into the stalk and pars nervosa of the pituitary gland.

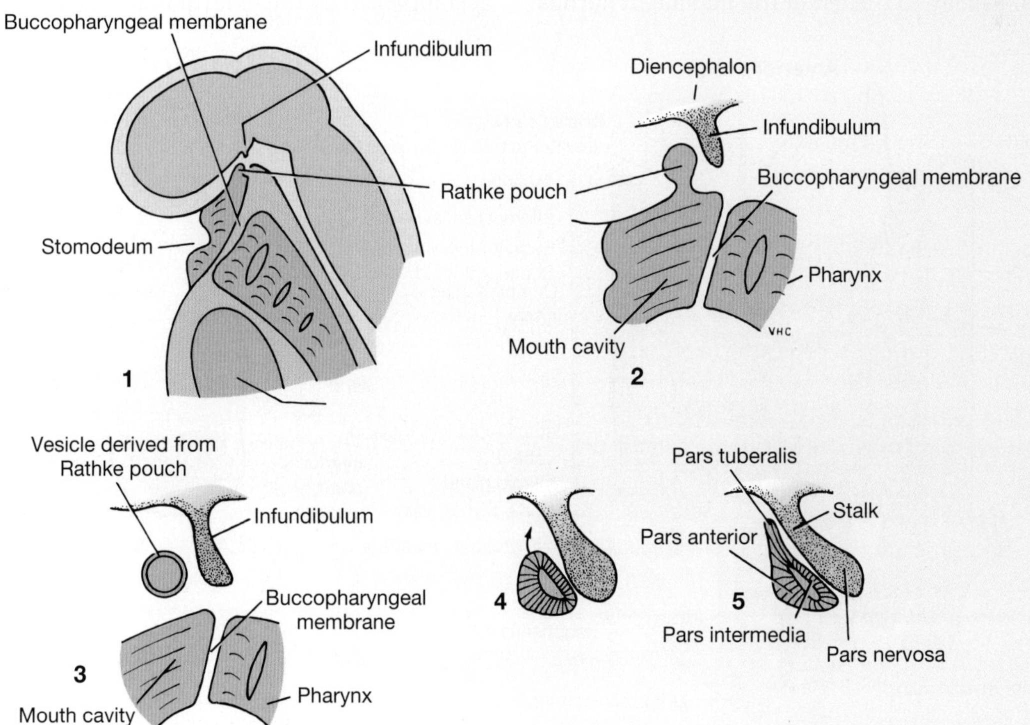

Figure 9.133 Sagittal sections showing different stages in the development of the pituitary gland.

Pineal Gland

The pineal gland is a small cone-shaped body that projects posteriorly from the posterior end of the roof of the third ventricle of the brain (see Fig. 9.33). The pineal consists essentially of groups of cells, the **pinealocytes**, supported by glial cells. The gland has a rich blood supply and is innervated by postganglionic sympathetic nerve fibers.

Pineal Gland Functions

The pineal gland influences the activities of the pituitary gland, islets of Langerhans of the pancreas, parathyroids, adrenals, and gonads. The pineal secretions, produced by the pinealocytes, reach their target organs via the bloodstream or through the CSF. Their actions are mainly inhibitory and either directly inhibit the production of hormones or indirectly inhibit the secretion of releasing factors by the hypothalamus.

Thyroid Gland

The thyroid gland consists of right and left lobes connected by a narrow isthmus (Fig. 9.134; see also Fig. 9.65). It is a vascular organ surrounded by a sheath derived from the pretracheal layer of the deep fascia. The sheath attaches the gland to the larynx and the trachea.

Each **lobe** is pear shaped, with its apex being directed upward as far as the oblique line on the lamina of the thyroid cartilage. Its base lies below at the level of the fourth or fifth tracheal ring.

The **isthmus** extends across the midline in front of the second, third, and fourth tracheal rings. A **pyramidal lobe** is often present, and it projects upward from the isthmus, usually to the left of the midline. A fibrous or muscular band frequently connects the pyramidal lobe to the hyoid bone; if it is muscular, it is referred to as the **levator glandulae thyroideae**.

Relations of Lobes

- **Anterolateral:** Sternothyroid, superior belly of the omohyoid, sternohyoid, and the anterior border of the SCM
- **Posterolateral:** Carotid sheath with the common carotid artery, internal jugular vein, and vagus nerve
- **Medial:** Larynx, trachea, pharynx, and esophagus (associated with these structures are the cricothyroid muscle and its nerve supply, the external laryngeal nerve; the recurrent laryngeal nerve is in the groove between the esophagus and the trachea)
- **Posterior:** Superior and inferior parathyroid glands and the anastomosis between the superior and inferior thyroid arteries

Isthmus Relations

- **Anterior:** Sternothyroids, sternohyoids, anterior jugular veins, fascia, and skin
- **Posterior:** Second, third, and fourth tracheal rings
- **Superior:** Terminal branches of the superior thyroid arteries anastomose along its upper border

Blood Supply

The **arteries** to the thyroid gland are the superior thyroid artery, inferior thyroid artery, and sometimes the thyroidea ima. The arteries anastomose profusely with one another over the surface of the gland.

The **superior thyroid artery**, a branch of the external carotid artery, descends to the upper pole of each lobe, accompanied by the **external laryngeal nerve**.

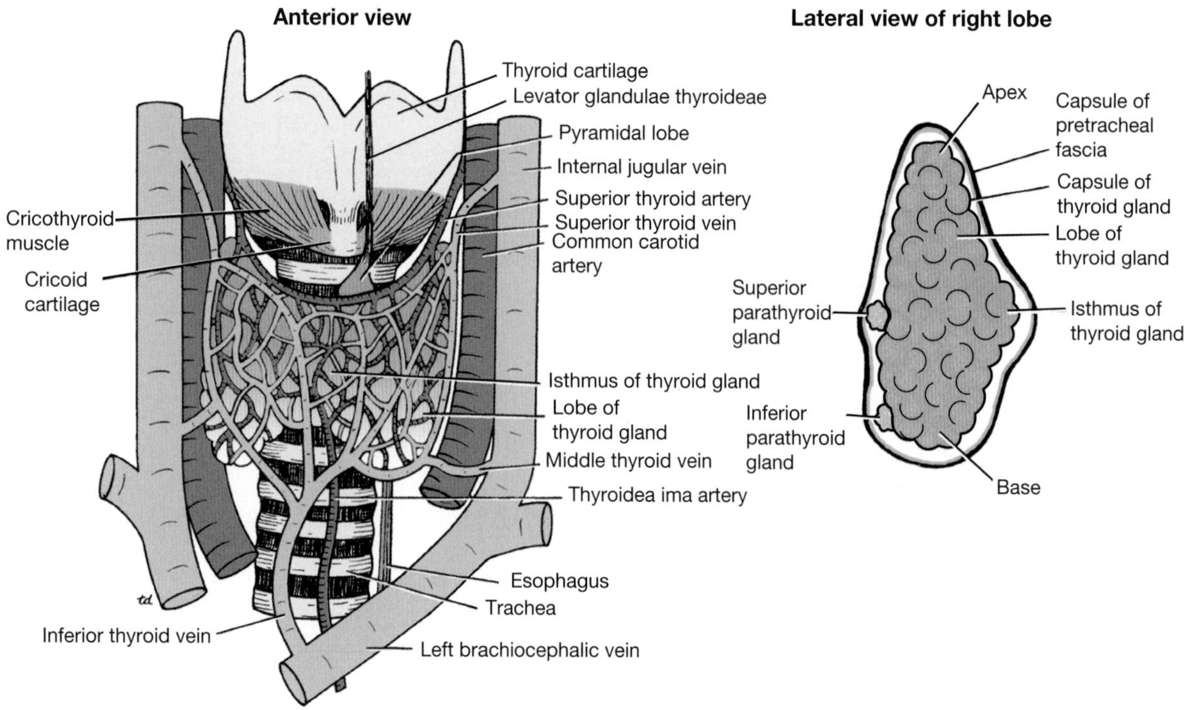

Figure 9.134 Structure and vascular supply of the thyroid gland.

The **inferior thyroid artery**, a branch of the thyrocervical trunk, ascends behind the gland to the level of the cricoid cartilage. It then turns medially and downward to reach the posterior border of the gland. The **recurrent laryngeal nerve** crosses either in front of or behind the artery, or it may pass between its branches.

The **thyroidea ima**, if present, may arise from the brachiocephalic artery or the arch of the aorta. It ascends in front of the trachea to the isthmus.

The **veins** from the thyroid gland are the **superior thyroid**, which drains into the internal jugular vein; the **middle thyroid**, which drains into the internal jugular vein; and the **inferior thyroid**. The inferior thyroid veins of the two sides anastomose with one another as they descend in front of the trachea. They drain into the left brachiocephalic vein in the thorax.

Lymph Drainage

Lymph from the thyroid gland drains mainly laterally into the **deep cervical lymph nodes**. A few lymph vessels descend to the paratracheal nodes.

Nerve Supply

Superior, middle, and inferior cervical sympathetic ganglia provide the nerve supply.

Thyroid Gland Functions

The thyroid hormones thyroxine and triiodothyronine increase the metabolic activity of most cells in the body. The parafollicular cells produce the hormone thyrocalcitonin, which lowers the level of blood calcium.

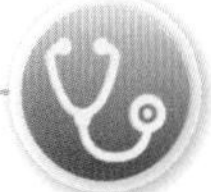

Clinical Notes

Thyroid Gland Swellings and Movement on Swallowing

The thyroid gland is invested in a sheath derived from the pretracheal fascia. This tethers the gland to the larynx and the trachea and explains why the thyroid gland follows the movements of the larynx in swallowing. Therefore, any pathologic neck swelling that is part of the thyroid gland will move upward when the patient is asked to swallow.

Thyroid Gland and the Airway

The close relationship between the trachea and the lobes of the thyroid gland commonly results in pressure on the trachea in patients with pathologic enlargement of the thyroid.

Retrosternal Goiter

The attachment of the sternothyroid muscles to the thyroid cartilage effectively limits upward expansion of the gland. With no limitation to downward expansion, it is not uncommon for a pathologically enlarged thyroid gland to extend downward behind the sternum. A retrosternal goiter (any abnormal enlargement of the thyroid gland) can compress the trachea and cause dangerous dyspnea; it can also cause severe venous compression.

Thyroid Arteries and Important Nerves

The two main arteries supplying the thyroid gland are closely related to important nerves that can be damaged during thyroidectomy operations. The **superior thyroid artery** on each side is related to the **external laryngeal nerve**, which supplies the cricothyroid muscle. The terminal branches of the **inferior thyroid artery** on each side are related to the **recurrent laryngeal nerve**. Damage to the external laryngeal nerve results in an inability to tense the vocal folds and in hoarseness. See the earlier discussion of the larynx for the results of damage to the recurrent laryngeal nerve.

Thyroidectomy and Parathyroid Glands

The parathyroid glands are usually four in number and are closely related to the posterior surface of the thyroid gland (see below). In **partial thyroidectomy**, the posterior part of the thyroid gland is left undisturbed so that the parathyroid glands are not damaged. The development of the inferior parathyroid glands is closely associated with the thymus. For this reason, it is not uncommon for the surgeon to find the inferior parathyroid glands in the superior mediastinum because they have been pulled down into the thorax by the thymus.

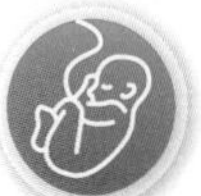

Embryology Notes

Thyroid Gland Development

The thyroid gland begins to develop during week 3 as an endodermal thickening in the midline of the floor of the pharynx between the **tuberculum impar** and the **copula** (Fig. 9.135). Later, this thickening becomes a diverticulum, the **thyroglossal duct**, that grows inferiorly into the underlying mesenchyme. As development continues, the duct elongates, and its distal end becomes bilobed. Soon, the duct becomes a solid cord of cells, and as a result of epithelial proliferation, the bilobed terminal swellings expand to form the thyroid gland.

The thyroid gland now migrates inferiorly in the neck and passes either anterior to, posterior to, or through

(continued)

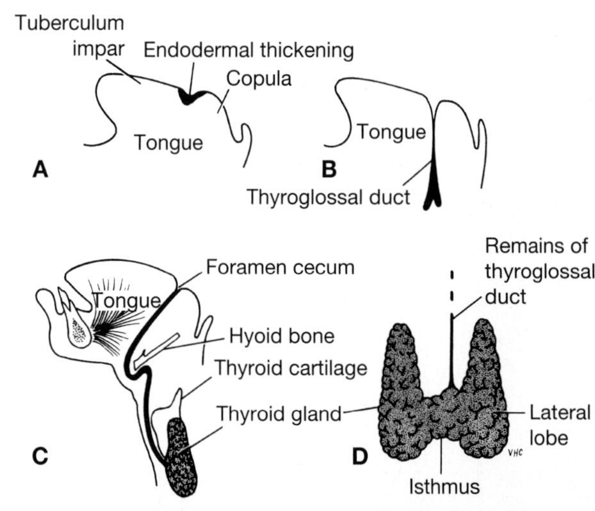

Figure 9.135 Different stages in the development of the thyroid gland. **A.** Sagittal section of the tongue showing an endodermal thickening between the tuberculum impar and the copula. **B.** Sagittal section of the tongue showing the development of the thyroglossal duct. **C.** Sagittal section of the tongue and neck showing the path taken by the thyroid gland as it migrates inferiorly. **D.** Frontal view of the fully developed thyroid gland. Note the remains of the thyroglossal duct above the isthmus.

the developing body of the hyoid bone. By week 7, it reaches its final position in relation to the larynx and trachea. Meanwhile, the solid cord connecting the thyroid gland to the tongue fragments and disappears. The site of origin of the thyroglossal duct on the tongue remains as a pit called the **foramen cecum**. The thyroid gland may now be divided into a small median **isthmus** and two large **lateral lobes**.

In the earliest stages, the thyroid gland consists of a solid mass of cells. Later, as a result of invasion by surrounding vascular mesenchymal tissue, the mass breaks up into plates and cords and finally into small clusters of cells. By month 3, colloid starts to accumulate in the center of each cluster so that **follicles** form. The **fibrous capsule** and connective tissue develop from the surrounding mesenchyme.

The **ultimobranchial bodies** (from the fifth pharyngeal pouch) and neural crest cells are believed to be incorporated into the thyroid gland, where they form the **parafollicular cells**, which produce **calcitonin**.

Thyroid Agenesis

Failure of development of the thyroid gland may occur and is the commonest cause of **congenital hypothyroidism** (formerly known as **cretinism**).

Incomplete Descent of the Thyroid

The descent of the thyroid may be arrested at any point between the base of the tongue and the trachea (Fig. 9.136).

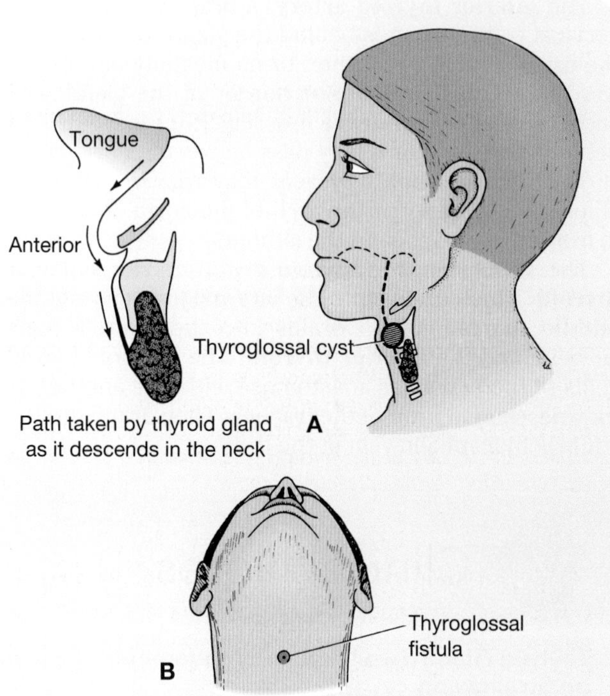

Figure 9.136 Thyroglossal cyst **(A)** in the midline in the neck and a thyroglossal fistula **(B)**.

Lingual thyroid is the most common form of incomplete descent (Fig. 9.137). The mass of tissue found just beneath the foramen cecum may be sufficiently large to obstruct swallowing in the infant.

Ectopic Thyroid Tissue

Ectopic thyroid tissue is occasionally found in the thorax in relation to the trachea or bronchi or even the esophagus. It is assumed that this thyroid tissue arises from endodermal cells displaced during the formation of the laryngotracheal tube or from endodermal cells of the developing esophagus.

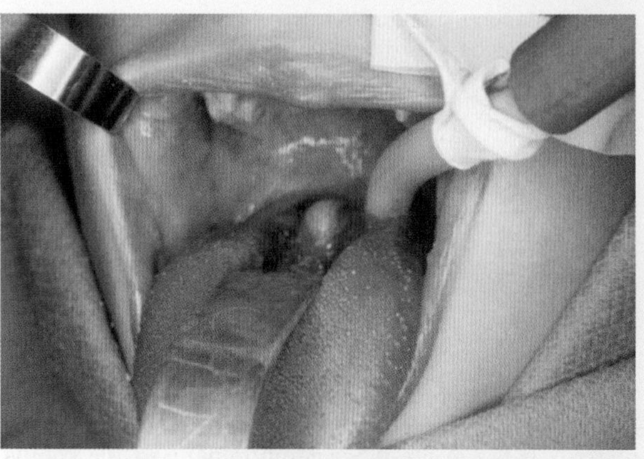

Figure 9.137 Lingual thyroid. (Courtesy of J. Randolph.)

Persistent Thyroglossal Duct

Conditions related to a persistence of the thyroglossal duct usually appear in childhood, in adolescence, or in young adults.

Thyroglossal Cyst

Cysts may occur at any point along the thyroglossal tract (Fig. 9.138; see also Fig. 9.136). They occur most commonly in the region below the hyoid bone. Such a cyst occupies the **midline** and develops as a result of persistence of a small amount of epithelium that continues to secrete mucus. As the cyst enlarges, it is prone to infection, so it should be removed surgically. Because remnants of the duct often traverse the body of the hyoid bone, this may have to be excised also to prevent recurrence.

Thyroglossal Sinus (Fistula)

Occasionally, a thyroglossal cyst ruptures spontaneously, producing a sinus (see Fig. 9.136). Usually, this is a result of an infection of a cyst. All remnants of the thyroglossal duct should be removed surgically.

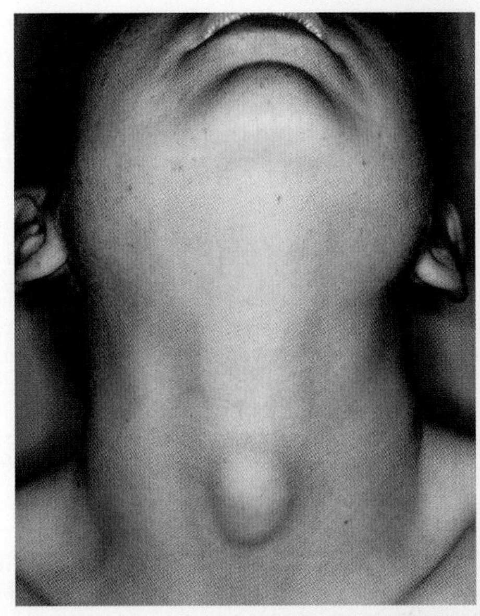

Figure 9.138 Thyroglossal cyst. (Courtesy of L. Thompson.)

Parathyroid Glands

The four parathyroid glands are ovoid bodies measuring about 6 mm long in their greatest diameter. They are closely related to the posterior border of the thyroid gland, lying within its fascial capsule (see Fig. 9.134).

The two **superior parathyroid glands** are more constant in position and lie at the level of the middle of the posterior border of the thyroid gland.

The two **inferior parathyroid glands** usually lie close to the inferior poles of the thyroid gland. They may lie within the fascial sheath, embedded in the thyroid substance, or outside the fascial sheath. Sometimes, they are found some distance caudal to the thyroid gland, in association with the inferior thyroid veins, or they may reside in the superior mediastinum in the thorax.

Blood Supply

The superior and inferior thyroid arteries supply blood to the parathyroid glands. The venous drainage is into the superior, middle, and inferior thyroid veins.

Lymph Drainage

Lymph drains to the **deep cervical** and **paratracheal lymph nodes**.

Nerve Supply

Superior or middle cervical sympathetic ganglia

Parathyroid Gland Functions

The chief cells produce **parathyroid hormone** (**PTH**), which stimulates osteoclastic activity in bones, thus mobilizing bone calcium and increasing calcium levels in the blood. PTH acts in bone to increase bone resorption, acts in the kidney nephrons to increase calcium reabsorption, and acts in the intestines to increase calcium absorption from food. The calcium levels in the blood control the secretion of PTH.

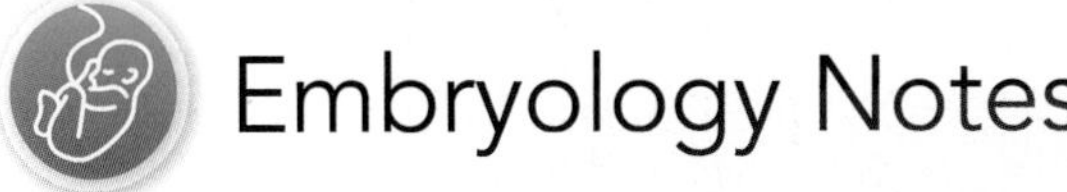

Embryology Notes

Parathyroid Gland Development

The pair of **inferior parathyroid glands** (**parathyroid III**) develop as the result of proliferation of endodermal cells in the **third pharyngeal pouch** on each side. As the thymic diverticulum on each side grows inferiorly in the neck, it pulls the inferior parathyroid with it, so that it finally comes to rest on the posterior surface of the lateral lobe of the thyroid gland near its lower pole and becomes completely separate from the thymus (Fig. 9.139).

The pair of **superior parathyroid glands** (**parathyroid IV**) develop as a proliferation of endodermal cells in the

(continued)

fourth pharyngeal pouch on each side. They loosen their connection with the pharyngeal wall and take up their final position on the posterior aspect of the lateral lobe of the thyroid gland on each side, at about the level of the isthmus. The final outcome is that the more caudal embryonic parathyroids take a more superior (cranial) final position because of their different relations to the embryonic thymus.

In the earliest stages, each gland consists of a solid mass of clear cells, the **chief cells**. In late childhood, acidophilic cells, the **oxyphil cells**, appear. The connective tissue and vascular supply are derived from the surrounding mesenchyme. It is believed that PTH is secreted early in fetal life by the chief cells to regulate calcium metabolism. The oxyphil cells are thought to be nonfunctioning chief cells.

Parathyroid Gland Absence and Hypoplasia

Agenesis or incomplete development of the parathyroid glands has been demonstrated in individuals with idiopathic hypoparathyroidism.

Ectopic Parathyroid Glands

The close relationship between the parathyroid III and the developing thymus explains the frequent finding of parathyroid tissue in the superior mediastinum of the thorax. If the parathyroid glands remain attached to the thymus, they may be pulled inferiorly into the lower part of the neck or thoracic cavity. Moreover, this also explains the variable position of the inferior parathyroid glands in relation to the lower poles of the lateral lobes of the thyroid gland.

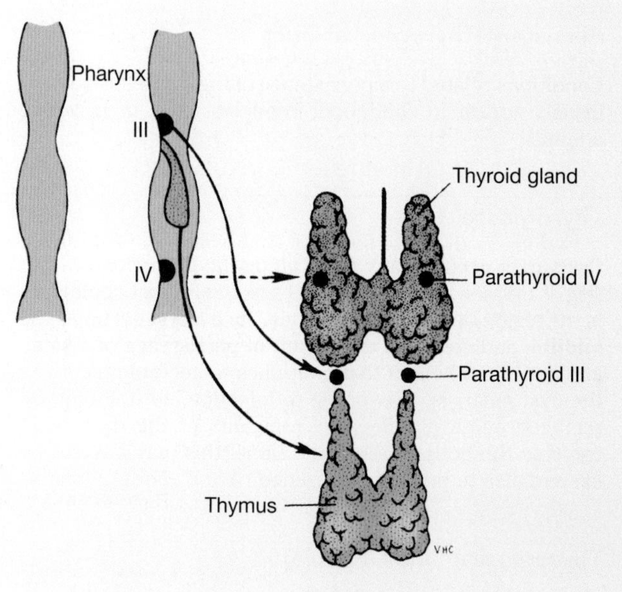

Figure 9.139 Parathyroid glands taking up their final positions in the neck.

SURFACE ANATOMY

Numerous structures in the head and neck are readily palpable and/or have distinctive surface landmarks that mark their underlying location. These lend themselves well for orientation in physical examination.

Surface Landmarks of the Head

Several distinct points in the head are reliable landmarks used in cranial references, measurements, and orientation for imaging. These are summarized in Table 9.3.

External Occipital Protuberance

This is a bony prominence in the middle of the squamous part of the occipital bone (Fig. 9.140). It lies in the midline at the junction of the head and neck and gives attachment to the **ligamentum nuchae**, which is a large ligament that runs down the back of the neck, connecting the skull to the spinous processes of the cervical vertebrae. A line joining the **nasion** to the external occipital protuberance over the superior aspect of the head indicates the position of the underlying **falx cerebri**, **superior sagittal sinus**, and the **longitudinal cerebral fissure**, which separates the right and left cerebral hemispheres.

Fontanelles

In infants, the **anterior fontanelle** lies between the two halves of the frontal bone in front and the two parietal bones behind. It is usually not palpable after age 18 months. The **posterior fontanelle** lies between the squamous part of the occipital bone and the posterior borders of the two parietal bones. It is usually closed by the end of the first year.

Superciliary Ridges

The superciliary ridges are two prominent ridges on the frontal bones above the upper margin of the orbit. The frontal air sinuses are situated within the frontal bone and lie deep to the superciliary ridge on each side (see Fig. 9.121).

Mastoid Process of the Temporal Bone

The mastoid process projects downward and forward from behind the ear (Fig. 9.141; see also Fig. 9.140). It is undeveloped in the newborn and grows as the result of the pull of the SCM, as the child moves their head. It can be recognized as a bony projection at the end of the second year.

Auricle and External Auditory Meatus

These structures lie in front of the mastoid process. The external auditory meatus is about 1 in. (2.5 cm) long and forms an S-shaped curve. To examine the outer surface of the tympanic membrane in the adult with an otoscope, the tube may be straightened by pulling the auricle upward and backward. In small children, the auricle is pulled straight back or downward and backward.

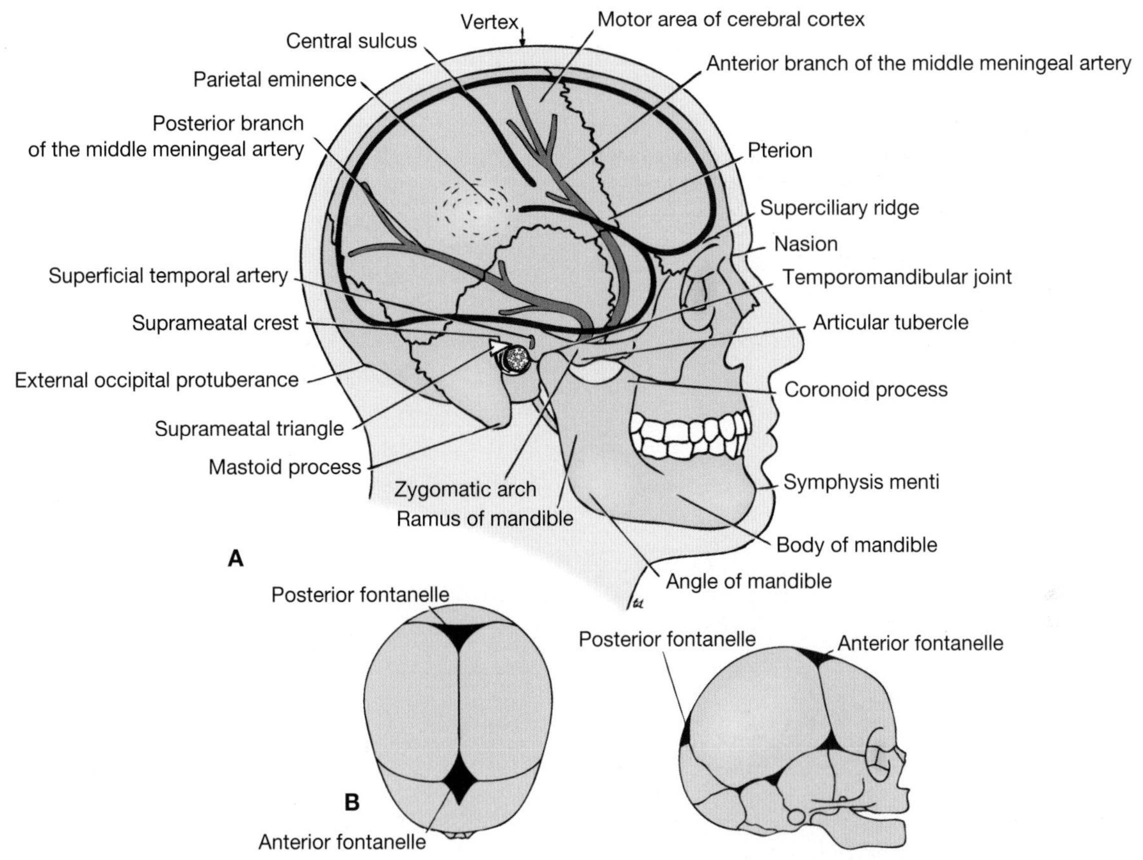

Figure 9.140 **A.** Right side of the head showing structures that have notable surface relations. **B.** Superior aspect and right side of the neonatal skull. Note the positions of the anterior and posterior fontanelles.

Zygomatic Arch

The zygomatic arch extends forward in front of the ear and ends in front in the zygomatic bone. The **temporal fossa**, which is filled with the temporalis muscle, lies above the zygomatic arch. The masseter muscle attaches to the lower margin of the zygomatic arch. Contraction of both the temporalis and masseter muscles can be felt by clenching the teeth. The pulsations of the **superficial temporal artery** can be felt as it crosses the zygomatic arch, immediately in front of the auricle.

Suprameatal Triangle

A small depression, the suprameatal triangle, is palpable above and behind the external auditory meatus, deep to the auricle (see Fig. 9.140). This is bounded behind by a line drawn vertically upward from the posterior margin of the external auditory meatus, above by the suprameatal crest of the temporal bone, and below by the external auditory meatus. The bony floor of the triangle forms the **lateral wall of the mastoid antrum**.

Temporomandibular Joint

The TMJ can be easily palpated in front of the auricle. Note that as the mouth is opened, the head of the mandible rotates and moves forward below the tubercle of the zygomatic arch.

Mandible

The **anterior border of the ramus** can be felt deep to the masseter muscle. The coronoid process of the mandible can be felt with the gloved finger inside the mouth, and the pterygomandibular ligament can be palpated as a tense band on its medial side.

The **posterior border of the ramus** is overlapped above by the parotid gland, but below, it is easily felt through the skin (see Figs. 9.140 and 9.141). The outer surface of the ramus is covered by the masseter muscle and can be felt on deep palpation when this muscle is relaxed.

The **body of the mandible** is best examined by having one finger inside the mouth and another on the outside. Thus, it is possible to examine the mandible from the **symphysis menti**, in the midline anteriorly, as far backward as the **angle**.

Masseter Muscle

The **anterior border of the masseter** can be easily felt by clenching the teeth (see Fig. 9.141). The pulsations of the **facial artery** can be felt as it crosses the lower

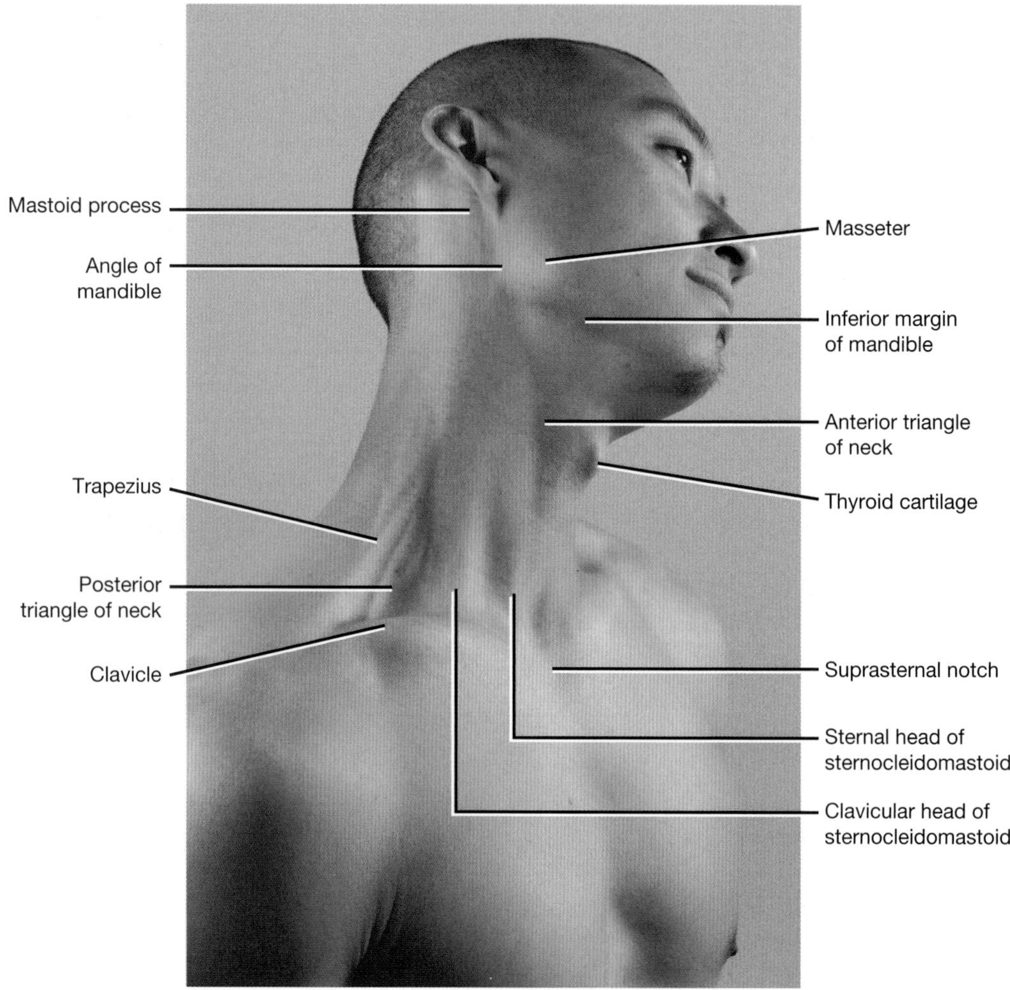

Figure 9.141 Anterior view of the neck of an adult male. Note that the head has been laterally rotated to the left at the atlantoaxial joints and at the joints of the cervical part of the vertebral column.

margin of the body of the mandible, at the anterior border of the masseter muscle. The **parotid duct** runs forward from the parotid gland one fingerbreadth below the zygomatic arch. It can be rolled beneath the examining finger at the anterior border of the masseter as it turns medially and opens into the mouth opposite the upper second molar tooth.

Orbital Margin

The frontal, zygomatic, and maxillary bones form the **orbital margin** (see Fig. 9.52). The **supraorbital notch**, if present, can be felt at the junction of the medial and intermediate thirds of the upper margin of the orbit. It transmits the supraorbital nerve, which can be rolled against the bone.

Infraorbital Foramen

The infraorbital foramen lies 5 mm below the lower margin of the orbit (see Fig. 9.1), on a line drawn downward from the supraorbital notch to the interval between the two lower premolar teeth. The **infraorbital nerve** emerges from the foramen and supplies the skin of the face.

Maxillary Air Sinus

The maxillary air sinus is situated within the maxillary bone and lies below the infraorbital foramen on each side (see Fig. 9.121).

Neck Surface Landmarks

The neck is more subject to individual variation in body form (eg, length, thickness, and fat content), and this may mask some surface landmarks. The following structures are usually discernable.

Anterior Aspect

The following structures can be palpated from above downward in the anterior midline (Figs. 9.142 and 9.143):

- **Symphysis menti:** The lower margin can be felt where the two halves of the body of the mandible unite in the midline.

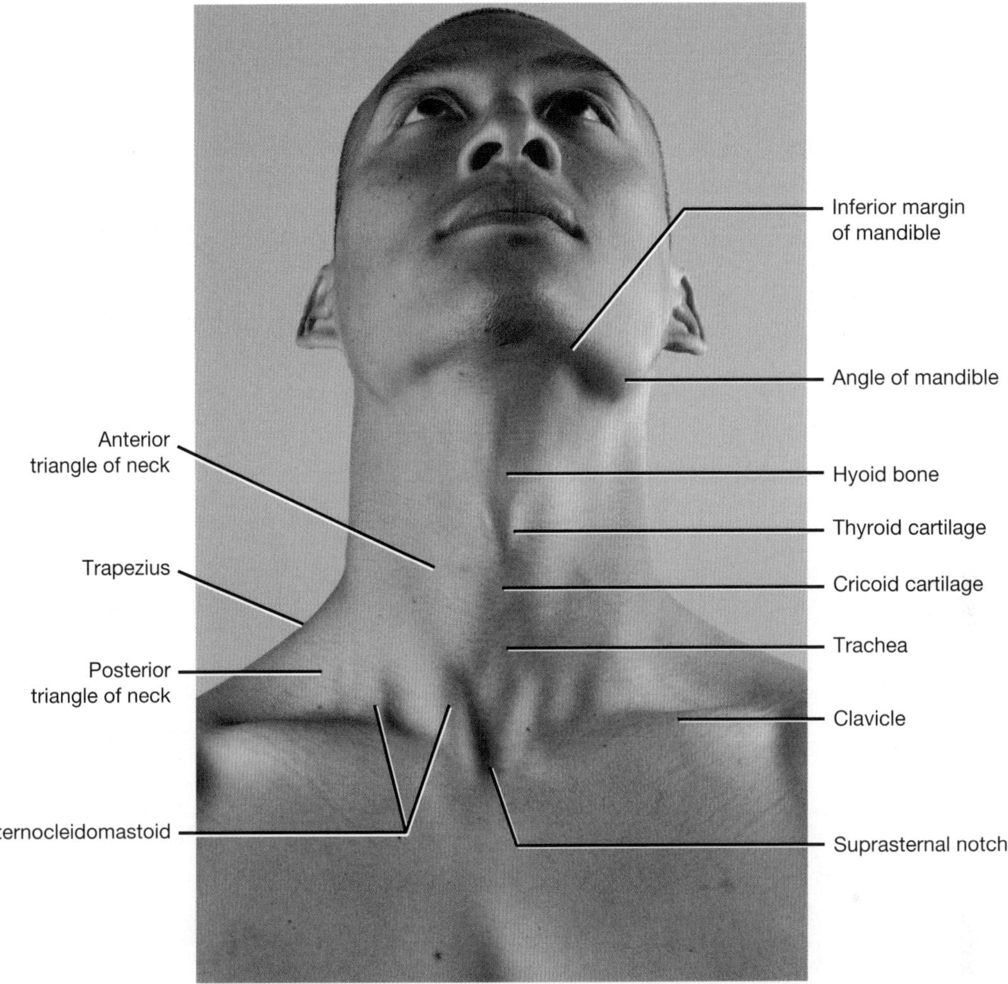

Figure 9.142 Anterior view of the head and neck of an adult male. Note that the atlanto-occipital joints and the cervical part of the vertebral column are partially extended for full exposure of the front of the neck.

- **Submental triangle:** This lies between the symphysis menti and the body of the hyoid bone. It is bounded anteriorly by the midline of the neck, laterally by the anterior belly of the digastric muscle, and inferiorly by the body of the hyoid bone. The mylohyoid muscle forms the floor. The submental lymph nodes are located in this triangle.
- **Body of the hyoid bone:** This lies above the thyroid cartilage of the larynx, opposite the C3 vertebra.
- **Thyrohyoid membrane:** This fills in the interval between the hyoid bone and the thyroid cartilage.
- **Upper border of the thyroid cartilage:** This notched structure lies opposite the C4 vertebra.
- **Cricothyroid ligament:** This structure fills in the interval between the cricoid cartilage and the thyroid cartilage.
- **Cricoid cartilage:** An important landmark in the neck, this lies at the level of the C6 vertebra, at the junction of the larynx with the trachea, at the level of the junction of the pharynx with the esophagus, at the level of the middle cervical sympathetic ganglion, and at the level where the inferior thyroid artery enters the thyroid gland.
- **Cricotracheal ligament:** This structure fills in the interval between the cricoid cartilage and the first tracheal ring.
- **First tracheal ring:** This can be felt by gentle palpation just above the isthmus of the thyroid gland.
- **Isthmus of the thyroid gland:** This lies in front of the second, third, and fourth tracheal rings.
- **Inferior thyroid veins:** The inferior thyroid veins lie in front of the fifth, sixth, and seventh tracheal rings.
- **Thyroidea ima artery:** When present, this artery ascends in front of the trachea to the isthmus of the thyroid gland, from the brachiocephalic artery.
- **Jugular arch:** This vein connects the two anterior jugular veins just above the suprasternal notch.
- **Suprasternal notch:** This can be felt between the medial ends of the clavicles. It is the superior border of the manubrium sterni and lies opposite the lower border of the body of the T2 vertebra.

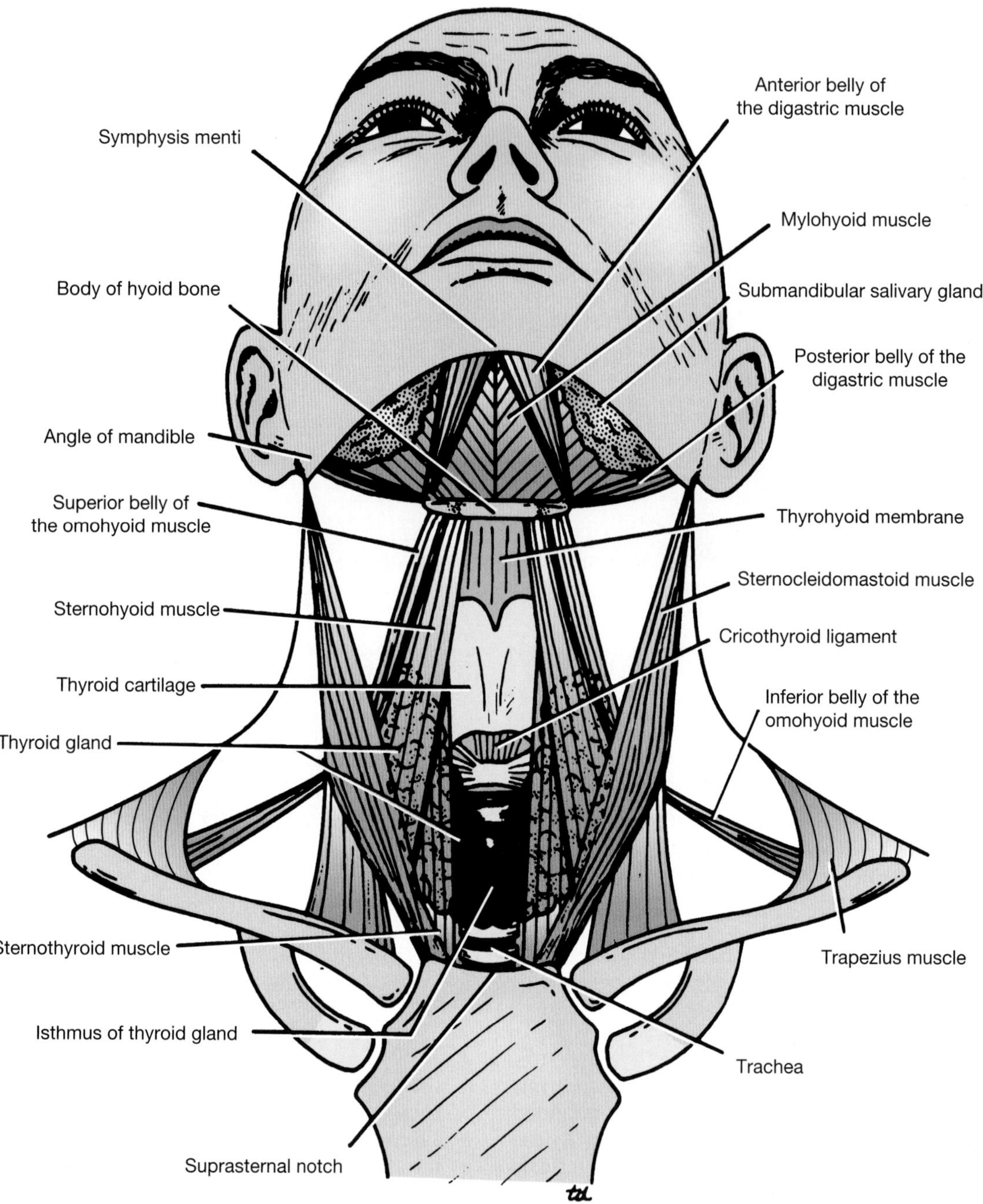

Figure 9.143 Surface anatomy of the neck from in front.

In the adult, the trachea may measure as much as 1 in. (2.5 cm) in diameter, whereas in an infant, it may be narrower than a pencil. In young children, the thymus gland may extend above the suprasternal notch as far as the isthmus of the thyroid gland, and the brachiocephalic artery and the left brachiocephalic vein may protrude above the suprasternal notch.

Posterior Aspect

The following structures can be palpated from above downward in the posterior midline.

The **external occipital protuberance** lies in the midline at the junction of the head and neck (Fig. 9.144). If the index finger is placed on the skin in the midline, it can be drawn downward in the **nuchal groove**. The first spinous process to be felt is that of the **C7 vertebra** (**vertebra prominens**). C1 to C6 spines are covered by the **ligamentum nuchae**.

Lateral Aspect

On the side of the neck, the SCM muscle can be palpated throughout its length as it passes upward from

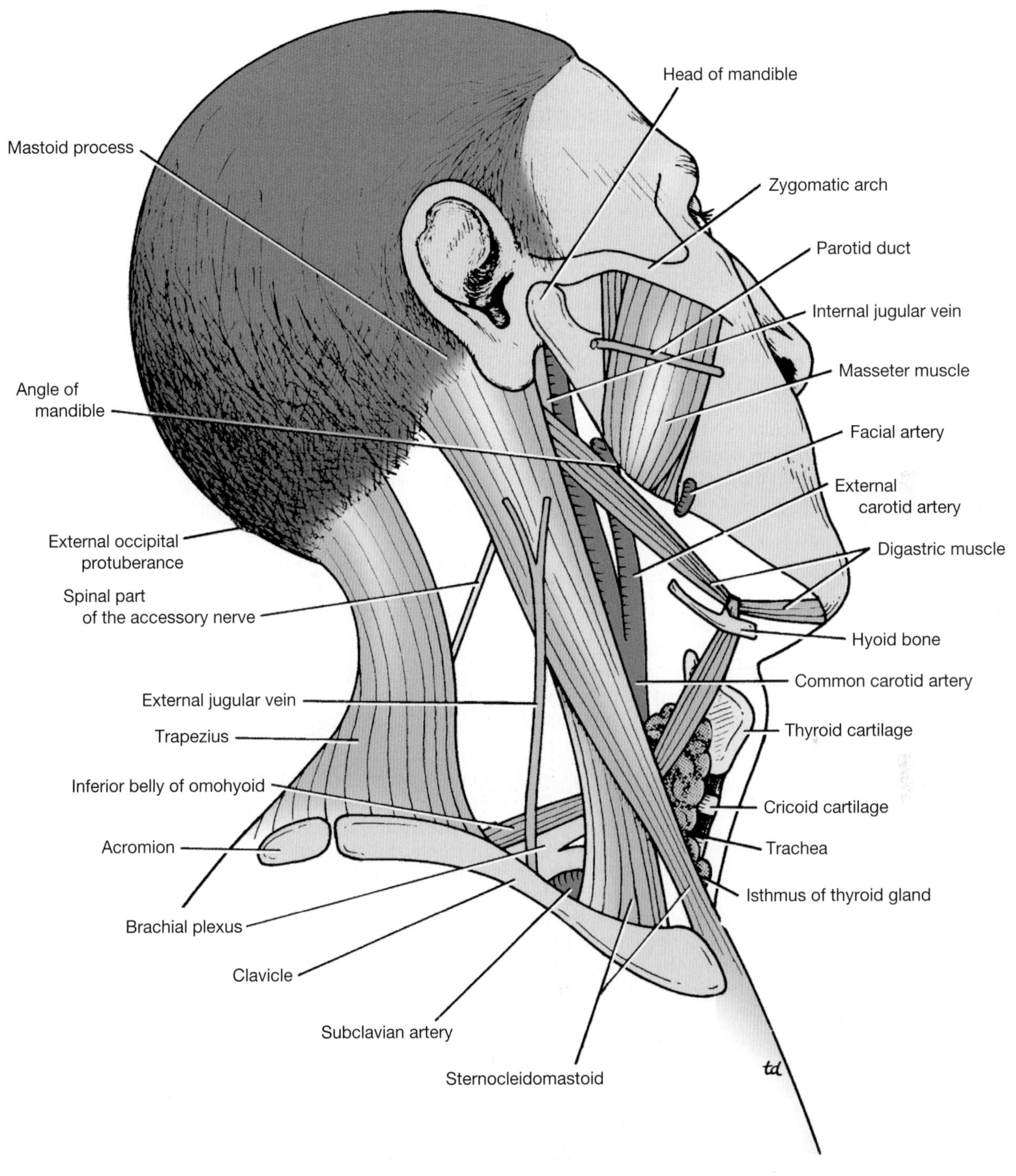

Figure 9.144 Surface anatomy of the neck from the posterolateral aspect.

the sternum and clavicle to the mastoid process (see Figs. 9.141 and 9.144). The muscle can be made to stand out by asking the patient to approximate the ear to the shoulder of the same side and at the same time rotate the head so that the face looks upward toward the opposite side. If the movement is carried out against resistance, the muscle will be felt to contract, and its anterior and posterior borders will be defined.

The SCM divides the neck into **anterior** and **posterior triangles**. The body of the mandible, SCM, and the anterior midline bound the anterior triangle. The anterior border of the trapezius, SCM, and the clavicle bound the posterior triangle.

Trapezius Muscle

The anterior border of the trapezius muscle can be felt by asking the patient to shrug their shoulders. It will be seen to extend from the superior nuchal line of the occipital bone downward and forward to the posterior border of the lateral third of the clavicle.

Platysma Muscle

The platysma can be seen as a sheet of muscle by asking the patient to clench the jaws firmly. The muscle extends from the body of the mandible downward over the clavicle to the anterior thoracic wall.

Root of the Neck

At the root of the neck are the suprasternal notch in the midline anteriorly and the clavicles. Each clavicle is subcutaneous throughout its entire length and can be easily palpated. It articulates at its lateral extremity with the **acromion of the scapula**. At the medial end of the clavicle, the **sternoclavicular joint** can be identified.

Anterior Triangle

The isthmus of the thyroid gland lies in front of the second, third, and fourth tracheal rings (see Figs. 9.142 and 9.143). The lateral lobes of the thyroid gland can be palpated deep to the sternocleidomastoid muscles. This is most easily carried out by standing behind the seated patient and asking the patient to flex their neck forward and so relax the overlying muscles. The observer can then examine both lobes simultaneously with the tips of the fingers of both hands.

Carotid Sheath

The carotid sheath, which contains the carotid arteries, internal jugular vein, vagus nerve, and deep cervical lymph nodes, can be marked out by a line joining the sternoclavicular joint to a point midway between the tip of the mastoid process and the angle of the mandible. At the level of the upper border of the thyroid cartilage, the common carotid artery bifurcates into the internal and external carotid arteries (see Fig. 9.144). The pulsations of these arteries can be felt at this level.

Posterior Triangle

At the posterior triangle of the neck, the accessory nerve is relatively superficial as it emerges from the posterior border of the SCM and runs downward and backward to pass beneath the anterior border of the trapezius (see Fig. 9.144). The course of this nerve may be indicated as follows: draw a line from the angle of the mandible to the tip of the mastoid process. Bisect this line at right angles and extend the second line downward across the posterior triangle; the second line indicates the course of the nerve.

Brachial Plexus Roots and Trunks

The roots and trunks of the brachial plexus occupy the lower anterior angle of the posterior triangle. A line drawn from the cricoid cartilage downward to the middle of the clavicle can indicate the upper limit of the plexus.

Third Part of the Subclavian Artery

The third part of the subclavian artery also occupies the lower anterior angle of the posterior triangle. Its course may be indicated by a curved line, which passes upward from the sternoclavicular joint for about 0.5 in. (1.3 cm) and then downward to the middle of the clavicle. Here, where the artery lies on the upper surface of rib 1, its pulsations can be felt easily. The subclavian vein lies behind the clavicle and does not enter the neck.

External Jugular Vein

The external jugular vein lies in the superficial fascia deep to the platysma. It passes downward from the region of the angle of the mandible to the middle of the clavicle. It perforates the deep fascia just above the clavicle and drains into the subclavian vein.

Salivary Glands

The three large salivary glands can be palpated. The **parotid gland** lies below the ear in the interval between the mandible and the anterior border of the SCM muscle (see Fig. 9.109). The **parotid duct** extends forward across the surface of the masseter (see Masseter Muscle, discussed earlier).

The **submandibular gland** has superficial and deep parts. The **superficial part** lies beneath the lower margin of the body of the mandible (see Fig. 9.110). The **deep part** of the submandibular gland, **submandibular duct**, and **sublingual gland** can be palpated through the mucous membrane covering the floor of the mouth in the interval between the tongue and the lower jaw. The submandibular duct opens into the mouth on the side of the frenulum of the tongue (see Fig. 9.94B).

Clinical Case Discussion

To diagnose this condition, the physician must understand the anatomy of the facial and laryngeal muscles and their nerve supply. The facial paralysis, slurred speech, high blood pressure, and absence of any other abnormal findings suggested a diagnosis of a left-sided cerebral hemorrhage (stroke), secondary to high blood pressure. However, a left-sided cerebral hemorrhage would cause paralysis of only the muscles of the lower part of the right side of the face, and so this was not the correct diagnosis.

This patient had paralysis of the muscles of facial expression across the entire right side of the face. Also, she could vocalize but not articulate well. Only a lesion of the right facial nerve, which supplies the facial muscles, could cause this. This patient was experiencing Bell palsy, the prognosis was excellent, and she had a complete recovery.

Key Concepts

Osteology

- The skeleton of the head and neck includes the skull, middle ear ossicles, hyoid bone, and cervical vertebrae. The skull bones join at fibrous sutural joints, except the mandible, which articulates with the skull via the synovial temporomandibular joint.
- Opening the mouth consists of both protrusion and depression of the mandible. Closing requires both retraction and elevation. The muscles of mastication include the masseter, temporalis, medial pterygoid, lateral pterygoid, and digastric.
- The neonatal skull has a small face relative to cranium and six fontanelles, which allow molding of the head during birth.

Scalp

- The scalp consists of five layers that spell out SCALP: Skin, Connective tissue, Aponeurosis, loose Areolar tissue, and Pericranium.
- The occipitofrontalis is the sole muscle of the scalp.
- Sensory nerves include branches of the trigeminal nerve anterior to the ear and cervical spinal nerves posterior to the ear.
- The external and internal carotid arteries provide blood to the scalp. Venous drainage is to the facial and external jugular veins. Lymph drainage is to the pericervical collar of nodes.

Face

- The ophthalmic, maxillary, and mandibular nerves, plus the great auricular nerve, contribute to the cutaneous innervation.
- The facial and superficial temporal arteries provide the primary blood supply. The facial vein is the main drainage route. The facial vein connects with the cavernous sinus via the superior ophthalmic vein. Lymph drainage is to the pericervical collar of nodes.
- The facial muscles (all supplied by cranial nerve [CN] VII) are organized around the facial orifices and act to regulate those openings.
- Five terminal branches of CN VII emerge from the parotid gland and spread across the face.

Interior of the Skull

- The meninges (dura, arachnoid, and pia mater) surround the brain. The dura has extensions (falx cerebri, falx cerebelli, tentorium cerebelli, diaphragma sellae) that partition the cranial cavity around parts of the brain. The subarachnoid space is filled with cerebrospinal fluid (CSF).
- The dura receives a rich sensory supply from the trigeminal nerve above the tentorium and from cervical nerves below the tentorium.
- The dural venous blood sinuses collect blood from the brain and run between the layers of the dura. Most blood in this system drains to the internal jugular veins.
- The cavernous sinuses sit on the sides of the sella turcica. The internal carotid artery and CNs III, IV, V1, V2, and VI pass through the sinus or its wall.
- The brain lies within the cranial cavity and has three main parts: forebrain, midbrain, and hindbrain. The internal carotid and vertebral arteries supply the brain.

Orbit and Eye

- The levator palpebrae superioris and the superior tarsal muscle insert into the upper eyelid and open the eye. The orbicularis oculi closes the eye. CN III supplies the levator, sympathetic fibers supply the superior tarsal, and CN VII supplies the orbicularis.
- The lacrimal apparatus consists of the structures that secrete and collect tears, that is, the lacrimal gland and the lacrimal ducts. The nasolacrimal duct drains into the inferior nasal meatus.
- The orbit has four walls and several openings. The optic canal and the superior orbital fissure are key in that they convey critical neurovascular structures.
- Six CNs (optic, oculomotor, trochlear, trigeminal, abducens, facial) plus additional autonomic components (including the ciliary ganglion) supply the orbit.
- The ophthalmic artery supplies the orbit and eye. Superior and inferior ophthalmic veins drain the orbit and empty into the cavernous sinus.
- The superior rectus, inferior rectus, medial rectus, lateral rectus, superior oblique, and inferior oblique are the extrinsic muscles that move the eye. CN IV controls the superior oblique, CN VI controls the lateral rectus, and CN III controls all the rest.
- The dilator pupillae, sphincter pupillae, and ciliary muscle are intrinsic smooth muscles. Sympathetic fibers control the dilator, whereas parasympathetic fibers affect the others.
- The eyeball has three layers: an external fibrous coat (sclera and cornea), a middle vascular coat (choroid, ciliary body, and iris), and an inner nervous coat (retina).

Temporal, Infratemporal, and Pterygopalatine Regions

- The temporal fossa is an oval area on the side of the head. The infratemporal fossa lies between the mandible and the pharynx. The pterygopalatine fossa sits deep and posterior–inferior to the orbit. Each region has several openings that communicate with adjoining areas.
- The superficial temporal artery supplies the temporal fossa. The maxillary artery and its branches supply the infratemporal and pterygopalatine fossae, plus areas that adjoin those.
- The maxillary and mandibular nerves run into the pterygopalatine and infratemporal fossae and distribute widely from those spaces. Autonomic nerves from other sources (CN VII, CN IX, carotid plexus) also enter these areas and distribute along certain trigeminal branches. CN VII also sends taste fibers into the oral cavity via its chorda tympani branch and the lingual branch of the mandibular nerve.

Neck

- Posterior rami of cervical nerves supply the skin on the back of the neck and scalp. Anterior rami of cervical nerves (via the cervical plexus) supply the skin over the front and sides of the neck. Cutaneous veins drain the head and neck into the external jugular vein network.
- The SCM muscle divides the neck into large anterior and posterior triangles. Each of these contains smaller triangular spaces defined by other muscles.
- The scalenus anterior and medius muscles form the interscalene triangle, which transmits the brachial plexus and subclavian artery.
- The root of the neck is above the thoracic inlet. The root conveys the subclavian vessels, brachial plexus, and thoracic duct (on the left).

Arteries, Veins, and Lymph

- Two arterial tracts supply blood to the head and neck: the carotid and subclavian systems. The carotid system delivers blood to the upper neck and the head. The subclavian system provides blood to the lower neck, deep neck, inside of the cranium, shoulder, upper limb, and thorax.
- The common carotid artery ascends the neck and divides into internal and external carotid arteries. The common carotid has no branches, except its two terminal branches. The internal carotid has no branches in the neck but has an extensive distribution in the cranial cavity. The external carotid has several branches in the neck and terminates in the head into the superficial temporal and maxillary arteries.
- The subclavian artery loops across the root of the neck and gives off multiple branches.
- The veins of the head and neck are organized in two groups: intracranial veins include the veins of the brain and the dural sinuses, and extracranial veins are those of the scalp, face, and neck. Several emissary veins connect the intra- and extracranial vessels.
- Lymph nodes form three groups: the pericervical collar, regional cervical group, and deep terminal group. The pericervical collar is a series of several regional groups of nodes arranged roughly in a ring around approximately the junction of the head and neck. The cervical regional nodes are regional groups of nodes located in a roughly vertical series in the neck proper. The deep cervical nodes form a vertical chain along the course of the internal jugular vein, within the carotid sheath, from the base of the skull to the root of the neck.

Nerves

- Twelve pairs of CNs branch off the brain and upper spinal cord and pass through the cranial foramina. The olfactory (CN I), optic (CN II), and vestibulocochlear (CN VIII) nerves are entirely sensory. The oculomotor (CN III), trochlear (CN IV), abducens (CN VI), accessory (CN XI), and hypoglossal (CN XII) nerves are entirely motor. The remaining nerves are mixed.
- The anterior rami of the C1 to C4 nerves form the cervical plexus. The cervical plexus supplies skin and muscles of the head, neck, and shoulder, plus the diaphragm and other thoracic structures. The phrenic nerve arises in the neck from the cervical plexus. It is the only motor nerve supply to the diaphragm. It also carries sensory branches from the pericardium, the mediastinal parietal pleura, and the pleura and peritoneum covering the upper and lower surfaces of the central part of the diaphragm.
- The brachial plexus forms in the posterior triangle of the neck by the union of the anterior rami of the C5 to C8 and the T1 spinal nerves. The plexus traverses the posterior triangle of the neck and supplies the upper limb.
- Sympathetic components originate in the upper thoracic spinal cord, ascend the cervical sympathetic trunks, and distribute from the cervical sympathetic ganglia. The superior cervical ganglion provides all sympathetic fibers to the head. Sympathetic targets include the superior tarsal and dilator pupillae muscles in the orbit.
- Parasympathetic components emerge with CNs III, VII, IX, and X. CN III projects to the ciliary ganglion and on to the sphincter pupillae and ciliary muscles in the orbit. CN VII projects to the pterygopalatine and submandibular ganglia and on to the lacrimal gland and the submandibular and sublingual

salivary glands. CN IX projects to the otic ganglion and then to the parotid gland. CN X has parasympathetic projections below the head, into the neck, thorax, and abdomen.

Ear

- The ear consists of three main parts: external, middle, and internal. The external and middle ear structures function for sound conduction and transmission, whereas the internal ear functions for sound perception and equilibrium.
- The external ear has an auricle and an external auditory meatus.
- The tympanic membrane (eardrum) forms the interface between the external and middle ears; it is extremely sensitive to pain. The auriculotemporal nerve and the auricular branch of the vagus nerve innervate its outer surface, and the tympanic plexus of the glossopharyngeal nerve supplies its inner aspect.
- The middle ear has four main components: the tympanic cavity, auditory ossicles and their muscles, auditory tube, and the mastoid area. The facial (CN VII) and glossopharyngeal (CN IX) nerves have significant relations to the middle ear.
- The internal ear consists of the bony labyrinth, comprising a series of cavities within the temporal bone, and the membranous labyrinth, comprising a series of membranous sacs and ducts contained within the bony labyrinth. CN VIII supplies the internal ear.

Digestive System

- The oral cavity, pharynx, and esophagus are the major components of the digestive system in the head and neck.
- The oral cavity includes the lips, teeth, tongue, palate, and salivary glands. It extends back to the palatoglossal folds, which form the boundary with the pharynx.
- The tongue has two parts: the anterior two thirds (body) and the posterior third (root). The lingual nerve carries general sensation from the body, and the chorda tympani branch of CN VII carries taste. CN IX provides both general sensation and taste for the root. The tongue has extrinsic and intrinsic muscles that are all (but one) supplied by CN XII.
- The palate has two parts, hard and soft. The tensor palatini and levator palatini muscles are the primary muscles of the soft palate. They also act on the auditory tube.
- The submandibular, sublingual, and parotid salivary glands empty into the oral cavity. The parotid duct crosses over the lateral surface of the masseter, pierces the buccinator muscle, and enters the vestibule of the mouth opposite the upper second molar tooth. The submandibular duct runs forward in the oral floor and opens at the side of the frenulum of the tongue. The sublingual gland opens by numerous small ducts. Parasympathetic nerves provide secretomotor fibers. CN VII innervates the submandibular and sublingual glands; CN IX supplies the parotid gland.
- The pharynx consists of three parts: nasopharynx, oropharynx, and laryngopharynx. These sit behind the nasal passages, oral cavity, and larynx, respectively. The superior, middle, and inferior constrictors are the main muscles of the pharynx. Three sets of tonsils (pharyngeal, palatine, and lingual) are fixed in the pharyngeal walls.
- The esophagus extends from the laryngopharynx to the stomach.

Respiratory System

- Components are the nose, paranasal sinuses, larynx, and trachea.
- The nose consists of the external nose and the nasal cavity, each divided in two by the nasal septum. The ophthalmic, maxillary, and facial arteries and the ophthalmic and maxillary nerves supply the external nose.
- Each nasal cavity has four walls. The lateral wall has nasal conchae and nasal meatuses, which are related to drainage of the paranasal sinuses and the nasolacrimal duct and to airflow. The roof area has the olfactory region. The sphenopalatine and facial arteries are the major vessels of the nasal cavity.
- The maxillary, frontal, sphenoid, and ethmoid sinuses are the paranasal sinuses. Each drains to a specific spot on the lateral wall of the nasal cavity.
- The major skeletal elements in the larynx are the thyroid, cricoid, arytenoid, and epiglottic cartilages. Extrinsic and intrinsic muscles act on the cartilages and produce abduction/adduction of the vocal folds or tension/relaxation of the vocal ligaments. CN X supplies the entire larynx via its superior laryngeal and recurrent laryngeal branches. The superior and inferior thyroid arteries supply the larynx.
- The trachea begins as a continuation of the larynx and descends into the thorax. It has incomplete cartilage rings in its wall. The esophagus fits against its posterior aspect. The recurrent laryngeal nerves and the inferior thyroid arteries supply the trachea.

Endocrine System

- Components are the pituitary, pineal, thyroid, and parathyroid glands.
- The pituitary has anterior and posterior lobes and is seated in the sella turcica. It has relations with the sphenoid air sinus and the venous cavernous sinus. Branches of the internal carotid artery supply the pituitary.

- The pineal projects from the roof of the third ventricle of the brain.
- The thyroid consists of two lobes and a connecting isthmus. It lies below the larynx and covers the trachea. The superior and inferior thyroid arteries supply the gland.
- There are two superior parathyroid and two inferior parathyroid glands. Each is closely related to the posterior aspect of the thyroid gland.

Radiographic and Surface Anatomy

- Many structures are visible through the various modes of medical imaging, including skeletal features, vascular structures, and soft tissues of the brain.
- Numerous structures in the head and neck are readily palpable and/or have distinctive surface landmarks that mark their underlying location. These lend themselves well to orientation in physical examination.

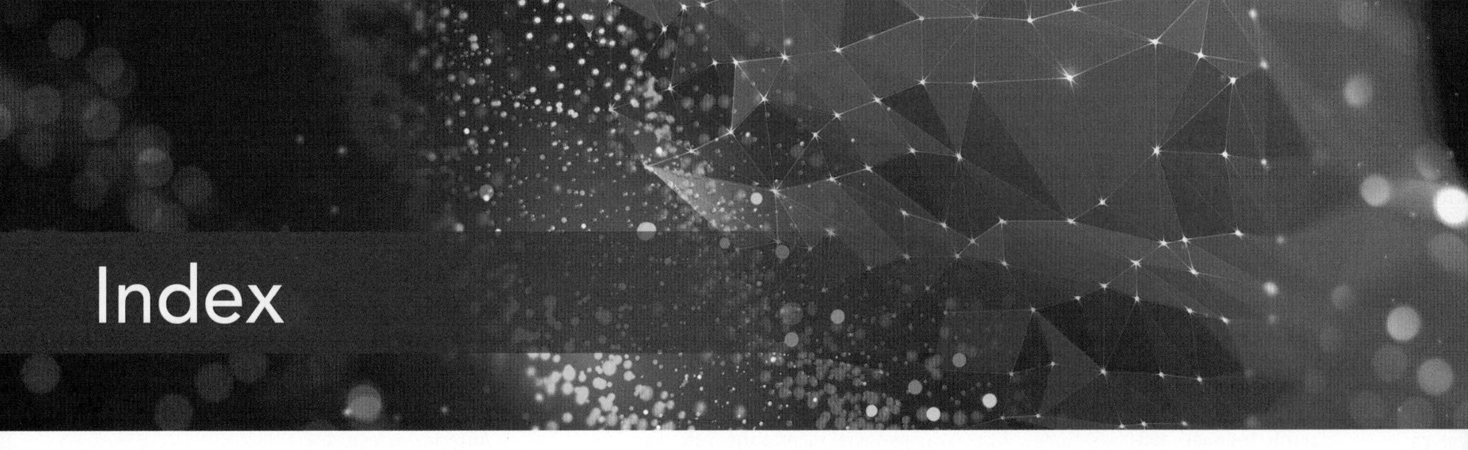

Index

Note: Page numbers followed by *f* indicate figures. Page numbers followed by *t* denote tables.